Asthma

Basic Mechanisms and Clinical Management

Asthma

Basic Mechanisms and Clinical Management

Edited by

Peter J. Barnes
National Heart and Lung Institute, London, UK

Ian W. Rodger
Merck Frosst Centre for Therapeutic Research,
Point Claire-Dorval, Quebec, Canada

Neil C. Thomson
Department of Respiratory Medicine,
Western Infirmary, Glasgow, UK

ACADEMIC PRESS
Harcourt Brace Jovanovich, Publishers
London   San Diego   New York
Boston   Sydney   Tokyo   Toronto

ACADEMIC PRESS LIMITED
24–28 Oval Road
LONDON NW1 7DX

United States Edition published by
ACADEMIC PRESS INC.
San Diego, CA 92101

A catalogue record for this book is available from
the British Library
ISBN 0-12-079026-2

Typeset by Paston Press, Loddon, Norfolk
Printed in Great Britain by The University Printing House, Cambridge

Foreword

Scientific, epidemiological and clinical information on asthma is expanding rapidly. In consequence, it has become necessary to revise *Asthma: Basic Mechanisms and Clinical Management* only four years after the first edition.

Asthma remains one of the most common and treatable conditions in medicine. It affects some 5% of the adult population in the Western world and around 10% of children. The condition is always distressing and occasionally lethal. It is therefore obligatory for every patient to receive the best possible treatment currently available.

One of the greatest challenges in modern medicine is the fact that, while the understanding of pathogenesis and proven improvements in therapy has developed rapidly, there is considerable evidence that morbidity from asthma is increasing and no reduction in mortality is occurring, in spite of attempts to identify and tackle factors which should prevent death. Thus, there is still much to learn. No doubt new information will emerge, but there may also be a need to re-evaluate some of our preconceived ideas and re-examine some of our previous treatment policies. In the meantime this radically revised and expanded second edition will help in this important re-evaluation process.

Peter Barnes, Ian Rodger and Neil Thomson must be congratulated in drawing together a group of specialist authors of international standing. Let us hope that their efforts to inform and educate both scientists and clinicians will be rewarded by a better quality of life for all asthmatic patients.

January 1992

Dame Margaret Turner-Warwick, DBE, DM, PhD, PRCP
President of the Royal College of Physicians, London NW1, UK

Preface

Asthma continues to be a major health problem throughout the world and affects over 5% of the population in industrialized countries. There is convincing evidence for increasing morbidity and mortality in many countries. That this is occurring despite increased awareness and amount of treatment prescribed is of particular concern, and underlines the need for greater understanding of this complex disease and its therapy. The first edition of this book appeared in 1988 and provided a comprehensive overview of asthma mechanisms and therapy. The book was widely acclaimed and has become a 'best seller' in its field. Because knowledge about asthma has advanced very rapidly, with new concepts and many new therapeutic agents developed, it has been necessary to produce a second edition after only four years. This new edition incorporates the many changes in our understanding of asthma which have occurred in recent years; this has involved radical revision of most chapters and the addition of several new chapters. We have selected internationally recognized experts who are at the forefront of research as contributors and we are very grateful to all of them for their outstanding and up-to-date contributions and for producing their manuscripts on time. Several books on asthma are now available, but this is the only book which brings together all the recent information on basic mechanisms of asthma and also covers in depth clinical aspects and therapy. This integrated approach should appeal to both basic researchers and to clinicians who need to keep abreast of recent developments in this rapidly expanding field.

We would like to thank Carey Chapman of Academic Press for all her help in putting together this second edition. We are very grateful to our secretaries for all their help in chasing up manuscripts and to our wives for their patience and understanding. We hope that the Second Edition will be even more successful than the first!

Peter Barnes
Ian Rodger
Neil Thomson

Contributors

Sandra D. Anderson Department of Respiratory Medicine, Royal Prince Albert Hospital, Camperdown, New South Wales, Australia 2050

Peter J. Barnes Department of Thoracic Medicine, National Heart and Lung Institute, Dovehouse Street, London SW3 6LY, UK

Frederick de Blay Hospices Tivils de Strasbourg, France

John R. Britton Respiratory Medicine Unit, City Hospital, Nottingham NG5 1PB, UK

William W. Busse University of Wisconsin Medical School, Madison, Wisconsin, USA

William J. Calhoun University of Wisconsin Medical School, Madison, Wisconsin, USA

Martin K. Church Immunopharmacology Group, Clinical Pharmacology and Medicine 1, Southampton General Hospital, Southampton SO9 4XY, UK

K. Fan Chung Department of Thoracic Medicine, National Heart and Lung Institute, Dovehouse Street, London SW3 6LY, UK

Marc Cluzel Department of Allergy and Allied Respiratory Diseases, 4th Floor, Hunt's House, Guy's Hospital, London SE1 9RT, UK

Donald W. Cockcroft Division of Respiratory Medicine, Department of Medicine, Royal University Hospital, Saskatoon, Saskatchewan S7N 0X0, Canada

Graham K. Crompton Respiratory Medicine Service, Northern General Hospital, Edinburgh EH5 2DR, UK

Douglas R. Corfield Department of Physiology, St George's Hospital Medical School, Cranmer Terrace, London SW17 0RE, UK

Christopher J. Corrigan Department of Allergy and Clinical Immunology, National Heart and Lung Institute, Dovehouse Street, London SW3 6LY, UK

Ronald Dahl University Hospital of Aarhus, Department of Respiratory Diseases, Section of Allergology, DK-8000, Aarhus, Denmark

Robert J. Davies   Academic Unit of Respiratory Medicine, Medical College of St Bartholomew's Hospital, University of London, London, UK

Jagdish L. Devalia   Academic Unit of Respiratory Medicine, Medical College of St Bartholomew's Hospital, University of London, UK

Jeffrey M. Drazen   Pulmonary Division, Brigham and Women's Hospital, 75 Francis Street, Boston MA 02115, USA

Roger Ellul-Micallef   Department of Medical Sciences, The University of Malta, Msida, Malta

Noemi M. Eiser   Lewisham Hospital, London SE13 6LH, UK

Kyeld Fredens   Institute of Anatomy B, University of Aarhus, Aarhus DK-8000, Denmark

Richard W. Fuller   Director of Clinical Research, Department of Respiratory Medicine, Glaxo Group Research, Greenford Road, Greenford, Middx, UB6 0HE, UK

D.C.K. Fung   Department of Physiology, St George's Hospital Medical School, Cranmer Terrace, London SW17 0RE, UK

Nicholas J. Gross   Departments of Medicine and Biochemistry, Stritch School of Medicine, Loyola University, Hines V A Hospital, Chicago IL 60141, USA

Mary Lou Hayden   Division of Allergy and Clinical Immunology, Box 225, University of Virginia Health Sciences Center, Charlottesville VA 22908, USA

James C. Hogg   Pulmonary Research Laboratory, St Paul's Hospital, Burrard Street, Vancouver, Canada

Stephen T. Holgate   Immunopharmacology Group, Southampton General Hospital, Southampton SO9 4XY, UK

A.B. Kay   Department of Allergy and Clinical Immunology, National Heart and Lung Institute, Dovehouse Street, London SW3 6LY, UK

Tak H. Lee   Department of Allergy and Applied Respiratory Disorders, 4th Floor, Hunt's House, Guy's Hospital, London SE1 9RT, UK

Anthony J. Newman-Taylor   Department of Occupational and Environmental Medicine, National Heart and Lung Institute, Emmanuel Kaye Building, Manresa Road, London SW3 6LR, UK

Wai H. Ng   Immunopharmacology Group, Clinical Pharmacology and Medicine I, Southampton General Hospital, Southampton SO9 4XY, UK

Paul M. O'Byrne   Asthma Research Group, Department of Medicine, McMaster University, Hamilton, Ontario, Canada

Clive P. Page   Department of Pharmacology, King's College, University of London, Manresa Road, London SW3 6LX, UK

Martyn R. Partridge   Consultant Physician, Whipps Cross Hospital, London E11 1NR, UK

Frederick L. Pearce   Chemistry Department, Christopher Ingold Laboratories, University College London, 20 Gordon Street, London WC1H 0AJ, UK

Søren Pedersen   Pediatric Department, Kolding Hospital, Skowangen 2-8, 600 Kolding, Denmark

Carl G.A. Persson   Pharmacological Laboratory, AB Draco Box 34, S-221 01 Lund, Sweden

Thomas A.E. Platts-Mills   Division of Allergy and Clinical Immunology, Box 225, University of Virginia Health Sciences Center, Charlottesville VA 22908, USA

Riccardo Polosa Immunopharmacology Group, Clinical Pharmacology and Medicine 1, Southampton General Hospital, Southampton SO9 4XY, UK

Neil B. Pride Department of Medicine, Royal Postgraduate Medical School, Hammersmith Hospital, Ducane Road, London W12 0NN, UK

David Proud Johns Hopkins University School of Medicine, Baltimore MD 21224, USA

Nigel J. Pyne Department of Physiology and Pharmacology, University of Strathclyde, Glasgow G1 1XW, UK

Paul Rafferty Dumfries and Galloway Royal Infirmary, Dumfries, UK

Paul S. Richardson Department of Physiology, St George's Hospital Medical School, Cranmer Terrace, London SW17 0RE, UK

Ian W. Rodger Director of Pharmacology, Merck Frosst Centre for Therapeutic Research, PO Box 1005, Point Claire-Dorval, Quebec H9R 4P8, Canada

Malcolm S. Sears Department of Medicine, McMaster University, Hamilton, Ontario, Canada

Bonnie Sibbald Department of General Practice, St George's Hospital Medical School, Cranmer Terrace, London SW17 0RE, UK

Dean Sheppard Chest Service Room 5KI, San Francisco General Hospital, 1001 Potrero Avenue, San Francisco CA 94110, USA

Nils Svedmyr Division of Clinical Pharmacology, Sahlgrenska University Hospital, Gothenburg, Sweden

Anne E. Tattersfield Respiratory Medicine Unit, City Hospital, Nottingham NG5 1PB, UK

Neil C. Thomson Department of Respiratory Medicine, Western Infirmary, Glasgow G11 6NT, UK

Per Venge Department of Clinical Chemistry, University of Upsala, Upsala, Sweden

George W. Ward, Jr Division of Allergy and Clinical Immunology, Box 225, University of Virginia Health Sciences Center, Charlottesville VA 22908, USA

Stephen E. Webber Department of Physiology, St George's Hospital Medical School, Cranmer Terrace, London SW17 0RE, UK

John G. Widdicombe Department of Physiology, St George's Hospital Medical School, Cranmer Terrace, London SW17 0RE, UK

Ann J. Woolcock Department of Thoracic Medicine, Royal Prince Albert Hospital, Missenden Road, Camperdown, NSW 2050, Australia

Contents

Contents

Contents

1

Epidemiology

MALCOLM R. SEARS

INTRODUCTION

Asthma is one of the commonest disorders encountered in clinical medicine. The prevalence, pathogenesis, and management of asthma have been extensively studied, but the fundamental cause of asthma and the factors inducing and inciting airway inflammation are still unclear; the optimum methods of prevention of disease or control of its manifestations have yet to be established; and the international differences in morbidity and increases in mortality have become subjects of intense investigation and debate.

Asthma defies precise definition, despite several carefully worded statements.[1,2] Perhaps the most concise and useful description of asthma is 'variable airflow obstruction'. The diagnosis is made by recognition of a pattern of one or more characteristic symptoms including wheeze, cough, chest tightness and dyspnoea, and is best confirmed by evidence of variable or reversible airflow obstruction accompanying symptoms.[3] In children, asthma causing nocturnal or post-exercise cough may be misdiagnosed as bronchitis or infection.[4,5] Increased responsiveness of the airways to non-allergic stimuli usually accompanies asthma symptoms[6] but is not synonymous with asthma. Airway hyperresponsiveness (AHR) is absent in some subjects with other clear evidence of asthma, and may be variably present in some children and adults without significant respiratory symptoms;[7–11] AHR is not sufficiently sensitive or specific for epidemiological purposes. Asthma is characterized by inflammation,[12] but present methods for detecting airway inflammation are not suitable for community studies. Evidence of variable or reversible airflow obstruction (a 20% increase in forced exhaled volume in 1 s (FEV_1) or peak expiratory flow rate (PEFR) occurring spontaneously or with treatment[13] is helpful if present. However, asthmatics who smoke, or work in highly

ASTHMA: BASIC MECHANISMS AND CLINICAL MANAGEMENT (2nd Edn)
ISBN 0-12-079026-2

polluted atmospheres, may develop less reversible disease, and some asthmatics develop irreversible disease despite being lifetime non-smokers.[14] A carefully constructed questionnaire is presently the most reliable tool for detecting current asthma in epidemiological surveys, but is less reliable for establishing cumulative prevalence rates for which longitudinal studies provide more accurate data.

ASTHMA IN CHILDREN

Between 1.6 and 20.5% of children in the United Kingdom,[5,8,15,24] Canada,[16,17] the United States,[18–20] Australia,[9,21–23] New Zealand,[25–27] and Scandinavia[28–30] have significant recurrent respiratory symptoms suggesting asthma (Table 1.1). The variations in questions asked, age groups studied, and local factors may all affect comparability of responses; a uniform approach is yet to be used to enable detection of true differences between countries.

The prevalence of wheezing in childhood has probably increased over the last decade;[31] however, differences in methodology, definitions, and use of the label 'asthma'

Table 1.1   Studies of prevalence of asthma and wheezing in children since 1980.

Location	Age (mean* or range)	Prevalence	Reference
Lower Hutt, NZ	11–13	13.5% asthma	25
Dunedin, NZ	9	18.1% wheezing (3/year or more)	26
Auckland, NZ	8–10	European 13.5% (symptoms + AHR) Maori 10.8%	27
Sydney, Australia	12.6* 8.9*	7.2% M, 4.2% F 8.6% M, 4.4% F	21
Queensland, Australia	8.1* 12.1*	20.5% wheeze 18.1% wheeze	22
South Australia	8	27.4% cumulative (asthma + wheeze)	23
New South Wales	8–10	12.4% asthma, 24.3% wheezing	9
Tyneside, UK	7	9.3% current, 11.1% cumulative	8
London, UK	9	11.1% current, 18.2% cumulative	15
National UK	7, 11, 16	Current 8.3%, 4.7%, 3.5% respectively Cumulative 18.3%, 21.9%, 24.7%	24
Southampton, UK	7, 11	Asthma 9.5%, wheeze 12.1% current	5
Boston, US	5–9	9.2% persistent wheeze	18
Baltimore, US	Grades 1, 6	7.2% current, 10.5% cumulative	20
National US	6–11	7.6% asthma and wheeze with colds	19
Hamilton, Canada	7–10	4.4% asthma, 21.2% wheezing most days	16
East Halton, Canada	9	20.5% wheezing (3/year or more)	17
Oslo, Norway	7–15	1.6% current, 3.7% cumulative, 9% wheeze	28
Sweden	4, 7, 10, 14	5.1% asthma	29
Sweden	7–16	4.0% asthma	30

have exaggerated any true increase in prevalence.[32,33] In Australia in 1969, 19.1% of 7-year-old children had had recurrent episodes of wheezing;[34] in New Zealand in 1973, 23% of 9-year-old children had a history of one or more attacks of wheezing,[35] while in 1981–82 18.1% had three or more wheezing episodes in a year.[26] In these and other studies, parents of half to two-thirds of the children reporting wheeze denied their child had 'asthma'; hence a change in use of that label in subsequent years could greatly alter the prevalence of reported asthma with little change in the burden of disease. Burney *et al.* found an increase in prevalence of asthma for English children of both sexes between 1973 and 1986;[31] however, the increase in prevalence of wheeze was much less and significant only in girls.

In the United States, however, reported prevalence among 6–11-year-old children increased significantly from 4.8 to 7.6% between the first (1971–74) and second (1976–80) National Health and Nutrition Examination Surveys.[19] In each of these surveys, 'asthma' included recurrent wheezing not associated with colds as well as physician-diagnosed asthma. The increase in prevalence cannot therefore be explained by a greater use of the label 'asthma', and is probably real. Similarly in Finland, the increase in asthma detected at medical examination in army conscripts rose from 0.08% in 1961 to 0.29% in 1966 and then 20-fold to 1.79% in 1989.[36] It seems unlikely that a change of this proportion relates to diagnostic fashion, as this would mean 95% of cases of asthma were undiagnosed before 1966.

Substantial increases in hospital admissions for asthma in children in many countries suggest that the prevalence of severe asthma has increased.[37–39] The rate of hospitalization for United States children under 15 years with asthma increased at least 145% between 1970 and 1984.[40] In England, admissions increased 167% in 5–14-year-olds over a period of 8 years.[41] The increase in hospital admissions for asthma has occurred despite falling admission rates for other respiratory conditions, and a considerable increase in the use of antiasthmatic medications,[42] and is in part due to a doubling of the re-admission rate.[42–44] In one New Zealand pediatric unit, admissions rose dramatically from 21 in 1965 to 186 in 1975 and 609 in 1985, while the severity on admission (based on wheezing, pulse rate and accessory muscle use) also increased considerably in the latter 10 years.[45] These facts all suggest that asthma has increased in severity, although there is some evidence of increased self-referral to hospital especially for nebulizer treatments for children.[46]

FACTORS INFLUENCING DEVELOPMENT OF CHILDHOOD ASTHMA

Sex

Studies of the prevalence of diagnosed asthma in children have usually found a male preponderance[20,47] which decreases with increasing age.[5,48] Male predominance may relate to a greater degree of bronchial lability and not to a greater prevalence of atopy in males,[49] although an Italian study found atopy was related to male sex.[50] In Boston children, the M:F ratio for 'asthma' was 1.8:1, but for 'recurrent wheeze most days or nights' was 1:1, suggesting a sex-related diagnostic bias in use of the label 'asthma'.[18]

Genetic and ethnic factors

Twin studies have shown serum IgE levels in adults and children are genetically influenced,[51] while other twin studies suggest a genetic effect on AHR, even when there is not clinical concordance for asthma.[52] However the slope of the dose–response curve to methacholine is not different between monozygotic and dizygotic twins, suggesting that environmental factors are more important than genetic factors in determining individual airway responsiveness.[53]

Differences in prevalence between races may be due to both genetic and environmental factors. Among children of different races living in the same environment, the prevalence of respiratory symptoms is similar. There were no significant differences in the proportions with a history of wheezing illness among London children of European (15%), African (18%) or Indian (17%) descent, although the European children reported a higher prevalence of croup, whooping cough and bronchitis.[54] In New Zealand, the prevalence of current respiratory symptoms accompanied by AHR to histamine was slightly higher in European (13.5%) than in Maori children (10.8%).[27] In the United States, the prevalence of asthma is consistently some 50% higher among black children than white children,[19,20] suggesting ethnic factors influence the expression of asthma, but differences in life-style may modify exposure to environmental factors despite residence in the same community.

Environment

Movement from a rural to an urban environment appears to increase substantially the likelihood of developing childhood asthma. In South Africa, 3.17% of Xhosa children resident in Cape Town, but only 0.14% of Xhosa children remaining in rural Transkei, demonstrated exercise-induced asthma.[55] Over 25% of children who moved to New Zealand from the Tokelauan Islands developed asthma, compared with 11% of those remaining in the islands.[56] These increases suggest environmental factors have provoked expression of asthma symptoms in susceptible individuals in the new location. The prevalence of rhinitis and eczema in Tokelauan Islanders living in New Zealand were 28.3 and 8.5% respectively compared with 13.7 and 0.1% in their peers living in the islands.[56] Hence allergens in the new environment were more potent sensitizing agents, and may be significant factors in inducing asthma as well as rhinitis and eczema. Among Swedish conscripts aged 17–20 years, the prevalence of asthma was significantly higher in city dwellers (3.3%) than rural residents (2.5%) suggesting again an influence of urbanization.[57]

Atopy

Development of asthma in children is related to atopy whether documented by positive skin tests[58] or elevated serum IgE levels.[59] Furthermore, the persistence of wheezing into later childhood is very strongly associated with atopy. Hayfever and eczema in a 7-year-old child with wheeze increased four-fold the risk of persistence of asthma to age 20.[60] Atopic children had an increased risk of developing AHR, especially those sensitive to more than one allergen group;[61,62] the severity of the AHR increased with the degree of atopy. House dust mite sensitivity is one of the more important risk factors for development of asthma in children and adults in the United States, Australia and New Zealand,[63,64] and probably in many other countries.

New Zealand studies have confirmed the relationship between serum IgE, clinical asthma and AHR; in children with serum IgE <32 IU/ml, asthma was not reported, while the prevalences of diagnosed asthma and of a methacholine $PC_{20}FEV_1 < 8$ mg/ml increased as serum IgE increased.[65] Furthermore, a clear relationship was found between serum IgE and AHR in children never admitting to asthma or wheezing.

Passive smoking

Parental, especially maternal, smoking is associated with reduction of pulmonary function,[66–69] lower respiratory tract illness[70–74] and with wheezing illness and asthma in children.[75] Cogswell et al.[76] followed a cohort of high-risk children born to parents at least one of whom was atopic. By age 5 years 62% of parents who smoked had children who had experienced episodes of wheeze compared with 37% of parents who did not smoke. Gortmaker et al.[77] found the prevalence of parent-reported asthma in children aged 0–17 years increased from 5.0 to 7.7% if the mother smoked, and the prevalence of 'functionally impairing' (i.e. severe) asthma doubled from 1.1 to 2.2%. In Boston children aged 5–9 years, persistent wheeze occurred in 1.85% of children from households where neither parent smoked, 6.85% of children from households with one parent currently smoking, and 11.8% of children from households with two parents currently smoking.[18] The trend was independent of parental wheezing, and was associated with a reduction in lung function in these children. Italian 9-year-old males had more than two-fold increase in AHR if one or other parent smoked.[78] The relationship between passive exposure to cigarette smoke and increased allergen sensitization in children remains somewhat uncertain.[79–81]

Early respiratory infection

Lower respiratory tract infections in early childhood may have a lasting effect on respiratory symptoms and pulmonary function in childhood.[74,82–91] Children with bronchiolitis due to the respiratory syncytial virus (RSV) had a greater exercise lability than control children with the same degree of atopy.[92] Wheezing and AHR were more common in Tyneside children after RSV bronchiolitis, although the prevalence of recognized and treated asthma, and of atopy, did not differ from that of a control group.[93] However, these studies beg the question of diagnosis; perhaps these children had had episodes of asthma misdiagnosed as bronchiolitis. Similar findings have been reported after 'croup'.[94]

Children with low respiratory tract infections in infancy[95,96] subsequently had an increased prevalence of cough, wheeze, colds going to the chest, use of medication, absences from school and medical consultations compared with controls, increased airway responsiveness to exercise and reduced pulmonary function, but no difference in the prevalence of atopy. Again it is possible that these children had pre-existing AHR which predisposed them to more severe and symptomatic lower respiratory tract infections.

Low lung function

Martinez et al. prospectively studied 124 newborn infants, and found that the risk of a wheezing illness was 3.7 times higher among infants whose airway conductance was in the lowest third compared with those in the highest two-thirds.[97] Girls whose lung volumes at end-expiration were in the lowest third had a 16-fold risk of a wheezing illness in the first year of life. Follow-up studies showed impaired airflow and lower lung volumes in those with repeated respiratory illness, further suggesting that diminished initial airway function may be a predisposing factor to recurrent wheezing illness.[98]

Socioeconomic status

Anderson et al.[24] found a striking similarity in the prevalence of asthma in different social classes in Britain. Likewise, Mitchell et al. found no relationship between socioeconomic status and asthma diagnosis, AHR or the combination.[99] However, while the prevalence of asthma may not be clearly associated with socioeconomic status, clinical manifestations, treatment and subsequent effects, e.g. school absenteeism and hospitalization, may differ among socioeconomic groups.[15,20,100]

CHILDHOOD ASTHMA AND AHR

Children with frequent symptoms of asthma almost invariably show AHR to histamine or methacholine,[6–9,101] and frequent variation in peak flow measurements. However, a substantial number of children show AHR to methacholine or histamine but have no current or past symptoms suggestive of asthma. This finding is consistent among studies in New Zealand,[7,27] Australia,[9] Canada,[17] the United States[102] and the United Kingdom,[8] and was similar in degree whether the challenge was performed using histamine,[8,9,27] methacholine[7,17] or hyperventilation with cold air.[102] On the other hand, some children with a history of current symptoms suggesting asthma (wheezing, cough, chest tightness on exercise) do not have demonstrable non-specific AHR.[7–9,17]

Among Australian children aged 8–11 years,[9,61,62] 17.9% had hyperresponsive airways, 6.7% of the cohort had hyperresponsiveness without current or past respiratory symptoms, and 5.6% had had a diagnosis of asthma yet did not show AHR. AHR was more prevalent than diagnosed asthma but less prevalent than wheezing or a report of any respiratory symptom. The association between symptoms and AHR was nevertheless highly significant ($P < 0.001$). Of children with a marked increase in airway responsiveness, all but one had diagnosed asthma. Factors associated with development of AHR included a history of early respiratory illness, a history of asthma in either parent, and atopy.[61,62] If all three factors were present, the risk of moderate or severe

AHR increased 6-fold. In New Zealand children, skin sensitivity to the house dust mite was associated with a 5-fold risk of developing AHR by age 13, while grass pollen sensitivity alone was not a significant risk factor either for hyperresponsiveness or for asthma symptoms.[64] Among Southampton children, AHR decreased with age from 29.1% at 7 years to 16.5% at 11 years, while prevalence of atopy increased from 26 to 31.6% over the same period.[103]

ASTHMA IN ADULTS

There are many fewer studies of the prevalence and characteristics of asthma in adults. The difficulties of obtaining a random sample in adults are greater than in childhood, and asthma may be confused with symptoms due to airway obstruction caused by smoking-related diseases.[104,105] Dodge and Burrows[106] found very different prevalence figures for physician-diagnosed asthma and wheezing, even in younger age groups; in 20–24-year-olds, 5% reported asthma, 12% had attacks of shortness of breath with wheeze, 25% had wheezed even without colds, and 42% had experienced wheezing with colds. As chronic bronchitis and emphysema are rare below age 35, the majority of the symptomatic subjects must have had asthma. In older subjects, however, many diagnosed as having asthma also carried the diagnosis of chronic bronchitis or emphysema. Differentiation may be difficult without detailed investigation and a prolonged test of reversibility. Asthma may be significantly under-diagnosed in adults, as well as over-diagnosed in those suffering from chronic bronchitis and emphysema.[107] Dyspnoea and poor lung function due to asthma may be incorrectly ascribed to chronic bronchitis or cardiac failure in the elderly.

Recent studies of the prevalence of 'asthma' in adulthood are summarized in Table 1.2. The same problems of differing methodologies as seen in childhood studies make comparisons between or even within countries difficult to intepret.

The incidence of asthma (new cases of the disease) in adult life is seldom measured. In the follow-up of 14-year-old Melbourne children, 15 of 82 'control' children had

Table 1.2 Studies of prevalence of asthma and wheezing in adults since 1980.

Location	Age (range)	Prevalence	Reference
Busselton, Australia	18–88	5.9% current (symptoms + AHR)	108
Tucson, US	>20	3.0–7.9% asthma, depend. age, sex >30% wheezing most ages	106
Lebanon, US	>7	5.6% asthma, 21.3% wheeze	109
NHANES National US	25–74	2.6% asthma	105
Saskatoon, Canada	20–29	2.7% current, 9.3% cumulative	110
Finland	18–64	1.84% asthma	111
Finland (army)	19	1.8% asthma	36
Sweden (army)	17–20	2.8% asthma	57

developed asthma symptoms by age 21, an incidence of 18.3% in 7 years or 2.6% per annum,[112] a much higher incidence than reported in the United States. The incidence in Connecticut was 1.4% in 6 years, or 0.2% per annum,[109] similar to the incidence of 1% in 4 years, or 0.25% per annum found in the Tecumseh study.[113] The National Health and Nutrition Survey follow-up study detected an incidence of 0.21% per annum; incidence was significantly higher in females than males.[105]

Measurements of airway responsiveness in adults are no more specific or sensitive than they are in children for confirming the diagnosis of asthma.[10] The difference in methacholine responsiveness between Italian adults with obvious histories of asthma and those with no history was not well defined, although the difference in mean airway responsiveness between the two groups was highly significant.[114] Among adults in England, AHR was associated with age, smoking (the effect of which increased with age) and atopy (the effect of which decreased with age).[115] AHR was least obvious in 35–44-year-olds and increased in older and younger subjects. In Norwegian adults, independent predictors for AHR included male sex, younger age, smoking, level of airway calibre (FEV_1) and rural residence.[116] While clear correlations exist between the presence of non-specific AHR and chronic respiratory symptoms in adults,[117,118] the presence of hyperresponsiveness is not specific for asthma.

The prevalence of asthma in adults in some developing countries is curiously much higher than the prevalence in children; the age of onset of asthma in such countries is often over 20 years. Among the South Fore people of Papua New Guinea, the point prevalence of asthma in children in the 1970s was nil, and the adult prevalence only 0.28%.[119] A decade later, the prevalence in children was 0.6%, but a striking 7.3% in adults.[120] Severe asthma, provoked by previously benign factors—exercise, stress, infection—now occurs in these people, who have a high level of allergy to the house dust mite[121] and a four-fold greater mite density in blanket dust than that found in a similar village which has not experienced the dramatic increase in asthma prevalence.[122]

The number of recognized occupational causes of asthma is ever increasing.[123] The prevalence of occupational asthma depends not only on the nature of the inciting agent, but also on the circumstances of exposure. In some industries, over 30% of workers develop asthma, e.g. animal handlers and workers with proteolytic enzymes, whereas lower rates occur with other agents, e.g. 5% with isocyanates and 4% with western red cedar. Occupational asthma may account for a significant part of the total burden of asthma in a population—some 15% of all cases of asthma in Japan are attributed to occupational causes.[124] 'Occupational' asthma may affect persons remote from the work site; a series of epidemics of asthma in Barcelona, resulting in considerable morbidity, was traced to exposure to soybean dust released during unloading of ships in the harbour.[125,126]

Epidemics of severe asthma and increased hospital admissions have occurred during or following weather changes. Outbreaks of asthma were associated with thunderstorms in Australia[127] and in England.[128] Asthma admissions in Birmingham correlated with daily spore counts measured 60 km away in Derby.[129] Some fungi depend on the weather for spore release (e.g. *Didymella*) hence fungal aeroallergens may cause epidemics of clinical asthma, similar to that seen in countries experiencing ragweed seasons.[130] The effects of weather changes on asthma are probably largely related to the indirect effects on local allergens, e.g. fungal spores, pollens, or house dust mite populations, rather than to direct cold or irritant effects on the airways. However, Bermuda has little air pollution and pollen counts are low all year, yet asthma attendances increased with lower humidity, cooler air temperature and winds from the northeast ocean with no appreciable aeroallergens, suggesting a direct effect of climatic factors on the expression of asthma.[131]

EVIDENCE FOR INCREASING SEVERITY OF ASTHMA

Data relating to hospital admissions for asthma,[37-45] and to the use of antiasthma drugs,[132,133] suggest that either the prevalence or severity of asthma, or both, have increased. The increase in admissions is not due to earlier presentation of patients with milder asthma[134] nor is there evidence for change in prevalence sufficient to account for the increase in hospitalization. An increase in the prevalence of severe asthma is therefore more likely.

The marked increase in use of bronchodilator drugs and inhaled corticosteroids in New Zealand, Australia and the United Kingdom between 1975 and 1981,[132] could reflect an increased severity of asthma, or improved treatment of asthma. However a 1984 New Zealand community survey of antiasthma drug use found 80% of prescriptions for salbutamol were for patients with asthma rather than chronic bronchitis and/or emphysema.[133] The same study found that inhaled corticosteroid therapy was still under-utilized; only 42% of subjects with daily symptoms of asthma were prescribed beclomethasone. Hence the increase in sales of antiasthma drugs was not necessarily the result of improved treatment of asthma. Given that total prevalence of asthma is not greatly changed, a considerable part of the increase in drug use must relate to an increase in the prevalence of more severe disease.

The observations suggesting an increase in chronic severity of asthma despite increased drug therapy raise the question of whether the increase in treatment could itself have increased severity of disease. In a randomized controlled year-long crossover study of 64 subjects, we found that the regular use of an inhaled β-agonist was associated with deterioration in control of asthma.[135] Surprisingly, the adverse effect of β-agonist was not diminished by any dose of inhaled corticosteroid; of eight subjects taking over 1500 μg beclomethasone daily, seven deteriorated on regular inhaled β-agonist and improved when β-agonist was used only on demand. Although this study of regular fenoterol is to date the only study designed to look specifically for this long-term adverse effect of β-agonists, other studies involving shorter periods of regular bronchodilator usage contain evidence suggesting that other β-agonists share this adverse effect, perhaps to a lesser degree.[136-139]

Hence the changing epidemiology of asthma is almost certainly related to an increase in severity of asthma. This may be due in part to environmental pollutants, house dust mite exposure, or occupational exposures, but there is also evidence to relate this change to use of pharmacological agents. β-Agonists are highly effective in relieving symptoms of asthma in the short term, but in the long term appear to maintain or increase the activity of the disease they treat, resulting in increased morbidity and increased mortality.

MORTALITY FROM ASTHMA

Changes in mortality rates are generally too small to be useful in studying the epidemiology of asthma. On two occasions in the last three decades, however, widely debated changes in reported asthma mortality have occurred.[140–144] Between 1964 and 1966, asthma mortality in England and Wales, Australia and New Zealand increased substantially, especially in young people. This increase was attributed to a direct toxic effect of high-dose sympathomimetic bronchodilator drugs,[144] to delay in obtaining more effective treatment due to over-reliance on symptomatic relief from bronchodilator therapy,[145] to increased exposure to aeroallergens,[146] or to diagnostic transfer.[141] The second 'epidemic' in New Zealand from 1977 took mortality in young people to over 4.0 per 100 000 in 5–34-year-olds.[147] Changes in asthma mortality in other countries over the last decade have been more gradual and more difficult to quantitate,[148–150] but appear to be real (Table 1.3).

A significant increase in mortality occurred in young people in the United Kingdom between 1974 and 1985.[151] In Canada, mortality in 5–34-year-olds more than doubled from 0.2 per 100 000 in 1974 to 0.5 per 100 000 in 1984.[152] In the United States asthma mortality rates also doubled from 0.15 to 0.36 per 100 000 in this age group.[150] The increase there, as in New Zealand, has been more obvious in non-Caucasians than Caucasians and in younger rather than older persons.[153,154]

The accuracy of certification of death due to asthma has been studied in England[155] and New Zealand,[156] with similar results. More false negatives and fewer false positives were identified in England than in New Zealand, although both countries had a net over-estimate of asthma mortality of 13% when age groups were matched,[157] indicating that the higher New Zealand mortality rate was not due to reduced accuracy of certification. In a regional study within New Zealand, a very low rate of false negative reporting of asthma deaths was found in young people, again verifying 5–34-year-olds as a suitable group for longitudinal study of trends.[143]

The introduction in 1979 of the 9th revision of the WHO International Classification of Diseases (ICD) caused problems in analysis of trends in mortality. Under the ICD9 rules, deaths certified as due to asthma, but with mention of bronchitis, previously coded under ICD8 to bronchitis, were now coded to asthma.[158] In older age groups, this caused an apparent increase in asthma mortality of 35% or more.[153–159] However in 5–34-year-olds, the effect of the introduction of ICD9 was negligible, and trends through 1979 in this groups can be accepted virtually without adjustment.[148] Furthermore, although the 1979 change in ICD produced a significant step-increase in reported asthma mortality in older age groups, this does not explain the continued upward trend in mortality rates in following years in many countries. An increase in total prevalence, an increase in prevalence of severe disease, a reduction in efficacy of treatment, or an adverse effect of treatment, must be proposed as the cause or causes of the increase in asthma mortality seen in many countries. Changes in diagnostic fashion, accuracy of certification or coding rules cannot explain the significant changes in mortality especially in young people.

Table 1.3   Annual mortality rates from asthma in persons aged 5–34 years in eight countries, 1970–88 (rate per 100 000 population).

	1970	1971	1972	1973	1974	1975	1976	1977	1978	1979	1980	1981	1982	1983	1984	1985	1986	1987	1988
USA	0.34	0.27	0.26	0.24	0.20	0.22	0.19	0.17	0.21	0.22	0.26	0.29	0.35	0.36	0.32	0.38	0.39	0.42	0.42
Canada	0.21	0.18	0.21	0.22	0.32	0.31	0.36	0.33	0.28	0.31	0.44	0.46	0.45	0.50	0.50	0.42	0.51	0.49	0.46
England/Wales	0.82	0.84	0.80	0.66	0.53	0.59	0.52	0.61	0.68	0.68	0.68	0.91	0.82	0.90	0.81	0.88	0.83	0.99	0.90
Australia	1.29	1.21	1.04	1.18	1.42	0.78	0.81	0.98	0.93	0.87	0.94	1.10	1.03	0.95	1.28	1.37	1.50	1.40	1.16
New Zealand	1.81	1.91	2.40	1.49	1.32	1.42	2.02	3.64	2.96	4.12	3.46	3.27	3.14	2.28	2.57	1.85	2.87	1.94	2.61
Japan	0.99	0.85	0.67	0.54	0.48	0.44	0.46	0.42	0.33	0.33	0.36	0.40	0.39	0.47	0.39	0.53	0.61	0.62	0.63
West Germany	0.41	0.41	0.50	0.54	0.49	0.49	0.66	0.63	0.70	0.78	0.85	0.83	0.86	0.84	0.80	0.86	0.73	0.73	0.56
France	0.15	0.21	0.23	0.18	0.17	0.26	0.26	0.20	0.28	0.19	0.27	0.29	0.31	0.26	0.37	0.53	0.50	0.50	0.45

RISK FACTORS FOR ASTHMA MORTALITY

Risk factors for death from asthma included age, ethnicity, psychosocial disturbances, a previous history of severe or life-threatening attacks, previous hospital admissions and emergency room visits and discontinuity of physician care.[160–162] Asthma mortality rates for Maori and Pacific Island polynesians in New Zealand in 1981–83 were respectively 5.6 and 2.8 times higher than the rate for Europeans.[147] Similar higher mortality rates are evident among black compared with white children in the United States.[153,154] Differing attitudes to medical care, and cultural and economic barriers to good-quality medical care, may explain part of this difference. In New Zealand, over twice as many persons died from asthma in low socioeconomic areas as from high socioeconomic areas.[163]

Half of the deaths in children under 15 years old identified in the New Zealand national study were associated with disturbed home and family relationships resulting in less attention being given to the child's asthma.[164] Similar findings have been reported in a case-control study of childhood asthma deaths in the United States.[165] Medical management risk factors included the prescription of several different classes of drugs for asthma, and inadequacy of prescribed drug therapy.[161]

Three recent case-control studies in New Zealand have associated prescription of fenoterol metered dose inhaler with a greater risk of mortality.[166–168] These studies have been difficult to interpret because of methodological issues: use of different information sources for drug exposure,[166] possible control selection bias[166,167] and difficulties in selecting appropriate markers for 'severe' asthma.[166–168] In the most recent of these studies,[168] risks for fenoterol were only slightly higher than for oral corticosteroids and theophylline. Risks were also associated with use of oral and nebulized salbutamol, but risks associated with salbutamol MDI cannot be assessed from the New Zealand studies, as salbutamol MDI was used by almost all asthmatics not using fenoterol. The low relative risk reported for salbutamol is therefore the inverse of the risk for fenoterol MDI, and is not measurable as an independent risk factor.

The dominant lesson from English,[169] American[170] and New Zealand[146,161,171,172] descriptive studies of asthma mortality was that a fatal outcome was associated with inadequate assessment and inappropriate treatment of severe asthma, with over-reliance on palliative bronchodilator therapy and insufficient use of corticosteroid therapy. However, these studies did not determine why those at risk had developed such severe asthma.

Recent findings indicate that regular β-agonist treatments may increase the severity of asthma,[135] and hence it seems plausible that both the 1960s epidemic and the recent New Zealand epidemic of asthma mortality reflect an overall increase in severity of asthma due to chronic use of high-dose inhaled bronchodilator. This effect increased the proportion of the population who, because of increased severity, were at risk of death from asthma when circumstances were less than ideal during an acute attack. The association between a specific potent β-agonist and mortality has two components; the selective prescription of a higher dose β-agonist for more severe asthma,[173] and the subsequent effect of that β-agonist in further increasing the severity of asthma.[135]

These findings, if confirmed by further studies, will result in a major shift in treatment of asthma, away from β-agonist therapy, and towards early use of anti-inflammatory drug treatment. The effects of such a change in treatment policy should have a favourable effect on the epidemiology of asthma, bringing about a measurable and sustained downward trend in both morbidity and mortality.

REFERENCES

1. Scadding JG: Definition and clinical categories of asthma. In Clark TJH, Godfrey S (eds) *Asthma.* London, Chapman and Hall, 1983, p 5.
2. Godfrey S: What is asthma? *Arch Dis Child* (1985) **60**: 997–1000.
3. Venables KM, Burge PS, Davison AG, Newman-Taylor AJ: Peak flow rate records in surveys: reproducibility of observers' reports. *Thorax* (1984) **39**: 828–832.
4. Konig P: Hidden asthma in childhood. *Am J Dis Child* (1981) **135**: 1053–1055.
5. Clifford RD, Radford M, Howell JB, Holgate ST: Prevalence of respiratory symptoms among 7- and 11-year-old schoolchildren and association with asthma. *Arch Dis Child* (1989) **64**: 1118–1125.
6. Hargreave FE, Ryan G, Thomson NC, *et al.*: Bronchial responsiveness to histamine or methacholine in asthma: measurement and clinical significance. *J Allergy Clin Immunol* (1981) **68**: 347–355.
7. Sears MR, Jones DT, Holdaway MD, *et al.*: The prevalence of bronchial reactivity to inhaled methacholine in New Zealand children. *Thorax* (1986) **41**: 283–289.
8. Lee DA, Winslow NR, Speight ANP, Hey EN: Prevalence and spectrum of asthma in childhood. *Br Med J* (1983) **286**: 1256–1258.
9. Salome CM, Peat, JK, Britton WJ, Woolcock AJ: Bronchial hyperresponsiveness in two populations of Australian schoolchildren. I. Relation to respiratory symptoms and diagnosed asthma. *Clin Allergy* (1987) **17**: 271–281.
10. Enarson DA, Vedal S, Schulzer M, Dybuncio A, Chan-Yeung M: Asthma, asthmalike symptoms, chronic bronchitis, and the degree of bronchial hyperresponsiveness in epidemiological surveys. *Am Rev Respir Dis* (1987) **136**: 613–617.
11. Pattemore PK, Asher MI, Harrison AC, *et al.*: The interrelationship among bronchial hyperresponsiveness, the diagnosis of asthma, and asthma symptoms. *Am Rev Respir Dis* (1990) **142**: 549–554.
12. Holgate ST, Beasley R, Twentyman OP: The pathogenesis and significance of bronchial hyperresponsiveness in airways disease. *Clinical Science* (1987) **73**: 561–572.
13. Editorial: Airflow limitation—reversible or irreversible? *Lancet* (1988) **1**: 26–27.
14. Brown PJ, Greville HW, Finucane KE: Asthma and irreversible airflow obstruction. *Thorax* (1984) **39**: 131–136.
15. Anderson HR, Bailey PA, Cooper JS, Palmer JC, West S: Morbidity and school absence caused by asthma and wheezing illness. *Arch Dis Child* (1983) **58**: 777–784.
16. Kerigan AT, Goldsmith CH, Pengelly LD: A three-year cohort study of the role of environmental factors in respiratory health of children in Hamilton, Ontario. *Am Rev Respir Dis* (1986) **133**: 987–993.
17. Fitzgerald JM, Sears MR, Roberts RS, Morris MM, Fester DA, Hargreave FE: Symptoms of asthma and airway hyperresponsiveness to methacholine in a population of Canadian schoolchildren. *Am Rev Respir Dis* (1988) **137**: 285.
18. Weiss ST, Tager IB, Speizer FE, Rosner B: Persistent wheeze. Its relation to respiratory illness, cigarette smoking, and level of pulmonary function in a population sample of children. *Am Rev Respir Dis* (1980) **122**: 697–707.
19. Gergen PJ, Mullally DI, Evans R: National survey of prevalence of asthma among children in the United States, 1976 to 1980. *Pediatrics* (1988) **81**: 1–7.
20. Mak H, Johnston P, Abbey H, Talamo RC: Prevalence of asthma and health service utilization of asthmatic children in an inner city. *J Allergy Clin Immunol* (1982) **70**: 367–372.
21. Peat JK, Woolcock AJ, Leeder SR, Blackburn CRB: Asthma and bronchitis in Sydney schoolchildren. I. Prevalence during a six-year study. *Am J Epidemiol* (1980) **111**: 721–727.

22. Mitchell C, Miles J: Lower respiratory tract symptoms in Queensland schoolchildren. The questionnaire: its reliability and validity. *Aust NZ J Med* (1983) **13**: 264–269.

23. Crockett AJ, Ruffin RE, Schembri DA, Alpers JH: The prevalence rate of respiratory symptoms in schoolchildren from two South Australian rural communities. *Aust NZ J Med* (1986) **16**: 653–657.

24. Anderson HR, Bland JM, Peckham CS: Risk factors for asthma up to 16 years of age: evidence from a national study. *Chest* (1987) **91**: 127S–130S.

25. Mitchell EA: Increasing prevalence of asthma in children. *NZ Med J* (1983) **96**: 463–464.

26. Jones DT, Sears MR, Holdaway MD, *et al.*: Asthma in New Zealand children. *Br J Dis Chest* (1987) **81**: 332–340.

27. Asher MI, Pattemore PK, Harrison AC, *et al.*: International comparison of the prevalence of asthma symptoms and bronchial hyperresponsiveness. *Am Rev Respir Dis* (1988) **138**: 524–529.

28. Skarpass IJK, Gulsvik A: Prevalence of bronchial asthma and respiratory symptoms in schoolchildren in Oslo. *Allergy* (1984) **40**: 295–299.

29. Holmgren D, Aberg N, Lindberg U, Engstrom I: Childhood asthma in a rural community. *Allergy* (1989) **44**: 256–259.

30. Braback L, Kalvesten L, Sundstrom G: Prevalence of bronchial asthma among schoolchildren in a Swedish district. *Acta Pediatr Scand* (1988) **77**: 821–825.

31. Burney PGJ, Chinn S, Rona RJ: Has the prevalence of asthma changed? Evidence from the national study of health and growth 1973–86. *Br Med J* (1990) **300**: 1306–1310.

32. Anderson HR: Is the prevalence of asthma changing? *Arch Dis Child* (1989) **64**: 172–175.

33. Hill R, Williams J, Tattersfield A, Britton J: Change in use of asthma as a diagnostic label for wheezing illness in schoolchildren. *Br Med J* (1989) **299**: 898.

34. Williams H, McNicol KN: Prevalence, natural history and relationship of wheezy bronchitis and asthma in children: an epidemiological study. *Br Med J* (1969) **4**: 321–325.

35. Anyon CP, Kiddle GB: The prevalence of wheezy children in Lower Hutt. *NZ Med J* (1974) **79**: 822–823.

36. Haahtela T, Lindholm H, Bjorksten F, Koskenvuo K, Laitinen LA: Prevalence of asthma in Finnish young men. *Br Med J* (1990) **301**: 266–301.

37. Mitchell EA: International trends in hospital admissions rates for asthma. *Arch Dis Child* (1985) **60**: 376–378.

38. Anderson HR: Increase in hospital admissions for childhood asthma: trends in referral, severity, and readmissions from 1970 to 1985 in a health region of the United Kingdom. *Thorax* (1989) **44**: 614–619.

39. Richards W: Hospitalization of children with status asthmaticus: a review. *Pediatr* (1989) **84**: 111–118.

40. Halfon N, Newacheck PW: Trends in the hospitalization for acute childhood asthma, 1970–84. *Am J Public Health* (1986) **76**: 1308–1311.

41. Anderson HR, Bailey P, West S: Trends in the hospital care of acute childhood asthma 1970–8: a regional study. *Br Med J* (1980) **281**: 1191–1194.

42. Mullally DI, Howard WA, Hubbard TJ, Grauman JS, Cohen SG: Increased hospitalizations for asthma among children in the Washington, DC area during 1961–1981. *Ann Allergy* (1984) **53**: 15–19.

43. Mitchell EA, Cutler DR: Paediatric admissions to Auckland Hospital for asthma from 1970 to 1980. *NZ Med J* (1984) **97**: 67–70.

44. Anderson HR: Increase in hospitalization for childhood asthma. *Arch Dis Child* (1978) **53**: 295–300.

45. Dawson KP: The severity of asthma in children admitted to hospital: a 20-year review. *NZ Med J* (1987) **100**: 520–521.

46. Storr J, Barrell E, Lenney W: Rising asthma admissions and self referral. *Arch Dis Child* (1988) **63**: 774–779.

47. Milne GA: The incidence of asthma in Lower Hutt. *NZ Med J* (1969) **70**: 27–29.

48. Dawson B, Horobin G, Illsley R, Mitchell R: A survey of childhood asthma in Aberdeen. *Lancet* (1969) **1**: 827–830.

49. Verity CM, VanHeule B, Carswell F, Hughes AO: Bronchial lability and skin reactivity in siblings of asthmatic children. *Arch Dis Child* (1984) **59**: 871–876.
50. Astarita C, Harris RI, de Fusco R, *et al*.: An epidemiological study of atopy in children. *Clin Allergy* (1988) **18**: 341–350.
51. Bazaral M, Orgel HA, Hamburger RN: Genetics of IgE and allergy: serum IgE levels in twins. *J Allergy Clin Immunol* (1974) **54**: 288–304.
52. Godfrey S, Konig P: Exercise-induced bronchial lability in atopic children and their families. *Annals Allergy* (1974) **33**: 199–205.
53. Zamel N, Leroux M, Vanderdoelen JL: Airway response to inhaled methacholine in healthy nonsmoking twins. *J Appl Physiol: Respirat Physiol* (1984) **56**: 936–939.
54. Johnston IDA, Bland JM, Anderson HR: Ethnic variation in respiratory morbidity and lung function in childhood. *Thorax* (1987) **42**: 542–548.
55. Van Niekerk CH, Weinberg EG, Shore SC, Heese HdeV, van Schalkwyk DJ: Prevalence of asthma: a comparative study of urban and rural Xhosa children. *Clin Allergy* (1979) **9**: 319–324.
56. Waite DA, Eyles EF, Tonkin SL, O'Donnell TV: Asthma prevalence in Tokelauan children in two environments. *Clin Allergy* (1980) **10**: 71–75.
57. Aberg N: Asthma and allergic rhinitis in Swedish conscripts. *Clin Exper Allergy* (1989) **19**: 59–63.
58. Zimmerman B, Feanny S, Reisman J, *et al*.: Allergy in asthma. 1. The dose relationship of allergy to severity of childhood asthma. *J Allergy Clin Immunol* (1988) **81**: 63–70.
59. Stempel DA, Clyde WA, Henderson FW, Collier AM: Serum IgE levels and the clinical expression of respiratory illness. *J Pediatrics* (1980) **97**: 185–190.
60. Giles GG, Gibson HB, Lickiss N, Shaw K: Respiratory symptoms in Tasmanian adolescents: a follow up of the 1961 birth cohort. *Aust NZ J Med* (1984) **14**: 631–637.
61. Peat JK, Britton WJ, Salome CM, Woolcock AJ: Bronchial hyperresponsiveness in two populations of Australian schoolchildren. II. Relative importance of associated factors. *Clin Allergy* (1987) **17**: 283–290.
62. Peat JK, Britton WJ, Salome CM, Woolcock AJ: Bronchial hyperresponsiveness in two populations of Australian schoolchildren. III. Effect of exposure to environmental allergens. *Clin Allergy* (1987) **17**: 291–300.
63. Platts-Mills TAE, de Weck AL (Chairmen): Dust mite allergens and asthma—a worldwide problem. *J Allergy Clin Immunol* (1989) **83**: 416–427.
64. Sears MR, Herbison GP, Holdaway MD, *et al*.: The relative risks of skin sensitivity to grass pollen, house dust mite and cat dander in the development of childhood asthma. *Clin Exper Allergy* (1989) **19**: 419–424.
65. Sears MR, Burrows B, Flannery EM, Herbison GP, Hewitt CJ, Holdaway MD: Relation between airway responsiveness and serum IgE in children with asthma and in apparently normal children. *New Engl J Med* (1991) **325**: 1067–1071.
66. O'Connor GT, Weiss ST, Tager IB, Speizer FE: The effect of passive smoking on pulmonary function and nonspecific bronchial responsiveness in a population-based sample of children and young adults. *Am Rev Respir Dis* (1987) **135**: 800–804.
67. Tager IB, Weiss ST, Rosner B, Speizer FE: Effects of parental cigarette smoking on the pulmonary function of children. *Am J Epidemiol* (1979) **110**: 15–26.
68. Weiss ST, Tager IB, Schenker M, Speizer FE: The health effects of involuntary smoking. *Am Rev Respir Dis* (1983) **128**: 933–942.
69. Tager IB, Weiss ST, Munoz A, Rosner B, Speizer FE: Longitudinal study of the effects of maternal smoking on pulmonary function in children. *New Engl J Med* (1983) **309**: 699–703.
70. Fergusson DM, Horwood LJ, Shannon FT, Taylor B: Parental smoking and lower respiratory illness in the first three years of life. *J Epidemiol Comm Health* (1981) **35**: 180–184.
71. Ware JH, Dockery DW, Spiro A, Speizer FE, Ferris BG: Passive smoking, gas cooking, and respiratory health of children living in six cities. *Am Rev Respir Dis* (1984) **129**: 366–374.
72. Harlap S, Davies AM: Infant admissions to hospital and maternal smoking. *Lancet* (1974) **1**: 529–532.

73. Colley JRT, Holland WW, Corkhill RT: Influence of passive smoking and paternal phlegm on pneumonia and bronchitis in early childhood. *Lancet* (1974) **2**: 1031–1034.
74. Leeder SR, Corkhill R, Irwig LM, Holland WW, Colley JRT: Influence of family factors on the incidence of lower respiratory illness during the first year of life. *Br J Prev Soc Med* (1976) **30**: 203–212.
75. Weitzman M, Gortmaker S, Walker DK, Sobol A: Maternal smoking and childhood asthma. *Pediatr* (1990) **85**: 505–511.
76. Cogswell JJ, Mitchell EB, Alexander J: Parental smoking, breast feeding, and respiratory infection in development of allergic diseases. *Arch Dis Child* (1987) **62**: 338–344.
77. Gortmaker SL, Walker DK, Jacobs FH, Ruch-Ross H: Parental smoking and the risk of childhood asthma. *Am J Public Health* (1982) **72**: 574–579.
78. Martinez FD, Antognoni G, Macri F, *et al.*: Parental smoking enhances bronchial responsiveness in nine-year-old children. *Am Rev Respir Dis* (1988) **138**: 518–523.
79. Murray AB, Morrison BJ: Passive smoking by asthmatics: its greater effect on boys than on girls and on older than younger children. *Pediatr* (1989) **84**: 451–459.
80. Ownby DR, McCullough J: Passive exposure to cigarette smoke does not increase allergic sensitization in children. *J Allergy Clin Immunol* (1988) **82**: 634–637.
81. Ronchetti R, Macri F, Ciofetta G, *et al.*: Increased serum IgE and increased prevalence of eosinophilia in 9-year-old children of smoking parents. *J. Allergy Clin Immunol* (1990) **86**: 400–407.
82. Samet JM, Tager IB, Speizer FE: The relationship between respiratory illness in childhood and chronic air-flow obstruction in adulthood. *Am Rev Respir Dis* (1983) **127**: 508–523.
83. Douglas JWB, Waller RE: Air pollution and respiratory infection in children. *Br J Prev Soc Med* (1966) **20**: 1–8.
84. Colley JRT, Douglas JWB, Reid DD: Respiratory disease in young adults: influence of early childhood lower respiratory tract illness, social class, air pollution, and smoking. *Br Med J* (1973) **3**: 195–198.
85. Kiernan KE, Colley JRT, Douglas JWB, Reid DD: Chronic cough in young adults in relation to smoking habits, childhood environment and chest illness. *Respiration* (1976) **33**: 236–244.
86. Leeder SR, Corkhill RT, Wysocki MJ, Holland WW: Influence of personal and family factors on ventilatory function of children. *Br J Prev Soc Med* (1976) **30**: 219–224.
87. Holland WW, Kasap HS, Colley JRT, Cormack W: Respiratory symptoms and ventilatory function: a family study. *Br J Prev Soc Med* (1969) **23**: 77–84.
88. Colley JR, Holland WW, Leeder SR, Corkhill RT: Respiratory function of infants in relation to subsequent respiratory disease: an epidemiological study. *Bull Eur Physiopathol Respir* (1976) **12**: 651–657.
89. Leeder SR, Corkhill RT, Irwig LM, Holland WW, Colley JRT: Influence of family factors on asthma and wheezing during the first five years of life. *Br J Prev Soc Med* (1976) **30**: 213–218.
90. Voter KZ, Henry MM, Stewart PW, Henderson FW: Lower respiratory illness in early childhood and lung function and bronchial reactivity in adolescent males. *Am Rev Respir Dis* (1988) **137**: 302–307.
91. Gold DR, Tager IB, Weiss ST, Tosteson TD, Speizer FE: Acute lower respiratory illness in childhood as a predictor of lung function and chronic respiratory symptoms. *Am Rev Respir Dis* (1989) **140**: 877–884.
92. Sims DG, Downham MAPS, Gardner PS, Webb JKG, Weightman D: Study of 8-year-old children with a history of respiratory syncytial virus bronchiolitis in infancy. *Br Med J* (1978) **1**: 11–14.
93. Pullan CR, Hey EN: Wheezing, asthma, and pulmonary dysfunction 10 years after infection with respiratory syncytial virus in infancy. *Br Med J* (1982) **284**: 1665–1669.
94. Gurwitz D, Corey M, Levison H: Pulmonary function and bronchial reactivity in children after croup. *Am Rev Respir Dis* (1980) **122**: 95–99.
95. Mok JYQ, Simpson H: Symptoms, atopy, and bronchial reactivity after lower respiratory infection in infancy. *Arch Dis Child* (1984) **59**: 299–305.

96. Mok JYQ, Simpson H: Outcome for acute bronchitis, bronchiolitis, and pneumonia in infancy. *Arch Dis Child* (1984) **59**: 306–309.

97. Martinez FD, Morgan WJ, Wright AL, *et al.*: Diminished lung function as a predisposing factor for wheezing respiratory illness in infants. *New Engl J Med* (1988) **319**: 1112–1117.

98. Martinez FD, Morgan WJ, Wright AL, *et al.*: Initial airway function is a risk factor for recurrent wheezing respiratory illness during the first three years of life. *Am Rev Respir Dis* (1991) **143**: 312–316.

99. Mitchell EA, Stewart AW, Pattemore PK, Asher MI, Harrison AC, Rea HH: Socioeconomic status in childhood asthma. *Int J Epidemiol* (1989) **18**: 888–890.

100. Wissow LS, Gittelsohn AM, Szklo M, Starfield B, Mussman M: Poverty, race, and hospitalization for childhood asthma. *Am J Public Health* (1988) **78**: 777–782.

101. Hopp RJ, Bewtra AK, Nair NM, Watt GD, Townley RG: Methacholine inhalation challenge studies in a selected pediatric population. *Am Rev Respir Dis* (1986) **134**: 994–998.

102. Weiss ST, Tager IB, Weiss JW, Munoz A, Speizer FE, Ingram RH: Airways responsiveness in a population sample of adults and children. *Am Rev Respir Dis* (1984) **129**: 898–902.

103. Clifford RD, Radford M, Howell JB, Holgate ST: Prevalence of atopy and range of bronchial response to methacholine in 7- and 11-year-old schoolchildren. *Arch Dis Child* (1989) **64**: 1126–1132.

104. Fletcher CM, Pride NB: Definitions of emphysema, chronic bronchitis, asthma, and airflow obstruction: 25 years on from the Ciba symposium. *Thorax* (1984) **39**: 81–85.

105. McWhorter WP, Polis MA, Kaslow RA: Occurrence, predictors, and consequences of adult asthma in NHANESI and follow-up survey. *Am Rev Respir Dis* (1989) **139**: 721–724.

106. Dodge RR, Burrows B: The prevalence of asthma and asthma-like symptoms in a general population sample. *Am Rev Respir Dis* (1980) **122**: 567–575.

107. Stellman JL, Spicer JE, Cayton RM: Morbidity from chronic asthma. *Thorax* (1982) **37**: 218–221.

108. Woolcock AJ, Peat JK, Salome CM, *et al.*: Prevalence of bronchial hyperresponsiveness and asthma in a rural adult population. *Thorax* (1987) **42**: 361–368.

109. Schachter EN, Doyle CA, Beck GJ: A prospective study of asthma in a rural community. *Chest* (1984) **85**: 623–630.

110. Cockroft DW, Berscheid BA, Murdock KY: Unimodal distribution of bronchial responsiveness to inhaled histamine in a random human population. *Chest* (1983) **83**: 751–754.

111. Vesterinen E, Kaprio J, Koskenvuo M: Prospective study of asthma in relation to smoking habits among 14 729 adults. *Thorax* (1988) **43**: 534–539.

112. Martin AJ, McLennan LA, Landau LI, Phelan PD: The natural history of childhood asthma to adult life. *Br Med J* (1980) **1**: 1397–1400.

113. Broder I, Higgins MW, Mathews KP, Keller JB: Epidemiology of asthma and allergic rhinitis in a total community, Tecumseh, Michigan. IV. Natural history. *J Allergy Clin Immunol* (1974) **54**: 100–110.

114. Cerveri I, Bruschi C, Zoia MC, *et al.*: Distribution of bronchial nonspecific reactivity in the general population. *Chest* (1988) **93**: 26–30.

115. Burney PGJ, Britton JR, Chinn S, *et al.*: Descriptive epidemiology of bronchial reactivity in an adult population: results from a community study. *Thorax* (1987) **38**: 38–44.

116. Bakke PS, Baste V, Gulsvik A: Bronchial responsiveness in a Norwegian community. *Am Rev Respir Dis* (1991) **143**: 317–322.

117. Ricjken B, Schouten JP, Weiss ST, Speizer FE, van der Lende R: The relationship of nonspecific bronchial responsiveness to respiratory symptoms in a random population sample. *Am Rev Respir Dis* (1987) **136**: 62–68.

118. Sparrow D, O'Connor G, Colton T, Barry CL, Weiss ST: The relationship of nonspecific bronchial responsiveness to the occurrence of respiratory symptoms and decreased levels of pulmonary function. The normative ageing study. *Am Rev Respir Dis* (1987) **135**: 1255–1260.

119. Anderson HR: The epidemiological and allergic features of asthma in the New Guinea Highlands. *Clin Allergy* (1974) **4**: 171–183.

120. Woolcock AJ, Dowse GK, Temple K, *et al.*: The prevalence of asthma in the South Fore people of Papua New Guinea. A method for field studies of bronchial reactivity. *Eur J Respir Dis* (1983) **64**: 571–581.

121. Dowse GK, Turner KJ, Stewart GA, Alpers MP, Woolcock AJ: The association between *Dermatophagoides* mites and the increasing prevalence of asthma in village communities within the Papua New Guinea highlands. *J Allergy Clin Immunol* (1985) **75**: 75–83.

122. Turner KJ: Changing prevalence of asthma in developing countries. In Michel FB, Bousqet J, Godard P (eds) *Highlights in Asthmology*. New York, Springer-Verlag, 1987, pp 37–43.

123. Chan-Yeung M, Lam S: Occupational asthma. *Am Rev Respir Dis* (1986) **133**: 686–703.

124. Kobayashi S: Different aspects of occupational asthma in Japan. In Fraser CA (ed.) *Occupational Asthma*. New York, Van Nostrand Reinhold, 1980, pp 229–244.

125. Anto JM, Sunyer J, Rodrigues-Roisin R, *et al.*: Community outbreaks of asthma associated with inhalation of soybean dust. *New Engl J Med* (1989) **320**: 1271–1273.

126. Sunyer J, Anto JM, Rodrigo MJ, *et al.*: Case-control study of serum immunoglobulin-E antibodies reactive with soybean in epidemic asthma. *Lancet* (1989) **1**: 179–182.

127. Egan P: Weather or not. *Med J Aust* (1985) **142**: 330.

128. Packe GE, Archer PStJ, Ayres JG: Asthma and the weather. *Lancet* (1983) **1**: 281.

129. Brown HM, Jackson F: Asthma and the weather. *Lancet* (1983) **2**: 630.

130. Salvaggio JE, Kundar VG: New Orleans epidemic asthma: relationship between outbreaks and influx of ragweed pollen. *J Allergy* (1968) **41**: 90.

131. Carey MJ, Cordon I: Asthma and climatic conditions: experience from Bermuda, an isolated island community. *Br Med J* (1986) **293**: 843–844.

132. Keating G, Mitchell EA, Jackson R, Beaglehole R, Rea H: Trends in sales of drugs for asthma in New Zealand, Australia and the United Kingdom, 1975–81. *Br Med J* (1984) **289**: 348–351.

133. Sinclair BL, Clark DWJ, Sears MR: Use of anti-asthma drugs in New Zealand. *Thorax* (1987) **42**: 670–675.

134. Rea H, Sears M, Mitchell E, Garrett J, Mulder J, Anderson R: Is asthma becoming more severe? *Thorax* (1987) **42**: 736.

135. Sears MR, Taylor DR, Print CG, *et al.*: Regular inhaled beta-agonist treatment in bronchial asthma. *Lancet* (1990) **336**: 1391–1396.

136. Beswick KBJ, Pover GM, Sampson S: Long-term regularly inhaled salbutamol. *Curr Med Res Opin* (1986) **10**: 228–234.

137. Van Arsdel PP, Schraffin RM, Rosenblatt J, Sprenkle AC, Altman LC: Evaluation of oral fenoterol in chronic asthmatic patients. *Chest* (1978) **73**: 6 (Suppl) 997–998.

138. van Schayck CP, Graafsma SJ, Visch MB, Dompeling E, van Weel C, van Herwaarden CLA: Increased bronchial hyperresponsiveness after inhaling salbutamol during 1 year is not caused by subsensitization to salbutamol. *J Allergy Clin Immunol* (1990) **86**: 793–800.

139. Harvey JE, Tattersfield AE: Airway response to salbutamol: effect of regular salbutamol inhalations in normal, atopic and asthmatic subjects. *Thorax* (1982) **37**: 280–287.

140. Speizer FE, Doll, R, Heaf P: Observations on recent increase in mortality from asthma. *Br Med J* (1968) **1**: 335–339.

141. Esdaile JM, Feinstein AR, Horwitz RI: A reappraisal of the United Kingdom epidemic of fatal asthma. *Arch Intern Med* (1987) **147**: 543–549.

142. Gandevia B: Pressurised sympathomimetic aerosols and their lack of relationship to asthma mortality in Australia. *Med J Aust* (1973) **1**: 273–277.

143. Jackson RT, Beaglehole R, Rea HH, Sutherland DC: Mortality from asthma: a new epidemic in New Zealand. *Br Med J* (1982) **285**: 771–774.

144. Stolley PD, Schinnar R: Association between asthma mortality and isoproterenol aerosols: a review. *Prev Med* (1978) **7**: 519–538.

145. Beaupre A: Death in asthma. *Eur J Respir Dis* (1987) **70**: 259–260.

146. Jenkins PF, Mullins J, Davies BH, Williams DA: The possible role of aero-allergens in the epidemic of asthma deaths. *Clin Allergy* (1980) **11**: 611–620.

147. Sears MR, Rea HH, Beaglehole R, *et al.*: Asthma mortality in New Zealand: a two-year national study. *NZ Med J* (1985) **98**: 271–275.

148. Jackson R, Sears MR, Beaglehole R, Rea HH: International trends in asthma mortality 1970 to 1985. *Chest* (1988) **94**: 914–918.
149. Buist AS: Is asthma mortality increasing? *Chest* (1988) **93**: 449–450.
150. Robin ED: Death from bronchial asthma. *Chest* (1988) **93**: 614–618.
151. Burney PGJ: Asthma mortality in England and Wales: evidence for a further increase, 1974–1984. *Lancet* (1986) **2**: 323–326.
152. Mao Y, Semenciw R, Morrison H, MacWilliam L, Davies J, Wigle D: Increased rates of illness and death from asthma in Canada. *Can Med Assoc J* (1987) **137**: 620–624.
153. Sly RM: Increases in deaths from asthma. *Ann Allergy* (1984) **53**: 20–25.
154. Sly RM: Mortality from asthma in children 1979–1984. *Ann Allergy* (1988) **60**: 433–442.
155. A subcommittee of the BTA Research Committee: Accuracy of death certificates in bronchial asthma. *Thorax* (1984) **39**: 505–509.
156. Sears MR, Rea HH, de Boer G, *et al.*: Accuracy of certification of deaths due to asthma. A national study. *Am J Epidemiol* (1986) **124**: 1004–1011.
157. Sears MR, Rea HH, Rothwell RPG, *et al.*: Asthma mortality: comparison between New Zealand and England. *Br Med J* (1986) **293**: 1342–1345.
158. World Health Organisation: Manual of the international statistical classification of diseases, injuries and cases of death: based on the recommendations of the ninth revision conference, 1975. Vol. 1. Geneva, World Health Organisation (1977).
159. Stewart CJ, Nunn AJ: Are asthma mortality rates changing? *Br J Dis Chest* (1985) **79**: 229–234.
160. British Thoracic Association: Death from asthma in two regions of England. *Br Med J* (1982) **285**: 1251–1255.
161. Rea HH, Scragg R, Jackson R, Beaglehole R, Fenwick J, Sutherland DC: A case-control study of deaths from asthma. *Thorax* (1986) **41**: 833–839.
162. Buist AS, Sears MR, Reid LM, Boushet HA, Spector SL, Sheffer AL: Asthma mortality: trends and determinants. *Am Rev Respir Dis* (1987) **136**: 1037–1039.
163. Jackson GP: Asthma mortality by neighbourhood of domicile. *NZ Med J* (1988) **101**: 593–595.
164. Sears MR, Rea HH, Fenwick J, *et al.*: Deaths from asthma in New Zealand. *Arch Dis Child* (1986) **61**: 6–10.
165. Strunk RC, Mrazek DA, Fuhrmann GSW, LaBrecque JF: Physiological and psychological characteristics associated with deaths due to asthma in childhood: a case-controlled study. *J Am Med Assn* (1985) **254**: 1193–1198.
166. Crane J, Pearce N, Flatt A, *et al.*: Prescribed fenoterol and death from asthma in New Zealand, 1981–83: case-control study. *Lancet* (1989) **1**: 918–922.
167. Pearce N, Grainger J, Atkinson M, *et al.*: Case-control study of prescribed fenoterol and death from asthma in New Zealand, 1977–81. *Thorax* (1990) **45**: 170–175.
168. Grainger J, Woodman K, Pearce N, *et al.*: Prescribed fenoterol and death from asthma in New Zealand, 1981–87: a further case-control study. *Thorax* (1991) **46**: 105–111.
169. Johnson AJ, Nunn AJ, Somner AR, Stableforth DE, Stewart CJ: Circumstances of death from asthma. *Br Med J* (1984) **288**: 1870–1872.
170. Barger LW, Vollmer WM, Felt RW, Buist AS: Further investigation into the recent increase in asthma death rates: a review of 41 asthma deaths in Oregon in 1982. *Ann Allergy* (1988) **60**: 31–39.
171. Rea HH, Sears MR, Beaglehole R, *et al.*: Lessons from the national asthma mortality study: circumstances surrounding death. *NZ Med J* (1987) **100**: 10–13.
172. Rothwell RPG, Rea HH, Sears MR, *et al.*: Lessons from the national asthma mortality study: deaths in hospitals. *NZ Med J* (1987) **100**: 199–202.
173. Garrett JE, Turner P: The severity of asthma in relation to beta agonist prescribing. *NZ Med J* (1991) **104**: 39–40.

2

Genetics

BONNIE SIBBALD

INTRODUCTION

The main obstacle to a better understanding of the genetic basis of asthma has been and continues to be the absence of unambiguous criteria for identifying and classifying asthma. Episodic wheeze and breathlessness are the principal symptoms of asthma, but patients vary so widely in their clinical presentation that it is difficult to find a set of diagnostic criteria that is both comprehensive and exclusive. Investigators cannot be certain of selecting homogeneous groups of patients for study, and the findings of one investigation cannot readily be compared with those of another.

In the work reported below, the diagnosis of asthma has generally been made by practising physicians on the basis of patients' presenting symptoms and history. Objective evidence of variable airflow obstruction has sometimes, but not always, been included as a diagnostic criterion. While this approach will rarely result in the incorrect labelling of individuals as asthmatic, underdiagnosis is common[1,2] and may be an important source of bias in genetic investigations.

MODE OF INHERITANCE OF ASTHMA

The occurrence of multiple cases of asthma in individual families was noted more than two centuries ago, but its significance was not appreciated until this century with the rapid development of genetics as a science. Among the most influential of the early family studies of asthma were those of Schwartz[3] and Leigh and Marley.[4] They provided convincing evidence of an increased prevalence of asthma and allergic disease in the

ASTHMA: BASIC MECHANISMS AND CLINICAL MANAGEMENT (2nd Edn)
ISBN 0-12-079026-2

relatives of asthmatic as compared with non-asthmatic subjects. A number of studies then followed, supporting these findings and showing also that the risk of asthma and allergic disease in offspring was higher when one or both parents were asthmatic than when neither parent was affected.[5] It remained for twin studies to show how much of this resemblance among family members was attributable to heredity and how much to a common environment.

Twin studies assess the relative magnitude of the genetic influence on a disorder by examining the concordance or degree of similarity in monozygotic (MZ) twins compared with dizygotic (DZ) twins. The assumption is made that the effect of a shared environment on the development of disease is the same for pairs of MZ twins as for pairs of DZ twins. Since MZ twins are genetically identical, whereas DZ twins share only half their genes, it follows that any significant increase in the concordance among the MZ twins is evidence of a genetic influence.

Early studies based on small numbers of twins suggested that the concordance for asthma was indeed higher in MZ that DZ twins.[5] These findings were later confirmed by Edfors-Lubs[6] in a much larger study involving 7000 twin pairs. Results showed that the concordance for asthma was 19% in MZ twins compared with 4.8% in DZ twins yeilding an overall heritability for asthma of 15%. More recently the twin studies of Hopp *et al.* give an estimated heritability for asthma of 50%.[7]

Although twin studies show clearly that asthma has an hereditary basis they tell us little about the mode of inheritance or genetic heterogeneity of asthma. Answers to these questions are best obtained through family studies. In family studies the proportion of relatives who are asthmatic is analysed according to their degree of genetic relatedness giving useful information about the number and nature of genes involved. Families are ascertained through an index case or proband and may be either nuclear or extended. Nuclear families include only the first-degree relatives of probands, such as parents, siblings, and offspring. Extended families or pedigrees normally span three or more generations of a family and therefore include relatives who are more distantly related to the proband. Nuclear family studies are most helpful in exploring whether asthma may be inherited differently in different families, but are of limited use in determining the mode of inheritance given the small numbers of relatives in any one family. Extended family studies are most useful in determining the mode of inheritance, but are limited by the possibility that the family under investigation may not reflect the inheritance of asthma generally.

The nuclear family study approach has been widely used to investigate the mode of inheritance of asthma. While all such studies suggest that asthma is heritable, many different hypotheses have been advanced regarding its genetic basis. A number of studies suggest that asthma is inherited as an autosomal dominant gene with incomplete penetrance.[3,8,9] This means that a single gene underlies the liability to asthma, but that the gene is not expressed in all individuals. Others have raised the possibility of polygenic inheritance[4,6,10] which means that a number of genes act together to determine the liability to asthma. More recently Greally *et al.*[11] have suggested that the mode of inheritance may vary between families, there being no one hypothesis to fit all observations. Some of this apparent confusion may be attributed to the lack of a precise and universally agreed definition of asthma. However this is unlikely to account in full for the observed differences among investigators. It seems probable that there may be considerable heterogeneity in the mode of inheritance of asthma.

BRONCHIAL HYPERRESPONSIVENESS

Bronchial hyperresponsiveness (BHR) is the cardinal feature of asthma. The airways of asthmatic subjects have both a decreased threshold and an increased response to a wide variety of specific and non-specific stimuli. Although almost all asthmatics exhibit BHR, not all individuals with BHR are asthmatic. Family studies show that there is an increased prevalence of BHR among the relatives of asthmatic compared with non-asthmatic individuals, but a high proportion of those with BHR have no clinical symptoms of asthma.[12,13] Community studies support these findings in showing that BHR has a high degree of sensitivity but only a moderate degree of specificity in identifying subjects with asthma.[14] In addition there appears to be a poor relationship between BHR and longitudinal changes in lung function and respiratory symptoms both in asthmatic[15] and non-asthmatic[16] subjects. BHR is therefore only one mechanism underlying airflow obstruction in asthma.

The possibility remains that, in some families at least, BHR underlies the development of asthma. Attention has therefore focused on elucidating the genetic basis of BHR in the hope that this will shed light on the inheritance of asthma. Twin studies suggest that BHR, as assessed by methacholine challenge, is under strong genetic control with an estimated heritability of 66%.[7] Family studies support the hypothesis that BHR is heritable, but give conflicting information about its genetic basis. Townley et al.[17] found a strongly bimodal distribution for BHR in 38 non-asthmatic parents of asthmatic children, suggesting that a single gene may underly BHR. However a later study of 83 families by the same authors suggested instead that more than one gene was involved.[18] Population studies of unrelated individuals show that BHR follows a unimodal distribution [19] which supports the idea that BHR has a polygenic or multifactorial mode of inheritance. The genetic relationship of BHR to asthma and atopy has yet to be assessed.

INHERITANCE OF ATOPY

Atopy undoubtedly plays an important part in the etiology of allergic disease. The term has no precise definition, but is most often used to describe a general liability to allergic disease as shown either by total serum IgE or allergen specific IgE. There is a close association between subjects' atopic status as shown by these measures and the presence of allergic diseases such as asthma, hayfever, and eczema.[20,21]

Family and twin studies show that atopy, as assessed by total serum IgE, is under strong genetic control, although its mode of inheritance is unclear.[22,23] In nuclear families, high serum IgE appears to be inherited as an autosomal recessive trait with an additional polygenic component. In contrast, studies of extended families show evidence of genetic heterogeneity, there being a major gene effect demonstrable in some families, but not in others. The disagreements can be attributed partly to the differences between investigators in their choice of analytic model, and partly to the difficulty of controlling for factors which affect serum levels of IgE such as age, sex, and recent allergen exposure.

The factors governing the specificity of the IgE-mediated response appear to be independent of those governing total serum IgE. Attention has focused on the human leucocyte antigen complex (HLA) which is known to govern histocompatibility and may additionally contain genes determining the specifity of immune responses (Ir genes). Both population and family study approaches have been used to explore the possibility that Ir genes are linked to HLA. Using the population study approach, investigators search for an HLA specificity which has a higher (or lower) prevalence in subjects with a particular antigenic sensitivity than in those without. Correction needs to be made for the number of HLA specificities examined since the chance of finding a spurious association increases with the number of tests carried out. The existence of a significant association suggests that HLA, or a gene tightly linked to the complex, may play a part in determining the specificity of the immune response.

Additional information is provided by family studies. Families are ascertained through a proband who has the specific antigenic sensitivity under investigation. The HLA haplotype (HLA genes on the same chromosome) of the proband is compared with that of his affected and unaffected relatives. If the affected relatives share the HLA haplotype of the index case more often than expected by chance alone, it may be inferred that HLA, or a gene tightly linked to the complex, plays a part in determining the specificity of the immune response. The technique is limited in that the families must have many affected individuals and, as such, may be genetically atypical.

Using the population study approach, Marsh et al. postulated a link between HLA-DW2 and skin test reactivity to Ra5, a highly purified component of ragweed pollen.[24] They found that 95% of persons who were Ra5 positive had DW2 compared with only 22% of those who were Ra5 negative. In addition they showed that the IgG response to desensitization with Ra5 was significantly better in those with DW2 than in those without this specificity. This suggested that DW2 itself or a gene tightly linked to DW2 might be responsible for determining the specificity of the IgE-mediated reaction to Ra5. Other studies have suggested that, in Caucasian populations, reactivity to a variety of allergens is closely linked to HLA haplotype (Table 2.1).

These findings are only partly supported by studies in nuclear and extended families. Blumenthal et al.[23] have shown that Ra5 ragweed sensitivity is linked to different HLA haplotypes in different families and that in some families no linkage with HLA is present. The production of specific IgE therefore cannot be related to any particular HLA antigen. Genes linked to HLA may govern the specificity of the response in some individuals, but in others, as yet unidentified genetic factors must be involved.

A potentially important new breakthrough in our understanding of the genetic basis of atopy was made recently by Cookson et al.[25,26] In contrast to the above work, Cookson et al. argued that both high total serum IgE and high specific IgE are evidence of an atopic constitution and likely to have a common underlying mechanism. They therefore defined atopy as fulfilling one or more of the following criteria: positive allergy skin test, high specific serum IgE, or high total serum IgE. Using these criteria they found that the distribution of atopic individuals in 40 nuclear and three extended families was consistent with autosomal dominant inheritance.[25]

This finding was later supported by a genetic linkage analysis of seven extended families.[26] Linkage analysis assumes that the farther apart two genes lie on the same chromosome, the more likely they are to become separated by the random cross-over of genetic material between pairs of chromosomes during meiosis. Genes which lie close together are less likely to become separated and are said to be tightly linked. The degree to which genes are linked is usually expressed as a Lod score which is the log of the odds

Table 2.1 Examples of associations between skin-test responses and combinations of specificities or single HLA antigens in HLA-A1,B8,Dw3 and HLA-A3,B7,Dw2.

	Strongest association		Relative risk		P values*	
Allergen	Combination	Single	Combination	Single	Combination	Single
Any	A1,Dw3	Dw3	2.6	2.5	0.026	0.002
allergen	A3,B7,Dw3	Dw2	3.2	1.9	0.030	0.020
Rye	A1,Dw3	B8	3.6	3.0	0.002	<0.001
pollen	A3,B7,Dw2	Dw2	3.7	2.4	0.010	0.004
Cat	A1,B8	B8	3.4	3.0	0.002	<0.001
dander	A3,B7,Dw2	B7	2.8	2.1	0.058	0.014
House	A1,B8	B8	2.5	2.3	0.024	0.018
dust	A3,B7,Dw2	Dw2	3.6	2.4	0.014	0.006

Relative risk $= (p1(1 - p2))/(p2(1 - p1))$ where $p1$ is the frequency of the phenotype in subjects with a positive skin test and $p2$ is the frequency in subjects with a negative test.

*by Fisher's exact test (two-tailed). The P values for associations with various HLA combinations were less significant than those for single HLA antigens because of the smaller numbers of subjects with combinations.

Reproduced from ref. 24, with permission.

that a person with disease gene 'A' will also have the marker gene 'B'. The linkage studies of Cookson showed a Lod score of 5.58 with the marker gene, p λ MS.51 on chromosome 11, which suggests that the putative atopy gene was located close to this marker. Studies are currently under way to determine whether other investigators can replicate these findings. If the work is confirmed, questions will arise as to what genetic factor may govern both total and specific IgE and how this can be reconciled with previous work which suggests that total and specific IgE are under separate genetic control.

ATOPY AND THE INHERITANCE OF ASTHMA

The majority of individuals with asthma are atopic as shown by allergy skin prick testing, but a substantial minority are not. Atopic and non-atopic asthmatics have been shown to differ in their personal and family history of allergy and their age at onset.[27-30] This wide variation in clinical presentation raises the issue of whether atopic and non-atopic forms of asthma are genetically distinct. Can asthma be inherited independently of atopy, or is it simply a manifestation of the atopic state?

Pepys[27] was among the first to suggest that there was a close association between the atopic status of asthmatic patients and the risk of asthma in their near relatives. His findings, and those of others (Table 2.2), showed that the greater a patient's skin test reactivity, the higher the prevalence of asthma in the first-degree relatives. However, the prevalences of hayfever and eczema in relatives also rose as patients' skin test reactivity increased. Therefore the influence of atopy on the expression of asthma could not be distinguished from its influence on allergic diseases in general.

Table 2.2 Prevalence of asthma, hayfever and eczema in the first degree relatives of asthmatic probands by probands' skin prick test response.

Proband's skin test response	Number of relatives	Number (%) of relatives with		
		Asthma	Hayfever	Eczema
Negative	669	36 (5.4)	14 (2.1)	12 (1.8)
1 or 2 positive	466	27 (7.9)	11 (2.4)	16 (33.4)
3 or more positive	1476	193 (13.1)	185 (12.5)	87 (5.9)

Reproduced from ref. 49, with permission.

The family studies of Gerrard[31] and Fergusson[32] helped to clarify these relationships. Their work showed that the prevalences of asthma, hayfever and eczema in offspring were all higher when parents had one or more of these disorders. However, children were more likely to develop the same allergic disorder as their parents than to manifest some other condition (Table 2.3). Therefore it seemed likely that the genetic predisposition to a specific condition could be inherited in addition to a general susceptibility to allergy.

Sibbald and Turner-Warwick[33,49] explored this hypothesis more fully. They examined the family histories of asthma, hayfever, and eczema among strictly defined groups of atopic 'extrinsic' and non-atopic 'intrinsic' asthmatic outpatients. The findings showed no important differences between the two groups, either in the proportion with a family history of asthma or in the relative prevalences of asthma among parents, siblings, and offspring. However, the relatives of extrinsic asthmatics had significantly higher overall prevalences of asthma, hayfever and eczema than did the relatives of intrinsic asthmatics. This suggested that there may be a genetic defect common to both forms of asthma, but that atopy could enhance the likelihood of its being expressed.

Additional support for this hypothesis came from family studies carried out in the community.[10,34] In these studies, the distribution of atopic and non-atopic asthma in the

Table 2.3 Table indicates the significance* of the prevalence of various allergic diseases in the child when the parent has an allergic disease.

Parents	Children		
	Asthma	Hayfever	Eczema
Asthma	38.84	0.00	1.74
Hayfever	12.88	15.38	4.77
Eczema	2.44	0.02	10.41

*Significance on Chi-square (χ^2) test with one degree of freedom, where: $\chi^2 = 10.83$, $P < 0.001$; $\chi^2 = 6.63$, $P < 0.01$; $\chi^2 = 3.84$, $P < 0.05$.

Reproduced from ref. 31, with permission.

Table 2.4 Distribution of atopic and non-atopic asthma in the relatives of asthmatic and control subjects.

Subject	Relatives at risk	Asthma prevalence (%) in relatives	
		Atopic	Non-atopic
Asthma (n = 135)			
Atopic	338	39 (12)	8 (2)
Non-atopic	99	5 (5)	4 (4)
Total	437	44 (10)	12 (3)
Control (n = 130)			
Atopic	164	6 (4)	4 (2)
Non-atopic	169	5 (3)	4 (2)
Total	333	11 (3)	8 (2)

Reproduced from ref. 34, with permission.

relatives of asthmatic probands was compared with that in the relatives of non-asthmatic probands matched for age, sex, and atopic status as shown by allergy skin testing. The results showed that in non-asthmatic subjects, there was no significant association between the atopic status of the probands and the prevalences of either atopic or non-atopic asthma in their first degree relatives (Table 2.4). Therefore the atopic status of non-asthmatic individuals did not influence the risk of asthma in their relatives.

This was in contrast to the findings among asthmatic subjects (Table 2.4). In these individuals, the overall prevalence of asthma was significantly higher in the relatives of atopic than non-atopic probands. More importantly the prevalence of non-atopic asthma did not vary with the probands' atopic status, whereas the prevalence of atopic asthma was higher in the relatives of atopic than non-atopic probands. These findings are best explained if asthma and atopy were inherited independently, but atopy enhanced the likelihood of a genetic predisposition to asthma being expressed. Relatives of atopic asthmatics could inherit a predisposition to both asthma and atopy, and so were more likely to develop asthma than were the relatives of non-atopic asthmatics, who could inherit only the predisposition to asthma.

SEX LINKAGE AND SEX INFLUENCE

In most populations childhood asthma is more prevalent in boys than girls, while the reverse is often true for adult asthma. Sex differences in the prevalence of asthma raise the possibility that asthma is either sex-linked or sex-influenced. The sex-linkage hypothesis assumes that the asthma gene is carried on the X chromosome leading to an excess of mother–son affected pairs and a deficit of father–daughter affected pairs. Family studies show, however, that the prevalence of mother–son affected pairs does not exceed that of father–daughter affected pairs.[11] Therefore asthma does not appear to be sex-linked.

Table 2.5   Prevalence of asthma among male and female relatives of male and female
asthmatics.

Probands	Prevalence (%) in relatives		Row significance
	Males	Females	
Atopic			
Male ($n = 171$)	49/464 (10.6)	40/466 (8.6)	NS
Female ($n = 127$)	30/388 (8.9)	35/394 (8.9)	NS
Column significance	NS	NS	
Non-atopic			
Male ($n = 35$)	4/96 (4.2)	4/107 (3.7)	NS
Female ($n = 59$)	9/169 (5.3)	13/176 (7.4)	NS
Column significance	NS	NS	

NS = Not significant.

Reproduced from ref. 35, with permission.

The sex-influence hypothesis assumes that females, the sex least often affected in atopic asthma, would need to inherit more predisposing genetic factors in order to develop asthma. This added genetic liability would be manifest as an increase in the overall prevalence of asthma among the relatives of female as compared with male asthmatics, but would be most visible in the female relatives. This is to say the prevalence among female relatives of female asthmatics would be higher than the prevalence among female relatives of male asthmatics. The reverse would be true for non-atopic asthma where males appear to be the sex least often affected. Family studies show, however, that there are no significant differences in the prevalence of asthma among the male and female relatives of male and female asthmatics with either atopic or non-atopic asthma (Table 2.5).[35] Therefore asthma does not appear to be a sex-influenced condition.

It may be that sex acts indirectly through a secondary factor, such as atopy, to influence the liability to asthma. At least two family studies have shown that there is a high prevalence of both skin test positivity and bronchial lability in the male compared with the female relatives of asthmatic children.[12,36] However in the more recent study of Verity *et al.*[37] no sex differences in skin test reactivity were found in the siblings of asthmatic children, although there was an increased tendency to bronchial lability among males.

HLA AND ASTHMA

The undoubted importance of HLA antigens in mediating the human immune response has led many investigators to search for an association between these genes and the clinical expression of asthma. Both population and family study approaches (as described above for atopy) have been used to investigate the possible linkage of asthma with HLA.

Using the population study approach, several investigators have found evidence of an increased frequency of specific HLA antibodies among asthmatic compared with non-asthmatic subjects. In 1971 Thorsby et al.[38] showed there was a trend toward an increased frequency of A1/B8 in asthmatic children. Hafez et al.[39] later demonstrated a significant increase in B8 in those with atopic asthma. Ostergaard and Eriksen[40] have also found an increased frequency of A1/B8, but only in children with both asthma and IgA deficiency. Brostoff et al.[41] found an increased frequency of BW6 in patients with non-atopic asthma, whereas Hafez et al.[39] showed there was a decrease in the frequency of this specificity in those with atopic asthma.

Family studies also show evidence of linkage. Hafez and colleagues[39] found that, in 18 families, 95% of the asthmatic siblings shared one or both of the haplotypes expressed by the index case (Table 2.6). This finding supports that of Wagatsuma et al.[42] who also found a significant association between HLA and asthma within families. In both studies there was no asthma-associated haplotype common to all families, suggesting that the expression of asthma was governed by genes linked to, but not identical with, the HLA complex.

In contrast to this body of work, there are a number of investigations showing no evidence of an association between HLA and asthma. No significant associations were found between HLA and either atopic or non-atopic asthma in the population studies of Rachelefsky[43], Turton[44], Flaherty[45], or Morris[46] and their coworkers. In addition no significant associations have been found with defined clinical subgroups, including patients with asthma and bronchopulmonary aspergillosis,[44] *Aspergillus*-sensitive asthmatics,[46] *Alternaria*-sensitive asthmatics,[45] or aspirin-sensitive asthmatics.[47]

A number of family studies also suggest that HLA has no role in asthma. The studies of Rachelefsky,[43] Turton,[44] and Brady[48] and their colleagues showed that the observed segregation of haplotypes among the asthmatic and non-asthmatic siblings of index patients did not differ from the predicted (Table 2.6). Therefore no evidence of linkage between HLA and asthma was found.

Table 2.6 HLA haplotype sharing in the families of asthmatic probands.

Siblings		Total	Haplotypes shared			Significance (Chi-square)
			2	1	0	
*Study showing linkage**						
Asthmatic	Observed	22	12	9	1	$P < 0.001$
	Expected		5.5	11	5.5	
Non-asthmatic	Observed	29	6	15	8	NS
	Expected		7.25	14.5	7.25	
*Study showing no linkage***						
Asthmatic	Observed	20	8	6	6	$0.1 < P < 0.5$
	Expected		5	10.25	4.75	
Non-asthmatic	Observed	19	2	11	6	$0.1 < P < 0.5$
	Expected		4.75	10	4.25	

*Reproduced from ref. 39, with permission.

**Reproduced from ref. 44, with permission.

NS = Not significant.

Table 2.7 Prevalence of asthma in the siblings of asthmatic subjects when neither, one, or both parents are affected.

Asthmatic subject	Number	Prevalence of asthma in siblings (%)		
		Neither parent affected	One parent affected	Both parents affected
Atopic	435	48/584 (8)	30/218 (14)	5/17 (29)
Non-atopic	116	11/341 (3)	11/66 (17)	—
Total	551	59/925 (6)	41/284 (14)	5/17 (29)

At least some of this disagreement is a reflection of the different methodologies used and their inherent weaknesses. However this is unlikely to account in full for the observed discrepancies. One possibility is that asthma is genetically heterogeneous with respect to its association with HLA. A more likely explanation is that clinical asthma is too complex or ill-defined for its association with HLA to be fairly evaluated using existing techniques.

GENETIC COUNSELLING

As our understanding of the pathophysiology of asthma improves, specific abnormalities may be detected whose genetic basis may prove easier to elucidate. In the interim, doctors must rely on empirical risks in the genetic counselling of patients.

Empirical risks are based on the observed prevalence of asthma in offspring when neither, one or both of their parents are affected. Such risks are valid only for the population from which the estimates were derived, since populations may vary in their liability to asthma. Studies carried out by Sibbald[50] in England suggest that the probability a non-atopic asthmatic parent will have an affected child is low, differing only slightly from the population frequency of 5 to 10%. On the other hand, the probability that the child of an atopic asthmatic parent will develop asthma is considerable varying from 14% when one parent is affected to 29% when both parents are affected. The risk of asthma therefore is two-fold or three-fold higher when a family history of asthma is accompanied by one of atopy (Table 2.7).

Estimates of the proportion of couples with at least one asthmatic partner can also be made. Assuming that mating is random and 10% of the population have asthma, 18% of couples will have at least one asthmatic partner and 1% will have two affected partners. It follows that over half of all asthmatic children will be born to families in which neither parent is affected because, although the risk to offspring is highest when one or both parents are asthmatic, the proportion of such partnerships is low.

CONCLUSION

Asthma is a multifactorial condition whose expression depends on both genetic and environmental controls. The genetic controls are not fully understood, but are thought to include the inheritance of a general susceptibility to allergic disease together with a specific liability to asthma.

Future advances in our understanding of the genetic basis of asthma depend on improvements in our knowledge of the pathophysiology of the condition. More needs to be learned about the genetic factors governing bronchial hyperresponsiveness, and the production and specificity of IgE. Only then can we begin to unravel the complex interactions underlying the inheritance of clinical allergic disease.

REFERENCES

1. Speight ANP: Is childhood asthma being underdiagnosed and undertreated? *Br Med J* (1978) **2**: 331–332.
2. Anderson HR, Bailey PA, Palmer JC, West S: Medical care of asthma and wheezing illness in children: a community survey. *J Epidemiol Comm Health* (1983) **37**: 180–186.
3. Schwartz M: *Heredity in Bronchial Asthma*. Copenhagen, Munksgaard Press, 1952.
4. Leigh D, Marley E: *Bronchial Asthma. A Genetic, Population and Psychiatric Study*. London, Pergamon Press, 1967.
5. Charpin J, Arnaud A: Facteurs genetiques dans l'asthme et les allergies respiratoire. *Poumon Coeur* (1971) **27**: 111–119.
6. Edfors-Lubs ML: Allergy in 7000 twin pairs. *Acta Allergol* (1971) **26**: 249–285.
7. Hopp RJ, Bewtra AK, Watt GD, Nair NM, Townley RG: Genetic analysis of allergic disease in twins. *J Allergy Clin Immunol* (1984) **73**: 265–270.
8. Cooke RA, Vander Veer A: Human sensitization. *J. Immunol* (1916) **1**: 201–305.
9. Weiner AS, Zieve, I, Fires JH: The inheritance of allergic disease. *Am Eugen* (1936) **7**: 141–162.
10. Sibbald B, Horn M, Brain E, Gregg I: Genetic factors in childhood asthma. *Thorax* (1980) **35**: 671–674.
11. Greally M, Jagoe WS, Greally J: The genetics of asthma. *Ir Med J* (1982) **75**: 403–405.
12. Konig P, Godfrey S: Prevalence of exercise-induced bronchial lability in families of children with asthma. *Arch Dis Child* (1973) **48**: 513–518.
13. Clifford RD, Pugsley A, Radford M, Holgate ST: Symptoms, atopy, and bronchial response to methacholine in parents with asthma and their children. *Arch Dis Child* (1978) **62**: 66–73.
14. Clough JB, Holgate ST: Natural history of bronchial hyperresponsiveness. *Clin Rev Allergy* (1989) **7**: 257–278.
15. Josephs LK, Gregg I, Mullee MA, Holgate ST: Nonspecific bronchial reactivity and its relationship to the clinical expression of asthma. *Am Rev Respir Dis* (1989) **140**: 350–357.
16. Redline S, Tager IB, Segal MR, Gold D, Speizer FE, Weiss ST: The relationship between longitudinal change in pulmonary function and nonspecific airway responsiveness in children and young adults. *Am Rev Respir Dis* (1989) **140**: 179–184.
17. Townley RG, Bewtra AK, Nair NM, Brodkey FD, Watt GD, Burke KM: Methacholine inhalation challenge studies. *J Allergy Clin Immunol* (1979) **64**: 569–574.
18. Townley RG, Bewtra AK, Wilson AF, *et al.*: Segregation analysis of bronchial response to methacholine inhalation challenge in families with and without asthma. *J Allergy Clin Immunol* (1986) **77**: 101–107.
19. Cockcroft DW, Berscheid BA, Murdock KY: Unimodal distribution of bronchial responsiveness to inhaled histamine in a random human population. *Chest* (1983) **83**: 751–754.
20. Burrows B, Lebowitz MD, Barbee RA: Respiratory disorders and allergy skin-test reactions. *Ann Int Med* (1976) **84**: 134–139.
21. Sparrow D, O'Connor G, Weiss ST: The relationship of airways responsiveness and atopy to the development of chronic obstructive lung disease. *Epidemiol Rev* (1988) **10**: 29–47.
22. Meyers D, Marsh D: Report on a national institute of allergy and infectious diseases sponsored workshop on the genetics of total immunoglobulin E levels in humans. *J Allergy Clin Immunol* (1981) **67**: 167–170.
23. Blumenthal MN, Bonnini S: Immunogenetics of specific immune responses to allergens in twins and families. In Marsh DG, Blumenthal MN (eds) *Genetic and Environmental Factors in Clinical Allergy*. Minneapolis, University of Minnesota Press, 1990, pp 132–142.

24. Marsh D, Meyers D, Bias W: The epidemiology and genetics of atopic allergy. *N Engl J Med* (1981) **305**: 1551–1559.
25. Cookson W, Hopkin J. Dominant inheritance of atopic immunoglobulin-E responsiveness. *Lancet* (1988) **1**: 86–88.
26. Cookson W, Sharp P, Faux J, Hopkin J: Linkage between immunoglobulin E responses underlying asthma and rhinitis and chromosome 11q. *Lancet* (1989) **1**: 1292–1295.
27. Pepys J: Types of allergic reaction. *Clin Allergy* (1973) **3**(Suppl): 491–509.
28. Gregg I: Epidemiological aspects. In Clark TJH, Godfrey S (eds) *Asthma*, 2nd edn. London, Chapman and Hall, 1983, pp 242–278.
29. Williams HE, McNicol KN: Prevalence, natural history and relationship of wheezy bronchitis and asthma in children. An epidemiological study. *Br Med J* (1969) **4**: 321–325.
30. Molina C, Brun J, Coulet M, Betail G, Delage J: Immunopathology of the bronchial mucosa in late onset asthma. *Clin Allergy* (1977) **7**: 137–145.
31. Gerrard J, Vickers P, Gerrard C: The familial incidence of allergic disease. *Ann Allergy* (1976) **36**: 10–15.
32. Fergusson D, Horwood L, Shannon F: Parental asthma, parental eczema, and asthma and eczema in early childhood. *J Chron Dis* (1983) **36**: 517–524.
33. Sibbald B, Turner-Warwick M: Factors influencing the prevalence of asthma among first degree relatives of extrinsic and intrinsic asthmatics. *Thorax* (1979) **34**: 332–337.
34. Sibbald B: Genetic basis of asthma. *Seminars Resp Med* (1986) **7**: 307–315.
35. Sibbald B: Genetic basis of sex-differences in the prevalence of asthma. *Br J Dis Chest* (1980) **74**: 93–94.
36. Davis JB, Bulpitt CJ: Atopy and wheeze in children according to parental atopy and family size. *Thorax* (1981) **36**: 185–189.
37. Verity CM, Vanheule B, Carswell F, Hughes AO: Bronchial lability and skin reactivity in siblings of asthmatic children. *Arch Dis Child* (1984) 871–876.
38. Thorsby E, Engeset A, Lie OK: HLA antigens and susceptibility to disease. *Tissue Antigens* (1971) **1**: 147–152.
39. Hafez M, Zedan M, El-Shennawy FA, Abd El-Hafez SA, El-Khyat H. HLA antigens and extrinsic bronchial asthma. *J Asthma* (1984) **21**: 259–263.
40. Ostergaard PA, Eriksen J: Association between HLA-A1/B8 in children with extrinsic asthma and IgA deficiency. *Eur J Paeditr* (1979) **2**: 263–270.
41. Brostoff J, Mowbray JF, Kapoor A, Hollowell SJ, Rudolf M, Saunders KB: 80% of patients with intrinsic asthma are homozygous for HLA-W6. Is intrinsic asthma a recessive disease? *Lancet* (1976) **2**: 872–873.
42. Wagatsuma Y, Yakura H, Nakayama E, *et al.*: Inheritance of asthma in families and its linkage to HLA haplotypes. *Acta Allergol* (1976) **31**: 455–462.
43. Rachelefsky G, Park MS, Seigal S, Terasaki PJ, Katz R, Saito S: Strong association between B-lymphocyte group-2 specificity and asthma. *Lancet* (1976) **2**: 1042–1044.
44. Turton CWG, Morris L, Buckingham JA, Lawler SD, Turner-Warwick M: Histocompatibility antigens in asthma: Population and family studies. *Thorax* (1979) **34**: 670–676.
45. Flaherty DK, Geller M, Surfus JE, Leo GM, Reed CE, Rankin J: HLA antigen frequencies and natural history of *Alternaria*-sensitive and perennial non-allergic asthmatics. *J Allergy Clin Immunol* (1980) **66**: 408–416.
46. Morris MJ, Faux JA, Ting A, Morris PJ, Lane DJ: HLA-A, B and C and HLA-DR antigens in intrinsic and allergic asthma. *Clin Allergy* (1980) **10**: 173–179.
47. Jones DH, May AG, Condemi JJ: HLA DR typing of aspirin sensitive asthmatics. *Ann Allergy* (1984) **52**: 87–89.
48. Brady RE, Glovsky MM, Opelz G, Terasaki P, Malish DM: The association of an HLA asthma-associated haplotype and immediate hypersensitivity in familial asthma. *J Immunogenet* (1981) **8**: 509–517.
49. Sibbald B: Extrinsic and intrinsic asthma: influence of classification on family history of asthma and allergic disease. *Clinical Allergy* (1980) **10**: 316.
50. Sibbald B: A family study approach to the genetic basis of asthma. PhD Thesis, University of London, 1981.

3

Airway Pathology in Asthma

JAMES C. HOGG

INTRODUCTION

The general features of the asthmatic state were well described in Osler's text[1] approximately a century ago. He stated that asthma tended to run in families, that paroxysms were often produced by a fresh cold and were sometimes associated with fright and violent emotions. Osler also wrote that asthmatic attacks could be precipitated by a dusty atmosphere, an unpleasant odour or the proximity of animals such as horses, cats and dogs. This clinical description of asthma has been confirmed many times and it is now well documented that asthmatics hyperreact to non-specific stimuli,[2,3] that upper respiratory tract infections reduce the threshold of airway responsiveness,[4] that attacks can be precipitated by antigen reacting with specific IgE antibodies on mast cells,[5] and that exercise[6] and breathing cold air[7] can produce asthmatic attacks in some people.

POST-MORTEM PATHOLOGY IN ASTHMA

The post-mortem changes in the lungs of patients with severe asthma were also known in Osler's time. These show that the lungs were hyperinflated due to air trapping caused by widespread plugging of segmental and subsegmental airways.[8-10] The cut surface of the lung shows that the parenchyma is well preserved and the lumen of most airways is occluded by tenacious plugs. Histologic examination of these airways (Figs 3.1,3.2) shows that the plugs consist of an inflammatory exudate that is made up primarily of plasma proteins, epithelial cells that have sloughed from the airway surface, and inflammatory cells, particularly eosinophils, that have migrated into the lumen.

ASTHMA: BASIC MECHANISMS AND CLINICAL MANAGEMENT (2nd Edn)
ISBN 0-12-079026-2

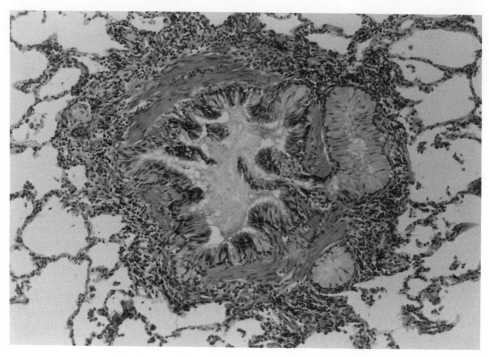

Fig. 3.1 A bronchiole from a patient with asthma where the lumen is filled with a plug, the epithelium shows many goblet cells, the muscle is increased, and there is a cuff of inflammatory cells around the airway.

Although the structure of the material occluding the airways is often referred to as a mucus plug, only a small amount of the material filling the lumen is actually mucus. The walls of the airways filled with the inflammatory exudate forming the plugs are also markedly abnormal. The epithelium is frequently missing and that which remains shows either an excess of goblet cells (goblet cell metaplasia) or squamous cells (squamous cell metaplasia). There is usually a marked thickening of the basement membrane upon which the epithelium sits (Fig. 3.2B) and some authors have attributed this increase in basement membrane to the deposition of immunoglobulins.[11] However, the change in the structure is due largely to an increase in the amount of Type IV collagen which is deposited in association with the proliferation of epithelial cells required to replace those which have been sloughed into the lumen. The airway wall beneath the basement membrane is also thickened due to the presence of the inflammatory exudate and an increase in the submucosal connective tissue. This increase is well documented for the airway smooth muscle which may show hyperplasia as well as hypertrophy.[12] More recent studies[10] have also shown that submucosal connective tissue elements other than muscle are also increased and that there is an expansion of the microvascular space.

The changes seen in the airway wall and lumen at autopsy are reflected in cytological examination of sputum during life where Creola bodies (sloughed epithelial clumps),[13,14] Charcot Leyden crystals (remnants of eosinophils)[13] and Curschman spirals (the casts of the airway filled by the exudate)[15] are frequently found. There is growing evidence[16,17] that similar though less severe changes are present in the airways

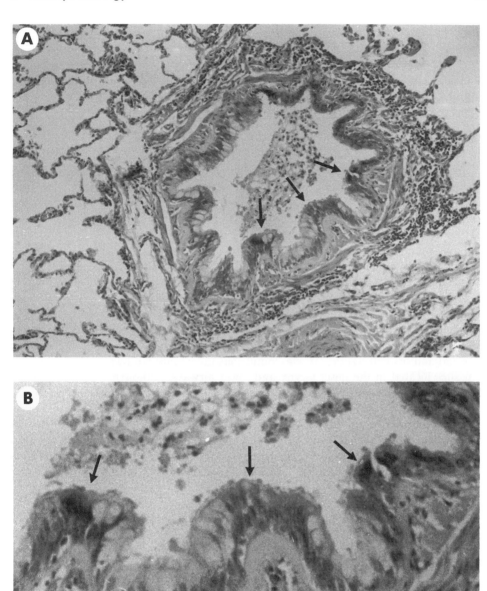

Fig. 3.2 Another bronchiole from a patient with asthma. The arrows in A are shown at higher magnification in B to demonstrate the marked increase in the epithelial basement membrane and the cellular infiltrate in the airway wall and lumen.

of asthmatics who have been biopsied during life and from post-mortem studies of patients who died from causes unrelated to their asthma.[18]

THE PATHOGENESIS OF THE STRUCTURAL CHANGES IN ASTHMATIC AIRWAYS

The structural changes found in the airways of asthmatic lungs are characteristic of a chronic inflammatory process involving tissue with a mucus-secreting surface.[19] The vascular dilatation, increased permeability of blood vessels with the formation of a plasma exudate, and the emigration of leucocytes from the vascular space into the interstitium and airway lumen, are common to all inflammatory reactions.[19] Others, such as the increased presence of mucus and desquamation of epithelial cells are specific for an inflammatory process involving tissue covered with a mucus-secreting surface.[19] Jennings and Florey[20] were among the first to show that irritation of the surface of the colon could cause the goblet cells to empty and that removing the irritant caused them to fill again within a few hours. Hulbert et al.[21] showed similar changes in guinea-pig airways irritated by cigarette smoke where goblet cell discharge followed by recovery were demonstrated. The early studies of Florey showing that stimulation of the vagus nerve produced secretion by the bronchial glands[22] have been confirmed and extended by Nadal and his colleagues[23-25] who found that the glands can be stimulated reflexly from sites located in the nose, larynx and lower airways. Although the mucus in the airway lumen can be attributed to excess discharge from goblet cells and bronchial glands, the cause of the epithelial shedding which is the second distinctive feature of an inflammatory response is much less clear. Gleich et al.[26] have suggested that this could be due to damage of the epithelial cells by toxins produced by eosinophils, particularly the major basic protein. However, the epithelial disruption might also be caused by a stripping off of the epithelial layer by an increase in pressure in the submucosa related to smooth muscle shortening.

PHYSIOLOGICAL CONSEQUENCES OF ABNORMAL AIRWAY STRUCTURE IN ASTHMA

A characteristic functional change in patients with asthma is an increase in bronchial responsiveness. This means that the airways are narrowed by stimuli which do not cause any change in normal airways. It has been postulated that this hyperresponsiveness is due to a lowering of the threshold for reflex bronchoconstriction by exposing the irritant receptors. Such a mechanism might explain how a number of agents such as nitrogen dioxide,[27] ozone,[28] cigarette smoke[29] and antigen challenge[30] enhance bronchial reactivity to histamine. Previous studies[21] have shown that a single exposure to an irritant such as cigarette smoke can produce an inflammatory reaction in guinea-pig airways. The early exudative phase of this inflammatory reaction is associated with an increased mucosal permeability that is maximum at half an hour following injury and then returns to normal. As the changes in airway permeability produced by cigarette smoke correlated with changes in airway responsiveness,[21] it was natural to hypothesize that exposure of the irritant receptors may have been responsible for the increase in airway responsiveness. However, this mechanism does not explain the very marked increase in airway hyperreactivity of chronic asthma where it has been difficult to demonstrate any increase in permeability even in patients with severe asthma. Indeed, studies from our laboratory[31] showed that the airway permeability in asthmatics was comparable to non-asthmatic controls who were very much less responsive to stimulants such as inhaled histamine.

A second possibility is that the increased airway responsiveness is due to the thickening of the airway wall produced by the inflammatory reaction.[10] Quantitative comparisons of airway dimensions between asthmatic and non-asthmatic patients have been confounded by the difficulties of matching airway size. In early studies Huber and Koessler[32] used the external diameter of the airway to compare normals to asthmatics and suggested that asthmatics had increased airway wall thickness. Most recent studies have shown that airway internal perimeter and wall area remain relatively constant despite changes in smooth muscle tone and lung volume[33–35] and this allows airway internal perimeter to be used as a marker of airway size. Studies using the approach here show that wall area was increased in both the large and small airways of asthmatic patients and that bronchial vascular congestion, exudation of fluid, connective tissue deposition, muscle hypertrophy, and epithelial hyperplasia all contribute to the increase in wall thickness.

Several authors[36–38] have suggested that similar amounts of smooth muscle shortening will cause greater narrowing of the airway lumen when the airway wall is thick. The relationship between airway wall area and changes in airway resistance that occur as muscle shortens has been discussed by Moreno et al.[38] Interestingly, baseline resistance appears to be only slightly increased even with severe thickening of the asthmatic airway walls because there is little encroachment on the lumen when the airway muscle is relaxed.[39] However, when muscle shortening occurs, even modest amounts of increased wall thickness produce an exaggerated effect on the airway lumen which markedly increases airway resistance.[10,38,39]

Wiggs et al.[39,40] have developed a computer model of airway function that allows calculation of total resistance as the airway muscle shortens. This analysis shows that airway resistance tends to reach a plateau in normal airways but progresses towards infinity in asthma because of airway closure.[40] This finding is consistent with Woolcock et al. observation[41] that the changes in FEV_1 reach a plateau in normal subjects that are maximally stimulated but continue to fall in patients with asthma. These effects of increased wall thickness also explain why less muscle shortening is required to close the airways of asthmatic as compared to non-asthmatic subjects.[39] Indeed, James et al. data[10] suggest that narrowing and closure of the airway lumen occurs in asthma because of the interaction between muscle shortening in the normal range and a thickened airway wall. This interrelationship also accounts for the rapid reversibility of the airway narrowing because muscle relaxation and lengthening results in a rapid increase in airway calibre and decrease in airway resistance.

In summary, the structural changes in the airways of patients with asthma are a result of an inflammatory process which has a complex aetiology relating to factors involving both the environment and the host. The resulting abnormal structure is predictable on the basis of what is known about the chronic inflammatory process in tissue covered with a mucus-secreting surface. These changes result in a generalized thickening of the airway wall which acts in series with airway smooth muscle lengthening and shortening to account for the rapidly reversible changes in airway calibre that characterize the asthmatic state.

REFERENCES

1. Osler W: *The Principles and Practice of Medicine*. New York, Appleton, 1892, p 497.
2. Itkin IH: Bronchial hypersensitivity to mecholyl and histamine in asthma subjects. *J Allergy* (1967) **40**: 245–256.
3. Nadel JA: Neurophysiological aspects of asthma. In Austen KF, Lichenstein LM (eds) *Asthma: Physiology, Immunopharmacology and Treatment*. New York, Academic Press, 1973, p 49.
4. Empey DW, Laitinen LA, Jacobs L, Gold WM, Nadel JA: Mechanisms of bronchial hyperreactivity in normal subjects after upper respiratory tract infection. *Am Rev Respir Dis* (1976) **113**: 131–139.
5. Ishizaka K, Ishizaka T: The significance of immunoglobulin E in reaginic hypersensitivity. *Ann Allergy* (1970) **28**: 189–202.
6. McFadden ER Jr: An analysis of exercise as a stimulus for production of airway obstruction. *Lung* (1981) **159**: 3–11.
7. McFadden ER Jr: Respiratory heat and water exchange: physiological and clinical implications. *J Appl Physiol* (1983) **54**: 331–336.
8. Dunnill MS: The pathology of asthma with special reference to changes in the bronchial mucosa. *J Clin Pathol* (1960) **13**: 27–33.
9. Dunnill MS, Massarella GR, Anderson JA: A comparison of the quantitative anatomy of the bronchi in normal subjects and status asthmaticus in chronic bronchitis and in emphysema. *Thorax* (1969) **24**: 176–179.
10. James AL, Pare PD, Hogg JC: The mechanics of airway narrowing in asthma. *Am Rev Respir Dis* (1989) **139**: 242–246.
11. Callerame ML, Condemi JJ, Bohrod MG, Vaughan JH: Immunological reaction of bronchial tissue in asthma. *N Engl J Med* (1971) **284**: 459.
12. Heard BE, Hossein S: Hyperplasia of bronchial muscle in asthma. *J Pathol* (1971) **110**: 319–331.
13. Dunnill MS: The pathology of asthma. In Middleton E, Reed CE, Ellis EE (eds) *Allergy, Principles and Practice*. St Louis, C. V. Mosby, 1978, pp 678–686.
14. Naylor B: The shedding of the mucosa of the bronchial tree in asthma. *Thorax* (1962) **17**: 69–72.
15. Curschman H: Unber bronchiolitis exuditive under uhr verhaltmis zum asthma nervosan. *Ptsch Arch Klin Med* (1883) **32**: 1.
16. Laitinen LA, Heino M, Laitinen A, Kava T, Hachtera T: Damage to the airway epithelium and bronchial reactivity in patients with asthma. *Am Rev Respir Dis* (1985) **131**: 599–606.
17. Beasley R, Roche WR, Roberts JA, Holgate ST: Cellular events in the bronchi in mild asthma and after bronchial provocation. *Am Rev Respir Dis* (1989) **139**: 806–817.
18. Sabonya RE: Concise clinical study: Quantitative structural alterations in long-standing allergic asthma. *Am Rev Respir Dis* (1984) **130**: 289–292.
19. Florey H: Secretion of mucus in the inflammation of mucus membranes. In Florey H (ed), *General Pathology*, 3rd edn. London, Lloyd Luke Medical Books, 1962, pp 167–196.
20. Jennings MA, Florey HW: Autoradiographic observations on mucus cells of stomach and intestine. *Q J Exp Physiol* (1956) **41**: 131–152.
21. Hulbert WC, Walker DC, Jackson A, Hogg JC: Airway permeability to horseradish peroxidase in guinea pigs: The repair phase after injury by cigarette smoke. *Am Rev Respir Dis* (1981) **123**: 320–326.
22. Florey H, Carleton HM, Wells AQ: Mucous secretion in the trachea. *Br J Exp Path* (1932) **13**: 269–284.

23. Nadel JA, Davis D, Phipps RJ: Control of mucous secretion and ion transport in airways. *Ann Rev Physiol* (1979) **41**: 369–381.
24. Nadel JA, Davis B: Parasympathetic and sympathetic regulation of secretion from submucosal glands in airways. *Fed Proc* (1980) **39**: 3075–3079.
25. Nadel JA: Autonomic control of airway smooth muscle and airway secretions. *Am Rev Respir Dis* (1977) **115**: 117–126.
26. Gleich GJ, Frigas E, Langering DA *et al.*: Cytotoxic properties of eosinophil major basic protein. *J Immunol* (1979) **123**: 2925.
27. Orehek J, Massari JE, Gayrard P, Grimaud C, Charpin J: The effect of short-term, low-level nitrogen dioxide exposure on bronchial sensitivity of asthmatic patients. *J Clin Invest* (1976) **57**: 301–307.
28. Golden JA, Nadel JA, Boushey HW: Bronchial hyperirritability in healthy subjects after exposure to ozone. *Am Rev Respir Dis* (1978) **118**: 287–294.
29. Gerrard JW, Cockcroft DW, Mink JT, Cotton DJ, Poonawala R, Dosman JA: Increased non-specific bronchial reactivity in cigarette smokers with normal lung function. *Am Rev Respir Dis* (1980) **122**: 577–581.
30. Cockcroft DW, Ruffin RE, Dolovitch J, Hargreave FE: Allergen-induced increase in non-allergic bronchial reactivity. *Clin Allergy* (1977) **7**: 503–513.
31. Elwood RK, Kennedy S, Belzberg A, Hogg JC, Pare PD: Respiratory mucosal permeability in asthma. *Am Rev Respir Dis* (1983) **128**: 523–527.
32. Huber HL, Koessler KK: The pathology of bronchial asthma. *Arch Int Med* (1922) **30**: 689.
33. James AL, Pare PD, Hogg, JC: Effects of lung volume, bronchoconstriction, and cigarette smoke on morphometric airway dimensions. *J Appl Physiol* (1988) **64**: 913–919.
34. James AL, Pare PD, Moreno RH, Hogg JC: Quantitative measurement of smooth muscle shortening in isolated pig trachea. *J Appl Physiol* (1987) **63**: 1360–1365.
35. James AL, Hogg JC, Dunn LA, Pare PD: The use of the internal perimeter to compare airway size and to calculate smooth muscle shortening. *Am Rev Respir Dis* (1988) **138**: 136–139.
36. Benson MK: Bronchial hyperreactivity. *Br J Dis Chest* (1975) **69**: 227–239.
37. Freedman BJ: The functional geometry of the bronchi. *Bull Physiopathol Respir* (1972) **8**: 545–551.
38. Moreno RH, Hogg JC, Pare PD: Mechanisms of airway narrowing. *Am Rev Respir Dis* (1986) **133**: 1171–1180.
39. Wiggs B, Moreno R, James A, Hogg JC, Pare PD: A model of the mechanics of airway narrowing in asthma. In Lenfant C (ed.) *Asthma: Its Pathology and Treatment. Lung Biology in Health and Disease*, vol 49. New York, Marcel Jebber, Inc. (1991). pp 73–101.
40. Wiggs BR, Moreno R, Hogg JC, Hilliam C, Pare PD: A model of the mechanics of airway narrowing. *J Appl Physiol* (1990) **69**: 849–860.
41. Woolcock AJ, Salome CM, Yan K: The shape of the dose-response curve to histamine in asthmatic and normal subjects. *Am Rev Respir Dis* (1984) **130**: 71–75.

4

Physiology

N.B. PRIDE

In this chapter some recent developments in understanding of overall airway, gas exchange and respiratory muscle function are discussed but no attempt is made to give a comprehensive description of applied physiology in asthma.

FACTORS RESTRICTING AND AMPLIFYING INDUCED AIRWAY NARROWING *IN VIVO*

Conventionally acute changes in airway function such as those occurring with bronchial challenge or in spontaneous asthma have been attributed to contraction or dilatation of airway smooth muscle (ASM); differences between normal and asthmatic responses have been explained largely in terms of enhanced contraction of ASM, whether due to enhanced mediator or neural stimulation of muscle contraction or an increased ASM response due to increased contractility or mass. Recent work however has emphasized that enhanced reductions in luminal calibre can occur with normal contractility of ASM either because (a) greater shortening can be produced for a given stimulus due to a reduction in restraining load on the muscle or (b) because a normal amount of shortening gives a disproportionate reduction in luminal calibre.[1] Because it is difficult to induce significant airway narrowing in normal subjects, a novel hypothesis has been that the abnormality leading to easily induced airway narrowing in asthma may be loss of normal mechanisms restricting the effects of ASM contraction, rather than amplification of contraction or its functional effects.[2]

Restriction of airway narrowing in normal subjects

In population studies of bronchial responsiveness there is a very wide range of responsiveness to inhaled histamine or methacholine; although only a minority of normal subjects produce significant narrowing in response to the largest doses of methacholine,

ASTHMA: BASIC MECHANISMS AND CLINICAL MANAGEMENT (2nd Edn)
ISBN 0-12-079026-2

it is believed that the distribution of responsiveness in the population is unimodal,[3] with a group of hyperresponsive individuals superimposed on a broadly normal distribution. If this model is correct, the hyperresponsiveness of identified asthma subjects merges imperceptibly into the normal range.

It has been difficult to explain these large differences in *in vivo* responsiveness by differences in the *in vitro* behaviour of human ASM;[4] *in vitro* human ASM from normal lungs invariably contracts in response to bronchoconstrictor drugs such as histamine and it has been difficult to demonstrate large interindividual differences in this response. Furthermore there is relatively little information on how much the *in vitro* mechanical properties of ASM in asthmatic subjects differ from those of normal subjects.[5–7]

These discrepancies focussed attention on factors restricting airway narrowing *in vivo*. In 1984 Woolcock *et al.*[8] suggested that dose–response curves to inhaled histamine in normal subjects differed from those in asthmatic subjects not only in position (much larger doses of histamine being required to induce airway narrowing in normal than in asthmatic subjects) but also in shape. Whereas progressive airway narrowing could be induced in subjects with asthma, only limited reduction in FEV_1 could be induced in normal subjects before a near-plateau of bronchial narrowing developed.[8,9] Convincing evidence of the development of a true plateau of airway narrowing in normal humans was subsequently obtained by others (Fig. 4.1).[10–12] These findings led to the alternative

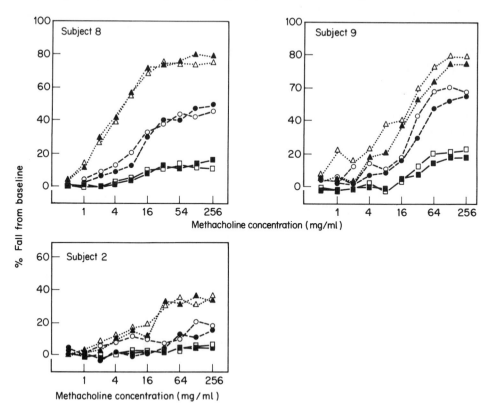

Fig. 4.1 Dose–response curves showing plateau of response developing to inhaled methacholine in three normal subjects on two separate days. Open symbols, day 1; closed symbols, day 2. Response assessed by FEV_1 (■ □), maximum expiratory flow at 40% vital capacity on complete (● ○) and partial (▲ △) forced exhalations. Reproduced from ref. 10, with permission.

hypothesis that the basic abnormality in asthma might be loss of normal mechanisms restricting airway narrowing rather than amplification of mechanisms of narrowing.[2]

Restraints on luminal narrowing are dependent on the mechanical properties of the total airway wall and of surrounding lung tissue. In central intrathoracic but extrapulmonary airways, cartilage restricts the extent of luminal narrowing. In the trachea, the attachments of the muscle to the cartilage rings, at least in cats and pigs,[13,14] result in the formation of complete cartilage rings encircling the lumen when the smooth muscle contracts. In the central conducting airways separate plates of cartilage are found but these are also brought closer together to 'fortify' the airway walls in the presence of ASM contraction. Contraction of ASM itself may directly decrease wall compliance[15] and occasional paradoxical decreases in maximum expiratory flow after bronchodilators in normal subjects have been attributed to enhanced collapsibility of central airways due to loss of the stabilization provided by contraction of ASM.[16]

For the intrapulmonary airways the most important factor stabilizing the airway wall against the effects of ASM contraction is the attachment of alveolar walls to the external perimeter of the airway wall. By these attachments the forces distending the alveoli are transmitted to the external airway wall, promoting airway distension as the alveoli expand. Theory and most experimental work suggests that these extra-airway forces would have their greatest stabilizing effect at large lung volumes, so that a given amount of activation of ASM would lead to greater shortening at small than at large lung volume.[17–19] Experiments in excised lobes of dogs have shown that while methacholine can induce complete airway closure in collapsed lung, this is not possible when the lungs are inflated.[20]

In vivo, the magnitude of maximum bronchoconstriction to inhaled methacholine is greater at small than at large lung volume[12,21,22] and is quite sensitive to relatively small changes in volume above and below functional residual capacity. However, the magnitude of airway narrowing produced by submaximal doses of methacholine appears to be unchanged by moderate changes in lung volume.[21,23] This suggests that ASM initially may contract freely and that the restraints applied by surrounding lung chiefly act to prevent extreme narrowing or closure.

Amplification of the luminal effects of ASM contraction in asthma

The conventional view of the enhanced constrictor responsiveness of asthmatic airways has been that the ASM is unduly 'twitchy' and primed to contract due to some undefined combination of an enhanced mediator or neural stimulation or an enhanced ASM response due to increased contractility or mass. Recent work has added to these possibilities by emphasizing that enhanced reductions in luminal calibre can occur with normal shortening of ASM.

The most obvious of these factors is the effect of thickening of the airway wall internal to the contracting muscle. The consequences of this on luminal narrowing were clearly set out by Freedman;[24] the analogous role of wall thickening in accounting for enhanced responsiveness of vascular smooth muscle in hypertension had been demonstrated earlier by Folkow.[25] Subsequently, Moreno et al. in Vancouver have modelled the effects of wall thickness[1] and James et al. developed methods to estimate this in collapsed human lungs at post-mortem.[26] They found on average a doubling of the thickness of the airway wall in lungs from 18 asthmatic subjects. These changes involved all sizes of airways. Calculations suggest these changes would not be sufficient to increase airway resistance at rest, but would greatly enhance the effects of challenge procedures (Fig. 4.2).[26] Of course it is impossible to know which of the observed changes were chronic and which associated with the final attack; intraluminal secretions would also amplify the effects of a given amount of shortening of ASM. It has also been hypothesized that rapid expansion of the blood volume in and around the airway wall might be responsible for the airway narrowing that occurs after exercise or isocapnic hyperventilation in asthmatic subjects.[27]

It is more difficult to examine the effects of changes in airway wall compliance and extra-airway forces in asthma. Airway conductance shows an abnormally small rise as lung volume is increased in asthmatic subjects.[28,29] Stiffening of the airway wall making it expand less in response to the usual distending forces associated with lung inflation might cause this change, but loss of parallel airways due to closure would have similar effects. Reduced compliance of the airway wall, due to inflammatory oedema, conceivably might increase the load against which ASM was operating, reducing shortening for a given amount of activation. In animal experiments, tracheal narrowing *in vitro* has been enhanced by prior treatment with intravenous papain.[30] Inducing emphysema by intratracheal elastase has enhanced airway response to methacholine in rats, and this change has been related to loss of lung elastic recoil.[31] There is probably also some loss of lung elastic recoil in human asthma[32] which would be expected to reduce the parenchymal forces distending the airway.

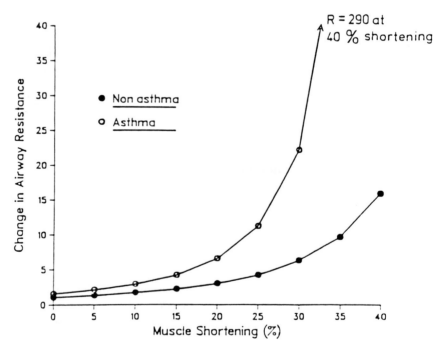

Fig. 4.2 Theoretical effects of the increase in airway wall thickening observed in asthmatic subjects on increase in airways resistance for a given degree of shortening of airway smooth muscle. The baseline resistance of the non-asthmatic airways is arbitrarily set as 1.0. Airway wall thickening in asthma only has a small effect on relaxed luminal diameter, but greatly enhances the rise in resistance in response to a given degree of smooth muscle shortening. Reproduced from ref. 26, with permission.

SITE OF AIRWAY NARROWING IN ASTHMA

There is no doubt that during an asthmatic attack, the severity of narrowing varies greatly between parallel airways. However, despite many investigations, attempts to determine the serial site of airway narrowing in asthma have been relatively inconclusive. Studies of the 'fixed' pathology of the airways, such as the studies of airway wall thickening discussed above[26] cannot provide the reference standard they provide in chronic obstructive pulmonary disease, because so much of the airway narrowing in asthma is likely to be due to the transient mechanisms of smooth muscle contraction, mucosal swelling and luminal secretions. Probably the first *in vivo* attempt to determine the serial site of narrowing was that of Koblett and Wyss in 1956[33] measuring pressures with an intrabronchial catheter. Subsequently less direct methods (changes during helium breathing or after a deep inflation) have been used to deduce this information.

Comparison of maximum expiratory flow–volume curves breathing air and helium–oxygen

In the 1970s there was considerable interest in trying to localize the serial site of airflow limitation in asthma by measuring the increase in maximum expiratory flow when density of the expired gas was reduced by breathing an He–O_2 mixture.[34] In some (but not all) asthmatic subjects, maximum expiratory flow does not show the normal increase when breathing HeO_2; this suggests that the major site of flow limitation is no longer in central airways as in normal subjects, but has moved to more peripheral airways where flow is presumed to be laminar and independent of density.[35] This change is usually attributed to increased frictional pressure losses in narrowed peripheral airways. Some asthmatic subjects consistently lose or consistently retain density dependence of maximum flow with repeated attacks, but this is not invariably the case; in general, loss of density dependence becomes more common as expiratory airflow limitation increases in severity[36,37] and is particularly observed in asthmatic subjects who smoke.[38] Lisboa *et al.*[39] have argued that measuring the density-dependence of airway resistance during ordinary tidal breathing gives a better indication of the site of predominant airway narrowing and have found a poor relation between the density-dependence of resistance and of maximum expiratory flow. Certainly studies in which density-dependence of maximum expiratory flow is reduced should not be interpreted as indicating *only* peripheral airways are involved even if they are the site of flow limitation.

Following this burst of activity in the 1970s, interest in the use of helium response on maximum expiratory flow waned. The method analysed the changes in the airways between the alveoli and the sites of expiratory flow limitation ('choke-points') but experimental studies in dogs showed that relatively small changes in geometry and position of choke-points could profoundly affect the helium response.[40] A review of experimental data obtained up to 1986 emphasized the considerable variation in size of the baseline helium response in the normal population and in disease; changes in helium response in an individual before and after an acute intervention may be more reliable.[41]

Effects of a deep inflation on airway function

More recently attempts have been made to localize the site of dominant airway narrowing by another indirect technique, the effects of a deep inflation (DI) on airway function. For 30 years it has been recognized that a DI may transiently affect airway dimensions when tidal breathing is resumed. The first studies demonstrated airway widening after DI in normal subjects when narrowing had been induced by inhaled histamine or methacholine. Later Gayrard *et al.*[42] pointed out that DI could lead to subsequent narrowing in subjects with acute asthma. Initially changes after DI were attributed to a change in bronchial muscle activity (direct or reflex) produced by stretch. An alternative hypothesis is that the relation between parenchymal and airway hysteresis explains the variable changes in airway function after DI.[43,44] When airway hysteresis exceeds that of parenchyma, DI results in temporary bronchial widening when tidal breathing is resumed. When parenchymal hysteresis exceeds that of the airways, DI results in bronchial narrowing. Equal degrees of hysteresis result in no effect of DI on resting airway calibre, as found in most normal subjects. A major interest of this idea is that it might localize the site of disease within the lung. Contraction of bronchial muscle in conducting airways would be expected to increase airway hysteresis without affecting parenchymal hysteresis. Increased tone in the extreme periphery of the lung (respiratory bronchioles and alveolar ducts) would be expected to increase parenchymal hysteresis with only a small increase in airway hysteresis.

The effects of DI can be examined by measuring the effects on airway resistance, or more simply by comparing maximal expiratory flow at 30–40% vital capacity above residual volume from forced expirations begun from just above functional residual capacity (partial curve, P) with isovolumic flow during manoeuvres started from total lung capacity (maximal curve, M) (Fig. 4.3). From these two expirations the results are expressed as M–P ratios. In normal subjects under basal conditions M–P ratios on average are a little greater than 1.0.[45] In spontaneous episodes of asthma M–P ratios are less than 1.0 (airway function worse after DI) and tend to fall as FEV_1 (% predicted) falls.[45,46] This suggests an important obstruction of the most peripheral airways in spontaneous asthma. In contrast, when acute obstruction is induced by challenge with inhaled short-acting drugs, M–P ratios rise—sometimes to very high values, indicating that DI removes obstruction. This is characteristic of a conducting airway response. Similar rises in M–P ratios have been found when airway narrowing is induced by

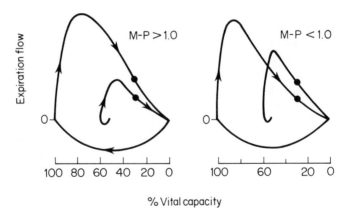

Fig. 4.3 Use of forced expirations started from about 60% vital capacity (partial curve) and full inflation (maximum curve) to derive isovolumic maximum expiratory flow at about 30% vital capacity on maximum (M) and partial (P) curves. Results expressed as M–P ratios in Fig. 4.4. Reproduced from ref. 44, with permission.

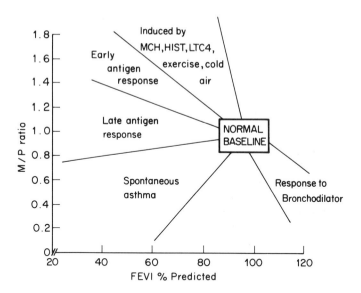

Fig. 4.4 Scheme of changes in isovolumic maximum expiratory flow on maximum and partial flow–volume curves (M–P ratios). In the normal subject this ratio is close to 1.0. With acute bronchoconstrictor challenges the ratio rises as FEV_1 falls but in spontaneous asthma, M–P ratios are <1.0 and fall as FEV_1 falls. Changes with antigen challenge are intermediate. Reproduced from ref. 44, with permission.

other acute, short-lived challenges such as exercise or hyperventilation; with antigen challenge however rises in M–P ratios are less pronounced for the impairment of FEV_1 in the early phase of the reaction and tend to be lower (although still more than 1.0) in the late phase.[44,47] Thus changes after allergen challenge are intermediate between those found with a simple pharmacological challenge and spontaneous asthma (Fig. 4.4). The results have been interpreted as providing evidence for the presence of inflammatory changes in the peripheral airways in spontaneous asthma and to a lesser extent in the late response to allergen. The tendency to airway narrowing after a DI has been shown to relate to elevated concentrations of eosinophils and histamine in bronchoalveolar lavage fluid in asthmatic subjects.[48] A similar response to DI to that found in spontaneous asthma is also found in smokers with airflow obstruction in whom the dominant role of peripheral airway changes is well established.

Direct intrabronchial measurements

There are obvious limits to deducing serial distribution of resistance from measurements at the mouth of gas flow and progress will probably depend on methods making more direct measurements of bronchial dimensions or the distribution of resistance. Unfortunately the acoustic reflection technique, which obtains a distance–area function of the airway, at present can only provide reliable data from the mouth to the main bronchi,[49] while hopes that tantalum dust could be used to obtain inhalation bronchograms *in vivo* have not been fulfilled. Several groups have returned to measuring pressures with intrabronchial catheters; these catheters may mechanically stimulate receptors in the airway mucosa and can only be used in central airways without compromising airflow through the catheterized airway. Another technique measures pressure–flow relations in the occluded lung beyond a bronchoscope wedged in a segmental bronchus. In asthmatic subjects in remission with normal total airways resistance and FEV_1, a considerable increase in peripheral lung resistance has been found (Fig. 4.5);[50] this technique measures the combined resistance of peripheral airways and collateral channels. These results directly confirm earlier suggestions from pathological and physiological studies that there are residual changes in the peripheral airways even in remission of asthma. They are relevant to arguments as to whether increased airway responsiveness is a primary abnormality in asthma or a consequence of altered geometry. Although airway hyperresponsiveness can be found commonly in asthma when overall airway function is normal, overall measurements may conceal considerable changes in peripheral airways. In addition, as discussed above, modest increases in airway wall thickness, which have a negligible effect on basal airways resistance, can greatly enhance the effect of a normal amount of shortening of airway smooth muscle in response to a constrictor stimulus.[26] These findings attenuate the distinction often made between the accepted importance of geometric factors in determining airway hyperresponsiveness in chronic obstructive pulmonary disease and its relative unimportance in the genesis of the hyperresponsiveness of asthma.[51]

In summary, functional abnormality of the peripheral airways is usually present in spontaneous asthma, even when in remission; the extent to which larger conducting airways are involved may vary between individuals and between attacks in an individual. Measurements before and after a DI suggest that easily reversible airway narrowing, such as that induced by histamine, methacholine or exercise, may chiefly involve central conducting airways while the less reversible changes of spontaneous asthma and the late reaction to allergens may be in more peripheral airways.

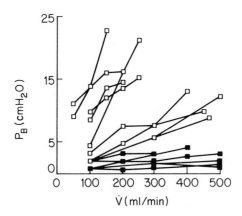

Fig. 4.5 Relation between intra-bronchial pressure (P_B) and inspiratory flow ($\dot{V}$) in the lung beyond a bronchoscope wedged in a segmental bronchus in six normal subjects (closed squares) and nine subjects with asthma studied at a time when they were asymptomatic and had normal FEV_1 and airway resistance (open squares). The steeper slope of the $P_B/\dot{V}$ relationship in the asthmatic subjects indicates an increased peripheral lung resistance (combination of peripheral airways and collateral channels). Reproduced from ref. 50, with permission.

FUNCTIONAL OBSTRUCTION OF THE EXTRATHORACIC AIRWAY

The dyspnoea and wheeze of asthma has to be distinguished from structural or functional obstruction of the extrathoracic airway. Structural narrowing of the larynx or trachea usually leads to persistent symptoms and well-recognized and distinctive changes in maximum expiratory and inspiratory flow–volume curves[52] which indicate the need for airway endoscopy. Functional obstruction of the upper airway in contrast is characteristically episodic and may mimic acute asthma. Two distinct patterns have been described. Most commonly, inspiratory stridor is associated with reduction in maximum inspiratory flow throughout the vital capacity and normal maximum expiratory flow; sometimes however there is reduction in both maximum inspiratory and expiratory flow. Limited endoscopic examinations suggest the obstruction is in the larynx. Typically patients are young women, some of whom are repeatedly admitted to hospital with recurrent attacks of noisy acute breathlessness. The second type of functional wheezing is mainly expiratory and is produced by forceful breathing close to residual volume;[53,54] this is associated with completely normal maximum flow–volume curves; the wheeze probably arises from excessive tidal narrowing of central intrathoracic airways during expiration. Other aspects of lung function such as blood gases, single breath N_2 test, and functional residual capacity are normal.

EFFECTS OF POSTURE ON AIRWAY FUNCTION

In normal subjects airways resistance during tidal breathing increases in the supine posture by about 50% compared to seated values. This increase is appropriate for the reduction in end-expired lung volume (functional residual capacity, FRC).[55]

In asthmatic subjects in remission, increases in resistance on lying down are a little greater than in normal subjects but there is a normal fall in FRC and resistance reverts to previous levels rapidly on sitting up. But when asthma is active, adopting the supine posture leads to absolute and proportionately larger increases in total respiratory resistance than in normal subjects (Fig. 4.6)[56] despite a smaller than normal reduction in FRC, implying a true rise in resistance at isovolume. This could be due to an increase in extrathoracic or chest wall resistance or a true decrease in isovolumic intrapulmonary airway dimensions; there are accompanying changes in maximum expiratory flow–volume curves which suggest a true decrease in airway dimensions.

The relevance of these changes to the development of nocturnal asthma is uncertain. Some studies have claimed that when the supine posture is maintained for several hours airway function progressively deteriorates in asthmatic but not in normal subjects;[57–59] but a controlled study in which groups of asthmatic subjects remained in either the sitting or supine posture showed similar deterioration in airway function in both groups.[60] In our own laboratory, airway function in some subjects with asthma does not revert to initial sitting values in the 10 min after lying supine; these subjects appear to be those with symptomatic asthma at the time of study (Fig. 4.6). Whatever the role of posture in the pathogenesis of nocturnal asthma, the supine posture exacerbates the degree of airway narrowing and discomfort; patients invariably seek relief by sitting up,

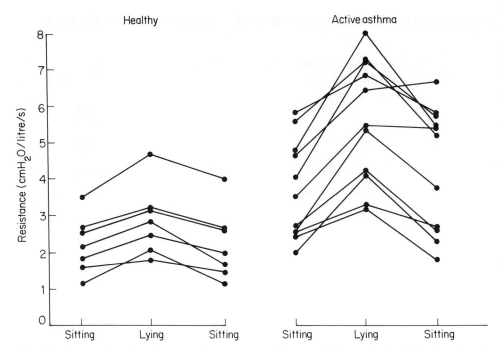

Fig. 4.6 Changes in total respiratory resistance measured by an oscillation method at 6 Hz when changing from sitting to the supine posture in seven normal subjects and 10 subjects with active asthma. Sitting values are higher in asthma and the absolute rise supine is greater. Two subjects with asthma failed to return to original sitting values after 10 min. Reproduced from ref. 56, with permission.

even although this leads to less dramatic improvement than in the orthopnoea of left heart failure.

HYPERINFLATION AND RESPIRATORY MUSCLE FUNCTION

FRC consistently rises during an attack of asthma. In the normal subject FRC is the volume at which the inward recoil of the lungs is equal to the opposing outward recoil of the chest cage. During a passive expiration, expiratory flow ceases at this volume. In an asthmatic attack the end-expired volume is larger than the relaxed volume of the chest. Several different mechanisms contribute to this increase in end-expired volume. First, there is usually a large increase in residual volume (RV), presumably due to enhanced airway closure or near closure; RV may sometimes be larger than the control FRC. Additional dynamic mechanisms maintain end-expired volume above that dictated by airway closure. Thus if there is expiratory flow limitation during tidal expiration, expiration may be then terminated by the initiation of the following inspiration rather than by the cessation of passive expiratory flow. But even in the absence of expiratory flow limitation, a large end-expiratory volume may be maintained by persistent inspiratory muscle activity throughout expiration.[61–63] Although we found hyperinflation was relatively well maintained when awake in the supine posture, this depends on appropriate respiratory muscle activity. A recent study has shown that hyperinflation tends to be reduced during sleep and particularly during rapid eye movement sleep[64] and this must contribute to the worsening of pulmonary function that occurs at night.

As airway size enlarges with increase in lung volume, breathing at a larger lung volume partially overcomes the effects of airway narrowing, but this compensation is achieved at the cost of the inspiratory muscles which have to contract starting at a shorter and less favourable resting length. The load on the right ventricle is probably also increased by hyperinflation. Recent studies with experimental bronchoconstriction suggest the degree of hyperinflation may be adjusted to minimize the total work of breathing. When moderate bronchoconstriction is induced by histamine, spontaneous hyperinflation reduces total work of breathing, a slight increase in total inspiratory work (the increase in elastic work outweighing the decrease in resistive work) above that at the original FRC being offset by a larger reduction in expiratory flow-resistive work (Fig. 4.7).[65] However, with severe spontaneous asthma hyperinflation is less likely to reduce airways resistance[28,46] sufficiently to prevent a considerable increase in total inspiratory work, which may account for much of the discomfort of the asthmatic attack and lead to eventual muscle fatigue.

The increased load on the inspiratory muscles in severe asthma has been recognized for many years, but it remains uncertain whether this leads to increased force and endurance in chronic asthma or to muscle fatigue in severe acute attacks. Gross inspiratory muscle weakness has been demonstrated in a few obese women with asthma who had been on chronic high doses of oral corticosteroids,[66] but smaller doses have not

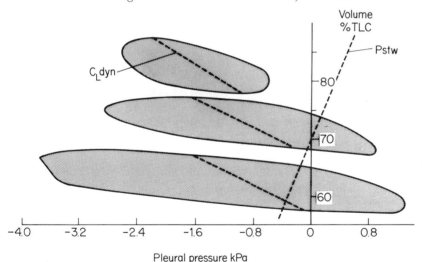

Fig. 4.7 Changes in pleural pressure–volume (PV) loops at three different degrees of hyperinflation during histamine-induced bronchial narrowing in an asthmatic subject. The middle PV loop shows the hyperinflation adopted spontaneously by the subject; to obtain the lower PV loop the subject voluntarily returned to control lung volumes before histamine inhalation; the upper PV loop was obtained by asking the subject to hyperinflate further. For each PV loop the slope ($\Delta V/\Delta P$) of the diagonal interrupted line indicates dynamic lung compliance ($C_L$dyn); stippled areas to the left and right of the $C_L$dyn line indicate work required to overcome inspiratory and expiratory airways resistance respectively. Inspiratory elastic work on lungs and chest wall is indicated by the area between the $C_L$dyn line and the chest wall relaxation (Pst_W vs volume) line. Spontaneous hyperinflation reduces inspiratory and expiratory flow resistance with only a moderate increase in inspiratory elastic work; further hyperinflation reduces flow resistive work but considerably increases inspiratory elastic work so that there is no change in total inspiratory work. Other abbreviations: TLC = total lung capacity; Pst_W = recoil pressure of relaxed chest wall. Reproduced from ref. 65, with permission.

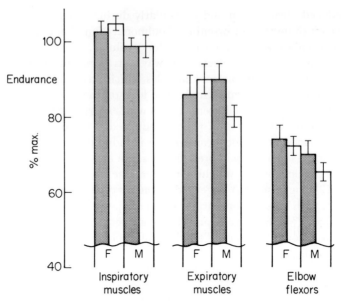

Fig. 4.8 Comparison of endurance of inspiratory and expiratory muscles and elbow flexors in 20 (10 M, 10 F) asthmatic subjects (shaded columns) and 20 (10 M, 10 F) control subjects. Endurance assessed following repetitive 15-s maximal static contractions, followed by 15-s rest over a 6-min period: assessed as ratio of final/initial force. Baseline strength of the asthmatic subjects did not differ significantly from that of control subjects for any of the three muscle groups tested. At time of testing asthmatic subjects had (FEV$_1$ 62% and FRC 142% of predicted). Reproduced from ref. 69, with permission.

been shown to have a definite effect.[67] Most studies that have taken account of the hyperinflation of the chest wall have concluded that the strength of both inspiratory and expiratory muscles is well preserved.[68–72] Indeed it has been suggested that endurance of the respiratory muscles is better in asthmatic than in control subjects (Fig. 4.8).[69] Almost all the patients in these studies had only modest hyperinflation and airway obstruction. Even if there is a training effect of chronic asthma on the inspiratory muscles, in the most severe attacks the load is so great that fatigue could well occur. Indeed the use of continuous positive airway pressure to relieve the need to overcome intrinsic positive end-expired pressure has been suggested.[73] Unfortunately no techniques are currently available for simply detecting fatigue in the presence of severe airway obstruction.

PULMONARY GAS EXCHANGE AND SHUNT

Pathological studies in fatal cases of asthma show multiple occlusions of airway by muco-inflammatory plugs, sometimes extending into major segmental or occasionally lobar airways. Presumably many airways are occluded by such plugs in less severe attacks, yet gross atelectasis on the chest radiograph is unusual. Fifteen years ago a detailed study of ventilation–perfusion inequality in asymptomatic asthmatic patients using the multiple inert gas elimination technique (MIGET) showed a striking bimodal distribution of ventilation–perfusion ratios with the majority of ratios in the normal range (close to 1.0) but a second population of very poorly ventilated units with ventilation–perfusion ratios around 0.1 or less; as much as 25% of the cardiac output could be perfusing these poorly ventilated units (Fig. 4.9). Furthermore there was no evidence that these poorly ventilated units collapsed and became sites of anatomical shunting of blood during breathing of 100% oxygen.[74] The most attractive explanation of these findings remains that the areas of low ventilation–perfusion ratio were receiving collateral ventilation and failed to collapse on oxygen breathing because obstructed airways kept the alveoli overdistended. Subsequently several similar studies have been made of ventilation–perfusion inequality in chronic, symptomatic asthma,[75–77] acute

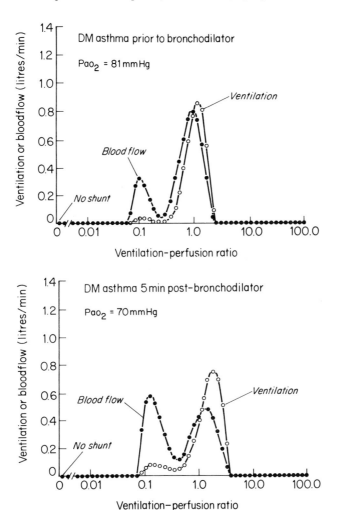

Fig. 4.9 Distribution of ventilation (○) and blood flow (●) against ventilation–perfusion ratio (log scale) in a subject with asthma before (top panel) and after (bottom panel) inhaled isoprenaline. Before isoprenaline distribution of blood flow was bimodal with about 20% of cardiac output going to low ventilation–perfusion ratio areas. Five minutes after isoprenaline blood flow to low ventilation–perfusion ratio areas has greatly increased leading to a 11 mmHg drop in arterial O_2 pressure. The before bronchodilator distribution is typical of mild asthma with no shunt. Ten minutes after isoprenaline administration baseline conditions had been restored. Reproduced from ref. 74, with permission.

severe asthma[78,79] and patients requiring mechanical ventilation.[80] In severe asthma there was often a bimodal distribution of ventilation–perfusion ratios, similar to, but more pronounced than, that found in patients in remission. Even when breathing increased concentrations of oxygen (30–50%) anatomical shunt was extremely small, although in patients receiving mechanical ventilation, breathing 100% oxygen did produce an average shunt of 8% of the cardiac output.[80] These results are surprising because significant shunts are known to develop in older normal subjects who breathe 100% oxygen[81] and the wedged bronchoscope technique suggests that collateral resistance at FRC is considerably increased even in remission of asthma. A possible explanation is that hyperinflation reduces collateral resistance and/or directly prevents areas of atelectasis developing. The MIGET technique has also been used to show that the transient deterioration in gas exchange sometimes found after intravenous salbutamol is due to increased blood flow to areas with low ventilation–blood flow ratios; this is not found when similar bronchodilation is produced by inhaled salbutamol,[77,79] although it can occur after inhaled isoprenaline (Fig. 4.9).

Overall these studies indicate that arterial oxygenation can be maintained by relatively modest increases in inspired oxygen even in severe asthma; apart from the absence of shunt, this is achieved by an increase in total ventilation and cardiac output.

CONCLUSIONS

In the last 20 years routine monitoring of the severity of asthma has been based on simple tests of airway function and, in the more severe attacks, arterial blood gases. Although 'exhaustion' is frequently cited as an indication for assisted ventilation, there are as yet no practical tests to assess the work of the inspiratory muscles and whether they are fatigued. Details of the serial site of airway narrowing, the nature of collateral pathways and the reasons why narrowing varies so greatly between parallel airways are hardly known. Abnormalities in the production and removal of airway secretions are poorly understood and it is not known whether there are abnormalities of control of airway mucosal blood flow. Our understanding of the physiology of the asthma attack remains very incomplete.

REFERENCES

1. Moreno RH, Hogg JC, Paré PD: Mechanics of airway narrowing. *Am Rev Respir Dis* (1986) **133**: 1171–1180.
2. Macklem PT: Bronchial hyporesponsiveness. *Chest* (1985) **87**: 158–159S.
3. Cockcroft DW, Berscheid BA, Murdock KY: Unimodal distribution of bronchial responsiveness in a random population. *Chest* (1983) **83**: 751–754.
4. Thomson NC: *In vivo* versus *in vitro* human airway responsiveness to different pharmacological stimuli. *Am Rev Respir Dis* (1987) **136**: S58–62.
5. Whicker SD, Armour CL, Black JL: Responsiveness of bronchial smooth muscle from asthmatic patients to relaxant and contractile agents. *Pulm Pharmacol* (1988) **1**: 25–30.
6. Bai TR: Abnormalities in airway smooth muscle in fatal asthma. *Am Rev Respir Dis* (1990) **141**: 552–557.

7. Bai TR: Abnormalities in airway smooth muscle in fatal asthma. A comparison between trachea and bronchus. *Am Rev Respir Dis* (1991) **143**: 441–443.
8. Woolcock AJ, Salome CM, Yan K: The shape of the dose–response curve to histamine in asthmatic and normal subjects. *Am Rev Respir Dis* (1984) **130**: 71–75.
9. Michoud, MC, Lelorier J, Amyot R: Factors modulating the interindividual variability of airway responsiveness to histamine. The influence of H_1 and H_2 receptors. *Bull Eur Physiopath Respir* (1981) **17**: 807–821.
10. Sterk PJ, Daniel, EE, Zamel N, Hargreave FE: Limited bronchoconstriction to methacholine using partial flow–volume curves in non-asthmatic subjects. *Am Rev Respir Dis* (1985a) **132**: 272–277.
11. Sterk PJ, Daniel EE, Zamel N, Hargreave FE: Limited maximal airway narrowing in nonasthmatic subjects. *Am Rev Respir Dis* (1985b) **132**: 865–870.
12. Kariya ST, Thompson, LM, Ingenito EP, Ingram RH Jr: Effects of lung volume, volume history and methacholine on lung tissue viscance. *J Appl Physiol* (1989) **66**: 977–982.
13. Olsen CR, Stevens AE, Pride NB, Staub NC: Structural basis for decreased compressibility of constricted trachea and bronchi. *J Appl Physiol* (1967) **23**: 35–39.
14. James AL, Paré PD, Moreno RH, Hogg JC: Quantitative measurement of smooth muscle shortening in isolated pig trachea. *J Appl Physiol* (1987) **63**: 1360–1365.
15. Olsen CR, Stevens AE, McIlroy MB: Rigidity of tracheal and bronchi during muscular constriction. *J Apply Physiol* (1967) **23**: 27–34.
16. Bouhuys A, Van de Woestijne KP: Mechanical consequences of airway smooth muscle relaxation. *J Appl Physiol* (1971) **30**: 670–676.
17. Mead J, Takishima T, Leith D: Stress distribution in lungs: a model of pulmonary elasticity. *J Appl Physiol* (1970) **28**: 596–608.
18. Hughes JMB, Jones HA, Wilson AG, Grant BJB, Pride NB: Stability of intrapulmonary bronchial dimensions during expiratory flow in excised lungs. *J Appl Physiol* (1974) **37**: 684–694.
19. Lai-Fook SJ, Hyatt RE, Rodarte JR: Effect of parenchymal shear modulus and lung volume on bronchial pressure–diameter behavior. *J Appl Physiol* (1978) **44**: 859–868.
20. Murtagh PS, Proctor DF, Permutt S, Kelly B, Evering S: Bronchial closure with mecholyl in excised dog lobes. *J Appl Physiol* (1971) **31**: 409–415.
21. Ding DJ, Martin JG, Macklem PT: The effects of lung volume on maximal methacholine-induced bronchoconstriction in normal humans. *J Appl Physiol* (1987) **62**: 1324–1330.
22. Sly PD, Brown KA, Bates JHT, Macklem PT, Milic-Emili J, Martin JG: Effect of lung volume on interruptor resistance in cats challenged with methacholine. *J Appl Physiol* (1988) **64**: 360–366.
23. Wang YT, Coe CI, Pride NB: The effect of reducing airway dimensions by altering posture on histamine responsiveness. *Thorax* (1990) **45**: 530–535.
24. Freedman BJ: The functional geometry of the bronchi. The relationship between changes in external diameter and calibre, and a consideration of the passive role played by the mucosa in bronchoconstriction. *Bull Eur Physiopathol Respir* (1972) **8**: 545–551.
25. Folkow B: The haemodynamic consequences of adaptive structural changes of the resistance vessels in hypertension. *Clin Sci* (1971) **41**: 1–12.
26. James AL, Paré PD, Hogg JC: The mechanics of airway narrowing in asthma. *Am Rev Respir Dis* (1989) **139**: 242–246.
27. McFadden ER, Jr: Hypothesis: exercise-induced asthma as a vascular phenomenon. *Lancet* (1990) **i**: 880–883.
28. Butler J, Caro CG, Alcala, R, DuBois A: Physiological factors affecting airway resistance in normal subjects and in patients with obstructive respiratory disease. *J Clin Invest* (1960) **39**: 584–591.
29. Colebatch HJH, Finucane KE, Smith MM: Pulmonary conductance and elastic recoil relationship in asthma and emphysema. *J Appl Physiol* (1973) **34**: 143–153.
30. Moreno RH, Paré PD: Intravenous papain-induced cartilage softening decreases preload of tracheal smooth muscle. *J Appl Physiol* (1989) **66**: 1694–1698.
31. Bellofiore S, Eidelman DH, Macklem PT, Martin JG: Effects of elastase-induced emphysema on airway responsiveness to methacholine in rats. *J Appl Physiol* (1989) **66**: 606–612.

32. Pride NB, Macklem PT: Lung mechanics in disease. In Macklem P, Mead J (eds) *Handbook of Physiology: Respiratory System*, Vol III. *Mechanics of Breathing*. Bethesda, MD, American Physiological Society, 1986, pp 678–679.

33. Koblett von H, Wyss F: Das klinische und funktionelle Bild des genuinen Bronchialkollapses mit Lungen emphysema. *Helv med Acta* (1956) **23**: 553–560.

34. Despas PJ, Leroux M, Macklem PT: Site of airway obstruction in asthma as determined by measuring maximal expiratory flow breathing air and a helium–oxygen mixture. *J Clin Invest* (1972) **51**: 3235–3243.

35. Ingram RH Jr, McFadden ER Jr: Localization and mechanisms of airway responses. *N Engl J Med* (1977) **197**: 596–600.

36. Fairshter RD, Wilson AF: Relationship between site of airflow limitation and localization of the bronchodilator response in asthma. *Am Rev Respir Dis* (1980) **122**: 27–32.

37. Partridge MR, Saunders KB: The site of airflow limitation in asthma: the effect of time, acute exacerbations of disease and clinical features. *Br J Dis Chest* (1981) **75**: 263–272.

38. Antic R, Macklem PT: The influence of clinical factors on site of airway obstruction in asthma. *Am Rev Respir Dis* (1976) **114**: 851–859.

39. Lisboa C, Macklem PT, Wood LDH: Density dependence of pulmonary pressure-flow curves and maximum expiratory flow. In Sadoul P, Milic-Emili J, Simonsson BG, Clark TJH (eds) *Small Airways in Health and Disease. Excerpta Medica*, 1979, pp 17–20.

40. Jadue C, Greville H, Coalson JJ, Mink SN: Forced expiration and HeO$_2$ response in canine peripheral airway obstruction. *J Appl Physiol* (1985) **58**: 1788–1801.

41. Teculescu DB, Pride NB: Density dependence of maximal expiratory flow: report on international workshop, 1986. *Bull Eur Physiopathol Respir* (1987) **23**: 663–666.

42. Gayrard P, Orehek J, Grimaud C, Charpin C: Bronchoconstrictor effects of a deep inspiration in patients with asthma. *Am Rev Respir Dis* (1975) **111**: 433–439.

43. Ingram RH Jr: Site and mechanism of obstruction and hyperresponsiveness in asthma. *Am Rev Respir Dis* (1987) **136**: S62–64.

44. Ingram RH Jr: Physiological assessment of inflammation in the peripheral lung of asthmatic patients. *Lung* (1990) **168**: 237–248.

45. Berry RB, Fairshter RD: Partial and maximal flow–volume curves in normal and asthmatic subjects before and after inhalation of metaproterenol. *Chest* (1985) **88**: 697–702.

46. Lim TK, Pride NB, Ingram RH, Jr: Effects of volume history during spontaneous and acutely induced air-flow obstruction in asthma. *Am Rev Respir Dis* (1987) **135**: 591–596.

47. Pellegrino R, Violante B, Crimi E, Brusasco V: Effects of deep inhalation during early and late asthmatic reactions to allergen. *Am Rev Respir Dis* (1990) **142**: 822–825.

48. Pliss IB, Ingenito EP, Ingram RH, Jr: Responsiveness, inflammation, and effects of deep breaths on obstruction in mild asthma. *J Appl Physiol* (1989) **66**: 2298–2304.

49. Molfino NA, McLean PA, Hoffstein V, *et al.*: Changes in central airway areas induced by methacholine, histamine and LTC$_4$ in asthmatic subjects. *Am Rev Respir Dis* (1991) **143**: A409.

50. Wagner EM, Liu MC, Weinmann GG, Permutt S, Bleecker ER: Peripheral lung resistance in normal and asthmatic subjects. *Am Rev Respir Dis* (1990) **141**: 584–588.

51. Yan K, Salome CM, Woolcock AJ: Prevalence and nature of bronchial hyperresponsiveness in subjects with chronic obstructive pulmonary disease. *Am Rev Respir Dis* (1985) **132**: 25–29.

52. Miller RD, Hyatt RE: Evaluation of obstructive lesions of the trachea and larynx by flow–volume loops. *Am Rev Respir Dis* (1973) **108**: 475–481.

53. Dekker E, Groen J: Asthmatic wheezing. Compression of the trachea and major bronchi as a cause. *Lancet* (1957) **272**: 1064–1068.

54. Rodenstein DO, Francis C, Stanescu DC: Emotional laryngeal wheezing: a new syndrome. *Am Rev Respir Dis* (1983) **127**: 354–356.

55. Linderholm H: Lung mechanics in sitting and horizontal postures studied by body plethysmographic methods. *Am J Physiol* (1963) **204**: 85–91.

56. Coe CI, Pride NB: Immediate changes in respiratory resistance on adopting the supine posture in normal and asthmatic subjects (abstract). *Eur Respir J* (1988) **1**: 600S.

57. Jonsson E, Mossberg B: Impairment of ventilatory function by supine posture in asthma. *Eur J Respir Dis* (1984) **65**: 496–503.

58. Larsson K, Bevegård S, Mossberg B: Posture-induced airflow limitation in asthma: relationship to plasma catecholamines and an inhaled anticholinergic agent. *Eur Respir J* (1988) **1**: 458–463.
59. Ballard RD, Saathoff MC, Patel DK, Kelly PL, Martin RJ: Effect of sleep on nocturnal bronchoconstriction and ventilatory patterns in asthmatics. *J Appl Physiol* (1989) **67**: 243–249.
60. Whyte KF, Douglas NJ: Posture and nocturnal asthma. *Thorax* (1989) **44**: 579–581.
61. Martin J, Powell E, Shore S, Emrich J, Engel LA: The role of respiratory muscles in the hyperinflation of bronchial asthma. *Am Rev Respir Dis* (1980) **121**: 441–447.
62. Muller N, Bryan AC, Zamel N: Tonic inspiratory activity as a cause of hyperinflation in histamine-induced asthma. *J Appl Physiol: Respirat Environ Exercise Physiol* (1980) **4**: 869–874.
63. Muller N, Bryan AC, Zamel N: Tonic inspiratory muscle activity as a cause of hyperinflation in asthma. *J Appl Physiol: Respirat Environ Exercise Physiol* (1981) **50**: 279–282.
64. Ballard RD, Irvin CG, Martin RJ, Pak J, Pandey R, White DP: Influence of sleep on lung volume in asthmatic patients and normal subjects. *J Appl Physiol* (1990) **68**: 2034–2041.
65. Wheatley JR, West S, Cala SJ, Engel LA: The effect of hyperinflation on respiratory muscle work in acute induced asthma. *Eur Respir J* (1990) **3**: 625–632.
66. Melzer E, Souhrada JF: Decrease of respiratory muscle strength and static lung volumes in obese asthmatics. *Am Rev Respir Dis* (1980) **121**: 17–22.
67. Picado C, Fiz JA, Montserrat JM, et al.: Respiratory and skeletal muscle function in steroid-dependent bronchial asthma. *Am Rev Respir Dis* (1990) **141**: 14–20.
68. Decramer M, Demedts M, Rochette F, Billiet L: Maximal transrespiratory pressures in obstructive lung disease. *Bull Europ Physiopath Resp* (1980) **16**: 479–490.
69. McKenzie DK, Gandevia SC: Strength and endurance of inspiratory, expiratory and limb muscles in asthma. *Am Rev Respir Dis* (1986) **134**: 999–1004.
70. Marks J, Pasterkamp H, Tal A, Leahy F: Relationship between respiratory muscle strength, nutritional status, and lung volume in cystic fibrosis and asthma. *Am Rev Respir Dis* (1986) **133**: 414–417.
71. Lavietes MH, Grocela JA, Maniatis T, Potulski F, Ritter AB, Sunderam G: Inspiratory muscle strength in asthma. *Chest* (1988) **93**: 1043–1048.
72. Weiner P, Suo J, Fernandez E, Cherniack RM: The effect of hyperinflation on respiratory muscle strength and efficiency in healthy subjects and patients with asthma. *Am Rev Respir Dis* (1990) **141**: 1501–1505.
73. Martin JG, Shore S, Engel LA: Effect of continuous positive airway pressure on respiratory mechanics and pattern of breathing in induced asthma. *Am Rev Respir Dis* (1982) **126**: 812–817.
74. Wagner PD, Dantzker DR, Iacovoni VE, Tomlin WC, West JB: Ventilation–perfusion inequality in asymptomatic asthma. *Am Rev Respir Dis* (1978) **118**: 511–524.
75. Corte P, Young IH: Ventilation–perfusion relationships in symptomatic asthma. Response to oxygen and clemastine. *Chest* (1985) **88**: 167–175.
76. Wagner PD, Hedenstierna G, Bylin G: Ventilation–perfusion inequality in chronic asthma. *Am Rev Respir Dis* (1987) **136**: 605–612.
77. Ballester E, Roca J, Ramis L, Wagner PD, Rodriguez-Roisin R: Pulmonary gas exchange in severe chronic asthma. Response to 100% oxygen and salbutamol. *Am Rev Respir Dis* (1990) **141**: 558–562.
78. Roca JR, Ramis L, Rodriguez-Roisin R, Ballester E, Montserrat JM, Wagner PD: Serial relationships between ventilation–perfusion inequality and spirometry in acute severe asthma requiring hospitalization. *Am Rev Respir Dis* (1988) **137**: 1055–1061.
79. Ballester E, Reyes J, Roca J, Guitart R, Wagner PD, Rodriguez-Roisin R: Ventilation–perfusion mismatching in acute severe asthma. Effects of salbutamol and 100% oxygen. *Thorax* (1989) **44**: 258–267.
80. Rodriguez-Roisin R, Ballester E, Roca J, Torres A, Wagner PD: Mechanisms of hypoxemia in patients with status asthmaticus requiring mechanical ventilation. *Am Rev Respir Dis* (1989) **139**: 732–739.
81. Wagner PD, Laravuso RB, Uhl RR, West JB: Continuous distributions of ventilation–perfusion ratios in normal subjects breathing air and 100% O_2. *J Clin Invest* (1974) **54**: 54–68.

5

Airway Smooth Muscle

IAN W. RODGER AND NIGEL J. PYNE

INTRODUCTION

It is well recognized that contraction of airway smooth muscle is the principal component underlying the bronchoconstriction that characterizes the acute phase of an asthmatic attack. It is also well accepted that the airway structure of asthmatic subjects is abnormal (see Chapter 3). Such abnormalities are thought to be consequent upon an exaggerated inflammatory process that thickens the airway wall, promotes interstitial oedema and induces hypersecretion of mucus into the airway lumen. Associated with these changes is an increase in airway smooth muscle mass which may also function abnormally as is evidenced by its hyperresponsiveness to a wide range of provoking stimuli. It is an apparent paradox that despite such an awareness we know little about the precise physiological role of airway smooth muscle.

The objective of this chapter is to provide an overview of airway smooth muscle with special reference to contractile mechanisms. Given the space constraints, this chapter is not an exhaustive review of the literature. Rather it is an attempt to 'paint the picture with a broad brush' and direct the interested reader to authoritative key references on particular aspects of the topic.

STRUCTURAL ASPECTS OF AIRWAY SMOOTH MUSCLE

In general, there are few studies concerning the structure of human airway smooth muscle, especially of the small airways that are the principal site of airways obstruction in asthma. In one of the few published studies[1] it has been shown that the musculature of the first and second order human bronchi closely resembles that of the trachea which is a much more extensively researched tissue. In contrast, that of the fourth to seventh order airways is substantially different in terms of the size and arrangement of the

ASTHMA: BASIC MECHANISMS AND CLINICAL MANAGEMENT (2nd Edn)
ISBN 0-12-079026-2

muscle bundles, number and size of gap junctions and appearance of the contractile myofilaments.[1] Interestingly, mast cells also appear to be more intimately associated with the smooth muscle of these smaller airways. Furthermore, innervation of the smaller airways is much denser than that of the trachea and large bronchi. It has been suggested[1] that the larger airways are adapted for myogenic control with a secondary neuromodulatory aspect, whereas the smaller bronchial airways are organized principally for control by neutral elements.

Generally, airway smooth muscle is regarded as being of the multi-unit type in that each cell is innervated and cell-to-cell communication is poor. This is because there is a paucity of so-called gap junctions which provide pathways of low resistance along which electrical signals can be transmitted. Spontaneous activity is rarely observed in such smooth muscle types. Action potentials are nearly always absent and the response to contractile agonists is via graded depolarization. In normal airway smooth muscle such a situation usually prevails. In asthmatic airway smooth muscle, however, pronounced action potential activity has been observed.[2] Such activity is indicative not of multi-unit, but of single-unit smooth muscle. This type of smooth muscle is generally poorly innervated and relies heavily upon gap junctions to provide cell-to-cell communication. Thus, it has been suggested[3,4] that asthmatic subjects with hyperresponsive airways may possess a greater degree of electrical coupling between smooth muscle cells due to an increased presence of gap junctions. Quite how multi-unit airway smooth muscle changes to become strongly single unit in nature is not yet known, although certain experimental observations[1,5–11] may provide useful pointers. For example, it has been shown in human and animal preparations that drugs which inhibit potassium efflux, and thus the electrical rectification capability of the plasma membrane, induce action potential discharge which results in contractile responses (see later). In effecting this change in cell behaviour, there is an accompanying rapid induction of gap junction formation, assembled from preformed proteins. Thus, multi-unit smooth muscle behaviour is converted into single-unit behaviour. Similar effects can be elicited by arachidonic acid metabolites.[3] Given that such metabolites may play an important role as chemical mediators of asthma, these observations may have far reaching implications with regard to bronchial hyperresponsiveness.

In terms of contraction of airway smooth muscle, two of the more important intracellular organelles are the sarcoplasmic reticulum (SR) and the mitochondrion. Generally, smooth muscles are regarded as possessing a paucity of SR, but that which exists is thought to play an important physiological role in that it is capable of sequestering and storing free calcium ions (Ca^{2+}) and releasing them, on demand, as so-called activator Ca^{2+}. It is these activator Ca^{2+} that initiate the biochemical events that ultimately generate contraction of airway smooth muscle[12] (see later). In contrast, mitochondria are thought not to pay a major role in Ca^{2+} homeostasis except in certain pathological conditions.[13,14]

THE CONTRACTILE PROTEINS AND THEIR REGULATION BY CALCIUM IONS

All smooth muscle cells contain the contractile proteins actin, myosin, tropomyosin and caldesmon.[15–18] They function by forming into filaments arranged in parallel such that they can slide past each other. Actin is a highly conserved molecule found in most eukaryotic cells and represents the major contractile protein of smooth muscle, being 10–20 times more abundant than myosin. Actin (thin) filaments are composed of two linear polymers of a 42-kilodalton (kDa) globular protein wrapped together in a helical configuration. Intertwined along its length, in the groove of the thin filament helix, lie tropomyosin and caldesmon. In contrast to the thin filaments of actin, myosin filaments are thick, bipolar and arranged asymmetrically in a hexameric structure. Myosin comprises one pair of heavy chains (each of 200 kDa) and two pairs of light chains (one pair of 17 kDa and the other of 20 kDa). The myosin molecule can essentially be divided into two components; a 'head' section attached to a long spine or 'tail' section. The globular head section of myosin is the region of the molecule that possesses both the binding sites for attachment to actin and the enzymatic (ATPase) sites which cleave ATP and so provide the energy necessary for the binding reactions to take place.[19,20] The two sets of myosin light chains are also located at the head of the myosin molecule. The 20-kDa light chains are considered to be essential regulators of the contractile process.

Intermediate filaments

Intermediate filaments consist of a group of relatively insoluble proteins that are considered by many to form the cytoskeleton of numerous cell types. In smooth muscle the cytoskeletal and contractile proteins are distributed in two cellular domains: (a) longitudinal intermediate filaments free of myosin, but containing α-actinin, desmin, filamin and actin, and (b) contractile protein filaments, i.e. actin, myosin, tropomyosin and caldesmon.[21–23] Elucidation of this assembly of proteins has led to the proposition that the intermediate filament domain may be responsible for the tonic phase of a smooth muscle contractile response with the initiation of contraction (phasic component) being the responsibility of the contractile protein domain.[22] A recent modification of this proposal has been advanced.[24] In this scheme, phosphorylation of different proteins (contractile and intermediate) is responsible for the different phases of the contractile response.[24]

Regulation of myosin by Ca^{2+}

When $[Ca^{2+}]_i$ reaches a threshold of between 0.5 and 1.0 μM, the free Ca^{2+} bind to calmodulin, a low molecular weight Ca^{2+}-binding protein with a high degree of specificity for Ca^{2+}.[25,26] Each calmodulin molecule has the capacity to bind up to a maximum of four molecules of Ca^{2+}. It is generally accepted that for activation of calmodulin at least three, and in all probability four, Ca^{2+} binding sites require to be occupied. Only then can calmodulin combine with and induce/augment the activity of a wide range of different proteins. Many of the substrates for calmodulin's action are enzymes, e.g. the ATPase responsible for Ca^{2+} efflux and cyclic nucleotide phosphodiesterase.[27–29] As far as contraction is concerned, the important enzyme is myosin light chain kinase (MLCK). Normally MLCK lies dormant within resting smooth muscle cells.[30–32] On combination with the Ca–calmodulin complex (activated

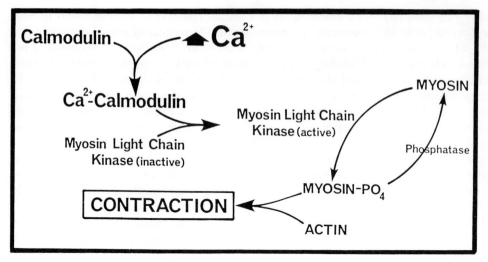

Fig. 5.1 Diagrammatic representation of the sequence of events involved in the regulation of myosin by Ca^{2+}. These events are widely regarded as being pivotal in inducing rapid tension generation following stimulation with a contractile agonist.

calmodulin), however, MLCK becomes active and responsible for the phosphorylation of a specific serine residue on the 20-kDa light chains of myosin. This phosphorylation step is generally, although not universally, regarded as a prerequisite for the activation of myosin ATPase by actin and hence contraction.[16,17,19,33–36] Dephosphorylation of myosin is achieved by a Ca^{2+}-independent phosphatase about which much less is known.[17] The sequence of events outlined in this section is illustrated diagrammatically in Fig 5.1.

Regulation of actin by Ca^{2+}

Whilst myosin phosphorylation/dephosphorylation reactions may be the dominant regulatory pathway for smooth muscle contraction, the co-existence of thin filament-linked regulation is regarded as likely. In recent times most attention has been focused upon the calmodulin- and actin-binding protein caldesmon.[37,38] In the absence of Ca^{2+}, caldesmon binds to filamentous actin and inhibits actin-activated myosin MgATPase so inhibiting contractile activation. Once Ca^{2+} levels are increased, however, caldesmon binds to calmodulin so relieving the inhibitory influence on actomyosin MgATPase and allowing contractile development.[37,38] An additional step in the actin regulatory process may involve caldesmon phosphorylation. Caldesmon is phosphorylated by a Ca^{2+}/calmodulin-dependent kinase (distinct from MLCK) and only the dephosphorylated form of caldesmon is inhibitory.[39,40]

Actin–myosin interaction

Contraction of smooth muscle is thought to occur via a mechanism similar to the sliding filament process first proposed for skeletal muscle.[41–46] The sliding of actin and myosin past each other is achieved by the cyclic attachment of the globular heads of the myosin molecules to actin (so-called crossbridge formation), a flexing change in the configuration of the myosin head with respect to actin, detachment of myosin from actin followed by subsequent re-attachment at another site further down the actin molecule. It is this rapid cyclical attachment and detachment of crossbridges between actin and myosin (crossbridge cycling) that is responsible for the active force development in smooth muscle. The process is fuelled by the energy derived from the breakdown of ATP by actin-activated myosin ATPase. Furthermore, the rate of force development is directly proportional to the rate of crossbridge cycling.[17,47] In the absence of ATP hydrolysis, i.e. when $[Ca^{2+}]_i$ is low and no activation of MLCK can occur, the orientation of the globular heads of myosin is such that crossbridge formation with actin is prohibited. Thus, at rest actin and myosin molecules can freely slide past each other and no active tension is developed.

THE AIRWAY SMOOTH MUSCLE CELL MEMBRANE

Calcium ion homeostasis

Contraction of airway smooth muscle is dependent upon the concentration of free (unbound) calcium ions ($[Ca^{2+}]_i$) within the cytoplasm of the cell.[48–53] In the resting (relaxed) state the $[Ca^{2+}]_i$ of airway smooth muscle cells is thought to lie somewhere between 0.05 and 0.25 μM.[50,51,53–56] This level of $[Ca^{2+}]_i$ is regarded as being insufficient to activate the contractile apparatus. In contrast, the concentration of Ca^{2+} in the extracellular fluid is of the order of 1–2 mM. It is evident, therefore, that there exists a large, inwardly-directed concentration gradient (a transmembrane concentration difference of approximately 10^4) down which Ca^{2+} will tend to flow. In the resting state, however, few Ca^{2+} gain admission to the cell. This is a testament to the functional integrity of the cell membrane which effectively, and efficiently, partitions the intra- and extra-cellular compartments. This partitioning is, however, not absolute. There is a small quantity of Ca^{2+} that enters the cell, albeit slowly, via a passive Ca^{2+} leak process. The intracellular Ca^{2+} levels, however, do not rise either sufficiently rapidly or to a sufficient magnitude to activate the contractile machinery.

Homeostatic regulation of Ca^{2+} is essential for the survival of smooth muscle cells since elevated intracellular concentrations of the cation are toxic to cellular metabolism. Reliance solely upon the relative impermeability of the cell membrane, as a means of controlling Ca^{2+} levels within the cells, would be both primitive and wholly inadequate. Thus the cells have developed several additional, sophisticated, homeostatic control mechanisms which, acting in concert with the plasma membrane, serve to ensure that any exposure to Ca^{2+} is as brief as possible. These auxiliary mechanisms are: (a) a sodium ion–calcium ion (Na^+–Ca^{2+}) exchange processes; (b) a Ca^{2+} efflux pump and (c) an intracellular Ca^{2+} uptake process. The first two processes are concerned with active extrusion of Ca^{2+} from the cell and, consequently, are sited in the cell membrane. The Ca^{2+} uptake process involves intracellular organelles, in particular the SR. Each of these processes is dealt with in more detail below.

Na$^+$–Ca^{2+} exchange

The existence of a Ca^{2+} removal mechanism linked to the inward movement of Na$^+$ was first postulated by Reuter *et al.*[57] for vascular smooth muscle. An essentially similar mechanism is thought to exist in airway smooth muscle.[58–60] Although the precise stoichiometry of the process remains a matter of some debate, the currently accepted view is that for each three Na$^+$ that enter the cell one Ca^{2+} is extruded. This view has developed largely as a result of experiments showing that the exchange process is sensitive to alterations in resting membrane potential and extracellular Na$^+$ concentration and is electrogenic in nature. Such observations highlight the fact that the exchange process is integrally linked to the activity of the plasmalemmal sodium pump (Na$^+$–K$^+$ ATPase) whose responsibility it is to maintain the inwardly directed Na$^+$ gradient upon which Ca^{2+} efflux depends.

The Ca^{2+} efflux pump

Most of the detailed characterization of the cellular calcium efflux process has been performed using erythrocytes. There is, however, considerable evidence that the efflux pump is similar in all vertebrate and invertebrate cells[61] and that such a mechanism exists in the plasmalemma of airway smooth muscle cells.[62–65]

Essentially, the membrane pump is an Mg^{2+}-dependent Ca^{2+}–H$^+$ ATPase that drives Ca^{2+} from the cell against its concentration gradient. The efflux of Ca^{2+} is currently throught to be an electrically neutral process with each extruded Ca^{2+} being exchanged for 2H$^+$. Any possible disruption to intracellular pH (the result of accumulation of H$^+$) is offset by the accompanying influx of Cl$^-$, HCO$_3^-$ or HPO$_4^{2-}$ from the extracellular fluid.

In unstimulated smooth muscle cells the Ca^{2+} pump exists in a low affinity state exhibiting an apparent K$_m$(Ca) of 10–20 μM.[25,66] Under such conditions the efflux of Ca^{2+} from cells is slow. Nevertheless, in conjunction with the Na$^+$–Ca^{2+} exchanger, this level of activity is estimated to be adequate to maintain the low [Ca^{2+}]$_i$ necessary to prevent activation of the contractile apparatus. In contrast, once the cell has been activated by a stimulus that increases the [Ca^{2+}]$_i$, the Ca^{2+} efflux pump responds accordingly by increasing its activity (by a factor up to seven-fold). This is achieved by virtue of the enzyme adopting a high affinity state in which it exhibits a K$_m$(Ca) of approximately 0.4 μM. If one assumes that the peak intracellular Ca^{2+} concentration attained during activation is in the region of 1 μM[56] then the rate of Ca^{2+} extrusion from the cell is likely to approach the V$_{max}$ of the enzyme. The conversion of the enzyme from a low to a high affinity state can be achieved by the action of activated calmodulin (see later), acidic phospholipids or certain fatty acids. Interestingly, certain acidic phospholipids, for example those derived from phosphatidylinositol (see later) stimulate the efflux pump to a higher degree than does activated calmodulin.[67]

Uptake of Ca^{2+} into intracellular organelles

Smooth muscles are generally regarded as possessing a paucity of SR. Notwithstanding, that which exists is thought to be capable of sequestering and storing Ca^{2+}.[68–70]

The SR, however, is not simply a 'sink' for Ca^{2+} removal. Ultrastructural studies of vascular smooth muscle have shown that the localization and Ca^{2+} content of junctional SR is consistent with it being the major source of so-called intracellular activator Ca^{2+}.[12,13,71,72]

To date, no similar studies have been performed in airway smooth muscle. However, subcellular and microsomal fractions of airway smooth muscle have been shown to accumulate Ca^{2+} via an ATP-dependent uptake mechanism.[62,63,73]

In contrast, mitochondria are thought unlikely to play a major role in the homeostatic control of $[Ca^{2+}]_i$ under normal circumstances.[13] They may, however, act in an important auxiliary capacity to sequester intracellular Ca^{2+}, in certain pathological conditions, when the cytoplasm experiences overload with the cation.[14]

From what has been said above, it is abundantly clear that the very process necessary to initiate contraction (the rise in $[Ca^{2+}]_i$) concomitantly activates homeostatic, regulatory mechanisms designed to protect the cell from the fatal consequences of prolonged exposure to elevated concentrations of the cation.

Membrane potential

Generally, the resting membrane potential of airway smooth muscle cells lies between -45 and -60 mV.[75] It is also largely true that, under normal circumstances, most species (the guinea-pig[75] and man[74] being notable exceptions) do not exhibit spontaneous oscillations of the membrane potential (slow waves), i.e. the cells are electrically quiescent.[75] A further characteristic feature is the membrane's remarkable propensity for outward electrical rectification consequent upon a depolarizing stimulus. This rectification behaviour is thought to be due to the opening of voltage-dependent, high conductance (260–290 pS) Ca^{2+}-activated K^+ channels that are present in the airway smooth muscle plasmalemma of several species.[11,76–79] This rectification ability, in addition to limiting the magnitude of any depolarization, effectively prevents the membrane potential from attaining the threshold necessary for eliciting opening of voltage-dependent Ca^{2+}-channels (see below). Conversely, drugs, such as tetraethylammonium and charybdotoxin, that block K^+ channels and reduce rectification, cause spike-like action potential discharge that is associated with contractile responses.[11,75,80] More detailed information on the electrophysiological aspects of airway smooth muscle is beyond the scope of this chapter. For such information the interested reader is directed to review articles by Giembycz and Rodger[81], Small and Foster[75] and Kotlikoff.[82]

Calcium ion channels

Given that the cell membrane effectively partitions the intra- and extracellular environments, it is self evident that activator Ca^{2+} originating in the extracellular compartment can only gain admission to the cell once the membrane has been rendered permeable to them. This is achieved by the opening of specific Ca^{2+} channels in the plasmalemma through which the Ca^{2+} flow down their electrochemical and concentration gradients. Two types of calcium channel have been proposed: (a) voltage-dependent (VDC) and (b) receptor-operated (ROC).[48] It is pertinent to this review that brief consideration be given to the existence and functional significance of these two types of calcium ion channels in airway smooth muscle. By necessity, this has been kept brief. For more comprehensive analyses of the subject, the interested reader is directed to selected review articles.[75,81–85]

Voltage-dependent Ca²⁺ channels (VDCs)

Of the two types of calcium channel that have been proposed, the characteristics and properties of the VDC are much better understood. As the name implies, the VDC possesses a Ca^{2+} conductance that is directly proportional to the potential difference that exists across the plasma membrane.[48,86,87] Hence, membrane depolarization increases both the probability of VDC opening and the duration of the open channel time.[86,87] Additionally, VDCs display a susceptibility to blockade by calcium entry blocking drugs, e.g. verapamil, nifedipine.

There is a substantial body of convincing evidence, from both electrophysiological and ion-flux studies, that supports the view that VDCs are present in airway smooth muscle and that they are true Ca^{2+} channels.[75,81–87] Similarly, with regard to contractile events, there is overwhelming evidence showing that VDCs are primarily responsible for contractions induced by KCl and tetraethylammonium (TEA). For example, in bovine,[88] canine,[89–92] and guinea-pig[93,94] airway smooth muscle KCl elicits a contraction that is accompanied by, and correlated with, both graded membrane depolarization and the influx of ^{45}Ca as assessed by the lanthanum technique.[93–96] Additionally, calcium antagonists not only suppress slow wave and action potential discharge evoked by both KCl and TEA, but also the associated uptake and tension changes in airway smooth muscle preparations.[74,92,95,97–101] Finally, the dihydropyridine Ca^{2+} agonist BAY K8644 has been shown to augment both ^{45}Ca uptake and KCl-induced contractions of airway smooth muscle.[102,103]

In summary, therefore, there is convincing evidence for the existence of true VDCs in airway smooth muscle. Opening of these channels is, in all likelihood, the principal mechanism that underlies the entry of extracellular Ca^{2+} into airway smooth muscle cells in response to substances such as TEA and KCl. In stark contrast, however, there is little evidence to support the involvement of VDCs in the mechanisms underlying contraction initiated by physiologically relevant agonists, for example, cholinomimetics, histamine and eicosanoids.[81,84,85]

Receptor-operated Ca²⁺ channels (ROCs)

Receptor-operated channels are ion channels opened, or operated, by a receptor for a stimulant substance.[48] It is envisaged that ROCs are not wholly selective for Ca^{2+}, have an ionic permeability determined by the controlling receptor, can be gated by either voltage-dependent or voltage-independent events and are not readily inhibited by organic calcium antagonists.[48,56]

Different pharmacological agonists (e.g. acetylcholine, methacholine, histamine, serotonin, leukotrienes C_4 and D_4) have been shown to elicit contraction of airway smooth muscle that is associated with graded depolarization of the cell membrane. Action potential discharge, however, is never observed.[89,91,92,104–110] Thus, VDC opening cannot occur in association with the upstroke of an action potential (since there is none), but, as in the case of KCl, graded depolarization may be responsible for VDC opening. This, however, is not the case since some of these same agonists have been shown to elicit contractions in fully depolarized airway preparations.[90,92,111,112] Furthermore, acetylcholine, histamine and leukotriene D_4 do not, apparently, induce increases in ^{45}Ca uptake into airway smooth muscle during the period associated with tension development.[95,108]

Collectively, therefore, these data argue against both the existence of ROCs in airway smooth muscle and the involvement of VDCs (to any significant extent) in the actions underlying receptor stimulation by pharmacological agonists. This latter view is strengthened by the many observations that calcium antagonists, in concentrations that block the contractile effects of KCl and TEA, fail to inhibit the contractions elicited by a wide range of agonists in airway preparations from several species including man.[92,95,97–101,113–117] Additionally, BAY K8644 does not potentiate contractions elicited by either acetylcholine or histamine in guinea-pig or human airway preparations.[102,103]

Given the corpus of evidence above, it is perhaps not unreasonable to dispel the notion that ROCs are present in the plasma membrane of airway smooth muscle. Notwithstanding, the results of a recent study,[56] using fura-2 fluorescence to measure $[Ca^{2+}]_i$ in cultured human airway smooth muscle cells, provide exciting new evidence concerning Ca^{2+} movements. The implications from this study[56] are that intracellular activator Ca^{2+} is responsible for the initiation of contraction but that the tonic (sustained) phase of contraction (see later) is associated with a low level of extracellular Ca^{2+} influx, via a mechanism that bears all the hallmarks of an ROC-mediated event. Furthermore, the compound SKF 96365, an inhibitor of ROC activity in non-excitable cells,[118] has been shown by Murray and Kotlikoff (personal communication) to block extracellular Ca^{2+} entry in experiments designed to extend their earlier observations.[56] Whilst these recent findings clearly require substantiation they may well signal for the first time not only the presence but also the active participation of ROCs in the excitation–contraction coupling process in airway smooth muscle. Unambiguous definition of such a role, through development of more selective inhibitors of Ca^{2+} influx via these ROCs, may very well lead to the development of novel therapeutic agents for use in asthma.

EXCITATION–CONTRACTION (E/C) COUPLING

Coupling mechanisms

Essentially two forms of E/C coupling are recognized: electromechanical and pharmacomechanical. Electromechanical coupling depends either upon electrical depolarization of the plasmalemma which opens calcium channels leading to Ca^{2+} influx and hence an increase in $[Ca^{2+}]_i$ or on a voltage-dependent release of stored intracellular Ca^{2+}. In contrast, the pharmacomechanical coupling mechanism is voltage-independent. It may involve either extracellular Ca^{2+} influx via ligand-gated calcium channels or release of activator Ca^{2+} from intracellular stores. The release mechanism is mediated either via ligand-generated intracellular second messengers or by direct action of a ligand on SR stores.

When a contractile agonist interacts with its receptor the $[Ca^{2+}]_i$ of airway smooth muscle cells rises abruptly from its resting level to between 0.3 and 1.0 μM.[50,51,53–56] This so-called activator Ca^{2+} can only be derived from two sources; from the extracellular compartment or from intracellular stores such as the SR. The relative contribution of activator Ca^{2+} from these two sources is dependent upon the nature and concentration of the agonist and the component (phasic or tonic) of the contractile response in question.[48,119–121]

The data presented in the section above highlight the fact that, at best, there is only a minor involvement of extracellular Ca^{2+} in the *initiation* (as opposed to *maintenance*) of contractions produced by pharmacological agonists interacting with their cell surface receptors. This being the case then such agonists must presumably rely principally upon activator Ca^{2+} released from intracellular stores for induction of contraction. This contention is sustained by the results of *in vitro* studies undertaken to examine the dependence of different agonists on extracellular Ca^{2+} for contraction. Thus, while contractions elicited by KCl and A23187 (the Ca^{2+}-ionophore) are readily inhibited in Ca^{2+}-free medium, those elicited by acetylcholine carbachol, methacholine, histamine, serotonin and the leukotrienes C_4 and D_4 are relatively unaffected.[54,88,92,95,100,101,112,114,116,122–128]

With the gradual acceptance that the SR in smooth muscle could act not only as a sink for Ca^{2+} but also as a physiologically important source of activator Ca^{2+} [12,73] there has developed an acute interest in the signal transduction mechanism responsible for the release of Ca^{2+} from such stores. The question that has been posed is how a contractile agonist, via interaction with its extracellularly located receptors, is able to communicate with the SR to induce it to release some of its stored Ca^{2+}. Whilst there is evidence for a Ca^{2+}-induced Ca^{2+} release mechanism[112] most attention has focused upon the pivotal role played by certain metabolites of cell membrane inositol phospholipids, acting as second messengers, in the control of intracellular Ca^{2+} release and the maintenance of the contractile state.

Receptor-G-protein interaction

Heterotrimeric guanine nucleotide regulatory proteins (G-proteins) are now widely regarded as critical elements that couple hormone and neurotransmitter receptors to ion channels and an array of cellular processes via modulation of the concentrations of intracellular second messengers.[129,130] These G-proteins possess α, β and γ subunits which, in the resting state, exist as an $\alpha\beta\gamma$ holomer (Fig. 5.2). In the inactive state the three subunits are combined because of the presence of GDP bound to the α subunit (Fig. 5.2). When an agonist binds to a receptor it promotes exchange of GDP for GTP in the α subunit. The binding of GTP to the α subunit induces a dissociation of the α,β,γ subunits to provide free activated, GTP-bound, α subunits and a $\beta\gamma$ dimeric complex (Fig. 5.2). In its GTP-attached mode the α subunits are capable of activating a range of appropriate effector molecules. An intrinsic GTPase activity of the α subunit hydrolyses the GTP to yield GDP. With GDP bound to it the α subunit loses its effector activating capability and is able to recombine with the $\beta\gamma$ complex to return the cycle to its ground state.

Different forms of the α, β and γ subunits are known to exist. This gives rise to a heterogeneity of G-proteins involved in signal transduction mechanisms in different systems. In the context of contraction of airway smooth muscle, receptors for contractile agonists are coupled to a G-protein termed Gp, the nature and characteristics of which are not yet known. Activation of Gp stimulates phospholipase C (PLC).[131] This enzyme

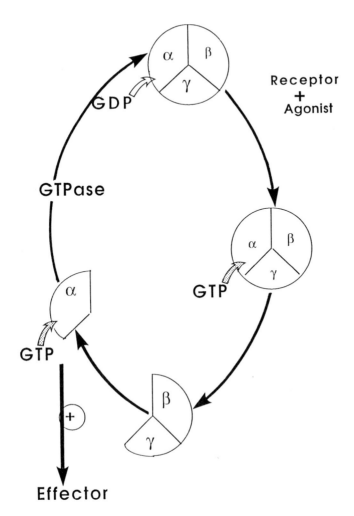

Fig. 5.2 Diagrammatic representation of the G-protein/GTP/GDP cycle that is regarded as critical in the receptor-mediated signal transduction process.

is responsible for cleaving a minor membrane phospholipid, phosphatidylinositol 4,5-bisphosphate (PIP_2), so generating inositol 1,4,5-trisphosphate (IP_3) and sn 1,2-diacylglycerol (DAG).[132,133] These two intracellular second messengers are widely regarded as having a pivotal role to play in controlling the contractile state of airway smooth muscle. IP_3 is regarded by many as the principal second messenger responsible for inducing the release of activator Ca^{2+} from intracellular stores.[133,134] DAG, on the other hand, has been implicated in the events underlying the tonic phase of airway smooth muscle contraction, via a protein kinase C (PKC)-dependent mechanism.[135,136]

Inositol-1,4,5-trisphosphate (IP_3) and intracellular Ca^{2+} release

With regard to airway smooth muscle, generation of inositol phospholipid metabolites in response to cholinergic agonists, histamine and leukotrienes has been demonstrated by several groups of workers in lung tissue from different species including man.[137–152] In these studies, however, either total inositol phosphates or total (unresolved) IP_3 was measured. Only the 1,4,5-isomer of IP_3 is active in mobilizing Ca^{2+} from non-mitochondrial intracellular stores.[133] Thus the reports [153–155] that this isomer is rapidly generated in airway tissues after contractile agonist stimulation are of paramount importance. It is also important to the hypothesis that the agonist-induced increases in the levels of IP_3 precede any detectable mechanical response. Additionally, IP_3 has been shown to elicit both Ca^{2+} release from SR stores and contraction of saponin-permeabilized airway smooth muscle.[138,156] Finally, it has been shown that there is a direct relationship between inositol phosphate accumulation and contraction using different muscarinic cholinoceptor agonists.[147,151] Taken together the above evidence is strongly supportive of the hypothesis that IP_3 is a second messenger responsible for the initiation of airway smooth muscle contraction via the mobilization of activator Ca^{2+} from intracellular stores. Precisely how IP_3 induces the liberation of Ca^{2+} from SR stores is not yet known although specific binding sites have been identified.[157,158] Recent evidence suggests that IP_3 directly activates a channel in the SR membrane that remains open only for as long as IP_3 is associated with its binding site.[159]

Understanding the mechanisms underlying pharmacomechanical coupling, however, is complicated by the fact that intracellular Ca^{2+} release in smooth muscle is not solely dependent upon IP_3 generation.[158–162] Furthermore, some release mechanisms require GTP-binding proteins whilst others do not. To complicate matters still further a GTP-activated intracellular Ca^{2+} translocation process has been identified which may allow Ca^{2+} to be moved between compartments without it entering the cytoplasm. It has been proposed that such a mechanism may be responsible for filling/refilling of the IP_3-releasable Ca^{2+} pool.[163–165] Further contradictory evidence to the IP_3 postulate exists. In the study of Langlands et al.[154] the cyclic guanosine monophosphate (cGMP) phosphodiesterase inhibitor M&B 22948 (zaprinast) prevented the histamine- and methacholine-induced generation of IP_3 without affecting the contractile response. Taken at face value this result indicates a dissociation between IP_3 generation and tension development and poses a question mark over the signal transduction pathways involving IP_3 as the principal chemical messenger involved in Ca^{2+} release in airway smooth muscle. In stark contrast, however, such an effect of zaprinast is absent in bovine airway smooth muscle.[155] Clearly a substantial amount of further work is required to unravel the intricacies of the mechanisms underlying pharmacomechanical coupling. One should also remain cognizant of the fact that convincing evidence exists[112] for the involvement of a Ca^{2+}-induced Ca^{2+} release mechanism in eliciting contraction of airway smooth muscle.

Diacylglycerol (DAG) and protein kinase C (PKC)

DAG is not implicated in the intracellular Ca^{2+} release process and, consequently the initial generation of tension. Instead, it has been suggested that DAG may be more intimately involved in those events that govern tension maintenance of smooth muscle via an effect on Ca^{2+}-activated, phospholipid-dependent protein kinase C.[24,121,135] Activation of protein kinase C is critically dependent upon the level of free Ca^{2+} within the myoplasm and upon certain phospholipids, notably phosphatidylserine. Under normal physiological conditions when a smooth muscle cell is at rest the basal levels of intracellular Ca^{2+} are insufficient to activate protein kinase C. However, upon stimulation with a contractile agonist, that mobilizes intracellular Ca^{2+}, two things happen that influence protein kinase C. Initially, the $[Ca^{2+}]_i$ increases abruptly, but transiently, and quickly returns towards baseline values. DAG then initiates the translocation of protein kinase C from the cytosol (where it exists in an inactive form) to the endoplasmic face of the plasmalemma. In this location the affinity of protein kinase C for Ca^{2+} is significantly enhanced such that the enzyme is capable of being maximally activated at a $[Ca^{2+}]_i$ that is less than 1 μM.[166–168] Thus, in the presence of DAG, protein kinase C is capable of being activated at the levels of intracellular Ca^{2+} that are thought to exist during the tonic (sustained) phase of a smooth muscle contraction.

Certain phorbol ester tumour promoters, most notably phorbol myristate acetate, 12-0-tetradecanoyl phorbol-13-acetate and phorbol dibutyrate, can substitute for DAG in the activation of protein kinase C. Whilst these agents are not wholly selective in activating protein kinase C they have, nevertheless, proved to be useful pharmacological tools. For example, it has been shown that these phorbol esters can induce slow monotonic contractions of airway smooth muscle, in some instances without increasing cytosolic Ca^{2+} levels.[52,135,169–172] Importantly, the time courses of the late-onset protein phosphorylation changes induced by cholinomimetic agonists and phorbol dibutyrate in airway preparations are very similar.[169] Furthermore, phorbol esters cause contraction of detergent-skinned smooth muscle when the free Ca^{2+} concentration is maintained at 0.1 μM, i.e. at a level beneath that required to induce a contraction in itself.[173,174] In not all instances, however, do phorbol esters induce contractile responses. Pretreatment of airway smooth muscle with phorbol esters inhibits agonist-induced contractions[175] and inhibits agonist-induced increases in $[Ca^{2+}]_i$.[54]

The precise physiological functions of protein kinase C are only slowly being unravelled. Exactly how the enzyme mediates its effects is also uncertain. What is known, however, is that there is more than one species of protein kinase C molecule; several discrete isoenzymes have been identified.[176] These proteins are derived both from multiple genes and from alternative splicing of a single mRNA transcript, yet they retain a primary structure containing conserved regulatory catalytic motifs with a high degree of sequence homology. To date seven isoenzymes have been identified. Each shows subtle differences in its mode of activation, sensitivity to Ca^{2+} and catalytic activity towards substrates. It is also known that the enzyme can phosphorylate a variety of different proteins, some of which are involved in the contractile mechanism. In general terms, such phosphotransferase activity is associated with an enhanced sensitivity to Ca^{2+}.[24,121,136] In spite of some contradictory results, protein kinase C is an attractive candidate mediator responsible for the enhanced sensitivity of contractile proteins to Ca^{2+}, a step regarded as essential for the generation and maintenance of the tonic phase of contraction.

Biochemical basis of airway smooth muscle contraction

It is widely accepted that myosin phosphorylation plays a major role in the contraction of airway smooth muscle. Adoption of this view stems from the results of numerous studies that have clearly shown that during contraction the levels of myosin light chain phosphorylation are significantly increased over resting levels.[17,34–36,47,51,53,177–179] Recently, however, it has been established that the magnitude of myosin light chain phosphorylation is not directly proportional to the development of tension *and* its maintenance, since myosin phosphorylation can decline whilst developed tension (the tonic phase of a contraction) is maintained (Fig. 5.3).[35,36,47,177,180]

The current interpretation of these events is that the level of myosin phosphorylation does not correlate with the absolute level of tension developed (i.e. the *number* of crossbridges formed). There is, however, a good correlation between the level of myosin phosphorylation and the rate of tension development (i.e. the *rate* of crossbridge cycling).[17,35,47] Interestingly, the time courses for myosin phosphorylation and dephosphorylation are closely paralled by agonist-induced changes in the intracellular free Ca^{2+} concentration in smooth muscle cells (the so-called Ca^{2+} transient) (Fig. 5.3).[50–56] Taken together, these two sets of observations have led to the suggestion that two Ca^{2+}-dependent pathways operate to control contraction of smooth muscle.[27,121,181,182]

In simplified terms, one current view of the sequence of biochemical events that underlies contraction of airway smooth muscle is as follows. Contractile agonists, on combining with their specific cell-surface receptors, activate phospholipase C via a G-protein. The activated phospholipase C cleaves PIP_2 creating the two second messengers IP_3 and DAG. The IP_3 promptly induces the release of Ca^{2+} from intracellular stores. As soon as the $[Ca^{2+}]_i$ increases, the free Ca^{2+} combine with the Ca^{2+}-binding protein calmodulin. The Ca^{2+}-calmodulin complex in turn activates myosin light chain kinase. This kinase then phosphorylates the 20-kDa light chain of myosin. The rate at which tension is then generated (the phasic component of the contraction) is determined by the rate at which crossbridges cycle, which in itself is determined by the magnitude of myosin light chain phosphorylation. The generation of IP_3 by a contractile agonist, however, is transient (Fig. 5.3).[153,154] Consequently, the second messenger-induced release of Ca^{2+} from the sarcoplasmic reticulum is not continuous. Thus, it would appear that IP_3 is adapted only to provide an initial burst of intracellular Ca^{2+} to induce rapid crossbridge cycling and thus tension development. In the absence of further release of intracellular Ca^{2+}, $[Ca^{2+}]_i$ returns towards (although not precisely to) resting levels (Fig. 5.3). This fall in $[Ca^{2+}]_i$ results in the dissociation of Ca^{2+} from calmodulin which consequently switches off the activity of myosin light chain kinase. Myosin phosphorylation must, therefore, decline and so too myosin ATPase activity (Fig. 5.3). Despite these events, which one might expect to uncouple the E/C sequence and

---

Fig. 5.3 Schematic representation of the time courses of several interlinked biochemical events involved in the generation of airway smooth muscle contraction. One of the first events to occur following receptor activation by a contractile agonist, added at the arrow (*bottom left*), is the rapid formation of 1,4,5-IP$_3$. IP$_3$ levels rise to a peak (a) and then rapidly wane to control values. Closely following this event there is a rapid elevation of $[Ca^{2+}]_i$ which peaks at (b). Like IP$_3$ the increase in $[Ca^{2+}]_i$ is only transient, levels returning to, or close to, basal values very quickly—a consequence of the protective homeostatic Ca^{2+} regulatory mechanisms operated by the smooth muscle cells. The shaded area illustrates the different $[Ca^{2+}]_i$ decay profiles measured by different investigators. Following the transient surge in $[Ca^{2+}]_i$ the 20-kDa light chain of myosin is phosphorylated (LC$_{20}$ phosphorylation) peaking at (c) and closely thereafter myosin is activated as an enzyme (myosin ATPase, peaking at (d)). This allows rapid crossbridge cycling between actin and myosin and hence the development of airway smooth muscle contraction. Note, however, that as tension develops LC$_{20}$ phosphorylation and myosin ATPase activity wane. Despite these events, and the very low $[Ca^{2+}]_i$ that exists at this time, the tonic contraction (e) is well-sustained. See text for further explanation. Reproduced from ref. 190, with permission.

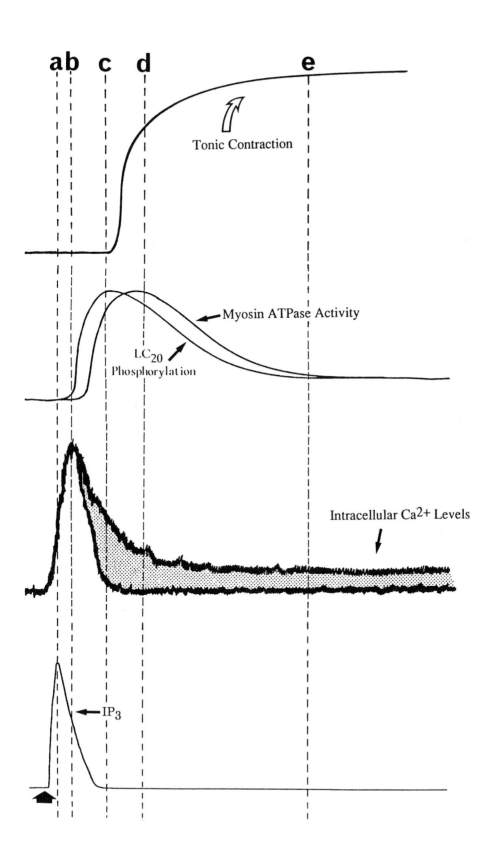

produce relaxation, the developed tension is well-sustained (Fig. 5.3; position e). It has been proposed, therefore, that such steady-state force maintenance does not require continued myosin light chain phosphorylation because of an alteration in the type of attachment formed between actin and myosin. Thus, instead of rapidly cycling cross-bridges, so-called latchbridges (dephosphorylated myosin crossbridges), which cycle slowly or not at all, are formed.[181-185] The maintenance of these latchbridges is Ca^{2+}-dependent, since a smooth muscle in the latch state can be relaxed by removal of Ca^{2+}. This does not necessarily imply that a latchbridge is directly regulated by Ca^{2+}. It does mean, however, that some Ca^{2+}-dependent process must be involved in the formation of latchbridges[182,185] possibly utilizing extracellular Ca^{2+}, entering the cell via ROCs[56], as discussed earlier. In view of the low $[Ca^{2+}]_i$ that exists during the tonic phase of contraction (Fig. 5.3) one of the characteristic features of the latchbridge state must be enhanced sensitivity of the contractile apparatus to Ca^{2+}. Precisely how this is achieved is not yet known although a possible role for protein kinase C has been proposed.[24,27,121] Interestingly, DAG is generated from more than one source during the sustained phase of contraction.[136] Initially, arachidonic acid-rich DAG is generated from PIP_2 by phospholipase C. Subsequently, DAG is derived from phosphatidylcholine (PC) by a PC-specific phospholipase C and also via the action of phospholipase D. The result of these events is a sustained increase in the total levels of DAG, within the airway smooth muscle cell and a consequent, persistent activation of protein kinase C. It has been proposed that phosphorylation of certain contractile proteins by protein kinase C brings about the enhanced sensitivity to Ca^{2+}.[24,27,121] Thus, it has been postulated that two separate, although in all likelihood interdependent, pathways exist to control contraction of airway smooth muscle. These are diagrammatically illustrated in Fig. 5.4. The first, a calmodulin/myosin light chain kinase pathway, is thought to be responsible for the initial rapid development of tension. The second pathway, via protein kinase C-mediated phosphorylations, is postulated to adapt the cell to accommodate sustained muscle contraction at minimum cost to itself, in terms of both energy expenditure (ATPase activity) and protection from the toxic consequences of intracellular Ca^{2+} overload.

There is another point that must be considered. The SR contains only a finite pool of activator Ca^{2+} and is, consequently, unable to maintain a prolonged low level of Ca^{2+} release in response to IP_3. Where, therefore, do the activator Ca^{2+} come from that enable the tonic phase of contraction to be maintained? One must presume that they come from the extracellular compartment entering the cell via some type of ion channel. The recent observations of Murray and Kotlikoff,[56] that were discussed earlier, would support this contention. Precisely how these putative ROCs are activated/regulated, or indeed how important they are to the overall contractile process remains to be determined. In terms of activation, however, one postulate is that emptying of the agonist/IP_3-sensitive Ca^{2+} pool can, in some cell types, cause enhanced permeability of the plasmalemma permitting Ca^{2+} entry.[186] This has been demonstrated, for example, in recent experiments using the non-phorbol ester tumour promoter thapsigargin.[187] Just how emptying of the Ca^{2+} pool in the SR influences the permeability of the plasmalemma is not yet known. It is not inconceivable, however, that yet another intracellular chemical signalling process is responsible for this capacitive process. Another postulate is that one of the metabolites of IP_3, namely myo-inositol-1,3,4,5-tetrakisphosphate (IP_4)[188,189] may act as an intracellular regulator of a plasmalemmal calcium channel

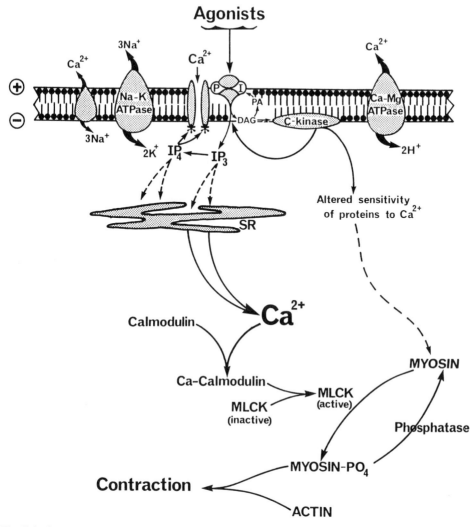

Fig. 5.4 Diagrammatic summary of the sequence of events thought to be involved in excitation–contraction coupling in airway smooth muscle. The cell membrane is shown containing the sodium–calcium exchange system, the sodium pump (Na–K ATPase), the Ca^{2+} efflux pump (Ca-Mg ATPase), protein kinase C (C-kinase) and a receptor complex coupled to the phosphatidylinositol (PI) system. On interacting with their cell surface receptors, agonists activate phospholipase C, via a G-protein linkage, which results in the formation of the intracellular second messengers inositol 1,4,5-trisphosphate (IP_3) and diacylglycerol (DAG). The initial tension development (phasic response) is determined by the activity of the calmodulin/myosin light chain kinase (MLCK) pathway which is turned on as a consequence of the release of activator Ca^{2+} from the sarcoplasmic reticulum (SR), probably by IP_3 and possibly via Ca^{2+}-induced Ca^{2+} release. Once generated, IP_3 is promptly phosphorylated to inositol 1,3,4,5-tetrakisphosphate (IP_4) by an IP_3 kinase. It has been suggested that IP_4 may be responsible for opening plasmalemmal ion channels (ROCs?) thus permitting a low level of influx of extracellular Ca^{2+}. These Ca^{2+} may be responsible for maintaining $[Ca^{2+}]_i$ at, or slightly above, basal levels during the period of maintained tension. The asterisks indicate the points on the inner surface of the plasmalemma at which IP_4 might act. Additionally, IP_4 may contribute to the process involved in replenishing the store of Ca^{2+} in the IP_3-releasable pool. It has been postulated that C-kinase may be responsible for enhancing the sensitivity of the contractile apparatus to Ca^{2+}. The C-kinase pathway may, therefore, be involved in the maintenance of developed tension (tonic phase of contraction) at a time when $[Ca^{2+}]_i$ is low. Diacylglycerol, the endogenous activator of PKC, is metabolized to phosphatidic acid (PA) which is then reincorporated into the membrane lipid pool.

(Fig. 5.4). IP_4 has been shown to be formed under the action of a specific *myo*-inositol-1,4,5-triphosphate-3-kinase which has a $K_m(Ca)$ around 1 μM. Since the $[Ca^{2+}]_i$ easily achieves such levels during the initial IP_3-triggered phase of a contraction, this is an attractive hypothesis. At the present time, however, such a process has not been demonstrated in muscle cells. There remains one further compelling reason for believing that extracellular Ca^{2+} must enter the cell during the plateau phase of a contraction. Numerous experiments have shown that repeated addition of contractile agonists to airway smooth muscle preparations bathed in Ca^{2+}-free medium causes a steady reduction in the size of the contractile response that can be elicited. The simple explanation for this effect is that the intracellular Ca^{2+} stores are not able to be refilled in the interval between successive additions of the contractile agonist. In all likelihood, therefore, entry of extracellular Ca^{2+} is essential both for the replenishment of the IP_3-releasable Ca^{2+} pool and for the maintained phase of a contractile response.

The overwhelming conclusion that can be drawn from the above description is that the initial events involved in E/C coupling and tension development in smooth muscle are fairly well understood. In stark contrast, the events involved in the maintenance of developed tension, which equates with the sustained bronchospasm of an asthmatic attack, remain to be determined. Unravelling the intricacies of the underlying mechanisms is one of the immediate challenges for the future.

ACKNOWLEDGEMENTS

The authors are grateful to the National Asthma Campaign, Scottish Home and Health Department, Scottish Hospitals Endowments Research Trust, Medical Research Council and Wellcome Trust, for financial support for their research.

REFERENCES

1. Daniel EE, Kannan M, Davis C, Posey-Daniel V: Ultrastructural studies on the neuromuscular control of human tracheal and bronchial muscle. *Resp Physiol* (1986) **63**: 109–128.
2. Akasaka K, Konno K, Ono Y, Mue S, Abe C: Electromyographic study of bronchial smooth muscle in bronchial asthma. *Tohoku J Exp Med* (1975) **117**: 55–59.
3. Barnes PJ: Pathogenesis of asthma: a review *J R Soc Med* (1983) **76**: 580–583.
4. Thomson NC: Neurogenic and myogenic mechanisms of nonspecific bronchial hyperreactivity. *Eur J Respir Dis* (1983) **64**: (Suppl 128): 206–211.
5. Kannan MS, Daniel EE: Structural and functional study of control of canine tracheal smooth muscle. *Am J Physiol* (1980) **328**: C27–C33.
6. Kannan MS, Jager LP, Daniel EE, Garfield RE: Effects of 4-aminopyridine and tetraethylammonium chloride on the electrical activity and cable properties of canine tracheal smooth muscle. *J Pharm Exp Ther* (1983) **227**: 706–715.
7. Berry JL, Elliott KRF, Foster RW, Green KA, Murray MA, Small RC: Mechanical biochemical and electrophysiological studies of RP 49536 and cromakalim in guinea-pig and bovine trachealis. *Pulm Pharmacol* (1991) **4**: 91–98.
8. Agrawal R, Daniel EE: Control of gap junction formation in canine trachea by arachidonic acid metabolites. *Am J Physiol* (1986) **250**: C495–C505.

9. Suzuki H, Morita K, Kuriyama H: Innervation and properties of the smooth muscle of the dog trachea. *Jpn J Physiol* (1976) **26**: 303–320.
10. Kroger EA, Stephens NL: Effect of tetraethylammonium ion on tonic airway smooth muscle: initiation of phasic electrical activity. *Am J Physiol* (1975) **228**: 633–636.
11. Green KA, Foster RW, Small RC: A patch-clamp study of K^+-channel activity in bovine isolated tracheal smooth muscle cells. *Br J Pharmacol* (1991) **102**: 871–878.
12. Somlyo AP, Somlyo AV, Kitazawa T, Bond M, Shuman H, Kowarski D: Ultrastructure, function and composition of smooth muscle. *Ann Biomed Engin* (1983) **2**: 579–588.
13. Kowarski D, Shuman H, Somlyo AP, Somlyo AV: Calcium release by noradrenaline from central sarcoplasmic reticulum in rabbit main pulmonary artery smooth muscle. *J Physiol* (1985) **366**: 153–175.
14. Daniel EE, Grover AK, Kwan CY: Calcium. In Stephens NL (ed) *Biochemistry of Smooth Muscle*. Boca Raton, CRC Press, 1983, pp 1–88.
15. Hartshore DJ, Gorecka A: Biochemistry of the contractile proteins of smooth muscle. In Bohr DF, Somlyo AP, Sparks HV (eds) *Handbook of Physiology*, Section 2, Vol II. Bethesda, MD, American Physiological Society (1980) pp 93–120.
16. Stull JT: Phosphorylation of contractile proteins in relation to muscle function. *Adv Cyclic Nucl Res* (1980) **13**: 39–93.
17. Kamm KE, Stull JT: The function of myosin and myosin light chain kinase phosphorylation in smooth muscle. *Ann Rev Pharmacol Toxicol* (1985) **25**: 593–620.
18. Kamm KE, Stull JT: Regulation of smooth muscle contractile elements by second messengers. *Ann Rev Physiol* (1989) **51**: 299–313.
19. Adelstein RS, Eisenberg E: Regulation and kinetics of the actin-myosin-ATP interaction. *Ann Rev Biochem* (1980) **49**: 956–969.
20. Adelstein RS: Regulation of contractile proteins by phosphorylation. *J Clin Invest* (1983) **72**: 1863–1866.
21. Small JV: Geometry of actin-membrane attachments in the smooth muscle cell: The localisations of vinculin and α-actinin. *EMBO J* (1985) **4**: 45–49.
22. Small JV, Furst DO, DeMey J: Localisation of filamin in smooth muscle. *J Cell Biol* (1986) **102**: 210–220.
23. Furst DO, Cross RA, DeMey J, Small JV: Caldesmon is an elongated, flexible molecule localized in the actomyosin domains of smooth muscle. *EMBO J* (1986) **5**: 251–257.
24. Rasmussen H, Takuwa Y, Park S: Protein kinase C in the regulation of smooth muscle contraction. *FASEB J* (1987) **1**: 177–185.
25. Manalan AS, Klee CB: Calmodulin. *Adv Cyclic Nucl Protein Phosphor Res* (1984) **18**: 227–278.
26. Cheung WY: Calmodulin plays a pivotal role in cellular regulation. *Science* (1980) **207**: 19–27.
27. Rasmussen H, Barrett PQ: Calcium messenger system: An integrated view. *Physiol Rev* (1984) **64**: 938–984.
28. Klee CB, Crouch TH, Richman PG: Calmodulin. *Ann Rev Biochem* (1980) **49**: 489–515.
29. Chau V, Huang CY, Chock PB, Wang JH, Sharma R: Kinetic studies of the activation of cyclic nucleotide phosphodiesterase by Ca^{2+} and calmodulin. In Kakiuchi K, Hidaka H, Means AR (eds) *Calmodulin and Intracellular Ca^{2+} Receptors*. New York, Plenum, 1982, pp 199–217.
30. Dabrowska R, Aromatoria D, Sherry JMF, Hartshorne DJ: Composition of the myosin light chain kinase from chicken gizzard. *Biochem Biophys Res Commun* (1977) **78**: 1263–1272.
31. Adelstein RS, Klee CB: Purification and characterisation of smooth muscle myosin light chain kinase. *J Biol Chem* (1981) **256**: 7501–7509.
32. Miller JR, Silver PJ, Stull JT: The role of myosin light chain kinase phosphorylation in β-adrenergic relaxation of tracheal smooth muscle. *Mol Pharmacol* (1983) **24**: 235–242.
33. DeLanerolle P, Stull JT: Myosin phosphorylation during contraction of tracheal smooth muscle. *J Biol Chem* (1980) **255**: 9993–10000.
34. DeLanerolle P, Condit JR, Tanenbaum M, Adelstein RS: Myosin phosphorylation, agonist concentration and contraction of tracheal smooth muscle. *Nature* (1982) **298**: 871–872.
35. Gerthoffer WT, Murphy RA: Myosin phosphorylation, agonist concentration and contraction of tracheal smooth muscle. *Nature* (1982) **298**: 871–872.

36. Gerthoffer WT: Calcium dependence of myosin phosphorylation and airway smooth muscle contraction and relaxation. *Am J Physiol* (1986) **250**: C597–C604.
37. Sobue K, Muramoto Y, Fujita M, Kakiuchi S: Purification of a calmodulin-binding protein from chicken gizzard that interacts with F-actin. *Proc Natl Acad Sci USA* (1981) **78**: 5652–5655.
38. Sobue K, Morimoto K, Inui M, Kanda K, Kakiuchi S: Control of actin–myosin interaction of gizzard smooth muscle by calmodulin- and caldesmon-linked flip-flop mechanism. *Biomed Res* (1982) **3**: 188–196.
39. Ngai PK, Walsh MP: Inhibition of smooth muscle actin-activated myosin Mg^{2+}-ATPase activity by caldesmon. *J Biol Chem* (1984) **259**: 13656–13659.
40. Ngai PK, Walsh MP: The effects of phosphorylation of smooth-muscle caldesmon. *Biochem J* (1987) **244**: 417–425.
41. Huxley H, Hanson J: Changes in the cross-striations of muscle during contraction and stretch and their structural interpretation. *Nature* (1954) **173**: 973–976.
42. Huxley AF, Niedergerke R: Structural changes in muscle during contraction. Interference microscopy of living muscle fibres. *Nature* (1954) **173**: 971–973.
43. Small JV, Sobieszek A: The contractile apparatus of smooth muscle. *Int Rev Cytol* (1980) **64**: 1–79.
44. Small JV, Sobieszek A: Contractile and structural proteins of smooth muscle. In Stephens NL (ed) *Biochemistry of Smooth Muscle*, Vol 1. Boca Raton, CRC Press, 1983, pp 1–84.
45. Gabella G: Structural apparatus for force transmission in smooth muscles. *Physiol Rev* (1984) **64**: 455–477.
46. Gabella G: Smooth muscle in the gut and airways. In Motta PM (ed) *Ultrastructure of Smooth Muscle. Electron Microscopy in Biology and Medicine. Current Topics in Ultrastructural Research*, Vol 8. Hingham, MA, Kluwer Academic, 1990, pp 137–151.
47. Kamm KE, Stull JT: Myosin phosphorylation, force and maximal shortening velocity in neurally stimulated tracheal smooth muscle. *Am J Physiol* (1985) **249**: C238–C247.
48. Bolton TB: Mechanisms of action of transmitters and other substances on smooth muscle. *Physiol Rev* (1979) **59**: 606–718.
49. Somlyo AP: Excitation–contraction coupling and the ultrastructure of smooth muscle. *Circ Res* (1985) **57**: 497–507.
50. Felbel J, Trockur B, Ecker T, Landgraf W, Hofman F: Regulation of cytosolic calcium by cAMP and cGMP in freshly isolated smooth muscle cells from bovine trachea. *J Biol Chem* (1988) **263**: 16764–16771.
51. Taylor DA, Stull JT: Calcium dependence of myosin light chain phosphorylation in smooth muscle cells. *J Biol Chem* (1988) **28**: 14456–14462.
52. Takuwa Y, Takuwa N, Rasmussen H: Measurement of cytoplasmic free Ca^{2+} concentration in bovine tracheal smooth muscle using aequorin. *Am J Physiol* (1987) **253**: C817–C827.
53. Taylor DA, Bowman BF, Stull JT: Cytoplasmic Ca^{2+} is a primary determinant for myosin phosphorylation in smooth muscle cells. *J Biol Chem* (1989) **264**: 6207–6213.
54. Kotlikoff MI, Murray RK, Reynolds EE: Histamine-induced calcium release and phorbol antagonism in cultured airway smooth muscle cells. *Am J Physiol* (1987) **245**: C561–C566.
55. Panettieri RA, Murray RK, DePalo LR, Yadvish PA, Kotlikoff MI: A human airway smooth muscle cell line that retains physiological responsiveness. *Am J Physiol* (1989) **256**: C329–C335.
56. Murray RK, Kotlikoff MI: Receptor-activated calcium influx in human airway smooth muscle cells. *J Physiol* (1991) **435**: 123–144.
57. Reuter, H, Blaustein MP, Haeusler G: Na–Ca exchange and tension development in arterial smooth muscle. *Phil Trans R Soc Land B* (1973) **265**: 78–94.
58. Bullock CG, Fettes JJF, Kirkpatrick CT: Tracheal smooth muscle—second thoughts on sodium–calcium exchange. *J Physiol* (1981) **318**: 46.
59. Chideckel EW, Frost JL, Mike P, Fedan JF: The effect of ouabain on tension in isolated respiratory tract smooth muscle of humans and other species. *Br J Pharmac* (1987) **92**: 609–614.
60. Gunst SJ, Stropp JQ: Effect of Na–K adenosinetriphosphate activity on relaxation of canine tracheal smooth muscle. *J Appl Physiol* (1988) **64**: 635–641.

61. Schatzmann HJ: Calcium extrusion across the plasma membrane by the calcium-pump and the Ca^{2+}–Na^+ exchange system. In Marme D (ed) *Calcium and Cell Physiology*. Berlin, Springer-Verlag, 1985, pp 18–52.
62. Grover AK, Kannan MS, Daniel EE: Canine trachealis membrane fractionation and characterization. *Cell Calcium* (1980) **1**: 135–146.
63. Hogaboom GK, Fedan JF: Calmodulin stimulation of calcium uptake and (Ca^{2+}–Mg^{2+})-ATPase activities in microsomes from canine tracheal smooth muscle. *Biochem Biophys Res Commun* (1981) **99**: 737–744.
64. Bryson SE, Rodger IW: Simultaneous measurement of agonist-induced ^{45}Ca efflux and contraction in isolated airway smooth muscle. *Br J Pharmac* (1987) **92**: 632P.
65. Goodman FR, Weiss GB, Karaki H, Nakagawa H: Differential calcium movements induced by agonists in guinea pig tracheal muscle. *Eur J Pharmac* (1987) **133**: 111–117.
66. Carafoli E: Calmodulin-sensitive calcium-pumping ATPase of plasma membranes: Isolation, reconstitution and regulation. *Fed Proc* (1984) **43**: 3005–3010.
67. Choquette D, Hakim G, Filoteo AG, Plishker GA, Bostwick JR, Penniston JT: Regulation of plasma membrane Ca^{2+} ATPases by lipids of the phosphatidylinositol cycle. *Biochem Biophys Res Commun* (1984) **125**: 908–915.
68. Devine CE, Somlyo AV, Somlyo AP: Sarcoplasmic reticulum and excitation–contraction coupling in mammalian smooth muscle. *J Cell Biol* (1972) **52**: 690–718.
69. Somlyo AP, Somlyo AV, Shuman H: Electron probe analysis of vascular smooth muscle: Composition of mitochondria, nuclei and cytoplasm. *J Cell Biol* (1979) **81**: 316–335.
70. Raeymaekers L, Hasselbach W: Ca^{2+} uptake, Ca^{2+}-ATPase activity, phosphoprotein formation and phosphate turnover in a microsomal fraction of smooth muscle. *Eur J Biochem* (1981) **116**: 373–378.
71. Bond M, Kitazawa T, Shuman H, Somlyo AV, Somlyo AP: Calcium release from and recycling by the sarcoplasmic reticulum in guinea pig smooth muscle. *J Physiol* (1984) **355**: 677–695.
72. Somlyo AP, Walker JW, Goldman YE, *et al.*: Inositol trisphosphate, calcium and muscle contraction. *Phil Trans R Soc Lond B* (1988) **320**: 399–414.
73. Sands H, Mascali J: Effects of cyclic AMP and of protein kinase on the calcium uptake by various tracheal smooth muscle organelles. *Arch Int Pharmacodyn Ther* (1978) **236**: 180–191.
74. Richards IS, Kulkarni A, Brooks SM: Human fetal tracheal smooth muscle produces spontaneous electromechanical oscillations that are Ca^{2+}-dependent and cholinergically potentiated. *Dev Pharmacol Ther* (1991) **16**: 22–28.
75. Small RC, Foster RW: Electrophysiology of the airway smooth muscle cell. In Barnes PJ, Rodger IW, Thomson NC (eds) *Asthma: Basic Mechanisms and Clinical Management*. London, Academic Press, 1988, pp 35–56.
76. McCann JD, Welsh MJ: Calcium-activated potassium channels in canine airways smooth muscle. *J Physiol* (1986) **372**: 113–127.
77. Huang HM, Dwyer TM, Farley JM: Patch-clamp recording of single Ca^{2+}-activated K^+-channels in tracheal smooth muscle from swine. *Biophys J* (1987) **51**: 50a.
78. Hisada T, Kurachi Y, Sugimoto T: Properties of membrane currents in isolated smooth muscle cells from guinea-pig trachea. *Pflugers Archiv* (1990) **416**: 151–161.
79. Kume H, Takagi K, Satake T, Tokuno H, Tomita T: Effects of intracellular pH on calcium-activated potassium channels in rabbit tracheal smooth muscle. *J Physiol* (1990) **424**: 445–457.
80. Jones TR, Charette L, Garcia ML, Kaczorowski GJ: Selective inhibition of relaxation of guinea-pig trachea by charybdotoxin, a potent Ca^{2+}-activated K^+-channel inhibitor. *J Pharmac Exp Ther* (1990) **255**: 697–703.
81. Giembycz MA, Rodger IW: Electrophysiological and other aspects of excitation–contraction coupling and uncoupling in mammalian airway smooth muscle. *Life Sci* (1987) **41**: 111–132.
82. Kotlikoff MI: Ion channels in airway smooth muscle. In Coburn RF (ed) *Airway Smooth Muscle in Health and Disease*. New York, Plenum Press, 1990, pp 169–182.

83. Rodger IW: Excitation–contraction coupling and uncoupling in airway smooth muscle. *Br J Clin Pharmac* (1985) **20**: 255S–266S.

84. Small RC, Foster RW: Airways smooth muscle: An overview of morphology, electrophysiology and aspects of the pharmacology of contraction and relaxation. In Kay AB (ed) *Asthma: Clinical Pharmacology and Therapeutic Progress.* Oxford, Blackwell, 1986, pp 101–113.

85. Rodger IW: Calcium channels in airway smooth muscle. *Amer Rev Resp Dis* (1987) **136**: S15–S17.

86. Marthan R, Martin C, Amedee T, Mironneau J: Calcium channel currents in isolated smooth muscle cells from human bronchus. *J Appl Physiol* (1989) **66**: 1706–1714.

87. Kotlikoff MI: Calcium currents in isolated canine airway smooth muscle cells. *Am J Physiol* (1988) **254**: C793–C801.

88. Kirkpatrick CT: Excitation and contraction in bovine tracheal smooth muscle. *J Physiol* (1975) **244**: 263–281.

89. Suzuki H, Morita K, Kuriyama H: Innervation and properties of the smooth muscle of the dog trachea. *Jpn J Physiol* (1976) **26**: 303–320.

90. Coburn RF, Yamaguchi T: Membrane potential-dependent and -independent tension in canine trachealis. *J Pharmac Exp Ther* (1977) **201**: 276–284.

91. Farley JM, Miles PR: Role of depolarisation in acetylcholine-induced contractions of dog trachealis muscle. *J Pharmac Exp Ther* (1977) **201**: 991–205.

92. Coburn RF: Electromechanical coupling in canine trachealis muscle: Acetylcholine contractions. *Am J Physiol* (1979) **236**: C177–C184.

93. Foster RW, Small RC, Weston AH: The spasmogenic action of potassium chloride in guinea-pig trachealis. *Br J Pharmac* (1983) **80**: 553–559.

94. Foster RW, Small RC, Weston AH: Evidence that the spasmogenic action of tetraethylammonium in guinea-pig trachealis is both direct and dependent upon the cellular influx of calcium ion. *Br J Pharmac* (1983) **79**: 225–263.

95. Raeburn D, Rodger IW: Lack of effect of leukotriene D_4 on Ca-uptake in airway smooth muscle. *Br J Pharmac* (1984) **83**: 499–504.

96. Weiss GB, Pang IH, Goodman FR: Relationship between ^{45}Ca movements, different calcium components and responses to acetylcholine and potassium in tracheal smooth muscle. *J Pharmac Exp Ther* (1985) **233**: 389–394.

97. Kannan MS, Jager LP, Daniel EE, Garfield RE: Effects of 4-aminopyridine and tetraethylammonium chloride on the electrical activity and cable properties of canine tracheal smooth muscle. *J Pharmac Exp Ther* (1983) **227**: 706–715.

98. Foster RW, Okpalugo BI, Small RC: Antagonism of Ca^{2+} and other actions of verapamil in guinea-pig isolated trachealis. *Br J Pharmac* (1984) **81**: 499–507.

99. Ahmed F, Foster RW, Small RC: Some effects of nifedipine in guinea-pig isolated trachealis. *Br J Pharmac* (1985) **84**: 861–869.

100. Baba K, Kawanishi M, Satake T, Tomita T: Effects of verapamil on the contractions of guinea-pig tracheal smooth muscle induced by Ca, Sr and Ba. *Br J Pharmac* (1985) **84**: 203–211.

101. Raeburn D, Roberts JA, Rodger IW, Thomson NC: Agonist-induced contractile responses of human bronchial muscle *in vitro*: Effects of Ca^{2+} removal, La^{3+} and PY 108068. *Eur J Pharmac* (1986) **121**: 251–255.

102. Allen SL, Foster RW, Small RC, Towart R: The effects of the dihydropyridine BAY K8644 in guinea-pig isolated trachea. *Br J Pharmac* (1985) **86**: 171–180.

103. Advenier C, Naline E, Renier A: Effects of BAY K8644 on contraction of the human isolated bronchus and guinea-pig isolated trachea. *Br J Pharmac* (1986) **88**: 33–39.

104. Kroeger EA, Stephens NL: Effect of tetraethylammonium on tonic airway smooth muscle: Initiation of phasic electrical activity. *Am J Physiol* (1975) **228**: 633–636.

105. Cameron AR, Kirkpatrick CT: A study of excitatory neuromuscular transmission in bovine trachea. *J Physiol* (1977) **270**: 733–745.

106. McCaig DJ, Souhrada JF: Alteration of electrophysiological properties of airway smooth muscle from sensitized guinea-pigs. *Resp Physiol* (1980) **41**: 49–60.

107. Kirkpatrick CT: Tracheobronchial smooth muscle. In Bulbring E, Brading AF, Jones AW, Tomita T (eds) *Smooth Muscle: An assessment of Current Knowledge*. London, Arnold, 1981, pp 385–395.
108. Ahmed F, Foster RW, Small RC, Weston AH: Some features of the spasmogenic actions of acetylcholine and histamine in guinea-pig isolated trachealis. *Br J Pharmac* (1984) **84**: 227–233.
109. McCaig DJ, Rodger IW: Electrophysiological effects of leukotriene D_4 in guinea-pig airway smooth muscle. *Br J Pharmac* (1988) **94**: 729–736.
110. Murlas CG, Doupnik CA: Electromechanical coupling of ferret airway smooth muscle in response to leukotriene D_4. *J Appl Physiol* (1989) **66**: 3533–3538.
111. Kirkpatrick CT, Jenkinson HA, Cameron AR: Interaction between drugs and potassium-rich solutions in producing contraction in bovine tracheal smooth muscle: Studies in normal and calcium depleted tissues. *Clin Exp Pharmac Pharmacol* (1975) **2**: 559–570.
112. Ito Y, Itoh T: The roles of stored calcium in contractions of cat tracheal smooth muscle produced by electrical stimulation, acetylcholine and high K^+. *Br J Pharmac* (1984) **83**: 667–676.
113. Jones TR, Davis C, Daniel EE: Pharmacological study of the contractile activity of leukotriene C_4 and D_4 on isolated human airway smooth muscle. *Can J Physiol Pharmacol* (1982) **60**: 638–643.
114. Cerrina J. Advenier C, Renier A, Floch A, Duroux P: Effects of diltiazem and other Ca^{2+}-antagonists on guinea-pig tracheal muscle. *Eur J Pharmac* (1983) **94**: 241–249.
115 Advenier C, Cerrina J, Duroux P, Floch A, Renier A: Effects of five different organic calcium antagonists on guinea-pig isolated trachea. *Br J Pharmac* (1984) **82**: 727–733.
116. Baba K, Satake T, Takagi K, Tomita T: Effects of verapamil on the response of the guinea-pig tracheal muscle to carbachol. *Br J Pharmac* (1986) **88**: 441–449.
117. Roberts JA, Giembycz MA, Raeburn D, Rodger IW, Thomson NC: *In vivo* and *in vitro* effect of verapamil on human airway responsiveness to leukotriene D_4. *Thorax* (1986) **41**: 12–16.
118. Merrit J, Armstrong WP, Hallam TJ, *et al*.: SK&F 96365, a novel inhibitor of receptor-mediated calcium entry and aggregation in Quin-2-loaded human platelets. *Br J Pharmacol* (1989) **98**: 674P.
119. Creese BR: Calcium ions, drug action and airways obstruction. *Pharmac Ther* (1983) **20**: 357–375.
120. Triggle DJ: Calcium, the control of smooth muscle function and bronchial hyperreactivity. *Allergy* (1983) **38**: 1–9.
121. Rodger IW: Calcium ions and contraction of airways smooth muscle. In Kay AB (ed) *Asthma: Clinical Pharmacology and Therapeutic Progress*. Oxford, Blackwell, 1986, pp 114–127.
122. Farley JM, Miles PR: The sources of calcium for acetylcholine-induced contractions of dog tracheal smooth muscle. *J Pharmac Exp Ther* (178) **207**: 340–346.
123. Creese BR, Denborough MA: Sources of calcium for contraction of guinea-pig isolated tracheal smooth muscle. *Clin Exp Pharmacol Physiol* (1981) **8**: 175–182.
124. Weiss EB, Mullick PC: Leukotriene effect in airways smooth muscle: Calcium dependence and verapamil inhibition. *Prostaglandins, Leukotrienes Med* (1982) **12**: 53–66.
125. Weichman BM, Tucker SS: Leukotriene D_4 elicits a non-sustained contraction of the guinea-pig trachea in calcium-free buffer. *Eur J Pharmac* (1984) **101**: 229–234.
126. Marthan RJ, Savineau JP, Mironneau J: Acetylcholine-induced contraction in human isolated bronchial smooth muscle: Role of an intracellular calcium store. *Resp Physiol* (1985) **67**: 127–135.
127. Marthan RJ, Armour CL, Johnson PRA, Black JL: Extracellular calcium and human isolated airway muscle: Ionophore A23187-induced contraction. *Resp Physiol* (1988) **71**: 157–168.
128. Nouailhetas VLA, Lodge NJ, Twort CHC, Van Breemen C: The intracellular calcium stores in rabbit trachealis. *Eur J Pharmac* (1988) **157**: 165–172.
129. Gilman AG: G-proteins: transducers of receptor-generated signals. *Ann Rev Biochem* (1987) **56**: 615–649.

130. Birnbaumer L: G-proteins in signal transduction. *Ann Rev Pharmacol Toxicol* (1990) **30**: 675–705.

131. Kitazawa T, Kobayashi S, Horiuti K, Somlyo AV, Somlyo AP: Receptor-coupled, permeabilised smooth muscle: Role of the phosphatidylinositol cascade, G proteins and modulation of the contractile response to Ca^{2+}. *J Biol Chem* (1989) **264**: 5339–5342.

132. Berridge MJ, Irvine RF: Inositol trisphosphate, a novel second messenger in cellular signal transduction. *Nature* (1984) **312**: 315–321.

133. Berridge MJ, Irvine RF: Inositol phosphates and cell signalling. *Nature* (1989) **341**: 197–203.

134. Somlyo AP, Walker JW, Goldman YE, *et al.*: Inositol trisphosphate, calcium and muscle contraction. *Phil Trans R Soc Lond B* (1988) **320**: 399–414.

135. Park S, Rasmussen H: Activation of tracheal smooth muscle contraction: Synergism between Ca^{2+} and activators of protein kinase C. *Proc Natl Acad Sci USA* (1986) **82**: 8835–8839.

136. Rasmussen H, Kelley G, Douglas JS: Interactions between Ca^{2+} and cAMP messenger systems in regulation of airway smooth muscle contraction. *Am J Physiol* (1990) **258**: L279–L288.

137. Baron CB, Cunningham M, Straus JF, Coburn RF: Pharmacomechanical coupling in smooth muscle may involve phosphatidylinositol metabolism. *Proc Natl Acad Sci USA* (1984) **81**: 6899–6903.

138. Hashimoto T, Hirata M, Ito Y: A role for inositol 1,4,5-trisphosphate in the initiation of agonist-induced contractions of dog tracheal smooth muscle. *Br J Pharmac* (1985) **86**: 191–199.

139. Grandordy BM, Cuss FM, Sampson AS, Palmer JB, Barnes PJ: Phosphatidylinositol response to cholinergic agonists in airway smooth muscle: Relationship to contraction and muscarinic receptor occupany. *J Pharmac Exp Ther* (1986) **238**: 273–279.

140. Grandordy BM, Barnes PJ: Phosphoinositide turnover in airway smooth muscle. *Amer Rev Resp Dis* (1987) **136**: S17–S20.

141. Takuwa Y, Takuwa N, Rasmussen H: Carbachol induces a rapid and sustained hydrolysis of polyphosphoinositide in bovine tracheal smooth muscle. Measurements of the mass of polyphosphoinositides, 1,2,-diacylglycerol and phosphatidic acid. *J Biol Chem* (1986) **261**: 14670–14675.

142. Duncan RA, Krzanowski JJ, Davis JS, Polson JB, Coffey RG, Szentivanyi A: Polyphosphoinositide metabolism in canine tracheal smooth muscle (CTSM) in response to a cholinergic stimulus. *Biochem Pharmacol* (1978) **36**: 307–310.

143. Kardasz AM, Langlands JM, Rodger IW, Watson J: Inositol lipid turnover in isolated guinea-pig trachealis and lung parenchyma. *Biochem Soc Trans* (1987) **15**: 474.

144. Mong S, Hoffman K, Wu H-L, Crooke ST: Leukotriene-induced hydrolysis of inositol lipids in guinea-pig lung. Mechanism of signal transduction for leukotriene D_4 receptors. *Mol Pharmacol* (1978) **31**: 35–41.

145. Mong S, Miller J, Wu H-L, Crooke ST: Leukotriene D_4 receptor-mediated hydrolysis of phosphoinositide and mobilization of calcium in sheep tracheal smooth muscle cells. *J Pharmac Exp Ther* (1988) **244**: 508–515.

146. Miller-Hance WC, Miller JR, Wells JN, Stull JT, Kamm KE: Biochemical events associated with activation of smooth muscle contraction. *J Biol Chem* (1988) **263**: 13979–13982.

147. Meurs H, Roffel AF, Postema JB, *et al.*: Evidence for a direct relationship between phosphoinositide metabolism and airway smooth muscle contraction induced by muscarinic agonists. *Eur J Pharmac* (1988) **156**: 271–274.

148. Hall IP, Hill SJ: β_2-Adrenoceptor stimulation inhibits histamine-induced inositol phospholipid hydrolysis in bovine tracheal smooth muscle. *Br J Pharmac* (1988) **95**: 1204–1212.

149. Hall IP, Hill SJ: Inhibition of histamine-stimulated inositol phospholipid hydrolysis by agents which increase cyclic AMP levels in bovine tracheal smooth muscle. *Br J Pharmac* (1989) **97**: 603–613.

150. Baron CB, Pring M, Coburn RF: Inositol lipid turnover and compartmentation in canine trachealis smooth muscle. *Am J Physiol* (1989) **256**: C375–C383.

151. Meurs H, Timmermans A, Van Amsterdam RGM, Brouwer F, Kauffman HF, Zaagsma J: Muscarinic receptors in human airway smooth muscle are coupled to phosphoinositide metabolism. *Eur J Pharmac* (1989) **164**: 369–371.

152. Coburn RF, Baron CB: Coupling mechanisms in airway smooth muscle. *Am J Physiol* (1990) **258**: L119–L133.

153. Chilvers ER, Challis RAJ, Barnes PJ, Nahorski SR: Mass changes of inositol(1,4,5)tris-phosphate in trachealis muscle following agonist stimulation. *Eur J Pharmac* (1989) **614**: 587–590.

154. Langlands JM, Rodger IW, Diamond J: The effect of M&B 22948 on methacholine- and histamine-induced contraction and inositol 1,4,5-trisphosphate levels in guinea-pig tracheal tissue. *Br J Pharmac* (1989) **98**: 336–338.

155. Chilvers ER, Giembycz MA, Challis RAJ, Barnes PJ, Nahorski SR: Lack of effect of zaprinast on methacholine-induced contraction and inositol 1,4,5-trisphosphate accumulation in bovine tracheal smooth muscle. *Br J Pharmacol* (1991) **103**: 1119–1125.

156. Twort CHC, Van Breemen C: Human airway smooth muscle in cell culture: control of the intracellular calcium store. *Pulm Pharmacol* (1989) **2**: 45–53.

157. Spat A, Bradford PG, McKinney JS, Rubin RP, Putney JW: A saturable receptor for ^{32}P-inositol-1,4,5-trisphosphate in hepatocytes and neutrophils. *Nature* (1986) **319**: 514–516.

158. Ross CA, Meldolesi J, Milner TA, Satoh T, Supattapone S, Snyder SH: Inositol 1,4,5-trisphosphate receptor localized to endoplasmic reticulum in cerebellar Purkinje neurons. *Nature* (1989) **339**: 468–470.

159. Ghosh TK, Eis PS, Mullaney JM, Ebert CL, Gill DL: Competitive reversible and potent antagonism of inositol 1,4,5-trisphosphate-activated calcium release by heparin. *J Biol Chem* (1988) **263**: 11075–11079.

160. Saida K, Twort CHC, Van Breemen C: The specific GTP requirement for inositol 1,4,5-trisphosphate-induced Ca^{2+} release from skinned vascular smooth muscle. *J Cardiovasc Pharmac* (1988) **12**: S47–S50.

161. Kobayashi S, Somlyo AV, Somlyo AP: Heparin inhibits the inositol 1,4,5-trisphosphate-dependent, but not the independent, calcium release induced by guanine nucleotide in vascular smooth muscle. *Biochem Biophys Res Commun* (1988) **153**: 625–631.

162. Kitazawa T, Kobayashi S, Horiuti K, Somlyo AV, Somlyo AP: Receptor-coupled, per-meabilized smooth muscle: Role of the phosphatidylinositol cascade, G-proteins and modulation of the contractile response to calcium. *J Biol Chem* (1989) **264**: 5339–5342.

163. Mullaney JM, Yu M, Ghosh TK, Gill DL: Calcium entry into the inositol 1,4,5-trisphosphate-releasable calcium pool is mediated by a GTP-regulatory mechanism. *Proc Natl Acad Sci USA* (1988) **85**: 2499–2503.

164. Thomas AP: Enhancement of the inositol 1,4,5-trisphosphate-releasable Ca^{2+} pool by GTP in permeabilised hepatocytes. *J Biol Chem* (1988) **263**: 2704–2711.

165. Ghosh TK, Mullaney JM, Tarazi FI, Gill DL: GTP-activated communication between distinct inositol 1,4,5-trisphosphate-sensitive and -insensitive calcium pools. *Nature* (1989) **340**: 236–239.

166. Nishizuka Y: Calcium, phospholipid turnover and transmembrane signalling. *Phil Trans Roy Soc Lond B* (1983) **302**: 101–102.

167. Nishizuka Y: The role of protein kinase C in cell surface signal transduction and tumour promotion. *Nature* (1984) **308**: 693–698.

168. Rasmussen H, Kojima I, Kojima K, Zawalich W, Appeldorf W: Calcium as intracellular messenger: Sensitivity modulation, C-kinase pathway, and sustained cellular response. *Adv Cyclic Nucl Protein Phosphor Res* (1984) **18**: 159–193.

169. Park S, Rasmussen H: Carbachol-induced protein phosphorylation changes in bovine tracheal smooth muscle. *J Biol Chem* (1986) **261**: 15373–15379.

170. Dale MM, Obianime AW: Phorbol myristate acetate causes in guinea pig lung parenchymal strip a maintained spasm resistant to isoprenaline. *FEBS Lett* (1985) **190**: 6–10.

171. Dale MM, Obianime AW: 4β-PDBu contracts parenchymal strip and synergises with raised cytosolic calcium. *Eur J Pharmac* (1987) **141**: 23–32.
172. Obianime AW, Hirst SJ, Dale MM: Interactions between phorbol esters and agents which increase cytosolic calcium in the guinea pig parenchymal strip: Direct and indirect effect on the contractile response. *J Pharmac Exp Ther* (1988) **247**, 262–270.
173. Chatterjee M, Tejada M: Phorbol ester-induced contraction in chemically skinned vascular smooth muscle. *Am J Physiol* (1986) **251**: C356–C361.
174. Miller JR, Hawkins DJ, Wells JN: Phorbol diesters alter the contractile responses of porcine coronary artery. *J Pharmac Exp Ther* (1986) **239**: 38–42.
175. Menkes H, Baraban JM, Snyder SH: Protein kinase C regulates smooth muscle tension in guinea-pig trachea and ileum. *Eur J Pharmac* (1986) **122**: 19–28.
176. Nishizuka Y: The molecular heterogeneity of protein kinase C and its implications for cellular regulation. *Nature* (1988) **334**: 661–665.
177. Silver PJ, Stull JT: Regulation of myosin light chain and phosphorylase phosphorylation in tracheal smooth muscle. *J Biol Chem* (1982) **257**: 6145–6150.
178. Kamm KE, Stull JT: Activation of smooth muscle contraction: Correlation between myosin phosphorylation and stiffness. *Science* (1986) **232**: 80–82.
179. Persechini A, Kamm KE, Stull JT: Different phosphorylated forms of myosin in contracting tracheal smooth muscle. *J Biol Chem* (1986) **261**: 6293–6299.
180. Silver PJ, Stull JT: Phosphorylation of myosin light chain and phosphorylase in tracheal smooth muscle in response to KC1 and carbachol. *Mol Pharmacol* (1984) **25**: 267–274.
181. Aksoy MO, Murphy RA, Kamm KE: Role of Ca^{2+} and myosin light chain phosphorylation in regulation of smooth muscle. *Am J Physiol* (1982) **242**: C109–C116.
182. Hai C-M, Murphy RA: Ca^{2+}, cross-bridge phosphorylation and contraction. *Ann Rev Physiol* (1989) **51**: 285–298.
183. Aksoy MO, Mras S, Kamm KE, Murphy RA: Ca^{2+}, cAMP and changes in myosin phosphorylation during contraction of smooth muscle. *Am J Physiol* (1983) **245**: C255–C270.
184. Hai C-M, Murphy RA: Cross-bridge phosphorylation and regulation of the latch state in smooth muscle. *Am J Physiol* (1988) **254**: C99–C106.
185. Murphy RA: Contraction in smooth muscle cells. *Ann Rev Physiol* (1989) **51**: 275–283.
186. Putney JW: A model for receptor-regulated calcium entry. *Cell Calcium* (1986) **7**: 1–12.
187. Putney JW, Takemura H, Hughes AR, Horstman DA, Thastrup O: How do inositol phosphates regulate calcium signalling? *FASEB J* (1989) **3**: 1899–1905.
188. Irvine RF, Letcher AJ, Heslop JP, Berridge MJ: The inositol tris/tetrakisphosphate pathway—demonstration of Ins(1,4,5)P$_3$-3-kinase activity in animal tissues. *Nature* (1986) **320**: 631–633.
189. Nahorski SR, Batty I: Inositol tetrakisphosphate: Recent developments in PI metabolism and receptor function. *Trends Pharmacol Sci* (1986) **7**: 83–85.
190. Rodger IW, Small RC: Pharmacology of airway smooth muscle. In Page CP, Barnes PJ (eds) *Pharmacology of Asthma, Handbook of Experimental Pharmacology*, Vol 98. Berlin, Springer-Verlag, 1991, pp 107–141.

6

Mast Cells and Basophils

F.L. PEARCE

INTRODUCTION

Human bronchial asthma is characterized by a widespread and variable intrathoracic airflow obstruction and an enhanced responsiveness of the airways to non-specific stimulation. Manifestation of the asthmatic response may be conveniently divided into three stages: a rapid spasmogenic phase, a late sustained phase and a subacute, chronic inflammatory phase.[1,2] The immediate response to inhaled allergen has traditionally been associated with the activation of pulmonary mast cells and the release of histamine and spasmogenic products of arachidonic acid metabolism, including prostaglandins and leukotrienes.[1,2] Recent studies have indicated that the IgE-dependent activation of alveolar macrophages[3] and platelets[4] may also be involved. The release of chemotactic factors may lead to the recruitment of further inflammatory cells including neutrophils, eosinophils and monocytes.[1,2] Activation of all three cell types may be involved in late phase responses and in the associated induction of non-specific bronchial hyperreactivity. Platelet-activating factor (PAF) may be essentially implicated in the latter phenomenon,[5] while the recruitment of eosinophils appears to be critical for the development of many of the features of chronic asthma, including desquamation of the surface respiratory epithelium.[1,2]

There is currently considerable interest in the cellular basis of acquired airway hyperresponsiveness and of the critical role of inflammation in the pathogenesis of asthma. The inflammatory changes in the chronic asthmatic include occlusion of the airways with viscid mucus, infiltration of the lumenal secretions and mucosa with inflammatory cells, thickening of the bronchial basement membrane, hypertrophy of the airway smooth muscle and breakdown of the bronchial epithelium.[6–8] The latter effect

ASTHMA: BASIC MECHANISMS AND CLINICAL MANAGEMENT (2nd Edn)
ISBN 0-12-079026-2

may expose afferent nerve endings and generate local axon reflexes to amplify and propagate the inflammatory response.[9]

From the above brief discussion, it is clear that no single cell type can be responsible for all of the manifestations of human bronchial asthma and that a diversity of inflammatory cells, mediators and neuronal mechanisms is likely to be involved. The present chapter will consider some of the properties of human pulmonary mast cells and discuss their possible role in asthma. In so doing, it should be appreciated than mast cells from different locations may exhibit marked variations in their morphological, histochemical and functional properties.[10–14] That is, they are biochemically heterogeneous.

MAST CELL HETEROGENEITY

The concept of mast cell heterogeneity has become firmly established over the last decade, largely as a result of the development of methods for the enzymic dispersion of free mast cells from diverse target tissues, including the lung, of experimental animals and man.[10–14] These preparations complement murine serosal mast cells, human basophil leucocytes and tissue culture derived mast cells which have been widely used in the study of mediator release.

The best example of mast cell heterogeneity derives from the pioneering work of Enerbäck and his colleagues on the distribution of this cell in the gastrointestinal tract of the rat.[15] Two distinct subpopulations may be identified. The mast cells in the lower layers of the intestinal wall resemble those found in other connective tissues (connective tissue mast cell(s), CTMC), whereas the cells in the mucosa (mucosal mast cell(s), MMC) show very different properties. They are smaller in size and more variable in shape than the CTMC, contain a unique proteolytic enzyme (rat mast cell protease (RMCP) II rather than RMCP I), have a lower content of histamine and 5-hydroxytryptamine and possess fewer granules. The latter contain the less highly sulphated glycosaminoglycan chondroitin sulphate di-B instead of heparin. These properties require that special conditions of fixation and staining be used to reveal this cell type. Most importantly, the granules may become resistant to metachromatic staining after routine processing in some common, formalin-based fixatives. The cells may also be distinguished by sequential staining with combinations of dyes such as alcian blue and safranin. The mature rat CTMC stains with safranin, whereas the MMC stains with alcian blue, consistent with the lower degree of sulphation of its proteoglycan matrix. Again, the fluorescent dye berberine stains only the CTMC. Finally, the two mast cell types differ grossly in their responses to histamine liberators and to anti-allergic drugs.[10–14]

It must be emphasized, however, that the above histochemical criteria for distinguishing between subpopulations of mast cells have been developed exclusively for the rat. The extent to which these findings may be extrapolated to other species, and especially to man, is by no means clear. It would currently appear that there are at least two types of histochemically distinct mast cell in both the intestine and lung of man.[16–18] However, the distinction between the cell types is more subtle and less striking than in the rodent.[18] Moreover, the subpopulations are no longer confined to particular anatomical areas of the target organ. Under these conditions, the terms CTMC and MMC, which are anatomical descriptions, may be incorrect and misleading.[14]

The observed histochemical differences may again reflect variations in the proteo-glycan content of the cells. This problem has not been unambiguously resolved in the human but chondroitin sulphate E has been associated with the intestinal cell, both chondroitin sulphate E and heparin with the lung cell, and heparin with the skin cell.[19,20]

A more distinct separation of human mast cells into two subtypes may be made on the basis of their neutral protease composition and the associated ultrastructure of their secretory granules. The predominant mast cell (MC) present in the mucosa of the bowel and the interalveolar septa of the lung contains tryptase with little, if any, chymase and has thus been designated MC_T. In contrast, the more abundant type in the submucosa of the intestine and in the skin contains both proteases and has been designated MC_{TC}.[19,21] The MC_T have varying numbers of irregularly shaped granules with discrete scrolls or particulate or beaded material, while the MC_{TC} have more regularly shaped, electron-dense granules with characteristic grating or lattice substructures.[21]

Evidence for the functional heterogeneity of human mast cells is also much less compelling than in the rodent. It would appear, however, that human skin mast cells differ from the lung and intestinal cells in producing prostaglandin D_2 (PGD_2) but little or no leukotriene C_4 (LTC_4) and in being uniquely responsive to basic histamine liberators such as morphine, compound 48/80, anaphylatoxins and substance P.[22,23]

DISTRIBUTION AND MORPHOLOGY OF HUMAN LUNG MAST CELLS

Mast cells are widely distributed throughout the human respiratory tract and are found in large numbers in the walls of the alveoli and airways. Most of the mast cells in the conducting airways are located below the bronchial epithelium but appreciable numbers of cells are found intercalated between the epithelial cells and adjacent to the surface of the lumen. These latter cells would come into immediate contact with inhaled antigens and might be expected to be of major importance in modulating the initial phases of the allergic response. More deeply situated mast cells and other cell types may then become progressively involved in the chronic disease as damage to the mucosal surface allows an increased penetration of inhaled antigen. Mast cells may be recovered from the mucosal, lumenal surface of the airways by bronchoalveolar lavage (BAL) and from the parenchyma of the tissue by enzymic dispersion.

Mast cells comprise (mean ± SEM, $n = 20$) $0.32 \pm 0.05\%$ of the total nucleated population recovered by BAL.[24] The majority of the cells obtained are alveolar macro-phages ($86.0 \pm 2.5\%$) with appreciable numbers of lymphocytes ($8.0 \pm 1.5\%$), neutro-phils ($4.0 \pm 1.0\%$) and eosinophils ($2.0 \pm 0.5\%$). In five experiments,[24] suspensions of cells obtained by enzymic dissociation of whole lung were again shown to contain large numbers of macrophages ($77.6 \pm 7.3\%$), significant numbers of lymphocytes ($5.7 \pm 2.3\%$) and neutrophils ($10.2 \pm 6.7\%$) and an increased proportion of mast cells ($3.9 \pm 1.2\%$) relative to the BAL fluid. In a further series of experiments, the histamine content of the parenchymal mast cell (2.6 ± 0.1 pg/cell, $n = 12$) was found to be

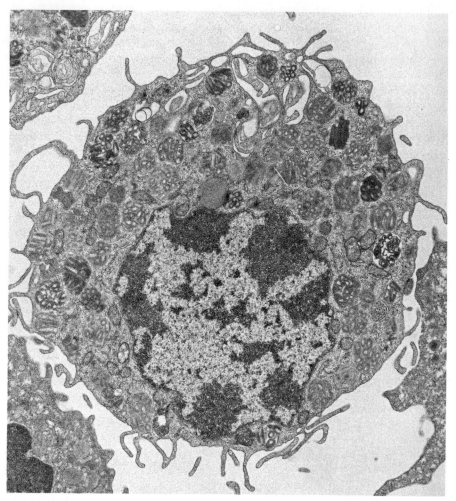

Fig. 6.1 Low power electron micrograph of a parenchymal mast cell obtained by enzymic dissociation of human lung. Reproduced from ref. 25, with permission.

significantly greater than that of the corresponding BAL cell ($1.2 \pm 0.3\%$ pg/cell, $n = 20$, $P < 0.01$).[24] Both populations stain with alcian blue dye, but do not counterstain with safranin, a property that seems to be characteristic of most human mast cells.[18]

The ultrastructure of the human parenchymal lung cell has been studied in some detail[21,25,26] and a representative example is shown in Fig. 6.1. The cytoplasm of the cell contains large numbers of secretory granules that can exhibit a variety of different ultrastructural patterns. The most common granule type contains cylindrical scrolls,[25] which may be characteristic of the MC_T phenotype,[21] while other mast cells contain granules whose matrices appear as highly ordered crystals or electron-dense particles. In addition, the cells also contain cytoplasmic lipid bodies. On activation, the granules became swollen and amorphous and their membranes fuse to produce chains that enlarge to form tortuous cytoplasmic channels. The latter eventually open to the exterior through multiple points on the cell surface, thereby permitting the release of histamine. These pores progressively widen, ultimately allowing the entry of extracellular markers. The opening of the degranulation channels is accompanied both by increasingly prominent filaments in the intervening cytoplasm and by the convolution of the plasma membrane into folds and projections.

The BAL cell broadly resembles that from the lung parenchyma. However, there are generally fewer granules, some of which are characteristically 'basket-shaped' or partially disrupted, and numerous lipid bodies and cytoplasmic folds and projections. Overall, the cell appears to be in a partially activated state.

BRONCHOALVEOLAR LAVAGE IN EXTRINSIC ASTHMA

The BAL fluid of 10 extrinsic asthmatic subjects contained a significantly ($P < 0.01$) higher proportion of both eosinophils ($8.0 \pm 2.7\%$) and mast cells ($1.41 \pm 0.27\%$) than that of normal controls.[25,27] The histamine content of the lavage increased in parallel with the number of mast cells. The forced expiratory volume in 1 s (FEV_1) and forced vital capacity (FVC) were measured in these subjects, together with the concentration of histamine required to produce a 20% reduction in FEV_1 (PC_{20} histamine). Strikingly, there was a highly significant correlation between the percentage of mast cells in the lavage and the severity of the disease as indicated by measured indices of both airway obstruction (FEV_1 expressed as a percentage of the predicted, and the FEV_1/FVC ratio) and of hyperresponsiveness (PC_{20} histamine).[27]

IMMUNOLOGICALLY INDUCED MEDIATOR RELEASE

Mast cells obtained by BAL of normal subjects and by enzymic dissociation of whole lung released histamine in a dose-dependent fashion on challenge with anti-human IgE (Table 6.1). The rate of release was rather more rapid for the BAL than for the parenchymal cell, requiring 2 and 5 min for completion, respectively. The spontaneous release of histamine was also greater for the BAL cell than the tissue cell.

In addition to histamine, anti-IgE induced a dose-dependent release of immunoreactive PGD_2 and LTC_4 from both mast cell populations (Table 6.1). The antiserum was more effective in inducing PGD_2 production than histamine release and maximal amounts of the prostanoid were generated at lower dilutions of antibody. As in the case of histamine, the spontaneous release of PGD_2 was higher for the BAL cells than for the dispersed lung cells. The spontaneous generation of LTC_4 was rather variable, particularly for the BAL cells, and higher concentrations of anti-IgE were required to evoke the *de novo* production of the eicosanoid. For both cell populations, PGD_2 was the predominant eicosanoid produced and exceeded the amount of LTC_4 formed by about one order of magnitude. As might be expected, the rates of release of the newly generated mediators were slower than for histamine for both BAL and parenchymal lung cells and required 10–15 min for completion.

Table 6.1 Immunologically induced release of mediators from BAL and dispersed lung (DL) cells.

Anti-IgE (Dilution)	Histamine (% release)		LTC$_4$ (ng/10^6 mast cells)		PGD$_2$ (ng/10^6 mast cells)	
	BAL	DL	BAL	DL	BAL	DL
100	39.0 ± 6.2	49.5 ± 6.5	18.2 ± 3.5	16.1 ± 5.0	242 ± 50	145 ± 49
300	34.8 ± 5.7	41.0 ± 9.0	10.5 ± 3.5	11.8 ± 3.2	251 ± 60	139 ± 39
1000	31.9 ± 4.9	31.7 ± 7.3	7.0 ± 2.5	8.8 ± 2.9	219 ± 47	142 ± 30
10 000	17.1 ± 10.2	10.0 ± 5.0	2.2 ± 1.2	2.9 ± 1.8	127 ± 34	63 ± 20
100 000	0 ± 2.0	0.5 ± 0.5	—	0.6 ± 0.3	61 ± 33	36 ± 20

All values are means ± SEM for 10 (BAL) or 8 (DL) experiments and are corrected for the spontaneous releases in the absence of inducer. Spontaneous releases for the BAL and DL cells, respectively, were: histamine 11.5 ± 2.0 and 4.4 ± 1.4, LTC$_4$ 11.0 ± 7.3 and 1.8 ± 0.6, and PGD$_2$ 55 ± 10 and 20 ± 14.

Reproduced from ref. 28, with permission.

The spontaneous release of histamine from the BAL mast cells of extrinsic asthmatic patients was 18.7 ± 3.7% ($n = 10$) as compared to 7.4 ± 0.8% ($n = 30$, $P < 0.01$) for control subjects.[27] The BAL cells of asthmatic individuals thus appear to be inherently unstable. Most interestingly, mast cells obtained by BAL of asthmatics showed an enhanced reactivity towards anti-IgE and exhibited a greater release of histamine at all effective dilutions of the antiserum (Fig. 6.2a). This effect was strikingly localized; it was confined to the BAL cells and not apparent in the basophil leucocytes of these individuals which behaved identically to the controls (Fig. 6.2b). Specific antigen also led to histamine release from BAL cells and basophils of asthmatic subjects but not controls (Fig. 6.2c).

HYPEROSMOLAR-INDUCED HISTAMINE RELEASE

In about three quarters of asthmatic subjects, vigorous exercise leads within 10 min to pronounced airflow obstruction. This is known as exercise-induced asthma (EIA). The precipitating event in this condition remains to be resolved but it is now recognized that the mechanism of bronchoconstriction may be related to the sensitivity of asthmatic airways to increased respiratory heat exchange and/or water loss consequent upon hyperventilation following exercise. The latter effect would act to increase the osmolarity of the fluid lining the lung, which could in turn lead to the activation of pulmonary mast cells. Consistently, increases in circulating levels of mast cell markers have been demonstrated during EIA,[1] and incubation in a hyperosmolar medium *in vivo* triggers histamine release from human basophils and potentiates immunological mediator release from isolated human lung cells.[29]

To test this hypothesis further, we examined the effect of hyperosmolar buffer solutions on BAL cells and dispersed lung cells.[30] In each case, raising the osmolarity of the incubation medium from 280 to 1270 mosm/kg by adding increasing concentrations of mannitol (0.1–1 M) led to a dose-dependent release of histamine. The kinetics of the

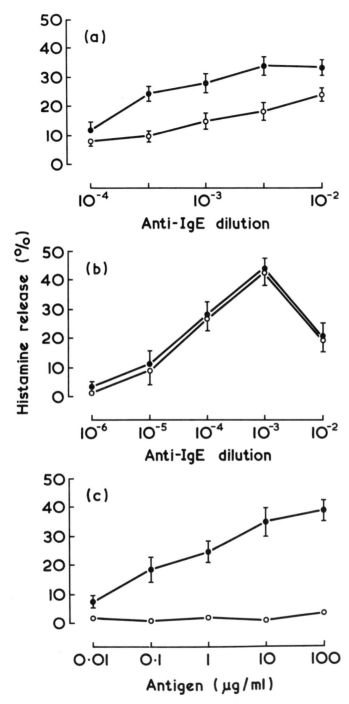

Fig. 6.2   Histamine release from BAL mast cells and basophil leucocytes from control (○) and asthmatic (●) subjects. (a) Release from BAL cells stimulated with anti-human IgE; (b) release from basophils stimulated with anti-human IgE, and (c) release from BAL cells stimulated with specific antigen to *Dermatophagoides pteronyssinus*. Values are means ± SEM. Reproduced from the data in ref. 27 and from unpublished results.

process were complex: there was an initial, fairly rapid release of the amine which reached a plateau after about 10 min. Thereafter, the release increased progressively and slowly over a 60-min period. After 10 min of incubation, the BAL cells were significantly more reactive than the dispersed lung cells, and the two populations gave optimal releases of histamine of $12.1 \pm 1.2\%$ ($n = 19$, BAL) and $2.7 \pm 0.5\%$ ($n = 7$, dispersed lung), respectively. Under the same conditions, isolated basophils were even more responsive and released $52.6 \pm 4.6\%$ ($n = 13$) of their total histamine. Similar but rather less marked effects were produced when the osmolarity was increased by adding increased amounts of buffer solutes. Interestingly, sodium cromoglycate attenuated the hyperosmolar release from the BAL cells with a maximum inhibition of about 40% at a concentration of 10 μM.[30]

BAL MAST CELLS AND STEROID THERAPY IN ASTHMA

Inhaled corticosteroids are one of the most effective groups of drugs available for the management of human bronchial asthma. Their action is undoubtedly complex and their efficacy probably arises from a number of anti-inflammatory effects. Corticosteriods reportedly inhibit histamine release from human basophils but not from lung parenchymal cells.[31] We therefore thought it to be of interest to study the effect of steroid treatment on BAL mast cells.

In a preliminary investigation,[32] seven asthmatic subjects were given a 2-week course of oral prednisolone (30 mg/day). This treatment led to a small improvement in lung function, with the FEV_1 rising from 70 ± 22 litres to 81 ± 23 litres, and a sharp drop in both the percentage of mast cells ($0.18 \pm 0.04\%$ to $0.11 \pm 0.03\%$) in, and the histamine content (6.6 ± 2.9 ng/10^6 cells to 3.3 ± 0.7 ng/10^6 cells) of, the lavage fluid. The spontaneous release of histamine from the isolated mast cells was also dramatically reduced ($17.1 \pm 2.7\%$ to $8.5 \pm 3.6\%$). These data then suggest that one effect of steroids in asthma therapy may be to reduce the number and suppress the spontaneous reactivity of the lumenal mast cells.

ANTIASTHMATIC DRUGS AND THE INHIBITION OF HISTAMINE RELEASE FROM PULMONARY MAST CELLS

Disodium cromoglycate has an established place in the treatment and prophylaxis of bronchial asthma. However, despite intensive research, the mode of action of the chromone is still uncertain. Its reactivity was originally attributed simply to the inhibition of mediator release from mast cells but it is now clear that the compound can attenuate the activity of a range of inflammatory cells including neutrophils, eosinophils and monocytes.[33] The drug can also inhibit reflex bronchoconstriction and influence C-fibre activity in the lungs and bronchi.[34] In addition, its effects on histaminocytes are very site-specific and vary strikingly from one mast cell subtype to another.[10–14] For these reasons, we examined the effect of sodium cromoglycate, together with its congener nedocromil sodium, on histamine release from BAL cells and lung parenchymal cells.

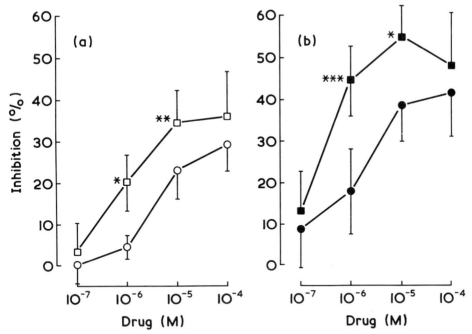

Fig. 6.3 Effect of sodium cromoglycate (O, ●) and nedocromil sodium (□, ■) on immunologically induced histamine release from (a) dispersed human lung mast cells and (b) human BAL mast cells. The drugs were added to the dispersed lung cells simultaneously with the secretory stimulus (open symbols) or preincubated with the lavage cells for 10 min before challenge (closed symbols). These conditions were shown to be optimal for activity in each case. Values are means ± SEM for eight (a) or five (b) experiments. Asterisks denote values which were significantly different, *$P < 0.05$, **$P < 0.01$, ***$P < 0.001$. Reproduced from ref. 35, with permission.

For comparison, the effects of the methylxanthine theophylline and the β-adrenoceptor agonist salbutamol were also tested.[24,35]

Immunologically induced histamine release from both cell types was comparably inhibited by the latter two drugs, the IC_{30} values (the concentrations required to produce 30% inhibition of release) for BAL and parenchymal cells being 500 μM and 300 μM for theophylline and 20 nM and 100 nM for salbutamol, respectively. However, both sodium cromoglycate and nedocromil sodium were strikingly more active against the BAL cell than the dispersed lung cell, and nedocromil sodium was about one order of magnitude more effective than sodium cromoglycate against both cell types (Fig. 6.3). The IC_{30} values for BAL and parenchymal cells were, respectively, 0.5 μM and 5 μM for nedocromil sodium and 7 μM and 420 μM for sodium cromoglycate.[35]

The characteristics of the inhibition produced by sodium cromoglycate and nedocromil sodium also varied according to the mast cell. A marked tachyphylaxis was observed with the parenchymal cell whereas the activity against the BAL cell increased with preincubation.[35] The latter observation is, of course, more in keeping with the clinical usage of the drug, where it is ideally administered prophylactically before antigen exposure. Given the superficial location of the BAL cell within the airways, and its greater exposure to drugs given by inhalation, there findings may have particular clinical significance.

THE ROLE OF BASOPHILS IN ALLERGY AND ASTHMA

The role of the basophil in the mediation of allergic inflammation has not been clearly elucidated. The basophil leucocyte has long been considered to be the circulating equivalent of the tissue mast cell but recent studies have emphasized the difference between these histaminocytes.[36] However, late phase reactions in the lung,[37] skin[38] and nose[39] are associated with an influx into the target organ of inflammatory leucocytes including basophils. A role for basophils rather than mast cells in the mediation of late phase reactions in the nose has been suggested by the finding of the basophil markers histamine and LTC_4, but not PGD_2 which is mast cell derived, in nasal washings in late antigen-induced rhinitis.[40] Clearly, the role of the basophil in other allergic conditions requires clarification.

THE ROLE OF MAST CELLS IN EARLY ASTHMATIC REACTIONS

Current evidence suggests that the immediate bronchoconstrictor response to inhaled allergens is largely mediated by mast cell products. Allergen challenge of extrinsic asthmatic subjects leads to a release of histamine into the systemic circulation[41] and a secretion of the amine, together with the other mast cell associated mediators tryptase and PGD_2, into the BAL fluid.[42,43] Pulmonary mast cells are then clearly activated in the course of the asthmatic response.

Elucidation of the exact role of histamine as a bronchoconstrictor mediator in asthma was originally rendered difficult by the central sedative action and questionable specificity of conventional antihistaminic drugs. The development of newer, non-sedative and more potent and selective histamine H_1-receptor antagonists such as cetirizine, astemizole and terfenadine has, however, rendered such a study possible. These findings have recently been reviewed.[44] In particular, administration of these agents prior to allergen challenge dramatically attenuates the immediate phase of bronchoconstriction. The available data indicate that about one half of this response is due to liberated histamine and the remainder to leukotrienes, thromboxanes and prostaglandins.

THE ROLE OF MAST CELLS IN LATE ASTHMATIC REACTIONS AND CYTOKINE PRODUCTION

Late phase asthmatic reactions have been intimately associated with the development of bronchial hyperreactivity and airway inflammation. As such, they may be more relevant to the situation in chronic clinical asthma. The role of mast cells in such reactions has been the subject of considerable debate. Release of histamine into the systemic circulation in late phase responses is controversial but has been reported by some authors.[2] However, as discussed above, allergen induced late phase reactions in the nose are accompanied by the release of histamine but not PGD_2 suggesting that the amine originates from basophils recruited into the nasal mucosa.[40]

The efficacy of sodium cromoglycate, which blocks immediate and late phase responses to inhaled allergens and the development of airway hyperreactivity has been widely used to implicate the mast cell in the progression of bronchial asthma. However, it is now clear that the activity of the chromone is not confined to the mast cell and that the drug may inhibit a range of inflammatory cells.[33] Moreover, a diversity of cromoglycate-like drugs have been developed, many of which are more potent than the chromone itself in preventing histamine release from lung mast cells.[45] However, with the exception of nedocromil sodium, none has proved to be clinically useful. Moreover, as shown above, β-adrenoceptor agonists such as salbutamol are much more potent than sodium cromoglycate in preventing histamine release from human pulmonary mast cells. However, these agents do not block late phase responses or the development of bronchial hyperreactivity.

The above data would then appear to mitigate against a role for the mast cell in chronic clinical asthma. However, interest in this field has been resurrected by several recent papers demonstrating the production of various cytokines by mast cells.[46–50] In total, these studies have shown that immunological activation of tissue culture derived murine mast cells leads to increased levels of mRNA and/or secretion of a large range of cytokines including tumour necrosis factor (TNF)-α, granulocyte/macrophage colony stimulating factor (GM-CSF), interferon (INF)-γ, interleukins (IL)-1,3,4,5 and 6, and four members of the macrophage inflammatory protein (MIP) gene family, namely T-cell activator (TCA)-3, JE, MIP-1α and MIP-1β.[46–50] Identification of these molecules raises the possibility of a wide range of potential roles for mast cells in pathological responses. Release of cytokines could recruit, prime and activate neutrophils, macrophages, basophils and eosinophils, increase immunoglobulin secretion and regulate the proliferation and phenotype of other mast cells. It should be recognized, however, that most of the available data are derived from murine mast cell lines and, given the heterogeneity already discussed, these results do not automatically translate to the human system. None the less, if it can be convincingly demonstrated that isolated human lung mast cells generate a comparable diversity of cytokines, then this cell would once again be firmly implicated in the ongoing inflammatory events of chronic asthma. In this event, drugs directed against the expression or release of cytokines may have tremendous clinical potential.

ACKNOWLEDGEMENTS

Work from the author's laboratory was supported by grants from The Asthma Research Council, Fisons plc, The Medical Research Council and The Wellcome Trust.

REFERENCES

1. Holgate ST, Kay AB: Mast cells, mediators and asthma. *Clin Allergy* (1985) **15**: 221–234.
2. Kay AB: Mediators and inflammatory cells in asthma. In Kay AB (ed) *Asthma: Clinical Pharmacology and Therapeutic Progress*. Oxford, Blackwell Scientific Publications, 1986, pp 1–10.
3. Joseph M, Tonnel AB, Torpier G, Capron A, Arnoux B, Benveniste J: Involvement of immunoglobulin E in the secretory processes of alveolar macrophages from asthmatic patients. *J Clin Invest* (1983) **71**: 221–230.
4. Morley J, Sanjar S, Page CP: The platelet in asthma. *Lancet* (1984) **2**: 1142–1144.

5. Page CP, Archer CB, Paul W, Morley J: Paf-acether: a mediator of inflammation and asthma. *Trends Pharmacol Sci* (1984) **5**: 239–241.
6. Barnes PJ, Fan Chung K, Page CP: Inflammatory mediators and asthma. *Pharmacol Rev* (1988) **40**: 49–84.
7. Holgate ST: The pathophysiology of bronchial asthma and targets for its drug treatment. *Agents Actions* (1986) **18**: 281–287.
8. Kay AB: Inflammatory cells in acute and chronic asthma. *Am Rev Respir Dis* (1987) **135**: S63–S66.
9. Barnes PJ: Airway neuropeptides. In Barnes PJ, Rodger IW, Thomson NC (eds) *Asthma: Basic Mechanisms and Clinical Management*. London, Academic Press, 1988, pp 395–413.
10. Pearce FL: Mast cell heterogeneity. *Trends Pharmacol Sci* (1983) **4**: 165–167.
11. Pearce FL, Ali H, Barrett KE, *et al.*: Functional characteristics of mucosal and connective tissue mast cells of man, the rat and other animals. *Int Arch Allergy Appl Immunol* (1985) **77**: 274–276.
12. Pearce FL, Ali H, Barrett KE, *et al.*: Mast cell heterogeneity: differential responsivity to histamine liberators and anti-allergic drugs. In Ganellin CR, Schwartz J-C (eds) *Advances in the Biosciences*, Vol 51, *Frontiers in Histamine Research*. Oxford, Pergamon Press, 1985, pp 411–421.
13. Pearce FL: Mast cell heterogeneity: an overview. In Kay AB (ed) *Asthma: Clinical Pharmacology and Therapeutic Progress*. Oxford, Blackwell Scientific Publications, 1986, pp 251–264.
14. Pearce FL: On the heterogeneity of mast cells. *Pharmacology* (1986) **32**: 61–71.
15. Enerbäck L: The gut mucosal mast cell. *Monog Allergy* (1981) **17**: 222–232.
16. Strobel S, Miller HRP, Ferguson A: Human intestinal mucosal mast cells: evaluation of fixation and staining techniques. *J Clin Pathol* (1981) **34**: 851–858.
17. Befus D, Goodacre R, Dyke N, Bienenstock J: Mast cell heterogeneity in man. I. Histologic studies in the intestine. *Int Arch Allergy Appl Immunol* (1985) **76**: 232–236.
18. Greenwood B: The histology of mast cells. In Engström I, Lindholm N (eds) *Current Views on Bronchial Asthma*. Stockholm, Fisons Sweden AB, 1985, pp 143–149.
19. Schwartz LB: Mediators of human mast cells and human mast cell subsets. *Anal Allergy* (1987) **58**: 226–135.
20. Thompson HL, Schulman ES, Metcalfe DD: Identification of chondroitin sulfate E in human lung mast cells. *J Immunol* (1988) **140**: 2708–2713.
21. Craig SS, Schwartz LB: Human MC_{TC} type of mast cell granule: the uncommon occurrence of discrete scrolls associated with focal absence of chymase. *Lab Invest* (1990) **63**: 581–585.
22. Lawrence ID, Warner JA, Cohan VL, Hubbard WC, Kagey-Sobotka A, Lichtenstein LM: Purification and characterization of human skin mast cells. Evidence for human mast cell heterogeneity. *J Immunol* (1987) **139**: 3062–3069.
23. Benyon RC, Lowman MA, Church MK: Human skin mast cells: their dispersion, purification, and secretory characterization. *J Immunol* (1987) **138**: 861–867.
24. Pearce FL, Flint KC, Leung KBP, *et al.*: Some studies on human pulmonary mast cells obtained by bronchoalveolar lavage and by enzymic dissociation of whole lung tissue. *Int Arch Allergy Immunol* (1987) **82**: 507–512.
25. Caulfield JP, Lewis RA, Hein A, Austen KF: Secretion in dissociated human pulmonary mast cells. Evidence for solubilization of granule contents before discharge. *J Cell Biol* (1980) **85**: 299–311.
26. Dvorak AM, Schulman ES, Peters SP, *et al.*: Immunoglobulin E-mediated degranulation of isolated human lung mast cells. *Lab Invest* (1985) **53**: 45–56.
27. Flint KC, Leung KBP, Hudspith BN, Brostoff J, Pearce FL, Johnson NMcI: Bronchoalveolar mast cells in extrinsic asthma: a mechanism for the initiation of antigen specific bronchoconstriction. *Br Med J* (1985) **291**: 923–926.
28. Leung KPB, Flint KC, Hudspith BN, *et al.*: Some further properties of human pulmonary mast cells recovered by bronchoalveolar lavage and enzymic dispersion of lung tissue. *Agents Actions* (1987) **20**: 213–215.
29. Eggleston PE, Kagey-Sobotka A, Schleimer RP, Lichtenstein LM: Interaction between hyperosmolar and IgE-mediated histamine release from basophils and mast cells. *Am Rev Respir Dis* (1984) **130**: 86–91.

30. Flint KC, Hudspith BN, Leung KBP, Pearce FL, Brostoff J, Johnson NMcI: The hyperosmolar release of histamine from bronchoalveolar mast cells and its inhibition by sodium cromoglycate. *Thorax* (1985) **40**: 717.

31. Fox CC, Kagey-Sobotka A, Schleimer RP, Peters SP, MacGlashan DW, Lichtenstein LM: Mediator release from human basophils and mast cells from lung and intestinal mucosa. *Int Arch Allergy Appl Immunol* (1985) **77**: 130–136.

32. Millar AB, Hudspith BN, Lau A, Pearce F, Johnson NMcI: A mechanism for the role of steroids in the treatment of asthma? *Thorax* (1989) **44**: 359P.

33. Kay AB, Walsh GM, Moqbel R, *et al.*: Disodium cromoglycate inhibits activation of human inflammatory cells *in vitro*. *J Allergy Clin Immunol* (1987) **80**: 1–8.

34. Richards IM, Dixon M, Jackson DM, Vendy K: Alternative modes of action of sodium cromoglycate. *Agents Actions* (1986) **18**: 294–300.

35. Leung KPB, Flint KC, Brostoff J, *et al.*: Effects of sodium cromoglycate and nedocromil sodium on histamine secretion from human lung mast cells. *Thorax* (1988) **43**: 756–761.

36. Henderson WR: Basophils. *Immunol Allergy Clinics N America* (1990) **10**: 273–282.

37. Pepys J, Hargreave FE, Chan M, McCarthy DS: Inhibitory effects of disodium cromoglycate on allergen-inhalation tests. *Lancet* (1968) **2**: 134–137.

38. Solley GO, Gleich GJ, Jordon RE, Schroeter AL: The late phase of the immediate wheal and flare reaction. Its dependence on IgE antibodies. *J Clin Invest* (1976) **58**: 408–420.

39. Bascom R, Wachs M, Naclerio RM, *et al.*: Basophil influx occurs after nasal antigen challenge: effects of topical corticosteroid pretreatment. *J Allergy Clin Immunol* (1988) **81**: 580–589.

40. Naclerio RM, Proud D, Togias AG, *et al.*: Inflammatory mediators in late antigen-induced rhinitis. *New Eng J Med* (1985) **313**: 65–70.

41. Holgate ST, Benyon RC, Howarth PH, *et al.*: Relationship between mediator release from human lung mast cells *in vitro* and *in vivo*. *Int Arch Allergy Appl Immunol* (1985) **77**: 47–56.

42. Murray JJ, Tonnel AB, Brasch AR, Roberts LJ, Gosset EP, Workman R: Release of prostaglandin D$_2$ into human airways during antigen challenge. *New Engl J Med* (1986) **315**: 800–804.

43. Wenzel SE, Fowler AA, Schwartz LB: Activation of pulmonary mast cells by brochoalveolar allergen challenge: *in vivo* release of histamine and tryptase in atopic subjects with and without asthma. *Am Rev Respir Dis* (1988) **137**: 1002–1008.

44. Wood-Baker R, Church MK: Histamine and asthma. *Immunol Allergy Clinics N America* (1990) **10**: 329–336.

45. Church MK: Cromoglycate-like anti-allergic drugs: a review. *Drugs Today* (1978) **14**: 281–341.

46. Wodnar-Filipowicz A, Heusser CH, Morani C: Production of the haemopoietic growth factors GM-CSF and interleukin-3 by mast cells in response to IgE-receptor-mediated activation. *Nature* (1989) **339**: 150–152.

47. Plaut M, Pierce JH, Watson CJ, Hanley-Hyde J, Nordan RP, Paul WE: Mast cell lines produce lymphokines in response to cross-linkage of F$_{CE}$RI or to calcium ionophores. *Nature* (1989) **339**: 64–67.

48. Young JD-E, Liu C-C, Butler G, Cohn ZA, Galli SJ: Identification, purification, and characterization of a mast cell-associated cytolytic factor related to tumor necrosis factor. *Proc Natl Acad Sci USA* (1987) **84**: 9175–9179.

49. Burd PR, Rogers HW, Gordon JR, *et al.*: Interleukin 3-dependent and independent mast cells stimulated with IgE and antigen express multiple cytokines. *J Exp Med* (1989) **170**: 245–257.

50. Gordon JR, Galli SJ: Mast cells as a source of both preformed and immunologically inducible TNF-α/catechin. *Nature* (1990) **346**: 274–276.

7

Macrophages

R.W. FULLER

INTRODUCTION

The human airway macrophage, otherwise called alveolar macrophage, like other tissue macrophages, is derived from circulating monocytes.[1–4] These cells have a physiological role as part of the host defence of the lung.[5–9] Unlike other residential macrophages, they may be less important as antigen-presenting cells but may retain important immune function.[10] The macrophage may well have an influence both as an activating cell of the immune process and as a cell which can terminate inflammatory responses. Thus the macrophage has been proposed as an initiating and perhaps perpetuating cell in asthma.[11] Of course, it is not possible to be absolutely certain which individual cell, or combination of cells, is responsible for the instigation of asthmatic inflammation. There is, however, compelling evidence to support the macrophage as a candidate cell and this will be outlined in this chapter.

ANATOMY

The airway macrophages are found throughout the respiratory tract from the alveolus to the larynx. They are found both in the lumen and the airway walls and are the most numerous cells in the airway lumen.[12] When surface and other markers are studied, there is a heterogeneity amongst the mononuclear phagocytes ranging from cells with monocyte-like markers to those which have markers associated with phagocytic cells and with antigen-presenting cells.[13–17] It is not known whether the cells in the resistance airways, which are important in asthma, arise in the alveoli and then ascend via the mucociliary escalator or whether they enter through the mucosa directly. Indeed, even if

ASTHMA: BASIC MECHANISMS AND CLINICAL MANAGEMENT (2nd Edn)
ISBN 0-12-079026-2

Table 7.1 Surface receptors/markers on human airway macrophages.

Histocompatibility antigens, e.g. MCH II, CD_{23}
Immunoglobulin receptors, e.g. IgA, IgG, IgE
Lectin-binding molecules
Pharmacological receptors, e.g. β_2, adenosine A_2
Complement receptors, e.g. C_3, C_5
Cytokine receptors, e.g. tumour necrosis factor, interleukin-1

cells in the normal airway are derived from the alveolus, in the disease state monocytes may still enter areas of inflammation directly. When the cells enter the airway lumen they will have the characteristics of monocytes and they will mature to macrophages during their residence in the lung. The airway macrophages have three fates under normal conditions. First, they may ascend the escalator and be expectorated, second, they may become resident long term as is the case in diseases caused by inhaled dust and third, they may leave the lung and reach at least the resident lymph nodes.[18] In the disease state a further fate, that of cell death, may also occur.

Except during infection, bronchoalveolar lavage studies show that in the airway of normal volunteers and asthmatic patients, the macrophage is the most numerous cell making up over 90% of the resident cells.[12] The surface morphology of the cells is altered by the disease[19-24] and does differ between normals and some asthmatics which may reflect differences in the activation state of the cells.[25-27] The reported surface receptors and markers on the human airway macrophage are listed in Table 7.1. The factors which control the numbers in the airways are not known. However, the numbers appear tightly controlled. In our studies in dog the reduction in macrophage number by lavage returned to control values by 24 h.[28] Thus, there appears to be active control of macrophage numbers by the lung and the increased numbers in some disease states reflect increased release of chemotactic activity by the lung.[29]

ACTIVATION OF THE AIRWAY MACROPHAGE

The airway macrophage can be activated by many stimuli (Table 7.2) including phagocytosis and immunological reactions. *In vitro* activation of the macrophage is associated with either the release of inflammatory mediators including cytokines, radicals, phospholipid products and enzymes listed in the next section, or priming which increases the likelihood of releasing products. *In vivo* the release of such substances could

Table 7.2 Reported *in vitro* challenges which lead to airway macrophage activation.

Particles, e.g. zymosan, opsonized red blood cells
Immunoglobulin, e.g. IgC, IgE
Bacterial products, e.g. lipopolysaccharide
Cytokines, e.g. tumour necrosis factor

come from a number of cells and, therefore, the expression of different surface markers[30] is used to infer activation.[31] It is unknown how these two indicators of cell activation are related *in vivo*. The activation of the cells and subsequent release of inflammatory mediators are of course important for the justification of the inflammatory role for the macrophage. *In vitro* activation occurs following phagocytosis,[32–36] immunological challenge,[37–41] exposure to cytokines and other pro-inflammatory substances such as bacterial products[42–47] as well as irritants and culture itself.[48,49] The activation that occurs uses the same 2° messenger pathways utilizing phosphotidyl inositol and diacyl glycerol as other cells.[50] However, the opening of a K^+ channel is also important.[51]

Phagocytosis

Exposure of the human airway macrophage *in vitro* to opsonized zymosan, opsonized erythrocytes[36] and latex particles[33] will cause dose-dependent release of mediators (Table 7.2). It is of interest that the macrophage will respond differently depending upon the phagocytic particle. For example, exposure to opsonized zymosan and opsonized sheep blood erythrocytes results in the release of thromboxane $(TX)B_2$ and N-acetylglucosaminidase but phagocytosis of equivalent numbers of neutrophils does not.[36] This may explain why in some circumstances phagocytosis of certain particulate matter, such as asbestos, is associated with lung inflammation while phagocytosis of other materials is not. The release of cytokine following phagocytosis has been less studied, although C_{3a} is released following zymosan challenge.[38] It is likely that phagocytosis of infecting organisms is followed by the release of cytokines as this is presumably the signal of neutrophil influx to the infected site but direct evidence is lacking.

Immunological

The macrophage has surface receptors for IgG, E and A that are identified by binding or the release of mediators following challenge *in vitro*.[37–40,53,54] Like phagocytosis, there appears to be differential release depending upon the class of immunoglobulin used in the challenge. IgG challenge is associated with radical release but not arachidonic acid metabolism or enzyme release, however, IgE challenge will release arachidonic acid products and enzyme but has little effect on oxygen radical release.[40,41] Whether the release is a result of activation of receptor dose or phagocytosis is not fully understood.[55]

The demonstration of IgE-dependent activation is important for determining the role of the airway macrophage in asthma which in some patients is entirely IgE-dependent. There is, however, debate as to the nature of the receptor.[39,56–58] Rosetting studies have suggested that it may be of low affinity and therefore not the same as the mast cell receptor. It has been suggested that it may be related to the CD_{23} antigen as is the case in the eosinophil and the B-lymphocyte.[59–61] However, the functional studies of cell activation when washing does not remove activity suggest a higher affinity. Indeed the airway macrophage is not likely to be activated through CD_{23} as no such activation could be determined in the U239 cells[58] or more recently in the human airway macrophage itself.[62]

Cytokine and other chemical mediators

As well as immunoglobulin receptors, these cells possess receptors for a number of inflammatory mediators and cytokines. Activation through complement receptors may indeed play a part in the response of the cells to phagocytosis. Of the mediators associated with asthma, including prostaglandins, leukotrienes, adenosine, platelet-activating factor, and neuropeptides, the macrophages are less responsive than other cells. Indeed, we have found little response to *in vitro* challenge of human airway macrophages to adenosine and substance P. As circulating monocytes they must respond to chemotactic agents in order to enter the lung and mature to airway macrophages. However, in mature cells such responses appear less. Some substances, such as the bacterial product lyphopolysaccharide, will change the profile of expression of messenger RNA within the cells and this marker of activation requires further study and may be the cause of the morphological change seen in immunocytochemistry.

PRODUCTS

The human airway macrophage can release a wide range of products, both pro- and anti-inflammatory, depending upon its response to activation and its anatomical situation and maturation. For example, the release of lysosymal enzymes and reactive oxygen species increases with maturation of monocytes to macrophages. The release is also subject to species differences. These products are listed in Table 7.3. There has been extensive study of the release of phospholipid-derived mediators, including platelet-activating factor, TXA_2 and leukotriene B_4 which are the most abundant, and the human cell appears not to make prostacyclin and only limited amounts of other products.

The release of cell products appears to change with the maturity of the cell, the site of residence of the cell and during disease stress. TXB_2 release is not changed, but leukotriene production, however, is greater from the mature cell.[63] Such increase is not seen with mature macrophages from other sites[64] suggesting differential activation. Lysosomal enzyme release and superoxide generation also increase with maturity.[65] Monocytes release more tumour necrosis factor and interleukins-1 and -6 than macrophages.[66–69] They also have greater capacity to kill[70] but less capacity to phagocytose particles[71] but have no difference in surface IgG receptors.[72] There are reported

Table 7.3   Release products from human airway macrophages.

Lipid products, e.g. thromboxane A_2, leukotriene B_4, platelet-activating factor
Reactive oxygen species
Enzymes, e.g. *N*-acetylglucosaminidase
Complement fractions, e.g. C_{3a}
Coagulation factors
Cytokines, e.g. tumour necrosis factor, granulocyte monocyte-colony
   stimulating factor
Enzyme inhibitors

changes in disease states such as increased LTB_4 generation in asbestosis.[73] The changes associated with smoking, however, may be related to change in maturation of the cell.[74]

Some studies have suggested that the human airway macrophage in asthma releases differing amounts of products especially those of arachidonic acid derivation compared to normal.[33] There are many explanations for this but there is no direct evidence *in vivo* and there is no truly specific mediator to the macrophage to use for this determination.

PHARMACOLOGY

The anatomical positioning and spectrum of product release from the airway macrophage clearly makes it a candidate for a primary cell in asthma. However, such data cannot be supported by depletion experiments in humans. Therefore the pattern of pharmacological response of the cell can be used to give further indirect evidence of similarity between its response and those in asthma.

Drugs that elevate intracellular cAMP levels

The alveolar macrophage, unlike the monocyte, has relatively few surface receptors that can be activated to cause elevation of intracellular cAMP to a sufficient level to cause inhibition[75] of release of mediators following phagocytosis of immunological challenge. For example, β_2-adrenoceptor agonists, which will inhibit both mast cell activation and monocyte activation,[76] are without functional inhibitory effects on the human airway macrophage.[77] There is evidence of β_2 receptors binding on the membrane and elevations of cAMP.[78,79] However, this increase in cAMP is trivial compared to the effects of fluoride, a direct stimulus of adenylyl cyclase, and is too small to alter the release of TXB_2.[79] It appears that the monocyte loses the majority of its β_2 receptors during maturation to the macrophage. The same is true of the adenosine A_2 inhibitory receptors which are fully active on the monocytes but not on the mature airway macrophage.[80] Other potential inhibitory agents, including prostacyclin, prostaglandin E_2, vasoactive intestinal peptide, etc., are also without inhibitory effect. On the other hand, the new long-acting β_2 agonist, salmeterol, will inhibit the human airway macrophage but this action is independent of β_2 agonism or adenylyl cyclase activation.[81]

In contrast, forskolin, which directly activates adenylyl cyclase and stable analogues of cAMP,[77] is inhibitory as are high concentrations of xanthines[80] which would inhibit phosphodiesterase in the cells. The human airway macrophage will therefore respond in a similar manner to other inflammatory cells if intracellular cAMP is increased. However, this is unlikely to occur following stimulation of surface receptors that are usually associated with such inhibition in other cells.

Drugs that alter membrane ion channels

The possibility that drugs that manipulate potassium channels may be anti-inflammatory and the demonstration of the opening of a potassium channel during the activation of the human airway macrophage led to pharmacological study of such mechanisms. Table 7.4 shows the drugs that inhibit potassium channels.[51] These will inhibit the activation of the human airway macrophage as will high concentrations of potassium solutions, implying that either the opening of such receptors is a prerequisite for the activation of the cell or that depolarization of the membrane will inhibit its activation. The ATP-sensitive potassium channel opener cromakalin was without effect as was the voltage-dependent calcium channel antagonist, nicardipine. These drugs which inhibit potassium channels may be potential anti-inflammatory drugs that may have specificity for the human airway macrophage but more information is required on the nature of the channel before this can be pursued further.

Anti-inflammatory agents

The human airway macrophage is inhibited by exposure to therapeutic concentrations of glucocorticosteroids for >8 h which is different from the response of the mast cell *in vitro*.[82–85] The effect is not permanent as the cells will recover activity following further incubation without the drug. There is, however, less evidence for such effect *in vivo*. High dose glucocorticosteroids will inhibit TXB_2 release from circulating monocytes *ex vivo* and human airway macrophages are also said to be more susceptible by some but not others.[84,85] However, it must be borne in mind that treatment with glucocorticosteroids may well alter the kinetics of monocytes from the bone marrow and may alter the population and maturity of the cells[86] within the lung which may give rise to the same results. *In vitro*, the range of inhibitory effects includes inhibition of phospholipid products and cytokines although lysosymal enzymes are not inhibited.[82] Further *in vivo* and *in vitro* studies are required to document the sensitivity of these cells to glucocorticosteroids.

In our hands sodium cromoglycate is without effect.[87] However, nedocromil sodium may have some inhibitory effect on the human airway macrophage under some conditions.[88] Ketotifen, in supertherapeutic concentrations, may be also inhibitory but these effects may be non-specific and act through inhibition of potassium channels.

Table 7.4   Drug targets of the human alveolar macrophage.

Drugs that increase intracellular cAMP		
β_2 agonists	—	
Adenosine A_2 agonists	($\downarrow$)	
Forskolin	$\downarrow$	
Phosphodiesterase inhibitor	$\downarrow$	(not all enzyme subtypes)
PGE_2	—	
VIP	—	
Drugs that alter membrane ion channels		
K^+ activators	—	
K^+ inhibitors	$\downarrow$	
Ca^{2+} inhibitors	—	
Anti-inflammatory		
Sodium cromoglycate/nedocromil sodium	($\downarrow$)	
Glucocorticosteroids	$\downarrow$	

$\downarrow$ = Inhibit; ($\downarrow$) = Minimal effect; — = No effect.

Cytokines

The activity of airway macrophages is also altered by biological products such as cytokines,[89] growth factor[90] and platelet-activating factor.[91] These effects are of undoubted importance in the pathophysiological action of the cells and may also have therapeutic potential.

CONCLUSIONS

The human airway macrophage is a good candidate for the initiating and perhaps perpetuating cell in asthma as it is present in the airway in large numbers. Further, it can release cytokines which are considered to be important in the generation of the inflammation. Finally, it has a similar pharmacology to that of asthmatic inflammation in that β_2-adrenergic agonists are without inhibitory effect, however, glucocorticosteroids do suppress such inflammation and macrophage production. Data on drugs that can specifically inhibit the activation of the airway macrophage, perhaps through potassium channel inhibition, are awaited with interest.

ACKNOWLEDGEMENTS

I thank the National Asthma Campaign and the Medical Research Council for their support.

REFERENCES

1. Crofton RW, Diesselhoff-den Dulk MMC, van Furth R: The origin, kinetics and characteristics of the Kupfer cells in the normal steady state. *J Exp Med* (1978) **148**: 1–17.
2. Van Furth R, Diesselhoff-den Dulk MMC: The kinetics of promonocytes and monocytes in the bone marrow. *J Exp Med* (1970) **132**: 813–828.
3. Meuret G, Schildknecht O, Joder P, Senn H: Proliferation activity and bacteriostatic potential of human blood monocytes, macrophages and pleural effusions, ascites, and of alveolar macrophages. *Blut* (1980) **40**: 17–25.
4. Meuret G: The kinetics of mononuclear phagocytes in man. In Schmalzl F, Huhn D, Schaefer HE (eds) *Haematology and Blood Transfusion*, Vol 27, *Disorders of the Monocyte Macrophage System*. Berlin, Springer-Verlag, 1981, pp 11–22.
5. Fels AOS, Cohn ZA: The alveolar macrophage. *J Appl Physiol* (1986) **60**: 353–369.
6. Sibille Y, Reynolds HY: Macrophages and polymorphonuclear neutrophils in lung defense and injury. *Am Rev Respir Dis* (1990) **141**: 471–501.
7. Hocking WG, Golde DW: The pulmonary–alveolar macrophage (First of Two Parts). *New Engl J Med* (1979) **301**: 580–588.
8. Hocking WG, Golde DW: The pulmonary–alveolar macrophage (Second of Two Parts). *New Engl J Med* (1979) **301**: 639–645.
9. Takemura R, Werb Z: Secretory products of macrophages and their physiological functions. *Am J Physiol* (1984) **246**: C1–C9.

10. Rich EA, Tweardy DJ, Fujiwara H, Ellner J: Spectrum of immunoregulatory functions and properties of human alveolar macrophages. *Am Rev Respir Dis* (1987) **136**: 258–265.

11. Fuller RW: The role of the alveolar macrophage in asthma. *Respir Med* (1989) **83**: 177–178.

12. Tomioka M, Ida S, Shindoh Y, Ishihara T, Takishima T: Mast cells in bronchoalveolar lumen of patients with bronchial asthma. *Am Rev Respir Dis* (1984) **29**: 1000–1005.

13. Kavai M, Laczko J, Csaba B: Functional heterogeneity of macrophages. *Immunology* (1979) **36**: 729–732.

14. Radzun HJ, Kreipe H, Parwaresch MR: Tartrate-resistant acid phosphatase as a differentiation marker for the human mononuclear phagocyte system. *Hematol Oncol* (1983) **1**: 321–327.

15. Schreiber AD, Kelley M, Dziarski A, Levinson AI: Human monocyte functional heterogeneity: monocyte fractionation by discontinuous albumin gradient centrifugation. *Immunology* (1983) **49**: 231–238.

16. Rossman MD, Chen E, Chien P, Rottem M, Cprek A, Schreiber AD: Fcgamma receptor recognition of IgG ligand by human monocytes and macrophages. *Am J Respir Cell Molec Biol* (1989) **1**: 211–220.

17. Brain JD: Lung macrophages: How many kinds are there? What do they do? *Am Rev Respir Dis* (1988) **137**: 507–509.

18. Harmsen AG, Muggenburg BA, Snipes MB, Bice DE: The role of macrophages in particle translocation from lungs to lymph nodes. *Science* (1985) **230**: 1277–1280.

19. Campbell DA, Poulter LW, du Bois RM: Phenotypic analysis of alveolar macrophages in normal subjects and in patients with intestinal lung disease. *Thorax* (1986) **41**: 429–434.

20. Campbell DA, du Bois RM, Butcher RG, Poulter LW: The density of HLA-DR antigen expression on alveolar macrophages is increased in pulmonary sarcoidosis. *Clin Exp Immunol* (1986) **65**: 165–171.

21. Kern JA, Lamb RJ, Reed JC, Elias JA, Daniele RP: Interleukin-1-beta gene expression in human monocytes and alveolar macrophages from normal subjects and patients with sarcoidosis. *Am Rev Respir Dis* (1988) **137**: 1180–1184.

22. Spiteri MA, Clarke SW, Poulter LW: Phenotypic and functional changes in alveolar macrophages contribute to the pathogenesis of pulmonary sarcoidosis. *Clin Exp Immunol* (1988) **74**: 339–346.

23. Sibille Y, Chatelain B, Staquet P, Merrill WW, Delacroix DL, Vaerman J-P: Surface IgA and Fc-alpha receptors on human alveolar macrophages from normal subjects and from patients with sarcoidosis. *Am Rev Respir Dis* (1989) **139**: 740–747.

24. Itoh A, Yamaguchi E, Kuzumaki N, Okazaki N, Furuya K, Abe S, Kawakami Y: Expression of granulocyte–macrophage colony-stimulating factor mRNA by inflammatory cells in the sarcoid lung. *Am J Respir Cell Mol Biol* (1990) **3**: 245–249.

25. Razma AG, Lynch JP, Wilson BS, Ward PA, Kunkel SL: Expression of Ia-like (DR) antigen on human alveolar macrophages isolated by bronchoalveolar lavage. *Am Rev Respir Dis* (1984) **129**: 419–424.

26. Norris AM, Poulter LW, Schmekel B, Burke CM: Comparison of bronchoalveolar lavage and endobronchial biopsies in the immunopathology of asthma. *Am Rev Respir Dis* **141**: A500.

27. Norris AM, Power C, Poulter LW, Burke CM: Immunopathology of bronchial asthma. *Am Rev Respir Dis* (1990) **141**: A501.

28. Dollery CT, Eady R, Fuller RW, Jackson DM, Norris A, Turner NC, Vendy K: Bronchial anaphylaxis in ascaris sensitive dogs. *Br J Pharmac* (1987) **90**: 34P.

29. Kelly J: Cytokines of the lung. *Am Rev Respir Dis* (1990) **141**: 765–788.

30. Gordon S, Perry VH, Rabinowitz S, Chung L-P, Rosen H: Plasma membrane receptors of the mononuclear phagocyte system. *J Cell Sci Suppl* (1988) **9**: 1–26.

31. Todd RF, Liu DY: Mononuclear phagocyte activation: activation-associated antigens. *Federation Proc* (1986) **45**: 2829–2836.

32. Hsueh W, Gonzelez-Crusi F, Hanneman E: Prostaglandin synthesis in different phases of phagocytosis in lung macrophages. *Nature* (1980) **283**: 80–82.

33. Damon M, Chavis C, Godard Ph, Michel FB, Crastes de Paulet A: Purification and mass spectrometry identification of leukotriene D_4 synthesized by human alveolar macrophages. *Biochem Biophys Res Comm* (1983) **111**: 518–524.

34. Scott WA, Rouzer CA, Cohn ZA: Leukotriene C release by macrophages. *Federation Proc* (1983) **42**: 129–133.

35. MacDermot J, Kelsey CR, Waddell KA, *et al.*: Synthesis of leukotriene B_4, and prostanoids by human alveolar macrophages: Analysis by gas chromatography/mass spectrometry. *Prostaglandins* (1984) **27**: 153–179.

36. Meagher L, Savill J, Baker A, Fuller R, Haslett C: Macrophage secretory responses to ingestion of aged neutrophils. *Biochem Soc Trans* (1989) **17**: 608–609.

37. Joseph M, Tonnel AB, Capron A, Voisin C: Enzyme release and superoxide anion production by human alveolar macrophages stimulated with immunoglobulin E. *Clin Exp Immunol* (1980) **40**: 416–422.

38. Rankin JA, Hitchcock M, Merrill W, Bach MK, Brashler JR, Askenase PW: IgE-dependent release of leukotriene C_4 from alveolar macrophages. *Nature* (1982) **297**: 329–331.

39. Joseph M, Tonnel A-B, Torpier G, Capron A, Arnoux B, Benveniste J: Involvement of immunoglobulin E in the secretory process of alveolar macrophages from asthmatic patients. *J Clin Invest* (1983) **71**: 221–230.

40. Pestel J, Dessaint JP, Joseph M, Bazin H, Capron A: Macrophage triggering by aggregated immunoglobulins. II. Comparison of IgE and IgG aggregates or immune complexes. *Clin Exp Immunol* (1984) **57**: 404–412.

41. Fuller RW, Morris PK, Richmond R, *et al.*: Immunoglobulin E-dependent stimulation of human alveolar macrophages: significance in type I hypersensitivity. *Clin Exp Immunol* (1986) **65**: 416–426.

42. Fu JY, Masferrer JL, Seibert K, Raz A, Needleman P: The induction and suppression of prostaglindin H_2 synthase (cyclooxygenase) in human monocytes. *J Biol Chem* (1990) **266**: 16737–16740.

43. Leslie CC, Detty DM: Arachidonic acid turnover in response to ipopolysaccharide and opsonized zymosan in human monocyte-derived macrophages. *Biochem J* (1986) **236**: 251–259.

44. Kemmerich B, Rossing TH, Pennington JE: Comparative oxidative microbicidal activity of human blood monocytes and alveolar macrophages and activation by recombinant gamma interferon. *Am Rev Respir Dis* (1987) **136**: 266–270.

45. Martin TR, Altman LC, Albert RK, Henderson WR: Leukotriene B_4 production by the human alveolar macrophage. A potential mechanism for amplifying inflammation in the lung. *Am Rev Respir Dis* (1984) **129**: 106–111.

46. Bach MK, Brashler JR, Hammarström, Samuelsson B: Identification of leukotriene C-1 as a major component of slow-reacting substance from rat mononuclear cells. *J Immunol* (1980) **125**: 115–117.

47. Polla B, de Rochemonteix B, Junod AF, Dayer J-M: Effects of LTB_4 and Ca^{++} ionophore A23187 on the release by human alveolar macrophages of factors controlling fibroblast functions. *Biochem Biophys Res Comm* **129**: 560–567.

48. Tardif J, Borgeat P, Laviolette M: Inhibition of human alveolar macrophage production of leukotriene B_4 by acute *in vitro* and *in vivo* exposure to tobacco smoke. *Am J Respir Cell Mol Biol* (1990) **2**: 155–161.

49. Kouzan S, Nolan RD, Fournier T, Bignon J, Eling TE, Brody AR: Stimulation of arachidonic acid metabolism by adherence of alveolar macrophages to a plastic substrate. *Am Rev Respir Dis* (1988) **137**: 38–43.

50. Hamilton TA, Adams DO: Molecular mechanisms of signal transduction in macrophages. *Immunology Today* (1987) **8**: 151–158.

51. Baker AJ, Turner NC, Fuller RW: Macrophage activation: role of potassium channels. *Am Rev Resp Dis* (1990) **141**: A647.

52. Baker AJ, Fuller RW: Human alveolar macrophages release C3a but not C5a when stimulated with opsonized zymosan. *Am Rev Resp Dis* (1989) **139**: A160.

53. Melewicz FM, Kline LE, Cohen AB, Speigelberg HL: Characterization of Fc receptors for IgE on human alveolar macrophages. *Clin Exp Immunol* (1982) **49**: 364–370.

54. Richards CD, Gauldie J: IgA-mediated phagocytosis by mouse alveolar macrophages. *Am Rev Respir Dis* (1985) **132**: 82–85.
55. Mantovani B, Rabinovitch M, Nussenzweig V: Phagocytosis of immune complexes by macrophages. Different roles of the macrophage receptor sites for complement (C3) and for immunoglobulin (IgG). *J Exp Med* (1972) **135**: 780–792.
56. Melewicz FM, Spiegelberg HL: Fc receptors for IgE on a subpopulation of human peripheral blood monocytes. *J Immunol* **125**: 1026–1031.
57. Anderson CL, Spiegelberg HL: Macrophage receptors for IgE: Binding of IgE to specific IgE Fc receptors on a human macrophage cell line, U937. *J Immunol* (1981) **126**: 2470–2473.
58. Storch J, Edwards RJ, MacDermot J: Thromboxane release by lymphokine-differentiated U937 human monocytic cells: Response to platelet-activating factor (PAF) and chemotactic peptide (FMLP) but not to low affinity IgE-receptor (FcεRII/CD23) occupation. *J Leuk Biol* (1990) **48**: 266–273.
59. Mayumi M, Kawabe T, Nishioka H, *et al.*: Interferon and (2'-5')oligoadenylate enhance the expression of low affinity receptors for IgE (FcRII/CD23) on the human monoblast cell line U937. *Mol Immunol* (1989) **26**: 241–247.
60. Yokata A, Kikutani H, Tanaka T, *et al.*: Two species of human Fc receptor II (Fc RII/CD023): specific and IL4-specific regulation of gene expression. *Cell* (1988) **55**: 611–618.
61. Vercelli D, Jabara HH, Lee BW, Woodland N, Geha RS, Leung DYM: Human interleukin 4 induced FcεRII/CD23 on normal human monocytes. *J Exp Med* (1988) **167**: 1406–1416.
62. Storch, J, MacDermot J: IgE and IgG are synergistic in antigen-mediated release of thromboxane from human lung macrophages. *Cell Immunol* (1991) **134**: 138–146.
63. Balter MS, Toews GB, Peters-Golden M: Different patterns of arachidonate metabolism in autologous human blood monocytes and alveolar macrophages. *J Immunol* (1989) **142**: 602–608.
64. Yokode M, Kita T, Kikawa Y, Ogorochi T, Narumiya S, Kawai C: Stimulated arachidonate metabolism during foam cell transformation of mouse peritoneal macrophages with oxidized low density lipoprotein. *J Clin Invest* (1988) **81**: 720–729.
65. Nakagawara A, Nathan CF, Cohn ZA: Hydrogen peroxide metabolism in human monocytes during differentiation *in vitro*. *J Clin Invest* **68**: 1243–1252.
66. Strieter RM, Remick DG, Lynch JP, *et al.*: Differential regulation of tumor necrosis factor-alpha in human alveolar macrophages and peripheral blood monocytes: A cellular and molecular analysis. *Am J Respir Cell Mol Biol* **1**: 57–63.
67. Sone S, Okubo A, Ogura T: Normal human alveolar macrophages have more ability than blood monocytes to produce cell-associated interleukin-1-alpha. *Am J Respir Cell Mol Biol* **1**: 507–515.
68. Elias JA, Schreiber AD, Gustilo K, *et al.*: Differential interleukin 1 elaboration by unfractionated and density fractionated human alveolar macrophages and blood monocytes: relationship to cell maturity. *J Immunol* (1985) **135**: 3198–3203.
69. Kotloff RM, Little J, Elias JA: Human alveolar macrophage and blood monocyte interleukin-6 production. *Am J Respir Cell Mol Biol* (1990) **3**: 497–505.
70. Weissler JC, Lipscomb MF, Lem VM, Toews GB: Tumour killing by human alveolar macrophages and blood monocytes. Decreased cytotoxicity of human alveolar macrophages. *Am Rev Respir Dis* (1986) **134**: 532–537.
71. Kunkel SL, Duque RE: The macrophage adherence phenomenon: its relationship to prostaglandin E_2 and superoxide anion production and changes in transmembrane potential. *Prostaglandins* (1983) **26**: 893–904.
72. Rossman MD, Chien P, Cassizzi-Cprek A, Elias JA, Holian A, Schreiber AD: The binding of monomeric IgG to human blood monocytes and alveolar macrophages. *Am Rev Respir Dis* (1986) **133**: 292–297.
73. Garcia JGN, Griffith DE, Cohen AB, Callahan KS: Alveolar macrophages from patients with asbestos exposure release increased levels of leukotriene B_4. *Am Rev Respir Dis* (1989) **139**: 1494–1501.
74. Wieslander E, Linden M, Hakansson L, *et al.*: Human alveolar macrophages from smokers have an impaired capacity to secrete LTB_4 but not other chemotactic factors. *J Respir Dis* (1987) **71**: 263–272.

75. Wirth JJ, Kierszenbaum F: Inhibitory action of elevated levels of adenosine-3':5'cyclic monophosphate on phagocytosis: effects on macrophage–*Trypanosoma cruzi* interaction. *J Immunol* (1982) **129**: 2759–2762.
76. Baker AJ, Fuller RW: Loss of beta receptor function during maturation of monocytes to macrophages. *Eur J Pharmacol* (1990) **183**: 876–877.
77. Fuller RW, O'Malley G, Baker AJ, MacDermot J: Human alveolar macrophage activation: inhibition by forskolin but not beta-adrenoceptor stimulation or phosphodiesterase inhibition. *Pulmonary Pharmacol* (1988) **1**: 101–106.
78. Liggett SB: Identification and characterization of a homogeneous population of β_2-adrenergic receptors on human alveolar macrophage. *Am Rev Respir Dis* (1989) **139**: 552–555.
79. Hjemdahl P, Larsson K, Johansson M-C, Zetterlund A, Eklund A: β-Adrenoceptors in human alveolar macrophages isolated by elutriation. *Br J Clin Pharmac* (1990) **30**: 673–682.
80. Baker AJ, Fuller RW: Effect of c'AMP, NECA and methylxanthines on the activation of human alveolar macrophages *in vitro. Br J Pharmac* (1991) in press.
81. Baker AJ, Fuller RW: Anti-inflammatory effect of salmeterol on human alveolar macrophages. *Am Rev Respir Dis* (1990) **141**: A394.
82. Fuller RW, Kelsey CR, Cole PJ, Dollery CT, MacDermot J: Dexamethasone inhibits the production of thromboxane B_2 and leukotriene B_4 by human alveolar and peritoneal macrophages in culture. *Clin Sci* (1984) **67**: 653–656.
83. Peters-Golden M, Thebert P: Inhibition by methylprednisolone of zymosan-induced leukotriene synthesis in alveolar macrophages. *Am Rev Respir Dis* (1987) **135**: 1020–1026.
84. Sebaldt RJ, Sheller JR, Oates JA, Roberts LJ, FitzGerald GA: Inhibition of eicosanoid biosynthesis by glucocorticoids in humans. *Proc Natl Acad Sci USA* (1990) **87**: 6974–6978.
85. Yoss EB, Spannhake EWm, Flynn JT, Fish JE, Peters SP: Arachidonic acid metabolism in normal human alveolar macrophages: Stimulus specificity for mediator release and phospholipid metabolism, and pharmacologic modulation *in vitro* and *in vivo. Am J Respir Cell Mol Biol* (1990) **2**: 69–80.
86. Rinehart JJ, Wuest D, Ackerman GA: Corticosteroid alterations of human monocyte to macrophage differentiation. *J Immunol* (1982) **129**: 1436–1440.
87. Fuller RW, MacDermot J: Stimulation of IgE sensitized human alveolar macrophages by anti-IgE is unaffected by sodium cromoglycate. *Clin Allergy* (1986) **16**: 523–526.
88. Thorel T, Joseph M, Tsicopoulos A, Tonnel AB, Capron A: Inhibition of nedcromil sodium of IgE-mediated activation of human mononuclear phagocytes and platelets in allergy. *Int Arcs Allergy Appl Immunol* (1988) **85**: 232–237.
89. Strieter RB, Chensue SW, Basha MA, *et al.*: Human alveolar macrophage gene expression of interleukin-8 tumor necrosis factor-α, lipopolysaccharid, and interleukin-1β. *Am J Respir Cell Mol Biol* (1990) **2**: 321–326.
90. Tsunawaki S, Sporn M, Ding A, Nathan C: Deactivation of macrophages by transforming growth factor-β. *Nature* (1988) **334**: 260–262.
91. Stewart AG, Phillips WA: Intracellular platelet-activating factor regulates eicosanoid generation in guinea-pig resident peritoneal macrophages. *Br J Pharmacol* (1989) **98**: 141–148.

8

Eosinophils

RONALD DAHL, PER VENGE AND KJELD FREDENS

INTRODUCTION

The eosinophil granulocyte was recognized by its special ability to stain with acidic dyes[1] because of its content of basic substances in the special granules. Much controversy has surrounded the function of this cell and opinions have varied from protective, tissue-preserving properties[2] to the opposite view of an aggressive tissue-damaging cell.[3] During recent years intensified interest has been focused on the eosinophil, which has revealed specific properties of the cell and a dynamic variation in its functional properties. An elevated number of blood eosinophils is found in a large number of diseases. Eosinophilia is invariably seen in diseases of tissue-invading helminthic parasites, especially when the larval stage migrates through the tissues. The number of blood eosinophils is correlated with the serum level of IgE, reflecting the common stimulus from the parasite. It seems a logical explanation that the eosinophils are attracted to the site where mast cell degranulation occurs, in this case at the site of the tissue parasite. As the eosinophil appears to be the major cytotoxic cell for parasitic larvae[4,5] this function seems highly beneficial.

THE EOSINOPHIL AND ASTHMA

The eosinophil is produced in the bone marrow and is distributed to the tissues via the bloodstream. It is primarily a tissue cell, and for every circulating eosinophil it has been estimated that there are about 200 mature eosinophil forms in the marrow and approximately 500 in connective tissues.[6] The concentration differences may be even greater in disease states with eosinophil tissue infiltration, such as in the bronchial mucosa in asthma, where the eosinophil seems to be the main infiltrating cell in this special

ASTHMA: BASIC MECHANISMS AND CLINICAL MANAGEMENT (2nd Edn)   ISBN 0-12-079026-2 inflammatory reaction.[7] The connection between asthma and the eosinophil granulocyte seems fundamental and is present irrespective of an allergic component of the disease. In groups of patients the disease severity correlates to the degree of blood eosinophilia,[8,9] and in an individual patient the blood eosinophil count varies in relation to the severity of the disease. Therefore, the eosinophil seems to be a marker of the inflammatory activity in the respiratory tract in asthma. Investigations have shown that the study of sputum samples is of even more value than studies of blood eosinophil numbers.[10] Also the study of bronchoalveolar lavage fluid demonstrated a correlation between the presence and activity of eosinophils and the severity of the asthmatic disease.[11] Although the eosinophil is related not only to allergic asthma but also to intrinsic asthma, valuable information has been gathered from patients with allergic bronchial asthma because their disease can be provoked by allergen challenge. Inhalation of a relevant allergen results in an early asthma reaction that subsides within 1–2 h. In 40–60% of the patients this early reaction after some hours is followed by a late asthmatic reaction, which usually subsides during the next 1–2 days. In patients who only react with an isolated early reaction, no changes are found in the number of blood eosinophils after 24 h[12] or in the number of eosinophils in bronchial lavage fluid after 6 h.[13] In contrast, patients who developed a late asthmatic reaction have a raised number of blood eosinophils after 24 h[12] and raised eosinophil number in bronchial lavage fluid after 6 h.[13] The rise in blood eosinophils has been found to correlate closely to the increase in non-specific bronchial reactivity which may follow allergen challenge.[14] Also natural exposure to allergens such as during the birch pollen season induces blood and lung eosinophilia.[15,16] These studies and the knowledge of the biochemical composition and function of the eosinophil provide increasing evidence that the eosinophil has a central position in the pathogenetic events in asthma.

BIOCHEMISTRY OF HUMAN EOSINOPHILS

In Table 8.1 our current knowledge of the biochemistry of the human eosinophil is summarized. The granules of eosinophils typically contain an abundance of heavily basic, medium-sized proteins, which are all more or less cytotoxic to both mammalian and non-mammalian cells. With the exception of EPX and EDN, which have been shown to be identical proteins, the other proteins are distinctive molecules. Several subpopulations of granules have been suggested from the morphology of the eosinophil and the density distribution of the granules. Thus the heavy crystalloid-containing granules appear to contain both ECP, EPX (EDN), EPO and MBP whereas another subpopulation of smaller and lighter granules only contain ECP and EPX(EDN),[17] with MBP making up the peculiar crystalloid structures in the granules and the other three proteins located in the matrix. The location of arylsulphatase B and other enzymes is uncertain (for reviews see refs 18 and 19).

Eosinophil cationic proteins

ECP was first isolated from the eosinophils of patients with chronic myeloid leukaemia but recently also from eosinophils of normal individuals.[20] From both sources ECP

Table 8.1 The biochemistry of human eosinophils.

Component	Characteristics	Major functions
Granule components		
Eosinophil cationic protein	18–21 kDa, single chain, pI > 11	Cytotoxic, neurotoxic (ECP) Interferes with coagulation and fibrinolysis Interferes with cell-mediated immunity Degranulates mast cells and basophils Ribonuclease activity Stimulant fibroblast activity
Eosinophil protein X or eosinophil-derived neurotoxin (EDN)	18 kDa, single chain, pI = basic	Cytotoxic, neurotoxic (EPX) Interferes with cell-mediated immunity Ribonuclease activity
Eosinophil peroxidase	67 kDa, light chain (15 kDa) heavy chain (52 kDa),	Peroxidase activity (EPO) Inactivates, e.g. LTC_4 pI > 11 Degranulates mast cells Cytotoxic Induces platelet aggregation
Major basic protein (MBP)	13.9 kDa, single chain, pI > 11	Cytotoxic Degranulates mast cells and basophils Induces platelet aggregation
Arylsulphatase B	70 kDa, tetramer, pI = acid	Unknown
Membrane component		
The Charcot–Leyden crystal protein (CLC)	13–17 kDa, single chain, pI = acidic	Lysophospholipase activity
Components formed upon activation		
Leukotriene C_4		Contraction of smooth muscle (LTC_4)
Platelet-activating factor (PAF-acether, AGEPC) Prostaglandins E_1 and E_2 (PGE_1 and PGE_2) (identical to eosinophil-derived inhibitor (EDI))		Contraction of smooth Chemotactic to eosinophils muscle (PAF) Inhibition of mast cell secretion
Oxygen-derived radicals (O_2^-, H_2O_2, OH·)		Cytotoxic Increases vascular permeability

displays some heterogeneity on SDS-polyacrylamide gel electrophoresis with molecular sizes varying from 18 to 21kDa. The heterogeneity is most likely the result of differences in carbohydrate contents, since no differences in amino acid composition were discernible and since measures to remove carbohydrate from the molecules resulted in one homogeneous band at 18 kDa. The cellular content of ECP in normal eosinophils is about 25 μg/10^6 cells.[18] In eosinophils of patients with various forms of eosinophila, the content varies enormously being only 0.025% of the normal content in some cell preparations. ECP is released from the cell upon exposure to serum protein opsonized particles.[21] Beside potent cytotoxic activities, which are dealt with in detail below, ECP has several other biological functions. Thus ECP enhances coagulation and kallikrein formation by a coagulation factor XII-dependent mechanism and preactivates plasminogen, rendering the plasminogen activator urokinase. ECP can inactivate the anticoagulant activity of heparin probably by complex formation.[22] Furthermore, ECP inhibits the T-lymphocyte response to phytohaemagglutinin in mixed lymphocyte reactions,[23] and also induces histamine release from human basophils.[24] In recent experiments ECP was shown to stimulate and alter fibroblast production of glycosaminoglycans.[25] It should be emphasized that all these effects are achieved at physiological or near physiological concentrations of ECP. Whether any of these reactions take place *in vivo* is, however, still uncertain, since specific inhibitor molecules to ECP have been identified in plasma.[26] ECP was recently cloned and the amino acid sequence showed a large degree of homology with EPX(EDN) and pancreatic ribonuclease.[27] ECP does exhibit some ribonuclease activity.[28,29]

EPX/EDN

EPX and EDN have been shown to be identical proteins.[30] The normal cellular content of EPX (EDN) is about 10 μg/10^6 eosinophils and is reduced to 20–50% in eosinophils of patients with various forms of eosinophilia.[18] EPX (EDN) has been purified from both normal eosinophils and eosinophils from patients with the hypereosinophilic syndrome.[31] The molecule appears to be identical from these various sources. EPX (EDN) also shows cytotoxic properties (see below). In addition EPX was shown to be as potent as ECP in inhibiting the T-lymphocyte response in mixed lymphocyte reactions or to the lectin phytohaemagglutinin.[23] As with ECP the amino-acid sequence of EPX (EDN) shows a high degree of homology with ribonuclease.[27] The ribonuclease activity of EPX (EDN) was 125-fold higher than that of ECP.[29] Furthermore, the amino acid sequences of EPX (EDN) and ECP show a 70% homology.[27] In addition, a monoclonal antibody EG2, prepared to ECP also picks up an epitope on EPX (EDN), as a further indication of a close relationship between the two proteins.[32]

Eosinophil peroxidase

EPO has so far only been purified and characterized from eosinophils of patients with eosinophilia.[33] The content in normal eosinophils has been estimated to be about 15 μg/10^6 eosinophils. The biological function of EPO is mainly related to its peroxidase activity, although some activities may be related to the heavily basic charge of the molecule. Thus EPO in the absence of H_2O_2 interferes with receptor-dependent events such as the chemotactic response of neutrophils and Fc and C3b-receptor dependent phagocytosis[34] and also induces platelet aggregation.[35]

Major basic protein

Major basic protein (MBP) is a low weight protein with a very high tendency to form aggregates. The biological activity of MBP is related to its basic charge and MBP has been shown to be cytotoxic to a variety of mammalian and non-mammalian cells. MBP does not seem to be restricted to the eosinophil, since antigenic material has been picked up in other cells such as basophils and trophoblastic cells.[19]

The Charcot–Leyden crystal protein

The Charcot–Leyden crystal protein (CLC), which makes up the Charcot–Leyden crystals found in tissues with heavy eosinophil infiltration, has recently been fully characterized and shown to be located to the membrane of the eosinophil.[36,37] However, the protein does not seem to be entirely specific to eosinophils, since basophils contain antigenically related material.[38] Interestingly, the CLC protein displays lysophospholipase activity. Thus the protein may be active in neutralization of toxic lysophospholipids, which are formed as a consequence of phospholipase A2 activity in stimulated cells.

Eosinophil mediators

Several products are formed by the eosinophil as a consequence of activation of the cell. Two such products of great potential interest are the leukotriene $C4(LTC_4)$[39,40] and platelet-activating factor (PAF).[41] The production of LTC_4 and PAF by eosinophils is comparable to any other cell, such as the mast cell. Both compounds are potent smooth muscle contracting agents, which may be relevant in diseases such as asthma. In addition PAF is, among other things, a potent and fairly selective chemoattractant for eosinophils.[42] Also, prostaglandins E_1 and E_2 are formed by the eosinophil and have been identified as the principles which inhibit histamine release from mast cells, eosinophil-derived inhibitor (EDI).[43] Oxygen radicals are also produced by the eosinophils upon stimulation by a number of compounds. The capacity of the eosinophil in this respect is fully comparable to that of the neutrophil.[44] These mediators may be active in the killing and destruction of parasites, but may be detrimental to the host if produced in large amounts inappropriately, as in asthma.

EOSINOPHIL FUNCTIONS

Apart from the fact that the eosinophil contains in its granules unique compounds, two other features in particular seem to distinguish the eosinophil from the neutrophil. The eosinophil is a poor phagocyte, although it may phagocytize immune complexes and bacteria.[45–50] The killing of microbes by the eosinophil is probably brought about by extracellular release of the cytotoxic compounds, in contrast to neutrophils, in which killing takes place within the phagolysosome. Thus the major function of the eosinophil is that of a secretory cell. A characteristic feature of eosinophils is their variability. Thus the state of activity of the cell may change dramatically as a consequence of exposure to various hormone-like substances produced mainly by T-lymphocytes and monocytes but also to a lesser extent by a whole variety of other cells. These substances are collectively called cytokines and some cytokines with particular relevance to eosinophil growth and activation are shown in Table 8.2.

The change in stage of activity includes increased number of receptors (receptor enhancement) and increased metabolic activity. The changes result in increased secretory activity, increased response to chemotactic principles, increased killing capacity, etc. The impact of this variability is obvious and reminiscent of the variability of the macrophage. Thus under normal conditions the eosinophil is a dormant and harmless cell but during various conditions, which involve the productions of the above compounds it is turned into an active and potentially dangerous cell. The extent of eosinophil accumulation at a specific site in the organism is governed by several mechanisms, some of which are related to the mechanisms described above (see Table 8.2). Thus one requirement is the availability of a sufficient number of cells in the blood pool. The mechanisms which govern the egress of eosinophils from the bone marrow are not understood but several mechanisms have been proposed which regulate eosinophilopoiesis. Some of these mechanisms may be independent of T-lymphocyte activity but others are T-lymphocyte dependent.[51] The second major requirement is the production of some factors at the specific site, which signals the eosinophil to leave the bloodstream. It is assumed that these signals involve specific eosinophil chemotactic factors, although few, if any, such factors have been demonstrated in man. In contrast it is quite obvious that most attractants for neutrophils *in vitro* will also attract eosinophils. So the question of how some processes become almost exclusively eosinophil-containing is still unsolved. Is it a matter of production of specific eosinophil chemoattractants, or of making the eosinophil more responsive to fairly unselective attractants, or of both? Or is the entire process governed at the endothelial cell level? A relative selective increased responsiveness of blood eosinophils has in fact been shown to be present in asthmatic patients.[52] An experiment, which may point to a role of the eosinophil–endothelial interaction, is the inhibition of eosinophil accumulation and the development of hyperreactivity in primates by the administration of antibodies to one of the adhesion molecules, ICAM-1, on

Table 8.2   Some eosinophil-activating factors and their characteristics.

Granulocyte-macrophage-CSF (GM-CSF)	MW 22.5 kDa	Eosinophilopoietic (GM-CSF) Enhances eosinophil-mediated killing Increases LTC$_4$ production
Eosinophil-enhancing factor (EAF)	MW 40 kDa	Enhances eosinophil-mediated killing Increases LTC$_4$ production
Tumour necrosis factor (TNF)	MW 17 kDa	Enhances eosinophil killing
Interleukin-3 (IL-3)		Eosinophilopoietic
Interleukin-5 (IL-5)		Increases degranulation Increases metabolism Increases the chemotactic and chemokinetic response

the endothelial cell.[53] The understanding of the processes that govern the selective accumulation of eosinophils in tissues will be crucial for our future pharmacological control of eosinophil-involving diseases such as asthma.

CELLULAR INJURY BY EOSINOPHILS

During an attack of asthma, eosinophils accumulate in the bronchial wall as well as in the airway lumen. During this inflammatory reaction various proteins from the eosinophil seem to be secreted. Some of these have a considerable potential for tissue damage. Thus MBP produces ciliostasis and varying degrees of damage to the respiratory epithelium at doses of 10 μg/ml. ECP, however, seems to be by far the most potent tissue-damaging protein of the eosinophils.[54] This was demonstrated in guinea-pig brains, where the so called Gordon phenomenon could be induced with ECP and EPX. ECP was 100 times more potent than EPX (EDN).[53] A single injection into the trachea of 0.2–5.0 μg of ECP reveals damage to the surface epithelium of the airway. The damage varies from detachment of the superficial part of the epithelium, leaving behind more or less intact basal cells, to a total removal of the surface epithelium in other places, especially those near the site of injection (Figs 8.1 and 8.2). Thus a high degree of cytotoxicity by ECP has been demonstrated in guinea-pigs and the ECP concentration tested seems easily obtained in asthmatic airways where up to 200 μg/ml ECP has been

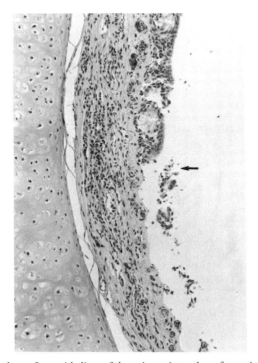

Fig. 8.1 Damage to the surface epithelium of the guinea pig trachea after a single injection of ECP.

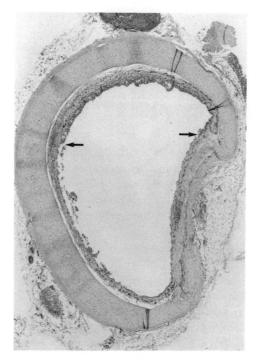

Fig. 8.2 Same section as Fig. 8.1. Damaged surface epithelium is seen below the two arrows.

found in the cell-free sputum supernatant (Virchow Jr C, Venge P, Virchow C, in preparation). In order to determine whether ECP has the same effect in humans, tissues with a known eosinophilic infiltration from different human organs were examined for a correlation between extracellular deposition of ECP and cellular injury. The ECP immunoreactivity was detected by immunofluorescence, the immunoperoxidase method and alkaline phosphatase conjugated antibodies. Both polyclonal and monoclonal antibodies were used.[55] In all cases where ECP immunoreactivity was restricted to the eosinophils, with no immunoreactivity in the extracellular space, no cellular injury was observed. In cases with signs of ECP degranulation, however, the extracellular-distributed ECP was always seen in or near necrotic areas. Similar results were seen in post-mortem lungs from asthmatics who died from severe asthma. Investigations here have revealed a clear correlation between ECP and cellular injury in lung tissue from severe asthma. Extracellular ECP immunoreactivity is seen throughout the bronchial wall as well as on the surface of the mucosa. A severe case is illustrated in Figs 8.3 and 8.4; a remnant of the surface epithelium is seen (arrows, Fig. 8.4) but most is totally removed. The wall is infiltrated with eosinophils, as seen from the distribution of ECP immunoreactivity in Fig. 8.3. Extracellularly deposited ECP is seen within a necrotic area with ulceration of the mucosa (asterisk, Fig. 8.3). The smooth muscle layer is also destroyed. It seems likely that eosinophils, through release of ECP, are responsible for much of the cellular injury related to asthma. This damage is mainly restricted to the surface epithelium, but damage may even be seen in deeper structures. This discussion has indicated that asthma may be the result of altered communication in a network of relations between inflammatory cells. It is likely that the eosinophil is at the very centre

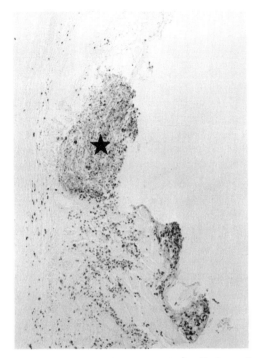

Fig. 8.3   ECP immunoreactivity (PAP) in a bronchial wall of an asthmatic patient.

of this network. This makes the eosinophil one of the primary targets of therapy and research.

PHARMACOLOGICAL CONTROL OF THE EOSINOPHIL

β-Agonists

In vivo studies have shown that β-adrenergic agonists decrease the number of circulating eosinophils[56] and the serum level of ECP in normal subjects and patients with bronchial asthma.[57] A weaker response in asthmatics than in normal subjects has been reported, but it is not known whether this is due to antiasthmatic therapy or a defect in β-receptors. Similar results have been reported after theophylline treatment. This indicates that the eosinophil in patients with bronchial asthma may respond less to bronchodilator drugs, and possibly there is an inverse relationship between the severity of the asthmatic disease and the responsiveness of the eosinophil to bronchodilators. β-Adrenergic antagonists give rise to bronchoconstriction when given to asthmatics by inhalation or orally. These drugs result in elevation of the blood eosinophil count and the serum ECP levels.[57–59] The long-acting β-agonist Salmeterol abolished the increase in serum ECP and bronchial reactivity to histamine after allergen-induced late-phase asthmatic reaction[60] and also reduced ECP in bronchoalveolar lavage.[61] This indicates an influence of this long-acting β_2-agonist on eosinophil activation and ECP release.

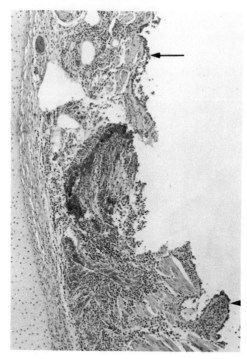

Fig. 8.4 Consecutive section of Fig. 8.3 demonstrating extensive damage to the bronchial wall. Haemotoxylin-eosin stain.

Steroids

Glucocorticosteroids decrease the number of eosinophils in blood and tissues[62] and decrease receptor numbers on the eosinophil surface.[63] Inhaled corticosteroids also decrease blood eosinophil number and serum ECP levels.[64] In patients with mild asthma, inhaled corticosteroids reduced ECP-levels in both bronchoalveolar lavage fluid and in serum without affecting the number of eosinophils.[65] Similarly, the expected rise in ECP-levels in bronchoalveolar lavage during a late asthmatic reaction was abrogated by a minimum dose of inhaled steroids in contrast to the number of eosinophils, which was unaffected (De Monchy JGR, Venge P, in preparation). This indicates that *in vivo* secretion of granule proteins, such as ECP, is more sensitive to glucocorticosteroids than eosinophil traffic. Nasal allergen challenge resulted in a late-oncoming increase in lavage fluid ECP and this increase was inhibited and the basal level of nasal lavage fluid ECP was decreased.[66] *In vitro*, eosinophil migration is virtually unaffected by even very high doses of steroids (Håkansson L, Venge P, in preparation) in contrast to degranulation which is potently inhibited.[64]

Sodium cromoglycate

Sodium cromoglycate may also influence the eosinophil. The main finding in a 4-week study of sodium cromoglycate was a decrease in the number of eosinophils in bronchial secretions in patients responding to the treatment.[67]

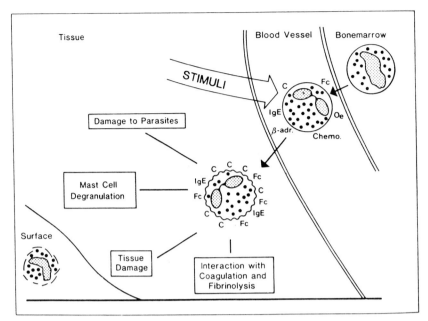

Fig. 8.5 The natural life and some of the proposed functions of the eosinophil when the cell is activated in the tissues.

In summary it seems possibly to conclude that the main drugs used for the treatment of asthma all affect the eosinophil in a way compatible with the hypothesis that the cell brings about damage to the airways in asthma.

SUMMARY

The eosinophil granulocyte in its activated state is a secretory cell. If extracellular release of its granule constituents of cytotoxic compounds takes place, this leads to damage of the surrounding cells. This can be of benefit if the target is an unwanted element such as a parasite, but it aggravates or creates tissue lesions in other inflammatory disease states. In asthma, eosinophils are numerous in the inflammatory infiltrates, and damage to the epithelium and mucosa of the bronchi can be caused by toxic eosinophil-derived proteins (Fig. 8.5). For the treatment of asthma it seems important to concentrate efforts to control the eosinophil, and drugs specific for that purpose could be a major contribution to the control of asthma.

REFERENCES

1. Ehrlich P: Über die specifischer granulationen des blutes. *Arch Anat Physiol* (1879) **3**: 571.
2. Weller PF, Wasserman SI, Austen KF: Selected enzymes preferentially present in the eosinophil. In Mahmoud AAD, Austen KF (eds) *The Eosinophil in Health and Disease*. New York, Grune & Stratton, 1980, p 115.

3. Frigas E, Gleich GJ: The eosinophil and pathophysiology of asthma. *J Allergy Clin Immunol* (1986) **77**: 527–537.

4. Butterworth AE, Wasson DL, Gleich GL, Loegering DA, David JR: Damage to schistosomula of *Schistosoma mansoni* induced directly by eosinophil major basic protein. *J Immunol* (1979) **122**: 211–229.

5. McLaren DJ, McKean JR, Olsson I, Venge P, Kay AB: Morphological studies on the killing of schistosomula of *Schistosoma mansoni* by human eosinophil and neutrophil cationic proteins *in vitro. Parasite Immunol* (1981) **3**: 359–373.

6. Kay AB: Eosinophils and neutrophils in the pathogenesis of asthma. In Weiss EB, Segal MS, Stein M (eds) *Bronchial Asthma, Mechanisms and Therapeutics*. Boston, Little, Brown and Company, 1985, pp 255–265.

7. Hogg JC: The pathology of asthma. In Middleton E, Reed CE, Ellis EE (eds) *Allergy, Principles and Practise*. St Louis, Mosby, 1983, pp 833–841.

8. Burrows B, Hasan FM, Barbee RM, Halonen M, Levowitz MD: Epidemiological observations on eosinophilia and its relation to respiratory diseases. *Am Rev Respir Dis* (1980) **122**: 709–719.

9. Honsinger RW, Silverstein D, Van Arsdel PP: The eosinophil and allergy. Why? *J Allergy Clin Immunol* (1972) **49**: 142–155.

10. Brown HM: Treatment of chronic asthma with prednisolone: Significance of eosinophils in the sputum. *Lancet* (1958) **2**: 1245–1247.

11. Bousquet J, Chanez P, Lacoste JY, *et al.*: Eosinophilic inflammation in asthma. *New Engl J Med* (1990) **323**: 1033–1039.

12. Booiy-Noord H, de Vries K, Sluiter HJ, Orie NGM: Late bronchial obstructive reaction to experimental inhalation of house-dust extract. *Clin Allergy* (1972) **2**: 43–61.

13. De Monchy JGR, Kauffman HF, Venge P, *et al.*: Broncho-alveolar eosinophilia during allergen-induced late asthmatic reactions. *Am Rev Respir Dis* (1985) **131**: 373–376.

14. Durham SR, Kay AB: Eosinophils, bronchial hyperreactivity and late asthmatic reactions. *Clin Allergy* (1985) **40**: 411–418.

15. Rak S, Löwhagen O, Venge P: The effect of immunotherapy on bronchial hyperresponsiveness and eosinophil cationic protein in pollen-allergic patients. *J Allergy Clin Immunol* (1988) **82**: 470–480.

16. Rak S, Håkansson L, Venge P: Immunotherapy abrogates the generation of eosinophil and neutrophil chemotactic activity during pollen season. *J Allergy Clin Immunol* (1990) **86**: 706–713.

17. Peterson CGB, Garcia RC, Carlsson MGC, Venge P. Eosinophil cationic protein (ECP), eosinophil protein x(EPX) and eosinophil peroxidase (EPO): Granule distribution, degranulation and characterization of released proteins. In Pederson C (ed) *Eosinophil granule proteins. Biochemical and functional studies*. Acta Universitas Uppsaliensis 125, Uppsala, 1987.

18. Venge P: The eosinophil in inflammation. In Venge P, Lindbom A (eds) *Inflammation. Basic Mechanisms, Tissue Injuring Principles and Clinical Models*. Stockholm, Almqvist & Wiksell International, 1985, pp 85–103.

19. Gleich GJ, Adolphson CR: The eosinophilic leukocyte: structure and function. *Adv Immunol* (1986) **39**: 177–253.

20. Peterson CGB, Jörnvall H, Venge P: Purification and characterization of eosinophil cationic protein from normal human eosinophils. *Eur J Haematol* (1988) **40**: 415–423.

21. Winqvist I, Olofsson T, Olsson I: Mechanisms for eosinophil degranulation; release of the eosinophil cationic protein. *Immunology* (1984) **51**: 1–8.

22. Fredens K, Dahl R, Venge P: *In vitro* studies of the interaction between heparin and eosinophil cationic protein. *Allergy* (1991) **46**: 27–29.

23. Peterson CGB, Skoog V, Venge P: Human eosinophil cationic proteins (ECP and EPX) and their suppressive effects on lymphocyte proliferation. *Immunobiology* (1985) **171**: 1–13.

24. Bergstrand H, Lundquist B, Peterson B-Å, Peterson C, Venge P: Eosinophil derived cationic proteins and human leukocyte histamine release. In Venge P, Lindbom A (eds) *Inflammation. Basic Mechanisms, Tissue Injuring Principles and Clinical Models*. Stockholm, Almqvist & Wiksell International, 1985, p 361.

25. Särnstrand B, Westergren-Thorsson G, Hernäs J, Peterson CGB, Venge P, Malmström A: Eosinophil cationic protein and transforming growth factor-A stimulates synthesis of hyaluronan and proteoglycan in human fibroblast cultures. 5th International Colloquium on Pulmonary Fibrosis, 1988: (Abstract).

26. Peterson CGB, Venge P: Interaction and complex formation between the eosinophil cationic protein (ECP) and alpha-2-macroglobulin. *Biochem J* (1987) **245**: 781–787.

27. Gleich GJ, Loegering DA, Bell MP, Checkel JL, Ackerman SJ, Kean DJ: Biochemical and functional similarities between human eosinophil-derived neurotoxin and eosinophil cationic protein: Homology with ribonuclease. *Proc Natl Acad Sci* (1986) **83**: 3146–3150.

28. Slifman NR, Loegering DA, McKean DJ, Gleich GJ: Ribonuclease activity associated with human eosinophil-derived neurotoxin and eosinophil cationic protein. *J Immunol* (1986) **137**: 2913–2917.

29. Gullberg U, Widegren B, Arnason U, Egesten A, Olsson I: The cytotoxic eosinophil cationic protein (ECP) has ribonuclease activity. *Biochem Biophys Res Comm* (1986) **139**: 1239–1242.

30. Slifman NR, Peterson CGB, Venge P, Dunette SL, Gleich GJ: Eosinophilderived neurotoxin and eosinophil protein-x: comparison of physicochemical, enzymatic and immunologic properties. *J Immunol* (1989) **143**: 2317–2322.

31. Peterson CGB, Venge P: Purification and characterization of a new cationic protein-eosinophil protein-x (EPX) from granules of human eosinophils. *Immunology* (1983) **50**: 19–26.

32. Tai PC, Spry CJF, Peterson C, Venge P, Olsson I: Monoclonal antibodies distinguish between storage and secreted forms of eosinophil cationic protein. *Nature* (1984) **309**: 182–184.

33. Carlson MGC, Peterson CGB, Venge P: Human eosinophil peroxidase: Purification and characterization. *J Immunol* (1985) **134**: 1875–1879.

34. Håkansson L: Anti-inflammatory effects of myeloperoxidase and eosinophil peroxidase. In Venge P, Lindbom A (eds) *Inflammation. Basic Mechanisms, Tissue Injuring Principles and Clinical Models*. Stockholm, Almqvist & Wiksell International, 1985, pp 319–322.

35. Rohrbach MS, Wheatley CL, Slifman NR, Gleich GJ: Activation of platelets by eosinophil granule proteins. *J Exp Med* (1990) **172**: 1271–1274.

36. Ackerman SJ, Loegering DA, Gleich GJ: The human eosinophil Charcot–Leyden crystal protein: biochemical characteristics and measurements by radioimmunoassay. *J Immunol* (1980) **125**: 2118–2126.

37. Weller PF, Goetzl, Austen KF: Identification of human eosinophil lysophospholipase as the constituent of Charcot–Leyden crystals. *Proc Natl Acad Sci USA* (1980) **77**: 7440–7443.

38. Ackerman SJ, Weil GJ, Gleich GJ: Formation of the Charcot–Leyden crystals by human basophils. *J Exp Med* (1982) **155**: 1597–1609.

39. Bruynzeel PLB, Kok PTM, Victor RJ, Verhagen J: On the optimal conditions of LTC$_4$ formation by human eosinophils *in vitro*. *Prostagl Leukotr Med* (1985) **20**: 11–22.

40. Shaw RJ, Cromwell O, Kay AB: Preferential generation of leukotriene C4 by human eosinophil. *Clin Exp Immunol* (1984) **70**: 716–722.

41. Lee T-C, Lenihan DJ, Malone B, Roddy LL, Wasserman SI: Increased biosynthesis of platelet-activating factor in activated human eosinophils. *J Biol Chem* (1984) **259**: 5526–5530.

42. Håkansson L, Westerlund D, Venge P: A new method for the measurement of eosinophil migration. *J Leucocyte Biol* (1987) **42**: 689–696.

43. Hubscher TT: Immune and biochemical mechanisms in the allergic disease of the upper respiratory tract; role of antibodies, target cells, mediators and eosinophils. *Ann Allergy* (1987) **38**: 83–90.

44. Pincus SH, Schooley WR, DiNapoli AM, Broder S: Metabolic heterogeneity of eosinophils from normal and hypereosinophilic patients. *Blood* (1981) **58**: 1175–1181.

45. Beeson PB, Bass DA: The eosinophil. In Smith LH (ed) *Major Problems in Internal Medicine*. Philadelphia, WB Saunders, 1977, pp 46–49.

46. Vadal MA, Varigos B, Nicola N, *et al.*: Eosinophil activation by colony-stimulating factor in man: metabolic effects and analysis by flow cytometry. *Blood* (1983) **61**: 1232–1241.

47. Veith MC, Butterworth AE: Enhancement of human eosinophil-mediated killing of *Schistosoma mansoni* larvae by mononuclear cell products *in vitro*. *J Exp Med* (1983) **157**: 1828–1843.

48. Silberstein DS, David JR: Tumor necrosis factor enhances eosinophil toxicity to *Schistosoma mansoni* larvae. *Proc Natl Acad Sci USA* (1986) **83**: 1055.
49. Silberstein DS, Ali MH, Baker SL, David JR: Human eosinophil cytotoxicity-enhancing factor: purification, physical characteristics, and partial amino acid sequence of an active polypeptide. *J Immunol* (1989) **143**: 979–983.
50. Carlson M, Garcia R, Hakansson L, Pederson CGB, Venge P: The mechanism of IL-5 induced priming of eosinophil degranulation. *J. Leucocyte Biol* (1990), suppl 1, 21.
51. Basten A, Beeson PB: Mechanisms of eosinophilia. II. Role of the lymphocyte. *J Exp Med* (1970) **131**: 1288–1305.
52. Håkansson L, Carlson M, Stålenheim G, Venge P: Migratory responses of eosinophil and neutrophil granulocytes from asthmatic patients. *J Allergy Clin Immunol* (1990) **85**: 743–750.
53. Wegner CD, Gundel RH, Reilly P, Haynes N, Letts LG, Rothlein R: Intercellular adhesion molecule-1 (ICAM-1) in the pathogenesis of asthma. *Science* (1990) **247**: 456–459.
54. Fredens K, Dahl R, Venge P: The Gordon phenomenon induced by the eosinophil cationic protein and eosinophil protein X. *J Allergy Clin Immunol* (1982) **70**: 361–366.
55. Fredens K, Dybdahl H, Dahl R, Baandrup V: Extracellular deposit of the cationic proteins ECP and EPX in tissue infiltrations of eosinophils related to tissue damage. *APMIS* (1988) **96**: 711–719.
56. Ohman JL, Lawrence M, Lowell FC: Effect of propranolol on the eosinophil, responses of cortisol, isoproterenol and aminophylline. *J Allergy Clin Immunol* (1972) **50**: 151–156.
57. Dahl R, Venge P: Blood eosinophil leucocyte and eosinophil cationic protein. *In vivo* study of the influence of β-2-adrenergic drugs and steroid medication. *Scand J Resp Dis* (1978) **59**: 319–322.
58. Reed CE, Cohen M, Enta T: Reduced effect of epinephrine on circulating eosinophils in asthma and after β-adrenergic blockade of *Bordella pertussis* vaccine. *J Allergy* (1970) **46**: 90–102.
59. Koch-Weser J: Beta-adrenergic blockade and circulating eosinophils. *Arch Int Med* (1968) **121**: 255–258.
60. Dahl R, Pedersen B: The influence of inhaled salmeterol on bronchial inflammation. A bronchoalveolar lavage study in patients with bronchial asthma. Joint Meeting SEP-SEPCR, London, 1990.
61. Pedersen B, Dahl R: The effect of salmeterol on the early and late phase reaction to bronchial allergen challenge and postchallenge variation in bronchial hyperreactivity blood eosinophils and serum ECP. EAACI, Glasgow, 1990.
62. Sabag N, Castrillon MA, Tchernitchin A: Cortisol-induced migration of eosinophil leucocytes to lymphoid organs. *Experientia* (1978) **34**: 666–667.
63. Oliver RC, Glauert AM, Throne KJI: Mechanisms of Fc-mediated interaction of eosinophils with immobilized immune complexes. I. Effects of inhibitors and activators of eosinophil function. *J Cell Sci* (1982) **56**: 337–356.
64. Venge P, Dahl R: Eosinophils in asthma. Is blood eosinophil number and activity important for the development of the late asthmatic reaction after allergen challenge? *Eur J Respir Dis* (1989) **2**(Suppl 6): 430s–434s.
65. Ädelroth E, Rosenhall L, Johansson S-Å, Linden M, Venge P: Inflammatory cells and eosinophilic activity in asthmatics investigated by bronchoalveolar lavage: The effects of antiasthmatic treatment with budesonide or terbutaline. *Am Rev Respir Dis* (1990) **142**: 91–99.
66. Bisgaard H, Grønborg H, Mygind N, Dahl R, Lindquist N, Venge P: Allergen induced increase of eosinophil cationic protein in nasal lavage fluid: Effect of the glucocorticoid budesonide. *J Allergy Clin Immunol* (1990) **85**: 891–895.
67. Diaz P, Galleguilles FR, Gonzales MC, Pantin CFA, Kay AB: Bronchoalveolar lavage in asthma: The effect of disodium cromoglycate (cromolyn) on leukocyte counts, immunoglobulins, and complement. *J Allergy Clin Immunol* (1984) **74**: 41–48.

T-lymphocytes

C.J. CORRIGAN AND A.B. KAY

INTRODUCTION

Over the years the course of asthma research has been marked by various vogues. In the early part of the century, the pathogenesis of asthma was regarded as explicable in terms of spasm of bronchial smooth muscle. Later, it became clear that asthmatic airways were not 'normal' between acute attacks in the sense that glucocorticoids could often 'open up' the airways even in relatively mild patients. Studies of bronchial histology in patients who had died of acute asthma confirmed that the bronchial mucosa of asthmatic patients was indeed inflamed. Thus, bronchospasm appeared to be superimposed on airways that were already chronically inflamed and, as a consequence, partially obstructed. Nowadays, bronchial mucosal inflammation is thought to play a key role in the genesis of asthma symptoms, despite the fact that the precise relationship of inflammation to accepted measures of asthma severity, such as non-specific bronchial hyperresponsiveness, remains unclear.

T-lymphocytes probably play a role in all inflammatory responses which are antigen driven since they are the cells which recognize and respond directly to such antigens. T-lymphocytes which express $\alpha\beta$ receptors can be divided into two major functional subgroups according to their expression of the phenotypic surface molecules CD4 and CD8. CD4 cells are now recognized as important mediators of inflammatory responses. The function of CD8 cells is to eliminate body cells expressing new surface antigens as a result of bacterial or viral infection or malignant transformation. They are also largely responsible for the host response to allografts. T-lymphocytes expressing $\gamma\delta$ receptors are relatively abundant at mucosal surfaces, but their precise function in both health and disease is presently unknown. This chapter contains a concise account of the functions of CD4 T-lymphocytes, a summary of the experimental observations which

ASTHMA: BASIC MECHANISMS AND CLINICAL MANAGEMENT (2nd Edn)
ISBN 0-12-079026-2

implicate them in asthma pathogenesis, and a discussion of the implications of these observations with respect to both current and future therapeutic strategies in asthma.

CD4 T-LYMPHOCYTES

Pro-inflammatory role of CD4 T-lymphocytes

T-lymphocytes respond to 'foreign' antigenic material after processing by antigen-presenting cells. It is now clear that CD4 T-lymphocytes, after activation by antigen, have the capacity to elaborate a wide variety of protein mediators called lymphokines. Lymphokines are believed to orchestrate the differentiation, recruitment, accumulation and activation of specific granulocyte effector cells at mucosal surfaces. A full account of the properties of individual lymphokines is provided in Chapter 20. The general properties of lymphokines that are responsible for their pro-inflammatory actions are shown in Table 9.1

To take as an example the case of eosinophils, CD4 T-lymphocytes are a major source of interleukin-5 which is known to (a) promote the differentiation of mature eosinophils from precursor cells;[1,2] (b) prolong the survival of eosinophils *in vitro* from days to weeks, especially in the presence of fibroblasts or endothelial cells;[3,4] (c) exhibit chemotactic activity for eosinophils but not neutrophils *in vitro*, although this effect was weak and requires confirmation;[5] (d) prime eosinophils for increased activity in a number of subsequent effector responses, including antibody-mediated killing of parasitic larvae, elaboration of lipid mediators and activation by platelet-activating factor (PAF).[4,6,7]

Similar effects on eosinophils were shown by interleukin-3[8] and granulocyte/macrophage colony stimulating factor (GM-CSF).[9,10] Interferon-γ can enhance eosinophil cytotoxicity.[11] The fact that T-lymphocyte clones from patients with the hypereosinophilic syndrome had interleukin-5-like activity[12] directly supports the hypothesis that eosinophil numbers and function may be regulated *in vivo* by T-lymphocytes.

Similarly, expansion and differentiation of mast cells in tissues have been shown to be dependent on interleukin-3 and interleukin-4.[13] A deficiency of mucosal (tryptase positive, chymase negative) mast cells was shown in the gastrointestinal tract of human patients with defective T-lymphocyte function.[14] In nude mice, interleukin-3 restored the intestinal mucosal mast cell response to *Strongyloides* infection and facilitated worm expulsion.[15]

Table 9.1 General pro-inflammatory functions of lymphokines.

Increasing the production of granulocytes from precursor cells both in the bone marrow and locally at sites of inflammation

Prolonging the survival of specific granulocytes, thereby causing their accumulation in tissues

Direct chemotaxis of specific granulocytes to sites of inflammation

Priming of specific granulocytes for an enhanced response to physiological activating stimuli

Influencing the activation of B-lymphocytes and the classes of antibodies that they produce in immune responses

These experiments emphasize the facts that activated CD4 T-lymphocytes have the propensity to bring about *selective* accumulation and activation of specific granulocytes in tissues (in contrast to lipid mediators such as leukotrienes and PAF which attract a variety of granulocytes non-specifically), and that T-lymphocyte mediated granulocyte accumulation and activation in asthma may occur independently of the presence or absence of IgE, thus providing a unifying hypothesis for the pathogenesis of asthma in both atopic and non-atopic patients. CD4 T-lymphocytes are therefore inflammatory cells *in their own right* and should not be regarded simply as 'helper' cells for the production of antibody.

It is worth noting that T-lymphocytes are the principal but not the sole source of pro-inflammatory lymphokines. For example, GM-CSF may be elaborated by macrophages and endothelial cells.[16] Mouse mast cell lines *in vitro* have been shown to produce interleukin-3, interleukin-4 and GM-CSF;[17] whether or not an analogous process occurs in human mast cells under physiological conditions remains to be seen, but the subject is clearly of great interest.

T-lymphocytes and the regulation of IgE synthesis

The precise role of IgE-dependent mechanisms in the pathogenesis of asthma is unclear, since not all sensitized atopic patients develop asthma, whilst not all asthmatic patients are obviously atopic. It has already been argued that activated CD4 T-lymphocytes have the capacity to generate eosinophil-rich inflammatory responses independently of the presence or absence of IgE. Nevertheless, it is clear that IgE-mediated reactions can exacerbate asthmatic symptoms in certain atopic individuals, and so to this extent at least the regulation of IgE synthesis is of relevance to a discussion of asthma pathogenesis.

Early observations showed that certain T-lymphocyte clones derived from both atopic and non-atopic individuals by activation with phytohaemagglutinin (PHA), when added to autologous or allogeneic B-lymphocytes, could enhance the synthesis of IgE by the B-lymphocytes.[18] It was later discovered that the amount of preferential IgE synthesis induced by T-lymphocyte clones was related to the amount of interleukin-4 secreted by the clones, and inversely related to the amount of interferon-γ secreted.[19,20] Anti-interleukin-4 antibodies and exogenous interferon-γ consistently inhibited IgE synthesis in these *in vitro* systems, with little effect on the synthesis of IgM or IgG.[19,21] Physical contact between the T- and B- lymphocytes is also essential, since exogenous interleukin-4 alone did not increase IgE synthesis by pure B-lymphocyte populations,[19] and no combination of lymphokines could replace the requirement for T-cell/B-cell contact.[22] The receptor(s) responsible for mediating this T-cell/B-cell contact are unknown. The fact that T-lymphocyte contact and interleukin-4 can induce preferential IgE synthesis in B-lymphocytes regardless of their antigen specificity may partly explain why polyclonal as well as allergen-specific IgE sythesis occurs in atopic individuals. Other lymphokines, including BCGF$_{low}$ and interleukin-2 can further enhance interleukin-4 induced IgE synthesis in these *in vitro* systems[23,24,] probably through their non-specific enhancement of B-lymphocyte proliferation.

Despite these observations, it is still not clear why certain individuals synthesize allergen-specific IgE and others do not. At the population level, atopy shows a strong tendency to be inherited, and recent data suggest that it may be inherited as an autosomal dominant trait with a high degree of penetrance.[25,26] For this reason, researchers have looked for global differences between atopic and non-atopic individuals, with particular regard to the synthesis of interleukin-4 and interferon-γ by their T-lymphocytes. Such differences have proven hard to find: one study of PHA-stimulated T-lymphocyte clones derived from patients with the hyper-IgE syndrome suggested that these cells were deficient in the production of interferon-γ,[27] whilst a second study suggested that a higher proportion of T-lymphocyte clones derived from atopic subjects synthesized interleukin-4 as compared to clones derived from non-atopics.[28] On the other hand, only one of three patients with atopic dermatitis demonstrated T-lymphocyte clones which were deficient in interferon-γ production,[28] whilst a second study of T-lymphocyte clones derived from a patient with the hyper-IgE syndrome failed to show distinct patterns of lymphokine production.[29] It has been shown that the ability of certain highly purified allergens to initiate a T-lymphocyte proliferative response depends on the presence of particular class II MHC molecules on the antigen-presenting cells. For example, the ability of subjects to respond to the *Lol pIII* allergen (one of the allergens of rye grass, *Lolium pratense*) is strongly associated with the presence of the amino acid sequence Glu-Tyr-Ser-Thr-Ser, found in the DRβ1 polypeptide chains of the class II molecules DR3, DR5 and DRw6.[30] Whilst such mechanisms may explain the heritability of IgE responses to *particular* allergens, they are unlikely to account for a global defect in the IgE response to a wide range of allergens.

Another possibility is that only allergen-specific T-lymphocytes in atopic individuals show such abnormalities. This has been regarded as unlikely, since allergens apparently show no particular structural features which distinguish them from other antigens. Nevertheless, it has recently been shown that *D. pteronyssinus*-specific T-lymphocyte clones from two atopic patients secreted large amounts of interleukin-4 and small amounts of interferon-γ on exposure to specific allergen, whereas stimulation of *D. pteronyssinus*-specific clones from an HLA-matched non-atopic donor resulted in the secretion of large amounts of interferon-γ and little interleukin-4.[31] Furthermore, T-lymphocyte clones from the same atopic patients specific for non-allergen antigens (*Candida albicans* or tetanus toxoid) produced small amounts of interleukin-4 and large amounts of interferon-γ. This variability of lymphokine profile appeared to be an inherent property of the T-lymphocytes, since stimulation of *D. pteronyssinus*-specific clones from the atopic patients with antigen-presenting cells from the non-atopic donor did not alter the preferential synthesis of interleukin-4. These observations, if found to be generally applicable in larger numbers of patients and with a wide variety of allergens, would support the hypothesis that atopic patients have regulatory abnormalities confined to T-lymphocytes specific for allergens, rather than a global abnormality of T-lymphocyte responses.

In summary, it is clear that products of activated CD4 T-lymphocytes, particularly interleukin-4 and interferon-γ, have important roles to play in the regulation of IgE synthesis by B-lymphocytes at the cellular level. Recent experiments suggest that abnormalities in IgE regulation may be confined to allergen-specific cells. Hopefully, future studies will determine whether this represents a fundamental abnormality of the atopic state or whether these abnormal clones arise as the result of some other genetic abnormality in atopic patients (for example in the microenvironment where the T-lymphocytes are first exposed to inhaled allergens). Other factors, such as the limiting dose quantity and repetitive nature of the exposure of individuals to allergens may also prove to be of importance.

Th1 and Th2 CD4 T-lymphocytes

Of the wide variety of lymphokines secreted by activated T-lymphocytes, interleukins-3 and -5 and GM-CSF are strongly implicated in allergic inflammation in that they can selectively recruit and activate mast cells and eosinophils, and interleukin-4 is implicated in the sense that it is responsible for the promotion of inappropriate IgE synthesis. The genes encoding all four of these lymphokines are located relatively close together in the human genome, on the long arm of chromosome 5,[32] raising the possibility that their expression may be at least in part coordinately regulated. There is now good evidence that this may be the case, at least in mouse T-lymphocytes. Antigen-activated murine CD4 T-lymphocyte clones can be divided into two broad types called Th1 and Th2, according to the pattern of lymphokines they secrete (Fig. 9.1).[33] Th1 cells secrete interleukin-2, interferon-γ and TNF-β, but not interleukin-4, -5 and -6. Th2 cells secrete interleukin -4, -5 and -6 but not interleukin-2, interferon-γ and TNF-β. Other lymphokines, including interleukin-3 and GM-CSF are secreted by both cell types. The

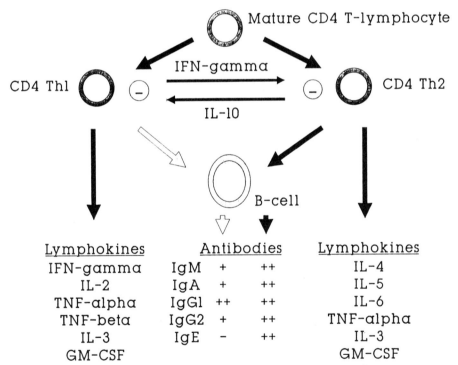

Fig. 9.1 Two functional types of CD4$^+$ T-lymphocyte in the mouse. Little is known about the factors that influence development of Th1 and Th2 cells from putative Th0 cells. Once formed, each can inhibit the proliferation of the other (through interferon-γ and interleukin-10) as shown. As a result of their different basic profiles of lymphokine synthesis, Th1 cells are better equipped to participate in DTH type reactions, whereas Th2 cells tend to promote an antibody response and allergic inflammation.

mechanisms that determine expression of Th1 or Th2 phenotypes are not completely understood. Exogenous lymphokines can favour the development of Th1 or Th2 cells: interferon-γ, when added to antigen-stimulated cultures of mouse CD4 T-lymphocytes favours the expression of the Th1 phenotype,[34] whilst a lymphokine secreted by Th2 cells, called 'cytokine synthesis inhibitory factor' or interleukin-10 inhibits Th1 clone proliferation.[35] Thus, products of Th1 clones have the capacity to inhibit the growth of Th2 clones, and vice versa (Fig. 9.1). In addition to lymphokines, the MHC haplotype of mouse strains has also been reported to influence the preferential development of Th1 and Th2 T-lymphocytes. Thus, mice of different MHC haplotypes, when immunized with the same antigen, may express predominantly a Th1 or Th2 type of lymphokine response in an antigen-specific fashion.[36]

The functional capacities of Th1 and Th2 CD4 T-lymphocyte clones reflect their respective patterns of lymphokine synthesis (Fig. 9.1). Th2 clones, through their secretion of interleukine-4 and -5, serve as excellent helper cells for Ig synthesis by B-lymphocytes *in vitro*,[37] since both these lymphokines non-specifically enhance B-lymphocyte activation. Addition of neutralizing anti-interleukin-4 and -5 antibodies to cultures of B-lymphocytes and Th2 clones causes a substantial inhibition of Ig synthesis.[38,39] In addition, by their secretion of interleukin-3, -4 and -5, Th2 clones favour the synthesis of IgE and the activation of mast cells and eosinophils (see p. 126), and are therefore strongly implicated in the pathogenesis of allergic and asthmatic inflammation. Enhancement of IgE production by interleukin-4 is effected through isotype switching.[40]

Some Th1-type clones have been shown to provide help for B-lymphocyte IgG synthesis, probably through their release of interleukin-2.[41] Th1 clones strongly suppress IgE production through their release of interferon-γ, which also suppresses B-lymphocyte proliferation in a non-specific fashion.[42] Th1 cells, but not Th2 cells, also have the capacity to elicit delayed type hypersensitivity (DTH) reactions *in vivo*. In an experimental system where T-lymphocytes and antigen were injected directly into mouse footpads, only Th1 clones were able to elicit antigen-specific swelling.[43] It is not clear why Th2 cells cannot elicit DTH reactions, but one obvious possibility is that the lymphokines produced by these cells are irrelevant to the pathogenesis of DTH.

In contrast to murine cells, human CD4 T-lymphocyte clones stimulated randomly using PHA do not fall cleanly into Th1 and Th2 patterns, and there are many examples of clones that secrete a mixture of lymphokines characteristic of both categories.[29,44] These results can be reconciled with the data from mice if it is assumed that precursors of Th1 and Th2 cells exist (Th0 cells) which secrete a mixture of Th1- and Th2-derived lymphokines, and that such precursors persist longer in cultures of human T-lymphocytes *in vitro*. Furthermore, evidence has already been presented that the lymphokine profiles of individual human T-lymphocyte clones might depend on their antigen specificity. Other factors, such as the site of antigen presentation and the nature of the antigen-presenting cells, may also be important.

The discovery of a functional dichotomy of activated CD4 T-lymphocytes, which have the propensity either to mediate DTH reactions and suppress IgE synthesis (Th1) or to mediate allergic and asthmatic inflammation and promote IgE synthesis (Th2), is likely to have a profound impact on our understanding of the pathogenesis of asthmatic bronchial inflammation and inappropriate IgE synthesis.

Activation markers on T-lymphocytes

Resting and activated T-lymphocytes

Some molecules appear or increase in numbers on the surface of T-lymphocytes after activation by specific antigen (Fig. 9.2). Expression of these molecules by

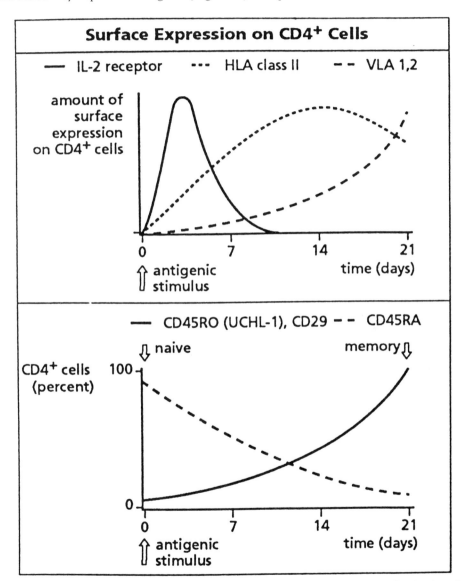

Fig. 9.2 *Upper panel.* Expression of activation markers on the surface of T-lymphocytes after they have been presented with specific antigen. These markers can be used to identify activated T-lymphocytes in tissue and body fluids. *Lower panel.* Reciprocal expression of CD45RA and CD45RO on T-lymphocytes. The functional significance of these changes is not known, but they do provide clues as to whether or not T-lymphocytes arriving at a given site have been previously exposed to antigen.

T-lymphocytes at sites of inflammation implies that they are activated and secreting lymphokines. The receptor for interleukin-2 (a lymphokine produced by activated T-lymphocytes which is essential for their own continued proliferation) appears on the surface of T-lymphocytes about 24 h after activation. In the absence of further antigenic exposure, it persists for several days and then declines.[45] Class II MHC molecules (HLA-DP, DQ and DR) appear on the surface of T-lymphocytes after activation by antigen. Their function on T-lymphocytes, which are not known to present antigen *in vivo*, is unknown but they are useful markers of cellular activation. The VLA family of molecules is concerned with binding of cells to tissue matrix substances such as laminin, fibronectin and collagen. VLA molecules are heterodimeric glycoproteins composed of a common (β_1) polypeptide chain non-covalently linked to a series of α chains (α_1-α_6) on the cell surface. T-lymphocytes begin to express VLA integrins after 2–3 weeks of chronic stimulation *in vitro*,[46] which is why they were originally termed 'Very Late Antigens'. The appearance of these molecules might be related to the need for T-lymphocytes to adhere to tissue at sites of chronic inflammation. Expression of VLA molecules by T-lymphocytes *in vivo* implies their chronic stimulation by specific antigen. VLA molecules are also expressed on granulocytes and a wide variety of other cells and tissues, either constitutively or in the context of inflammation.

Many other molecules are increased in numbers on the T-lymphocyte surface after activation, such as the cellular receptors for transferrin and glucocorticoids.

Naive and memory T-lymphocytes

The CD45 surface molecule is found on all leucocytes. Several structural variants of this molecule have been described, including two of molecular weight 220 and 205 kDa, called CD45RA and CD45RB because of their restricted distribution on B-lymphocytes, T-lymphocytes and NK cells. In addition, a smaller molecular weight species (180 kDa) called CD45RO may also be expressed on T-lymphocytes.[47] All these forms are produced by differential splicing of the mRNA transcript of the CD45 gene,[48] and can be recognized by their binding to specific monoclonal antibodies such as 2H4 (which binds to CD45RA/B but not CD45RO) and UCHL1 (CD45RO only).[49,50] CD45RA and CD45RO are expressed on peripheral blood T-lymphocytes in a reciprocal fashion: CD45RA 'high' cells are CD45RO 'low', and vice versa. CD45RO cells also show increased expression of the surface marker CD29,[51] which can be recognized by monoclonal antibodies such as 4B4. Analysis of CD45 expression by T-lymphocyte clones *in vitro* has shown that individual CD4 CD45RA T-lymphocytes, after activation, progressively lose surface expression of CD45RA and acquire CD45RO and CD29 (Fig. 9.2).[52] These changes do not revert when the activating antigen is removed, in contrast to the activation markers described above. CD45RO, CD29 'high' T-lymphocytes in the laboratory show enhanced help for IgE synthesis, enhanced responses to recall antigens and greater cytotoxicity as compared to CD45RA "high" cells.[53] Furthermore, CD29 'high' cells constitute 40–50% of adult peripheral blood T-lymphocytes but <5% of neonatal umbilical cord T-lymphocytes.[51] For these reasons CD45RO, CD29 'high' cells are thought to be memory cells which have previously been activated by exposure to specific antigen. Arrival of such cells at sites of experimental antigen challenge implies specific recruitment of T-lymphocytes that have previously been exposed to the initiating antigen.

Experimental observations implicating activated CD4 T-lymphocytes in the pathogenesis of asthmatic bronchial inflammation

Relationship of numbers and activation status of CD4 T-lymphocytes to asthma severity

The classical studies of bronchial histopathology in patients having died of asthma,[54] showed an intense invasion of the bronchial mucosa with inflammatory cells, particularly eosinophils and mononuclear cells. More recent studies have concentrated on living asthmatics with milder disease, utilizing the techniques of bronchoalveolar lavage (BAL) and bronchial biopsy through the fibreoptic bronchoscope. These studies have shown that many of the inflammatory changes observed in asthma deaths are also a feature of milder, apparently well-controlled disease. In such studies, attempts are often made to correlate T-lymphocyte numbers and activation status with asthma severity, thus providing circumstantial evidence for involvement of activated T-lymphocytes in the disease. Notwithstanding the fact that its precise cause is unknown, bronchial hyperresponsiveness is widely utilized to measure asthma severity since it is invariably observed in asthmatics and its degree can be correlated with both the severity of symptoms and the amount of therapy required for disease control.[55,56]

In two recent studies of bronchial biopsies obtained from mild atopic asthmatics,[57,58] the numbers and activation status of mucosal T-lymphocytes were assessed by immunostaining with monoclonal antibodies directed against T-lymphocyte phenotypic and activation markers. Interestingly, the total numbers of both CD4 and CD8 T-lymphocytes in the bronchial mucosa of these mild asthmatics was not significantly elevated as compared with the normal controls; CD4 cells predominated over CD8 in both cases. In contrast, only cells in the biopsies from asthmatics showed evidence of interleukin-2 receptor expression, suggesting activation. Furthermore, in the biopsies from asthmatics, the numbers of activated T-lymphocytes could be correlated with both the total numbers of eosinophils and the numbers of activated eosinophils. Finally, the degree of activation could be correlated with the degree of disease severity, as assessed by measurement of bronchial hyperresponsiveness. These observations provide circumstantial evidence supporting the hypotheses that activated CD4 T-lymphocytes control the numbers and activation status of eosinophils in asthmatic bronchial inflammation, and that the degree of activation is one factor which determines disease severity. Using the techniques of immunostaining and flow cytometry, it has been shown that a proportion of CD4 T-lymphocytes, but not CD8 cells, in the peripheral blood of patients with acute severe asthma are activated, as assessed by expression of interleukin-2 receptor, HLA-DR and VLA-1.[59] The degree of activation of these cells decreased after therapy to an extent that could be correlated with the degree of clinical improvement.[60] Fibreoptic bronchoscopy of such patients is not of course clinically or ethically practicable.

Some studies have demonstrated an increase in the relative numbers of lymphocytes found in BAL fluid obtained from patients with mild, stable asthma,[61] whereas others have shown similar numbers in asthmatics and normal controls.[62] Studies on the activation status of these lymphocytes are eagerly awaited. In a further study employing bronchial allergen challenge of sensitized atopic asthmatics,[63] a selective increase in CD4 T-lymphocytes in BAL fluid was observed 48 h after allergen challenge in those subjects who had previously been shown to develop a late-phase reaction. These findings complement those of decrease in CD4 T-lymphocyte numbers in the peripheral blood following allergen inhalation by atopic asthmatics,[64] and together suggest that a process of selective recruitment of CD4 T-lymphocytes to the lung may occur in association with the late phase asthmatic reaction to allergen bronchial challenge. The possible relevance (or otherwise) of this model to the pathogenesis of 'real' asthma has already been discussed. The activation status of these CD4 T-lymphocytes is not known at present, although in a study employing cutaneous allergen challenge of atopic subjects,[65] activated (interleukin-2 receptor bearing) CD4 T-lymphocytes were selectively recruited during the course of the late phase reaction.

Lymphokine secretion by activated CD4 T-lymphocytes in asthma

Despite the fact that sensitive ELISA and radioimmunoassays for many lymphokines are now available, measurement of lymphokine secretion by activated CD4 T-lymphocytes *in vivo* is very difficult owing to their low concentrations and rapid metabolism. Furthermore, the concentrations of lymphokines in the peripheral blood and BAL fluid of asthmatics may only dimly reflect those concentrations released locally in the inflamed bronchial mucosa. In a study referred to above,[60] serum concentrations of interferon-γ were shown to be elevated in a group of acute severe asthmatics as compared with mild asthmatics and normal controls. Interferon-γ secretion is characteristic of a 'Th1 type' response, but since 'Th2 type' lymphokines were not measured in this study it is impossible to assess the relative contributions of each type of response. Furthermore, Th1-type CD4 T-lymphocyte activation might be a superimposed phenomenon in *acute severe* asthma, owing for example to concurrent infection.

One useful alternative to the direct measurement of lymphokine concentrations is the detection of the synthesis of their mRNA using the technique of *in situ* hybridization with lymphokine-specific cDNA probes or riboprobes. Although this is not a strictly quantitative technique, it does have the advantage that it can localize the secretion of lymphokines within cells and tissues. Using this technique it has recently been shown that interleukin-5 mRNA was elaborated by cells in the bronchial mucosa of a majority of mild asthmatics but not normal controls.[66] The amount of mRNA detected correlated broadly with the numbers of activated CD4 T-lymphocytes and eosinophils in biopsies from the same subjects, providing direct evidence supporting the hypothesis that activated CD4 T-lymphocytes secrete interleukin-5 in the asthmatic bronchial mucosa which regulates the numbers and activation status of eosinophils. In a further study using *in situ* hybridization, the cutaneous inflammatory responses to challenge with allergen and tuberculin were compared in atopic subjects.[67] Both types of response (late-phase allergic and DTH) were associated with an influx of activated CD4 T-lymphocytes, but whereas mRNA molecules encoding interleukin-2 and interferon-γ were abundant within the tuberculin reactions, very little mRNA encoding these lymphokines was observed in the late phase allergic reactions. Conversely, mRNA encoding interleukin-4 and -5 was abundant in the late phase allergic but not the tuberculin reactions. In effect, the profiles of lymphokine secretion in the allergic and tuberculin reactions closely parallelled those of Th2 and Th1 CD4 T-lymphocytes, respectively (see page 129). The detection of mRNA does not necessarily equate with protein synthesis, and it will need to be shown that translation and secretion of these lymphokines also occurs. Furthermore, as discussed above, T-lymphocytes are not the only possible sources of these lymphokines. Nevertheless, these observations provide direct evidence in support of the hypothesis that activated CD4 T-lymphocytes, through their patterns of lymphokine secretion, regulate the types of granulocyte which participate in inflammatory reactions. Furthermore, they demonstrate that Th1 and Th2 CD4 T-lymphocyte responses can be detected in humans under physiological conditions, and that the antigen specificity of the T-lymphocyte might be one factor which determines which type of response is initiated.

T-lymphocytes and asthma therapy

Glucocorticoids are the only antiasthma drugs which have been shown unequivocally to reduce the degree of bronchial hyperresponsiveness in asthma of wide-ranging severity and aetiology. The effects of glucocorticoids are dose dependent and cumulative over months.[68,69] Although glucocorticoids are classified as 'anti-inflammatory', their precise mechanism of action is unknown. One possibility is that glucocorticoids act at least in part through a direct inhibitory effect on inflammatory leucocytes. There is now a large body of evidence (reviewed in ref. 70) suggesting that, whereas T-lymphocytes and antigen-presenting cells are exquisitely sensitive to glucocorticoid inhibition in the majority of subjects, B-lymphocytes and granulocytes, particularly eosinophils and mast cells, are insensitive to inhibition by glucocorticoids at therapeutic concentrations. Taken together, these observations allow the hypothesis that the activated CD4 T-lymphocyte may be one primary target of glucocorticoid therapy in asthma (and indeed other inflammatory diseases). Support for this hypothesis has been provided by the observation that resistance to the therapeutic effect of glucocorticoids in groups of difficult-to-manage asthmatics was accompanied by resistance of both T-lymphocytes and antigen-presenting cells isolated from these patients to the inhibitory effects of glucocorticoids *in vitro*.[71–74] Clinical glucocorticoid resistance in these patients was not attributable to abnormal absorption or metabolism of glucocorticoids.[72] Furthermore, other "anti-inflammatory' drugs, such as methotrexate[75] and gold salts[76] have been shown to be effective in asthma therapy, although how far this reflects an inhibitory action on T-lymphocytes is unknown.

Cyclosporin A and the newer compound FK-506 are potent anti-inflammatory reagents whose principal actions are to inhibit T-lymphocyte proliferation and lymphokine secretion. Apart from their widespread use in suppression of allograft rejection, they have been shown to be efficacious in a wide variety of inflammatory diseases such as Crohn's disease.[77] It would seem eminently justifiable to appraise drugs like cyclosporin A for their possible therapeutic effects in asthma, particularly in those patients with chronic, severe disease who are poorly controlled even with oral glucocorticoid therapy.

CONCLUSIONS—THE DIRECTION OF FUTURE RESEARCH

The pathogenesis of asthma—a hypothesis

CD4 T-lymphocytes can respond directly to antigens encountered at mucosal surfaces and, by the secretion of lymphokines, bring about the accumulation and activation of

Mechanisms in asthma

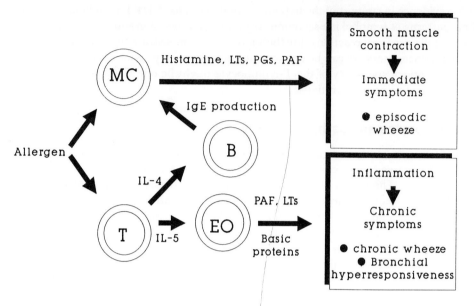

Fig. 9.3   Two pathways for antigen-mediated bronchial mucosal inflammation in asthma. Antigens (including allergens) may activate T-lymphocytes directly, leading to release of lymphokines which subsequently activate granulocytes such as eosinophils. This mechanism need not involve antigen-specific IgE. Antigens may also activate granulocytes (such as mast cells and eosinophils) directly if the latter possess surface-bound antigen-specific IgE which is cross-linked after antigen exposure. This mechanism is not obviously applicable to non-atopic subjects. The first mechanism (which is inhibited by glucocorticoids) may be more important in chronic disease, whilst the second (which is partly inhibited by granulocyte-stabilizing drugs such as cromoglycate) might be responsible for acute exacerbations following exposure of atopic subjects to allergens. MC, mediator cell; B, B-lymphocyte; T, T-lymphocyte; EO, eosinophil.

particular granulocytes. The direct activation of T-lymphocytes by antigen and their subsequent effects on granulocytes form one possible mechanism for the genesis of asthmatic bronchial inflammation, which is independent of the presence or absence of antibodies including IgE (Fig. 9.3).

B-lymphocytes in atopic subjects may secrete IgE in response to airborne allergens and other antigens. The control of this process is in part influenced by CD4 T-lymphocyte products. Allergen-specific IgE bound to granulocyte F_c receptors may activate these cells directly on exposure to allergens, with release of inflammatory mediators. This forms a second possible mechanism for the genesis of asthmatic inflammation which depends upon the presence of allergen-specific antibodies (Fig. 9.3).

It will be important in future studies to delineate the relative contributions of these two parallel mechanisms to the pathogenesis of asthma. Whereas direct degranulation of mast cells and eosinophils on exposure to allergens may be important in producing acute exacerbations of disease in atopic subjects, inflammation orchestrated by activated CD4 T-lymphocytes may be more important in maintaining chronic ongoing disease.

The direction of future studies

If the thesis that mucosal inflammation is important in asthma is to stand the test of time, the precise relationship of inflammation to symptoms of bronchial asthma must be better defined. Every effort must be made to appraise the relevance of 'bronchial hyperresponsiveness' to the pathogenesis of asthma and its precise relationship to inflammation. Finally the validity, or otherwise, of clinical models of asthma must be critically assessed. It would undoubtedly be of value to document the types and amounts of lymphokines present in the bronchial mucosa of asthmatics with disease of varying aetiology and severity. This may be a first step towards defining the pathogenesis of asthma in terms of functional abnormalities at the cellular level, and may uncover variability in asthma pathogenesis according to its aetiology.

Nothing is known about the nature of the activating antigen(s). In cases where a particular provoking antigen can be implicated (e.g. in experimental allergen challenge and occupational asthma), it should be possible to test whether or not antigen-specific T-lymphocytes can be implicated in disease pathogenesis by determining the cloning frequency of allergen-specific T-lymphocytes retrieved from bronchial biopsies or BAL fluid. In other cases (e.g. asthma not associated with atopy) the task is much more difficult, since there is no clue as to the nature of the provoking antigen(s). In such cases the antigens might originate from an external source (aeroallergens, viruses); alternatively, it is possible that CD4 T-lymphocytes in asthmatics may inappropriately recognize antigens within the bronchial mucosa; in other words, asthma may be an 'auto-immune' disease. One indirect approach to this problem might be to examine the usage of antigen receptor $V\beta$ genes by T-lymphocytes in the bronchial mucosa of 'intrinsic' asthmatics. Limited usage of $V\beta$ genes would suggest that the T-lymphocytes are responding to a single antigen (although it is unlikely that the particular antigen could then be identified). This approach has been used to demonstrate, for example, that the T-lymphocyte response in a subset of patients with Crohn's disease was relatively oligoclonal, suggesting a response to a single (unknown) antigen.[78]

In summary, it seems clear that a better understanding of the antigen specificity and functional capacity of CD4 T-lymphocytes in the asthmatic bronchial mucosa will play a large part in our further understanding of the pathogenesis of the disease.

REFERENCES

1. Sanderson CJ, Warren DJ, Strath M: Identification of a lymphokine that stimulates eosinophil differentiation *in vitro. J Exp Med* (1985) **162**: 60–74.
2. Campbell HD, Tucker WQJ, Hort Y, *et al.*: Molecular cloning, nucleotide sequence and expression of the gene encoding human eosinophil differentiation factor (interleukin-5). *Proc Natl Acad Sci USA* (1987) **84**: 6629–6633.
3. Rothenberg ME, Owen WF, Silberstein DS, Soberman RJ, Austen KF, Stevens RL. Eosinophils cocultured with endothelial cells have increased survival and functional properties. *Science* (1987) **237**: 645–647.
4. Rothenberg ME, Petersen J, Stevens RL, *et al.*: IL-5 dependent conversion of normodense human eosinophils to the hypodense phenotype uses 3T3 fibroblasts for enhanced viability, accelerated hypodensity and sustained antibody-dependent cytotoxicity. *J Immunol* (1989) **143**: 2311–2316.

5. Wang JM, Rambaldi A, Biondi A, Chen ZG, Sanderson CJ, Mantovani A: Recombinant human interleukin-5 is a selective eosinophil chemoattractant. *Eur J Immunol* (1989) **19**: 701–705.

6. Lopez AF, Sanderson CJ, Gamble JR, Campbell HD, Young IG, Vadas MA: Recombinant human interleukin-5 is a selective activator of human eosinophil function. *J Exp Med* (1988) **167**: 219–224.

7. Numao T, Fukuda T, Akutsu I, Makino S, Enokihara H, Honjo T: Selective enhancement of eosinophil chemotaxis by recombinant human interleukin-5. *J Allergy Clin Immunol* (1989) **83**: 298.

8. Rotheberg ME, Owen WF, Silberstein DS, *et al.*: Human eosinophils have prolonged survival, enhanced functional properties and become hypodense when exposed to human interleukin-3. *J Clin Invest* (1988) **81**: 1986–1992.

9. Silberstein DS, Owen WF, Gasson JC, *et al.*: Enhancement of human eosinophil cytotoxicity and leukotriene synthesis by biosynthetic (recombinant) granulocyte-macrophage colony stimulating factor. *J Immunol* (1986) **137**: 3290–3294.

10. Lopez AF, Williamson DJ, Gamble JR, *et al.*: Recombinant human granulocyte–macrophage colony stimulating factor stimulates *in vitro* mature human neutrophil and eosinophil function, surface receptor expression and survival. *J Clin Invest* (1986) **78**: 1220–1228.

11. Valerius T, Repp R, Kalden JR, Platzer E. Effects of IFN on human eosinophils in comparison with other cytokines. *J Immunol* (1990) **145**: 2950–2958.

12. Raghavachar A, Fleischer S, Frickhofen N, Heimpel H, Fleischer B: T lymphocyte control of human eosinophilic granulopoiesis. *J Immunol* (1987) **139**: 3753–3758.

13. Stevens RL, Austen KF: Recent advances in the cellular and molecular biology of mast cells. *Immunol Today* (1989) **10**: 381–386.

14. Irani AA, Craig SS, De Blois G, Elson CO, Schechter NM, Schwartz LB: Deficiency of tryptase-positive, chymase-negative mast cell type in gastrointestinal mucosa of patients with defective T lymphocyte function. *J Immunol* (1987) **138**: 4381–4386.

15. Abe T, Nawa Y: Worm expulsion and mucosal mast cell response induced by repetitive IL-3 administration in *Strongyloides ratti* infected nude mice. *Immunology* (1988) **63**: 181–185.

16. Sieff CA: Haematopoietic growth factors. *J Clin Invest* (1987) **79**: 1549–1557.

17. Gordon JR, Burd PR, Galli SJ: Mast cells as a source of multifunctional cytokines. *Immunol Today* (1990) **11**: 458–464.

18. Romagnani S, Maggi E, Del Prete GF, Ricci M: Activation through CD3 molecule leads a number of human T-cell clones from allergic and non-allergic individuals to promote IgE synthesis. *J Immunol* (1987) **138**: 1744–1749.

19. Del Prete GF, Maggi E, Parronchi P, *et al.*: IL-4 is an essential factor for the IgE synthesis induced *in vitro* by human T-cell clones and their supernatants. *J Immunol* (1988) **140**: 4193–4198.

20. Maggi E, Del Prete GF, Macchia D, *et al.*: Profile of lymphokine activities and helper function for IgE in human T cell clones. *Eur J Immunol* (1988) **18**: 1045–1050.

21. Pene I, Rousset F, Briere F, *et al.*: IgE production by normal human lymphocytes is induced by interleukin-4 and suppressed by interferons γ and α and prostaglandin E_2. *Proc Natl Acad Sci USA* (1988) **85**: 6880–6884.

22. Vercelli D, Jabara HH, Arai K, Geha RS: Induction of human IgE synthesis requires IL-4 and T/B cell interactions involving the T cell receptor/CD3 complex and MHC class II antigens. *J Exp Med* (1989) **169**: 1295–1308.

23. Parronchi P, Tiri A, Macchia D, *et al.*: Noncognate contact-dependent B-cell activation can promote IL-4 dependent *in vitro* human IgE synthesis. *J Immunol* (1990) **144**: 2102–2108.

24. De Kruyff RH, Turner T, Abrams JS, Palladino MA, Umetsu DT: Induction of human IgE synthesis by CD4+ T cell clones. Requirement for interleukin-4 and low molecular weight B Cell growth factor. *J Exp Med* (1989) **170**: 1477–1493.

25. Cookson WOCM, Hopkin JM: Dominant inheritance of atopic IgE responsiveness. *Lancet* (1988) **1**: 86–88.

26. Cookson WOCM, Sharp PA, Faux JA, Hopkin JM: Linkage between IgE responses underlying asthma and rhinitis and chromosome 11q. *Lancet* (1989) **1**: 1292–1295.

27. Del Prete G, Tiri A, Maggi E, *et al.*: Defective *in vitro* production of γ-interferon and tumour necrosis factor-α by circulating T-cells from patients with hyper-immunoglobulin E syndrome. *J Clin Invest* (1989) **84**: 1830–1835.

28. Romagnani S, Del Prete G, Maggi E, *et al.*: Role of interleukins in induction and regulation of human IgE synthesis. *Clin Immunol Immunopathol* (1989) **50**: 513–518.

29. Quint DJ, Bolton EJ, MacNamee LA, *et al.*: Functional and phenotypical analysis of human T-cell clones which stimulate IgE production *in vitro*. *Immunology* (1989) **67**: 68–74.

30. Ansari AA, Freidhoff LR, Meyers DA, Bias WB, Marsh DG: Human immune responsiveness to *Lolium perenne* allergen *Lol pIII* (*rye III*) is associated with HLA-DR3 and DR5. *Human Immunol* (1989) **25**: 59–71.

31. Wierenga EA, Snoek M, de Groot C, *et al.*: Evidence for compartmentalisation of functional subsets of CD4+ T-lymphocytes in atopic patients. *J Immunol* (1990) **144**: 4651–4656.

32. Chandraseknarappa SC, Rebelsky MS, Firak TA, Le Beau MM, Westbrook CA: A long-range restriction map of the interleukin-4 and interleukin-5 linkage group on chromosome 5. *Genomics* (1990) **6**: 94–99.

33. Mosmann TR, Coffman RL: Th1 and Th2 cells: different patterns of lymphokine secretion lead to different functional properties. *Annu Rev Immunol* (1989) **7**: 145–173.

34. Gajewski TF, Joyce J, Fitch FW: Antiproliferative effect of interferon-γ in immune regulation. III. Differential selection of Th1 and Th2 murine helper T-lymphocyte clones using recombinant IL-2 and recombinant IFN-γ. *J Immunol* (1989) **143**: 15–20.

35. Fiorentino D, Bond HW, Mosmann TR: Two types of mouse T helper cells. IV. Th2 clones secrete a factor that inhibits cytokine production by Th1 clones. *J Exp Med* (1989) **170**: 65–80.

36. Murray JS, Madri J, Tite J, Carding SR, Bottomly K: MHC control of CD4+ T cell subset activation. *J Exp Med* (1989) **170**: 2135–2140.

37. Stevens TL, Bossie A, Sanders VM, *et al.*: Regulation of antibody isotype secretion by subsets of antigen-specific helper T Cells. *Nature* (1988) **334**: 255–258.

38. Boom WH, Liano D, Abbas AK: Heterogeneity of human helper/inducer T-lymphocytes. II. Effects of interleukin-4 and interleukin-2-producing T cell clones on resting B-lymphocytes. *J Exp Med* (1988) **167**: 1352–1363.

39. Rasmussen R, Takatsu K, Harada N, Takahashi T, Bottomly K: T cell-dependent hapten-specific and polyclonal B cell responses require release of interleukin-5. *J Immunol* (1988) **140**: 705–712.

40. Lebman DA, Coffman RL: Interleukin-4 causes isotype switching to IgE in T-cell-stimulated clonal B cell cultures. *J Exp Med* (1988) **168**: 853–862.

41. Coffman RL, Seymour BW, Lebman DA, *et al.*: The role of helper T cell products in mouse B cell differentiation and isotype regulation. *Immunol Rev* (1988) **102**: 5–28.

42. Reynolds DS, Boom WH, Abbas AK: Inhibition of B-lymphocyte activation by interferon-γ. *J Immunol* (1987) **139**: 767–773.

43. Cher DJ, Mosmann TR: Two types of murine helper T cell clone: 2. Delayed-type hypersensitivity is mediated by Th1 clones. *J Immunol* (1987) **138**: 3688–3694.

44. Paliard X, de Waal Malefijt R, Yssel H, *et al.*: Simultaneous production of IL-2, IL-4 and IFN-γ by activated human CD4+ and CD8+ T cell clones. *J Immunol* (1988) **141**: 849–855.

45. Hemler ME, Brenner MB, McLean JM, Strominger JL: Antigenic stimulation regulates the level of interleukin-2 receptor expression on human T cells. *Proc Natl Acad Sci USA* (1984) **81**: 2172–2176.

46. Hemler ME, Huang C, Schwarz L: The VLA protein family: characterisation of five distinct cell surface heterodimers each with a common 130 000 Mr beta subunit. *J Biol Chem* (1987) **262**: 3300–3309.

47. Beverley PCL, Merkenschlager M, Terry L: Phenotypic diversity of the CD45 antigen and its relationship to function. *Immunology* (1988) (Suppl 1) 3–5.

48. Ralph SJM, Thomas ML, Morton CC, Trowbridge IS: Structural variants of human T200 glycoprotein (leukocyte common antigen). *EMBO J* (1987) **6**: 1251–1257.

49. Morimoto C, Letvin NL, Distaso JA, Aldrich WR, Schlossman SF: The isolation and characterisation of the human suppressor inducer T cell subset. *J Immunol* (1985) **134**: 1508–1515.

50. Terry LA, Brown MH, Beverley PCL: The monoclonal antibody UCHL1 recognises a 180 000 MW component of the human leukocyte common antigen, CD45. *Immunology* (1988) **64**: 331–336.
51. Sanders ME, Makgoba MW, Sharrow SO, *et al.*: Human memory T-lymphocytes express increased levels of three cell adhesion molecules (LFA-3, CD2 and LFA-1) and three other molecules (UCHL1, CDw29 and Pgp-1) and have enhanced IFN-γ production. *J Immunol* (1988) **140**: 1401–1407.
52. Akbar AN, Terry L, Timms A, Beverley PCL, Janossy G: Loss of CD45R and gain of UCHL1 reactivity is a feature of primed T-cells. *J Immunol* (1988) **140**: 2171–2178.
53. Sanders ME, Makgoba MW, Shaw S: Human naive and memory T Cells: reinterpretation of helper-inducer and suppressor-inducer subsets. *Immunol Today* (1988) **9**: 195–198.
54. Dunnill MS. The pathology of asthma with special reference to the bronchial mucosa. *J Clin Pathol* (1960) **13**: 27–33.
55. Hargreave FE, Ryan G, Thomson NC, *et al.*: Bronchial responsiveness to histamine or methacholine in asthma: measurement and clinical significance. *J Allergy Clin Immunol* (1981) **68**: 347–355.
56. Juniper EF, Frith PA, Hargreave FE: Airway responsiveness to histamine and methacholine: relationship to minimum treatment to control symptoms of asthma. *Thorax* (1981) **36**: 575–579.
57. Azzawi M, Bradley B, Jeffery PK, *et al.*: Identification of activated T-lymphocytes and eosinophils in bronchial biopsies in stable asthma. *Am Rev Respir Dis* (1990) **142**: 1407–1413.
58. Bradley BL, Azzawi M, Jacobson M, *et al.*: Eosinophils, T-lymphocytes, mast cells, neutrophils and macrophages in bronchial biopsies from atopic asthma: comparison with atopic non-asthma and normal controls and relationship to bronchial hyperresponsiveness. *J Allergy Clin Immunol* (1991) **88**: 661–674.
59. Corrigan CJ, Hartnell A, Kay AB: T-lymphocyte activation in acute severe asthma. *Lancet* (1988) **1**: 1129–1131.
60. Corrigan CJ, Kay AB: CD4 T-lymphocyte activation in acute severe asthma. Relationship to disease severity and atopic status. *Am Rev Respir Dis* (1990) **141**: 970–977.
61. Graham DR, Luksza AR, Evans CC: Bronchoalveolar lavage in asthma. *Thorax* (1985) **40**: 717.
62. Wardlaw AJ, Dunnette S, Gleich GJ, Collins JV, Kay AB: Eosinophils and mast cells in bronchoalveolar lavage fluid in mild asthma: relationship to bronchial hyperreactivity. *Am Rev Respir Dis* (1988) **137**: 62–69.
63. Metzger WJ, Zavala D, Richerson HB, *et al.*: Local allergen challenge and bronchoalveolar lavage of allergic asthmatic lungs. Description of the model and local airway inflammation. *Am Rev Respir Dis* (1987) **135**: 433–440.
64. Gerblich AA, Campbell AE, Schuyler MR: changes in T-lymphocyte subpopulations after antigenic bronchial provocation in asthmatics. *N Engl J Med* (1984) **310**: 1349–1352.
65. Frew AJ, Kay AB. The relationship between infiltrating CD4+ T-lymphocytes, activated eosinophils and the magnitude of the allergen-induced late-phase cutaneous reaction. *J Immunol* (1988) **141**: 4158–4164.
66. Hamid Q, Azzawi M, Ying S, *et al.*: Expression of mRNA for interleukin-5 in mucosal bronchial biopsies from asthma. *J Clin Invest* (1991) **87**: 1541–1546.
67. Kay AB, Ying S, Varney V, *et al.*: Messenger RNA expression of the cytokine gene cluster IL-3, IL-5 and GM-CSF in allergen-induced late-phase reactions in atopic subjects. *J Exp Med* (1991) **173**: 775–778.
68. Kraan J, Koeter GH, Van der Mark W, *et al.*: Dosage and time effects of inhaled budesonide on bronchial hyperreactivity. *Am Rev Respir Dis* (1988) **137**: 44–48.
69. Kerrebijn KF, Van Essen-Zandvliet EEM, Niejens HJ: Effect of long-term treatment with inhaled corticosteroids and beta-agonists on the bronchial responsiveness in children with asthma. *J Allergy Clin Immunol* (1987) **79**: 653–659.
70. Various authors in: Schleimer RP, Claman HN, Oronsky A (eds) *Anti-inflammatory Steroid Action: Basic and Clinical Aspects*. London, Academic Press, 1989.
71. Poznansky MC, Gordon ACH, Grant IWB, Wyllie AH: A cellular abnormality in glucocorticoid resistant asthma. *Clin Exp Immunol* (1985) **61**: 135–142.

72. Corrigan CJ, Brown PH, Barnes NC, *et al.*: Clucocorticoid resistance in chronic asthma: glucocorticoid pharmacokinetics, glucocorticoid receptor characteristics and inhibition of peripheral blood T-lymphocyte proliferation by glucocorticoids *in vitro*. *Am Rev Respir Dis* (1991) **144**: 1016–1025.

73. Corrigan CJ, Brown PH, Barnes NC, Tsai J-J, Frew AJ, Kay AB: Glucocorticoid resistance in chronic asthma: activation of peripheral blood T-lymphocytes in glucocorticoid resistant asthmatics, and a comparison of the *in vitro* inhibitory effects of glucocorticoids and cyclosporin A. *Am Rev Respir Dis* (1991) **144**: 1026–1032.

74. Wilkinson JRW, Crea AEG, Clark TJH, Lee TH: Identification and characterisation of a monocyte-derived neutrophil-activating factor in corticosteroid-resistant bronchial asthma. *J Clin Invest* (1989) **84**: 1930 1941.

75. Mullarkey MF, Blumenstein BA, Andrade WP, Bailey GA, Olason I, Wetzel CE: Methotrexate in the treatment of corticosteroid-dependent asthma. A double blind crossover study. *N Engl J Med* (1988) **318**: 603–607.

76. Bernstein DI, Bernstein IL, Bodenheimer SS, Pietrusko RG: An open study of auranofin in the treatment of corticosteroid-dependent asthma. *J Allergy Clin Immunol* (19988) **81**: 6–16.

77. Brynskov J, Trede N: Plasma interleukin-2 and a soluble/shed interleukin-2 receptor in the serum of patients with Crohn's disease. Effect of cyclosporin. *Gut* (1990) **31**: 795–799.

78. Posnett DN, Schmelkin I, Burton DA, August A, McGrath H, Mayer LF: T cell antigen receptor V gene usage: increases in Vβ8+ T cells in Crohn's disease. *J Clin Invest* (1990) **85**: 1770–1776.

Epithelial Cells

ROBERT J. DAVIES AND JAGDISH L. DEVALIA

INTRODUCTION

Recent evidence suggests that the airway epithelium plays a critical role, not only in the pathogenesis of the inflammation that characterizes asthma but also in its aetiology. Traditionally the airway epithelium has been regarded as a physical barrier, playing an important role in mucociliary clearance and preventing entry of noxious agents into the underlying tissues. This is not difficult to envisage when the cell types are considered (Fig. 10.1). The upper airway is lined by a pseudostratified ciliated columnar epithelium containing columnar and basal cells, of which the latter type gradually decreases in number distally in the lower airways, until there are none in the terminal and respiratory bronchioles. The basal cells are thought to play a role in the attachment of the columnar cells to the airway basement membrane[1] and contrary to popular belief, do not appear to be the progenitor cells for the airway epithelium. The columnar cells, on the other hand are composed of ciliated and non-ciliated cells. Of these, the non-ciliated cells (also referred to as the mucous cells) comprise the goblet, serous, Clara and presecretory cell types and are involved primarily in the production of airway secretions. These cells are also thought to be the progenitor cells for the terminally differentiated ciliated cells.[2] Electron microscopic studies of the airways have demonstrated that the ciliated cells are joined to each other at the luminal surface by tight junctions, which serve to present a permeability barrier[3,4] and to maintain the integrity of the epithelium (Fig. 10.2).[5] The ciliated cells additionally play a central role in mucociliary clearance which is an integral component of defence against infectious agents and inhaled toxic materials in the respiratory system.[4] Studies of mucociliary clearance have demonstrated that efficient transport of mucus is determined by synchronized beating of the

ASTHMA: BASIC MECHANISMS AND CLINICAL MANAGEMENT (2nd Edn)
ISBN 0-12-079026-2

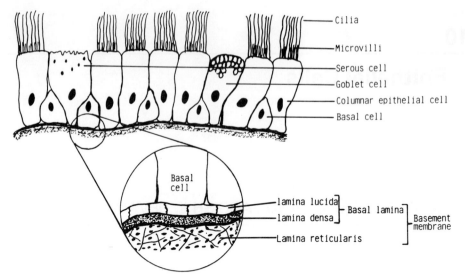

Fig. 10.1 Schematic view of the major epithelial cell types in airway epithelium.

ciliated cells and may be influenced by the autonomic nervous system, since both adrenergic and cholinergic agents[6,7] stimulate ciliary beat frequency of these cells.

AIRWAY EPITHELIUM AND HYPERREACTIVITY

The bronchial epithelium acts as both a physically and a metabolically active barrier, which under normal circumstances regulates and maintains a chemical homeostasis necessary for the functional integrity of the airways.[8] Damage to the epithelium results in an imbalance of this homeostasis and consequently plays an important role in the development of airway disease.

Although it has been suggested that mediator release and the response of the airways to these mediators are important in the clinical manifestation of asthma, the nature of the important cells and the mediators involved remain to be fully elucidated. Whilst some studies have suggested an increase in inflammatory cells such as neutrophils,[9] eosinophils[10,11] and mast cells[12] as being important, others have implicated that damage to the epithelial cells may be more important.[13-15]

Although several histopathological studies have demonstrated that epithelium damage is a characteristic feature of fatal status asthmaticus,[5,16,17] others have demonstrated that epithelial derangement may also be present during remissions[13] or be absent altogether, as found in mild asthmatic subjects.[18] It is not yet clear whether the loss of epithelial integrity contributes to the increased bronchial responsiveness or whether it is itself a result of the airway inflammation and the consequential hyperreactivity. Due to the role of the epithelium as a physicochemical barrier, it is possible that several mechanisms, including (a) increased permeability to allergen;[19,20] (b) changes in osmolarity of the bronchial surface lining fluid;[19] (c) exposure of sensory nerve fibres and potentiation of local axon reflexes;[21] (d) production of inflammatory[22-25] and reduction

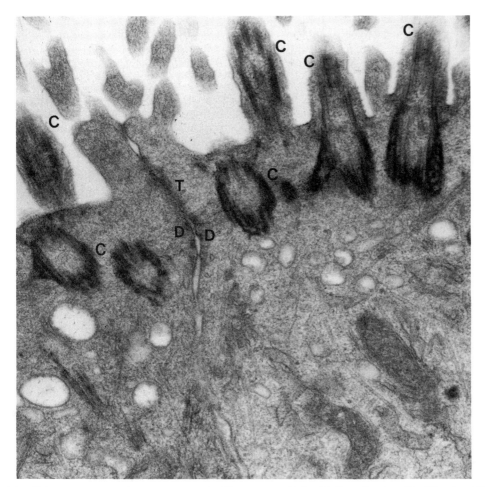

Fig. 10.2   Transmission electron micrograph of human bronchial epithelium showing cilia (C), microvilli (M), tight junction (T) and desmosomes (D) (magnification × 33 600).

of putative 'protective' (both anti-inflammatory and relaxing)[26–30] epithelium-derived mediators; (e) production of specifically 'inflammatory' cytokines and their interactions with other cytokines[31–32] and (f) modulation of the immune system[33] may explain how epithelial abnormalities could lead to increased bronchial reactivity. Of these mechanisms, those involving synthesis and release of agents with either inflammatory or protective properties and immunoregulation by the epithelial cells have been the most widely studied and will be discussed in greater detail.

MEDIATOR RELEASE

Animal tracheal epithelial cells have been shown to generate leukotrienes B_4 and C_4 (LTB$_4$ and LTC$_4$) and prostaglandins D_2, E_2, $F_{2\alpha}$ and 6-keto-$F_{1\alpha}$ (PGD$_2$, PGE$_2$, PGF$_{2\alpha}$

and PG6-keto-$F_{1\alpha}$).[22,34] Recently, it has been found that ozone (O_3), which may have a mechanism similar to that of nitrogen dioxide (NO_2), augments eicosanoid metabolism in bovine tracheal epithelial cells, with significant increases in PGE_2, $PGF_{2\alpha}$, 6-keto-$F_{1\alpha}$ and LTB_4.[35] Studies with cultured human tracheal and bronchial epithelial cells have demonstrated that these cells can also generate PGE_2 and $PGF_{2\alpha}$ and additionally 12- and 15-lipoxygenase metabolites, such as 12- and 15-hydroxyeicosotetraenoic acids (12-HETE and 15-HETE).[23,25,36] We have recently demonstrated that human bronchial epithelial cells exposed to NO_2 at concentrations as low as 0.4 p.p.m., occasionally found at the kerb side in heavy summer traffic, generate PGE_2, 15-HETE and 12-HETE and additionally LTC_4.[37]

The generation of these mediators and indeed their relevance in the initiation of hyperreactivity in asthma remain questionable. There are species differences with respect to both the stimulus required and the mediator/s released. Although animal studies have demonstrated that tracheal epithelial cells are capable of generating LTB_4,[22] an eosinophil chemoattractant, this has not been shown to be the case for the human cells which have been shown to synthesize 15-HETE, another potential eosinophil chemoattractant.[23] Also most investigations have concentrated on compounds of arachidonic acid origin and it is possible that the bronchial epithelium may preferentially generate other mediators such as PAF, a more potent and selective eosinophil chemoattractant[38] and activator,[39] in vivo. Although human tracheal epithelial cells have been shown to contain both linoleic acid and arachidonic acid, which are similarly distributed and available for metabolism via the oxidative pathways,[40] most in vitro studies have looked at metabolism of arachidonic acid, which has been exogenously added to the test system and which itself may lead to its preferential metabolism. Indeed, studies of ω-6-lipoxygenase, a naturally occurring enzyme in leucocytes, have demonstrated that the normally preferred metabolism of linoleic acid by this enzyme, becomes altered in favour of exogenously added arachidonic acid.[41]

The possibility that epithelial cells produce 'protective' compounds which have either relaxing or chemorepellant properties, has recently been explored. Flavahan and co-workers[26,27] originally reported that mechanical removal of epithelium from canine bronchial rings rendered these hyperresponsive to histamine, 5-hydroxy tryptamine and acetylcholine and thus suggested that this bronchoconstrictive response was a consequence of the removal of a naturally occurring relaxing factor being released by the epithelium. Although others have since demonstrated a similar effect of epithelium removal on the underlying airway smooth muscle in vitro,[28–30,42–44] the nature of the putative factor/s still remains to be elucidated. It has, however, been suggested that the epithelium-dependent attenuation of airway reactivity to bronchoconstrictors in guinea-pigs,[42] dogs[26] and rabbits[44] may involve an inhibitory cyclooxygenase metabolite of arachidonic acid since indomethacin reverses this attenuation.

In a system involving the use of human umbilical vein-derived endothelial cell cultures, Buchanan et al.[45] have demonstrated that 13-hydroxyoctadecadiene (13-HODE), a metabolite of linoleic acid having chemorepellant activity towards neutrophils, is generated under normal conditions. These authors have further demonstrated that in this model linoleic acid is metabolized in preference to arachidonic acid, under 'basal' or unstimulated conditions.

Quite separately from synthesizing specifically the 'protective mediators', it has been suggested that airway epithelial cells may also play a protective role against the various adverse effects of the tachykinins, by modulating their degradation by an epithelium-associated endopeptidase.[46] Indeed, we have recently demonstrated that human cultured bronchial epithelial cells contain the mRNA coding for neutral endopeptidase (NEP), and are therefore capable of synthesizing this enzyme (unpublished data).

It is possible that concentrations of compound/s produced by the epithelium under normal conditions, and which act directly or indirectly as airway smooth muscle relaxants and have anti-inflammatory properties, could be diminished following epithelial cell damage and rendering the airways inflamed and hyperresponsive.

CYTOKINE SYNTHESIS

The cytokines have received a great deal of attention in the last decade and their role particularly in inflammatory responses has been reviewed.[31,47] Studies in both rodents and humans have demonstrated that interleukin-3 (IL-3, Multi-CSF), interleukin-5 (IL-5) and the colony stimulating factors (CSF), granulocyte-macrophage-CSF (GM-CSF) and granulocyte-CSF (G-CSF) which closely resemble IL-3, are capable of stimulating the growth, differentiation and activation of basophil/mast cells, neutrophils and eosinophils either individually or in conjuction with one another.[31,48] More recently, it has been demonstrated that GM-CSF and other factors enhance the viability and the functional activation of eosinophils *in vitro*,[49] and it has been suggested that similar effects induced by IL-3 and IL-5 may also predominate in allergy and hypereosinophilic syndromes, *in vivo*.[50]

Although the production of these cytokines has generally been attributed to fibroblasts, lymphocytes, macrophages and endothelial cells, recent evidence suggests that airway epithelial cells are also capable of synthesizing some of these compounds. Studies with human nasal,[51] bronchial[52] and tracheal epithelial cells[53] in culture have demonstrated that these cells are capable of synthesizing GM-CSF. It has, however, been suggested that other cytokines such as interleukin-1 (IL-1) and tumour necrosis factor (TNF), which have also been shown to be produced by human bronchial epithelial cell cultures[32] and epithelial tumour cell lines,[54] may induce the production of CSFs[55] and other inflammatory cytokines such as interleukin-8 (IL-8; also known as neutrophil chemotactic factor).[56]

With the advent of highly specialized molecular biology techniques and availability of specific molecular probes and monoclonal antibodies, interest has recently focused on the role of the cytokines in induction of specific ligands and receptors which may play an important role in the development of inflammation of the airways. Several investigators have reported that the expression of one such ligand, intercellular adhesion molecule-1 (ICAM-1), a member of the immunoglobulin superfamily, which is active in the recruitment and migration of neutrophils[57,58] and eosinophils[59] and which has also been shown to be the surface receptor for the major group of Rhinoviruses,[60–63] is upregulated by IL-1, interferon-γ (IFN-γ) and TNF.[63–64] Although ICAM-1 has been reported to be expressed on several human epithelial cell types,[63] to our knowledge there are no reports of ICAM-1 expression on human airway epithelial cells, to date. Using a cell culture system,[65] we have recently demonstrated that human bronchial epithelial cells are capable of expressing ICAM-1, at least *in vitro* (Fig. 10.3).[66] This may have important

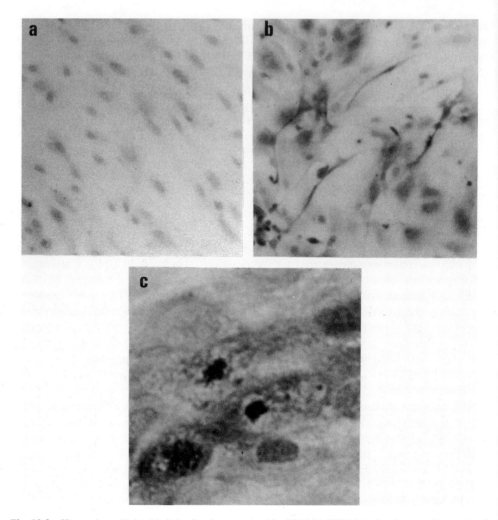

Fig. 10.3 Human bronchial epithelial cell cultures stained for ICAM-1 (CD54) in the absence of monoclonal antibody MCA 532 (Serotec, England) (a = negative control; magnification × 175) and in the presence of monoclonal antibody MCA 532 (b = magnification × 175; c = magnification × 875).

implications regarding infiltration of the bronchus by eosinophils and neutrophils, as is seen in the airways of asthmatics during exacerbation.

IMMUNOREGULATION

Cytokines have been shown to influence expression of the major histocompatibility complex (MHC) class II antigens on the surface of epithelial cells, thereby conferring upon these cells a potentially important role of antigen processing and presentation to the T-lymphocytes. Studies of cultured human retinal pigment epithelial cells[67] and foetal pancreatic duct epithelial cells[68] have demonstrated that these cells are capable of expressing the HLA DR antigens, following exposure to IFN-γ. Of more relevance to airway diseases, however, immunohistochemical studies of human fibrotic lung[69] and human bronchial tissue, obtained from patients with peripheral lung cancer,[70] have reported that the Type II alveolar epithelial cells and ciliated bronchial epithelial cells, respectively, express the HLA DR antigens and the genes encoding these antigens.

The putative mechanisms and consequences of the interaction between antigen-presenting cells (APCs) and T-lymphocytes have been reviewed recently.[33] It has been suggested that preferential binding of specific allergenic peptides to the HLA-class II antigens may lead to recognition by—and activation—and proliferation—of specific T-cell clones (either Th1 or Th2 clones), which predispose the individual to the development of certain diseases. Th1-lymphocytes produce predominantly interleukin-2 (IL-2) and/or IFN-γ and are thought to be involved in delayed-type hypersensitivity reactions and in the synthesis of IgM and some IgG subclasses. The Th2-lymphocytes, on the other hand, have been shown to synthesize interleukins-4, -5, -6 and more recently -10, and are thought to be important in allergic-type inflammatory reactions and defence against parasites. Of the various cytokines produced by the different sets of T-cells, it has been suggested that whilst IFN-γ is capable of inhibiting growth and proliferation of the Th2-lymphocytes, IL-4 and IL-10, also known as cytokine synthesis inhibitory factor (CSIF), are capable of influencing the growth and function of the Th1-lymphocytes.

CULTURE OF HUMAN AIRWAY EPITHELIAL CELLS, *IN VITRO*

In spite of increasing evidence for an important physicochemical role of the airway epithelium *in vivo*, it has not proved easy to assign a specific pathogenic role to the airway epithelium *in vivo*, due to the presence of other cell types and underlying tissues. Human airway epithelial cell cultures offer an ideal *in vitro* model system for the study of the epithelium in the aetiology of airway diseases and the underlying mechanism/s of inflammation and hyperresponsiveness. Although nasal and bronchial epithelial cells have been cultured *in vitro* by several groups,[71–74] a major difficulty experienced by many of the workers in the field has been to get these cells to grow consistently to confluency, such that large numbers can subsequently be harvested for further study. Also the epithelial cells have often been isolated from enzyme-dispersed tissue, which in itself is known to bring about detrimental morphological and biochemical changes and in the case of the earlier studies investigating bronchial cells, the bronchial tissue has been obtained 8–12 h post-mortem, again questioning the physiological status of the cells. Indeed, Farber and Young[75] and others have demonstrated that anoxic conditions lead to accelerated degradation of membrane phospholipids and consequently cause irreversible cell injury. We have addressed these difficulties and have recently demonstrated that it is possible to culture to confluency, both nasal and bronchial epithelial cells to the fully differentiated ciliated cell types (Fig. 10.4).[65] To our knowledge there are no reports of any form of a comparison between cells of asthmatic and non-asthmatic subjects *in vitro*, details of which may give a better insight into the role of these cells in the aetiology of asthma.

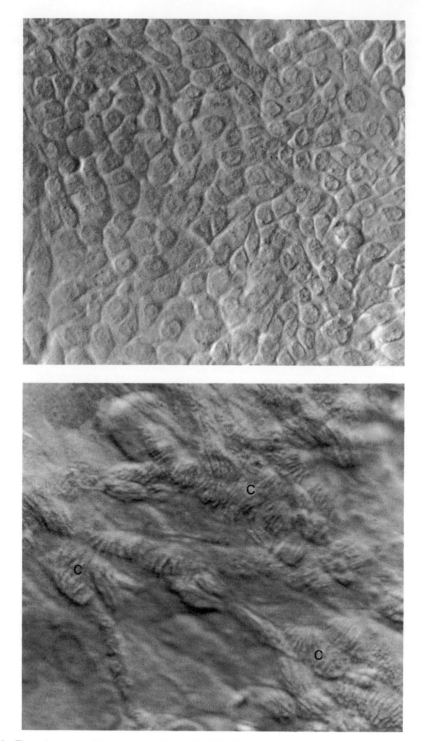

Fig. 10.4 Typical culture of human bronchial epithelial cells, viewed by light microscopy incorporating Hoffman Modulation Contrast optics at (a) low power (magnification × 300) and (b) high power, showing ciliated cells (C) (magnification × 600).

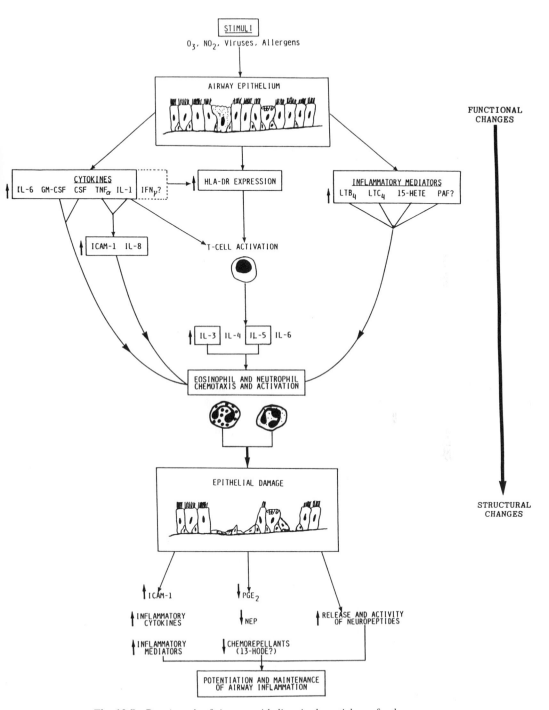

Fig. 10.5 Putative role of airways epithelium in the aetiology of asthma.

SUMMARY

Taken together, these studies indicate that human epithelial cells have the capacity to generate a range of inflammatory compounds and to regulate the expression of others such as the cytokines and cell-adhesion molecules. In view of the importance of the airway epithelium as the first line of defence against airborne dusts, vapour, gases and fumes and its capacity to play a role in the maintenance of a physicochemical homeostasis, it is not difficult to envisage how perturbation of this barrier, and particularly the epithelial cells which predominate within this barrier, may bring about adverse changes in and around the surrounding tissues and possibly help to explain the pathogenesis of asthma.

It is tempting to hypothesize that in bronchial asthma dysfunction of the bronchial epithelium, as a result of acute exposure to irritants such as air pollutants, cigarette smoke, viruses, bacteria, etc. or as a consequence of genetic predisposition to a specific allergen, itself results in the initiation, maintenance and potentiation of inflammation at the site/s of exposure (Fig. 10.5). This may be expressed either in the form of generation of potent eosinophil and neutrophil chemoattractants and activators or else in the form of compounds such as the cytokines which have profound effects either directly or indirectly on growth, differentiation and maintenance and inter-tissue trafficking of these and other 'inflammatory' cell types, such as the Th2-lymphocytes. Alternatively, depletion of any naturally occurring anti-inflammatory mediators and smooth-muscle relaxing agents, which help to maintain the integrity of the bronchus and the surrounding tissues, may ensue.

In view of advances that have been made in the understanding of the putative mechanisms that may be of importance in the aetiology of asthma it should be possible to formulate specific therapies that counteract not only the bronchoconstriction that is so characteristic of asthma, but the events leading to bronchoconstriction. It is probable that this new generation of therapeutic agents will address the question of the specific inflammatory cell types involved and ways of downregulating their growth and activation, and may take the form of specific monoclonal antibodies directed against specific cytokines and cell-adhesion molecules.

REFERENCES

1. Evans MJ, Plopper CG: The role of basal cells in adhesion of columnar epithelium to airway basement membrane. *Am Rev Respir Dis* (1988) **138**: 481–483.
2. Evans MJ, Shami SG, Cabral-Anderson LJ, Dekker NP: Role of nonciliated cells in renewal of the bronchial epithelium of rats exposed to NO_2. *Am J Pathol* (1986) **123**: 126–133.
3. Farquhar MG, Palade GE: Junctional complexes in various epithelia. *J Cell Biol* (1963) **17**: 375–412.
4. Carson JL, Collier AM, Boucher RC: Ultrastructure of the respiratory epithelium in the human nose. In Mygind N, Pipkorn U (eds) *Allergic and Vasomotor Rhinitis. Pathological Aspects.* Copenhagen, Munksgaard, 1987, pp11–27
5. Elia C, Bucca C, Rolla G, Scappaticci E, Cantino, D: A freeze-fracture study of human bronchial epithelium in normal, bronchitic and asthmatic subjects. *J Submicrosc Cytol Pathol* (1988) **20**: 509–517.
6. Wong LB, Miller IF, Yeates DB: Regulation of ciliary beat frequency by autonomic mechanisms: *in vitro. J Appl Physiol* (1988) **65**: 1895–1901.

7. Sanderson MJ and Dirksen ER: Mechanosensitive and beta adrenergic control of the ciliary beat frequency of mammalian respiratory tract cells in culture. *Am Rev Respir Dis* (1989) **139**: 432–440.

8. Allegra L, Fabbri LM, Picotti G, Mattoli, S: Bronchial epithelium and asthma. *Eur Respir. J* (1989) **2** (Suppl 6): 460s–468s.

9. Stelzer J, Bigby BG, Stulbarg, *et al.*: Ozone-induced changes in bronchial reactivity to methacholine and airway inflammation in humans. *J Appl Physiol* (1986) **60**: 1321–1325.

10. Filley WV, Holley KE, Kephart GM, Gleich GJ: Identification by immunofluorescence of eosinophil granule major basic protein in lung tissues of patients with bronchial asthma. *Lancet* (1982) **2**: 11–15.

11. De Monchy JGR, Kauffman HF, Venge P, *et al.*: Bronchoalveolar eosinophils during allergen-induced late asthmatic reactions. *Am Rev Respir Dis* (1985) **131**: 373–376

12. Flint KC, Leung KBP, Hudspith BN, Brostoff J, Pearce FL, Johnson NM: Bronchoalveolar mast cells in extrinsic asthma: a mechanism for the initiation of antigen-specific bronchocon-striction. *Br Med J* (1985) **291**: 923–926.

13. Laitinen LA, Heino M, Laitinen A, Kava T, Haahtela T: Damage of the airway epithelium and bronchial reactivity in patients with asthma. *Am Rev Respir Dis* (1985) **131**: 599–606.

14. Beasley R, Roche WR, Robers JA, Holgate ST: Cellular events in the bronchi in mild asthma and after bronchial provocation. *Am Rev Respir Dis* (1989) **139**: 806–817.

15. Jeffery PK, Wardlaw AJ, Nelson FC, Collins JV, Kay, AB: Bronchial biopsies in asthma: an ultrastructural, quantitative study and correlation with hyperreactivity. *Am Rev Respir Dis* (1989) **140**: 1745–1753.

16. Dunnill MS: The pathology of asthma with special reference to changes in the bronchial mucosa. *J Clin Pathol* (1960) **13**: 27–33.

17. Cutz E, Levison H, Cooper, DM: Ultrastructure of airways in children with asthma. *Histopathology* (1978) **2**: 407–421.

18. Lozewicz S, Wells C, Gomez E, *et al.*: Morphological integrity of the bronchial epithelium in mild asthmatics. *Thorax* (1990) **45**: 12–15.

19. Hogg JC, Eggleston PA: Is the asthma an epithelial disease? *Am Rev Respir Dis* (1984) **129**: 207–208.

20. Hogg JC: Mucosal permeability and smooth muscle function in asthma. *Med Clin N Am* (1990) **74**: 731–740

21. Barnes PJ: Asthma is an axon reflex. *Lancet* (1986) **1**: 242–245.

22. Holtzman MJ, Aizawa H, Nadel JA, Goetzl EJ: Selective generation of leukotriene B4 by tracheal epithelial cells from dogs. *Biochem Biophys Res Commun* (1983) **114**: 1071–1076.

23. Hunter JA, Finkbeiner WE, Nadel JA, Goetzl EJ, Holtzman MJ: Predominant generation of 15-lipoxygenase metabolites of arachidonic acid by epithelial cells from human trachea. *Proc Natl Acad Sci USA* (1985) **82**: 4633–4637.

24. Lazarus SC: Role of inflammation and inflammatory mediators in airways disease. *Am J Med* (1986) **81** (Suppl 5A): 2-7.

25. Churchill L, Chilton FH, Resau JH, Bascom R, Hubbard WC, Proud D: Cyclooxygenase metabolism of endogenous arachidonic acid by cultured human tracheal epithelial cells. *Am Rev Respir Dis* (1989) **140**: 449–459.

26. Flavahan NA, Aarhus LL, Rimete TJ, Vanhoutte PM: Respiratory epithelium inhibits bronchial smooth muscle. *J Appl Physiol* (1985) **58**: 834–838.

27. Flavahan NA, Vanhoutte PM: The respiratory epithelium releases a smooth muscle relaxing factor. *Chest* (1985) **87**: 189s–190s.

28. Barnes PJ, Cuss FM, Palmer JB: The effect of airway epithelium on smooth muscle contracti-bility in bovine trachea. *Br J Pharmacol* (1985) **86**: 685–691.

29. Vanhoute PM: Epithelium-derived relaxing factor(s) and bronchial reactivity. *Am Rev Respir Dis* (1988) **138**: S24–S30.

30. Wilkens JH, Wilkens H, Forstermann U, Frolich JC: The effect of bronchial epithelium on bronchial contractility. *Pneumologie* (1990) **44**: 373–374.

31. Denberg JA, Dolovich J, Harnish D: Basophil, mast cell and eosinophil growth and differen-tiation factors in human allergic disease. *Clin Expt Allergy* (1989) **19**: 249–254.

32. Mattoli S, Miante S, Calabro F, Mazzetti M, Allegra L: Human bronchial epithelial cells exposed to isocyanates potentiate the activation and proliferation of T cells induced by antigen receptor triggering through the release of IL-1 and IL-6. In Johanssen SGO (ed) *Pharmacia Allergy Research Foundation, Award Book 1990*. Upssala, AW Grafiska, 1990, pp 25–35.

33. Ricci M, Rossi O: Dysregulation of IgE responses and airway allergic inflammation in atopic individuals. *Clin Exp Allergy* (1990) **20**: 601–609.

34. Eling TE, Danilowicz RM, Henke DC, Sivarajah K, Yankaskas JR, Boucher RC: Arachidonic acid metabolism by canine tracheal epithelial cells. Product formation and relationship to chloride secretion. *J Biol Chem* (1986) **261**: 12841–12849.

35. Leikauf GD, Driscoll KE, Wey HE: Ozone-induced augmentation of eicosanoid metabolism in epithelial cells from bovine trachea. *Am Rev Respir Dis* (1988) **137**: 435–442.

36. Robinson C, Campbell A, Herbert CA, Sapsford RJ, Devalia JL, Davies RJ: Calcium-dependent release of eicosanoids in human cultured bronchial epithelial cells. *Br J Pharmacol* (1990) **100**: 471P (abstract).

37. Sapsford RJ, McCloskey DT, Devalia JL, Cundell DR, Davies RJ: Nitrogen dioxide (NO_2): Effects on human bronchial epithelial cell function *in vitro*. *Thorax* (1991) **46**: 306P (Abstract).

38. Wardlaw AJ, Moqbel R, Cromwell O, Kay, AB: Platelet-activating factor: a potent chemotactic and chemokinetic factor for human eosinophils *J Clin Invest* (1986) **78**: 1701–1706.

39. Kroegel C, Yukawa T, Dent G, Chanez P, Chung KF, Barnes PJ: Platelet-activating factor induces eosinophil peroxidate release from purified human eosinophils. *Immunology* (1988) **64**: 559–562.

40. Holtzman MJ, Grunberger D, Hunter JA: Phospholipid fatty acid composition of pulmonary airway epithelial cells: potential substrates for oxygenation. *Biochem Biophys Acta* (1986) **877**: 459–464.

41. Soberman RJ, Harper TW, Betteridge D, Lewis RA, Austen KF: Characterisation and separation of arachidonic acid 5-lipoxygenase and linoleic acid ω-6-lipoxygenase (arachidonic acid 15-lipoxygenase) of human polymorphonuclear leukocytes. *J Biol Chem* (1985) **260**: 4508–4515.

42. Hay DWP, Farmer SC, Raeburn D, Robinson VA, Flemming WW, Feaden JS: Airway epithelium modulates the reactivity of guinea pig respiratory smooth muscle. *Eur J Pharmacol* (1986) **129**: 11–18.

43. Farmer SG: Airway smooth muscle responsiveness: modulation by the epithelium. *Trends in Pharmacol Sci* (1987) **8**: 8–10.

44. Butler GB, Adler KB, Evans JN, Morgan DW, Szarek JL: Modulation of rabbit airway smooth muscle responsiveness by respiratory epithelium: involvement of an inhibitory metabolite of arachidonic acid. *Am Rev Respir Dis* (1987) **135**: 1099–1104.

45. Buchanan MR, Hass TA, Legarde M, Guichardant M: 13-hydroxyoctadecadienoic acid is the vessel wall chemorepellant factor, LOX. *J Biol Chem* (1985) **260**: 16056–16059.

46. Frossard N, Rhoden KJ Barnes PJ: Influence of epithelium removal on guinea pig airway responses to tachykinins: role of endopeptidase and cyclooxygenase. *J Pharmacol Exp Therap* (1989) **248**: 292–297.

47. Strober W, James SP: The interleukins *Pediatr Res* (1988) **24**: 549–557.

48. Lopez AF, Sanderson CJ, Gamble JR, Campbell HD, Young IG, Vadas MA: Recombinant human interleukin 5 is a selective activator of human eosinophil function. *J Exp Med* (1988) **167**: 219–224.

49. Owen WF, Rothenberg ME, Silberstein DS, *et al.*: Regulation of human eosinophil viability, density and function by granulocyte/macrophage colony-stimulating factor in the presence of 3T3 fibroblasts. *J Exp Med* (1987) **166**: 129–141.

50. Rothenberg ME, Owen WF, Silberstein DS, *et al.*: Cytokine regulation of human eosinophil viability, density and function. *J Allergy Clin Immunol* (1988) **81**: 209 (Abstract).

51. Denburg JA, Jordana M, Gibson P, Hargreave F, Gauldie J, Dolovich J: Cellular and molecular basis of allergic airways inflammation. In Johanssen SGO (ed) *Pharmacia Allergy Research Foundation, Award Book 1990*. Upssala, AW Grafiska, 1990, pp 15–22.

52. Cox G, Vancheri C, Otoshi T, Gauldie J, Dolovich J, Jordana M, Denburg JA: Human bronchial epithelial cell derived granulocyte macrophage-colony stimulating factor (GM-

CSF) prolongs survival of human eosinophils *in vitro. J Allergy Clin Immunol* (1990) **85**: 233 (Abstract).

53. Churchill L, Friedman B, Schleimer RP, Proud D: Granulocyte macrophage-colony stimulating factor (GM-CSF) production by cultured human tracheal epithelial cells. *J Allergy Clin Immunol* (1990) **85**: 233 (Abstract).

54. Spriggs DR, Imamura K, Rodriguez C, Sariban E, Kufe DW: Tumor necrosis factor expression in human epithelial tumor cell lines. *J Clin Invest* (1988) **81**: 455–460.

55. Sieff CA, Niemeyer C, Tsai S, Clark SC, Faller DV: Monocytes regulate hematopoiesis by stimulating the production of hematopoietic growth factor by mesenchymal cells. *Blood* (1986) **68**: 180a.

56. Elner VM, Strieter RM, Elner SG, Baggiolini M, Lindley, Kunkel SL: Neutrophil chemotactic factor (IL-8) gene expression by cytokine-treated retinal pigment epithelial cells. *Am J Pathol* (1990) **136**: 745–750.

57. Smith CW, Rothlein R, Hughes BJ, *et al.*: Recognition of an endothelial determinant for CD18-dependent human neutrophil adherence and transendothelial migration. *J Clin Invest* (1988) **82**: 1746–1756.

58. Kyan-Aung U, Haskard DO, Lee TH: The role of ELAM-1 and ICAM-1 in eosinophil and neutrophil adhesion to endothelium. *J Allergy Clin Immunol* (1990) Abstract 552 in abstracts book from 46th annual meeting of American Academy of Allergy and Immunology.

59. Wegner CD, Gundel RH, Reilly P, Haynes N, Letts G, Rothlein R: Intercellular adhesion molecule-1 (ICAM-1) in the pathogenesis of asthma. *Science* (1990) **247**: 456–459.

60. Grave JM, Davis G, Meyer AM, *et al.*: The major human Rhinovirus receptor is ICAM-1. *Cell* (1989) **56**: 819–847.

61. Tomassini JE, Graham D, Dewitt CM, Lineburger DW, Rodkey JA, Colonno, RJ: cDNA cloning reveals that major group Rhinovirus receptor on HeLa cells is ICAM-1. *Proc Natl Acad Sci (USA)* (1989) **86**: 4907–4911.

62. Staunton DE, Merluzzi VJ, Rothlein R, Barton R, Martin SD, Springer TA: A cell adhesion molecule, ICAM-1, is the major receptor for Rhinoviruses. *Cell* (1989) **56**: 849–853.

63. Springer TA: Adhesion receptors of the immune system. *Nature* (1990) **346**: 425–434.

64. Dustin ML, Rothlein R, Bhan AK, Dinarello CA, Springer TA: Induction by IL-1 and interferon-γ: Tissue distribution, biochemistry and function of a natural adherence molecule (ICAM-1). *J Immunol* (1986) **137**: 245–254.

65. Devalia JL, Sapsford RJ, Wells C, Richman P, Davies RJ: Culture and comparison of human bronchial and nasal epithelial cells *in vitro. Respiratory Medicine* (1990) **84**: 303–312.

66. Sapsford RJ, Devalia JL, McAulay AE, d'Ardenne AJ, Davies RJ: Expression of α 1-6 integrin cell-surface receptors in normal human bronchial biopsies (HBB) and cultured bronchial epithelial cells (HBE). *J Allergy Clin Immunol* (1991) **87**: 303 (Abstract).

67. Liversidge JM, Sewell HF, Forrester JV: Human retinal pigment epithelial cells differentially express MHC class II (HLA, DP, DR and DQ) antigens in response to *in vitro* stimulation with lymphokine or purified IFN-γ. *Clin Exp Immunol* (1988) **73**: 489–494.

68. Motojima K, Matsuo S, Mullen Y: DR antigen expression on vascular endothelium and duct epithelium in fresh or cultured human fetal pancreata in the presence of gamma-interferon. *Transplantation* (1989) **48**: 1022–1025.

69. Komatsu T, Yamamoto M, Shimokata K, Nagura H: Phenotypic characterisation of alveolar capillary endothelial cells, alveolar epithelial cells and alveolar macrophages in patients with pulmonary fibrosis, with special reference to MHC class II antigens. *Virchows-Arch-(A)* (1989) **415**: 79–90.

70. Rossi GA, Sacco O, Lapertosa G, Corte G, Ravazzoni C, Allegra L: Human ciliated bronchial epithelial cells express HLA DR antigens and HLA DR genes. *Am Rev Res Dis* (1988) **137**: 5 (Abstract).

71. Lechner JF, Haugen A, McClendon IA, Pettis EW: Clonal growth of normal adult human bronchial epithelial cells in serum-free medium. *In Vitro* (1982) **18**: 633–642.

72. Wiesel JM, Gamiel H, Vlodavsky I, Gay I, Ben-Bassat H: Cell attachment, growth characteristics and surface morphology of human upper-respiratory tract epithelium cultured on extracellular matrix. *Eur J Clin Invest* (1983) **13**: 57–63.

73. Wu R, Yankaskas J, Cheng E, Knowles MR, Boucher R: Growth and differentiation of human nasal epithelial cells in culture. *Am Rev Respir Dis* (1985) **132**: 311–320.
74. Ayars GH, Altman LC, McManus MM, *et al.*: Injurious effect of the eosinophil peroxidase–hydrogen peroxidase–halide system and major basic protein on human nasal epithelium *in vitro*. *Am Rev Respir Dis* (1989) **140**: 125–131.
75. Farber JL, Young EE: Accelerated phospholipid degradation in anoxic rat hepatocytes. *Arch Biochem Biophys* (1981) **211**: 312–320.

11

Mucus and Mucus-secreting Cells in Asthma

P.S. RICHARDSON AND D.C.K. FUNG

SECRETORY CELLS OF THE AIRWAY

The respiratory epithelium contains eight or more different cell types, of which at least five are involved in secretion. In the surface epithelium these are goblet cells, Clara cells and ciliated cells, while in the submucosal glands they comprise serous and mucous cells. Surface epithelial serous cells are present in some species, but not, so far as we know, in adult man.

Goblet cells

The surface epithelial cells, which from their microscopic appearance and staining properties clearly store and secrete mucus, are referred to as *goblet cells* because of their shape when distended by vesicles of mucus in chemically fixed preparations.[1] However, Sandoz *et al.*[2] have challenged this picture of these cells on the basis of their appearance in rapidly frozen sections; here the secretory granules are smaller, more electron dense and more discrete, thus the whole cell has a less bloated (or goblet-like) appearance. Perhaps we should call them 'surface epithelial mucous cells'; but 'goblet cell' is a traditional term which skips from the tongue, a misnomer, perhaps, but likely to persist. These cells exist in the airways of all species so far studied.[3] In man, goblet cells are common in the trachea and main bronchi with a density of $6800/mm^2$,[4,5] which may increase to $10000/mm^2$ in chronic bronchitis. The frequency of goblet cells is less in the bronchioles in health, and reports conflict as to whether their number increases in chronic obstructive airway disease.[6]

Goblet cells, and the related mucous cells of the submucosal glands (see below), contain mucins.[7] Even in dissociating conditions, these molecules are up to 8 μm in

ASTHMA: BASIC MECHANISMS AND CLINICAL MANAGEMENT (2nd Edn)
ISBN 0-12-079026-2

length,[8] so they must be extensively folded or coiled to fit into secretory granules of 500 nm diameter. Secretory vesicles pass from the Golgi apparatus to the apex of the cell where they fuse with the apical membrane, discharging their contents.[3,9] Verdugo[7] has recently reviewed the packing of mucins, large polyanions, into secretory vesicles and their subsequent swelling on secretion.

Epithelial serous cells

Serous cells have been well reviewed recently.[10] Surface epithelial serous cells resemble those found in the submucosal glands. So far, serous cells have only been found in any number in the epithelium of specific pathogen-free (SPF) animals and the human foetus.[1] They give the periodic acid/Schiff reaction (PAS stain) and thus contain glycoconjugate, the nature of which is uncertain.[10] Jeffery and Reid[11] have demonstrated that in the airways of SPF rats the number of serous cells fell and the number of goblet cells rose with exposure to tobacco smoke. They concluded that serous cells may transform to goblet cells as a result of exposure to tobacco smoke and possible other irritants. Further evidence for this conclusion is reviewed in ref. 10. It is also likely that serous cells in submucosal glands can transform to mucous cells.

Clara cells (non-ciliated bronchiolar secretory cells)

These cells are apparently secretory in nature, as they contain two types of electron-dense secretory granules,[3] but, depite considerable investigation, the nature of their secretory product remains elusive. From histochemical evidence they probably contain a mixture of glycoprotein, protein and lipid,[12] but the mixture may vary from one species to another. They only occur in airways <1 mm in diameter, so can only contribute to small airway secretions.[13] It has been suggested that one of the Clara cell's secretory products may be a bronchiolar surfactant which helps maintain the patency of small airways.[14] Evans et al.[15] suggested that they may transform into ciliated and brush cells in rats exposed to NO_2.

Ciliated cells

Ciliated cells are the commonest cells in the respiratory tract, even in the large airways outnumbering goblet cells by five times.[3,16] They lack secretory granules and have fewer ribosomes than other secretory cells,[17] and their main function is to maintain the co-ordinated movement of cilia.[18] Ciliated cells, however, possess a glycocalyx along their luminal border at the base of the cilia, but also this extends along other epithelial cells which line the airway lumen.

Airway glycocalyx

This layer stains with Alcian blue even at pH1, suggesting that it consists of a substance made acid by sulphate radicals. It has been described in the large airways of several species, including man.[19–21] There is increasing evidence that this surface layer can be released and can thus contribute to airway mucus. Evidence comes both from epithelial cells in culture and *in vivo*.

Evidence from cultured cells

Varsano *et al.*[22] cultured cells from canine trachea. These lost cilia before becoming confluent, but had a clear glycocalyx and lacked secretory granules. After incubation with ^{35}S-sulphate, the radiolabelled molecules in the culture fluid were mainly in the totally included volume of a Sepharose CL 4B gel filtration column, though with a small quantity of macromolecular material in the void volume (Vo). Treatment of the cells with trypsin released a large amount of macromolecular material with one peak in the Vo (implying a molecular mass of $>10^6$ Da) and another in the partially included volume. The macromolecules released by trypsin resisted digestion with chondroitinase ABC or heparan-sulphate-lyase, but were degraded by keratanase and endo-β-galactosidase, suggesting a polylactosamine type of molecular structure. Kim *et al.* have studied the release of the secretory material from cultured epithelial cells taken from the hamster trachea.[23] These have a glycocalyx as well as secretory granules. Treatment with human neutrophil elastase caused thinning of the glycocalyx as well as release of secretory granules.

Evidence in vivo

Autoradiographic studies on cat trachea *in vivo* have shown that the glycocalyx layer takes up radiolabelled sugars, amino acids and sulphate precursors.[19,24] The precursors are taken up initially over the cell bodies but then migrate to the apical surface so that much of the radioactivity coincides with the surface membrane. ^{35}S-sulphate was taken up preferentially by submucosal gland cells while ^{3}H-glucose labelled the surface epithelium more intensely. After dual radiolabelling with these two precursors, treatment of the tracheas with repeated high doses of pilocarpine, which selectively releases material from the submucosal glands,[24] gives a secretion rich in ^{35}S-labelled glycoconjugates and relatively poor in their ^{3}H-labelled counterparts. This is consistent with the known action of muscarinic agonists in releasing the contents of submucosal glands and leaving little stainable glycoconjugate in the submucosa.[19,24] Subsequent passage of dilute ammonia vapour through the trachea releases mucin-like material with a high ^{3}H to ^{35}S ratio; Gallagher *et al.*[26] have argued that the glycocalyx is the most likely source.

Nature of the glycocalyx

Spicer *et al.*[25] have suggested, on histochemical grounds, that the glycocalyx consists of proteoglycan. It has been considered an integral part of the epithelial cells, but as epithelial cells rapidly incorporate radioactivity from radiolabelled sulphate, sugars and amino acids, and as these radiolabels can then be recovered as macromolecules in airway secretion, it is possible that the glycocalyx may release macromolecules into mucus. Bhaskar et al.[25] have identified a proteoglycan in mucus from the airways of man and dog which, they suggest, is largely chondroitin sulphate from the epithelial surface (probably the glycocalyx). Davies et al.[27] have demonstrated autoradiographically that ^{3}H from ^{3}H-glucose, given for 2 h into the trachea of the cat, labels predominantly the microvillus border of the ciliated epithelium, with little radiolabel being taken up by goblet cells. Mucus rich in ^{3}H-labelled macromolecules is released in response to ammonia vapour even after the submucosal glands have been virtually emptied with repeated high doses of pilocarpine.[28] Unstimulated mucus contains a radiolabelled macromolecular species of high molecular weight (excluded from Sepharose CL-2B and Superose 6) with a buoyant density of 1.6 g/ml in caesium chloride gradient, unusually high for a glycoprotein. This radiolabelled macromolecule is partially degraded by trypsin (so that it runs as glycopeptides in the partially included volume of Superose 6) but not by chondroitinase ABC or by hyaluronidase so, despite its high buoyant density, it appears to be a glycoprotein rather than a typical proteoglycan.[29] Treatment of the trachea with pilocarpine does not increase the output of this component, while treatment with ammonia vapour or rhamnolipids does (unpublished results).

It remains uncertain whether release of macromolecules from the glycocalyx requires energy, thus justifying the name *secretion,* or if it is simple *release,* a process of molecular shedding, without energy expenditure.

Submucosal glands

In man, there are numerous glands in the submucosa of the trachea and bronchi.[30] They consist of a duct lined with ciliated epithelium (the ciliated duct) opening into the airway lumen; further upstream the lining consists of columnar cells and becomes the collecting duct, from which a number of branches arise. These are lined with mucus-secreting cells and terminate in a short serous tubule[30]. The arrangement of the mucous and serous cells in each gland is such that the serous secretions must pass over mucus-secreting cells before they enter the collecting duct.

Serous cells

Serous cells (see above) in the submucosal glands have been well reviewed recently.[10] They contain discrete electron-dense granules, which are smaller, and exhibit greater variety than those in mucous cells. Recently serous cells have been cultured. Immuno-cytochemical studies show that the serous cells contain lysozyme and lactoferrin, as well as glycoconjugate.[32,33]

Mucous cells (see above and Verdugo[7])

The mucous cells resemble the goblet cells of the surface epithelium, as they contain, in conventionally fixed tissues, a large number of electron-lucent granules that enlarge towards the apex of the cell, where they appear to fuse with the luminal cell membrane before secretion.[34] Their mucus content consists of a mixture of acid and neutral glycoprotein.[1,30] Until recently it has been difficult to study the secretions of these cells in isolation as, unlike serous cells, they are difficult to culture.

MUCUS COMPOSITION

Mucus is a mixture, consisting mainly of water (about 95%), with 1% salts, 1–3% proteins and glycoproteins including mucins.[35] Some recent reports stress the presence of proteoglycans and lipids in airway mucus (see below).

Mucins

Mucins are high molecular weight mucus glycoproteins consisting of a peptide core with regions that are densely covered with sugar sidechains alternating with sparsely glyco-sylated regions.[36] The sugar sidechains are characteristically oligosaccharides, O-linked to serine and threonine residues on the peptide core. The peptide core is also rich in proline, an amino acid which gives the mucin rods their flexibility. Typically mucins have molecular weights ranging from 5 to 50×10^6 Da. Reduction of mucins, e.g. by dithiothreitol, characteristically lessens their size, so disulphide bonds are believed to link adjacent regions of peptide core. Mucins are thought to be the chief molecules responsible for conferring the properties of viscosity and elasticity upon mucus, though other molecules may modify this. The chief evidence for this is that agents that reduce the disulphide bonds, characteristically part of mucin structure, also greatly diminish the viscoelastic properties of mucus.[37,38].

Proteoglycans

Mucus, including that collected from the healthy airways of human subjects,[39] that secreted by airways in organ culture,[26] and by cultured secretory cells,[22,40] has been found to contain proteoglycans. Bhaskar et al. have reported that mucus collected via a fibreoptic bronchosope from non-smoking healthy human volunteers contains proteogly-cans but is devoid of typical mucins, and argue that proteoglycans are, in these circumstances, the main gel-forming macromolecules.[39] Mucins, they report, only begin to appear in mucus when submucosal gland secretion is stimulated by, for example, cholinergic drugs or when secretion is augmented by chronic irritation.[26,41] On the other hand, Thornton et al. have reported that mucus collected via tracheal tubes from the healthy respiratory tracts of children undergoing dental extraction contained typical mucins and, apparently, little proteoglycan.[8]

These reports are difficult to reconcile. Possible reasons for the differences include the following: In Thornton's study, the tracheal tube was passed through the larynx without local anaesthesia, and irritation from this may have excited reflexes releasing typical mucins from the submucosal glands.[42] On the other hand bronchoscopy[39] is normally done on the airways after treatment with local anaesthetic. While this would prevent reflex stimulation of mucin output from submucosal glands, local anaesthetic itself releases large quantities of mucus macromolecules (of unspecified chemical type, but possibly including proteoglycans) into the airway.[43] Another difference between the two studies is that, in Bhaskar's study,[39] the mucus samples were dissolved directly in caesium bromide solution in preparation for density gradient centrifugation; in Thornton's study,[8] however, mucus was first dissolved in 6M guanidine hydrochloride buffer, a strong dissociating agent. It is possible that, in the former study,[39] the solvent failed to bring mucins into solution.

It is now clear that the airway mucus may contain proteoglycans. Their role in forming of mucus gels, however, remains in doubt.

Other mucus constituents

Although mucins and, possibly, other high molecular weight glycoconjugates appear to be the main molecules determining the visco-elasticity of mucus, there are significant quantities of non-mucin proteins in airway mucus. The picture emerging suggests that:

(1) Many of the non-mucin proteins so far identified are involved in antimicrobial defence of the respiratory tract.
(2) The main source of these 'defence' proteins is the serous cells of the submucosal gland.[10] This, coupled with the absence of the precursors of mucin core peptides from bronchial serous cells in man,[44] suggests that a major role of the serous cell is defensive.
(3) Non-mucin proteins can interact with the mucin molecules to alter the viscoelastic properties of the mucus gel.[45,46]

Serum proteins

Serum proteins, such as albumin and immunoglobulins, may be present in airway mucus, particularly in the inflamed airway. These may be derived from airway secretory cells as well as plasma exudate from the local vasculature. The most abundant serum protein is albumin. Sequences of albumin mRNA in the airways[47] suggest that, in addition to plasma exudation, this protein may be locally synthesized and secreted. Active transport of albumin into the lumen by epithelial cells of ferret and rabbit trachea *in vitro* has been demonstrated.[48,49] This transport mechanism has not yet been shown in man. The role of albumin in mucus is unknown, but it can modify the rheological properties of mucus.[50] Another function of transport of albumin from the submucosa into the lumen may be to reduce submucosal oedema which could encroach into the airway lumen. Accumulation of extravascated albumin in the submucosa would exert a colloid osmotic pressure, making the submucosal tissues swollen and oedematous; transport of the albumin to the airway lumen would lessen this. In asthma, albumin concentration in mucus increases, but it is possible that the increase might be even greater were it not for epithelial damage which may compromise transepithelial albumin transport.

Locally produced proteins

Lysozyme and lactoferrin are both cationic proteins that play important roles in host-defence mechanisms. Both have anti-bacterial properties: lysozyme hydrolyses the cell walls of some bacteria, hence causing lysis; lactoferrin chelates iron and hence limits growth of iron-dependent micro-organisms.[51] Other 'defence proteins' present include immunoglobulins, of which secretory IgA is most abundant (see ref. 52 for review); antileukoprotease (bronchial inhibitor) which is responsible for most of the inhibitory actions of bronchial secretions against leucocyte proteases,[53] and a family of peroxidases which may also contribute to the defence against invading organisms. Recently, a family of proteins collectively known as proline-rich proteins has been reported to be present in respiratory tract fluid.[54,55] Their funtions are not known, but a role of regulating the viscoelastic properties of the mucus gel has been suggested.[54,55]

Lipids

In addition to proteins, lipids are also present in significant amounts in respiratory tract fluid, including mucus from the normal human respiratory tract.[26,39] Phospholipids such as phosphatidylcholine are present in significant quantities in patients with asthma and cystic fibrosis.[56,57] The relative quantities of lipids from different sources (alveolar vs. tracheobronchial secretions) and their physiological significance are not clear at present. It is possible that lipids and mucins may interact to alter the physical properties of the mucus gel network.[57]

REGULATION OF MUCUS SECRETION

Innervation of the secretory apparatus

Innervation of airway submucosal glands has been studied mainly in animal species, particularly the cat, but there are now some studies in man. Studies of cat trachea and bronchi by light and electron microscopy have shown that the submucosal glands receive a rich innervation from the autonomic nervous system, with nine times more cholinergic than adrenergic varicosities being in close contact with them.[58] This study did not demonstrate any differential innervation of serous and mucous cells (e.g. with mucous cells receiving more adrenergic nerves and serous cells more cholinergic nerves or vice versa), but did note that serous cells received a denser innervation with axons of both types than mucous cells. Despite this apparent lack of differential innervation of secretory cells, specific effects of nervous activity are still possible if the receptors to particular neurotransmitters are concentrated on one cell type rather than another. There is evidence for this, at least in the ferret: serous cells contain more α-adrenoceptors than mucous cells, while the latter contain more β-adrenoceptors, while both cell types are richly endowed with muscarinic receptors.[59]

In man, the submucosal glands also receive a dual innervation from the sympathetic and parasympathetic systems, again with the parasympathetic (cholinergic) nerve terminals predominating.[60,61]

Immunofluorescence studies have shown that there are nerve terminals that react with antibodies to peptidergic transmitters: vasoactive intestinal peptide (VIP), substance P, galanin, peptide histidine isoleucine (PHI) or, in man, peptide histidine methionine (PHM), gastrin-releasing peptide and neuropeptide Y.[62,63,64] There are nerves in which peptides coexist with classical (adrenergic or cholinergic) transmitters, but probably others that are entirely peptidergic, e.g collateral branches of afferent nerves containing substance P.

Nervous mechanisms controlling airway mucus secretion

Most studies of secretion concentrate on one of three aspects of mucus secretion: the amount of macromolecular secretion, the volume of secretion released per unit time (reflecting mainly water flow) or the physical properties of the secretions. Several recent studies have measured particular macromolecules in mucus to indicate the cellular origin of the secretion; for example, lysozyme and lactoferrin come only from serous cells,[32,33] so an increased rate of lysozyme output indicates serous cells secretion.[65,66] There is no convenient equivalent for mucous cell secretion; typical high molecular weight mucin[36,67] probably comes from these cells; but, so far, we lack a simple, selective assay for this. Another approach to determining the cell type a particular agent stimulates has been to examine control and stimulated tissues under the EM. Morphometry may reveal which cell type the stimulus has emptied. This has proved easier in serous that in mucous cells where fusion of granules, in conventionally fixed tissue, makes a simple count of remaining secretory granules unreliable. Recently Gashi *et al.* have attempted to overcome this problem by comparing the volume of mucous cells in stimulated and control tissues.[68]

Cholinergic control of airway secretion

Muscarinic agonists increase the output of mucus and radiolabelled mucins from submucosal glands in most species and preparations studied, including human bronchial mucosa *in vitro*.[69,70] Atropine blocks this action, which therefore depends upon muscarinic receptors.[24,69,71–74] Autoradiographic evidence from experiments involving radioligand binding to submucosal glands in human airways suggest the presence of both M1 and M3 muscarinic receptor subtypes.[75] Evidence based on the effects of functional antagonism of secretion in the cat trachea, however, did not allow straightforward classification of the muscarinic receptors in terms of known receptor subtypes.[76]

Parasympathetic (vagal) nerve stimulation also increases mucus output,[24,72] but atropine typically blocks only part of this effect (see below).[77,78] Shimura *et al.* have shown that part of the effect of nerve stimulation can be explained by contraction of the myoepithelial cells in the submucosal gland ducts.[79,80] They dissected individual glands from the cat trachea, and measured the tension generated by the contraction of myoepithelial cells. Electrical field stimulation caused gland contraction by a nervous mechanism, inhibited by TTX. α-Adrenoceptor blockade with phentolamine prevented about 15% of the action, whereas atropine blocked it entirely. They suggest that both cholinergic and, to some extent, adrenergic sympathetic nerves can expel mucus from submucosal glands by actively contracting their ducts.

So far, in human bronchus *in vitro*, atropine appears to block the entire effect of electrical field stimulation which releases secretions via TTX-blockable (thus presumably nervous) pathways.[81] The scatter of results reported, however, was such that the experiments might well have failed to demonstrate any but the most powerful of nervous controls.

Adrenoceptor control of airway secretion

In the cat and the ferret, both α- and β-adrenoceptor agonists stimulate secretion from submucosal glands.[72,82–84] There is more disagreement over the role of adrenoceptors in controlling secretion into human bronchi; probably both α- and β-receptors stimulate secretion,[85,86] but others have found either no adrenoceptor actions[69,70] or that only α-adrenoceptor agonists stimulate secretion.[74] Autoradiographs of human bronchi treated with radioligands for specific adrenoceptors have demonstrated the presence of β-receptors on submucosal glands. The majority of the β-adrenoceptors are of the β_2 subtype, but about 10% are β_1, consistent with responses to both circulation and nerve-released catecholamines.[87,88]

In the cat, electrical stimulation of sympathetic nerves to the airway increases glycoconjugate output into the trachea; propranolol largely prevents this, while thymoxamine and phentolamine are ineffective, suggesting that sympathetic nerves act mainly via β-adrenoceptors.[42,83] In the ferret, however, α-adrenoceptors play the larger part in mediating sympathetic nervous control of secretion.[82] In man, experiments to test the effect of sympathetic control of airway secretion are more difficult. Field stimulation of human bronchi has given negative results, not necessarily convincing, that atropine abolished the effect of electrical stimulation. As pointed out above, however, these results had such a large scatter that they cannot rule out sympathetic effects. Adrenergic nerves end in varicosities near the bronchial submucosal glands in man.[60,61] Calculations, based on the likely release of noradrenaline by such nerves, suggest that the nerves are sufficiently near submucosal glands to cause secretion.[86]

Differential responsiveness of cells to adrenergic stimuli has been described. Basbaum et al.[89] noted that, in the ferret, serous cells discharged their granules more readily in response to α-adrenoceptor agonists than to β-agonists, while later studies by the same group[68,84] showed that the opposite was true for mucous cells. This can be explained by the demonstration that α-adrenoceptors predominate on serous cells while β-adrenoceptors predominate on mucous cells.[59]

King and Viires[90] examined the effect of a range of concentrations of methacholine on the rheology and transport of tracheal mucus in the dog. They found that low doses of methacholine increased the rate of secretion, producing mucus of low elastic modulus, but not so low as to delay its transport on the frog palate. High doses also accelerated secretory rate, but produced mucus of high elastic modulus, transported more slowly on the frog palate. One interpretation of this is that separate mechanisms control water and mucin secretion, with the one controlling the output of water having a lower threshold of response to cholinergic stimulation than that which controls mucin secretion. However, Leikauf et al.[91] have since found that a single concentration of methacholine caused no change in the viscoelasticity of secretions collected directly from the gland duct into a micropipette. They studied only one point on the dose–response curve. One explanation for their finding of unchanged visco-elasticity is that their dose of methacholine was sufficient to stimulate water and mucin secretion equally; another is that glandular mucus (collected by Leikauf) and whole mucus (collected by King) somehow respond differently to cholinergic agonists. It is remarkable that the later paper[91] nowhere refers to the earlier[90] and the apparent contradiction between the two sets of results passes without comment. Leikauf *et al.*[91] also demonstrated that an α-adrenoceptor agonist produced secretions of low viscosity, while a β-agonist stimulated secretions of high viscosity.

The results of King, Basbaum and Leikauf (reviewed above) raise the possibility that the different autonomic mechanisms controlling airway secretion could adjust the composition of secreted mucus to give it physical properties suitable for different functions. For example, mucus with the optimum properties for cough is likely to be different from that best suited for mucociliary transport.[92] Could the autonomic nervous system adjust the composition and properties of mucus to satisfy particular requirements in different conditions? This attractive possibility remains unproven. It is also possible that pathophysiological mechanisms could pervert the system to give poorly cleared mucus, something which must be considered in asthma.

Non-adrenergic, non-cholinergic neurotransmitters and secretion

Stimulation of autonomic nerves supplying the airways augments secretion via adrenergic and cholinergic pathways as outlined above; but administration of large doses of muscarinic and adrenergic antagonists fails to block completely the autonomic control, so in addition there appear to be non-adrenergic, non-cholinergic (NANC) control mechanisms.[77,78,83] A number of peptide neurotransmitters, known to be present in airway nerves can influence mucus secretion.[62] Potential peptide neurotransmitters have been found in three functionally distinct classes of nerve, any of which may be important in NANC control of secretion: in parasympathetic nerves (often co-localized with acetylcholine), in sympathetic nerves (often co-localized with noradrenaline), and in afferent nerves. Peptide transmitters in parasympathetic nerves include vasoactive intestinal peptide (VIP), peptide histidine isoleucine or, in man, peptide histidine methionine (PHI or PHM), and gastrin-releasing peptide (GRP); those in sympathetic nerves include neuropeptide Y (NPY), while those in afferent nerves include substance P (SP) and calcitonin gene related peptide (CGRP). For convenience, the putative NANC transmitters considered below have been grouped according to possible nerve origins. This may be misleading, however, as a particular peptide transmitter could exist in more than one type of nerve.

Parasympathetic nerve peptide transmitters

Vasoactive intestinal peptide (VIP) has been reported to *inhibit* glycoprotein secretion into non-bronchitic human airway *in vitro*. This inhibition is much weaker, even absent, in the hypertrophied submucosal glands of the bronchitic airway. VIP *stimulates* secretion into the airways of the ferret and dog.[93,94]

VIP also manifests mixed stimulatory and inhibitory actions in its interactions with other neurotransmitters. Webber and Widdicombe[66] have demonstrated VIP's interactions with α-adrenergic and cholinergic mechanisms which control the flow of secretions into the lumen of ferret trachea *in vitro*. VIP shifted the dose-response curve to methacholine to the *right*, lessening the secretory response to a given concentration of the muscarinic agonist. With phenylephrine, VIP shifted the dose–response curve to the *left*.

Shimura *et al.*[205] on the other hand, working on glycoconjugate output from isolated feline submucosal glands, found that VIP shifted the dose–response curve to methacholine to the *left*. There are obviously a large number of possible interactions between transmitters still to be tested and many different species where interactions may differ.

PHI, while it has no direct effect on mucus secretion into the ferret trachea, causes a moderate inhibition of secretion evoked by methacholine, while not affecting that in response to phenylephrine.[95]

Gastrin-releasing peptide (GRP) has been found in the airways of several species. This includes man, where GRP-immunoreactive nerves are present in the nasal mucosa, with some endings near the submucosal gland acini. Radiolabelled GRP binds to the submucosal gland cells, suggesting the presence of receptors, and exogenous GRP releases lactoferrin (from serous cells) and other glycoconjugates.[63] Some postganglionic nerves, presumably parasympathetic, in cat trachea show GRP immunoreactivity; in this tissue as well as in the human nose GRP stimulates release of mucus glycoconjugates.[96]

Sympathetic neurotransmitters

NPY is found in many sympathetic nerves. Where tested, it has lacked a clear direct action on airway secretions.[64,95] However, NPY somewhat enhances the effects of cholinergic and α-adrenoceptor agonists on mucus volume output in the ferret trachea, while inhibiting their actions on lysozyme and hence, presumably, serous cell secretions.[95]

Afferent neurotransmitters

Substance P stimulates secretion of radiolabelled glycoconjugates into dog trachea.[97] Coles *et al.*[93,98] have confirmed this, showing that at least part of its action is to contract myoepithelial cells around the submucosal gland duct, squeezing mucus from the ducts without necessarily releasing fresh material from secretory cells. Shimura's group have elegantly confirmed this on individual glands dissected from the feline trachea,[99] as well as showing that this transmitter has a small direct effect on the release of secretory granules from cells. The effect of substance P on cellular secretion has been confirmed on serous cells in culture.[100] In the ferret trachea, SP augments mucus volume output (essentially water), the secretion of Na^+ and Cl^- into the lumen, and the secretion of macromolecules, effects potentiated by enkephalinase inhibition.[101,102] There is also evidence that SP acts on human bronchi to release mucus glycoproteins, and that inhibition of enzymatic peptide degradation with phosphoramidon potentiates this effect.[103] There is now somewhat stronger circumstantial evidence that SP may be a neurotransmitter releasing mucus in human airways. Capsaicin, a releaser of neuronal SP,[104] increases the rate of secretion of mucus glycoprotein from human airways *in vitro*. Morphine pretreatment, which would inhibit neuronal SP release, abolishes capsaicin's effect, while pretreatment with naloxone, an opioid antagonist, strengthens it.[105] Clearly, these effects could be explained in terms of neural release of SP by capsaicin, though rival explanation may be possible, too.

CGRP, another peptide seen in afferent nerves, has a weak stimulatory action on the volume output of mucus and the lysozyme output (hence serous cell secretion) from ferret trachea, effects somewhat enhanced by the enkephalinase inhibitor, thiorphan.[106]

Despite its stimulation of lysozyme output, CGRP inhibited the stimulations of lysozyme produced by methacholine and phenylephine. These actions on the submucosal glands in the ferret trachea may play little role in the human airway where submucosal glands lack CGRP receptors.[107] However, the stimulatory effect of CGRP on albumin transport across the surface epithelium into ferret trachea[106] may have a parallel in man, where the epithelium has CGRP receptors.[107]

Classical vs. NANC neurotransmission and airway secretion

So much has been written recently about the NANC innervation, peptide neurotransmitters and their role in airway secretion that it is difficult to review the subject briefly. The length of this section of the review, which is certainly not comprehensive, should not obscure an important truth: that, in the species so far studied, the classical nerves and transmitters (adrenergic and cholinergic) exercise a more powerful control over secretion than do their peptidergic couterparts. Peptide transmitters may modulate the actions of classical transmitters (see the papers by Webber reviewed above), or have some other action such as regulating the growth of secretory tissues or the relative numbers of different secretory cell types; but, in terms of gross output of secretions, classical mechanisms are probably the more powerful.

FUNCTIONS OF MUCUS

One of the main functions of mucus is to clear inhaled particles and other debris from the respiratory tract.[3,108,109] During health, this is almost entirely achieved by interaction of mucus with cilia to produce mucociliary flow. The cilia beat within a periciliary fluid layer with their tips engaging the overlying mucus blanket only during the power stroke and therefore propelling the mucus with its trapped debris in one direction.[110] Glycoproteins give mucus viscosity and elasticity,[37] properties essential for mucociliary transport.[111] Bhaskar and colleagues have recently suggested that there are circumstances under which proteoglycans and lipids, rather than glycoproteins, may be the molecules determining the physical properties of mucus,[26,39,112] but this remains open to question.

Cilia on the mucus-depleted frog palate can transport gels formed by a number of chemically distinct polymers, such as guaran, polyacrylamide, agarose, and gelatin.[113] Their function as mucus substitutes seems to depend on their combining gel and fluid properties, with the macromolecules just beginning to form a network. The concentration of macromolecules is also important in determining the rate of transport; in experiments with reconstituted canine tracheal mucus on the frog palate, mucociliary transport was fastest with concentrations of non-dialysable solids between 1.5 and 2.5%. Below this concentration the mucus has little elasticity and transport rates are low, while at greater concentrations the increase in elasticity also appears to slow transport.[114]

In normal quiet breathing, in a healthy respiratory tract, airflow does not appreciably alter mucus transport, but if the mucus layer is abnormally thick or if airflow is rapid (e.g. during high-frequency ventilation) then the air stream can interact with the mucus layer to alter its velocity.[115,116] Scherer has estimated the velocity of the serous layer in various generations of the bronchial tree during cough. He concluded that, in healthy individuals, cough would significantly accelerate serous (i.e. the watery periciliary fluid) flow down to the 12th airway generation.[117] The magnitude of cough-induced serous layer velocities depended on the thickness and viscosity of the serous layer and increased linearly with the ratio of thickness to viscosity.

Mucus also has antibacterial and antiviral functions. Some of these depend on antibacterial substances, most of which are secreted by serous cells: lysozyme and peroxidase are active against some bacteria, while lactoferrin may prevent bacterial growth by chelating iron.[10] In addition serous cells synthesize secretory IgA by combining IgA from submucosal lymphocytes with secretory piece, a glycoprotein. Secretory IgA is important in local epithelial immunity. Bacteria and viruses adhere to specific epitopes on the epithelial surface. Mucus glycoproteins can, if they possess similar epitopes, inhibit the binding of pathogens to cell surfaces.[118,119]

THE NATURE AND EFFECT OF MUCUS PLUGGING IN ASTHMA

Post-mortem examinations of lungs from those dying in *status asthmaticus* typically shows that mucus plugs narrow many airways from the trachea to the bronchioles, with the smaller airways being particularly affected.[120] Keal and Reid[121] have pointed out that some asthmatics die in *status* without such plugging , but this is unusual. More recently it has become clear that stagnant and abnormal mucus may narrow some of those airways of asthmatics patients in whom the disease is far milder, even those in remission who have died in accidents unconnected with their airway function.[122] What is the nature of the material blocking or narrowing the airways of asthmatic patients? Why does it accumulate?

Histology of airway mucus in asthma

Evidence on this comes from two main sources: the appearance of the airways in sections of lungs taken from asthmatic patients, usually those dying in *status asthmaticus*,[120,122] and study of sputum from asthmatic patients.[123] Mucus and exudate from patients with mild asthma resemble that from patients with more severe disease. In either case microscopic examination shows that layers of eosinophilic material, containing proteins such as plasma albumin, fibrin and immunoglobulins, alternate with layers positive for mucus stains. There are eosinophils, neutrophils and shed epithelial cells in profusion along with the ground substances.

Chemical properties of mucus in asthma

Little is known of the chemical abnormality of airway mucus from asthmatic patients. It is clear, though, that asthmatic sputum contains plasma proteins,[124,125] though in concentrations apparently no higher than those found in other diseases involving airway inflammation. Both albumin and immunoglobulins increase the viscosity of mucus, possibly by cross-linking neighbouring molecules of glycoprotein,[50,126] but we do not know the extent to which these proteins account for the apparently abnormal physical properties of asthmatic mucus (see below). Another inadequately tested possibility is that airway mucins are abnormal in asthma.

Effect of mucus plugging

Airway hyperreactivity

Mucus in the airway lumen will reduce the space available for conduction of air. Plainly this will raise the resistance to airflow for, according to Poiseuille's law, the resistance to laminar flow in a tube increases as $1/r^4$ (where r is the radius). But Freedman[127] has pointed out that the effect is more radical than that; any material within the ring of airway smooth muscle exaggerates the effect of smooth muscle contraction in raising airway resistance. In the asthmatic airway, where the airway wall is thickened by hypertrophied submucosal gland, oedema, and basement membrane thickening,[128,129] and a smear of stagnant mucus/exudate in the lumen,[128] this effect could be profound; it takes less shortening of bronchial smooth muscle to close the airway completely or to cause any given degree of luminal narrowing.[129] This geometric argument might explain at least part of the excessive response (airway *hyperreactivity* or *hyperresponsiveness*) to bronchoconstrictor stimuli typically seen among asthmatic subjects.[35] It could not, however, explain the reduced threshold to bronchoconstriction seen in asthmatics.[130]

Although this simple application of Poiseuille's law appears straightforward, there is little experimental evidence to confirm it as a cause of airway hyperresponsiveness. One set of experiments to test the hypothesis involved injection of about 40 ml of mucus simulant ('mucus') into the airways of sheep weighing ~35 Kg.[131] This volume of 'mucus', combined with lignocaine (lidocaine) to prevent coughing, was instilled via a bronchoscope and spread in the airways by artificial ventilation with an inspiratory bias. By analogy with man (~70 Kg body weight, ~150 ml airway deadspace), this volume of 'mucus' should have occupied an appreciable fraction of the volume of the conducting airways, so it is surprising that it did not increase resting airway resistance. After the 'mucus' instillation, an intravenous dose of carbachol increased airway resistance by no more than it had beforehand, a result which appears to contradict Freedman's hypothesis of hyperreactivity but can probably be explained. Lignocaine (lidocaine), present in the instilled 'mucus', inhibits contraction of airway smooth muscle in response to cholinergic agonists.[132] This was probably sufficient to offset the hyperreactivity predicted by simple physical principles. Another test of the Freedman hypothesis involved acute exposure of guinea-pigs to cigarette smoke to cause airway inflammation, with subsequent testing of airway reactivity to histamine[133] and measurement of airway dimensions[134] in both smoke-exposed animals and air-exposed controls. The smoke-exposed guinea-pigs exhibited hyperreactivity, but there was no evidence of swelling of the airway walls to explain this. The experiment was not designed to measure intraluminal mucus; the authors concluded either an increase in this or augmented contraction of airway smooth muscle could explain the observed hyperreactivity.[134]

Ventilation–Perfusion mismatch

Plugs of mucus/exudate form in some airways but not in others. This must contribute to the unevenness of alveolar ventilation seen in the asthmatic lung.[135] In extreme cases scattered regions of the lung, presumably those normally ventilated by airways which have become plugged, may collapse. This is commoner in young children, where collateral ventilation is less well developed.[136]

WHY DO MUCUS PLUGS FORM IN THE ASTHMATIC AIRWAY?

There are several likely reasons for airways becoming blocked with mucus and exudate in asthma, some better established than others. Secretory rate almost certainly increases in the asthmatic airway, exudate and cells augment the mucus in the airway lumen, the resulting mixture is physically abnormal, and clearance of the lumen by ciliary action and coughing is slowed. This section reviews the evidence on these points.

Increased mucus secretion in asthma

Almost all the evidence for increased mucus secretion in asthma is indirect. Most powerful of the accumulated circumstantial evidence is that many of the reflexes, mediators released and cells present in the asthmatic airway are known to stimulate secretion. These are reviewed after the more direct evidence, namely the coughing up of sputum, the hypertrophy of submucosal glands and the hyperplasia of the surface goblet cells.

Sputum

In a healthy person, perhaps 10 ml of mucus converges each day on the larynx from all the peripheral airways.[137,138] Cilia waft this to the pharynx, where it is swallowed. In health we produce no sputum. Asthmatics, on the other hand, usually expectorate sputum at some or all stages of an attack. By itself this is only weak evidence that their airways are hypersecreting; the normal daily volume of secretion might be trapped in the airway during the first few days of an attack and then be released rapidly during recovery. Some sufferers, however, cough up large volumes of sputum, far more than the duration of their illness would warrant at 10 ml/day.

Overgrowth of the secretory cells

More powerful evidence comes from the enlargment of the submucosal glands, seen in the bronchi of asthmatic dying in *status asthmaticus,* which suggests a work hypertrophy.[128] In addition there is often goblet cell hyperplasia.[139]

The drives to mucus secretion in asthma

The most extensive evidence, also indirect, comes from the finding that many of the mechanisms involved in asthma — trigger factors, reflexes, mediators and cells — can also drive airway secretion.

Reflexes

Cough is an important symptom of most asthmatic attacks; mechanical and chemical stimulation of the larynx and lower airways sufficient to cause coughing also elicits secretion from submucosal glands in the trachea and presumably from those in the bronchi too.[42,140,141] Phipps and Richardson[42] argued that mucus secretion is a part of the cough mechanism (see also ref. 3). So far, all stimuli tested which cause coughing also accelerate airway secretion; a blast of air shears a thick layer of mucus more effectively than a thin one, so an increase in secretory rate makes a cough more effective.[115,142]

There are two distinct types of airway nerve fibres that might form the afferent limb of the reflex response to irritation of the lower airway.[143] One is the myelinated rapidly adapting fibre with epithelial endings ('cough' and 'irritant') receptors,[144] exquisitely sensitive to mechanical stimuli; the other is the non-myelinated or C-fibre with endings that respond to several chemical irritants, including low doses of bradykinin, but which appear less sensitive to mechanical stimuli.[143,145] There is evidence that activity in either drives secretion; injection of small doses of bradykinin into the bronchial arteries of dogs, sufficient to stimulate non-myelinated fibres selectively, increases gland secretion by a reflex.[146] Inhalation of dust aerosols, which excite myelinated nerves in the airway epithelium and is unlikely to drive the mechanically less sensitive unmyelinated endings, also triggers secretion via a reflex in the cat.[141] Both types of receptor, then, can probably promote secretion, and there is evidence also that both may cause coughing.[143]

Mediators

A variety of inflammatory mediators is involved in the processes leading to an attack of asthma. Most of these have multiple actions including the ability to influence mucus output into the airways.

Histamine. Histamine enhances secretion into the tracheas of ferret, cat and goose *in vivo*.[147,148] It causes secrection into human airways both *in vivo*[149] and *in vitro* via H_2-receptors.[74]

Arachidonic acid stimulates the output of glycoconjugates from pieces of human bronchus in tissue culture, an action which probably depends on its metabolism to active mediators via both cyclooxygenase and lipoxygenase pathways.[150]

Cyclooxygenase products of arachidonic acid. Several prostaglandins (A_2, E_1, E_2, F_1, $F_{2\alpha}$) stimulate the secretion of glycoconjugates into cat trachea *in vivo*.[148] In human bronchus, $PGF_{2\alpha}$ stimulates secretion,[151,152] as do PGA_2 and D_2,[151] but there is disagreement over the action of PGE_2; Marom *et al.*[151] found an inhibitory action on mucus release from the human bronchus in tissue culture over a period of up to 7 days, particularly at a concentration of 1 μM, while other concentrations had smaller effects. On the other hand, Rich *et al.*[152] working on preparations of human bronchus cultured for up to 6 h, reported that PGE_2, over a similar range of concentrations, failed to inhibit glycoconjugates into secretion of radiolabelled glycoconjugates, and there was some evidence of stimulation. PGE_2 may act on two sets of prostaglandin receptors, one exciting and the other inhibiting secretion. Differences in the state of the tissues, so far undefined, may determine which action predominates.

Lipoxygenase products of arachidonic acid. Peatfield *et al.*[153] found that leukotriene C_4 stimulated the secretion of radiolabelled glycoconjugates into the cat trachea *in vivo* and showed evidence of inhibition by the leukotriene inhibitor FPL 55712. *In vitro*, however, they could find no evidence of activity of this mediator. Maron *et al.*[150] showed that leukotrienes C_4 and D_4, at concentrations of 0.4 nM and upwards, both enhance secretion from human bronchus *in vitro*. FPL 55712, a leukotriene receptor antagonist, inhibited these responses. HETEs also stimulate secretion from human bronchi.[150]

Platelet-activating factor (PAF). PAF, released from macrophages and eosinophils in response to allergen challenge,[154,155] releases mucus glycoconjugates from the respiratory tract at least under some circumstances. This was first shown in ferret trachea *in vitro*, where it had an action at concentrations of 10^{-6} M and upwards, effects that could be prevented by plasma proteins in the incubation medium.[156] Since then this has been extended to secretions from explants of airways from rabbit, rat and guinea-pig, but effects were not seen at concentrations less than 10^{-4} M,[157] Adler *et al.*[157] found that a specific PAF antagonist (Ro 19-3704) blocked these effects, as did a combined blocker of the lipoxygenase/cyclooxygenase pathways, so they reasoned that the effects of PAF depended on secondary mediators.

Goswami *et al.* have investigated the effects of PAF on secretion from explants of human bronchus in organ culture.[158] They found that low concentrations of PAF (20 nM and upwards) stimulated the output of airway glycoconjugates and that they could inhibit (but not abolish) this effect with high concentrations of Ro 19-3704. PAF caused bronchial explants to release leukotrienes, and a specific LTD_4 antagonist completely prevented PAF's stimulation of secretory glycoconjugates. Indomethacin, given to block the cyclooxygenase pathway, actually enhanced the effect of PAF suggesting a diversion of arachidonic acid products from the cyclooxygenase to the more effective lipoxygenase pathway. Lundgren *et al.* have performed similar experiments on explants from feline trachea and human bronchus, demonstrating that PAF causes secretion of glycoconjugates, and confirming that Ro 19-3704 blocks at least a part of these effects.[159] The results agreed well with those of Goswami except that the minimum effective concentrations of PAF were much higher (10 μM rather than 20 nM). Evidence for the role of secondary mediators in the secretory response to PAF came from their findings that simultaneous administration of arachidonic acid enhanced the effects of PAF.

Another study has given somewhat different results on the relative roles of lipoxygenase and cyclooxygenase products; Sasaki *et al.* examined the effects of PAF on the output of glycoconjugates from individual submucosal glands dissected from feline trachea.[160] They showed that PAF had no effect on secretion unless platelets were also present in the preparation (a finding which does not contradict the results of Lundgren *et al.*, as platelets may have been present in their preparation). However, inhibitors of the cyclooxygenase pathway and a thomboxane receptor antagonist blocked the secretory response, suggesting that, in this preparation, cyclooxygenase products had the major effect.

Histamine, prostaglandins, leukotrienes and PAF are all released in the asthmatic airway, so the ability of these mediators to release mucus glycoconjugate output gives further reason to suppose that airway secretion increases during attacks of asthma. This may well be the basis for the response to antigen challenge (see below).

Antigen challenge

In the anaesthetized dog, airway challenge with antigen increases the rate at which respiratory tract fluid reaches the point in the trachea from which it can be collected.[161] Phipps *et al.*[162] took tracheas from sheep sensitive to *Ascaris suum,* mounted them in Ussing chambers and studied both the secretion of radiolabelled glycoconjugates and the ion fluxes across the tissues. Exposure to *Ascaris* antigen increased the output of radiolabelled glycoproteins and, after a lag during which ions were absorbed from luminal to submucosal aspect, secretion of Na^+ and Cl^- ions into the lumen also increased. This suggests that initially there was secretion of concentrated mucus, poor in water and ions; later the volume was also augmented as water followed the passage of ions. Control proteins, to which the sheep was insensitive, had only minor effects on the secretion of mucus, probably the non specific action shown by many proteins on airway secretion.[163] Sodium cromoglycate reduced the effect of antigen challenge to a size similar to that of the non-specific effect, so the authors concluded that mediator release accounted for the major part of the response.[162]

King *et al.*[164] tested the effects of *Ascaris suum* antigen given by aerosol to conscious dogs with skin sensitivity to *Ascaris.* They collected mucus on to a cytology brush inserted through a port in the tracheal wall and measured the volume collected over a given time and also its physical properties. The extent to which the rate of mucus collection increased on challenge depended on the dose of antigen; with low doses, mucus elasticity tended to lessen but at higher doses it recovered and even increased to above the control level. Atropine and H_1 histamine antagonists lessened these responses both in terms of secretory rate and physical properties of mucus, though they did not abolish them; but H_2 blockers were ineffective.

There are few investigations of the effect of antigen challenge on secretion in human airway. Shelhamer *et al.* tested how antigens affected the secretion of radiolabelled glycoconjugates from passively sensitized bronchi, taken from human lungs removed at operation.[74] Antigen challenge augmented the release of radiolabelled glycoconjugates. Moreover, the medium in which challenged bronchus had been incubated increased the output of glycoconjugates from other airways, not passively sensitized; this suggests that mediators released during the original challenge persisted and could elicit further secretion. One doubt in the interpretation of these results is that there were no controls for the non-specific effects of proteins on secretion, but in view of the clear actions of antigens on secretion into the airways of sheep[162] and dog,[164] it is likely that antigen challenge in man does increase the output of airway mucus.

Loss of epithelium and airway secretion

A clear feature of the asthmatic airway is damage to the epithelium and the shedding of epithelial cells.[128,165] Isolated submucosal gland from the cat trachea slow their glyco-conjugate secretion when airway epithelium is added to their incubation medium,[166] suggesting that epithelial loss or damage might increase secretory rate, perhaps by loss of epithelial relaxing factors or enkephalinase. *In vivo*, exposure of afferent nerve endings might also augment the reflexes which cause secretion.

Drugs used in the treatment of asthma

Sufferers from asthma often take drugs to alleviate symptoms and these may alter the quantity or quality of mucus secreted into the airways. This in turn might affect the accumulation of mucus in patients' airways.

In several animal species, adrenoceptor agonists stimulate secretion. Both α- and β-adrenoceptor agonists stimulate glycoconjugate secretion in cat and ferret.[72,82,83,167] In the cat, selective β_1-agonists have a stronger effect on glycoconjugate secretion than their β_2-counterparts.[83] There is now evidence that, at least in the ferret, α-adrenoceptor agonists stimulate secretions of low viscosity, mainly from serous cells, while β-adrenoceptor agonists act mainly on mucous cells and release mucus of a higher viscosity.[59,91] So far, evidence for a parallel in human airway is lacking, but it would be surprising if there were not some mechanism for differential control over serous and mucous cell secretion in man; it may not be based on adrenoceptors, however.

In the human airway, early studies failed to show any action of adrenoceptor agonists on secretion,[69] but recent studies suggest that they do affect it. Shelhamer *et al.* found that α-agonists stimulated the secretion of radiolabelled glycoconjugates from human airway, though in this study β-agonists did not.[74] Phipps *et al.* found that both α- and β-agonists (including salbutamol, a relatively selective β_2-agonist) would stimulate secretion of radiolabelled glycoconjugates from human bronchus *in vitro*, and that their respective antagonists prevented such effects.[85] The reason for the contradiction between the results of these two sets of experiments is not clear, but the methods used gave a scatter of results, and it is usually necessary to perform a number of experiments to establish an effect; perhaps two experiments each with adrenaline and isoprenaline were too few on which to discount the action of β-receptors.[74] Richardson and Phipps[138] suggested that the spate of deaths from asthma, which coincided with the use of isoprenaline aerosols in the late 1960s,[168,169] may have resulted from the drug's repeated stimulation of mucus secretion into airways where clearance had ceased.[148.] Accumulation of mucus in the airways could also play a part in the exacerbation of asthma apparently produced by regular inhalation of the β_2-agonist fenoterol.[170]

At least in the ferret, tracheal epithelium transports albumin from submucosal tissues into the lumen. This is a receptor-controlled process, powerfully stimulated by β-adrenoceptor agonists including salbutamol.[48] If human airway epithelium behaves in the same way, this routine drug treatment of asthma attacks may increase the protein content of mucus and, as a result, its viscosity.[50]

Leucocytes

In health the macrophages form the main resident population of leucocytes in the airway lumen. In asthma neutrophils and, particularly, eosinophils, move into the airway lumen. Each of these leucocytes can, given the right stimulus, release substances which augment airway secretion.

Macrophages. Once macrophages are activated, for instance by exposure to zymogen granules or complement (C3)-coated Sepharose beads, they release monocyte-derived mucus secretagogue (MMS). This has a molecular weight of about 2000 Da, and releases glycoconjugates from human airway tissue culture.[171,172]

Neutrophils. Neutrophils can release several proteolytic enzymes, including neutrophil elastase and cathepsin G. Neutrophil elastase has been tested on cultured cells from the dog trachea where the enzyme releases glycoconjugate from the cell surface glycocalyx.[22] This glycoconjugate is susceptible to degradation with keratanase, suggesting a keratan sulphate or polylactosamine structure. Neutrophil elastase also releases lectin-reactive glycoconjugate from the glycocalyx on epithelial cells cultured from the hamster trachea.[23] Material released from the hamster trachea is predominantly mucus glycoprotein rather than proteoglycan.[173] More recent results show that both neutrophil elastase and cathepsin G, at concentrations of 10^{-9} M and upwards, cause secretion of proteoglycan-like material (degraded by chondroitinase ABC) from the granules of bovine serous cells in culture. These effects were particularly intense, causing increases in secretory rate of up to 2000% over baseline.[174] Thus it appears that proteolytic enzymes from neutrophils can release glycoconjugates from at least two cellular sources.

Activated neutrophils have been reported to produce a substance ($\sim$100 kDa) which releases glycoconjugates from human airway cultures *in vitro*. Inhibition of proteinases failed to prevent this response, so the authors suggested a secretagogue protein from neutrophils, independent of proteinases.[175]

Eosinophils. Eosinophils, typically the most numerous cell in the airway lumen during asthma attacks,[6] produce, when activated, several proteins that could influence mucus secretion; these include major basic protein and eosinophil cationic protein.[176] Eosinophils also release low molecular weight mediators such as PAF (see above). The effects of some of the proteins purified from eosinophil granules have recently been tested on the release of mucus glycoconjugates from human and feline airway explants.[177] Major basic protein at 50 μg/ml (a concentration which has been reported in sputum from asthmatic patients).[178] inhibited release of mucus glycoconjugate from feline airway, but was not tested on human bronchus. Eosinophil cationic protein, on the other hand, stimulated glycoconjugate output from both feline and human airway at a concentration of 2.5 μg/ml; whether this concentration occurs in the asthmatic airway appears not to be known.

Major basic protein (10^{-6} M, or $\sim$12 μg/ml, and upwards added to the luminal side of the epithelium) also stimulates the short circuit current across canine tracheal epithelium by stimulating chloride secretion into the lumen.[179] Water would be likely to follow by osmosis.

Other influences

Airway osmolarity. A number of other factors may increase airway secretion before or during an asthma attack. The breathing of chilled air, or hyperpnoea (e.g. during exercise), increases the heat and water loss from the walls of the lower airway. This is one of the triggers for asthma.[180] In cat trachea, flow of poorly conditioned air through the tracheobronchial tree results in secretion of mucus, possibly via the release of mediators.[181] It is the raised osmolarity rather than cooling, both of which result from drying the airway surface, which appears to be at the root of this effect.

Proteins including serum. When serum enters the airway it stimulates secretion by the non specific action of proteins. This was first shown in cat trachea, but also applies in human bronchus, where one part of serum in 100 volumes of Krebs–Henseleit is sufficient to trigger secretion.[163,182] Higher concentrations of serum are frequently found in asthmatic sputum.[125] There is now evidence for active transport of serum proteins across the epithelium into the lumen, increased by drugs such as β-adrenoceptor agonists.[48]

  This section has reviewed the evidence that mucus secretion increases in the asthmatic airway, and examined the processes which are likely to drive such an increase. A remarkable number of such drives may participate during an asthmatic attack. The accountancy of the system, the task of deciding which of the many mechanisms are likely to be important, may be daunting, but it is important to tackle it if there is to be any hope of developing rational therapies to control hypersecretion in asthma.

The evidence that mucus is abnormal in asthma

Sputum expectorated by asthmatics is often jelly-like, apparently with an abnormally high viscoelasticity.[139] There are remarkably few objective measurements of the physical properties of mucus from the airways of asthmatic patients, perhaps because it is difficult to obtain samples large enough to allow easy investigation. Charman and Reid used a cone and plate viscometer to demonstrate the viscosity of sputum expectorated by patients with several airway diseases (cystic fibrosis, chronic bronchitis, bronchiectasis and asthma). There was a large scatter of viscosities within each disease group, and much overlap in values between groups, but the asthmatics had the highest mean value.[183] It would be interesting to repeat these tests with measurements of viscosity at a lower shear rate (nearer to that imposed by the cilia)[92] and to add measurements of elasticity. It is likely that the physical properties of mucus secreted during an asthma attack vary from one airway to another and from one day to the next. The most abnormal secretions may stagnate in the airways while more normal ones, capable of being moved by cilia and cough, might appear as sputum. Ideally, then, such a study should measure the physical properties of plugs collected directly from the lower airway at different stages of an attack as well as those of sputum.

  The physical abnormality of mucus in asthma is poorly documented, then, but clinical observation suggests that it is one of the roots of bronchial and bronchiolar plugging. Certainly one would expect mucus with extremely high viscoelasticity to resist movement either by cough or ciliary action.[92]

Failure of the mucociliary escalator in asthma

Mucus transport in asthma

Even in the asymptomatic asthmatic patient, the speed at which cilia move radio-opaque particles placed on the tracheal surface (tracheal mucus velocity or TMV) is about half that in the normal subject (6.3 mm/min vs. 11.6 mm/min).[184] Subsequent challenge with inhaled antigen slowed TMV again, by a further 25 to 50%.[184,185] Sluggish mucociliary transport probably extends into the smaller airways. Bateman *et al.*[186] had subjects breathe an aerosol of polystyrene particles, 5 µm in diameter and labelled with 99Tc, a gamma-emitting radioisotope, so that the dust settled in many airways, large and small. This allowed them to follow the clearance of radiolabelled dust from the lung fields with a gamma camera. In asthmatic subjects the radiolabelled dust tended to settle in more central airways (and thus had a shorter distance to travel before quitting the chest) than in the normals; but, once allowance had been made for this, the normals cleared the dust faster.

Slowing of mucociliary transport by antigen and leukotrienes

Wanner and his colleagues (see ref. 187) have analysed the deficit in the mucociliary transport in asthma by attempting to block the effects of airway antigen challenge in man and animals with drugs of specific action. This approach has given useful insights into the nature of the airway dysfunction. The first antigen challenge experiment involved anaesthetized dogs, sensitive to *Ascaris suum* on skin test, being given an aerosol of that antigen.[188] The immediate effect was, in half the dogs, a rise in airway resistance which peaked in 5 min and returned to normal within an hour. In all dogs, whether or not airway resistance had altered, TMV began to slow after 15 min and had still not recovered by the end of the experiment, 2 h after challenge. Control challenge with ragweed pollen, to which the dogs were insensitive, altered neither airway resistance nor TMV. Treatment of the dogs before *Ascaris* challenge with a leukotriene antagonist, FPL 55712, made little difference to the rise in airway resistance, but converted the slowing of TMV into an acceleration. This suggested the hypothesis that leukotrienes or SRS-A were at the root of the slowing of mucociliary transport. In agreement with this, it has been found that histamine and acetylcholine, two other mediators believed to be important in the response to airway challenge, both accelerate TMV.[188,189]

Equivalent tests in man gave similar results.[185] Asthmatic subjects, sensitive to ragweed pollen, were challenged with an aerosol of that antigen after receiving either placebo or FPL 55712. Airway conductance (the reciprocal of resistance) and TMV were measured at intervals. After placebo, challenge slowed TMV to 74% of baseline, while after the leukotriene antagonist, challenge accelerated TMV (to 130% of baseline). As in the dog, airway conductance waxed and waned more quickly than did TMV.

Subsequent experiments with leukotriene aerosols in conscious sheep go some way to confirm the role of leukotrienes suggested by the earlier experiments.[190] Two groups of sheep, one with and the other without specific *Ascaris* sensitivity, were given aerosols of leukotriene D_4 (LTD_4) at different concentrations. Allergic sheep showed rises in specific airway resistance in response to aerosols of LTD_4 at concentrations of 100 and 150 µg/ml; FPL 55712 (an LT inhibitor) inhibited this bronchoconstriction. Non-allergic sheep failed to bronchoconstrict in response to aerosols of the mediator at these concentrations. In the allergic sheep, an aerosol of 25 µg/ml LTD_4 was sufficient to slow TMV, though in the non-allergic animals only the highest concentration (150 µg/ml) was effective. Thus far the results agree with the idea that leukotrienes are crucial to allergic inhibition of mucus transport, but another observation fails to fit this scheme: FPL 55712 did not prevent the slowing of transport induced by LTD_4. This is unexpected; possibly FPL 55712 does not block all leukotriene receptors. This observation, however, does not discredit the idea that leukotrienes may be involved in slowing of mucociliary transport after antigen challenge to the airways.

The delay between antigen challenge and slowing of mucociliary transport suggest an indirect response, involving a cascade of mediators or cells, but with leukotrienes being important in the later part of the pathway. Abraham *et al.*[191] have shown that the delayed rise in airway resistance in response to allergen challenge can be prevented by either WEB 2086 (PAF antagonist) or by FPL 55712 (LT antagonist), suggesting involvement of both PAF and leukotrienes. The reaction of mucociliary transport to PAF appears not to have been tested *in vivo* in sheep, but *in vitro* PAF slows transport of airway surface liquid (e.g. 10^{-5} M PAF slowed transport velocity to 40% of control).[192]

Wanner's group has also tried to analyse how antigens, PAF and leukotrienes inhibit mucociliary transport.[193] They tested the reaction of ciliated cells brushed from the airways of sheep, allergic and non-allergic, to leukotriene D_4 and prostaglandins. Both classes of mediators accelerated ciliary beat frequency in the cells, irrespective of the allergic status of their providers. A direct action of leukotrienes on ciliated cells, then, cannot explain their impairment of mucociliary transport nor that produced by antigen inhalation. More evidence that direct depression of ciliary beat frequency is not the mechanism of slowed mucociliary transport in response to PAF and antigen comes from recent *in vitro* experiments[192] which demonstrated a startling dissociation between mucociliary transport velocity and ciliary beat. PAF, at a concentration of 10^{-5} M, slowed ciliary transport of airway surface liquid by 60%, while diminishing ciliary beat frequency by only ~5%. Antigen challenge, in this preparation, accelerated ciliary beat frequency by 10% while halving mucociliary transport velocity.

If ciliary beat frequency is not the sole, or even possibly the main determinant of mucus clearance in the airways, what other factors could be? Alternative explanations of slowed mucociliary transport in asthma, antigen challenge, and allied mediator treatments include the following:

(1) *Force of ciliary beat.* In the heart, force of ventricular contraction, as well as heart rate, determines cardiac output. By analogy, the force of ciliary contraction might determine mucus transport velocity independently of beat frequency. This does not appear to have been tested.

(2) *Abnormal physical properties of mucus.* When the viscoelastic properties of mucus depart an optimal range, mucociliary transport slows.[92,108] Although the physical properties of mucus probably deviate from the ideal in asthma (see above), mucus transport slowed without apparent change in its physical properties after allergen and PAF challenges to sheep airways *in vitro.*[192] Physical properties of mucus, while they may be important, are not the only factors involved.

(3) *Sloughing of ciliated cells.* Asthma itself damages the epithelium sufficiently to slough ciliated cells,[120,165] but the rapid recovery, in about 3 h, after impairment of mucociliary transport by LTD_4 suggests that here loss of ciliated cells is not the mechanism. After antigen challenge, however, the impairment of mucociliary transport has a more leisurely time course, with a maximum at 8 h and a duration of up to 22 days;[194] sloughing and regrowth of ciliated cells could underlie this process.

The evidence reviewed here suggests that several distinct processes slow mucociliary transport in asthma.

Other mechanisms that may impair mucociliary transport in asthma

Eosinophils are one of the cells found in large numbers in the lumen and submucosa of the asthmatic airway. Frigas *et al.*[178,195] have measured the concentration of major basic protein, an eosinophil product with a molecular mass of ~12 000 Da, in secretions from asthmatic patients. They identified it in sputa from virtually all asthmatics with a mean concentration of 7 μg/ml and a maximum of 96 μg/ml, while those from patients suffering other diseases of the airway, with two exceptions, contained none. At a concentration of 10 μg/ml it caused ciliostasis and a patchy shedding of epithelial cells from guinea-pig trachea kept in organ culture. At 100 μg/ml it caused rapid shedding of the epithelium. Major basic protein paralyses isolated axonemes from human cilia.[196]

Dulfano and Luk[197] centrifuged sputa from patients with intrinsic and extrinsic asthma into sol and gel. They tested the sols on the beating of human bronchial ciliated cells, and found that most asthmatic sol preparations inhibited ciliary beating with a maximal effect 60 min after application. Gel chromatographic separation of the sputum sols demonstrated a ciliostatic substance eluting as a peak with molecular mass of 8000–9000 Da. Assay of the peak for major basic protein proved negative. There may be several substances (proteins?) in the asthmatic airway capable of inhibiting or damaging ciliated cells.

CAN DRUG TREATMENT HELP TO CLEAR MUCUS AND EXUDATE FROM THE AIRWAY?

Leukotriene antagonists

Results from studies on antigen challenge to the airways of dogs and of human asthmatic subjects show that leukotriene antagonists can improve mucociliary transport after airway antigen challenge.[185,188] This suggests that a safe leukotriene antagonist might have a place in the therapy of asthma. A recent report suggests that treatment of stable chronic asthmatic patients with an oral leukotriene antagonist (ICI 204,219) increases FEV_1,[198] but no one appears yet to have tested whether this antagonist accelerates mucociliary transport.

Sodium cromoglycate

Sodium cromoglycate also helped prevent the slowing of mucociliary transport in Wanner *et al's.* canine model of asthma,[188] but the possible role of this drug, or the pharmacologically related nedocromil, in accelerating mucociliary transport in asthmatic man has not, it seems, been tested.

Glucocorticoids

Several aspects of the action of glucocorticoids on airway secretion and clearance have now been investigated. Dexamethasone administered in the drinking water of rats prevents goblet-cell hyperplasia in the tracheal epithelium which develops in response to instillation of activated or lysed neutrophils (or to purified neutrophil elastase) into the lower airways.[199] It would be interesting to see whether inhaled glucocorticoids prevent, or even reverse, the goblet-cell metaplasia and submucosal gland hypertrophy seen in the airways of human asthmatics.

Glucocorticoids slow the secretion of airway mucus, and the mechanism of this has recently been reviewed by Lundgren *et al.*[200] Marom *et al.* first showed that dexamethasone treatment slows the basal secretion rate of glycoconjugates from explants of human airways.[201] Dexamethasone, at 10^{-9}M and upwards, inhibits glycoconjugate release from explants of feline airway in organ culture, and treating the explants with antibodies against lipocortin prevented this inhibition, evidence that glucocorticoids act via this intermediate.[202] Shimura *et al.* examined the effects of glucocorticoids on the release of glycoconjugates from individual submucosal glands, dissected from the cat trachea.[203] They confirmed the inhibitory action of dexamethasone, at concentrations as low as 10^{-9}M, on the basal rate of secretion and also showed that this drug inhibits release of mucus glycoconjugates in response to both α- and β-adrenoceptor agonists. There was no clear evidence for inhibition of uptake of a radiolabelled precursor and its synthesis into mucus glycoconjugates.

There is evidence that treatment of asthmatics with glucocorticoids accelerates the movement of radiolabelled particles from peripheral airways of asthma sufferers, but does not restore clearance to normal.[204]

CONCLUSIONS

The mucus and exudate that cling to the airway walls in many who suffer asthma obstruct airflow, cause airway hyperresponsiveness and lead to ventilation–perfusion mismatch. This is one of the major lesions in the asthmatic lung, certainly in severe asthma, but also probably in milder forms of the disease. Increased mucus production, abnormal mucus which resists movement by cilia or coughing, and other defects in the mucociliary system, combine to frustrate the clearance mechanisms and so lead to the plugging of airways with mucus and exudate. Therapy to relax airway smooth muscle in those who suffer asthma is now effective, but treatment to clear stagnant mucus is rudimentary; such therapies as exist (e.g. glucocorticoids) have developed by chance rather than through systematic search. This is an area where thoughtful and energetic research gives real hope of improving the treatment of asthma.

REFERENCES

1. Jeffery PK, Reid LM: The respiratory mucus membrane. In Brain J, Proctor D, Reid L (eds), *Respiratory Defence Mechanisms*, Part 1. New York, Marcel Dekker, 1977, 193–245.
2. Sandoz D, Nicholas G, Laine MC: Two mucus cell types revisited after quick freezing and cryosubstitution. *Biol Cell* (1985) **54:** 79–88.
3. Nadel JA, Widdicombe JH, Peatfield AC: Regulation of airway secretions, ion transport and water movement, In Fishman AP (ed) *Handbook of Physiology:* section 3, Vol 1, Bethesda, MD, American Physiological Society, 1985, pp 419–446.

4. Ellefson P, Tos M: Goblet cells in the human trachea. Quantitative studies of normal tracheae. *Anat Anz* (1972) **130:** 501–520.

5. Ellefson P, Tos M: Goblet cells in the human trachea. Quantitative studies of pathophysiological biopsy material. *Arch Otolaryngol* (1972) **95:** 547–555.

6. Thurlbeck WM: Chronic airflow obstruction in lung disease. In Bennington JL (ed) *Major Problems in Pathology*. Philadelphia, WB Saunders, 1976, p 45.

7. Verdugo P: Goblet cell secretion and mucogenesis. *Ann Rev Physiol* (1990) **52:** 157–176.

8. Thornton DJ, Davies JR, Kraayenbrink M, Richardson PS, Sheehan JK, Carlstedt I: Mucus glycoproteins from 'normal' human tracheobronchial mucus. *Biochem J* (1990) **256:** 179–186.

9. Neutra MR, Leblond CP: Synthesis of the carbohydrate of mucus in the Golgi complex as shown by electron microscope radioautography of goblet cells injected with glucose-3H. *J Cell Biol* (1966) **30:** 119–136.

10. Basbaum CB, Jany B, Finkbeiner WE: The serous cell. *Ann Rev Physiol* 1990 **52:** 97–113.

11. Jeffery PH, Reid L: The effect of tobacco smoke with or without phenylmethyloxadiazole (PMO) on rat bronchial epithelium: a light and electron microscopic study. *J. Pathol* (1981) **133:** 341–359.

12. Widdicombe JG, Pack RG: The Clara cell. *Eur J Respir Dis* (1982) **63:** 202–220.

13. Plopper CG: Comparative morphologic features of bronchiolar epithelial cells. The Clara cell. *Am Rev Respir Dis* (1983) **128:** 537–541.

14. Smith P, Heath D, Moosavi H: The Clara cell. *Thorax* (1974) **29:** 147–163.

15. Evans MJ, Cabral-Anderson LJ, Freeman G: Role of the Clara cell in renewal of the bronchial epithelium. *Lab Invest* (1978) **38:** 648–653.

16. Breeze RG, Wheeldon EB: The cells of pulmonary airways. *Am Rev Respir Dis* (1977) **116:** 705–770.

17. Rhodin JAG: The ciliated cell. Ultrastructure and function of the human tracheal mucosa. *Am Rev Respir Dis* (1966) **93:** (3), 1–15.

18. Sleigh MA: Mucus transport by cilia. *Chest* (1981) **80** (Suppl): 791–795.

19. Jeffery PK: Structure and function of mucus-secreting cells of cat and goose airway epithelium. In *Respiratory Tract Mucus. Ciba Foundation Symposium* 54, Elsevier, (1978), 5–20.

20. Korhonen LK, Holopainen E, Paavolainen M: Some histochemical characteristics of the tracheobronchial tree and pulmonary neoplasms. *Acta Histochem Bd* (1969) **32:** 57–73.

21. Spicer SS, Chakrin LW, Wardell SR, Kendrick W: Histochemistry of mucosubstances in the canine and human respiratory tract. *Lab Invest* (1971) **25:** 483–490.

22. Varsano S, Borson DB, Gold M, Forsberg LS, Basbaum C, Nadel JA: Proteinases release 35SO4-radiolabelled macromolecules from cultured airway epithelial cells. *Fed Proc* (1986) **45:** 786.

23. Kim KC, Wasano K, Niles RM, Schuster JE, Stone PJ, Snider GL: Human neutrophil elastase releases cell surface mucins from primary cultures of hamster tracheal epithelial cells. *Proc Natl Acad Sci USA* (1987) **84:** 9304–9308.

24. Florey H, Carleton HM, Wells AW: Mucus secretion in the trachea. *Br J Exp Path* (1932) **13:** 269–284.

25. Spicer SS, Mochizuki I, Setser ME, Martinez JR: Complex carbohydrates of rat tracheobronchial surface epithelium visualized ultrastructurally. *Am J Anat* (1980) **158:** 93–109.

26. Bhaskar KR, O'Sullivan DD, Opaskar-Hincman H, Reid LM, Coles SJ: Density gradient analysis of secretions produced *in vitro* by human and canine airway mucosa: identification of lipids and proteoglycans in such secretions. *Exp Lung Res* (1986) **10:** 401–422.

27. Davies JR, Corbishley CM, Richardson PS: The uptake of radiolabelled precursors of mucus glycoconjugates by secretory tissues in the feline trachea. *J Physiol* (1990) **420:** 10–30.

28. Gallagher JT, Hall RL, Phipps RJ, Jeffery PK, Kent PW, Richardson PS: Mucus glycoproteins (mucins) of the cat trachea: Characterisation and control of secretion. *Biochem Biophys Acta* (1986) **886:** 243–254.

29. Davies JR, Gallagher JT, Richardson PS, Sheehan JK, Carlstedt I: Mucins in cat airway secretions; *Biochem J* (1991) **275:** 663–669.

30. Spicer SS, Chakrin LW, Wardell SR: Respiratory mucus secretion. In Dulfano M (ed) *Sputum, Fundamentals and Clinical Pathology*. Illinois, Springfield, 1973, pp 22–68.

31. Meyrick B, Sturgess JM, Reid LM: A reconstruction of the duct system and secretory tubules of the human bronchial submucosal gland. *Thorax* (1969) **24**: 729–736.

32. Bowes D, Corrin B: Ultrastructural immunocytochemical localisation of lysozyme in human bronchial glands. *Thorax* (1977) **32**: 163–170.

33. Bowes D, Clark AE, Corrin B: Ultrastructural localisation of lactoferrin and glycoprotein in human bronchial gland. *Thorax* (1981) **36**: 108–115.

34. Meyrick B, Reid LM: Ultrastructure of cells in the human bronchial submucosal glands. *J Anat* (1970) **107**: 281–299.

35. Richardson PS: The control of mucus secretion in the airways. In Saunders KB (ed) *Advanced Medicine* 19. London, Pitman, 1983, pp 336–348.

36. Carlstedt I, Sheehan JK: Macromolecular structure and polymeric structure of mucus glycoproteins. In *Mucus and Mucosa. Ciba Foundation Symposium* **109**, Pitman (1984), 157–166.

37. Sheffner AL: The reduction *in vitro* in viscosity of mucoprotein solutions by a new mucolytic agent, *n*-acetylcysteine. *Ann NY Acad Sci* (1936) **106**: 721–729.

38. Sheffner AL, Medler EM, Jacobs LW, Sarrett HP: The *in vitro* reduction in viscosity of human tracheobronchial secretions by acetylcysteine. *Am Rev Respir Dis* (1964) **90**: 721–729.

39. Bhaskar KR, O'Sullivan DD, Seltzer J, Rossing TH, Drazen JM, Reid LM: Density gradient study of bronchial mucus aspirates from healthy volunteers (smokers and non-smokers) and from patients with tracheostomy. *Exp Lung Res* (1985) **9**: 298–308.

40. Paul A, Picard J, Mergey M, Veissiere D, Finkbeiner WE, Basbaum CB: Glycoconjugates secreted by bovine tracheal serous cells in culture. *Arch Biochem Biophys* (1988) **260**: 75–84.

41. Bhaskar KR, Drazen JM, O'Sullivan DD, Scanlon PM, Reid LM: Transition from normal to hypersecretory bronchial mucus in a canine model of bronchitis: changes in yield and composition. *Exp Lung Res* (1988) **14**: 101–120.

42. Phipps RJ, Richardson PS: The effects of irritation at various levels of the airway upon mucus secretion into the cat trachea. *J Physiol* (1976) **261**: 563–581.

43. Somerville M, J-A Karlsson, Richardson PS: The effect of local anaesthetic agents upon mucus secretion in feline trachea *in vivo*. *Pulm Pharmacol* (1990) **3**: 93–101.

44. Perini J-M, Marianne T, LaFitte J-J, Lamblin G, Roussel P, Mazzuca M: Use of antisera against deglycosylated human mucins for cellular localization of their peptide precursors: antigenic similarities between bronchial and intestinal mucins. *J Hishochem Cytochem* (1989) **37**: 869–875.

45. Snyder CE, Nadziejko CE, Herp A: Binding of basic proteins to glycoproteins in human bronchial secretions. *Int J Biochem* (1982)**14**: 895–898.

46. Creeth JM, Bridge JL, Horton JR: An interaction between lysozyme and mucus glycoprotein. *Biochem J* (1979) **181**: 717–724.

47. Nahon J-L: The regulation of albumin and a-fetoprotein gene expression in mammals. *Biochemie* (1987) **69**: 445–459.

48. Webber SE, Widdicombe JG: The transport of albumin across the ferret *in vitro* whole trachea. *J. Physiol* (1989) **408**: 457–472.

49. Price AM, Webber SE, Widdicombe JG: Transport of albumin by the rabbit trachea *in vitro*. *J Appl Physiol* (1990) **68**: 726–730.

50. List SJ, Findley BP, Forstner GG, Forstner JF: Enhancement of the viscosity of mucin by serum albumin. *Biochem J* (1978) **75**: 565–571.

51. Clamp JR, Creeth JM: Some non-mucin components of mucus and their possible biological roles. In *Ciba Foundation Symposium* **109** (1984) 121–131.

52. Daniels RP: Immunoglobulin secretion in the airways. *Annu Rev Physiol* (1990) **52**: 177–195.

53. Franken C, Meijer CJLM, Dijkman JH: Tissue distribution of antileukoproteases and lysozyme in humans. *J Histochem Cytochem* (1989) **37**: 493–498.

54. Bailleul V, Richet C, Hayem A, Degand P: Propriétés rhéologiques des sécrétions bronchiques: mise in evidence et rôle de polypeptides riches en proline (PRP). *Clin Chimica Acta* (1977) **74**: 115–123.

55. Warner TF, Azen EA: Proline-rich proteins are present in serous cells of submucosal glands in the respiratory tract. *Am Rev Respir Dis* (1984) **130**: 115–118.

56. Sahu S, Lynn WS: Lipid composition in patients with asthma and patients with cystic fibrosis. *Am Rev Respir Dis* (1977) **115**: 233–239.

57. Galabert C, Jacquot J, Zahm JM, Puchelle E: Relationship between lipid content and rheological properties of airway secretions in cystic fibrosis. *Clin Chim Acta* (1987) **164:** 139–149.

58. Murlas C, Nadel JA, Basbaum CB: A morphometric analysis of the autonomic innervation of cat tracheal glands. *J Auton Nerv Syst* (1980) **2:** 23–37.

59. Basbaum CB, Barnes PJ, Grillo MA, Widdicombe JH, Nadel JA: Adrenergic and cholinergic receptors in submucosal glands of the ferret trachea: autoradiographic localisation. *Eur J Respir Dis* (1983) **128** (Suppl): 433–435.

60. Partanen M, Laitinen A, Hervonen A, Toivanen M, Laitinen LA: Catecholamine- and acetylcholinesterase-containing nerves in human lower respiratory tract. *Histochemistry* (1982) **76:** 175–188.

61. Pack RJ, Richardson PS: The aminergic innervation of the lower respiratory tract: a light and electron microscopic study. *J Anat* (1984) **138:** 493–502.

62. Richardson P, Webber S: The control of mucous secretion in the airways by peptidergic mechanisms. *Am Rev Respir Dis* (1987) **136** (Suppl): S72–S76.

63. Baraniuk JN, Lundgren JD, Goff J, Peden D, Merida M, Shelhamer J, Kaliner MA: Gastrin-releasing peptide (GRP) in human nasal mucosa. *J Clin Invest* (1990) **85:** 998–1005.

64. Baraniuk JN, Catellino S, Goff J, *et al.*: Neuropeptide Y (NPY) in human nasal mucosa. *Am J Respir Cell Mol Biol* (1990) **3:** 165–173.

65. Tom-Moy M, Basbaum CB, Nadel JA: Localization and release of lysozyme from ferret trachea: effect of adrenergic and cholinergic drugs. *Cell Tiss Res* (1983) **228:** 549–562.

66. Webber SE, Widdicombe JG: The effect of vasoactive intestinal polypeptide on smooth muscle tone and mucus secretion from the ferret trachea. *Br J Pharmacol* (1987) **91:** 1139–148.

67. Gum JR, Byrd JC, Hick JM, Toribara NW, Lamport DTA, Kim YS: Molecular cloning of human intestinal mucin cDNAs. *J Biol Chem* (1989) **237:** 527–532.

68. Gashi AA, Nadel JA, Basbaum CB: Tracheal gland mucous cells stimulated *in vitro* with adrenergic and cholinergic drugs. *Tissue Cell* (1989) **21:** 59–67.

69. Sturgess J, Reid L: An organ culture study of the effect of drugs on the secretory activity of the human bronchial submucosal gland. *Clin Sci* (1972) **43:** 533–543.

70. Boat TF, Kleinerman JI: Human respiratory tract secretions 2. Effect of cholinergic and adrenergic agents on *in vitro* release of protein and mucus glycoprotein. *Chest* (1975) **67:** 32S–34S.

71. Chakrin LW, Baker AP, Christian P, Wardell JR: The effect of cholinergic stimulation on the release of macromolecules by canine trachea *in vitro*. *Am Rev Respir Dis* (1973) **108:** 69–76.

72. Gallagher JT, Kent PW, Passatore M, Phipps RJ, Richardson PS: The composition of tracheal mucus and the nervous control of its secretion in the cat. *Proc R Soc London Ser B* (1975) **192:** 49–76.

73. Davis B, Marin M, Fischer S, Graf P, Widdicombe JG, Nadel JA: New method for study of canine mucous gland secretion *in vivo*: cholinergic regulation. *Am Rev Respir Dis (Abstr)* (1976) **113:** 257.

74. Shelhamer JH, Marom Z, Kaliner M: Immunologic and neuropharmacologic stimulation of mucous glycoprotein release from human airways *in vitro*. *J Clin Invest* (1980) **66:** 1400–1408.

75. Mak JCW, Barnes PJ: Autoradiographic visualisation of muscarinic receptor subtypes in human and guinea pig lungs. *Am Rev Respir Dis* (1990) **141:** 1559–1568.

76. Gater PR, Alabaster VA, Piper I: A study of muscarinic receptor subtype mediating mucus secretion in the cat trachea *in vitro*. *Pulm Pharmacol* (1989) **2:** 87–92.

77. Borson DB, Charlin M, Gold BD, Nadel JA: Neural regulation of $^{35}SO_4$-macromolecule secretion from tracheal glands of ferrets. *J Appl Physiol* (1984) **57:** 457–466.

78. Peatfield AC, Richardson PS: Evidence for non-cholinergic, non-adrenergic nervous control of mucus secretion into the cat trachea. *J Physiol* (1983) **342:** 335–345.

79. Shimura S, Sasaki T, Okayama H, Sasaki H, Takishima T: Neural control of contraction in isolated submucosal gland from feline trachea. *J Appl Physiol* (1987) **62:** 2404–2409.

80. Shimura S, Sasaki T, Sasaki H, Takishima T: Contractility of isolated single submucosal glands from trachea. *J Appl Physiol* (1986) **60:** 1237–1247.

81. Baker B, Peatfield AC, Richardson PS: Nervous control of mucin secretion into human bronchi. *J Physiol* (1985) **365:** 297–305.
82. Phipps RJ, Nadel JA, Davis B: Effect of alpha-adrenergic stimulation on mucus secretion and on ion transport in cat trachea *in vitro*. *Am Rev Resp Dis* (1980) **121:** 359–365.
83. Peatfield AC, Richardson PS: The control of mucin secretion into the lumen of the cat trachea by α- and β-adrenoceptors, and their relative involvement during sympathetic nerve stimulation. *Eur J Pharmacol* (1982) **81:** 617–626.
84. Basbaum CB: Regulation of secretion from serous and mucous cells in the trachea. In *Ciba Foundation Symposium* **109** (1984), 4–19.
85. Phipps RJ, Williams IP, Richardson PS, Pell J, Pack RJ, Wright N: Sympathomimetic drugs stimulate the output of secretory glycoproteins from human bronchi *in vitro*. *Clin Sci* (1982) **63:** (1), 23–28.
86. Pack RJ, Richardson PS, Smith ICH, Webb SR: The functional significance of the sympathetic innervation of mucous glands in the bronchi of man. *J Physiol* (1988) **403:** 211–219.
87. Carstairs JR, Nimmo AJ, Barnes PJ: Autoradiographic localisation of β-adrenoceptors in human lung. *Eur J Pharmacol* (1984) **103:** 189–190.
88. Sharma RK, Jeffery PK: Airway β-receptor number in cystic fibrosis and asthma. *Clin Sci* (1990) **78:** 409–417.
89. Basbaum CB, Ueki I, Brezina L, Nadel JA: Tracheal submucosal gland serous cells stimulated *in vitro* with adrenergic and cholinergic agonists. A morphometric study. *Cell Tiss Res* (1981) **220:** 481–498.
90. King M, Viires N: Effect of methacholine chloride on rheology and transport of canine tracheal mucus. *J Appl Physiol* (1979) **47:** 26–31.
91. Leikauf GD, Ueki IF, Nadel JA: Autonomic regulation of viscoelasticity of cat tracheal gland secretions. *J Appl Physiol* (1984) **56:** 426–430.
92. King M: Rheological requirements for optimal clearance of secretions: ciliary transport versus cough. *Eur J Respir Dis* (1980) **61** (Suppl 110): 39–45.
93. Coles SJ, Bhaskar KR, O'Sullivan DD, Neill KH, Reid LM: Airway mucus: composition and regulation of its secretion by neuropeptides *in vitro*. In *Ciba Foundation Symposium* **109** (1984), 40–60.
94. Peatfield AC, Barnes PJ, Bratcher C, Nadel JA, Davis B: Vasoactive intestinal peptide stimulates tracheal submucosal gland secretion in ferret. *Am Rev Respir Dis* (1983) **128** (1): 89–93.
95. Webber SE: The effects of peptide histidine isoleucine and neuropeptide Y on mucus volume output from the ferret trachea. *Br J Pharmacol* (1988) **95:** 49–54.
96. Lundgren JD, Baraniuk JN, Ostrowski NL, Kaliner MA, Shelhamer JH: Gastrin-releasing peptide stimulates glycoconjugate release from feline trachea. *Am J Physiol* (1990) **258:** L68–L74.
97. Baker AP, Hillegass LM, Holden DA, Smith WJ: Effect of Kallidin, substance-P and other basic polypeptides on the production of respiratory macromolecules. *Am Rev Respir Dis* (1977) **115:** 811–817.
98. Coles SJ, Neil KH, Reid LM: Potent stimulation of glycoprotein secretion in canine trachea by substance P. *J Appl Physiol* (1984) **57:** 1323–1327.
99. Shimura S, Sasaki T, Okayama H, Sasaki H, Takishima T: Effect of substance P on mucus secretion of isolated submucosal gland from feline trachea. *J Appl Physiol.* (1987) **63:** 646–653.
100. Lundgren JD, Wiedermann CJ, Logun C, Plutchok J, Kaliner M, Shelhamer JH: Substance P mediated secretion of respiratory glycoconjugates from feline trachea *in vitro*. *Exp Lung Res* (1989) **15:** 17–29.
101. Mizoguchi H, Hicks CR: Effects of neurokinins on ion transport and sulfated macromolecule release in the isolated ferret trachea. *Exp Lung Res* (1989) **15:** 837–848.
102. Webber SE: Receptors mediating the effects of substance P and neurokinin A on mucus secretion and smooth muscle tone of the ferret trachea: potentiation by an enkephalinase inhibitor. *Br J Pharmacol* (1989) **98:** 1197–1206.

103. Rogers DF, Aursudkij B, Rogers DF: Effects of tachykinins on mucus secretion in human bronchi *in vitro*. *Eur J Pharmacol* (1989) **174:** 283–286.
104. Jessel TM, Iversen LL: Opiate analgesics inhibit substance P release from rat trigeminal nucleus. *Nature* (1977) **268:** 549–551.
105. Rogers DF, Barnes PJ: Opioid inhibition of neurally mediated mucus secretion in human bronchi. *Lancet* (1989) **1:** 930–932.
106. Webber SE, Lim JCS, Widdicombe JG: The effects of calcitonin gene-related peptide on submucosal gland secretion and epithelial albumin transport in the ferret trachea *in vitro*. *Br J Pharmacol* (1991) **102:** 79–84.
107. Mak JC, Barnes PJ: Autoradiographic localization of calcitonin gene-related peptide binding sites in human and guinea pig lung. *Peptides* (1988) **9:** 957–963.
108. Meyer FA: Mucus structure: relation to biological transport function. *Biorheology* (1976) **13:** 49–58.
109. Sade J, Eliezer N, Silberberg A, Nevo AC: The role of mucus in transport by cilia. *Am Rev Respir Dis* (1970) **102:** 48–52.
110. Sleigh MA, Blake JR, Liron N: The propulsion of mucus by cilia. *Am Rev Respir Dis* (1988) **137:** 726–741.
111. Sadé J, Eliezer N, Silberberg A, Nevo AC: The role of mucus in transport by cilia. *Am Rev Respir Dis* (1970) **102:** 48–52.
112. Bhaskar KR, O'Sullivan DDF, Coles SJ, Kozakevich H, Vawter GP, Reid LM: Characterization of airway mucus from a fatal case of status asthmaticus. *Pediat Pulmonol* (1988) **5:** 176–182.
113. King M, Gilboa A, Meyer FA, Silberberg A: On the transport of mucus and its rheologic simulants in ciliated systems. *Am Rev Respir Dis* (1974) **110:** 740–745.
114. Shih CK, Litt M, Khan MA, Wolf DP: Effect of nondialyzable solids concentration and viscoelasticity on ciliary transport of tracheal mucus. *Am Rev Respir Dis* (1977) **115:** 989–996.
115. Kim CS, Rodriguez CR, Eldridge MA, Sackner MA: Criteria for mucus transport in the airways by two-phase gas–liquid flow mechanism. *J Appl Physiol* (1986) **60:** 901–907.
116. Kim CS, Greene MA, Sankaran S, Sackner MA: Mucus transport in the airways by two-phase gas–liquid flow mechanisms: continuous flow model. *J Appl Physiol* (1986) **60:** 908–917.
117. Scherer PW: Mucus transport by cough. *Chest* (1981) **80:** 830–833.
118. Ramphal R, Pyle M: Evidence for mucins and sialic acid as receptors for *Pseudomonas aeruginosa* in the lower respiratory tract. *Infect Immun* (1983) **41:** 339–344.
119. Ramphal R, Pyle M: Adherence of mucoid and nonmucoid *Pseudomonas aeruginosa* to acid-injured tracheal epithelium. *Infect Immun* (1983) **41:** 345–351.
120. Dunnill MS: The pathology of asthma, with special reference to changes in the bronchial mucosa. *J Clin Pathol* (1960) **13:** 27–33.
121. Keal EE, Reid L: Pathological alteration in mucus in asthma within and without the cell. In Stein M (ed) *New Directions in Asthma*. Park Ridge, Il, American College of Chest Physicians, 1975, pp 223–239.
122. Dunnill MS: The morphology of the airways in bronchial asthma. In Stein M (ed) *New Directions of Asthma*. Park Ridge, Il, American College of Chest Physicians, 1975, pp 213–221.
123. Sanerkin NG, Evans DMD: The sputum in bronchial asthma, pathognomic patterns. *J Path Bact* (1965) **89:** 535–541.
124. Bhaskar KR, Reid L: Application of density gradient methods for the study of mucus glycoprotein and other macromolecular components in the sol and gel phases of asthmatic sputa. *J Biol Chem* (1981) **256:** 7583–7585.
125. Brogan TD, Ryley HC, Allen L, Hutt M: Relation between sputum sol phase composition and diagnosis in chronic chest diseases. *Thorax* (1971) **26:** 418–423.
126. Puchelle E, Zahm JM, Havez R: Donnees biochimiques et rheologiques dans l'expectoration III-relation des proteines et mucines bronchiques avec les proprietes rheologiques. *Bull Physiopathol Resp* (1973) **9:** 237–256.
127. Freedman BJ: The functional geometry of the bronchi. *Bull Physiopathol Resp* (1971) **8:** 545–552.

128. Dunnill MS, Massarella GR, Anderson JL: A comparison of the quantitative anatomy of the bronchi in normal subjects, in status asthmaticus, in chronic bronchitis and emphysema. *Thorax* (1969) **24:** 176–170.

129. James AL, Paré PD, Hogg JC: The mechanics of airway narrowing in asthma. *Am Rev Respir Dis* (1989) **139:** 242–246.

130. Woolcock AJ, Salome CM, Yan K: The shape of the dose-response curve to histamine in asthmatic and normal subjects. *Am Rev Respir Dis* (1984) **130:** 71–75.

131. Kim CS, Eldridge MA, Wanner A: Airway responsiveness to inhaled and intravenous carbachol in sheep: effect of airway mucus. *J Appl Physiol* (1988) **65:** 2744–2751.

132. Weiss EB, Hargreaves WA, Viswanath SG: The inhibitory action of lidocaine in anaphylaxis. *Am Rev Respir Dis* (1978) **117:** 859–869.

133. Hulbert WC, McClean T, Hogg JC: The effect of acute airway inflammation on bronchial reactivity in guinea pigs. *Am Rev Respir Dis* (1985) **131:** 7–11.

134. James AL, Pare PD, Hogg JC: Effects of lung volume, bronchoconstriction and cigarette smoke on morphometric airway dimensions. *J Appl Physiol* (1988) **64:** 913–919.

135. Wagner PD, Dantzker DR, Iacovani VE, Tomlin WC, West JB: Ventilation–perfusion inequality in asymptomatic asthma. *Am Rev Respir Dis* (1978) **118:** 511–524.

136. Maxwell GM: The problem of mucus plugging in children with asthma. *J Asthma* (1985) **22:** 131–137.

137. Toremalm NG: The daily amount of tracheo-bronchial secretions in man. *Acta Otolaryngol (Suppl)* (1960) **158:** 43–53.

138. Richardson PS, Phipps RJ: The anatomy, physiology, pharmacology and pathology of tracheobronchial mucus secretion and the use of expectorant drugs in human disease. *Pharmacol Therap* (1978) **3:** 441–479.

139. Hilding AC: The relation of ciliary insufficiency to death from asthma and other respiratory diseases. *Ann Otol* (1943) **52:** 5–19.

140. German VF, Ueki IF, Nadel JA: Micropipette measurement of airway submucosal gland secretion: laryngeal reflex. *Am Rev Respir Dis* (1980) **122:** 413–416.

141. Peatfield AC, Richardson PS: The action of dust in the airways on secretion into the trachea of the cat. *J Physiol* (1983) **342:** 327–334.

142. King M, Brock G, Lundell C: Clearance of mucus by simulated cough. *J Appl Physiol* (1985) **58:** 1776–1782.

143. Karlsson J-A, Sant'Ambrogio G, Widdicombe JG: Afferent neural pathways in cough and bronchoconstriction. *J Appl Physiol* (1988) **65:** 1007–1023.

144. Sant'Ambrogio G: Information arising from the tracheobronchial tree of mammals. *Phys Rev* (1982) **62:** 531–569.

145. Coleridge JCG, Coleridge HM: Afferent vagal C fibre innervation of the lungs and airways and its functional significance. *Rev Physiol Biochem Pharmac* (1984) **99:** 1–110.

146. Davis B, Roberts AM, Coleridge HM, Coleridge JC: Reflex tracheal gland secretion evoked by stimulation of bronchial C-fibers in dogs. *J Appl Physiol* (1982) **53:** 985–991.

147. Kyle H, Widdicombe JG: The effects of peptides and mediators on mucus secretion rate and smooth muscle tone in the ferret trachea. *Agents Actions* (1987) **22:** 86–90.

148. Richardson PS, Phipps RJ, Balfre K, Hall RL: The role of mediators, irritants and allergens in causing mucin secretion from the trachea. In *Respiratory Tract Mucus Ciba Foundation Symposium* **54,** Elsevier (1978), 111–126.

149. Lopez-Vidriero MT, Das I, Picot R, Smith AP, Reid L: Bronchial secretion from normal human airways after inhalation of prostaglandin F2α, acetylcholine, histamine and citric acid. *Thorax* (1977) **32:** 734–739.

150. Marom Z, Shelhamer JH, Back MK, Morton DR, Kaliner M: Slow reacting substances, leukotrienes C4 and D4 increase the release of mucus from human airway *in vitro*. *Am Rev Respir Dis* (1982) **126:** 449–451.

151. Marom Z, Shelhamer JH, Kaliner M: Effects of arachidonic acid, monohydroxyeicosatetranoic acid and prostaglandins on the release of mucous glycoproteins from human airways *in vitro*. *J Clin Invest* (1981) **67:** 1695–1702.

152. Rich B, Peatfield AC, Williams IP, Richardson PS: Effects of prostaglandins E1, E2, and F2α on mucin secretion from human bronchi *in vitro*. *Thorax* (1984) **39:** (6), 420–423.

153. Peatfield AC, Piper PJ, Richardson PS: The effect of leukotriene C4 on mucin release into the cat trachea *in vivo* and *in vitro*. *Br J Pharmacol* (1982) **77**(3): 391–393.
154. Page CP: Platelet activating factor. Chapter 19 of this volume.
155. Lee TC, Lenihan DJ, Malone BJ, Roddy LL, Wasserman SI: Increased biosynthesis of platelet activating factor in activated human eosinophils. *J Biol Chem* (1984) **259**: 5526–5530.
156. Hahn HL, Purnama I, Lang M, Sannwald U, Stenzel H: Effects of platelet activating factor on release of mucus from tracheal submucosal gland in the ferret. *Am Rev Respir Dir* (1985) **131**: A27 (Abstract).
157. Adler KB, Schwarz JE, Anderson WH, Welton AF: Platelet activating factor stimulates secretion of mucin by explants of rodent airways in organ culture. *Exp Lung Res* (1987) **13**: 25–43.
158. Goswami SK, Ohashi MO, Stathas P, Marom ZM: Platelet-activating factor stimulates secretion of respiratory glycoconjugate from human airways in culture. *J Allergy Clin Immunol* (1989) **84**: 726–734.
159. Lundgren JD, Kaliner M, Logun C, Shelhamer JH: Platelet activating factor and tracheo-bronchial respiratory glycoconjugate release in feline and human explants: involvement of the lipoxygenase pathway. *Agents & Actions* (1990) **30**: 329–337.
160. Sasaki T, Shimura S, Ikeda K, Sasaki H, Takishima T: Platelet-activating factor increases platelet-dependent glycoconjugate secretion from tracheal submucosal gland. *Am J Physiol* (1989) **257**: L373–L378.
161. Yamatake Y, Sasagawa S, Yanaura S, Kobayashi N: Involvement of histamine H_1- and H_2-receptors in induced asthmas in dogs. *Jpn J Pharmac* (1977) **27**: 791–797.
162. Phipps RJ, Denas SM, Wanner A: Antigen stimulates glycoprotein secretion and alters ion fluxes in sheep trachea. *J Appl Physiol* (1983) **55**: 1593–1602.
163. Peatfield AC, Hall RL, Richardson PS, Jeffery PK: The effect of serum on the secretion of radiolabelled mucous macromolecules into the lumen of the cat trachea. *Am Rev Respir Dis* (1982) **125**: (2), 210–215.
164. King M, El AJ, Phillips DM, Angus GE: Antigen challenge and canine tracheal mucus. *Int Arch Allergy Appl Immunol* (1985) **77**: (3), 337–342.
165. Laitinen LA, Heino M, Laitinen A, Kava T, Haahtela T: Damage of the airway epithelium and bronchial reactivity in patients with asthma. *Am Rev Respir Dis* (1985) **131**: 599–606.
166. Sasaki T, Shimura S, Sasaki H, Takishima T: Effects of epithelium on mucus secretion from feline tracheal submucosal glands. *J Appl Physiol* (1989) **66**: 764–770.
167. Borson DB, Chinn RA, Davis B, Nadel JA: Adrenergic and cholinergic nerves mediate secretion from tracheal glands of ferrets. *J Appl Physiol* (1980) **49**: 1027–1031.
168. Speizer FE, Doll R, Heaf P, Strang LB: Investigation into use of drugs preceding death in asthma. *Br Med J* (1968) **1**: 335–339.
169. Anon: Beta-adrenergic bronchodilators and sudden death in asthmatics. *Drug Ther Bull* (1976) **14**: 21–22.
170. Sears MR, Taylor DR, Print CG, *et al.*: Regular inhaled beta-agonist in treatment of bronchial asthma. *Lancet* (1990) **336**: 1391–1396.
171. Marom Z, Shelhamer JH, Kaliner M: Human pulmonary macrophage-derived mucus secretagogue. *J Exp Med* (1984) **159**(3): 844–860.
172. Marom Z, Shelhamer JH, Kaliner M: Human monocyte-derived mucus secretagogue. *J Clin Invest* (1985) **75**(1): 191–198.
173. Niles RM, Christensen TG, Breuer R, Stone PJ, Snider GL: Serine proteases stimulate mucous glycoprotein release from hamster tracheal ring organ culture. *J Lab Clin Med* (1986) **108**: 489–497.
174. Sommerhoff CP, Nadel JA, Basbaum CB, Caughey GH: Neutrophil elastase and cathepsin G stimulated secretion from cultured bovine airway gland serous cells. *J Clin Invest* (1990) **85**: 682–689.
175. Logun C, Rieves RD, Lundgren JD, Marom Z, Kaliner M, Shelhamer JH: Activated human neutrophils release a high molecular weight protein which stimulates respiratory glyco-conjugate release from human airways *in vitro*. *Am Rev Respir Dis* (1988) **137**: A14 (Abstract).

176. Gleich GJ: The eosinophil and bronchial asthma: current understanding. *J Allergy Clin Immunol* (1990) **85:** 422–436.

177. Lundgren JD, Davey RT, Lundgren B, *et al.*: Eosinophil cationic protein stimulates and major basic protein inhibits airway mucus secretion. *J Allergy Clin Immunol* (1991) **87:** 689–698.

178. Frigas E, Loegering DA, Solley GO, Farrow GM, Gleich GJ: Elevated levels of eosinophil major basic protein in the sputum of patients with bronchial asthma. *Mayo Clin Proc* (1981) **56:** 345–353.

179. Jacoby DB, Ueki I, Widdicombe JH, Loegering DA, Gleich GJ, Nadel JA: Effect of eosinophil major basic protein on ion transport in dog tracheal epithelium. *Am Rev Respir Dis* (1988) **137:** 13–16.

180. McFadden ER: Respiratory heat and water exchange: physiological and clinical implications. *J Appl Physiol* (1983) **54:** 331–336.

181. Peatfield AC, Richardson PS, Wells UM: The effects of airflow on mucus secretion into the trachea of the cat. *J Physiol* (1986) **380:** 429–439.

182. Williams IP, Rich B, Richardson PS: Action of serum on the output of secretory glycoproteins from human bronchi *in vitro*. *Thorax* (1983) **38:** 682–685.

183. Charman J, Reid LM: Sputum viscosity in chronic bronchitis, bronchiectasis, asthma and cystic fibrosis. *Biorheology* (1972) **9:** 185–199.

184. Mezey RJ, Cohn MA, Fernandez RJ, Januszkiewicz AJ, Wanner A: Mucociliary transport in allergic patients with antigen-induced bronchospasm. *Am Rev Respir Dis* (1978) **118:** 677–684.

185. Ahmed T, Greenblatt DW, Birch S, Marchette B, Wanner A: Abnormal mucociliary transport in allergic patients with antigen-induced bronchospasm: role of slow reacting substance of anaphylaxis. *Am Rev Respir Dis* (1981) **124:** 110–114.

186. Bateman JRM, Pavia D, Sheahan NF, Agnew JE, Clarke SW: Impaired tracheobronchial clearance in patients with mild stable asthma. *Thorax* (1983) **38:** 463–467.

187. Wanner A: Allergic mucociliary dysfunction. *J Allergy Clin Immunol* (1983) **72:** 347–350.

188. Wanner A, Zarzecki S, Hirch J, Epstein S: Tracheal mucus transport in experimental canine asthma. *J Appl Physiol* (1975) **39:** 950–957.

189. Garrard CS, Mussatto DJ, Loutenço RV: Lung mucociliary transport in asymptomatic asthma: effects of inhaled histamine. *J Lab Clin Med* (1989) **113:** 109–195.

190. Russi W, Abraham WM, Chapman G, Stephenson J, Codias E, Wanner A: Effects of leukotriene D4 on mucociliary and respiratory function in allergic and non-allergic sheep. *J Appl Physiol* (1985) **59:** 1416–1422.

191. Abraham WA, Stevenson JS, Garrido R: A possible role for PAF in allergen-induced late response: modification by a selective antagonist. *J Appl Physiol* (1989) **66:** 2351–2357.

192. Seybold ZV, Mariassy AT, Stroh D, Kim CS, Gazeroglu H, Wanner A: Mucociliary interaction *in vitro*: effects of physiological and inflammatory stimuli. *J Appl Physiol* (1990) **68:** 1421–1426.

193. Wanner A, Sielczak M, Mella JF, Abraham WM: Ciliary responsiveness in allergic and non-allergic airways. *J Appl Physiol* (1986) **60:** 1967–1971.

194. Allegra L, Abraham WM, Chapman GA, Wanner A: Duration of mucociliary dysfunction following antigen challenge in allergic sheep. *J Appl Physiol* (1983) **55:** 726–730.

195. Frigas E, Loegering BS, Gleich GJ: Cytotoxic effect of the guinea-pig eosinophil major basic protein on tracheal epithelium. *Lab Invest* (1980) **42:** 35–43.

196. Hastie AT, Loegering DA, Gleich GJ, Kneppers F: The effect of purified human eosinophil major basic protein on mammalian ciliary activity. *Am Rev Respir Dis* (1987) **135:** 848–853.

197. Dulfano MJ, Luk CK: Sputum and ciliary inhibition in asthma. *Thorax* (1982) **37:** 646–651.

198. Hui K, Barnes N: Lung function impairment in asthma with a cysteinyl-leukotriene receptor antagonist. *Lancet* (1991) **337:** 1062–1063.

199. Lundgren JD, Kaliner MA, Logun C, Shelhamer JH: Dexamethasone reduces rat tracheal goblet cell hyperplasia produced by human neutrophil products. *Exo Lung Res* (1988) **14:** 853–863.

200. Lundgren JD, Kaliner MA, Shelhamer JH: Mechanisms by which glucocorticoids inhibit secretion of mucus in asthmatic airways. *Am Rev Respir Dis* (1990) **141:** S52–S58.
201. Marom Z. Shelhamer J, Alling D, Kaliner M: The effects of corticosteroids on mucous glycoprotein secretion from human airways *in vitro*. *Am Rev Respir Dis* (1984) **129:** 62–65.
202. Lundgren JD, Hirata F, Marom Z, *et al*. Dexamethasone inhibits respiratory glycoconjugate secretion from feline airways by the induction of lipocortin (lipomodulin) synthesis. *Am Rev Respir Dis* (1988) **137:** 353–357.
203. Shimura S, Sasaki T, Ikeda K, Yamauchi K, Sasaki H, Takishima T: Direct inhibitory action of glucocorticoid on glycoconjugate secretion from airway submucosal gland. *Am Rev Respir Dis* (1990) **141:** 1044–1049.
204. Agnew JE, Bateman JR, Pavia D, Clarke SW: Peripheral airways mucus clearance in stable asthma is improved by oral corticosteroid therapy. *Bull Eur Physiopathol Respir* (1984) **20** (3): 295–301.
205. Shimura S, Sasaki T, Ikeda K, Sasaki H, Takishima T: VIP augments cholinergic-induced glycoconjugate secretion in tracheal submucosal glands *J Appl Physiol* (1988) **65:** 2537–2544.

12

The Tracheobronchial Circulation

J.G. WIDDICOMBE, D.R. CORFIELD AND S.E. WEBBER

INTRODUCTION

The airway mucosa is reddened in asthma, indicating hyperaemia. Asthma is a disease of inflammation of the airways, and hyperaemia is a characteristic of all inflammation. The role of the airway vasculature in this phenomenon has only recently been studied, and this research has been associated with a general interest in the physiology and pathology of the lesser circulation of the lungs.

STRUCTURE OF THE TRACHEOBRONCHIAL CIRCULATION

Arterial supply

Blood flow to the cervical trachea and intrathoracic airways is approximately 2% of cardiac output but is hard to measure accurately due to the anatomy of the circulation. The origin of the circulation is highly variable from species to species. The bronchial arteries can arise from multiple sites on the aorta and subclavian, internal mammary and intercostal arteries and supply not only the intrathoracic airways and lung parenchyma but also the vasa vasorum of the pulmonary vessels and other intrathoracic structures.[1,2] The sheep is a favoured experimental model and the anatomy is shown in Fig. 12.1. Arterial anastamoses exist between the bronchial and both the coronary and pulmonary circulations in most species.[3]

Arteries supplying the cervical trachea originate largely from the common carotid arteries, in sheep from vessels almost exclusively on the left side of the neck and in dogs from the superior thyroid artery on both sides.[4,5]

ASTHMA: BASIC MECHANISMS AND CLINICAL MANAGEMENT (2nd Edn)
ISBN 0-12-079026-2

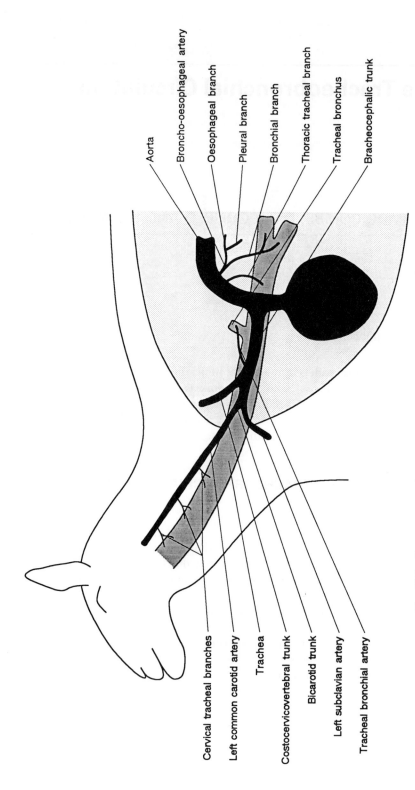

Fig. 12.1 Gross anatomy of the tracheobronchial circulation of the sheep. Redrawn from ref. 1.

Aorta

Broncho-oesophageal artery

Oesophageal branch

Pleural branch

Bronchial branch

Thoracic tracheal branch

Tracheal bronchus

Bracheocephalic trunk

Cervical tracheal branches

Left common carotid artery

Trachea

Costocervicovertebral trunk

Bicarotid trunk

Left subclavian artery

Tracheal bronchial artery

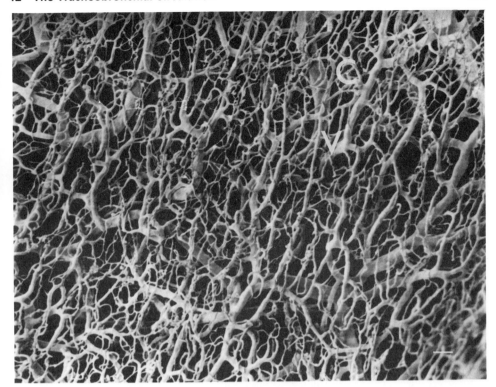

Fig. 12.2 Scanning electron microscopy picture taken from the luminal side of a vascular cast from the lateral wall of the trachea over the fifth cartilage half-ring of a dog. A rich vascular network is shown in the tracheal mucosa. Small superficial capillaries (C) are draining into deeper veins (V). Magnification × 75; bar = 100 μm. Reproduced from ref. 5.

The microvascular network

Blood flow to the airway mucosa is among the highest to any tissue, 100–150 ml/min/ 100 g of tissue. There is a dense subepithelial capillary network along the airway of all species studied (Fig. 12.2) except the rabbit where the network is sparse.[6–8] The endothelium, unlike that in the nose, is non-fenestrated. In the larger bronchi a second capillary network lies outside the smooth muscle connected by branches penetrating the layer.[9] Blood flow to airway smooth muscle itself is relatively sparse. The capillary network drains into an extensive submucosal venous plexus. The size of the plexus varies between species; it is most marked in the sheep and rabbit, of intermediate size in man and least evident in the dog.[10] In the sheep trachea the plexus is formed from thin-walled sinuses up to 0.5mm in diameter (Fig. 12.3) with little or no vascular smooth muscle; in man and rabbit smooth muscle is generally present. Anastomoses with pulmonary vessels occur at precapillary, capillary and postcapillary levels of the bronchial vasculature[3] but are not present in the tracheal circulation.[9] Arterio-venous anastomoses, such as in the nose and skin, have not been found in the tracheobronchial circulation.

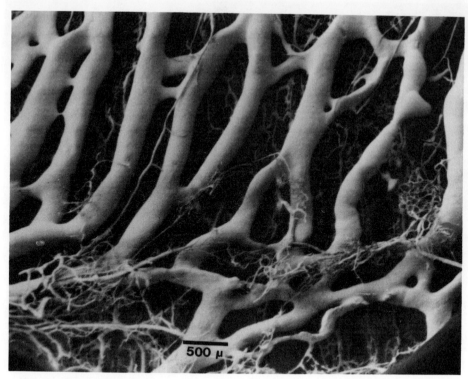

Fig. 12.3 Low-power scanning electron micrograph of tracheal vasculature of the sheep. The blood vessels have been filled with anatomical corrosion compound and the soft tissue digested away; view from the abluminal (submucosal) surface showing network of sinuses, with subepithelial capillaries lying deeper. The transverse direction of the trachea is across the figure, the sinuses running mainly longitudinally. The intercartilaginous space is transverse at the bottom of the picture, showing connecting vessels joining the sinuses. Reproduced from ref. 7.

Venous drainage

Blood returns from the bronchial circulation to both right and left sides of the heart via bronchial and pulmonary veins.[3,9] The tracheal circulation drains via systemic veins; in sheep the venous drainage matches the arterial input and is mostly via vessels on the left side of the neck.

INNERVATION AND NEURAL CONTROL OF THE CIRCULATION

Parasympathetic cholinergic control

The role of the parasympathetic cholinergic nervous system in the control of the tracheobronchial circulation is unclear and whether there are changes in the cholinergic innervation of the vasculature during asthma, as suggested for smooth muscle, is not known. Cutting the vagi decreases resting bronchial blood flow in some species[11] and tracheal vascular resistance is decreased in dogs when the superior laryngeal nerves supplying the trachea are cut.[12] However, other studies have reported no changes in resting blood flow or even an increase when the vagi are cut.[13] Nerve section experiments are difficult to interpret since profound changes in systemic blood pressure are produced by sectioning and the vagi contain a mixed population of nerves, not only parasympathetic but sensory and sympathetic motor fibres as well.

Vegal nerve stimulation increases bronchial blood flow in several species[14,15] and stimulation of the superior laryngeal nerve increases tracheal blood flow in pigs[15] and reduces tracheal perfusion pressure in dogs.[12] The increased bronchial blood flow in cats and pigs on vagal nerve stimulation is not affected by atropine[15,16] suggesting a non-cholinergic mechanism (see below); however, vasodilation of the tracheal circulation in dogs and increased tracheal blood flow in pigs on stimulation of the superior laryngeal artery are substantially reduced by atropine suggesting, at least in part, a cholinergic mechanism.[12,15] The difference in results could be a species difference, a difference between the tracheal and bronchial circulations, or a difference in methodology. Whatever the reason nerve stimulation studies, like nerve sectioning, are not strongly definitive.

Injections of acetylcholine or other muscarinic agonists directly into the bronchial or tracheal circulation of several species produces large concentration-dependent increases in blood flow when the circulation is perfused at constant pressure[17–19] and large decreases in tracheal vascular pressure when perfused at constant flow.[20,21] Also, aerosolized muscarinic agonists increase bronchial blood flow. The increased bronchial blood flow in dogs with aerosolized methacholine[22] and the increased tracheal blood flow with close-arterial acetylcholine[18] are greatly reduced by pretreatment with atropine, suggesting mediation via muscarinic cholinergic receptors. It seems likely that the muscarinic agonists are not acting directly on receptors on the vascular smooth muscle to induce vasodilation, but rather are inducing release of endothelium-derived relaxing factors (EDRF) as occurs in other vascular beds.[23]

It is clear that exogenous application of muscarinic agonists potently dilates the tracheobronchial vasculature; however it is still not clear if the parasympathetic cholinergic nervous system plays a role in the physiological regulation of tracheobronchial blood flow.

Sympathetic adrenergic control

Physiological and pharmacological studies suggest that the main nervous control of the tracheobronchial circulation is by the sympathetic nervous system. Stimulation of sympathetic nerves innervating the bronchial circulation of the dog produces a potent reduction in blood flow,[24] and stimulation of sympathetic nerves to the tracheal vasculature of the dog perfused at constant flow greatly increases perfusion pressure indicating vasoconstriction.

Exogenous application of adrenergic receptor agonists has potent effects on the tracheobronchial circulation. Local injections of adrenaline or noradrenaline into the bronchial circulation of dogs and sheep markedly reduce bronchial blood flow.[18,19] The reduced bronchial blood flow produced by adrenaline in the dog is blocked by phentolamine suggesting it is mediated by α-receptors.[18] Further evidence for an important role of α-receptors comes from exogenous application of the relatively specific α-agonist phenylephrine which, when aerosolized, strongly reduces blood flow in sheep,[25] an effect blocked by phentolamine, and increases tracheal perfusion pressure in dogs.[20] Thus there is evidence that α-receptors mediate the potent vasocontriction produced by sympathetic nerve stimulation. However, there are also β-receptors present in large numbers on bronchial arteries,[26] and these receptors will respond to noradrenaline released from sympathetic nerves and, perhaps more importantly, to increased levels of circulating adrenaline. Close-arterial injections of isoprenaline, a relatively specific β-agonist, into the bronchial circulation[19,27] potently increases blood flow and this response is blocked by propranolol indicating a β-receptor effect. Furthermore salbutamol, a specific β_2-agonist, reduces tracheal perfusion pressure suggesting vasodilation.[20,21] Presumably a vasoconstriction of the tracheobronchial circulation is observed with stimulation of sympathetic nerves because noradrenaline is a more potent agonist on α-receptors than on β-receptors.

Non-adrenergic, non-cholinergic control

There is now a wealth of evidence from anatomical, histological and some physiological studies that both parasympathetic and sympathetic nerves to the airways, including to the tracheobronchial circulation, store and release transmitters which are non-adrenergic and non-cholinergic (NANC) in nature. The NANC transmitters are peptides.

Vasoactive intestinal polypeptide (VIP) and peptide histidine isoleucine (PHI: PHmethionine in man) are thought to co-exist with acetylcholine in parasympathetic motor nerves to the airway vasculature[28] and are vasodilator.[29,30] In sympathetic motor nerves neuropeptide Y, a vasoconstrictor,[30] probably co-exists with noradrenaline.[31] Sensory or C-fibre nerves, which also innervate the vasculature, contain several peptides, all vasodilator,[29,30] including substance P (SP), neurokinin A (NKA), neurokinin B (NKB) and calcitonin gene-related peptide (CGRP).[32] All of these peptides have been identified immunohistochemically to be localized to nerves in and around airway blood vessels,[33] and results from physiological and pharmacological studies suggest they are important in the regulation of the vasculature.

REFLEX CONTROL OF THE CIRCULATION

The tracheobronchial circulation is under reflex control, probably acting mainly by changes in sympathetic nervous tone, although the role of the parasympathetic system has not been properly evaluated. Stimulation of peripheral and probably central chemo-receptors vasoconstricts the tracheal vasculature[34] but the effects on the bronchial circulation are less clear, both constriction and dilation having been described.

Vasodilator reflexes to the tracheobronchial circulation can be demonstrated by irritation of many sites in the respiratory tract. The larynx and the pulmonary C-fibre reflex have been most studied, activation of each of which causes vasodilation.[35] Pharmacological excitation of cardiac C-fibre receptors as part of the Bezold–Jarisch reflex also causes tracheal vasodilation in the dog.[35]

Other reflexes of importance in respiratory and cardiovascular control have little effect on the tracheobronchial vasculature. For example stimulation of slowly adapting pulmonary stretch receptors has no effect on the tracheal circulation but relaxes the tracheal smooth muscle.[35] The same applies to carotid sinus baroreceptors assessed by carotid artery occlusion.

The reflex control of the tracheal circulation shows marked asymmetry. Thus, stimulation of the superior laryngeal or vagal nerves on one side produces a more pronounced ipsilateral than contralateral response.[36] It is difficult to see the advantage of this asymmetry but it may be an evolutionary remnant; similar asymmetrical changes are seen in the nose.

RESPONSES TO NON-NEURAL MEDIATORS

Histamine

Histamine is probably the best characterized of the non-neural mediators in the airways. It is released from mast cells or basophils in response to a number of stimuli including cold air and allergen. When released it has potent, if complex, effects on the tracheobronchial circulation. In sheep close-arterial application of histamine can produce either vasoconstriction, vasodilation or a combination of the two;[4] the vasodilations are either short-lived (30 s) or prolonged (4–5 min). The prolonged dilation is prevented by bilateral cervical vagotomy although the mechanism of this effect is unknown. The rapid dilation and the constriction are both unaffected by histamine H_2-receptor blockade by cimetidine but are both prevented by mepyramine, an H_1-receptor antagonist. Histamine has a much simpler action on the bronchial circulation producing only vasodilations whether injected intravenously,[37] directly into the bronchial artery[38] or administered as an aerosol.[39] There is some debate concerning the receptors mediating the effects of histamine on the bronchial circulation and both H_1- and H_2-receptors have been implicated depending on the method used to measure blood flow and the route of administration of histamine.[4,39]

5-Hydroxytryptamine

5-Hydroxytryptamine (5HT) is formed by the decarboxylation of dietary tryptophan and in man is principally localized to epithelial neuroendocrine cells and the dense secretory granules of platelets. Recently the role of platelets in the pathogenesis of asthma has been reappraised with the identification of a platelet-activating factor (PAF, see below). The potent effects of PAF on the airways, including the tracheobronchial circulation, may be due to the release of 5HT from platelets.[40]

Like histamine, 5HT has a complex action on the tracheal circulation when perfused at constant flow.[41] It produces either a constriction or a constriction followed by a dilation. This vasodilation is unusual since only constrictor responses to 5HT have been observed in the pulmonary circulation. The vasoconstriction and dilation seem to be

mediated by different 5HT-receptors. The constriction is blocked by ketanserin suggesting a $5HT_2$-receptor effect. In contrast the dilation is not affected by ketanserin but is
prevented by methysergide suggesting a role for $5HT_1$-receptors. The relatively selective
$5HT_3$-receptor agonist 2-methyl 5HT had no effect on the tracheal vasculature suggesting a lack of involvement of $5HT_3$-receptors in this tissue. Despite one early report
indicating that 5HT increases bronchial blood flow when injected into the aorta,[11] the
effects of 5HT on the bronchial circulation and the receptors mediating these effects
have not been systematically studied.

Bradykinin

Bradykinin is generated from kininogens in plasma by the action of kininogenase
enzymes produced by the liver and other tissues. It potently increases tracheal blood
flow in the sheep[23] and pig[42] and reduces tracheal perfusion pressure in the dog.[43]
Bradykinin also increases bronchial blood flow in the pig.[42] Bradykinin is slightly more
potent than lys-bradykinin at increasing tracheal blood flow in sheep suggesting this
vasodilation is mediated by B_2-receptors.[23] The vasodilations to bradykinin are extremely long-lasting suggesting an indirect mechanism. However, indomethacin is
without effect ruling out the release of prostaglandins by bradykinin. The vasodilations
to bradykinin are prevented by pretreatment with haemoglobin which inactivates
preformed endothelium-derived relaxing factor (EDRF). Thus bradykinin stimulates
B_2-receptors to release EDRF which dilates the tracheal blood vessels.

Lipid mediators

The action of phospholipase A_2 on cell membrane phospholipids leads to the production
of arachidonic acid which is the precursor for prostaglandins, thromboxanes, leukotrienes and several hydroxyacids.[44] Prostaglandins and thromboxanes are produced by a
cascade system following the action of cyclooxygenase enzymes on arachidonic acid, and
leukotrienes and hydroxyacids are formed by a similar cascade following the action of
lipoxygenase enzymes on arachidonic acid. All of these mediators can be produced and
released from a large number of different cells in the airways including mast cells,
basophils, neutrophils, macrophages, eosinophils and endothelial and epithelial cells.
When released they all have effects on the tracheobronchial circulation.

   The prostaglandins are all potent tracheobronchial vasodilators. PGE_1, $PGF_{2\alpha}$ and
PGD_2 strongly vasodilate the dog tracheal circulation when injected close-arterially[43]
and $PGF_{2\alpha}$ and PGI_2 increase bronchial blood flow when given by inhalation or as an
infusion into the bronchial artery.[22,45] Although thromboxane A_2 is a potent vasoconstrictor of the pulmonary circulation its effects on tracheobronchial blood flow have not
been investigated. LTC_4 and LTD_4 reduce bronchial blood flow in the sheep[46] and
LTC_4 is a weak constrictor of the sheep tracheal circulation when injected close-
arterially.[21] The effects of LTB_4 and LTE_4 have not been examined.

   By an alternative pathway phospholipase A_2 can act on membrane phospholipids to
produce lyso-PAF which is converted to PAF by acetyl transferase. PAF is also released
by a large number of cells in the airways and is considered to be an important mediator

in asthma principally because it can mimic several aspects of the disease and in particular bronchial hyperresponsiveness. Despite this it is only recently that the effects of PAF on the tracheobronchial circulation have been examined. PAF is a weak vasodilator in the dog tracheal circulation[43] but is much more potent at increasing tracheal blood flow in the sheep.[47] This effect in the sheep is not due to secondary release of histamine, prostaglandins or leukotrienes but seems to be due to a direct effect of PAF on its own receptors on the vascular smooth muscle.

Other mediators

There are other mediators such as endothelins, adenosine, complement fragments and oxygen radicals that are released in the airways particularly when there is inflammation and may be important regulators of airway blood flow both in health and inflammatory disease. However, the effects of these mediators on tracheobronchial blood flow have, in general, not been examined. In addition blood-borne hormones may also affect the airway vasculature. Adrenaline is a potent vasoconstrictor (see above) as is also exogenous vasopressin. Whether these hormones are active endogenously is not known.

TRACHEOBRONCHIAL CIRCULATION AND ASTHMA

The tracheobronchial circulation may play an important role in the pathogenesis of asthma in several ways. Firstly, large increases in blood flow may cause engorgement of blood vessels (particularly the sinuses described above) to such an extent that this increases mucosal thickness enough to increase airway resistance. Secondly, the circulation may be involved in oedema formation during the inflammatory phase of the disease. This will correspond to increased release of inflammatory cells and mediators into the mucosa and eventually into the airway lumen and thus perpetuate the disease; the oedema itself may also produce significant increases in airway resistance. Thirdly, the circulation will play a major role in the regulation of the penetration and clearance both of inflammatory mediators released in the airway, and of drugs such as β-agonists administered as aerosols to treat the disease. Several studies have investigated the effects on the tracheobronchial circulation of the external stimuli which can trigger asthma.[21] Furthermore, the role of changing mucosal thickness on airway resistance and the effects of changing tracheal blood flow on the penetration of drugs have been examined.[48]

The effects of allergen

Sheep and pigs are spontaneously sensitive to *Ascaris suum* antigen and so provide an excellent model with which to examine the effects of allergen on the tracheobronchial circulation. Ascaris delivered as an aerosol produces a rapid increase in bronchial blood flow in sheep[49] and pigs[50] which lasts for up to 1 h. In sheep this is followed by a second increase in blood flow 5 h after challenge which persists for several hours.[49] Similarly, in young (1-year-old sheep) ascaris produces a rapid tracheal vasodilation when injected close-arterially; in contrast a vasoconstriction is observed in older sheep (5 years).[21] The vasodilation and vasoconstriction in young and older sheep with ascaris, and the increase in sheep bronchial blood flow, are not significantly affected by antihistamines ruling out antigen-induced release of histamine from mast cells. However both prostaglandins and leukotrienes are implicated in the tracheal responses as both the dilation in young sheep and the constriction in older sheep are attenuated by indomethacin and the leukotriene receptor antagonist FPL55712. The increase in bronchial flow in the sheep is also blocked by indomethacin. The difference in response of the trachael vasculature of young and older sheep to antigen is probably due to a different combination of mediators being released in the two groups of sheep with dilators dominant in young sheep and constrictors in older sheep. In contrast to sheep, the increased bronchial blood flow with ascaris in pigs[50] is abolished by pretreatment with capsaicin implicating the release of sensory neuropeptides by allergen challenge. The role of these peptides in the responses of the sheep airway vasculature to antigen has not been studied.

The effects of cold air

Hyperventilation, inhalation of cold air and exercise can all cause bronchoconstriction; the common underlying mechanisms are cooling of the airway mucosa and hypertonicity of the airway surface liquid. It has been postulated that the bronchoconstriction is related to abnormal changes in the airway vascular bed, which one would expect to have an important role in determining mucosal temperature.

Cooling of the airways increases tracheobronchial blood flow in experimental animals.[51] Not only does cooling the mucosa cause a vasodilation, but application of hypertonic solutions has a similar effect.[52] The responses are not affected by α- or β-adrenoceptor blockade or by vagotomy, and are therefore presumably a 'local' effect. There is a difference of opinion as to whether local sensory nerves and axon reflexes are important in the responses.

Thus mucosal cooling and hypertonicity cause airway vasodilation, although the mechanisms of this response have not been fully worked out. The hypothesis that abnormal responses of the airway vasculature underlie the bronchoconstriction due to hyperventilation, cold-air inhalation and exercise is an attractive one, but further work is required to test or establish it.

The effects of the circulation on mucosal thickness and airway resistance

It has been recognized for some time that airway resistance can be substantially affected by the thickness of the airway wall or mucosa. Small changes in the thickness of the mucosa, which may have little effect on baseline airways calibre, can greatly amplify changes in airway resistance produced by smooth muscle shortening.[53,54] Increased blood flow is a feature of the inflammatory response in asthma and may change the thickness of the mucosa and hence airway resistance both directly, by changing the blood volume of the mucosa and indirectly, by modulating the magnitude of plasma exudation and oedema formation in the tissues.

As we described earlier the vascular bed of the mucosa is dense. In sheep capillaries and small vessels within 55 μm of the epithelium occupy up to 20% of the tissue volume,[55] and beneath these lies an extensive network of large venous sinuses;[7] changes in blood volume could therefore markedly alter mucosal thickness. Experimentally, however, it is difficult to separate the effect of hyperaemia on airway resistance from that of smooth muscle contraction for most of the agents that contract smooth muscle are also vasodilators.

Anatomical studies have shown that vascular congestion can double the blood volume of the subepithelial microvasculature but these changes are hard to relate to overall changes in airways resistance.[55] Nitroglycerine is a vasodilator which only weakly relaxes airway smooth muscle; instilled directly into the airways of sheep it increases peripheral airways resistance by nearly 300%.[56] However it is uncertain on which vascular bed, pulmonary or bronchial, the drug is acting.

Changes in the thickness of the tracheal mucosa can be measured *in vivo* using a surface probe. A single cartilaginous ring is clamped to exclude the actions of the trachealis muscle and to provide a fixed reference point. The probe is driven down until it contacts the luminal surface. Repeated measurements detect changes in the thickness of the mucosa underlying the probe. In dogs vasoactive agents alter the thickness of the mucosa over a range of 135 μm or by about 20% of the overall mucosal thickness.[5] Drugs which decrease vascular resistance increase mucosal thickness and similarly drugs that increase vascular resistance decrease mucosal thickness. In sheep, with an airway vasculature more like that of man than is the dog's, the changes are substantially greater. The vasoconstrictor phenylephrine decreases mucosal thickness by 100 μm; the largest increase in thickness, of over 300 μm, is produced by bradykinin. The changes are rapid in onset and of limited duration paralleling the changes in vascular resistance and blood flow; this suggests that changes in mucosal thickness are predominantly due to changes in blood volume. The increases in thickness are certainly fast enough to occur alongside the smooth muscle contraction produced by inhaled agonists. In sheep maximal smooth muscle contraction is estimated to double tracheal airways resistance; superimposing a simultaneous increase in mucosal thickness of 300 μm increases resistance by 2.6 times.[48] It is hard to extrapolate the effects seen in the trachea to other airways but changes in mucosal thickness would have proportionately greater effects in smaller airways. One can only speculate on the proportion of the airway narrowing present in asthma and produced with inhalation challenge that is due to mucosal hyperaemia.

The interaction of blood flow and oedema formation in the airways has not been investigated. Increasing blood flow will increase hydrostatic pressure in capillaries and venules but by what amount this will enhance plasma leakage and oedema formation is unknown.

At present much remains unknown of the effects of the tracheobronchial circulation on airway resistance. Most speculative of all is the possible role of vasoconstrictor agents as a treatment to reduce airway inflammation and bronchoconstriction.

Removal of inhaled drugs and inflammatory mediators

The distribution and removal of drugs and mediators from the airway wall is potentially important in asthma since it will influence the life of active mediators in the mucosa and also the distribution and activity of aerosolized agents used to treat or test asthma. A clear clue to the importance of airway blood flow in affecting mediator concentration was seen in the study of Kelly et al.[57] They showed that the peripheral airway broncho-constriction seen in dogs with inhalation of a histamine aerosol is prolonged when bronchial blood flow is decreased. Csete et al.[56] varied tracheal blood flow in the sheep with vasoactive drugs and measured the effects of antigen challenge on tracheal smooth muscle tone; vasodilation decreases the smooth muscle response to antigen and vasoconstriction prolongs it. Thus airway blood flow plays an important role in the strength and duration of mediator actions on airway smooth muscle.

Using the perfused sheep tracheal vascular preparation, we have changed blood flow by drugs or directly by controlling a perfusion pump, and measured ^{99m}Tc-DTPA uptake from the lumen into venous drainage.[58,59] Surprisingly when blood flow is increased, DTPA uptake is less, and vice versa when blood flow is decreased,[58,59] and this was true for changes in blood flow induced both by vasoactive drugs and by altering perfusion flow rate. The explanation for these paradoxical results is uncertain, but increases in blood flow increase microvascular pressure and result in more interstitial fluid and a greater interstitial barrier to diffusion by DTPA. Alternatively there may be a redistribution of blood flow between the subepithelial capillary network, presumably the main site of drug uptake, and deeper vessels. Another possibility is that changes in blood flow could alter the release of endothelial agents such as EDRF and endothelins, which in turn might affect epithelial permeability. In vitro PAF increases epithelial permeability, but the drugs that alter DTPA uptake in the sheep trachea in vivo have little or no effect. Thus the barrier to drug uptake and action depends on epithelium, interstitium and vasculature, and changes in mucosal blood flow affect drug uptake and mediator actions. In view of the potential clinical importance of the subject, more investigations are clearly needed.

CONCLUSIONS

The tracheobronchial vascular bed is dilated by many of the inflammatory mediators known to be released in asthma, and by antigen in sensitive animals. It is under nervous control and dilator reflexes can be set up in experimental asthma. Thus its dilation may correspond to the hyperaemia of the mucosa seen in asthmatic patients. The effects of this dilation may include oedema and thickening of the mucosa, and an abnormal removal of mediators and take up of aerosolized drugs by the mucosa. Potentially the airway vascular bed has an important role to play in the pathophysiology of asthma, and further studies on this role in human asthmatics are needed.

REFERENCES

1. Magno M: Comparative anatomy of the tracheobronchial circulation. Eur J Pharmacol (1990) **3** (Suppl 12): 557s–563s.
2. McLaughlin RF: Bronchial artery distribution in various mammals and in humans. Am Rev Respir Dis (1983) **128**: S57–S58.

3. Daly I de B, Hebb C. *Pulmonary and Bronchial Vascular Systems*. London, Edward Arnold, 1966.
4. Webber SE, Salonen RO, Widdicombe JG: H_1- and H_2-receptor characterization in the tracheal circulation of sheep. *Br J Pharmacol* (1988) **95**: 551–561.
5. Laitinen A, Laitinen LA, Moss R, Widdicombe JG: Organization and structure of the tracheal and bronchial blood vessels in the dog. *J Anat* (1989) **165**: 133–140.
6. Hughes T: Microcirculation of the tracheobronchial tree. *Nature* (1965) **206**: 425–426.
7. Hill P, Goulding D, Webber SE, Widdicombe JG: Blood sinuses in the submucosa of the large airways of the sheep. *J Anat* (1989) **162**: 235–247.
8. Salassa JR, Pearson BW, Payne WS: Gross and microscopical blood supply of the trachea. *Ann Thorac Surg* (1977) **24**: 100–107.
9. Deffebach ME, Charan NB, Lakshminarayan S, Butler J: The bronchial circulation. Small, but a vital attribute of the lung. *Am Rev Respir Dis* (1987) **135**: 463–481.
10. Widdicombe JG: Comparison between the vascular beds of upper and lower airways. *Eur Resp J* (1990) **3** (Suppl 12): 564s–571s.
11. Horisberger B, Rodbard S: Direct measurement of bronchial artery flow. *Circ Res* (1960) **8**: 1149–1156.
12. Laitinen LA, Laitinen MV, Widdicombe JG: Parasympathetic nervous control of tracheal vascular resistance in the dog. *J Physiol (Lond)* (1987) **385**: 135–146.
13. Jindal SK, Lakshminarayan S, Kirk W, Butler J: Effect of cervical vagotomy on anastomotic bronchial blood flow after pulmonary artery obstruction in dogs. *Indian J Med Res* (1985) **81**: 83–85.
14. Martling CR, Anggard A, Lundberg JM: Non-cholinergic vasodilation in the tracheobronchial tree of the cat induced by vagal nerve stimulation. *Acta Physiol Scand* (1985) **125**: 343–346.
15. Matran R, Alving K, Martling CR, Lacroix JS, Lundberg JM: Vagally mediated vasodilatation by motor and sensory nerves in the tracheal and bronchial circulation of the pig. *Acta Physiol Scand* (1989) **135**: 29–37.
16. Martling CR, Gazelius B, Lundberg JM: Nervous control of tracheal blood flow in the cat measured by the laser Doppler technique. *Acta Physiol Scand* (1987) **130**: 409–417.
17. Bruner HD, Schmidt CF: Blood flow in the bronchial artery of the anaesthetized dog. *Am J Physiol* (1947) **148**: 648–666.
18. Himori N, Taira N: A method for recording smooth muscle and vascular responses of the blood-perfused dog trachea *in situ*. *Br J Pharmacol* (1976) **56**: 293–299.
19. Parsons GH, Kramer GC, Link DP, *et al*: Studies of reactivity and distribution of bronchial blood flow in sheep. *Chest* (1985) **87**: 180S–182S.
20. Laitinen LA, Laitinen MA, Widdicombe JG: Dose-related effects of pharmacological mediators on tracheal vascular resistance in dogs. *Br J Pharmac* (1987) **92**: 703–709.
21. Webber SE, Salonen RO, Deffebach ME, Widdicombe JG: Effects of antigen on tracheal circulation and smooth muscle in sheep of different ages. *J Appl Physiol* (1989) **67**: 1256–1264.
22. Lakshminarayan S, Jindal SK, Kirk W, Butler J: Increases in bronchial blood flow following bronchoconstriction with methacholine and prostaglandin $F_{2\alpha}$ in dogs. *Chest* (1985) **5**: 183S–184S.
23. Corfield DR, Webber SE, Hanafi Z, Widdicombe JG: The actions of bradykinin and lys-bradykinin on tracheal blood flow and smooth muscle in anaesthetized sheep. *Pulmonary Pharmacol* (1991) **4**: 85–90.
24. Murao H: Nervous regulation of the bronchial vascular system. *Jpn Circ J* (1965) **29**: 855–865.
25. Barker JA, Chediak AD, Baier HJ, Wanner A: Tracheal mucosal blood flow responses to autonomic agonists. *J Appl Physiol* (1988) **65**: 829–834.
26. Carstairs JR, Nimmo AJ, Barnes PJ: Autoradiographic localisation of beta-receptors in human lung. *Eur J Pharmacol* (1984) **103**: 189–190.
27. Lung MA, Wang JCC, Cheng KK: Bronchial circulation: an autoperfusion method for assessing its vasomotor activity and the study of alpha adrenoceptors in the bronchial artery. *Life Sci* (1976) **19**: 557–580.
28. Lundberg JM, Fahrenkrug J, Hokfelt T, *et al*: Co-existence of peptide HI (PHI) and VIP in nerves regulating blood flow and bronchial smooth muscle tone in various mammals including man. *Peptides* (1984) **5**: 593–606.

29. Laitinen LA, Laitinen A, Salonen RO, Widdicombe JG: Vascular actions of airway neuropeptides. *Am Rev Respir Dis* (1987) **135**: S71–75.

30. Salonen RO, Webber SE, Widdicombe JG: Effects of neuropeptides and capsaicin on the canine tracheal vasculature *in vivo. Br J Pharmacol* (1988) **95**: 1262–1270.

31. Lundberg JM, Lundblad L, Martling C-R, Saria A, Stjärne P, Ängård A: Coexistence of multiple peptides and classic neurotransmitters in airway neurones: functional and pathophysiological aspects. *Am Rev Respir Dis* (1987) **136**: (Suppl 1): S16–S22.

32. Hua XY, Theodorsson-Norheim E, Brodin E, Lundberg JM, Hedqvist T: Multiple tachykinins (neurokinin A, neuropeptide K, and substance P) in capsaicin-sensitive sensory neurones in the guinea-pig. *Regul Pep* (1985) **13**: 1–19.

33. Uddman R, Sundler F: Neuropeptides in the airways: a review. *Am Rev Respir Dis* (1987) **136**: S3–8.

34. Sahin G, Webber SE, Widdicombe JG: Chemical control of tracheal vascular resistance in dogs. *J Appl Physiol* (1987) **63**: 988–995.

35. Sahin G, Webber SE, Widdicombe JG: Lung and cardiac reflex actions on the tracheal vasculature in anaesthetized dogs. *J Physiol* (1987) **387**: 47–57.

36. Sahin G, Webber SE, Widdicombe JG: Nervous control of tracheal vascular resistance. *Clin Respir Physiol* (1987) **23**: 384s.

37. Parsons GH, Villablanka A, Colbert S, Nichol GM, Chung KF: Dose of histamine determines whether bronchial blood flow increases via H-1 or H-2 receptor stimulation. *Am Rev Respir Dis* (1989) **139**: A451.

38. Link DP, Parsons GH, Lantz BM, Gunther RA, Green JF, Cross CE: Measurement of bronchial blood flow in the sheep by video dilution technique. *Thorax* (1985) **40**: 143–149.

39. Long WM, Sprung CL, El-Fawal H, *et al.*: Effects of histamine on bronchial artery blood flow and bronchomotor tone. *J Appl Physiol* (1985) **59**: 254–261.

40. Morley J, Sanjar S, Page CP: The platelet in asthma. *Lancet* (1984) **2**: 1142–1144.

41. Webber SE, Salonen RO, Widdicombe JG: Receptors mediating the effects of 5-hydroxytryptamine on the tracheal vasculature and smooth muscle of sheep. *Br J Pharmacol* (1990) **99**: 21–26.

42. Matran R, Alving K, Lundberg JM: Cigarette smoke, nicotine and capsaicin aerosol-induced vasodilation in pig respiratory mucosa. *Br J Pharmacol* (1990) **100**: 535–541.

43. Laitinen LA, Laitinen A, Widdicombe J: Effects of inflammatory and other mediators on airway vascular beds. *Am Rev Respir Dis* (1987) **135**: S67–70.

44. Barnes PJ, Chung KF, Page CP: Inflammatory mediators and asthma. *Pharmacol Rev* (1988) **40**: 49–84.

45. Deffebach ME, Lakshminarayan S, Kirk W, Butler J: Bronchial circulation and cyclooxygenase products in acute lung injury. *J Appl Physiol* (1987) **63**: 1083–1088.

46. Long WM, Yerger LD, Sprung CL, Wanner A, Abraham WM: Differential effects of lipoxygenase and cycloxygenase products on antigen-induced late phase increases on bronchomotor tone and bronchial artery blood flow. *Am Rev Respir Physiol* (1986) **133**: 175.

47. Corfield DR, Webber SE, Widdicombe JG: Mechanisms of platelet activating factor-induced changes in tracheal blood flow. *Br J Pharmacol* (1991) **103**: 1740–1744.

48. Corfield DR, Hanafi Z, Webber SE, Widdicombe JG: Changes in tracheal mucosal thickness and blood flow in sheep. *J Appl Physiol* (1991) **71**: 1282–1288.

49. Long WM, Yerger LD, Martinez H, *et al.*: Modification of bronchial blood flow during allergic airway responses. *J Appl Physiol* (1988) **65**: 272–282.

50. Alving K, Matran R, Lacroix JS, Lundberg JM: Allergen challenge induces vasodilatation in pig bronchial circulation via a capsaicin-sensitive mechanism. *Acta Physiol Scand* (1988) **134**: 571–572.

51. Salonen RO, Deffebach ME, Widdicombe JG: Cold dry air-induced smooth muscle and vascular responses in the trachea of the anaesthetized dog. *J Physiol* (1988) **407**: 35.

52. Deffebach ME, Salonen RO, Webber SE, Widdicombe JG: Cold and hyperosmolar fluids in canine trachea: vascular and smooth muscle tone and albumin flux. *J Appl Physiol* (1989) **66**: 1309–1315.

53. Hogg JC, Paré PD, Moreno R: The effects of submucosal edema on airways resistance. *Am Rev Respir Dis* (1987) **135**: S54–S56.

54. Moreno RH, Hogg JC, Paré PD: Mechanics of airway narrowing. *Am Rev Respir Dis* (1986) **133**: 1171–1180.
55. Mariassy AT, Gazeroglu H, Wanner A: Morphometry of the subepithelial circulation in sheep airways: effects of vascular congestion. *Am Rev Respir Dis* (1991) **143**: 162–166.
56. Csete ME, Abraham WM, Wanner A: Vasomotion influences airflow in peripheral airways. *Am Rev Respir Dis* (1990) **141**: 1490–1413.
57. Kelly L, Kolbe J, Mitzner W, Spannhake EW, Bromberger BB, Menkes H: Bronchial blood flow affects recovery from constriction in dog lung periphery. *J Appl Physiol* (1986) **60**: 1954–1959.
58. Corfield DR, Webber SE, Hanafi Z, Widdicombe JG: Clearance of ^{99m}Tc-DTPA from the tracheal lumen in anaesthetized sheep. *J Physiol* (1989) **415**: 85P.
59. Corfield DR, Webber SE, Hanafi Z, Widdicombe JG: Tracheal clearance of ^{99m}Tc-DTPA at controlled arterial perfusion flow rates in anaesthetized sheep. *J Physiol* (1990) **423**: 20P.

13

Plasma Exudation into Airway Tissue and Lumen

CARL G.A. PERSSON

INTRODUCTION

The role of the tracheobronchial circulation in health and disease is now attracting worldwide interest. Several reports and discussions have been published on the anatomy of the bronchial circulation and blood flow in different species,[1-14] on the relationship between bronchial and pulmonary circulations[2,3,6,11,14-16] and on the vascularization of the airway mucosa/submucosa[1,2,8,17,18] and its role in the regulation of temperature and humidity of inspired air. An extensive update on the bronchial circulation can be found in a recent publication.[19] Despite the fact that inflamed airways have for a long time been considered a prominent feature in asthma, specific roles of the bronchial circulation in this disease (Table 13.1) have only recently been emphasized.[12,20,21] (The exception being Hyde Salter who saw a role for the bronchial circulation in haemoptysis and in the hypersecretion/exudation that occurred in asthma.[22]) Studies of inflammation in asthma

Table 13.1 Tracheobronchial microcirculation in asthma.

Nurtures airways, nerves and vessels

Humidifies inspired air

Clears inflammatory mediators

Clears inhaled drugs

Distributes drugs and mediators from large to small airways?

Supplies airway tissue and lumen with inflammatory cells

Supplies airway tissue and lumen with plasma exudate

ASTHMA: BASIC MECHANISMS AND CLINICAL MANAGEMENT (2nd Edn)
ISBN 0-12-079026-2

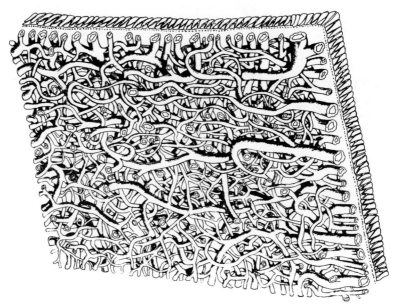

Fig. 13.1(a)   Schematic illustration of a profuse subepithelial plexus of microvessels

have rather focused on inflammatory cells and the airway epithelium. The inflammatory process, its acute, intermittent, and sustained aspects, must nevertheless involve significant airway microvascular events.

The present overview deals particularly with plasma exudation from tracheobronchial microvessels (Figs. 13.1a and 13.1b). Plasma exudation is not an exaggeration of the normal capillary–mucosal exchange of fluid and solutes but a specific inflammatory response of subepithelial postcapillary venules. The exudation is not dependent on uncertain disease characteristics as airway oedema, shedded epithelium, or increased absorption ability, nor is it dependent on which particular cellular mechanisms happen to be fuelling the inflammatory process. The basic purpose of airway exudation of plasma would be to neutralize offending stimuli on the mucosal surface be it allergen, occupational agents or other inflammatory factors. Exuded plasma and plasma-derived peptides contribute to the pathogenesis of asthma,[21] and exudative indices on the surface of the bronchial mucosa may quantitatively reflect the inflammatory process in this disease.

THE SUBEPITHELIAL MICROCIRCULATION

Since the first mention of bronchial arteries over two thousand years ago these vessels have obviously been discovered and forgotten, or their existence denied, several times.[2,3] Daly and Hebb[3] have given an interesting account of the contribution by Leonardo da Vinci to this field. This great artist illustrated the distribution of the bronchial arteries and their accompanying nerves, and discussed the fact that 'Nature duplicated artery

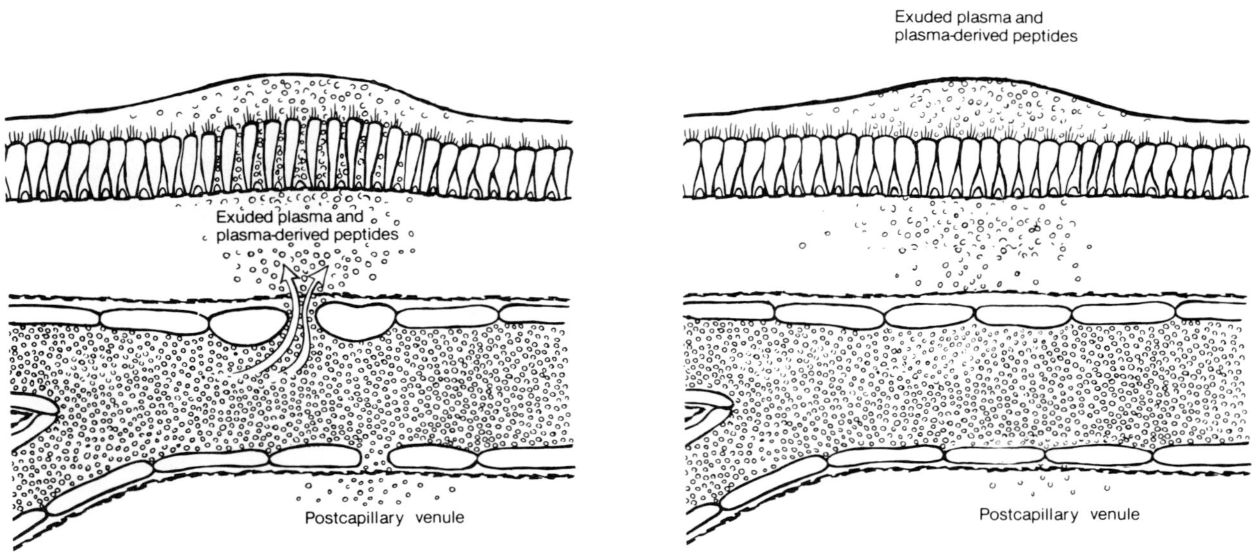

Exuded plasma and
plasma-derived peptides

Postcapillary venule

Exuded plasma and
plasma-derived peptides

Postcapillary venule

Fig. 13.1(b) Scheme illustrating the concept of inflammatory stimulus-induced exudation of plasma macromolecules across the vessel wall and the mucosal barrier. Note that the luminal entry of unfiltered exudate occurs across a normal epithelium (see text).

and vein in such an instrument'.[3] The bronchial circulation receives 1–5% of the cardiac output.[3,9,11,12] This fraction can readily be measured in species like the pig and the sheep, where a single bronchial artery supplies almost the whole bronchial circulation.[3,9,12] (In man, dog and ox a number of bronchial arteries originate from the aorta, the intercostal and other arteries.)[2,3,5,6,18] Bronchial arteries nurture not only bronchi but also nerves, pulmonary vessels, pleura and some other tissues.[2,3] Venous drainage of the extrapulmonary airways and the first new generations of bronchi goes to the right heart via the azygous and hemiazygous veins.[2,3,11] A major part of the venous blood from the bronchial circulation goes to the pulmonary vein via tributaries along the airways and peripherally through anastomoses between bronchial capillaries and pulmonary capillaries or precapillaries.[2,3,11] Laitinen et al.,[18] employing light and electron microscopy of vascular casts, have demonstrated the organization of an impressive microvasculature in the tracheobronchial wall of dogs and man, confirming the extending earlier work by Miller and others who used these species and guinea-pigs.[2,8,17] (Figs 13.1, 13.2). Most especially, just beneath the epithelium there is a copious capillary–venular network, which is continuous along the airways (Fig. 13.2). There are also deeper-lying plexuses, including a peribronchial microvascular network.[2,8,19]

The subepithelial microvascular network must have a role in the elimination and distribution of drugs, mediators and other factors deposited or released on the airway surface or in mucosal tissues. An efficient elimination capacity of blood flow in the abundant subepithelial microvessels will attenuate or prevent mucosal mediators from reaching the deeper-lying airway smooth muscle. Antagonizing and additive interactions between different bronchoconstrictive and bronchodilating agents given simultaneously, or in sequence, may not only relate to their actions on bronchial smooth muscle. A drug that increases bronchial mucosal blood flow, and potentially increases elimination of an inhaled mediator, may be difficult to distinguish from a drug that attenuates mediator-induced bronchoconstriction at the level of bronchial smooth muscle, and vice versa. The possibility that topically applied drugs may have to pass a vascular compartment before reaching the bronchial smooth muscle is compatible with some observations on inhaled xanthines, showing bronchodilation only when clinically effective systemic blood levels were attained (Svedmyr, Johannesson, Persson, unpublished; cf ref. 23). In contrast, inhaled β-receptor agonists are locally effective in the

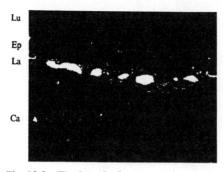 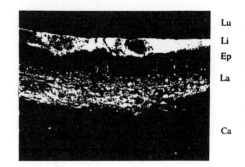

Fig. 13.2 The fate of a fluorescent plasma tracer (MW 150 000) given intravenously is illustrated in these graphs of guinea-pig trachea. Left, the control airway where only the abundant subepithelial vessels contain the tracer. Right, 10 min after inflammatory provocation of the mucosa plasma is exuded into the lamina propria (La) and constitutes much of the airway liquid (Li) in the Lumen (Lu). Note that the epithelium is non-fluorescent (see text).

airways at exceedingly low plasma levels.[24] As with other drugs, few details are known about the pathways for these substances in the airway wall.

The subepithelial network of microvessels is continuous throughout the lower airways,[2,19] and may accordingly distribute locally released or applied agents from airway to airway. Kröll et al.[25] demonstrated the effectiveness of such a microvascular flow along the airways (as well as of the pulmonary–bronchial anastomizing microcirculations) by the finding that even the extrapulmonary tracheobronchial microvessels were well perfused in guinea-pig isolated lungs where only the pulmonary artery was perfused. Presumably, this was due to a retrograde flow in airway microvascular plexuses. The subepithelial capillary–venular vessels as a distribution system may facilitate the spreading of inflammatory reactions but may also distribute inhaled drugs to small airways, where deposit of aerosols is difficult to achieve. Whether such distributions are operating in asthmatic airways to any significant extent now remains speculative.

The microvessels may be divided into four kinds depending on function: resistance vessels, exchange vessels, capacitance vessels and exudation vessels. The corresponding anatomical parts are arteries with precapillary 'sphincters', capillaries, sinus vein and postcapillary venules. Both plasma exudation and white cell diapedisis take place in the venules. The mechanisms for extravasation of plasma and cells are distinct. Indeed, cells may migrate into the tissue without any concomitant leak of plasma. Also, plasma is exuded through endothelial gaps through which cells may not pass. The present overview deals exclusively with airways plasma exudation and the emphasis is on luminal entry of plasma exudates. This latter process may be called mucosal exudation.

DEFINITIONS AND DISTINCTIONS

(1) 'Mucosal or airway exudation' is the bulk flow of plasma, plasma-derived mediators, and the associated additional fluid across microvascular (venular endothelial) and mucosal (epithelial) barriers into the airway lumen.
(2) The mucosal exudate may have attracted substantial amounts of fluid on its way to the mucosal surface. However, in contrast to the 'transudation' of protein-poor fluid, the mucosal exudate is little filtered and contains also the large plasma proteins.
(3) Airway exudation of unfiltered plasma proteins reflects dramatic increases in the microvascular and mucosal permeabilities. However, the airway absorption ability remains unaltered during and after the plasma exudation process (see below).
(4) The mechanisms involved and the largely unfiltered nature of the plasma exudate distinguish mucosal exudation from airway secretory processes.
(5) The mucosal exudation of plasma is also distinct from and independent of the migration of white cells across venular and mucosal barriers into the airway lumen.

CONDITIONING OF INSPIRED AIR

During quiet oronasal breathing the heating (or cooling) and humidifying of incoming air takes place in the upper airways. Clearly, the tracheobronchial passages, with their profuse subepithelial microvessels, have a role in the conditioning of inspired air when demands are high.[19,26–30] Hence, when the thermal burden was increased by rapid inspirations at subfreezing conditions, a large part of the respiratory tree participated in heating the inspired air.[27] Exercise and cooling of upper and lower airways may either not change or increase the mucosal/submucosal blood flow.[28,29]

Exercise or hyperventilation of dry cold air is known to induce significant bronchoconstriction in about three-quarters of the asthmatic population.[30] Humidification of the dry air, with ensuing hyperosmolarity of bronchial surface liquids, may be a major initiating stimulus[30,31] causing the release of bronchoconstrictory and inflammatory mediators.[31] Cole[32] has listed several sources which supply water vapour to the inspiratory air in healthy subjects: 'water content of ambient air, recovery from expiratory air, lachrymation via the nasolacrymal duct, secretion from the paranasal sinuses, salivation, secretions of the goblet cells and seromucinous glands of the respiratory mucosa'. Under inflammatory conditions, substantial amounts of vessel fluid must reach the mucosal surface and this is also supported by a range of observations.[33–34] Fluid emanating directly from tracheobronchial microvessels may, therefore, contribute to the humidification of inspired air, particularly in asthma. Cellular mediators, including histamine and arachidonic products, which have been demonstrated to be released in response to airway challenges with cold dry air,[31,44] may have increased plasma exudation into the airways. The volume of fluid that reaches the airway surface as a result of exudation may be substantial. After extravasation, an abundance of plasma-derived peptides will be produced and the increased number of solutes will attract additional fluid to the exudate. The expansion of the volume of the exudate will go on in the lamina propria as well as on the mucosal surface. The fluid of the exudate is a potentially important factor in the conditioning of incoming air. The plasma-derived mediators of the exudate may further be involved in the airway obstruction that follows from hyperventilation and exercise in asthma.

TRACHEOBRONCHIAL BLOOD FLOW AND EXUDATION

Angiograms in 15 patients with chronic obstructive lung disease showed that the bronchial arteries were larger than normal, and it was concluded that bronchial blood flow was elevated in this disease.[45] Bronchial arterial proliferation and enlargement may occur in bronchiectasis, pneumonia and tuberculosis.[11] There has also been a debate as to the role of bronchial–pulmonary arterial anastomoses in a number of lung diseases.[3–6] However, the focus has not been on asthma.

The richly vascularized mucosa of the airways receives a large fraction of the bronchial blood flow.[13] If the intratracheobronchial pressure is increased, this will decrease the bronchial blood flow, due to a compressing effect on the superficial vascular network. Pulmonary over-inflation and positive end-expiratory pressure have accordingly been demonstrated to decrease bronchial blood flow.[46,47] Nordin et al.,[48] who studied the effects on intubation on rabbit trachea, demonstrated significant decreases in mucosal/submucosal blood flow at increasing cuff pressures.

Blood gas changes that occur in asthma may affect bronchial blood flow. Experimental hypoxaemia in animals has been associated with variable effects,[10,11] however, an increased vascular resistance may be induced in the bronchial as well as in the pulmonary circulation.[10] Hypercarbia seems to decrease the bronchial vascular resistance whereas the pulmonary vascular resistance is increased by it.[10]

Work in animals shows that the neural, hormonal and pharmacological regulation of bronchial and tracheal blood flow has the characteristics of a systemic vascular bed (see Chapter 12). It has been speculated[49] that the increased bronchial blood flow produced by many mediators could in part be secondary to a bronchoconstriction-induced decrease in interstitial pressure.

In theory, many facets of inflammation are dependent on changes in the blood flow. Alterations in bronchial blood flow will affect the delivery of plasma and the perfused surface area. Hence the degree of plasma exudation under high-permeability conditions may also be affected. The flow may be increased through tissue that is affected by inflammation.[50,51] However, it is unclear to what extent the hydrostatic pressure in the venules is increased by an increased blood flow. This is the crucial aspect because when venular gap formation has been induced by inflammation (see below) it is the hydrostatic pressure inside the postcapillary venules that determines the extent of plasma exudation.

Increased blood flow cannot be considered a specific inflammatory response because many non-inflammatory factors may produce this effect. Furthermore, baseline blood flow in the airway mucosa is high and appears to be more than sufficient to fuel inflammatory processes. Airways plasma exudation has been shown to be little dependent on moderate changes in mucosal/submucosal blood flow.[43] Even a 50% reduction in flow may not reduce inflammatory stimulus-induced mucosal exudation.[53]

INCREASED VASCULAR PERMEABILITY

Under physiological conditions fluid equilibrium is maintained by a balance between the hydrostatic pressure in the capillary bed, which tends to drive fluid out of the vascular compartment, and the counteracting force of the transmural colloid osmotic pressure gradient upheld by plasma proteins. Inflammatory stimuli have dramatic effects on the postcapillary venule. They separate endothelial cells and produce large holes in the wall (Fig. 13.1). The ensuing extravasation of unfiltered plasma will practically abolish the colloid osmotic pressure gradient.[53] The vascular exudation of large molecules is secondary to an active endothelial process which is subject to physiological and pharmacological control.[50,53]

The proposed bronchoconstrictory mediators of asthma (amines, peptides, lipid products, etc.) have, with few exceptions, the additional capacity of increasing microvascular permeability and hence inducing plasma exudation (Table 13.2). Neurogenic, possibly substance P- or other tachykinin-mediated, mucosal exudation occurs in rodents but appears not to operate in human airways.[54–56] The cholinergic transmitter acetylcholine, a potent bronchoconstrictor and secretagogue, is also without effect on vascular permeability.[54] However, a large variety of non-neural mediators remains to account for plasma exudation in human asthma. Some examples are given in Table 13.2.

The vascular target cells responsible for increased permeability to macromolecules in inflammation are the endothelial cells of postcapillary venules (8–30 μm in diameter).[8,53,57] These cells harbour receptors for agents known to mediate and modulate

Table 13.2 Microvascular effects of a variety of cellular, neural and humoral mediators. (From refs 12, 19, 20, 21, 47, 53, 70 and refs cited therein.)

Source	Mediator	Blood flow	Vascular permeability
Inflammatory cells, epithelium and other cellular sources	Histamine	↑	↑
	PGE_1, D_2, $F_{2\alpha}$	↑	↑ (weak)
	LTC_4, D_4	↓ ↑	↑
	PAF-acether	↑	↑
	Adenosine	↑	—
Neural	Acetylcholine	↑	—
	Substance P	↑	(↑ guinea-pigs, rats)
	Neurokinin A	↑	(↑ guinea-pigs, rats)
Plasma	Bradykinins	↑	↑
	Anaphylatoxins: C3a, C5a	↓	↑
	Fibrin degradation peptides	↓ ↑	↑
	Other plasma protein degradation peptides	?	↑

vascular permeability. They also have an intriguing organization of filaments and myoid proteins that could exert contractile activity.[53,57] Majno and Palade[57] suggested that the mediator-induced deformation of endothelial cells resulting in the gaps (Fig. 13.1) was due to a contractile effect. Although direct proof of the validity of this hypothesis is lacking, it has been widely accepted. It is attractive because, as a corollary, relaxation of endothelial cells could explain the closure of the gaps that so readily takes place spontaneously after, or even during, an attack of an immediate-type inflammatory mediator such as histamine.[53,58] Spontaneous closure of venular gaps is an important mechanism of the permeability-regulating endothelial cells. The amount of extravasated plasma is determined by the number of venular leakage sites, the time period during which they are kept open, and the hydrostatic pressure difference across the venular wall.

PLASMA EXUDATION IN ASTHMA

Exposure of the airway mucosa to inflammatory factors produces plasma exudation not only into the airway wall but also into the lumen[38–43] (Figs 13.1, 13.2). Guinea-pig tracheobronchial data thus show excellent correlation between luminal and tissue exudative indices for immediate, biphasic, and sustained airways inflammation and for dose response to inflammatory challenges.[38,59] Hence, it is likely that the occurrence of plasma exudation in asthma can be studied by sampling and analysing airway surface liquids. The composition of sputum, mucus plugs, and lavage liquids suggests that mucosal exudation is a common, if not characteristic, feature of asthmatic airways.[21,39–41,60–65]

Nasal and tracheobronchial endothelial–epithelial barriers exhibit similarities with respect to inflammatory stimulus-induced plasma exudations.[66] In human nasal airways, it seems clear that rhinitis symptoms induced by infection, exposure to allergen or cold dry air, are associated with plasma exudation and activation of exuded mediators.[31,34,37,42] The bronchoalveolar lavage (BAL) is a much more restricted technique than the nasal lavage and it is less specific. The relatively large contribution of alveolar liquids may complicate the use of BAL for studies of bronchial liquids.[67] Furthermore, the most commonly analysed plasma protein, albumin, is normally entering the airway and alveolar lining fluids and may accumulate there. This poses a problem in BAL studies whereas in nasal experiments the mucosa can be repeatedly lavaged to create a low and consistent baseline level of albumin. Grönneberg et al.,[40] employing a novel BAL technique, have demonstrated that allergen-induced plasma exudation in allergic asthma is detected by increases in the large plasma proteins, such as fibrinogen, rather than by changes in the albumin levels. Due to a high and variable background level of albumin in bronchial lavage fluids, this protein may not be a reliable index of bronchial mucosal exudation. The unfiltered nature of the mucosal exudation process[38,59,68] suggests that large plasma proteins, which are not transuded or secreted, may be preferable indices of tracheobronchial plasma exudation.

Sticking of white cells to endothelium and their subsequent emigration across the vascular wall are characteristic of many inflammatory processes and are acknowledged events in asthmatic airways. As with protein exudation, the leucocyte–endothelium interactions occur mainly in postcapillary venules, and the diapedesis is through endothelial intercellular junctions.[69,70] However, leucocytes have a protein-tight seal during emigration, and mediator-induced exudation of plasma macromolecules occurs without cellular escape,[50,53,57,69,70] showing that different mechanisms are involved in the two types of exudative process.

MUCOSAL OEDEMA IN ASTHMA?

In the current literature it is taken for granted that airway oedema is an immediate result of tracheobronchial extravasation of plasma. Oedema is also consistently mentioned in discussions of airway pathology in asthma. Histology illustrating, but not quantitating, increased interstitial spaces has been interpreted to demonstrate the presence of oedema in asthma.[60,71] The airway narrowing, as seen in the bronchoscope, is also uncritically reported as airway oedema. However, the distinction between narrowing due to oedema or bronchial constriction, respectively, is not clear by intraluminal inspection only. The recent demonstration that luminal entry is a major elimination route of plasma extravasated from subepithelial microvessels[38,59,72] provides a mechanism that may prevent the formation of airway mucosal oedema. Indeed, it was the observation that no oedema occurred in response to exudative mucosal provocations that prompted my own and Erjefält's investigations into the luminal entry of plasma exudates.[38] A general presence of mucosal oedema in asthmatic airways is not well supported by histopathologic findings nor is it an obligatory result of airway exudation of plasma.

Mucosal thickening may occur in asthma even if plasma exudation does not produce a proper oedema. Accumulation of cells may contribute to increased thickness and so may structural changes, including enlargement of epithelial basement membrane and fibrosis and fibrin formation in the lamina propria. Unlike luminal mucous material, the tissue components will not be moved away from critical sites of resistance. They can be deformed by constriction of deeper lying airway smooth muscle but will not be compressed and will therefore exaggerate the reduction in airway lumen that occurs during bronchoconstriction. Mucosal thickening might be a substantial factor in bronchial hyperresponsiveness,[21] the proposed clinical hallmark of asthma.[73]

When plasma enters the airway lumen, many potential consequences relating to mucus viscosity and plug formation can be listed. Mucociliary transport would be reduced by addition of too much fluid to the periciliary fluid layer.[74] The transepithelial passage of plasma has been suggested to cause sloughing of epithelium,[60,71] but recent data suggest that this may not be so.[59,75–77] The mucosal crossing of exudate now appears as a non-injurious process (see below). Plasma proteins may increase mucus production,[78] prevent its normal hydration.[79] and increase its viscocity by mucin–albumin complexes[80] and by activation of the coagulation system with fibrin formation.[59,81]

Since 1986[21] it has been increasingly realized that peptides derived from the exuded plasma protein systems may contribute to the asthmatic diathesis. The kinin, complement, clotting, fibrinolysis and other systems would be activated to produce a great variety of inflammatory and bronchoconstrictive mediators, capable also of causing further recruitment of inflammatory cells. The presence of plasma proteins may be necessary for conditioning of inflammatory cells, abundant in asthma. Thus, stimulated macrophages have been demonstrated to release inflammatory factors only after being primed for a period of time by plasma proteins.[82] Although plasma exudation may not produce airway oedema, epithelial sloughing or increased absorption permeability (see below) it may be a major factor in the asthmatic diathesis (Fig. 13.3).

ANTIASTHMA DRUGS AND PLASMA EXUDATION

It is an intriguing observation that several antiasthma drugs may reduce inflammatory stimulus-induced airway exudation of plasma.[21,83–85] A part of this action, at least in experimental systems, is produced by direct effects of the drugs on venular endothelial cells. With the exception of glucocorticoids, airway antiexudative effects of antiasthma drugs have so far been demonstrated only in small numbers of patients. In 1940, Menkin[86] observed that adrenal cortex extract inhibited vascular permeability. The latency time before a vascular antipermeability effect of topical glucocorticosteroids is manifested in the hamster cheek pouch is about 1 h and these drugs need to affect the vascular target only for a short period of time, exerting a 'hit and run' effect.[87,88] However, in human airways this direct vascular tightening action may not be readily induced (Greiff, Alkner, Andersson, Persson, unpublished). Hence, in airway diseases glucocorticoids may affect a range of earlier steps in the inflammatory process that fuel the exudation (Fig. 13.4).

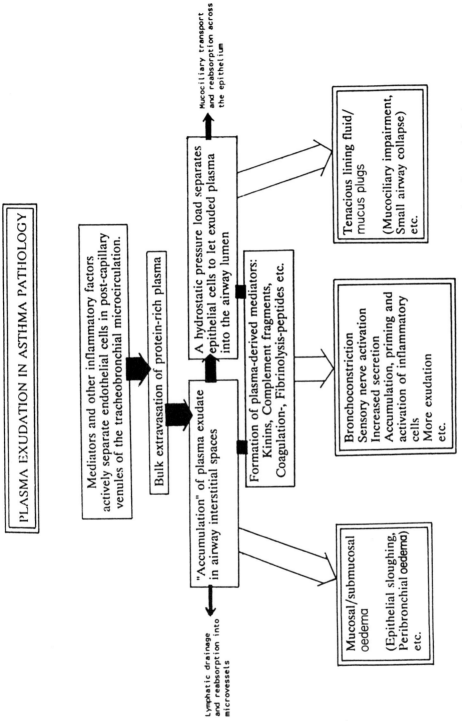

PLASMA EXUDATION IN ASTHMA PATHOLOGY

Mediators and other inflammatory factors
actively separate endothelial cells in post-capillary
venules of the tracheobronchial microcirculation.

Bulk extravasation of protein-rich plasma

"Accumulation" of plasma exudate
in airway interstitial spaces

Lymphatic drainage
and reabsorption into
microvessels

A hydrostatic pressure load separates
epithelial cells to let exuded plasma
into the airway lumen

Mucociliary transport
and reabsorption across
the epithelium

Formation of plasma-derived mediators:
Kinins, Complement fragments,
Coagulation-, Fibrinolysis-peptides etc.

Mucosal/submucosal
oedema

(Epithelial sloughing,
Peribronchial oedema)
etc.

Bronchoconstriction
Sensory nerve activation
Increased secretion
Accumulation, priming and
activation of inflammatory
cells
More exudation
etc.

Tenacious lining fluid/
mucus plugs

(Mucociliary impairment,
Small airway collapse)
etc.

Fig. 13.3 Plasma exudates in the airway wall and lumen may contribute in several ways to the pathogenesis of asthma.

Glucocorticoids inhibit airways plasma exudation

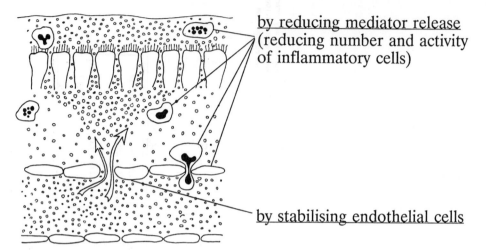

by reducing mediator release (reducing number and activity of inflammatory cells)

by stabilising endothelial cells

Fig. 13.4 When glucocorticoids reduce plasma exudation in human airways this probably reflects inhibition of cellular mechanisms that fuel the inflammatory process (above) rather than a direct vascular antipermeability effect (below).

Studies in animals[84,88] and human subjects with allergic rhinitis[89,90] or asthma[41,91] have shown that glucocorticoids reduce plasma exudation and its entry into the lumen of inflamed airways.[92,93] Moreover, a close relationship between glucocorticoid-induced clinical improvement and reduction of plasma exudation has been observed. It has been suggested that the attenuation of plasma exudation by glucocorticoids may halt a vicious circle and thus contribute to the general efficacy of these drugs in asthma.[92]

Antiasthma xanthines may be subdivided into adenosine blockers such as theophylline (and caffeine) and enprofylline (3-propylxanthine), which does not exert specific antagonism of the effects of adenosine.[94,95] Both enprofylline and theophylline relax large and small airways,[95] and they may produce several anti-inflammatory effects, including a vascular antiexudative effect.[84,85] An antiexudative effect may have contributed to the protection provided by these two xanthines against late phase airway responses occurring after allergen challenge in atopic asthmatic subjects.[96] Xanthines may reduce both symptoms and plasma exudation in inflammatory stimulus provocated human nasal mucosa.[97] Again, symptom induction and pharmacological prevention correlated nicely with plasma proteins and plasma-derived mediators, whereas levels of cellular mediators such as histamine correlated less well.[97,98] Chromones are the third type of drug, known to reduce late-phase asthmatic responses. These drugs, too, may attenuate plasma exudation and its entry into airways.[85,99,100] In experimental animal studies chromones exert direct vascular antipermeability effects. However, in human airways the antiexudative effects of these drugs probably reflect inhibition of earlier steps of the inflammatory process and not an end-organ vascular effect (cf. Fig. 13.4).[101]

An anti-oedema action of sympathomimetics has long been recognized and this is generally believed to reflect the α-adrenoceptor-mediated vasoconstrictor action of these drugs. However, experimental work suggests that sympathomimetics have a capacity to reduce exudation through another mechanism. Despite the fact that β_2-receptor agonists increase blood flow they reduce plasma exudation in guinea-pig airways.[85,102] The postcapillary venular endothelium harbours β_2-receptors.[53,83] Hence, β_2-receptor agonists may reduce plasma exudation through direct effects on the microvascular wall. The importance of a vascular antipermeability effect of β_2-agonists in asthmatic airways remains to be established.

Mucosal exudation of plasma specifically reflects the active inflammation of airway tissue. Accordingly, any antiasthma drug that attenuates airway inflammation would, as a result, also reduce the plasma exudation process.[103,104] The antiexudative effect can thus be produced by stopping the inflammation at any crucial level; for example by reducing the presence and actions of exudative mediators in the airway (cf. Fig. 13.4). As discussed above, it is also possible that antiexudative effects in part reflect drug actions directly on the venular wall. Particularly if the venules are abnormally prone to exude plasma the venular endothelium would be an important target site for antiasthma drugs. However, drugs which completely inhibit the ability of venular endothelial cells to separate are probably not warranted. Airway mucosal exudation is primarily a defence mechanism[66,105] which would be needed also in asthmatic bronchi. The observation that mucosal exudation can always be induced by a greater stimulus in the presence of either glucocorticoids, xanthines, chromones or β_2-agonists[85](and Greiff, Alkner, Andersson, Persson, unpublished) may be a safeguard mechanism of the presently available antiasthma drugs.

MUCOSAL ABSORPTION AND MUCOSAL EXUDATION

The hypothesis that 'mucosal absorption hyperpermeability' may characterize allergic airway diseases has been widely disseminated during the last 25 years.[106–109] This notion apparently prevails despite the fact that it has been criticized and that reliable data from asthmatic or rhinitic airways to support it are now largely lacking. Indeed, observations in subjects with atopic airway disease rather suggest that the mucosa has an unchanged, or even reduced, capacity to absorb allergenic material.[105] The reputed perviousness of the mucosal absorption barrier in airway disease seems to me to be a subject where the attraction of a hypothesis has received greater weight than actual data.

A series of studies involving guinea-pig tracheobronchial airways and human nasal airways is now supporting the proposal[110] that airway exudation may not be associated with an increased ability of the mucosa to absorb luminal solutes. Neither during the exudation of unfiltered plasma nor in the postexudation phase is the absorption of small or large solutes changed.[111–114] This separation between exudation- and absorption-'permeabilities' may explain the fact that there is now compelling evidence to support that plasma exudation does occur in asthma and rhinitis whereas an increased airway mucosal absorption has not been demonstrated in these diseases.

How is it possible then that unfiltered plasma can traverse the mucosa without affecting absorption? It was hypothesized that the luminal entry of exudate was induced by an increased hydrostatic pressure in the subepithelial space.[110] By affecting the lateral aspects of epithelial cells this pressure would transiently open interepithelial pathways. Through these, a burst of unfiltered exudate would be moved unidirectionally into the lumen by the elevated subepithelial pressure. Promptly after luminal entry of the exudate the epithelial junctions would resume their tightness, so that the absorption barrier of the mucosa remains uncompromised both during and after the exudation process. By simple *in vitro* experiments essential functional aspects of this hypothesis have been demonstrated.[76,112] The airway luminal entry of macromolecules *in vitro* is thus induced by elevating the subepithelial pressure by only 5 cm H_2O.[76] The pressure-induced epithelial passage is reversible, repeatable, and non-injurious, and it does not increase the rate of absorption of luminal solutes.[76,112] Furthermore, as also was shown under *in vitro* conditions, the pressure-induced luminal entry of macromolecules is not affected by agents which are exudative or antiexudative *in vivo*.[76] Taken together, the *in vitro* and *in vivo* data indicate that the plasma exudate itself creates the pathways for its entry into the airway lumen. By the persistent luminal entry the exudate fulfils its role in first line mucosal defence. Another conclusion is that antiexudative drugs are not active on the epithelial barrier when they reduce mucosal exudation. Indeed, a selective tightening of the epithelium by drugs would be a mucosal-oedema promoting effect and, therefore, not desirable.

REFERENCES

1. Reisseissen FD: *Über den Bau der Lungen*. Berlin, Rücker, 1805, pp 1–28.
2. Miller WS: *The Lung*, 2nd edn. Springfield, Charles Thomas, 1947, pp 74–88.
3. Daly I de B, Hebb C: *Pulmonary and Bronchial Vascular Systems*. London, Edward Arnold, 1966, pp 42–88.
4. Marchand P, Gilroy JC, Wilson VH: An anatomical study of the bronchial vascular system and its variation in disease. *Thorax* (1950) **5**: 207–221.
5. Cudkowicz L, Armstrong JB: Observations on the normal anatomy of the bronchial arteries. *Thorax* (1951) **6**: 343–358.
6. McLaughlin RF, Tyler WS, Canada RO: Subgross pulmonary anatomy in various mammals and man. *JAMA* (1961) **175**: 694–697.
7. Florange W: Anatomie und Patologie der Arteria Bronchialis. In Cohrs P, Giese W, Meesen H (eds) *Ergebnisse der allgemeinen Patologie und patologische Anatomi*, Berlin, Springer, 1960, pp 152–224.
8. Pietra GG, Szidon JP, Leventhal MM, Fishman AP: Histamine and interstitial pulmonary edema in the dog. *Circ Res* (1971) **29**: 323–337.
9. Magno MG, Fishman AP: Origin, distribution and blood flow of bronchial circulation in anesthetized sheep. *J Appl Physiol* (1982) **53**: 272–279.
10. Baile EM, Paré PD: Response of the bronchial circulation to acute hypoxemia and hypercarbia in the dog. *J Appl Physiol* (1983) **55**: 1474–1479.
11. Charan NB: The bronchial circulatory system: Structure, function, and importance. *Respiratory Care* (1984) **29**: 1226–1135.
12. Baier H, Long WM, Wanner A: Bronchial circulation in asthma. *Respiration* (1985) **48**: 199–205.
13. Parsons GH, Kramer GC, Link DP, *et al.*: Studies of reactivity and distribution of bronchial blood flow in sheep. *Chest* (1985) **87**: 180S–182S.
14. Kelly L, Kolbe J, Mitzner W, Spannhake EW, Bromberger-Barnea B, Menkes H: Bronchial blood flow affects recovery from constriction in dog lung periphery. *J Appl Physiol* (1986) **60**: 1954–1959.
15. Ghoreyeb AA, Karsner HT: A study of the relation of pulmonary and bronchial circulation. *J Exp Med* (1913) **18**: 500–506.

16. Modell HJ, Beck K, Butler J: Functional aspects of canine bronchial–pulmonary vascular communications. *J Appl Physiol* (1981) **50**: 1045–1051.
17. Sobin SS, Frasher WG, Tremer HM, Hadley GM: The microcirculation of the tracheal mucosa. *Angiology* (1963) **14**: 165–170.
18. Laitinen LA, Laitinen A, Salonen RO, Widdicombe JG: Vascular actions of airway neuropeptides. *Am Rev Respir Dis* (1987) **136**: 559–564.
19. Butler J (ed): *The Bronchial Circulation*. Dekker, New York, 1991.
20. Persson CGA, Svensjö E: Airway hyperreactivity and microvascular permeability to large molecules. *Eur J Respir Dis* (1983) **64**(Suppl 131): 183–214.
21. Persson CGA: Role of plasma exudation in asthmatic airways. *Lancet* (1986) **2**: 1126–1129.
22. Salter HH: *Asthma: its Pathology and Treatment*, 2nd edn. Churchill, London, 1868.
23. Kröll F, Karlsson J-A, Nilsson E, Ryrfeldt Å, Persson CGA: Rapid clearance of xanthines from airway and pulmonary tissues. *Am Rev Respir Dis* (1990) **141**: 1167–1171.
24. Davies DS: Pharmacokinetic studies with inhaled drugs. *Eur J Respir Dis* (1982) **63**(Suppl 119): 67–72.
25. Kröll F, Karlsson J-A, Persson CGA: Bronchial circulation perfused via the pulmonary artery in guinea-pig isolated lungs. *Acta Physiol Scand* (1987) **129**: 437–440.
26. Ingelstedt S: Studies on the conditioning of air in the respiratory tract. *Acta Oto-Laryngol* (1956) **131**(Suppl): 1–80.
27. McFadden ER Jr, Denison DM, Waller JF, Assoufi B, Peacock A, Sopcoith T: Direct recordings of the temperatures in the tracheobronchial tree in normal man. *J Clin Invest* (1982) **69**: 700–705.
28. Paulson B, Bende M, Ohlin P: Nasal mucosal blood flow at rest and during exercise. *Acta Otolaryngol* (1985) **99**: 140–143.
29. Baile EM, Dahlby RW, Wiggs BR, Paré PD: Role of tracheal and bronchial circulation in respiratory heat exchange. *J Appl Physiol* (1985) **58**: 217–222.
30. Andersson SD: Issues in exercise-induced asthma. *J Allergy Clin Immunol* (1985) **76**: 763–772.
31. Togias AG, Naclerio RM, Proud D, *et al*: Nasal challenge with cold, dry air results in release of inflammatory mediators. *J Clin Invest* (1985) **76**: 1375–1381.
32. Cole P: Modification of inspired air. In Proctor DF, Andersen (eds) *The Nose*. Amsterdam, Elsevier, 1982, pp 351–376.
33. Florey H, Carleton HM, Wells AQ: Mucus secretion in the trachea. *Br J Exp Pathol* (1932) **13**: 269–284.
34. Ingelstedt S, Ivstam B: The source of nasal secretion in infectious allergic and experimental conditions. *Acta Otolaryngol* (1949) **37**: 451–456.
35. Rossen RD, Butler WT, Cate TR, Szwed CF, Couch RB: Protein composition of nasal secretion during respiratory virus infection. *Proc Soc Exp Biol Med* (1965) **119**: 1169–1179.
36. Hanicki Z, Koj A: Plasma albumin loss due to bronchopathy. *Clin Chim Acta* (1965) **11**: 581–583.
37. Baumgarten CR, Togias AG, Naclerio RM, Lichtenstein LM, Normal PS, Proud D: Influx of kininogens into nasal secretions after antigen challenge of allergic individuals. *J Clin Invest* (1985) **76**: 191–197.
38. Persson CGA, Erjefält I: Inflammatory leakage of macromolecules from the vascular compartment into the tracheal lumen. *Acta Physiol Scand* (1986) **126**: 615–616.
39. Persson CGA: Plasma exudation and asthma. *Lung* (1988) **166**: 1–23.
40. Grönneberg R, Gilljam H, Salomonsson P, *et al.*: Local allergen challenge increases bronchovascular permeability in asthmatics. *J Allergy Clin Immunol* (1991) **87**: 214.
41. Van der Graaf EA, Out TA, Roos CM, Jansen H: Respiratory membrane permeability and bronchial hyperreactivity in patients with stable asthma. *Am Rev Respir Dis* (1991) **143**: 362–368.
42. Svensson C, Andersson M, Persson CGA, Alkner U, Venge P, Pipkorn U: Albumin, bradykinins and eosinophil cationic protein on the nasal mucosal surface in hay fever patients during natural allergen exposure. *J Allergy and Clin Immunol* (1990) **85**: 828–833.
43. Persson CGA: Plasma exudation from tracheobronchial microvessels in health and disease. In Butler J (ed) *The Bronchial Circulation*. New York, Dekker, 1991, in press.

44. Togias AG, Naclerio RM, Peters SP, *et al*.: Local generation of sulfidopeptide leukotrienes upon nasal provocation with cold dry air. *Am Rev Respir Dis* (1986) **133**: 1133–1137.

45. Boushy SF, North LB, Trice JA: The bronchial arteries in chronic obstructive pulmonary disease. *Am J Med* (1969) **46**: 506–515.

46. Baile EM, Albert RK, Kirk W, Lakshaminarayan B, Wiggs BJR, Paré PD: Positive end-expiratory pressure decreases bronchial blood flow in the dog. *Appl Physiol* (1984) **56**: 1289–1293.

47. Baier H, Yerger L, Moas R, Wanner A: Vascular and airway effects of endogenous cyclooxygenase products during lung inflation. *J Appl Physiol* (1985) **59**: 884–889.

48. Nordin U, Lindholm GE, Wolgast M: Blood flow in the rabbit tracheal mucosa under normal conditions and under the influence of tracheal intubation. *Acta Anaesth Scand* (1977) **21**: 81–94.

49. Lakshaminarayan S, Jindal SK, Kirk W, Butler J: Increases in bronchial blood flow following bronchoconstriction with methacholine and prostaglandin $F_{2\alpha}$ in dogs. *Chest* (1985) **5**: 183S–184S.

50. Zweifach BW: Microvascular aspects of tissue injury. In Zweifach BW, Grant L, McCluskey (eds) *The Inflammatory Process*, 2nd edn. New York, Academic Press, 1973, pp 3–46.

51. Long WM, Yerger LD, Codias EK, *et al*.: Early and late antigen-induced changes in bronchial artery blood flow and bronchomotor tone in allergic sheep. *Fed Proc* (1986) **44**: 1756.

52. Svensson C, Baumgarten CR, Alkner U, Pipkorn U, Persson CGA: Topical α-adrenoceptor stimulation may not reduce histamine-induced plasma leakage in human nasal airways. *Clin Exp Allergy* in press.

53. Grega GJ, Persson CGA, Svensjö E: Endothelial cell reactions to inflammatory mediators assessed *in vivo* by fluid and solute flux analyses. In Ryan US (ed) *Endothelial Cells*. Boca Raton, CRC (1988) pp 103–119.

54. Persson CGA, Erjefält I: Non-neural and neural regulation of plasma exudation in airways. In Kaliner M, Barnes P (eds) *Neural Regulation of Airways in Health and Disease (Lung Biology in Health and Disease)*. New York, Dekker, 1988, pp 523–549.

55. Persson CGA: Mucosal exudation in respiratory defence. Neural or nonneural control? *Int Arch Allergy Appl Immunol* (1991) **94**: 222–226.

56. Greiff L, Erjefält I, Wollmer P, *et al*: Nicotine evokes neurogenic mucosal exudation of plasma into guinea-pig but not into human airways. In Thesis, Lund (1991) 109–123.

57. Majno G, Palade GE: Studies on inflammation I. *J. Biophys Biochem Cytol* (1961) **11**: 571–605.

58. Greiff L, Pipkorn U, Alkner U, Persson CGA: The nasal pool-device applies controlled concentrations of solutes on human nasal airway mucosa and samples its surface exudation/secretions. *Clin Exp Allergy* (1990) **20**: 253–259.

59. Erjefält I, Persson CGA: Inflammatory passage of plasma macromolecules into airway tissue and lumen. *Pulm Pharmacol* (1989) **2**: 93–102.

60. Dunnill MS: The pathology of asthma with special reference to changes in the bronchial mucosa. *J Clin Pathol* (1960) **13**: 27–33.

61. Ryley HC, Brogan TD: Variation in the composition of sputum in chronic chest diseases. *Br J Exp Path* (1968) **49**: 625–633.

62. Guirgis HA, Townley RG: Biochemical study on sputum in asthma and emphysema. *J Allergy Clin Immunol* (1973) **51**: 86.

63. Brogan TD, Ryley HC, Neale L, Yassa J: Soluble proteins of bronchopulmonary secretions from patients with systic fibrosis, asthma, and bronchitis. *Thorax* (1975) **30**: 72–79.

64. Fabbri LM, Boschetto P, Zocca E, *et al*.: Bronchoalveolar neutrophilia during late asthmatic reactions induced by toluene diisocyanate. *Am Rev Respir Dis* (1987) **136**: 36–42.

65. Mattoli S, Mattoso VL, Soloperto M, Allegra L, Fasoli A: Cellular and biochemical characteristics of bronchoalveolar lavage fluid in symptomatic nonallergic asthma. *J Allergy Clin Immunol* (1981) **87**: 794–802.

66. Persson CGA: Plasma exudation in tracheobronchial and nasal airways: a mucosal defence mechanism becomes pathogenic in asthma and rhinitis. *Eur Respir J* (1990) **3**(Suppl 12): 652s–657s.

67. Venge P, Brattsand R, Laitinen L, Persson CGA: Which markers of inflammation should be used in therapeutic intervention studies of CB/COAD. In Persson CGA, *et al.* (eds) *Inflammatory Indices in Chronic Bronchitis.* Basel, Birkhäuser, 1990, pp 289–294.

68. Alkner U, Svensson C, Andersson M, Pipkorn U, Persson CGA: Fibrinogen and albumin on the surface of allergen- and histamine-exposed human nasal mucosa. *Abstract J Allergy Clin Immunol* (1991) **87**: 217.

69. Marchesi VT: The site of leukocyte emigration during inflammation. *Quart J Exp Physiol* (1961) **46**: 115–133.

70. Hurley JV: *Acute Inflammation,* 2nd edn. Edinburgh, Churchill Livingstone, 1983.

71. Hogg JC, Walker DC: Pathology of the airway epithelium in asthma. *Clin Resp Physiol* (1986) **22**(Suppl 7): 12–19.

72. Erjefält I, Luts A, Persson CGA. The appearance of airway absorption- and exudation-tracers in guinea-pig tracheobronchial lymph nodes. (1991), *Clin Exp Allergy* in press.

73. Boushey HA, Holzman MJ, Sheller JR, Nadel JA: Bronchial hyperreactivity. *Am Rev Respir Dis* (1980) **121**: 389–413.

74. Wanner A: Mucociliary function in bronchial asthma. In Weiss EB, Segal MS, Stein M (eds) *Bronchial Asthma,* 2nd edn. Boston, Little Brown, 1985, pp 270–279.

75. Persson CGA, Erjefält I, Sundler F: Airway microvascular and epithelial leakage of plasma induced by PAF-acether and capsaicin. *Am Rev Respir Dis* (1987) **135**: A401.

76. Persson CGA, Erjefält I, Gustafsson B, Luts A: Subepithelial hydrostatic pressure may regulate plasma exudation across the mucosa. *Int Arch Allergy Appl Immunol* (1990) **92**: 148–153.

77. Luts A, Sundler F, Erjefält I, Persson CGA: The airway epithelial lining is intact promptly after the mucosal crossing of a large amount of plasma exudate. *Int Arch Allergy Appl Immunol* (1990) **91**: 385–388.

78. Williams JP, Rich B, Richardson PS: Action of serum on the output of secretory glycoproteins from human bronchi *in vitro. Thorax* (1983) **38**: 682–685.

79. Aitken ML, Verdugo P: Donnan mechanism of mucus hydration: Effect of soluble proteins. *Am Rev Respir Dis* (1986) **133**: A294.

80. List SJ, Findlay BP, Forstner GG, Forstner JF: Enhancement of the viscosity of mucin by serum albumin. *Biochem J* (1978) **175**: 565–571.

81. Hirsch SR: The role of mucus in asthma. In Stein M (ed) *New Directions in Asthma.* Park Ridge, American College Chest Physicians, 1975, pp 351–363.

82. Gerberick GF, Jaffe HA, Willoughby JB, Willoughby WF: Relationships between pulmonary inflammation, plasma transudation, and oxygen metabolite secretion by alveolar macrophages. *J Immunol* (1986) **137**: 114–121.

83. Persson CGA, Svensjö E: Vascular responses and their suppression: drugs interfering with vascular permeability. In Bonta IL, Bray MA, Parnham MJ (eds) *Handbook of Inflammation, 5. The Pharmacology of Inflammation.* Amsterdam, Elsevier, 1985, pp 61–81.

84. Erjefält I, Persson CGA: Antiasthma drugs attenuate inflammatory leakage of plasma into airway lumen. *Acta Physiol Scand* (1986) **128**: 653–654.

85. Erjefält I, Persson CGA: Pharmacological control of plasma exudation in guinea-pig lower airways. *Am Rev Respir Dis* (1991) **143**: 1008–1014.

86. Menkin V: Effect of adrenal cortex extract on capillary permeability. *Am J Physiol* (1940) **129**: 691–697.

87. Svensjö E, Roempke K: Time-dependent inhibition of bradykinin- and histamine-induced increase in microvascular permeability by local glucocorticosteroid treatment. *Progr Resp Res* (1985) **19**: 173–180.

88. Brattsand R: Development of glucocorticoids with lung selectivity. In Hargreave F (ed) *Glucocorticoids and Mechanisms of Asthma.* Amsterdam, Excerpta, Medica, 1989, pp 17–38.

89. Svensson C, Klementsson H, Alkner U, Pipkorn U, Persson CGA: A topical glucocorticoid reduces the levels of fibrinogen and bradykinins on the allergic mucosa during natural pollen exposure. *J Allergy Clin Immunol* (1991) **87**: 147.

90. Pipkorn U, Proud D, Schleimer RP, *et al*: Effects of systemic glucocorticoid treatment on human nasal mediator release after antigen challenge. *J Allergy Clin Immunol* (1986) **77**(Suppl): 180.

91. Moretti M, Giannico G, Marchioni CF, Bisetti A: Effects of methylprednisolone on sputum biochemical components in asthmatic bronchitis. *Eur J Respir Dis* (1984) **65**: 365–370.
92. Andersson PT, Persson CGA: Developments in anti-asthma glucocorticoids. In O'Donnell SR, Persson CGA (eds) *Directions for New Antiasthma Drugs*. Basel, Birkhäuser, 1988, pp 239–260.
93. Persson CGA, Pipkorn U. Glucocorticoids. In Waksman BH (ed) *Fifty Years' Progress in Allergy*. Basel, Karger, 1990, pp 264–277.
94. Persson CGA, Andersson K-E, Kjellin G: Effects of enprofylline and theophylline may show the role of adenosine. *Life Sci* (1986) **38**: 1057–1072.
95. Persson CGA: Development of safer xanthine drugs for treatment of obstructive airway disease. *J Allergy Clin Immunol* (1986) **78**: 817–824.
96. Pauwels R, Van Reuterghem D, Van Der Straeten M, Johannesson N, Persson CGA: The effect of theophylline and enprofylline on allergen induced bronchoconstriction. *J Allergy Clin Immunol* (1985) **76**: 583–590.
97. Naclerio RM, Bartenfelder D, Proud D, *et al*: Theophylline reduces the response to nasal challenge with antigen. *Am J Med* (1985) **79**(Suppl 6A): 43–47.
98. Persson CGA: Xanthines as airway anti-inflammatory drugs. *J Allergy Clin Immunol* (1988) **81**: 615–617.
99. Heilpern S, Rebuck, AS: Effect of disodium cromoglycate (Intal) on sputum protein composition. *Thorax* (1972) **27**: 726–728.
100. Persson CGA: Cromoglycates, plasma exudation and asthma. *Trends Pharmacol Sci* (1987) **8**: 202–203.
101. Svensson C, Baumgarten C, Pipkorn U, Persson CGA: Nedocromil may not attenuate histamine-induced plasma exudation in the human nasal airways. *Clin Exp Allergy* (1991) in press.
102. Erjefält I, Persson CGA: Long duration and high potency of antiexudative effects of formoterol in guinea-pig tracheobronchial airways. *Am Rev Respir Dis* (1991) **144**: 788–791.
103. Persson CGA: Airway plasma exudation in detection of anti-asthma drugs. In Morley J, Andersson G (eds) *New Drugs for Asthma*. Basel, Birkhäuser, 1991, in press.
104. Persson CGA: Role of plasma exudation in asthmatic airways. *Lancet* (1986) **2**: 1126–1129.
105. Persson CGA, Erjefält I, Alkner U, *et al*.: Plasma exudation as a first line respiratory mucosal defence. *Clin Exp Allergy* (1991) **21**: 17–24.
106. Salvaggio JE, Cavanaugh JA, Lowell FC, Leskowitz SO: A comparison of the immunologic responses of normal and atopic individuals to intranasally administered antigen. *J Allergy* (1982) **35**: 62–69.
107. Boucher RC, Ranga V, Paré PD, Inoue S, Moroz LA, Hogg JC: Effect of histamine and methacholine on guinea pig tracheal permeability to HRP. *J Appl Physiol: Respir Environ Exercise Physiol* (1978) **45**: 939–948.
108. Boucher RC, Ranga V: Fate and handling of antigens by the lung. In Daniele RP (ed) *Immunology and Immunological Diseases*. Boston, Blackworth, 1988, pp 55–78.
109. Ranga V, Powers MA, Padilla M, Strope GL, Fowler L, Kleinerman J: Effects of allergic bronchoconstriction to large polar solutes in the guinea-pig. *Am Rev Resp Dis* (1983) **128**: 1065–1070.
110. Persson CGA: Permeability changes in obstructive airway diseases. In Sluiter HJ, Van Der Lende R (eds) *Bronchitis IV*. Assen, Van Corcum, 1989, pp 236–248.
111. Erjefält I, Persson CGA: Allergen, bradykinin, and capsaicin increase outward but not inward macromolecular permeability of guinea-pig tracheobronchial mucosa. *Clin Exp Allergy* (1991) **21**: 217–224.
112. Gustafsson B, Persson CGA: Assymetrical effects of increase in hydrostatic pressure on macromolecular movement across the airway mucosa. *Clin Exp Allergy* (1990) **21**: 121–126.
113. Greiff L, Erjefält I, Wollmer P, Pipkorn, Persson CGA: Different patterns of inflammatory effects on guinea pig airway barriers *in vivo*: Plasma exudation with and without increased absorption of small and large solutes. *Thorax* (1991) **46**: 700–705.
114. Greiff L, Wollmer P, Pipkorn U, Persson CGA: Unaffected absorption of ^{51}Cr-EDTA across the human nasal airway barriers in the presence of topical histamine. *Thorax* (1991) **46**: 630–632.

14

Prostaglandins and Thromboxane

PAUL M. O'BYRNE

INTRODUCTION

Asthma is a common disease, with a cumulative prevalence in a varitey of countries where statistics have been compiled of at least 10–15%.[1] While dyspnoea, wheeze, chest tightness and cough with or without sputum are the usual presenting symptoms in asthma, these symptoms can also occur in other conditions and are not specific for asthma. However, a diagnosis of asthma can be made by objectively documenting reversible airflow obstruction which improves either spontaneously or after treatment. In addition, the presence of airway hyperresponsiveness to a variety of inhaled stimuli is characteristic of asthma.[2]

Events occurring in the airways as a result of acute and chronic airway inflammation are important in the pathogenesis of asthma.[3] This has been known for more than 100 years in patients with severe fatal asthma.[4] In these patients, a large number of inflammatory cells along with epithelial desquamation, mucosal oedema and excess secretions are present in the airways.[5] It is now recognized that airway inflammation is also important in milder asthma. For example, studies have demonstrated increases in airway eosinophils and mast cells in patients with very mild, stable asthma.[6] The severity of airway hyperresponsiveness correlates with the numbers of these inflammatory cells in the airways. The mechanisms by which airway inflammation may cause airway hyperresponsiveness and airway narrowing in asthma are still largely unknown. It is likely, however, that mediators released from effector cells in the airways cause the influx of inflammatory cells, and subsequent activation of these cells. Further release of mediators from activated cells causes the bronchoconstriction, airway hyperresponsiveness and other manifestations of inflammation such as airway oedema and excess airway secretions.

ASTHMA: BASIC MECHANISMS AND CLINICAL MANAGEMENT (2nd Edn)
ISBN 0-12-079026-2

   The investigation of the potential role of a mediator in the pathogenesis of asthma has, to date, depended on three pieces of evidence. Firstly, the inhaled mediator mimics a component of the asthmatic response. Secondly, the mediator (or its metabolite) can be measured in a biological fluid following induction of an asthmatic response. Thirdly, a selective mediator receptor antagonist or synthetase inhibitor inhibits some component of an asthmatic response. These studies tend to be performed initially in animal models and eventually in asthmatic subjects. While several mediators have been proposed as playing a role in the pathogenesis of asthma, problems have existed which have prevented convincing evidence being obtained for a role for any mediator. The problems include (a) the difficulties in measuring the mediator or its metabolite at its site of action in the airways; (b) the lack of potent, specific mediator antagonists; (c) the absence of an animal model of asthma. Several animal models of airway hyperresponsiveness exist[7-9], and studies using these models have lead to interesting and potentially important insights into the pathogenesis of airway hyperresponsiveness. However, definitive studies can only be performed in human subjects, which imposes major limitations on the interventions which can be done, for example, to measure mediator release.

   The purpose of this review is to examine the evidence that one group of mediators, cyclooxygenase products of arachidonic acid metabolism, are released in human airways and are involved in the pathogenesis of asthmatic responses. In addition, evidence will be considered which suggests that some members of this group of mediators provide a protective function in asthmatic airways.

ARACHIDONIC ACID METABOLISM

The release of arachidonic acid from cell membrane phospholipids through the action of a family of phospholipases can result in the production of a wide variety of mediators which may be relevant in the pathogenesis of asthma (Fig. 14.1). These lipid mediators have traditionally been considered in two classes: mediators which result from the action of the enzyme cyclooxygenase on arachidonic acid, which are prostaglandins (PGs) or thromboxane (Tx); and mediators which result from the action of the enzyme 5-lipooxygenase or arachidonic acid, which are leukotrienes (LT). More recently, however, other products have been identified which result from the activity of different enzymes, such as 12- and 15-lipooxygenase. Lastly, platelet-activating factor (PAF) has been recognized to be a mediator derived from arachidonic acid metabolism.

   The oxidative metabolism of arachidonic acid by cyclooxygenase produces the cyclic endoperoxides PGG_2 and PGH_2. The subsequent action of prostaglandin isomerases produces either PGD_2 or PGE_2, reductive cleavage produces $PGF_{2\alpha}$ while one or two terminal synthetases on the endoperoxide produces PGI_2 and TxA_2. Cyclooxygenase appears to be present in most cells; however, the cyclooxygenase metabolite(s) released from a particular cell are quite specific (for example TxA_2 from platelets, and PGI_2 from endothelial cells). This suggests that terminal synthestases are cell specific.

   The effect of 5-lipooxygenase on arachidonic acid is to produce 5-hydro-peroxyeicosatetraenoic acid (5-HPETE), which is converted by dehydrase to LTA_4. This intermediate metabolite can be acted upon by epoxide hydrolase resulting in LTB_4, or by glutathione-s-transferase resulting in LTC_4, which is further metabolized to LTD_4

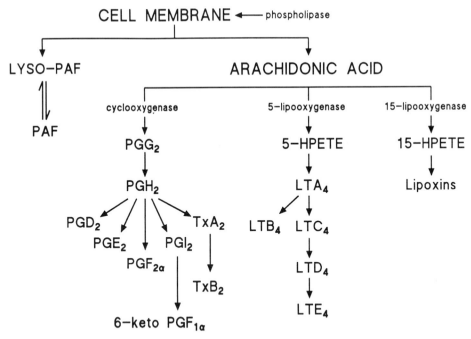

Fig. 14.1   The spectrum of eicosanoids produced as a consequence of arachidonic acid metabolism.

and LTE_4. It is now recognized that the biological activity of previously called slow-reacting substance of anaphylaxis (SRS-A) is made up by the sulphidopeptide leukotrienes LTC_4, LTD_4 and LTE_4.[10]

PAF is derived from the activity of phospholipase A_2 on membrane phospholipids which cleaves arachidonic acid from a glycerol backbone to form an inactive precursor, lyso-PAF. Subsequent incorporation of an acetyl group by acetyltransferase results in the active PAF. The half-life of PAF is very short, being less than 1 min; interestingly, PAF is inactivated by removal of the acetyl group to produce the inactive precursor, lyso-PAF.

ROLE OF CYCLOOXYGENASE PRODUCTS IN ASTHMA

All of the cyclooxygenase products of arachidonic acid metabolism have been synthesized and, with the exception of thromboxane, are available for study. Thromboxane has an exceedingly short half-life (about 30 s) and studies with thromboxane have been limited to a few, very limited, experimental preparations, none of them in the airways. Fortunately, several stable thromboxane mimetics have been synthesized. These are endoperoxides which activate the thromboxane receptor and mimic the biological actions of thromboxane. In addition, while a wide variety of cyclooxygenase inhibitors exist and have been extensively studied; again with the exception of thromboxane, no selective synthetase inhibitors or receptor antagonists are available for the other prostaglandins.

Despite the above limitations, prostaglandins are believed to have a variety of effects on airway function in asthma. The prostaglandins are most easily considered in two classes. These are stimulatory prostaglandins, such as PGD_2 and $PGF_{2\alpha}$, which are potent bronchoconstrictors, and inhibitory prostaglandins, such as PGE_2, which can reduce bronchoconstrictor responses and attenuate the release of bronchoconstrictor mediators, such as acetylcholine, from the airway nerves.

Evidence has been obtained in both animal models of airway hyperresponsiveness and in human subjects with asthma that cyclooxygenase metabolites are involved in causing bronchoconstriction and also airway hyperresponsiveness after inhalation of stimuli, such as allergens. There is, however, little convincing evidence that cyclooxygenase metabolites are important in causing the ongoing, persisting airway hyperresponsiveness that is characteristic of asthma. This is because several studies have failed to demonstrate any effect of cyclooxygenase inhibitors on stable airway hyperresponsiveness in asthmatic subjects.

The initial studies examining the role of cyclooxygenase metabolites in the pathogenesis of transient airway hyperresponsiveness after an inflammatory stimulus were carried out using the cyclooxygenase inhibitor, indomethacin in dogs with airway hyperresponsiveness after inhaled ozone. Indomethacin did not alter baseline airway responsiveness to inhaled acetylcholine, but did prevent the development of airway hyperresponsiveness after inhaled ozone.[11] Despite the absence of airway hyperresponsiveness, the magnitude of the inflammatory response, as measured by the numbers of neutrophils in the airway epithelium, was not altered by indomethacin. This suggested that a cyclooxygenase product was not responsible for the chemotaxis of acute inflammatory cells into the airways after inhaled ozone; however, a cyclooxygenase product was released during the inflammatory response which caused airway hyperresponsiveness. Subsequently, a reputed combined cyclooxygenase and lipooxygenase inhibitor, BW775c was also demonstrated to prevent the development of airway hyperresponsiveness after inhaled ozone in dogs.[12] Inhibition of cyclooxygenase by indomethacin also prevents the development of airway hyperresponsiveness in other species; for example, after C_{5a} des arg in rabbits,[13] and after inhaled allergen in sheep.[14] The importance of cylooxygenase products in these responses may be species dependent. For example, BW775c but not indomethacin, prevents airway hyperresponsiveness after inhaled ozone in guinea-pigs,[15] suggesting that a lipooxygenase rather than a cyclooxygenase product was causing airway hyperresponsiveness in this species.

Cyclooxygenase products have been implicated in the pathogenesis of allergen-induced early asthmatic[16] as well as late asthmatic responses[17] in human subjects. This has been done by pretreating subjects with several different cyclooxygenase inhibitors. For example, Joubert et al.[18] reported that pretreatment with indomethacin inhibited the late response in 10 out of 11 subjects studied, without having a major effect on the early response. A more recent study, however, has not confirmed these observations on either allergen-induced early or late responses. Pretreatment with indomethacin (100 mg/day) did not influence either the early or late asthmatic responses.[19] These results suggested that cyclooxygenase products were not important mediators in causing these asthmatic responses. However, in this study, indomethacin significantly inhibited the development of allergen-induced airway hyperresponsiveness,[19] which suggests that a cyclooxygenase product is involved in the pathogenesis of this response. The most likely candidates are the stimulatory prostaglandins PGD_2, $PGF_{2\alpha}$ or TxA_2.

STIMULATORY PROSTAGLANDINS AND THROMBOXANE

PGD_2 is known to be released from stimulated dispersed human lung cells *in vitro*[20] and from the airways of allergic human subjects which have been stimulated by allergen.[21] PGD_2 is a bronchoconstrictor of human airways,[22] and is more potent when inhaled by human subjects than $PGF_{2\alpha}$. PGD_2 causes bronchoconstriction directly through stimulation of specific contractile receptors and indirectly through acting presynaptically to release acetylcholine from airway cholinergic nerves.[23] Subthreshold contractile concentrations of PGD_2 have been demonstrated to increase airway responsiveness to inhaled histamine and methacholine in asthmatic subjects.[24] Thus, PGD_2 released in human airways after allergen inhalation has the potential to both cause acute bronchoconstriction and increase airway hyperresponsiveness to other constrictor mediators. However, specific receptor antagonists for PGD_2 or inhibitors of its production are not available to allow a precise evaluation of the importance of this cyclooxygenase metabolite in causing asthmatic responses.

As with PGD_2, $PGF_{2\alpha}$ has the potential for being important in causing bronchoconstriction and airway hyperresponsiveness after inhaled allergen in human subjects. This is because it is released from human lungs, is a potent bronchoconstrictor in asthmatic airways,[25] and inhaled subthreshold constrictor concentrations can increase airway responsiveness in dogs[26] and human subjects.[27,28] Again as with PGD_2, there are no selective $PGF_{2\alpha}$ receptor antagonists available, that would allow identification of the importance of these metabolites in causing these responses. Indeed, it has been suggested that all contractile prostaglandins act via a single TP_1-receptor.[29] Therefore, differentiation of the relative importance of the contractile prostaglandins in causing asthmatic responses may prove to be extremely difficult.

Both PGD_2 and $PGF_{2\alpha}$ cause bronchoconstriction in human subjects through a direct effect on airway receptors and indirectly through cholinergic-mediated bronchoconstriction.[30] It is not known, however, whether the cholinergic component occurs through a cholinergic reflex or through a direct presynaptic effect causing the release of acetylcholine.

TxA_2 is a potent constrictor of smooth muscle. TxA_2 was originally described as being released from platelets,[31] but is now known to be released from other cells, including macrophages and neutrophils.[32] As the biological half-life of TxA_2 is very short, implicating TxA_2 in disease processes has depended on measurement of its more stable metabolite thromboxane B_2 (TxB_2) in biological fluids; on the use of the stable endoperoxides U44069 or U46619, which mimic most of the biological effects of TxA_2 and have been used as TxA_2 analogues; and on the use of inhibitors of TxA_2 synthesis and antagonists of the TxA_2 receptor. Using these techniques, TxA_2 has been implicated in the pathogenesis of airway hyperresponsiveness in dogs[33-35] and primates;[36] of the late cutaneous response to intradermal allergen[37] in humans; of the immediate response to inhaled allergen in dogs;[38] of the late asthmatic response after inhaled allergen in humans;[39] and of airway hyperresponsiveness in asthmatic subjects.[40]

The mechanism by which TxA_2 causes airway hyperresponsiveness is not yet known, but possible mechanisms include presynaptic modulation of acetylcholine release, or an effect on airway smooth muscle. TxA_2 was initially demonstrated to modulate acetylcholine release in airways by Munoz *et al.* using the TxA_2 mimetic U46619, which increased the responses to field stimulation in trachealis muscle. No increase in the responses to exogenous acetylcholine by U46619 was demonstrated, suggesting that the augmentation was occurring presynaptically, through increased acetylcholine release in response to field stimulation. Further support for this hypothesis was provided by Tamaoki et al.,[42] who demonstrated that aggregated platelets in an organ bath released TxA_2. The TxA_2 transiently increased the responses to field stimulation and this effect was prevented by a TxA_2 receptor antagonist. Once again, the responses to an exogenous cholinergic agonist was not altered by the released TxA_2.

Attempts to measure the stable metabolite TxB_2 in human subjects during asthmatic episodes or following allergen challenge have lead to conflicting results. Both Shephard et al.[39] and Manning et al.[43] have demonstrated increased levels of TxB_2 in plasma following allergen challenge. However, plasma TxB_2 measurements must be viewed with caution because of the possibility of local platelet generation of TxB_2 and measurements should be confirmed by assaying the 2,3-dinor metabolite of TxB_2 which cannot come from platelet activation alone.

The TxA_2 synthetase inhibitor, OKY 046, administered orally, reduces acetylcholine airway hyperresponsiveness in stable asthmatic subjects (although these studies were uncontrolled), while a lipooxygenase inhibitor had no effect in these subjects.[40] Thus, TxA_2 may be an important mediator in the pathogenesis of airway hyperresponsiveness either in stable asthma or after inhaled allergens. Recent studies, however, have examined the effect of the thromboxane synthetase inhibitor, CGS 13080, on airway responses after allergen challenge. CGS 13080 slightly but significantly inhibited the magnitude of the early but not the late responses after inhaled allergen. In addition, there was no effect on airway hyperresponsiveness to inhaled histamine measured 24 h post allergen.[43] These studies taken together suggest that thromboxane may be released following allergen challenge and be partly responsible for the early asthmatic response but, in contrast to dogs, it is not important in causing airway hyperresponsiveness following allergen inhalation.

INHIBITORY PROSTAGLANDINS

The differentiation of the prostaglandins into stimulatory and inhibitory classes is somewhat inappropriate. For example, both PGE_2 and $PGF_{2\alpha}$ can have different effects on the airways depending on the time after inhalation when the response is measured.[44,45] However, the main action of PGE_2 and PGI_2 on airway function is to relax airway smooth muscle and to antagonize the contractile responses of other bronchoconstrictor agonists. In addition PGE_2 is extremely potent at inhibiting the release of acetylcholine from airway cholinergic nerves.[46] This effect is thought to occur through stimulation of presynaptic receptors.

The evidence that inhibitory prostaglandins play a role in modulating the contractile responses of agonists such as histamine and acetylcholine in asthmatic subjects comes from studies which have demonstrated that tachyphylaxis (a decreased response to repeated stimulation) occurs following repeated challenges with exercise or inhaled histamine, when challenges are separated by up to 6 h.[47,48] In addition, both exercise refractoriness[47,49] and histamine tachyphylaxis[48] are prevented by pretreatment with indomethacin, which suggests that tachyphylaxis occurs through release of inhibitory prostaglandins in the airways. Lastly pretreatment of asthmatic subjects with oral PGE_1, in doses which do not cause bronchodilation, reduces airway responsiveness to both histamine and methacholine.[50] These results are consistent with studies of airway smooth muscle *in vitro*, where histamine tachyphylaxis occurs through inhibitory prostaglandin release,[51] and with studies in dogs *in vivo* where histamine tachyphylaxis is inhibited by indomethacin.[52] In addition, histamine tachyphylaxis in asthmatic subjects is blocked by pretreatment with cimetidine in asthmatics,[53] suggesting that H_2 receptor stimulation is involved with the development of histamine tachyphylaxis. Stimulation of H_2 receptors in the lung *in vitro* has previously been shown to be associated with PGE_2 release in guinea-pigs,[20] and PGE_2 release from canine trachealis by histamine is antagonized by cimetidine.[54]

Contraction of asthmatic airways by histamine also reduces airway responsiveness to acetylcholine[55] and exercise.[56] This lack of specificity suggests that either receptor downregulation or an alteration of the contractile properties of airway smooth muscle is occurring. Indeed, PGE causes heterologous receptor desensitization in some isolated cell systems and airway smooth muscle has specific PGE receptors[29] mediating inhibitory effects such as relaxation. However, there is no current evidence from either *in vivo* or *in vitro* preparations to support this speculation.

CONCLUSIONS

Despite more than 20 years of research on the release, metabolism, and clinical relevance of prostaglandins and thromboxane in lung disease, no definitive role has been identified for any one of these mediators. In airway diseases, such as asthma, it is likely that PGD_2 and TxA_2 are involved in causing acute bronchoconstriction after stimuli such as inhaled allergen in asthmatic patients. Also, there is evidence that indicates that inhibitory prostaglandins can be released by normal or asthmatic airways, which reduces bronchoconstrictor responses to stimuli such as exercise and histamine. However, it is unlikely that prostaglandins are directly involved in causing the influx and maturation of the effector inflammatory cells, or are involved in causing the ongoing airway hyperresponsiveness in asthma.

REFERENCES

1. Sears MR: Epidemiology of Asthma. In O'Byrne PM (ed) *Asthma is an Inflammatory Disease.* New York, Marcel Dekker, 1990, pp 1–34.
2. Hargreave FE, Ramsdale EH, Dolovich J: Measurement of airways responsiveness in clinical practice. In Hargreave FE, Woolcock AJ (eds) *Airway Responsiveness Measurement and Interpretation.* Mississauga, Astra Pharmaceuticals, 1985, pp 122–126.
3. O'Byrne PM, Kirby JG, Hargreave FE: Airway inflammation and hyperresponsiveness. *Am Rev Respir Dis* (1987) **136**: S35–S37.
4. Osler W: In *The Principles and Practice of Medicine.* New York, Appleton, 1892, 497.
5. Dunhill MS, Massarell GR, Anderson JA: A comparison of the quantitive anatomy of the bronchi in normal subjects, in status asthmaticus, in chronic bronchitis and in emphysema. *Thorax* (1969) **24**: 176–179.

6. Kirby JG, Hargreave FE, Gleich GJ, O'Byrne PM: Bronchoalveolar cell profiles of asthmatic and nonasthmatic subjects. *Am Rev Respir Dis* (1987) **136**: 379–383.

7. Lee L-Y, Bleeker ER, Nadel JA: Effect of ozone on bronchomotor reponse to inhaled histamine in dogs. *J Appl Physiol* (1977) **43**: 626–631.

8. Murphy KR, Wilson MC, Irvin CG, *et al.*: The requirement for polymorphonuclear leukocytes in the asthmatic response and heightened airways reactivity in an asthmatic model. *Am Rev Respir Dis* (1986) **134**: 62–68.

9. Abraham WM, Delehunt JC, Yerger L, Marchette B: Characterization of a late phase pulmonary response after antigen challenge in allergic sheep. *Am Rev Respir Dis* (1984) **128**: 839–844.

10. Lewis RA, Austen KF: The biologically active leukotrienes. Biosynthesis, metabolism, receptors, functions and pharmacology. *J Clin Invest* (1984) **73**: 889–897.

11. O'Byrne PM, Walters EH, Aizawa H, Fabbri LM, Holtzman MJ, Nadel JA: Indomethacin inhibits the airway hyperresponsiveness but not the neutrophil influx induced by ozone in dogs. *Am Rev Respir Dis* (1984) **130**: 220–224.

12. Fabbri LM, Aizawa H, O'Byrne PM, *et al.*: An anti-inflammatory drug (BW755c) inhibits airway responsiveness induced by ozone in dogs. *J Allergy Clin Immunol* (1985) **76**: 162–166.

13. Berend N, Armour CL, Black JL: Indomethacin inhibits C5a des arg-induced airway hyperresponsiveness in the rabbit. *Am Rev Respir Dis* (1985) **131**: 24A.

14. Lanes S, Stevenson JS, Codias E, *et al.*: Indomethacin and FPL 55321 inhibit antigen-induced airway hyperresponsiveness in sheep. *J Appl Physiol* (1986) **61**: 864–872.

15. Lee HK, Murlas C: Ozone-induced bronchial hyperreactivity in guinea pigs is abolished by BW 755C or FPL 55712 but not by indomethacin. *Am Rev Respir Dis* (1985) **132**: 1005–1009.

16. Fish JE, Ankin MG, Adkinson NF, Peterman VI: Indomethacin modification of immediate-type immunologic airway responses in allergic asthmatic and non-asthmatic subjects. *Am Rev Respir Dis* (1982) **123**: 609–614.

17. Fairfax AJ: Inhibition of the late asthmatic response to house dust mite by non-steroidal anti-inflammatory drugs. *Prostaglandins, Leukotrienes and Medicine* (1982) **8**: 239–248.

18. Joubert JR, Shephard E, Mouton W, Van Zyk L, Viljoen I: Non-steroid anti-inflammatory drugs in asthma: dangerous or useful therapy? *Allergy* (1985) **40**: 202–207.

19. Kirby JG, Hargreave FE, Cockcroft DW, O'Byrne PM: The effect of indomethacin on allergen-induced asthmatic responses. *J Appl Physiol* (1989) **66**: 578–583.

20. Yen SS, Mathe AA, Dugan JJ: Release of prostaglandins from healthy and sensitized guinea-pig lung and trachea by histamine. *Prostaglandins* (1976) **11**: 227–239.

21. Murray JJ, Tonnel AB, Brash AR, *et al.*: Release of prostaglandin D_2 into human airways during acute antigen challenge. *N Engl J Med* (1986) **315**: 800–804.

22. Hardy CC, Robinson C, Tattersfield AE, Holgate ST: The bronchoconstrictor effect of inhaled prostaglandin D_2 in normal and asthmatic men. *N Engl J Med* (1984) **311**: 209–213.

23. Tamaoki J, Sekizawa K, Graf PD, Nadel JA: Cholinergic neuromodulation by prostaglandin D_2 in canine airway smooth muscle. *J Appl Physiol* (1987) **63**: 1396–1400.

24. Fuller RW, Dixon CMS, Dollery CT, Barnes PJ. Prostaglandin D_2 potentiates airway responsiveness to histamine and methacholine. *Am Rev Respir Dis* (1986) **133**: 252–254.

25. Thomson NC, Roberts R, Bandouvakis J, Newball H, Hargreave FE: Comparison of bronchial responses to prostaglandin $F_{2\alpha}$ methacholine. *J Allergy Clin Immunol* (1981) **68**: 392–398.

26. O'Byrne PM, Aizawa H, Bethel RA, Chung KF, Nadel JA, Holtzman MJ: Prostaglandin $F_{2\alpha}$ increases airway responsiveness of pulmonary airways in dogs. *Prostaglandins* (1984) **28**: 537–543.

27. Walters EH, Parrish RW, Bevan C, Smith AP: Induction of bronchial hypersensitivity: evidence for a role for prostaglandins. *Thorax* (1981) **36**: 571–574.

28. Fish JE, Jameson A, Albright A, Norman PS: Modulation of bronchomotor effects of chemical mediators by $PGF_{2\alpha}$. *Amer Rev Respir Dis* (1984) **129**: A2.

29. Gardiner PJ: Eiconsanoids and airway smooth muscle. *Pharm Ther* (1989) **44**: 1–62.

30. Beasley R, Varley J, Robinson C, Holgate ST: Cholinergic-mediated bronchonconstriction induced by prostaglandin D_2, its initial metabolite $9_\alpha,11_\beta$-$PGF_{2\alpha}$, and $PGF_{2\alpha}$ in asthma. *Am Rev Respir Dis* (1987) **136**: 1140–1144.

31. Hamberg M, Svensson J, Samuelsson B: Thromboxanes: a new group of biologically active compounds derived from prostaglandin endoperoxides. *Proc Natl Acad Sci USA* (1975) **72**: 2994–2998.

32. Higgs GA, Moncada S, Salmon JA, Seager K: The source of thromboxane and prostaglandins in experimental inflammation. *Br J Pharmac* (1983) **79**: 863–868.

33. Aizawa H, Chung KF, Leikauf GD, *et al.*: Significance of thromboxane generation in ozone-induced airway hyperresponsiveness in dogs. *J Appl Physiol* (1985) **59**: 1918–1923.

34. Chung KF, Aizawa H, Becker AB, Frick O, Gold WM, Nadel JA: Inhibition of antigen-induced airway hyperresponsiveness by a thromboxane synthetase inhibitor (OKY 046) in allergic dogs. *Am Rev Respir Dis* (1986) **134**: 258–261.

35. O'Byrne PM, Leikauf GD, Aizawa H, *et al.*: Leukotriene B4 induced airway hyperresponsiveness in dogs. *J Appl Physiol* (1985) **59**: 1941–1946.

36. McFarlane CS, Ford-Hutchinson AW, Letts LG: Inhibition of thromboxane (TXA$_2$)-induced airway hyperresponsiveness to aerosolized acetylcholine by the selective TXA$_2$ antagonist L655,240 in the conscious primate. *Am Rev Respir Dis* (1985) **137**: 100A.

37. Dorsch WD, Ring J, Melzer H: A selective inhibitor of thromboxane biosynthesis enhances immediate and inhibits late cutaneous allergic reactions in man. *J Allergy Clin Immunol* (1983) **72**: 168–174.

38. Kleeberger SR, Kolbe J, Adkinson NF Jr, Peters SP, Spannhake EW: Thromboxane contributes to the immediate antigenic response of canine peripheral airways. *J Appl Physiol* (1987) **62**: 1589–1595.

39. Shephard EG, Malan L, Macfarlane CM, Mouton W, Joubert JR: Lung function and plasma levels of thrombane B$_2$, 6-ketoprostaglandin F$_{1\alpha}$ and B-thromboglobulin in antigen-induced asthma before and after indomethacin pretreatment. *Br J Clin Pharm* (1985) **19**: 459–470.

40. Fujimura M, Sasaki F, Nakatsumi Y, *et al.*: Effects of a thromboxane synthetase inhibitor (OKY-046) and a lipoxygenase inhibitor (AA-861) on bronchial responsiveness to acetylcholine in asthmatic subjects. *Thorax* (1986) **41**: 955–959.

41. Munoz NM, Shioya T, Murphy TM, *et al.*: Potentiation of vagal contractile response by thromboxane mimetic U-46619. *J Appl Physiol* (1986) **61**: 1173–1179.

42. Tamaoki J, Sekizawa K, Osborne ML, Ueki IF, Graf PD, Nadel JA: Platelet aggregation increases cholinergic neurotransmission in canine airway. *J Appl Physiol* (1987) **62**: 2246–2251.

43. Manning PJ, Stevens WH, Cockcroft DW, O'Byrne PM: The role of thromboxane in allergen-induced asthmatic responses. *Am Rev Respir Dis* (1990) **141**: A395.

44. Walters EH, Parrish RW, Bevan C, Parrish RW, Smith BH, Smith AP: Time-dependent effect of prostaglandin E$_2$ inhalation on airway responses to bronchoconstrictor agents in normal subjects. *Thorax* (1982) **37**: 438–442.

45. Fish JE, Newball HH, Norman PS, Peterman VI: Novel effects of PGF$_{2\alpha}$ on airway function in asthmatic subjects. *J Appl Physiol* (1983) **54**: 105–112.

46. Walters EH, O'Byrne PM, Fabbri LM, Graf PD, Holtzman MJ, Nadel JA: Control of neurotransmission by prostaglandins in canine trachealis smooth muscle. *J Appl Physiol* (1984) **57**(1): 129–134.

47. O'Byrne PM, Jones GL: The effect of indomethacin on exercise-induced bronchoconstriction and refractoriness after exercise. *Am Rev Respir Dis* (1986) **134**: 60–72.

48. Manning PJ, Jones GL, O'Byrne PM: Tachyphylaxis to inhaled histamine in asthmatic subjects. *J Appl Physiol* (1987) **63**: 1572–1577.

49. Margolskee DJ, Bigby BG, Boushey HA: Indomethacin blocks airway tolerance to repetitive exercise but not to eucapnic hyperpnea in asthmatic subjects. *Am Rev Respir Dis* (1988) **137**: 842–846.

50. Manning PJ, Lane CG, O'Byrne PM: The effect of oral prostaglandin E$_1$ on airway responsiveness in asthmatic subjects. *Pulmonary Pharmacology* (1989) **2**: 121–124.

51. Anderson WH, Krzanowski JJ, Polson JB, Szentivanyi A: Characteristics of histamine tachyphylaxis in canine tracheal smooth muscle. *Naunyn-Schiedeberg Arch Pharmacol* (1977) **308**: 117–125.

52. Shore S, Martin JG: Tachyphylaxis to inhaled aerosolized histamine in anesthetized dogs. *J Appl Physiol* (1985) **59**: 1355–1363.

53. Jackson PA, Manning PJ, O'Byrne PM: A new role for histamine H_2-receptors in asthmatic airways. *Am Rev Respir Dis* (1988) **138**: 784–788.
54. Manning PM, Jones GL, Lane CG, O'Byrne PM: Histamine-induced prostaglandin E_2 release from canine tracheal smooth muscle is inhibited by H_2-receptor blockade. *Am Rev Respir Dis* (1988) **137**: 373A.
55. Manning PJ, O'Byrne PM: Histamine bronchoconstriction reduces airway responsiveness in asthmatic subjects. *Am Rev Respir Dis* (1988) **137**: 1323–1325.
56. Hamilec CM, Manning PJ, O'Byrne PM: Exercise refractoriness post histamine bronchoconstriction in asthmatic subjects. *Am Rev Respir Dis* (1988) **138**: 794–798.

15

Cysteinyl Leukotrienes

JEFFREY M. DRAZEN

FORMATION AND METABOLISM

The leukotrienes (LTB$_4$, LTC$_4$, LTD$_4$ and LTE$_4$) and lipoxins (LxA and LxB) are molecules derived by lipoxygenation of arachidonic acid. Although each of these molecules is potentially important in the pathogenesis of asthma, most evidence suggests that among these molecules, LTC$_4$, LTD$_4$ and LTE$_4$ play the major role in initiating and maintaining an asthmatic response; this chapter will focus primarily on these molecules.

Arachidonic acid is a normal component of many cell membrane phospholipids; it is commonly found esterified to such phospholipids in the *sn*2 position. In the presence of appropriately activated phospholipase A$_2$, free arachidonic acid is cleaved from the cell membrane (Fig. 15.1). Alternatively phospholipase C, which is activated in the course of a number of transmembrane signalling events,[1] cleaves membrane phospholipids to form a phosphorylated base, such as phosphatidyl-serine, -choline or -inositol, and diacylglycerol. The latter moiety, which has a role in transmembrane signalling itself, is cleaved by diglyceride lipase resulting in the formation of a monoacylglycerol and arachidonic acid.

The arachidonic acid, cleaved from cell membrane phospholipids, interacts with a specific 5-lipoxygenase activating protein,[2] which allows it to serve as a substrate for the enzyme 5-lipoxygenase (Fig. 15.2).[3,4] 5-Lipoxygenase sequentially catalyses the addition of oxygen to arachidonic acid to form 5-hydroperoxy eicosatetraenoic acid and leukotriene A$_4$ (LTA$_4$) respectively; LTA$_4$ is a major branch point in the formation of the leukotrienes.[5] A variety of cells, most notably neutrophilic polymorphonuclear leukocytes (PMNs), possess a specific epoxide hydrolase that catalyses the formation of LTB$_4$ from LTA$_4$. It is also possible for multiple lipoxygenases to act sequentially on arachidonic acid to form the lipoxins.[6,7] In distinction to the neutrophil, other cells, including

ASTHMA: BASIC MECHANISMS AND CLINICAL MANAGEMENT (2nd Edn)
ISBN 0-12-079026-2

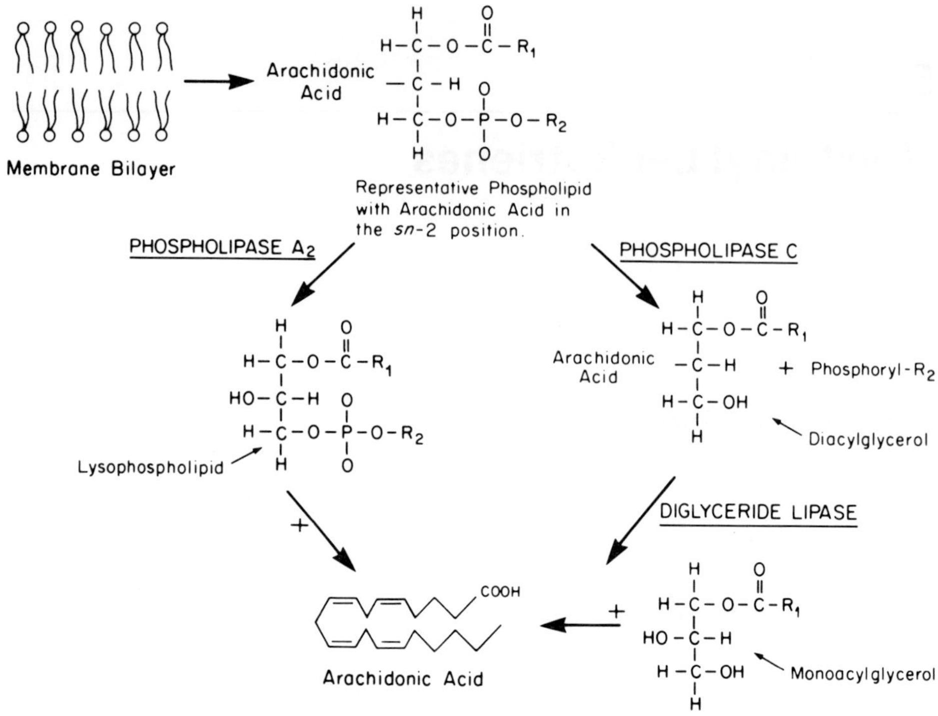

Fig. 15.1 Schematic representation of arachidonic acid mobilization from cell membrane phospholipids during cellular activation.

eosinophils and mast cells, not only have the capacity to form LTA_4 from arachidonic acid, but they also possess a specific glutathionyl-S-transferase, LTC_4 synthase, which catalyses the conjugation of glutathione to LTA_4, at carbon 6, to form leukotriene C_4 (LTC_4). LTC_4 serves as a substrate for γ-glutamyl transpeptidase which cleaves the glutamic acid moiety from its peptide chain to form leukotriene D_4 (LTD_4); LTD_4 is further processed by the removal of the glycine moiety from its peptide chain to form leukotriene E_4 (LTE_4)[5,8-10] LTC_4, LTD_4 and LTE_4 make up the material formerly known as slow-reacting substance of anaphylaxis or SRS-A.

Once formed, and in the presence of appropriately activated PMNs, cysteinyl leukotrienes are degraded to their respective sulphoxides and 6-*trans* diastereoisomers of LTB_4.[11] In the absence of such cells the major degradation and excretion products of the cysteinyl leukotrienes are native LTE_4, N-acetyl LTE_4, or the products resulting from ω-oxidation and β-elimination of LTE_4.[12-14]

LEUKOTRIENES IN ASTHMA

In the decade since the structural identification of the leukotrienes a number of lines of evidence have accrued indicating that the cysteinyl leukotrienes may be involved in the asthmatic response; these are reviewed below.

The pathology of chronic mild asthma and production of cysteinyl leukotrienes by cells found in the asthmatic lesion.

Airway biopsies in patients with chronic mild asthma demonstrate mast cells in increased numbers and in various states of activation, eosinophils with granular patterns indicative of activation, lymphocytes bearing the CD25 phenotype, loss of epithelial integrity and deposition of types III and V collagen.[15–19] The cysteinyl leukotrienes are synthesized and exported [20] into the microenvironment by constitutive and infiltrating cells including mast cells and eosinophils.[21–24] Furthermore, since plasma leakage is prominent in more severe asthma,[25] it is likely that the vascular endothelium will be exposed to cells capable of donating LTA_4. It is well established that the cysteinyl leukotrienes are also formed when LTA_4-exporting cells such as polymorphonuclear leukocytes provide LTA_4 for effector cells such as vascular endothelial cells or

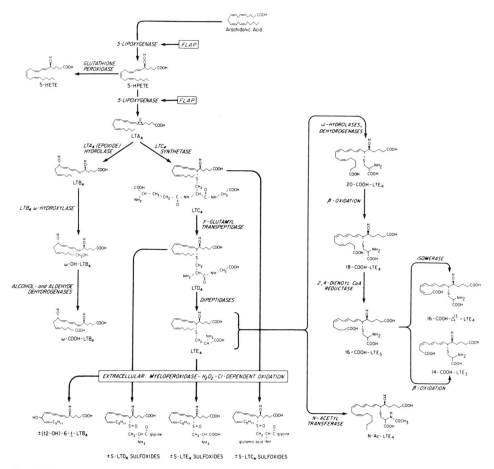

Fig. 15.2   An overview of the 5-lipoxygenase pathway. Note that 'FLAP' indicates the 5-lipoxygenase activating protein[2] and that the stereochemistry at the 13–14 double bond in $16\text{-COOH-}\Delta^{13}\text{-LTE}_4$ is not defined.

platelets.[26–31] These data clearly establish that the cells implicated in the asthmatic response have the capacity to produce cysteinyl leukotrienes.

Biological effects of the cysteinyl leukotrienes relevant to the asthmatic response.

The leukotrienes are known to have profound biochemical and physiological effects, even in picomolar concentrations, including induction of airway obstruction, tissue oedema, and expression of bronchial mucus from submucosal glands;[32–34] these pathobiological effects make them important potential mediators of asthmatic responses. Prominent among the effects of the cysteinyl leukotrienes are their ability to mediate airway narrowing in normal individuals and persons with asthma. When aerosols of leukotrienes are inhaled by normal subjects, airway obstruction, as manifested by a decrease in flow rates during a forced exhalation, occurs;[35–48] the specific results obtained depend on the index of airway obstruction used in a particular circumstance.

When flow rates at 30% of vital capacity from partial flow–volume curves ($\dot{V}_{30}P$) are used as the outcome indicator, it has been established that LTC_4 and LTD_4 have airway effects that are prolonged compared to those induced by histamine or methacholine. The duration of effect of histamine and methacholine is on the order of 3–5 min when a 30% decrease in the $\dot{V}_{30}P$ is induced. In contrast, the duration of effect resulting from the sulphidopeptide leukotrienes, when an equivalent magnitude of effect is achieved, is on the order of 25–30 min. More important than differences in the duration of effect is the relative potency of the cysteinyl leukotrienes compared to reference agonists such as histamine or methacholine. The range of nebulizer concentrations required to achieve roughly a 30% decrease in the $\dot{V}_{30}P$ due to inhalation of LTD_4 in normal subjects varies about 100-fold from approximately 3 μM to 300 μM. On average, normal subjects are about 3000 times more responsive to leukotrienes than they are to histamine. Among normal subjects there is a relationship between responsiveness to the leukotrienes and responsiveness to reference agonists such as histamine or methacholine[38,41] such that the subjects that are more responsive to histamine are those that are more responsive to the leukotrienes. In contrast, when the FEV_1 is used as the outcome indicator, approximately five times greater leukotriene concentrations in the nebulizer are required to achieve a 15–20% decrease in this airway response index compared to the nebulizer concentrations required to reduce the $\dot{V}_{30}P$ by 30 to 40%. Although these data are consistent with the hypothesis that the airways which narrow in order to reduce the FEV_1 are less sensitive to the cysteinyl leukotrienes than the airways that narrow to decrease the $\dot{V}_{30}P$, this hypothesis has never been established by direct experiment.

In subjects with asthma, LTD_4 is a potent bronchoconstrictor agonist when administered by aerosol as indicated by decrements in the forced expiratory volume in the first second (FEV_1), forced expiratory flow rates such as the $\dot{V}_{30}P$, or specific conductance.[38,40,41,45,48,49] When the $\dot{V}_{30}P$ or the $\dot{V}_{40}P$ is used as the outcome indicator nebulizer concentrations of LTD_4 on the order of 0.3 to 30 μM are required to decrease airflow rates by approximately 30%; when compared to normal subjects these concentrations are approximately 10% of those required by normal subjects to achieve the same effect. In contrast the relative sensitivity to histamine in normal versus asthmatic subjects is approximately 100-fold. Therefore even though asthmatic subjects are hyperresponsive compared to normal subjects to the cysteinyl leukotrienes, the relative degree of hyperresponsiveness is less that that observed when histamine or methacholine is used as the contractile agonist.

LTE$_4$ is also a potent bronchoactive agonist; the potency of LTE$_4$ relative to histamine differs among normal and asthmatic subjects. In normal subjects LTE$_4$ is about 30 times more potent than histamine[48] whilst in subjects with asthma LTE$_4$ is about 300 times more potent than histamine,[50] regardless of whether flow rates low in the vital capacity from partial flow–volume curves[48] or specific conductance[50] are used as the outcome indicators. An increment in hyperresponsiveness to LTE$_4$ occurs in aspirin-induced asthma as compared to other asthmatic subjects,[51] indicating a potentially unique role for this cysteinyl leukotriene in the pathogenesis of this form of asthma.

Leukotriene recovery in asthma

Cysteinyl leukotrienes have been recovered after experimental challenges which elicit clinical symptoms similar to those that occur in spontaneously occurring asthmatic conditions. Leukotrienes have been recovered in the nasal lavage fluid after intranasal challenge with either antigen or cold air.[52,53] Leukotrienes are recovered in significantly greater amounts in the bronchoalveolar lavage fluid (BAL) from subjects with symptomatic asthma compared to subjects with asymptomatic asthma or normal subjects [54–57] suggesting that the leukotrienes are produced locally in the lungs of patients with asthma. Although leukotrienes can be recovered in BAL from patients with active asthma or after airway challenge, because of the invasive nature of the procedure required to obtain the fluid, it is unlikely that the extensive clinical use of BAL leukotriene levels will occur.

In this regard, indices of leukotriene production that rely on measurements made on blood or urine samples offer potential utility in the assessment of which asthmatic responses represent states in which the leukotrienes are among the effector molecules mediating bronchoconstriction. A number of studies have detected cysteinyl leukotrienes in the plasma during asthma attacks[58–62] but the methods used to assure the authenticity of the materials identified have been suboptimal and the findings have not been widely reproduced probably for technical reasons.[63] In contrast, it has been shown that accurate and quantitative measurements of LTE$_4$ can be made in urine samples.[64–66] In normal human subjects, after intravenous administration of radio-labelled LTC$_4$, 12–48% of the counts are recovered in the urine with 4–13% as intact LTE$_4$.[67,68] Not only can exogenously adminstered leukotrienes be recovered in the urine but it is now clear that leukotriene recovery can serve as an index of endogenous release of leukotrienes.[64,65,69] For example, it has been shown that there is an increase in the recovery of LTE$_4$ in the urine of asthmatic subjects early after antigen challenge; the magnitude of the fall in the FEV$_1$ and the amount of LTE$_4$ in the urine are well correlated.[69,70] Furthermore, native LTE$_4$ is the major metabolite recovered in the urine after acute antigen challenge.[71] Taylor *et al.*[65] used Varian MCH-10 solid phase extraction followed by RP-HPLC and RIA to measure LTE$_4$ in the urine. To allow quantitative determination of the amounts of LTE$_4$ in the urine, they used recovery of radiolabel added as an internal standard. In normal subjects they recovered 23.8 ng of LTE$_4$ per mmol of creatinine; while in 20 asthmatic subjects during acute spontaneous attacks they recovered slightly over three times as much LTE_4, 78.3 ng/mmol creatinine. There was no relationship observed between the severity of the attack as measured by the FEV_1 and the amount of LTE_4 recovered in the urine. In six of the eight subjects in whom urinary LTE_4 measurements were available both before and after treatment for an acute asthmatic exacerbation (all received prednisolone) there was a decrease in the LTE_4 excretion rate. They found no differences in the LTE_4 excretion between normal subjects and subjects with symptomatic or asymptomatic rhinitis. Wescott et al.[66] confirmed these findings by demonstrating that subjects with asthma had higher LTE_4 excretion than a normal reference group. These data clearly indicate that both spontaneous and induced asthma, at least in some individuals, are accompanied by an increase in the rate of urinary LTE_4 excretion and, by inference, increased cysteinyl leukotriene production.

Leukotriene receptor blockade and synthesis inhibition

It is well established in the guinea pig that there are at least two distinct receptors for the cysteinyl leukotrienes in airway contractile tissues;[72] in contrast only a single leukotriene receptor subtype has been clearly identified in human tissues.[73] Although over a dozen chemically distinct antagonists at the LTD_4 receptor have been recognized, only a few have been shown to be effective antagonists at the LTD_4 in man[74–78] (Table 15.1). The importance of these agents derives from their use as probes for the role of the leukotrienes in the pathobiology of asthma. For example, a number of LTD_4 receptor antagonists have been tested for their effects on the bronchospasm that accompanies experimental antigen-, cold air-, or exercise-induced asthma.[79–83] In subjects with antigen-induced bronchospasm the LTD_4 receptor antagonists L649,923 and LY171,883 had a limited but statistically significant positive effect on the early but not the late asthmatic response.[79,82] Intravenous administration of MK-571, an LTD_4 receptor antagonist with proven efficacy,[78] resulted in over a 50% decrease in the bronchospasm accompanying exercise.[83] In contrast to these positive studies, it has been shown that the inhaled leukotriene antagonist L-648,051 had no significant protective

Table 15.1 Effects of leukotriene receptor antagonists on the bronchoconstrictor response to inhaled LTD_4 in intact man.

Agent	Dose and route	Effects on the LTD_4 response	Ref.
L-649,923	1000 mg p.o.	3.8-fold decrease in LTD_4 responsiveness	74
LY-171,883	400 mg p.o.	4.5-fold decrease in LTD_4 responsiveness	75
L-648,051	12 mg by inhalation	Decrease in LTD_4 response in duration and magnitude by $\approx 50\%$	76 76
ICI-204,219	40 mg p.o.	117-fold decrease in LTD_4 responsiveness	77
MK-571	28 mg i.v.	44-fold decrease in LTD_4 responsiveness	78

effect against either the early or the late asthmatic response[81] resulting from exposure to inhaled antigen. The negative data have been interpreted to suggest that the leuko-trienes have only a minor role in allergen-induced airway obstruction. However such a statement cannot be made with great confidence because the adequacy of leukotriene receptor antagonism at the time of antigen presentation and in the subjects studied was not established by the investigators.

Another strategy to investigate the role of leukotrienes in asthma has been to study the effects of inhibitors of the enzyme, 5-lipoxygenase, on experimentally induced asthmatic responses.[84–86] The advantage of this approach is that if the inhibition of 5-lipoxygenase is effective then the formation of all leukotrienes (as well as lipoxins that derive from initial 5-lipoxygenation) including LTB_4 and the cysteinyl leukotrienes will be pre-vented. Thus if leukotrienes act other than through the stimulation of the LTD_4 receptor their effects will be prevented. Initial studies with two chemically distinct 5-lipoxygenase inhibitors, piriprost (U-60,257)[84] and nafazatrom,[85] were inconclusive in that these agents did not alter the asthmatic response to inhaled antigen or exercise but adequate inhibition of 5-lipoxygenase was not demonstrated. In contrast, administration of A-64077, a novel 5-lipoxygenase inhibitor,[86] resulted in specific, potent and selective inhibition of 5-lipoxygenase as well as an amelioration of the asthmatic response to the hyperventilation of cold, dry air. The magnitude of the effect achieved in the cold air model was similar to the effects of theophylline,[87] inhaled terbutaline[88] or high-dose inhaled atropine[89] in this model.

In subjects with spontaneously occurring asthma, LT171883, an LTD_4 receptor antagonist,[75] had a positive effect on lung function as indicated by a small, ≈ 0.3 litre, but significant improvement in FEV_1 and resulted in decreased inhaler use in mild chronic asthmatic subjects.[90] The effects on FEV_1 took approximately 6 weeks to manifest, suggesting that the leukotrienes may effect asthma in part by altering airway responsiveness (see below). An important point demonstrated by this study is that it may take weeks to months, rather than days to weeks, to appreciate an antiasthmatic effect of agents acting on the 5-lipoxygenase pathway.

Leukotrienes and airway hyperresponsiveness

Asthma is characterized by increased 'irritability' of the airways to a variety of distinct stimuli in the environment, such as air pollutants, viral infections, strong odours, allergens, cold air, and exercise.[91–94] Current data suggest that the airway 'inflam-mation' observed in subjects with asthma and hyperreactivity are closely linked.[95–98] Although cellular infiltration and hyperresponsiveness are widely recognized as com-mon features of asthma, the precise pathophysiological mechanisms linking bronchial hyperreactivity and inflammation remain unclear. Numerous mechanisms have been proposed, including enhanced autonomic or axon[99–101] reflexes, enhanced smooth muscle contractile responses,[102–104] defects in heat regulation,[105–107] altered epithelial function[108,109] and release of bronchoactive mediators.[110,111] Among these mechanisms, the release of mediators of inflammation has received much attention, and among mediators particular importance has been assigned to the leukotrienes. In subjects with asthma, inhalation of LTC_4 results in an enhanced response to inhaled prostaglandin D_2 and histamine.[112] However the effects are ephemeral, noted only during the first 9 min after exposure to LTC_4, a time when LTC_4 itself does not have significant effects on airway function. The mechanism of this enhanced response is not known.

In normal subjects LTD_4 inhalation has been shown to induce prolonged hyper-responsiveness to inhaled methacholine;[113] inhalation of an aerosol generated from a solution containing 1–500 $\mu g/ml$ of LTD_4 by normal subjects was associated with an enhanced response to inhaled methacholine (measured as $PC_{35}SGaw$) which peaked at 7 days and persisted in some subjects for up to 2 weeks. The magnitude of the enhanced response was an approximate 35% decrease in the $PC_{35}SGaw$ for methacholine. A similar effect of LTE_4 on airway hyperresponsiveness *in vivo* has been demonstrated in asthmatic but not normal subjects.[50] In particular, inhalation of LTE_4, at doses that induce a small but significant contractile response, enhances the response to subsequent administration of inhaled histamine. This enhancement is on the order of a four-fold shift in the histamine dose response curve with the effect lasting approximately 24 h; however small effects persist for up to a week. The ability of LTD_4 and LTE_4 to enhance airway responsiveness but over a time course on the order of weeks is consistent with the need for prolonged treatment with antagonists at the LTD_4/LTE_4 receptor in order to effect a significant decrease in airway responsiveness in spontaneous asthma.

CONCLUSIONS

These data support the following assumptions as to the role of cysteinyl leukotrienes in bronchial asthma: (a) they are produced by constitutive (mast cells/macrophages) and infiltrating (eosinophils) cells implicated in the asthmatic response; (b) they are potent bronchoconstrictors; (c) laboratory-induced and spontaneous asthma is associated with an enhanced recovery of leukotrienes in the urine of subjects with asthma; (d) asthma is somewhat ameliorated by agents capable of interfering with leukotriene action or synthesis, and (e) the formation of the cysteinyl leukotrienes may not only trigger bronchospasm, but may also sensitize the airways to the effects of irritants and/or mediators, leading to bronchial hyperreactivity. Although initial data are encouraging that the leukotrienes may play a pivotal role in the asthmatic response, the final test of this hypothesis awaits the results of large-scale clinical trials in spontaneously occurring asthma.

REFERENCES

1. Omann GM, Allen RA, Bokoch GM, Painter RG, Traynor AE, Sklar LA: Signal transduction and cytoskeletal activation in the neutrophil. *Physiol Rev* (1987) **67**: 285–322.
2. Dixon RA, Diehl RE, Opas E, *et al.*: Requirement of a 5-lipoxygenase-activating protein for leukotriene synthesis. *Nature* (1990) **18** (343): 282–284.
3. Matsumoto T, Funk CD, Radmark O, Hoog JO, Jornvall H, Samuelsson B: Molecular cloning and amino acid sequence of human 5-lipoxygenase. *Proc Natl Acad Sci USA* (1988) **85**: 26–30.
4. Soberman RJ: Enzymes of the 5-lipoxygenase pathway. *Prog Clin Biol Res* (1989) **297**: 30–43.
5. Samuelsson B, Dahlen SE, Lindgren JA, Rouzer CA, Serhan CN: Leukotrienes and lipoxins: structures, biosynthesis, and biological effects. *Science* (1987) **237**: 1171–1176.

6. Serhan CN, Nicolaou KC, Webber SE, *et al.*: Lipoxin A. Stereochemistry and biosynthesis. *J Biol Chem* (1986) **15**(261)16340–16345.

7. Serhan CN, Hamberg M, Samuelsson B, Morris J, Wishka DG: On the stereochemistry and biosynthesis of lipoxin B. *Proc Natl Acad Sci USA* (1986) **83**: 1983–1987.

8. Orning L, Bernstrom K, Hammarstrom S: Formation of Leukotrienes E3, E4 and E5 in rat basophilic leukemia cells. *Eur J. Biochem* (1981) **120**: 41–45.

9. Lewis RA, Drazen JM, Austen KF, Clark DA, Corey EJ: Identification of the C(6)-S-conjugate of leukotriene A with cysteine as a naturally occurring slow reacting substance of anaphylaxis (SRS-A). Importance of the 11-*cis*-geometry for biological activity. *Biochem Biophys Res Commun* (1980) **96**: 271–277.

10. Parker CW, Koch D, Huber MM, Falkenhein SF: Formation of the cysteinyl form of slow reacting substance (leukotriene E4) in human plasma. *Biochem Biophys Res Commun* (1980) **97**: 1038–1046.

11. Lee CW, Lewis RA, Tauber AI, Mehorta M, Corey EJ, Austen KF: The myeloperoxidase-dependent metabolism of leukotrienes C_4, D_4 and E_4 to 6-*trans*-leukotriene B_4 diasteroisomers and the subclass-specific S-diastereomeric sulfoxides. *J Biol Chem* (1983) **258**: 15004–15010.

12. Delorme D, Foster A, Girard Y, Rokach J: Synthesis of B-oxidation products as potential leukotriene metabolites and their detection in bile of anesthetized rat. *Prostaglandins* (1988) **36**: 291–302.

13. Rokach J, Foster A, Delorme D, Girard Y: Metabolism of peptide leukotrienes in the rat. *Adv Prostaglandin Thromboxane Leukotriene Res* (1989) **19**: 102–107.

14. Stene DD, Murphy RC: Metabolism of leukotriene E4 in isolated rat hepatocytes. Identification of beta-oxidation products of sulfidopeptide leukotrienes. *J Biol Chem* (1988) **263**: 2773–2778.

15. Laitinen LA, Heino M, Laitinen A, Kava T, Haahtela T: Damage of the airway epithelium and bronchial reactivity in patients with asthma. *Am Rev Respir Dis* (1985) **131**: 599–606.

16. Beasley R, Roche WR, Roberts JA, Holgate ST: Cellular events in the bronchi in mild asthma and after bronchial provocation. *Am Rev Respir Dis* (1989) **139**: 806–817.

17. Roche WR, Beasley R, Williams JH, Holgate ST: Subepithelial fibrosis in the bronchi of asthmatics. *Lancet* (1989) **1**: 520–524.

18. Jeffery PK, Wardlaw AJ, Nelson FC, Collins JV, Kay AB: Bronchial biopsies in asthma. An ultrastructural, quantitative study and correlation with hyperreactivity. *Am Rev Respir Dis* (1989) **140**: 1745–1753.

19. Heard BE, Nunn AJ, Kay AB: Mast cells in human lungs. *J Pathol* (1989) **157**: 59–63.

20. Lam BK, Owen WF, Austen KF, Soberman RJ. The identification of a distinct export step following the biosynthesis of leukotriene C4 by human eosinophils. *J Biol Chem* (1989) **264**: 12885–12889.

21. MacGlashan DW, Schleimer RP, Peters SP, *et al.*: Comparative studies of human basophils and mast cells. *Fed Proc* (1983) **42**: 2504–2509.

22. Fox CC, Kagey-Sobotka A, Schleimer RP, Peters SP, MacGlashan DW, Lichtenstein LM: Mediator release from human basophils and mast cells from lung and intestinal mucosa. *Int Arch Allergy Appl Immunol* (1985) **77**: 130–136.

23. Weller PF, Lee CW, Foster DW, Corey EJ, Austen KF, Lewis RA: Generation and metabolism of 5-lipoxygenase pathway leukotrienes by human eosinophils: predominant production of leukotriene C4. *Proc Natl Acad Sci USA* (1988) **80**: 7626–7630.

24. Heavey DJ, Ernst PB, Stevens RL, Befus AD, Bienenstock J, Austen KF: Generation of leukotriene C4, leukotriene B4, and prostaglandin D2 by immunologically activated rat intestinal mucosa mast cells. *J Immunol* (1988) **140**: 1953–1957.

25. Persson CG: Plasma exudation and asthma. *Lung* (1988) **166**: 1–23.

26. MacLouf JA, Murphy RC: Transcellular metabolism of neutrophil-derived leukotriene A4 by human platelets. A potential cellular source of leukotriene C4. *J Biol Chem* (1988) **263**: 174–181.

27. Feinmark SJ, Cannon PJ: Endothelial cell leukotriene C4 synthesis results from intercellular transfer of leukotriene A4 sythesized by polymorphonuclear leukocytes. *J Biol Chem* (1986) **261**: 16466–16472.

28. Grimminger F, Menger M, Becker G, Seeger W: Potentiation of leukotriene production following sequestration of neutrophils in isolated lungs: indirect evidence for intercellular leukotriene A4 transfer. *Blood* (1988) **72**: 1687–1692.

29. Fradin A, Zirrolli JA, MacLouf J, Vausbinder L, Henson PM, Murphy RC: Platelet-activating factor and leukotriene biosynthesis in whole blood. A model for the study of transcellular arachidonate metabolism. *J Immunol* (1989) **143**: 3680–3685.

30. Bigby TD, Meslier N: Transcellular lipoxygenase metabolism between monocytes and platelets. *J Immunol* (1989) **143**: 1948–1954.

31. Grimminger F, Becker G, Seeger W: High yield enzymatic conversion of intravascular leukotriene A4 in blood-free perfused lungs. *J Immunol* (1988) **141**: 2431–2436.

32. Piper PJ: Formation and actins of leukotrienes. *Physiol Rev* (1984) **64**: 744–761.

33. Raible DG, Lichtenstein LM: The role of leukotrienes in human pathophysiology. *Ann NY Acad Sci* (1988) **524**: 334–344.

34. Schwartz LB, Austen KF: Structure and function of the chemical mediators of mast cells. *Prog Allergy* (1984) **34**: 271–321.

35. Holroyde MC, Altounyan REC, Cole M, Dixon M, Elliott EV: Bronchoconstriction produced in man by leukotrienes C & D. *Lancet* (1981) **ii**: 17–18.

36. Weiss JW, Drazen JM, Coles N, *et al*.: Bronchoconstrictor effects of leukotriene C in humans. *Science* (1982) **216**: 196–198.

37. Barnes NC, Piper PJ, Costello JF: Comparative effects of inhaled leukotriene C_4, leukotriene D_4 and histamine in normal human subjects. *Thorax* (1984) **39**: 500–504.

38. Smith LJ, Greenberger PA, Patterson R, Krell RD, Bernstein PR: The effect of inhaled leukotriene D_4 in humans. *Am Rev Respir Dis* (1985) **131**: 368–372.

39. Bisgaard H, Groth S, Masden F: Bronchial hyperreactivity to leukotriene D_4 in exogenous asthma. *Br Med J* (1985) **290**: 1468–1471.

40. Roberts SA, Giembycz MA, Raeburn D, Rodger IW, Thomson NC: *In vitro* and *in vivo* effect of verapamil on human airway responsiveness to leukotriene D_4. *Thorax* (1986) **41**: 12–16.

41. Adelroth E, Morris MM, Hargreave FE, O'Byrne PM: Airway responsiveness to leukotrienes C_4 and D_4 and to methacholine in patients with asthma and normal controls. *New Eng J Med* (1986) **315**: 480–484.

42. Bisgaard H, Groth S, Dirksen H: Leukotriene D_4 induces bronchoconstriction in man. *Allergy* (1983) **38**: 441–443.

43. Bisgaard H, Poulsen L, Sondergaard I: Nebulization and selective deposition of LTD_4 in human lungs. *Allergy* (1987) **42**: 336–342.

44. Smith LJ, Kern R, Patterson R, Krell RD, Bernstein PR: Mechanism of leukotriene D_4-induced bronchoconstriction in normal subject. *J Allergy Clin Immunol* (1987) **80**: 340–347.

45. O'Byrne PM: Leukotrienes, airway responses, and asthma. *An New York Acad Sci* (1988) **524**: 282–288.

46. Drazen JM: Inhalation challenge of humans with sulfidopeptide leukotrienes. *Chest* (1986) **89**: 414–419.

47. Weiss JW, Drazen JM, McFadden ER Jr, *et al*.: Airway constriction in normal humans produced by inhalation of leukotriene D: potency, time course, and effect of acetylsalicylic acid. *J Am Med Assoc* (1983) **249**: 2814–2817.

48. Davidson AB, Lee TH, Scanlon PD, *et al*.: Bronchoconstrictor effects of leukotriene E_4 in normal and asthmatic individuals. *Amer Rev Respir Dis* (1987) **135**: 333–337.

49. Griffin M, Weiss JW, Leitch AG, *et al*.: Effects of leukotriene D on the airways in asthma. *N Engl J Med* (1983) **308**: 436–439.

50. Arm JP, Spur BW, Lee TH: The effects of inhaled leukotriene E4 on the airway responsiveness to histamine in subjects with asthma and normal subjects. *J Allergy Clin Immunol* (1988) **82**: 654–660.

51. Arm JP, O'Hickey SP, Spur BW, Lee TH: Airway responsiveness to histamine and leukotriene E_4 in subjects with aspirin-induced asthma. *Am Rev Resp Dis* (1989) **140**: 148–153.

52. Silber G, Proud D, Warner J, *et al*.: *In vivo* release of inflammatory mediators by hyperosmolar solutions. *Am Rev Respir Dis* (1988) **137**: 606–612.

53. Togias AG, Naclerio RM, Peters SP, *et al*.: Local generation of sulfidopeptide leukotrienes upon nasal provocation with cold, dry air. *Am Rev Respir Dis* (1986) **133**: 1133–1137.

54. Zehr BB, Casale TB, Wood D, Floerchinger C, Richerson HB, Hunninghake GW: Use of segmental airway lavage to obtain relevant mediators from the lungs of asthmatic and control subjects. *Chest* (1989) **95**: 1059–1063.
55. Wardlaw AJ, Hay H, Cromwell O, Collins JV, Kay AB: Leukotrienes, LTC4 and LTB4, in bronchoalveolar lavage in bronchial asthma and other respiratory diseases. *J Allergy Clin Immunol* (1989) **84**: 19–26.
56. Lam S, Chan H, LeRiche JC, Chan-Yeung M, Salari H: Release of leukotrienes in patients with bronchial asthma. *J Allergy Clin Immunol* (1988) **81**: 711–717.
57. Diaz P, Gonzalez MC, Galleguillos FR, *et al.*: Leukocytes and mediators in bronchoalveolar lavage during allergen-induced late-phase asthmatic reactions. *Am Rev Respir Dis* (1989) **139**: 1383–1389.
58. Iwasaki E: Leukotriene C4 in children with atopic asthma. I. Plasma levels in acute asthma. *Acta Paediatr Jpn Overseas Ed* (1989) **31**: 286–294.
59. Iwasaki E: Leukotriene C4 in children with atopic asthma. II. Plasma levels in bronchial challenge with specific allergen. *Acta Paediatr Jpn Overseas Ed* (1989) **31**: 295–302.
60. Isons T, Koshihara Y, Murota S, Fukada Y, Furukawa S: Measurement of immunoreactive leukotriene C4 in blood of asthmatic children. *Biochem Biophys Res Commun* (1985) **130**: 486–492.
61. Okubo T, Takahashi H, Sumitomo M, Shindoh K, Suzuki S: Plasma levels of leukotrienes C4 and D4 during wheezing attack in asthmatic patients. *Int Arch Allergy Appl Immunol* (1987) **84**: 149–155.
62. Schwartzberg SB, Shelov SP, Van Praag D: Blood leukotriene levels during the acute asthma attack in children. *Prostaglandins Leukot Med* (1987) **26**: 143–155.
63. Heavey DJ, Soberman RJ, Lewis RA, Spur B, Austen KF: Critical considerations in the development of an assay for sulfidopeptide leukotrienes in plasma. *Prostaglandins* (1987) **33**: 693–708.
64. Tagari P, Ethier D, Carry M, *et al.*: Measurement of urinary leukotrienes by reversed-phase liquid chromatography and radioimmunoassay. *Clin Chem* (1989) **35**: 388–391.
65. Taylor G, Black P, Turner N, *et al.*: Urinary leukotriene E4 after antigen challenge and in acute asthma and allergic rhinitis. *Lancet* (1989) **1**: 584–588.
66. Westcott JY, Johnston K, Batt RA, Wenzel SE, Voelkel NF: Measurement of peptiodoleukotrienes in biological fluids. *J Appl Physiol* (1990) **68**: 2640–2648.
67. Orning L, Kaijser L, Hammarstrom S: *In vivo* metabolism of leukotriene C4 in man: urinary excretion of leukotriene E4. *Biochem Biophys Res Commun* (1985) **130**: 214–220.
68. Maltby NH, Taylor GW, Ritter JM, Fuller RW, Dollery CT: Leukotriene C4 elimination and metabolism in man. *J All Clin Immunol* (1990) **85**: 3–9.
69. Sladek K, Dworski R, Fitzgerald GA, *et al.*: Allergen-stimulated release of thromboxane A2 and leukotriene E4 in humans. *Am Rev Resp Dis* (1990) **141**: 1441–1445.
70. Manning PJ, Rokach J, Malo J, *et al.*: Urinary leukotriene E4 levels during early and late asthmatic responses. *J All Clin Immunol* (1990) **86**: 211–220.
71. Tagari P, Rasmussen JB, Delorme D, *et al.*: Comparison of urinary leukotriene E4 and 16-carboxytetranordihydro leukotriene E4 excretion in allergic asthmatics after inhaled antigen. *Eicosanoids* (1990) **3**: 75–80.
72. Snyder DW, Krell RD: Pharmacological evidence for a distinct leukotriene C4 receptor in guinea-pig trachea. *J Pharmacol Exp Ther* (1984) **231**: 616–622.
73. Buckner CK, Krell RD, Laravuso RB, Coursin DB, Bernstein PR, Will JA: Pharmacological evidence that human intralobar airways do not contain different receptors that mediate contractions to leukotriene C4 and leukotriene D4. *J Pharmacol Exp Ther* (1986) **237**: 558–562.
74. Barnes N, Piper PJ, Costello J: The effect of an oral leukotriene antagonist L-649,923 on histamine and leukotriene D4-induced bronchoconstriction in normal man. *J Allergy Clin Immunol* (1987) **79**: 816–821.
75. Phillips GD, Rafferty P, Robinson C, Holgate ST: Dose-related antagonism of leukotriene D4-induced bronchoconstriction by p.o. administration of LY-171883 in nonasthmatic subjects. *J Pharmacol Exp Ther* (1988) **246**: 732–738.
76. Evans JM, Barnes NC, Zakrzewski JT *et al.*: L-648,051, a novel cysteinyl leukotriene antagonist is active by the inhaled route in man. *Br J Clin Pharm* (1989) **28**: 125–135.

77. Smith LJ, Geller S, Ebright L, Glass M, Thyrum PT: Inhibition of leukotriene D4-induced bronchoconstriction in normal subjects by the oral LTD4 receptor antagonist ICI 204,219. *Am Rev Respir Dis* (1990) **141**: 988–992.

78. Kips, JC, GF Koos, I DeLepeleire, *et al.*: MK-571: A potent antagonist of LTD$_4$-induced bronchoconstriction in the human. *Am Rev Resp Dir* (1991) **144**: 617–621.

79. Britton JR, Hanley SP, Tattersfield AE: The effect of an oral leukotriene D4 antagonist L-649,923 on the response to inhaled antigen in asthma. *J Allergy Clin Immunol* (1987) **79**: 811–816.

80. Israel E, Juniper EF, Callaghan JT, *et al.*: Effect of a leukotriene antagonist, LY171883, on cold air-induced bronchoconstriction in asthmatics. *Am Rev Respir Dis* (1989) **140**: 1348–1353.

81. Bel EH, Timmers MC, Dijkman JH, Stahl EG, Sterk PJ: The effect of an inhaled leukotriene antagonist, L-648,051, on early and late asthmatic reactions and subsequent increase in airway responsiveness in man. *J All Clin Immunol* (1990) **85**: 1067–1075.

82. Fuller RW, Black PN, Dollery CT: Effect of the oral leukotriene D$_4$ antagonist LY171883 on inhaled and intradermal challenge with antigen and leukotriene D$_4$ in atopic subjects. *J Allergy Clin Immunol* (1989) **83**: 939–944.

83. Manning PJ, Watson RM, Margoleskee DJ, Williams VC, Schwartz JI, O'Byrne PM: Inhibition of exercise-induced bronchoconstriction by MK-571, a potent leukotriene D$_4$-receptor antagonist. *New Eng J Med* (1990) **323**: 1736–1740.

84. Mann JS, Robinson C, Sheridan AQ, Clement P, Bach MK, Holgate ST: Effect of inhaled piriprost (U-60,257) a novel leukotriene inhibitor, on allergen and exercise induced bronchoconstriction in asthma. *Thorax* (1986) **41**: 746–752.

85. Fuller RW, Maltby N, Richmond R, *et al.*: The effects of a 5-lipoxygenase inhibitor on asthma induced by cold, dry air. *New Eng J Med* (1990) **323**: 1740–1744.

86. Israel, E, Dermarkarian RD, Rosenberg M, *et al.*: The effects of a 5-lipoxygenase inhibitor on asthma induced by cold, dry air. *New Eng J Med* (1990) **323**: 1740–1744.

87. Merland N, Cartier A, L'Archeveque J, Ghezzo H, Malo JL: Theophylline minimally inhibits bronchoconstriction induced by dry cold air inhalation in asthmatic subjects. *Am Rev Resp Dis* 137: **137**: 1304–1308.

88. Latimer KM, O'Byrne PM, Morris MM, Roberts R, Hargreave FE: Bronchoconstriction stimulated by airway cooling: Better protection with combined inhalation of terbutraline sulfate and cromolyn sodium than with either alone. *Am Rev Resp Dis* (1983) **128**: 440–443.

89. O'Byrne P, Thomson NC, Morris M, Roberts RS, Daniel EE, Hargreave FE: The protective effect of inhaled chlorpheniramine and atropine on bronchoconstriction induced by airway cooling. *Am Rev Resp Dis* (1983) **128**: 611–617.

90. Cloud ML, Enas GC, Kemp J, *et al.*: A specific LTD4/LTE4-receptor antagonist improves pulmonary function in patients with mild, chronic asthma. *Am Rev Respir Dis* (1989) **140**: 1336–1339.

91. O'Byrne PM: Allergen-induced airway hyperresponsiveness. *J Allergy Clin Immunol* (1988) **81**: 119–127.

92. McFadden, ER: Exercise-induced asthma. Assessment of current etiologic concepts. *Chest* (1987) **91**: 151S–157S.

93. Sheppard D: Airway hyperresponsiveness. Mechanisms in experimental models. *Chest* (1989) **96**: 1165–11680.

94. Liekauf GD, Doupnik CA, Leming LM, Wey HE: Sulfidopeptide leukotrienes mediate acrolein-induced bronchial hyperresponsiveness. *J Appl Physiol* (1989) **66**: 1838–1845.

95. Barnes NC, Costello JF: Airway hyperresponsiveness and inflammation. *Br Med Bull* (1987) **43**: 445–459.

96. Hargreave FE, Gibson PG, Ramsdale EH, Fitzgerald JM, Hepperle MJ: Airway hyperresponsiveness and asthma. *Agents Actions* (1989) **28**(Suppl): 205–211.

97. Pauwels R: The relationship between airway inflammation and bronchial hyperresponsiveness. *Clin Exp Allergy* (1989) **19**: 395–398.

98. Magnussen H, Nowak D: Roles of hyperresponsiveness and airway inflammation in bronchial asthma. *Respiration* (1989) **55**: 65–74.

99. Barnes PJ: Cholinergic control of airway smooth muscle. *Am Rev Respir Dis* (1987) **136**: S42–45.
100. Barnes PJ: Asthma as an axon reflex. *Lancet* (1986) **1**: 424–425.
101. Andersson RG, Grundstrom N: Innervation of airway smooth muscle. Efferent mechanisms. *Pharmacol Ther* (1987) **32**: 107–130.
102. DeMarzo N, DiBlasi P, Boschetto P, *et al.*: Airway smooth muscle biochemistry and asthma. *Eur Respir J* (1989) **2**(Suppl): 473s–476s.
103. Torphy TJ: Action of mediators on airway smooth muscle: functional antagonism as a mechanism for bronchodilator drugs. Agents Actions (1988) **23**(Suppl): 37–53.
104. Svedmyr N: Airway smooth muscle and disease workshop: theophylline. *Am Rev Respir Dis* (1987) **136**: 568–571.
105. Zawadski DK, Lenner KA, McFadden ER: Comparison of intraairway temperatures in normal and asthmatic subjects after hyperpnea with hot, cold, and ambient air. *Am Rev Respir Dis* (1988) **138**: 1553–1558.
106. Ingenito E, Solway J, Lafleur J, Lombardo A, Drazen JM, Pichurko B: Dissociation of temperature-gradient and evaporative heat loss during cold gas hyperventilation in cold-induced asthma. *Am Rev Respir Dir* (1988) **138**: 540–546.
107. McFadden ER, Lenner KA, Strohl KP: Postexertional airway rewarming and thermally induced asthma. New insights into pathophysiology and possible pathogenesis. *J Clin Invest* (1986) **78**: 18–25.
108. Nadel JA: Role of airway epithelial cells in the defense of airways. *Prog Clin Biol Res* (1988) **263**: 331–339.
109. Goldie RG, Fernandes LB, Rigby PJ, Paterson JW: Epithelial dysfunction and airway hyperreactivity in asthma. *Prog Clin Biol Res* (1988) **263**: 317–329.
110. Henderson WR: Lipid-derived and other chemical mediators of inflammation in the lung. *J Allergy Clin Immunol* (1987) **79**: 543–553.
111. Drazen JM, Austen KF: Leukotrienes and airway responses. *Am Rev Respir Dis* (1987) **136**: 985–998.
112. Phillips GD, Holgate ST: Interaction of inhaled LTC_4 with histamine and PGD_2 on airway caliber in asthma. *J Appl Physiol* (1989) **66**: 304–312.
113. Kaye MG, Smith LJ: Effects of inhaled leukotriene D_4 and platelet-activating factor on airway reactivity in normal subjects. *Am Rev Resp Dis* (1990) **141**: 993–997.

16

Histamine

NOEMI M. EISER

INTRODUCTION

Histamine was the first of the mediators of hypersensitivity and inflammation to be investigated and described. The brief history on Table 16.1 includes its synthesis in 1907, its isolation from decomposing ergot, as well as an outline of the extensive research into its properties and its association with mast cells in man.[1-11] Detailed documentation is available elsewhere.[12-14] Mast cells are found both in upper and lower respiratory tracts—in submucosal connective tissue, alveoli and bronchial lumen.[15,17] They comprise up to 2% of alveolar tissue.[17] Many stimuli, including antigen bridging of membrane-bound IgE, can activate these mast cells. A complex series of events culminates in their degranulation, with the release of intracellular histamine from their granules and its extrusion through channels composed of the fused granule walls and the cell membrane.[18,19]

THREE TYPES OF HISTAMINE RECEPTORS

When Black et al.[11] developed specific H_2-receptor agonists and antagonists, it became clear that there were at least two types of histamine receptors. Further investigations soon revealed 'atypical' H_2-receptors, stimulated by histamine and 4-methyl histamine but not protected by known H_2-receptor antagonists.[20,21] Radioligand binding studies have now confirmed the presence of H_3-receptors in the brain,[22-24] in the autonomic nervous system, as well as in bronchial airways and on mast cells.[25-28] H_3-receptors are located presynaptically on histamine-synthesising nerve terminals and are involved in

ASTHMA: BASIC MECHANISMS AND CLINICAL MANAGEMENT (2nd Edn)
ISBN 0-12-079026-2

Table 16.1 History of histamine.

1907	Synthesis	Windaus & Vogt[1]
1910	Isolation from decomposing ergot	Barger & Dale[2]
1910–19	Tissue and species differences in sensitivity recognized	Dale & Laidlaw[3,4]
1927	Intracutaneous histamine produces .triple response	Lewis[5]
1928	Histamine i.v. produces dyspnoea, wheeze and fall in vital capacity in asthmatics	Weiss et al.[6]
1932	Antigen-induced histamine release from sensitized guinea-pig lung in vitro	Bartosch et al.[7]
1951	Antigen-induced histamine release and bronchoconstriction in human asthmatic lung challenged in vitro	Schild et al.[8]
1953–55	Histamine release associated with degranulation of mast cells	Riley & West[9]
1966	Two types of histamine receptor ?	Ash & Schild[10]
1972	Specific H_2-receptor agonists and antagonists developed	Black et al.[11]

Table 16.2 Histamine receptors.

	Agonist	Antagonist	Relative pA2 value	Potencies :K1 value
H_1-receptor	histamine	diphenhydramine		14
	2-methyl histamine	chlorpheniramine	9.0	2.6
	2-[pyridyl]ethylamine	mepyramine		0.2
	2-[2-thiazolyl]ethylamine	clemastine		0.3
	betahistine	terfenadine	8.2	52
		astemazole		8.0
		azelastine		6.4
		ketotifen		0.3
H_2-receptor	histamine	burinamide	5.11	
	4-methyl histamine	metiamide	6.04	
	dimaprit	cimetidine	6.10	
	impromidine	ranitidine	7.20	
H_3-receptor	histamine			
	R-α methyl histamine	thioperamide	8.96	

K1 value is proportional to the concentration of antagonist responsible for 50% inhibition of specific binding from displacement experiments. pA2 is the value which shifts the dissociation curve for histamine to its receptor by 2 log units.

the negative feed back control of histamine synthesis and release.[25] Some of the known agonists and antagonists of these receptors are listed on Table 16.2.

EFFECTS OF HISTAMINE AND ITS RECEPTORS ON THE LUNG (Table 16.3)

Tracheobronchial smooth muscle

Species and site differences

The prevailing pattern of histamine receptors determines the effect of histamine on airway smooth muscle. Since it varies considerably between species and even between different sites in the same airway,[29] extrapolation of results from animal models to man has created considerable confusion. In most species, the predominance of broncho-constricting H_1-receptors over bronchodilating H_2-receptors ensures that histamine produces bronchoconstriction. Nevertheless, in a few species the preponderance of H_2-receptors results in histamine-induced bronchodilatation whereas in others, H_2 receptors are not demonstrable. While the role of H_3-receptors remains undetermined, recent evidence indicates that they modulate both cholinergic and non-cholinergic non-adrenergic (NANC)-induced bronchoconstriction in the lung.[26–28]

Human tracheobronchial tree

In man, inhaled histamine induces bronchoconstriction. Changes in airway resistance and maximum flow at low lung volumes reflects constriction of large and small airways.[30] H_1-receptor antagonists prevent histamine-induced bronchoconstriction in a

Table 16.3 Histamine—effects in human lung.

Tissue	Receptor
Bronchial smooth muscle	
Bronchoconstriction	H_1
Inhibition of cholinergic	
bronchoconstriction	H_3
Blood vessels	
Pulmonary arteries	
Constriction	H_1
Dilatation	H_2
Bronchial arteries	
Constriction (high dose histamine)	H_1
Dilatation (low dose histamine)	H_1
Nasal vessels—dilatation	$H_1 + H_2$
Permeability increase	
Pulmonary epithelial	H_1
Vascular	?
Sputum	
Volume	H_1
Glycoprotein content	H_2

dose-dependent way in normal and asthmatic subjects alike, whether given orally, intravenously or by inhalation.[31–42] The effect of H_2-receptor antagonists is more controversial.[34–39,43–46] A preliminary report concerning human bronchus *in vitro* suggested the presence of bronchodilating H_2-receptors[47] and implied that H_2-receptor antagonists might be harmful to asthmatics. It was further suggested by Chand[48] that an absence of H_2-receptors might be the cause of bronchial hyperresponsiveness. However, in most *in vivo* studies of normal and asthmatic subjects cimetidine, a specific and potent H_2-receptor antagonist, did not alter the bronchial response to histamine significantly.[34,35,43,44,46] Nevertheless, a few groups reported minor changes in histamine responsiveness. Our own group initially found that cimetidine produced a small, though statistically significant, rightward shift of the histamine dose–response curve in normals and asthmatics.[36,37] By contrast, three American groups reported that the histamine response of asthmatics but not of normal subjects was slightly enhanced by cimetidine.[38,39,45] All effects attributed to cimetidine were small and could have been spurious; relatively few subjects were studied in each series and the local concentrations of antagonist may have been inadequate in some studies.

In vitro, the relationship between bronchial smooth muscle length or tension and dose of histamine is relatively simple. *In vivo*, response to stimulation can only be assessed by exceedingly indirect means. Airway calibre is usually estimated by measuring either airway resistance or the rate of airflow during forced expiration. It is determined not only by bronchial smooth muscle tone but also by pulmonary vascular tone and by bronchial inflammation, oedema and secretions. All of these may be modified by local neural reflex activity and by interactions with other mediators. The ease with which histamine reaches its receptors in the presence of secretions, oedema and any changes in pulmonary epithelial permeability may also affect the bronchial response. Finally any measure of airway function *in vivo* reflects the product of effects in a complex branching system of airways, with resistances in series and in parallel. Thus, it may be misleading to extrapolate results from *in vivo* studies to events at the bronchial smooth muscle level.

Unfortunately, it is hard to secure sufficient lung specimens and technically difficult to perform the *in vitro* studies. Consequently, relatively few have been performed. None the less, it is clear that human lung parenchyma is 16–28 times more sensitive to histamine than bronchus.[49,50] Brompheniramine, an H_1-receptor antagonist, prevents histamine-induced bronchoconstriction[51] while cimetidine, an H_2-receptor antagonist, has no effect on the histamine dose–response curves of lobar, segmental, or subsegmental bronchi.[52] Surprisingly, relaxation precedes contraction at low doses of histamine, dimiprit and impromidine.[53] These findings are difficult to reconcile with the partial inhibition of histamine-induced contraction and relaxation by mepyramine and the lack of effect of cimetidine and metiamide on any part of the response.[49,50,53]

We have re-examined the role of histamine receptors more directly *in vivo*.[30] In normal and asthmatic subjects we compared the effects on specific airways conductance and flow at low lung volumes of histamine and specific agonists of H_1-receptors (betahistine) and H_2-receptors (impromidine). Suitable doses for inhalation were chosen from the *in vitro* potency characteristics. Both histamine and betahistine induced reproducible, dose-dependent constriction in large and small airways, while impromidine was without effect. Normals and asthmatics behaved similarly (Fig. 16.1a+b). Ipratropium bromide (120 μg), inhaled by three normal subjects after the final dose of impromidine, produced significant bronchodilatation (Fig. 16.1c). Thus impromidine's impotence was due to an

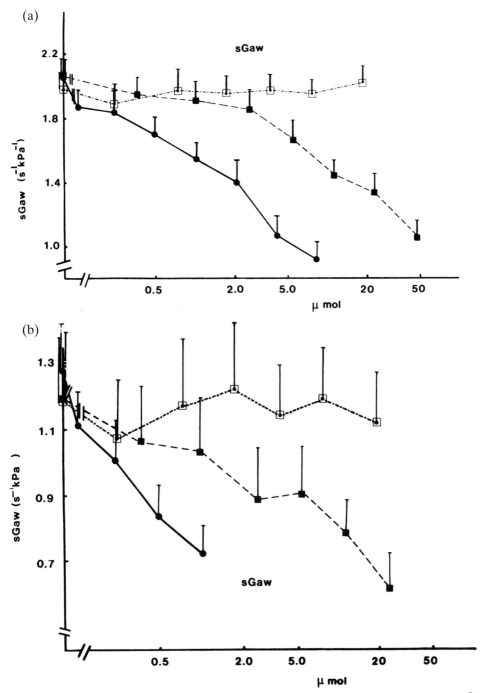

Fig. 16.1 Log dose–response curves in 10 normal (a) and five asthmatic subjects (b) for histamine (●), betahistine (■) and impromidine (□). Each point represents the mean response with standard error bar for all subjects to each dose of agonist aerosol. (c) shows the lack of effect of increasing doses of impromidine in three normal subjects and bronchodilatation following ipratropium bromide 120 μg. Reproduced from ref. 20, with permission. (*continued*)

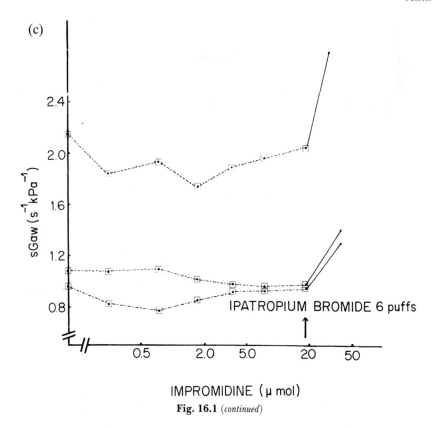

IMPROMIDINE (μ mol)

Fig. 16.1 (*continued*)

absence of H_2-receptors on large and small human airways rather than a lack of bronchodilating potential. In conclusion, the balance of evidence from both *in vitro* and *in vivo* work suggests that in man, the predominant effect of histamine in large and small airways is bronchoconstriction mediated by H_1-receptors. There is little to support the notion of a significant population of bronchodilating H_2-receptors on human airways or of any imbalance of histamine receptors as a cause for asthma.

Pulmonary epithelial permeability

It has been postulated that non-specific bronchial hyperresponsiveness might be due to an abnormally permeable pulmonary epithelium allowing the access of non-specific irritants, antigen and mediators to the underlying vagal, irritant receptors and bronchial smooth muscle.[54] Histamine increases epithelial permeability.[55–58] However, there is no significant difference in permeability between normal and asthmatic subjects, no correlation between permeability and bronchial responsiveness and no difference in the effect of histamine on the permeability of normal and asthmatic subjects.[55,57–60] Results from a small study of five normal subjects pretreated with histamine antagonists, suggested that H_2-receptors mediated histamine-induced increases in pulmonary epithelial permeability.[56] We have since performed a larger study using the same technique—the half-time clearance from lung to blood of inhaled 99mTc-DTPA.[60] Both inhaled histamine and the H_1-receptor agonist, betahistine, produced bronchoconstriction and increased permeability in all seven normal and five asthmatic subjects. By contrast, the H_2-receptor agonist, impromidine, was without effect in either group (Fig. 16.2). Since histamine-induced increases in permeability and bronchoconstriction were also prevented by oral terfenadine 120 mg but not by cimetidine 400 mg, we concluded that in human lung both these properties of histamine are mediated via H_1-receptors alone.

Pulmonary vasculature

There is relatively little information concerning the effects of histamine on human pulmonary vessels. However, Boe et al. demonstrated that in segmental pulmonary arteries histamine-induced vasoconstriction is mediated via H_1-receptors and vasodilatation via H_2-receptors.[61,62] In addition, Lui and colleagues have recently described histamine's biphasic action on human bronchial arteries—vasodilatation at low concentrations and vasoconstriction at higher concentrations, both mediated via H_1-receptors (Barnes, personal communication). In the nose, histamine-induced increases in nasal airway resistance predominantly represent vasodilatation. The effects can be partly prevented by pretreatment with either H_1- or H_2-receptor antagonists[63] and can be reproduced by nasal instillation of betahistine and impromidine.[64] Thus, in the nose, histamine-induced vasodilatation is mediated via both H_1-and H_2-receptors.

Vascular permeability is discussed elsewhere. There is little information pertaining to human lung; in the dog histamine-induced peribronchial oedema and in the sheep increases in lymph flow and protein content are attributed to enhanced permeability of postcapilliary venules in the bronchial circulation when gaps develop between the endothelial cells.[65,66] In guinea-pigs, histamine-induced permeability is mediated via H_1-receptors and NANC-induced plasma exudation can be prevented by H_3-receptor stimulation.[67] In the normal human nose, histamine also induces plasma leakage by increasing vascular permeability.[68] Since prior treatment with terfenadine can partially prevent antigen-induced increases in albumen concentrations in nasal lavage fluid of rhinitic patients,[69] it is probably mediated via H_1-receptors also. Further work is needed on the lower human airways.

Sputum

In the dog, histamine instillation produces a net flux of Cl and Na ions into tracheal lumen—an effect prevented by prior treatment with an H_1-receptor antagonist,[70] whereas antigen-induced bronchorrhoea is significantly inhibited both by H_1-and H_2-receptor antagonists.[71] In humans the bronchial mucus glycoprotein content can be increased by exogenous histamine and H_2-receptor agonists in vitro.[72] Unfortunately, the only relevant study in asthma was uncontrolled.[73] Nevertheless, in five of eight acute asthmatic episodes, H_1-receptor but not H_2-receptor antagonists reduced bronchorrhoea. It is possible that both H_1- and H_2-receptors are involved in sputum production and content in asthma.

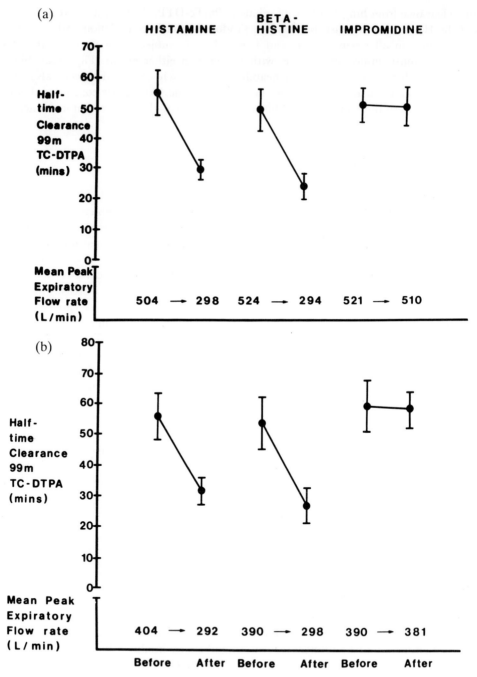

Fig. 16.2 The effect of histamine, betahistine and impromidine in seven normal (a) and five asthmatic (b) subjects on pulmonary epithelial permeability, as measured by half-time clearance of inhaled 99mTc-DTPA, and on airway calibre, as measured by peak expiratory flow rate (PEFR). Each line joins the mean baseline value with that achieved after inhalation of the agonist. (c) shows the mean effect in four normal subjects of pretreatment with terfenadine 120 mg and cimetidine 400 mg on histamine-induced changes in pulmonary epithelial permeability and lung function. Reproduced from ref. 60, with permission.

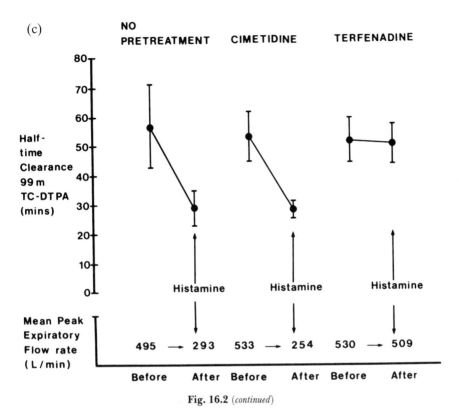

Fig. 16.2 (*continued*)

HISTAMINE TACHYPHYLAXIS

In 1951 Hawkins and Schild demonstrated histamine tachyphylaxis in human airways *in vitro*.[74] While the histamine response of normal and asthmatic subjects is reproducible when repeated on separate days,[75–79] there is doubt about responses performed on the same day. Some groups have found no evidence of systematic sensitization or tachyphylaxis[80–82] while others have reported tachyphylaxis in asthmatics when histamine challenges are repeated within 1–6 h.[46,83–87] This tachyphylaxis is said to be specific for histamine and not simply a result of bronchoconstriction since neither acetyl choline, cold air nor exercise challenge reduce the response to subsequent histamine inhalation.[84,86,87] Conversely, exercise-induced asthma is reduced by preceding histamine challenge.[86] The putative histamine tachyphylaxis is thought to be dependent on prostaglandin release mediated via the histamine H_2-receptor since it can be prevented by pretreatment with the cyclooxygenase inhibitor, indomethacin, and by the H_2-receptor antagonist, cimetidine.[46,83] In one study, histamine tachyphylaxis was demonstrated only in the more hyperresponsive asthmatics, with PD_{20} values of more than 25–100 μg.[85] It was suggested that those unable to demonstrate tachyphylaxis had studied asthmatics with particularly responsive airways. This is unlikely and certainly not the case in Kung's patients.[82] They had mild asthma requiring no prophylactic medication and their histamine responsiveness was comparable to that of Manning's patients.[83] Furthermore, the location of these H_2-receptors is uncertain; as mentioned before, none have been identified either on human bronchial smooth muscle or on pulmonary mast cells.[88,89] Currently, the existence of histamine tachyphylaxis remains in some doubt.

NEURAL CONTROL (Table 16.4)

While this topic is addressed in detail elsewhere (see Chapter 22), a few points particularly referrable to histamine are highlighted here.

Cholinergic nervous system

The role of the cholinergic nervous system in many animal species has been reviewed.[14] Briefly, histamine stimulates lung irritant receptors in intact and vagotomized animals. Both histamine- and antigen-induced bronchoconstriction is mediated, in part, via the vagus nerve; it is amplified by vagal stimulation and reduced by vagotomy. Chlorpheniramine, but not cimetidine, inhibits the effect of histamine on sensory and motor

Table 16.4   Histamine interactions in man.

Agent	Subjects	Histamine response	References
Prostaglandins			
PGF$_{2\alpha}$			
PGE$_2$	Normal subjects	Increased	161–164
PGD$_2$	Normals (given with histamine)		
PGD$_2$	Normals (given before histamine)	No effect	164,165
Leukotrienes			
LTB$_4$,LTC$_4$	Normal subjects	No effect	
LTD$_4$,LTE$_4$			165–167
LTB$_4$,LTC$_4$	Asthmatics	Increased	
LTD$_4$,LTE$_4$			
Cholinergic nervous system			
Blockade	Normal subjects	Controversial varies between subjects	93–103, 105,106
	Asthmatics		
Adrenergic nervous system			
α Blockade	Normal/asthmatic	Decreased	109–111
α Stimulation	Normal	No effect	112
	Asthmatic	Increased	
β Stimulation	Asthmatic	Decreased	94, 99, 103–106
β Blockade	Asthmatic	Increased	107, 108
NANC (non-adrenergic, non-cholinergic) system			
VIP (putative neurotransmitter)	Asthmatic	Decreased	115
Stimulation	Normal/asthmatic	Decreased	113, 114

components of the canine vagus nerve.[90–92] Thus, histamine, via the H_1-receptor, mediates and augments the effect of the cholinergic system. In addition, H_3-receptors may have an inhibitory function in guinea-pig trachea since low concentrations of histamine inhibit cholinergic neurotransmission in the presence of both H_1- and H_2- receptor antagonists.[26] In man, the role of the parasympathetic nervous system remains controversial; anticholinergic agents have reduced histamine- and antigen-induced bronchoconstriction in some studies[54,93–96] but not in others.[97–101] While it may be argued that either the dose or local concentrations of anticholinergic agents may have been inadequate in some studies, it is more likely that histamine acts both directly on bronchial smooth muscle and indirectly via the cholinergic nervous system, and that the contribution of the vagus nerve varies widely between individuals (Fig. 16.3) — both normal and asthmatic.[93,99,101] Furthermore, there is recent *in vitro* evidence that H_3-receptors can inhibit cholinergic contraction of human bronchi.[27] Possibly the balance between H_1- and H_3-receptors determines the importance of the cholinergic system in man.

Adrenergic nervous system

β_2-Adrenergic agonists are functional antagonists of bronchial smooth muscle contraction *in vitro* regardless of the bronchoconstrictor.[102] Many studies of normal and asthmatic subjects have confirmed the protection afforded by β_2-adrenergic agonists against histamine-induced bronchoconstriction *in vivo*[103–106] and have shown how β-blockers enhance this response in asthmatics. By contrast, α-adrenergic antagonists reduce histamine responsiveness in normal and asthmatic subjects[109–111] and α-adrenergic stimulants enhance the histamine response in asthmatics; they have no effect in normal subjects.[112]

Non-adrenergic non-cholinergic (NANC) nervous system

Little data is available. However, recent studies demonstrate that activation of the NANC nervous system by stimulation of the vocal cords can reduce the histamine responsiveness of normals and asthmatics alike.[113,114] Similar effects are produced in asthmatics by vasoactive intestinal peptide, a putative neurotransmitter for the system.[115] Thus, the NANC nervous system probably inhibits the effects of histamine on human tracheobronchial smooth muscle.

IMPORTANCE OF HISTAMINE IN ASTHMA

Histamine release in asthma

Plasma and bronchoalveolar lavage (BAL) histamine levels

The problems inherent in plasma histamine analyses have been reviewed by Ind *et al.*[116] Concentrations of histamine are low and, since histamine metabolism is fast, plasma histamine may not reflect local lung levels. Plasma histamine represents only 0.5% of

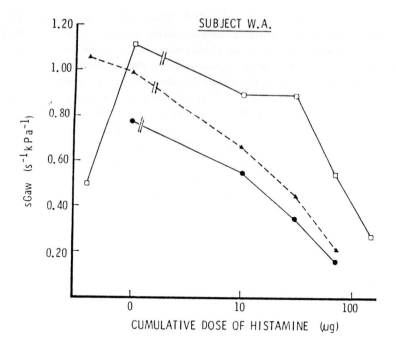

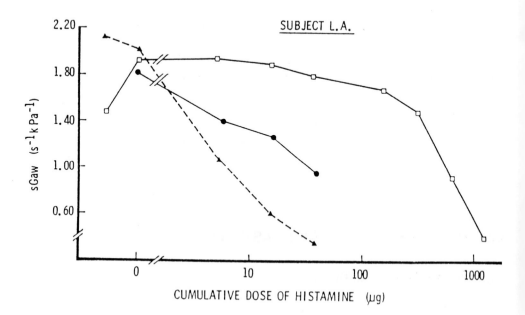

Fig. 16.3 Comparison of the effects of placebo (▲ – – – ▲) and atropine (□——□) on the original histamine dose–response curves (●——●) in two asthmatic subjects. Cumulative dose of histamine is plotted against specific airway conductance. Reproduced from ref. 93, with permission.

whole blood histamine, the rest residing in basophils. Thus, plasma concentrations are crucially dependent on the care taken in the sampling and separation of plasma. Of equal importance is the sensitivity and specificity of the histamine assay. Early bioassays and fluorimetric assays produced conflicting results. The more recent, double-isotope modifications of radioenzymatic assays appear more sensitive and specific. Table 16.5 summarizes the results from recent studies.[116-136] Plasma histamine is raised in acute asthma, correlates with the severity of asthma and falls after immunotherapy.[116-121] However, there is some debate whether either plasma or BAL histamine levels are raised in stable asthma.[116-120,130-134] Despite the controversies surrounding these measurements, the raised plasma and BAL histamine levels obtained during exercise-, antigen- and cAMP-induced asthma have been regarded as evidence of mast cell degranulation.[118,122-128,130,135] Levels are not altered by isocapnic hyperventilation, hypertonic saline or methacholine challenge.[118,123,125,129]

Perhaps more exciting is the identification from BAL fluid of cytokines which promote histamine release from basophils and mast cells (HRF) and others (HRIF) which specifically inhibit HRF.[136-138] These are discussed in more detail elsewhere. Briefly, BAL fluid from asthmatics contains less HRF than that of normal subjects but asthmatics spontaneously produce more HRF from mononuclear cells than normal subjects.[139,140] The quantity of HRF correlates with non-specific bronchial responsiveness and with clinical symptoms.[140] It falls in patients who improve on immunotherapy.[141] While the role of these cytokines needs clarification, it is possible that both may contribute to the pathogenesis of asthma. For instance, an impaired production of HRIF might allow unbridled HRF activity to promote histamine release from mast cells.

Table 16.5 Histamine in plasma and bronchoalveolar lavage (BAL).

Asthmatics vs normal subjects	Induced asthma
Plasma histamine	
Stable asthma — Not raised[116,117] / Raised[118-120]	Antigen-raised — Early response[122-126] / Late response[123]
Acute asthma raised[116,117]	Exercise raised[118,127,128]
Correlation with severity of asthma[119,120]	Isocapnic hyperventilation — not raised[118]
Levels after immunotherapy reduced[121]	Hypertonic saline — not raised[129]
	Methacholine — not raised[123,125]
	cAMP-raised[125]
Histamine level in BAL fluid	
Stable asthma — Not raised[130,131] / Raised[132-134]	Antigen-raised — Early response[130] / Late response only[135]
Reduced level of histamine releasing factor in asthmatics[136]	

Table 16.6 Effect of H_1-receptor antagonists on bronchial tone in asthmatics.

Drug	References	Rise in FEV$_1$	Rise in sGaw	Comment
Chlorpheniramine				
10–25 mg i.v.	142	15%		Effect depends on baseline
20 mg i.v.	37		40%	No effect in normal subjects
5 mg inhaled	32	12%	35%	Children
4 mg inhaled	147	No effect		Children
8 mg oral	35, 38, 39	No effect		
Clemastine				
1.5 mg inhaled	33	7%	22%	Stable outpatient asthmatics
0.05% inhaled	143	21%		Recovering from acute asthma
20 μg inhaled	144	15%		
200 μg inhaled		24%		
0.5 g/l	34			
0.5 mg inhaled	148			
0.05% inhaled	149			Stable outpatients
0.6 mg	41	No effect		
2 mg oral				
1 mg i.v.				
Terfenadine				
60–180 mg oral	150	No Effect		
60–180 mg oral	42	9–10%		
60 mg oral	145	32%		Great variation between children
				Similar to salbutamol
120 mg	146	30% ($\dot{V}$25p)		

Histamine tone (Table 16.6)

Not surprisingly, H_2-receptor antagonists have no effect on the airway calibre of normal and asthmatic subjects.[34–39,43,44] H_1-receptor antagonists are similarly ineffectual in normal subjects. Nevertheless, if given in adequate dosage, they can produce significant bronchodilatation in asthmatics whether given orally, intravenously or by inhalation.[32,33,37,42,142–146] However, not all studies have shown this,[34,38,39,41,147–150] particularly those concerned with stable asthmatics. The bronchodilatation is most marked in asthmatics recovering from acute asthma[143] and in those with the most initial airways obstruction.[142] Up to 32% improvements in FEV_1 have been documented in children after oral terfenadine.[145] In some studies the effects were comparable to those produced by inhaled salbutamol[143,146] and intravenous theophyllines.[142] Since the drugs concerned, chlorpheniramine, clemastine and terfenadine have no significant anticholinergic properties *in vivo*[33,36,42] the bronchodilatation is due solely to H_1-receptor antagonism. The modern H_1-receptor antagonists, such as terfenadine, are specific, potent and do not cross the blood–brain barrier.[151,152] Although it is possible to give large doses safely, no consistent dose–response relationship for bronchodilation has been demonstrated. Nevertheless, these findings have given rise to the concept that 'histamine tone' is present in the airways of patients with uncontrolled asthma due to a constant outpouring of histamine from pulmonary mast cells.

Comparison and interaction with other mediators

In man, inhaled histamine produces maximum bronchoconstriction within 1–4 min. The mean duration of action (19 min) depends on the dose given and the degree of bronchoconstriction produced.[153,154] The leukotrienes, whose speed of onset of action is similar to that of histamine, act for 2.5–3.0 times longer. They are also much more potent bronchoconstrictors. In normal subjects 700–6000-fold differences have been found for LTC_4 and LTD_4, respectively whilst 60 and 145-fold differences were found for LTE_4 in normal and asthmatic subjects.[155–159] Unexpectedly, one group reported that equivalent molar quantities of histamine and leukotrienes produced comparable bronchoconstriction in asthmatics.[160] However, evaluation of the relative importance of these mediators in asthma is difficult because of their complex interactions (Table 16.4); pretreatment with prostaglandins $F_{2\alpha}$ and E_2 enhances histamine responsiveness in normal subjects while leukotrienes produce similar effects in asthmatics only.[161–167]

Histamine and induced asthma (Table 16.7)

The pathogenesis of various types of induced asthma has been investigated recently. H_1-receptor antagonists provide partial protection against the early asthmatic response to inhaled antigen,[37,40,148,168–174] but the extent varies between subjects. Although 40–50% protection is possible, it is only apparent in the first 15 min of the early response.[170,171] No dose-dependent effect has been demonstrated with 60–180 mg terfenadine p.o (Fig.16.4).[40] By contrast, neither 10 mg p.o. chlorpheniramine nor terfenadine 120 mg p.o. significantly alter the late response to antigen (Fig.16.5).[169,175] However, both these and other H_1-receptor antagonists offer 30–50% protection against exercise-induced

Table 16.7 Effect of H_1-receptor antagonists on bronchoconstriction.

Drug	Dose/route	Reference	Comment
INDUCED ASTHMA			
Antigen—early response			**Partial protection**
Phenergan	25–50 mg	168	Small effect and degree varies between patients
Chlorpheniramine	10–20 mg i.v.	37, 169	
Clemastine	0.5% inhaled	148	40–80% protection for first 2–15 min only
Astemazole	10 mg oral	170	1.5–2-fold protection
Terfenadine	60–180 mg oral	40	40–50% protection only
		171, 172, 173, 174	5–8 min only
Antigen—late response			**No effect**
Chlorpheniramine	10 i.v.	169	
Terfenadine	120 mg oral	175	
Exercise-induced asthma			**Partial protection**
Clemastine	0.5 mg inhaled	176	48% protection
Chlorpheniramine	20 mg i.v.	177	40–50% protection
Terfenadine	60 mg oral	145	
	60–180 mg oral	150	30% protection
	180 mg oral	178	
Other challenges			**Variable protection**
Terfenadine 120–240 mg	Non-isotonic aerosols	129, 179–182	Significant protection very variable between subjects
	Cold air hyperventilation		
	Hyperventilation		
CLINICAL ASTHMA			**NO EFFECT**
Clemastine	0.2 mg qds inhaled for 2 weeks; 11 stable asthmatics	149	No difference vs placebo aerosol
Astemazole	10 mg oral daily for 2 weeks in pollen season; 30 asthmatics	170	Marginal effect at start of season
Terfenadine	60–180 mg nocte for 2 weeks in 18 patients with nocturnal asthma	184	No difference vs placebo tablets
	120 mg—single blind, nonrandomized	185	

asthma[145,150,176–178] and can partly attenuate bronchoconstriction induced by hyperventilation, cold air hyperventilation and inhalation of non-isotonic aerosols[129,179–182] Thus, mast cell degranulation is probably involved in these induced asthmas. While histamine plays a significant role in the pathogenesis of these conditions, the extent varies between subjects.

Histamine and spontaneously occurring asthma (Table 16.7)

The interpretation of early clinical trials with H_1-receptor antagonists is hampered by inadequate control of the studies, a lack of objective measurements of response and also by the non-specificity of most of the 'antihistamines'. There was little evidence to support their efficacy in asthma and central nervous system side effects limited their use.[183] Some of the recently developed H_1-receptor antagonists, such as ketotifen and azelastine, have pronounced mast cell stabilizing properties *in vitro*. This complicates interpretation of results in asthma. There are few clinical studies[149,170,184,185] with the more specific new H_1-receptor antagonists, whose potencies are compared on Table 16.2.[186] Although relatively specific, terfenadine 60 mg b.d. for 1 week decreases histamine release from nasal antigen challenge in rhinitic patients.[69,187] *In vivo*, therefore, it has some mast cell stabilizing properties. Nevertheless, the results in clinical asthma with these agents are no more encouraging than those from earlier studies. Two weeks of regular inhaled clemastine did not significantly improve 11 stable asthmatics,[149] while astemazole 10 mg daily p.o. for 2 weeks marginally improved 30 asthmatics, but only at the beginning of the pollen season.[170] Since plasma histamine is high at night, two groups investigated the effects of oral terfenadine 60–180 mg *nocte* on nocturnal asthma.[184,185] Neither demonstrated any significant benefit when compared with placebo.

CONCLUSIONS

Current data suggest that histamine is released in asthma—both acute and induced. There is significant 'histamine tone' in asthma. The potency of histamine is low compared with that of other mediators and it may be further diminished by tachyphylaxis. H_1-receptors mediate histamine-induced bronchoconstriction and pulmonary epithelial permeability in man. There is no evidence of a significant population of H_2-receptors on bronchial smooth muscle nor of any imbalance in H_1- and H_2-receptors producing bronchial hyperresponsiveness. However, both types of receptor are involved in pulmonary vascular responses and in sputum production. The role of H_3-receptors needs further clarification in normal and asthmatic lungs but it can inhibit cholinergic bronchoconstriction. The role of the cholinergic nervous system remains controversial; it probably varies between individuals.

As would be expected, H_2-receptor antagonists have no significant effect on either spontaneous or on induced asthma. H_1-receptor antagonists partially block many types of induced asthma but the effect is small. They do not attenuate the late response to

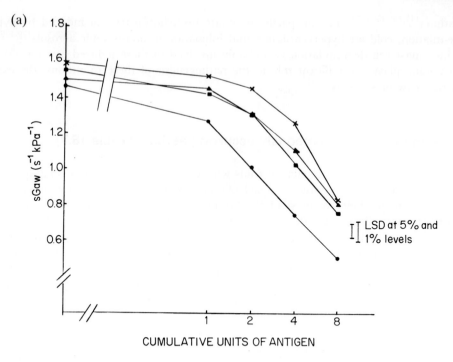

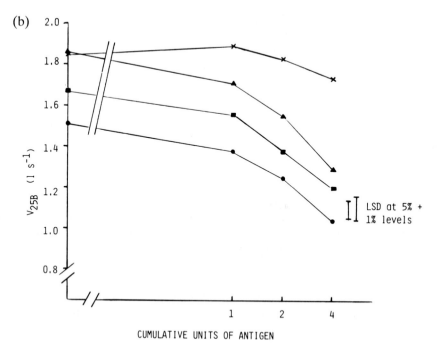

Fig. 16.4 Mean antigen dose–response curves of nine asthmatics following premedication with placebo (●) and with terfenadine 60 mg (▲), 120 mg (×) and 180 mg (■). In (a) cumulative antigen dose is plotted against specific airway conductance and in (b) against flow at 25% vital capacity above baseline residual volume. Reproduced from ref. 40, with permission.

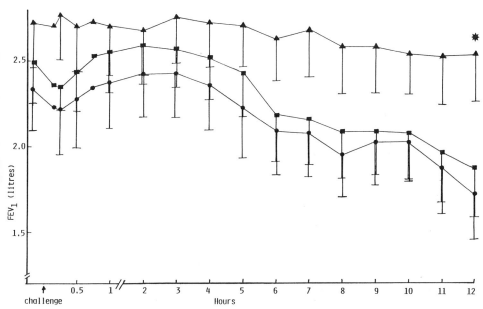

Fig. 16.5 The effect of oral terfenadine 120 mg (■) and repeated inhalation of salbutamol 200 μg (▲) compared with placebo (●) premedication on the early and late responses to inhaled antigen in nine atopic patients with dual responses. Salbutamol, but not terfenadine, significantly protects against the late response. Reproduced with permission from ref. 175.

inhaled antigen, considered a useful model for naturally occurring asthma and even the recent, more specific and potent H_1-receptor antagonists have failed to improve clinical asthma. Consequently, histamine, despite its diverse actions in the human lung, is relatively unimportant in the pathogenesis of asthma.

REFERENCES

1. Windaus A, Vogt H: Synthese des Imidazolyl-Athylamins. *Ber D Deutsch Chem Gesell* (1907) **XL**: 3691–3695.
2. Barger F, Dale HH: The presence in ergot of physiological activity of b-imidazolylethylamine. *J Physiol (Lond)* (1910) **40**: 38.
3. Dale HH, Laidaw PP: The physiological action of b-imidazolylethylamine. *J Physiol (Lond)* (1910) **41**: 318–344.
4. Dale HH, Laidaw PP: Histamine shock. *J Physiol (Lond)* (1919) **52**: 355–390.
5. Lewis T: The blood vessels of the human skin and their responses. London, Shaw, 1927.
6. Weiss S, Robb GP, Blumgart HL: The velocity of blood flow in health and disease as measured by the effect of histamine on minute vessels. *Am J Heart* (1928) **4**: 664–691.
7. Bartosch R, Feldberg W, Nagel E: Das Freiwerden eines histaminahnlichen stoffes bei der anaphylaxie des meerschweinchens. *Pflug Arch ges Physiol* (1932) **230**: 129–153.
8. Schild HO, Hawkins DF, Mongar JL, Herxheimer H: Reactions of isolated human asthmatic lung and bronchial tissue to a specific antigen. *Lancet* (1951) **ii**: 376–382.
9. Riley JF, West GB: The presence of histamine in tissue mast cells. *J Physiol (Lond)* (1953) **120**: 528–537.
10. Ash ASF, Schild HO: Receptors mediating some actions of histamine. *Brit J Pharmacol* (1966) **27**: 427–439.

11. Black JW, Duncan WAM, Durant GJ, Ganellin CR, Parsons ME: Definition and antagonism of histamine H2-receptors. *Nature* (1972) **236**: 385–390.
12. Beaven MA: Histamine. *N Eng J Med* (1976) **294**: 30–36; 320–325.
13. Forman JC: Histamine: In Buckle DR, Smith H (eds) *Development of antiasthma drugs.* Butterworth, London, 1984, pp 29–53.
14. White MV, Slater JE, Kaliner MA: Histamine and asthma. *Am Rev Respir Dis* (1987) **135**: 1165–1176.
15. Tomita A, Patterson R, Suszko IM: Respiratory mast cells and basophiloid cells. *Int Arch Allergy* (1974) **47**: 261–272.
16. Wasserman SI: The lung mast cell: its physiology and potential relevance to the defence of the lung. *Environ Health Perspect* (1980) **35**: 153–164.
17. Fox B, Bull TB, Guz A: Mast cells in human alveolar wall: an electron microscopic study. *J Clin Pathol* (1981) **34**: 1333–1342.
18. Freidman MM, Kaliner MA: *In situ* degranulation of nasal mucosal mast cells: ultrastructure features and cell to cell associations. *J Allergy Clin Immunol* (1985) **76**: 70–82.
19. Caulfield JP, Lewis RA, Hein A, Austin KF: Secretion in dissociated human pulmonary mast cells. *J Cell Biol* (1980) **85**: 299–311.
20. Fleisch J, Calkins PJ: Comparison of drug-induced responses in rabbit trachea and bronchus. *J Appl Physiol* (1976) **41**: 62–66.
21. Eyre P, Chand N: Preliminary evidence for two subclasses of histamine H2-receptors. *Agents Actions* (1979) **9**: 1–3.
22. Arrang JM, Garbarg M, Schwartz J-C: Auto-inhibition of brain histamine release mediated by a novel class (H3) of histamine receptor. *Nature* (1983) **302**: 832–837.
23. Arrang JM, Garbarg M, Lancelot JC, *et al.*: Highly potent and selective ligands for histamine H3-receptors. *Nature* (1987) **327**: 117–123.
24. Arrang JM, Garbarg M, Lancelot JC *et al.*: The third histamine receptor. Highly selective and potent ligands. *Int Arch Allergy Immunol* (1989) **88**: 79–81.
25. Ishikawa S, Sperelakis N: A novel class (H3) of histamine receptors on perivascular nerve terminals. *Nature* (1987) **327**: 158–160.
26. Ichinose M, Barnes PJ: Histamine H3-receptors modulate nonadrenergic noncholinergic neural bronchoconstriction in guinea pig *in vivo*. *Eur J Pharmacol* (1989) **174**: 49–55.
27. Ichinose M, Barnes PJ: Inhibitory histamine H3-receptors on cholinergic nerves in human airways. *Eur J Pharmacol* (1989) **163**: 383–386.
28. Ichinose M, Stretton CD, Schwartz JC, Barnes PJ: Histamine H3-receptors inhibit cholinergic neurotransmission in guinea pig airways. *Brit J Pharmac* (1989) **97**(1): 13–15.
29. Chakrin LW, Krell RD: Histamine receptors in the respiratory system: a review of current evidence. In Torsoli A, Lucchelli PE, Brimblecombe RW (eds) H2-antagonists in peptic ulcer disease and progress in histamine research. *Exerpta Medica* (1980) 338–346.
30. White JP, Mills J, Eiser NM: Comparison of the effects of histamine H1- and H2-receptor agonists on large and small airways in normal and asthmatic subjects. *Brit J Dis Chest* (1987) **81**: 155–169.
31. Casterline CL, Evans R: Further studies on the mechanism of human histamine-induced asthma. *J Allergy Clin Imunol* (1976) **58**: 607–612.
32. Woenne R, Kattan M, Orange RP, Levison H: Bronchial hyperreactivity to histamine and methacholine in asthmatic children after inhalation of SCH1000 and chlorpheniramine maleate. *J Allergy Clin Immunol* (1978) **62**: 119–124.
33. Nogrady SG, Bevan C: Inhaled antihistamines-bronchodilatation and effects on histamine and methacholine-induced bronchoconstriction. *Thorax* (1978) **33**: 700–704.
34. Thomson NC, Kerr JW: Effects of inhaled H1- and H2-receptor antagonists in normal and asthmatic subjects. *Thorax* (1980) **35**: 428–434.
35. Maconochie J, Woodings EP: Effects of H1- and H2-receptor blocking agents on histamine-induced bronchoconstriction in nonasthmatic subjects. *Brit J Clin Pharmac* (1979) **7**: 231–236.
36. Eiser NM, Mills J, McRae KD, Snashall PD, Guz A: Histamine receptors in normal human bronchi. *Clin Sci* (1980) **58**: 537–544.
37. Eiser NM, Mills J, Snashall PD, Guz A: The role of histamine receptors in asthma. *Clin Sci* (1981) **60**: 363–370.

38. Nathan RA, Segall N, Glover GC, Schocket AL: The effects of H1 and H2 antihistamines on histamine inhalation challenges in asthmatic patients. *Am Rev Respir Dis* (1979) **120**: 1251–1259.

39. Schacter EN, Brown B, Lach E, Gerstenhaber B: Histamine blocking agents in healthy and asthmatic subjects. *Chest* (1982) **82**: 143–147.

40. Chan TB, Shelton DM, Eiser NM: Effect of an oral H1-receptor antagonist, terfenadine, on antigen-induced asthma. *Brit J Dis Chest* (1986) **80**: 375–384.

41. Hartmann V, Magnussen H, Holle JP, Schuler E: Modulation of histamine-induced bronchoconstriction with inhaled, oral and intravenous clemastine in normal and asthmatic subjects. *Thorax* (1981) **36**: 737–740.

42. Rafferty P, Holgate ST: Terfenadine is a potent and selective H1-receptor antagonist in asthmatic airways. *Am Rev Respir Dis* (1987) **135**: 181–184.

43. Nogrady SG, Bevan C: H2-receptor blockade and bronchial hyperreactivity to histamine in asthma. *Thorax* (1981) **36**: 268–271.

44. Michoud MC, Lelorier J, Amyot R: Factors modulating the interindividual variability of airway responsiveness to histamine. The influence of H1- and H2-receptors. *Bull Eur Physiopath Resp* (1981) **17**: 807–821.

45. Tashkin DP, Ungerer R, Wolfe R, Mendosa G, Calvarese B: Effect of orally administered cimetidine on histamine- and antigen-induced bronchospasm in subjects with asthma. *Am Rev Respir Dis* (1982) **125**: 691–695.

46. Jackson PJ, Manning PK, O'Byrne PM: A new role for histamine H2-receptors in asthmatic airways. *Am Rev Respir Dis* (1988) **138**: 784–788.

47. Dunlop LS, Smith AP: The effect of histamine antagonists on antigen-induced contractions of sensitised human bronchus *in vitro*. *Brit J Pharmacol* (1977) **59**: 475 p.

48. Chand N: Is airway hyperreactivity in athma due to histamine H2-receptor deficiency? *Medical Hypotheses* (1980) **6**: 1105–1112.

49. Vincenc K, Black J, Yan C, Armour C, Donnelly PD, Woolcock AJ: Comparison of *in vivo* and *in vitro* responses to histamine in human airways. *Am Rev Respir Dis* (1983) **128**: 875–879.

50. Goldie RG, Paterson JW, Wale JL: Pharmacological responses of human and porcine lung tissue: comparison of parenchyma, bronchus and pulmonary artery. *Brit J Pharmacol* (1982) **76**: 515–521.

51. Persson CGA, Ekman M: Contractile effects of histamine in large and small respiratory airways. *Agents Actions* (1976) **614**: 389–393.

52. Armour CL, Lazar NM, Schellenberg RR *et al.*: A comparison of *in vivo* and *in vitro* human airway reactivity to histamine. *Am Rev Respir Dis* (1984) **129**: 907–910.

53. Vincenc K, Black J, Shaw R: Relaxation and contraction responses to histamine in the human lung parenchymal strip. *Eur J Pharmacol* (1984) **98**: 201–210.

54. Simonsson BG, Jacobs FM, Nadal JA: The role of the autonomic nervous system and the cough reflex in the increased responsiveness of airways in patients with obstructive airways disease. *J Clin Invest* (1967) **46**: 1812–1818.

55. Elwood RK, Kennedy S, Belzberg A, Hogg JC, Paré PD: Respiratory mucosal permeability in asthma. *Am Rev Respir Dis* (1983) **128**: 523–527.

56. Braude S, Coe C, Royston D, Barnes PJ: Histamine increases lung permeability by an H2-receptor mechanism. *Lancet* (1984) **ii**: 372–374.

57. Rees PJ, Shelton D, Chan TB, Eiser NM, Clark TJH, Maisey MN: Effects of histamine on lung permeability in normal and asthmatic subjects. *Thorax* (1985) **40**: 603–606.

58. O'Byrne PM, Dolovich M, Duvall A, Newhouse MT: Lung epithelial permeability after histamine challenge. *Am Rev Respir Dis* (1982) **125**: 281–285.

59. Kennedy SM, Elwood RK, Wiggs BJR, Paré PD, Hogg JC: Increased airway mucosal permeability of smokers. *Am Rev Respir Dis* (1984) **129**: 143–148.

60. Chan TB, Eiser N, Shelton D, Rees PJ: Histamine receptors and pulmonary epithelial permeability. *Brit J Dis Chest* (1987) **81**: 260–267.

61. Boe J, Simonsson BG, Stahl E: Effect of histamine, 5-hydroxytryptamine and prostaglandins on isolated human pulmonary arteries. *Eur J Respir Dis* (1980) **61**: 12–19.

62. Boe J, Boe M-A, Simonsson BG: A dual action of histamine on isolated human pulmonary arteries. *Respiration* (1980) **40**: 117–122.

63. Mygind N, Secher C, Kirkegaard J: Role of histamine and antihistamines in the nose. *Eur J Respir Dis* (1983) **64**(Suppl 128): 16–20.

64. Shelton D, Eiser N: Histamine receptors in the normal nose. *Bull Europ Physiopath Resp* (1987) **23**(Suppl 12): 343.

65. Pietra GG, Szidon JP, Leventhal MM, Fishman AP: Histamine and interstitial oedema. *Circ Resp* (1971) **29**: 323–337.

66. Hutchison AA, Bernard GR, Snapper JR, Brigham KL: Effect of aerosol histamine on lung lymph in awake sheep. *J Appl Physiol* (1984) **56**: 1090–1098.

67. Ichinose M, Belvisi MG, Barnes PJ: Histamine H3-receptors inhibit neurogenic microvascular leakage in airways. *J Appl Physiol* (1990) **68**: 21–25.

68. Svenson C, Baumgarten CR, Pipkorn U, Alkner U, Persson CG: Reversibility and reproducibility of histamine-induced plasma leakage in nasal airways. *Thorax* (1989) **44**: 13–18.

69. Naclerio RM, Kagey-Sobotka, Lichtenstein LM, Freidhoff L, Proud D: Terfenadine, an H1 antihistamine, inhibits histamine release *in vivo* in the human. *Am Rev Respir Dis* (1990) **142**: 167–171.

70. Marin MG, Davis B, Nadel JA: Effect of histamine on electrical and ion transport properties of tracheal epithelium. *J Appl Physiol* (1977) **42**: 735–738.

71. Yamatake Y, Sasagawa S, Yanaura S, Kobayashi N: Involvement of histamine H1-and H2-receptors in induced asthma in dogs. *Jap J Pharmacol* (1977) **27**: 791–797.

72. Shelhamer JH, Maran Z, Kaliner MA: Immunologic and neuropharmacologic stimulation of mucus glycoprotein from human airways *in vivo*. *J Clin Invest* (1980) **66**: 1400–1408.

73. Shimura S, Sasaki T, Sasaki H, Takishima T: Chemical properties of bronchorrhea sputum in bronchial asthma. *Chest* (1988) **94**: 1211–1215.

74. Hawkins DF, Schild HO: The actions of drugs on isolated human bronchial chains. *Brit J Pharmacol* (1951) **6**: 682–690.

75. Juniper EF, Frith PA, Dunnett C, Cockcroft DW, Hargreave FE: Reproducibility and comparison of responses to inhaled histamine and methacholine. *Thorax* (1978) **33**: 705–710.

76. Eiser NM, MacRae KD, Guz A: Evaluation and expression of bronchial provocation tests. *Bull Europ Physiopath Resp* (1981) **17**: 427–440.

77. Schoeffel RE, Anderson SD, Gillam I, Lindsay DA: Multiple exercise and histamine challenge in asthmatic patients. *Thorax* (1980) **35**: 164–170.

78. Ruffin RE, Alpers JH, Crockett AJ, Hamilton R: Repeated histamine tests in asthmatic patients. *J Allergy Clin Immunol* (1981) **67**: 285–289.

79. Hariparsad D, Wilson N, Dixon C, Silverman M: Reproducibility of histamine challenge tests in asthmatic children. *Thorax* (1983) **38**: 258–260.

80. Lemire I, Cartier A, Malo JL, Pineau H, Ghezzo H, Martin RR: Effect of sodium cromoglycate on histamine inhalation tests. *J Allergy Clin Immunol* (1984) **73**: 234–239.

81. Polosa R, Finnery JP, Holgate ST: Lack of tachyphylaxis to histamine in both moderate and mild asthmatics. *Agents Actions* (1990) **30**: 281–283.

82. Kung M, Scott GC, Burki NK: Airway responsiveness determined by consecutive histamine challenges in asymptomatic asthmatics. *J Appl Physiol* (1989) **67**: 2622–2626.

83. Manning PJ, Jones GL, O'Byrne PM: Tachyphylaxis to inhaled histamine. *J Appl Physiol* (1987) **63**: 1572–1577.

84. Manning PJ, O'Byrne PM: Histamine bronchoconstriction reduces airway responsiveness in asthmatic subjects. *Am Rev Respir Dis* (1988) **137**: 1323–1325.

85. Connolly MJ, Stenton SC, Avery AJ, Walters EH, Hendrick DJ: Refractory period following bronchoconstriction provoked by histamine in asthmatic subjects. *Thorax* (1989) **44**: 146–150.

86. Hammielec CM, Manning PJ, O'Byrne PM: Exercise refractoriness after histamine inhalation in asthmatic subjects. *Am Rev Respir Dis* (1988) **138**: 794–798.

87. Carpentiere G, Castello F, Marino S: Airway responsiveness to histamine in patients refractory to repeated exercise. *Chest* (1988) **93**: 933–936.

88. Kaliner MA: Human lung tissue and anaphylaxis. The effect of histamine on the immunological release of mediators. *Am Rev Respir Dis* (1978) **118**: 1015–1023.

89. Platshon LF, Kaliner MA: The effects of immunological release of histamine upon human lung cyclic nucleotide levels and prostaglandin generation. *J Allergy Clin Immunol* (1978) **62**: 1113–1121.

90. Sampson SR, Vidruk DH: The nature of the receptor mediating effects of histamine on rapidly adapting vagal afferents in the lung. *J Physiol (Lond)* (1979) **287**: 509–518.

91. Dixon M, Jackson DM, Richard IM: The effects of H1-and H2-receptor agonists on total lung resistance, dynamic lung compliance and irritant receptor discharge in the anaesthetised dog. *Brit J Pharmacol* (1979) **66**: 203–209.

92. Bradley SL, Russell JA: Distribution of H1-and H2-receptors in dog airway smooth muscle. *Physiologist* (1977) **20**: 11.

93. Eiser NM, Guz A: Effect of atropine on experimentally-induced airways obstruction in man. *Bull Eur Physiopath Resp* (1982) **18**: 449–460.

94. Cockcroft DW, Killian DN, Mellon AJJ, Hargreave FE: Protective effect of drugs on histamine-induced asthma. *Thorax* (1977) **32**: 429–437.

95. Holtzman MJ, Sheller JR, Dimeo M, Nadel JA, Boushey HA: Effect of ganglionic blockade on bronchial reactivity in atopic subjects. *Am Rev Respir Dis* (1980) **122**: 17–22.

96. Yu DYC, Galant SP, Gold WM: Inhibition of antigen-induced bronchoconstriction by atropine in asthmatic patients. *J Appl Physiol* (1972) **32**: 823–828.

97. Schiller IW, Lowell FC: The effects of drugs in modifying the response of asthmatic subjects to inhalation of pollen extracts, as determined by vital capacity measurements. *Ann Allergy* (1947) **5**: 564–566.

98. Itkin IH, Anand SC: The role of atropine as a mediator blocker of induced bronchial obstruction. *J Allergy* (1970) **45**: 178–186.

99. Casterline CL, Evans R, Ward GW: The effect of atropine and albuterol on the human bronchial response to histamine. *J Allergy Clin Immunol* (1976) **58**: 607–613.

100. Rosenthal RR, Norman PS, Summer WR, Permutt S: The role of parasympathetic system in antigen-induced bronchospasm. *J Appl Physiol* (1977) **42**: 600–606.

101. Thomson NC: The effect of different pharmacological agents on respiratory reflexes in normal and asthmatic subjects. *Clin Sci* (1979) **56**: 235–241.

102. Barnes PJ: Neural control of human airways in health and disease. *Am Rev Respir Dis* (1986) **134**: 1289–1314.

103. Bandouvakis J, Cartier A, Roberts R, Ryan G, Hargreave FE: The effect of ipratropium and fenoterol on methacholine- and histamine-induced bronchoconstriction. *Brit J Dis Chest* (1981) **75**: 295–305.

104. Salome CM, Schoeffel RE, Yan K, Woolcock AJ: Effect of aerosol and oral fenoterol on histamine and methacholine challenge in asthmatic subjects. *Thorax* (1981) **36**: 580–584.

105. Chung F, Morgan B, Keyes SJ, Snashall PD: Histamine dose–response relationships in normal and asthmatic subjects. *Am Rev Respir Dis* (1982) **126**: 849–854.

106. Britton J, Hanley SP, Garrett HV, Hadfield JW, Tattersfield AE: Dose related effects of salbutamol and ipratropium bromide on airway calibre and reactivity in subjects with asthma. *Thorax* (1988) **43**: 300–305.

107. Ruffin RE, Frith PA, Anderton RC, Kumana CR, Newhouse MT, Hargreave FE: Selectivity of beta adrenoceptor antagonist drugs assessed by histamine bronchial provocation. *Clin Pharmac Ther* (1879) **25**: 536–540.

108. Ruffin RE, McIntyre ELM, Latimer KM, Ward HE, Crockett AJ, Alpers JH: Assessment of β-adrenoceptor antagonists in asthmatic patients. *Brit J Clin Pharmac* (1982) **13**: 325S–335S.

109. Bianco S, Griffin JP, Kamburoff PL, Prime FJ: The effect of thymoxamine on histamine induced bronchospasm in man. *Brit J Dis Chest* (1972) **66**: 27–32.

110. Kerr KW, Govindaraj M, Patel KR: Effect of alpha-receptor blocking drugs and disodium cromoglycate on histamine hypersensitivity in bronchial asthma. *Brit Med J* (1970) **ii**: 139–141.

111. Gaddie J, Legge JS, Petrie G, Palmer KNV: The effect of an alpha-adrenergic receptor blocking drug on histamine sensitivity in bronchial asthma. *Brit J Dis Chest* (1972) **66**: 141–146.

112. Dinh Xuan AT, Regnard R, Matran R, Mantrand P, Adventier C, Lockhart A: Effects of clonidine on bronchial responses to histamine in normal and asthmatic subjects. *Eur Respir J* (1988) **1**: 345–350.

113. Michoud MC, Amyot R, Jeanneret-Grosjean A, Couture J: Reflex decrease of histamine-induced bronchoconstriction after laryngeal stimulation in humans. *Am Rev Respir Dis* (1987) **136**: 618–622.

114. Michoud MC, Jeanneret-Grosjean A, Cohen A, Amyot R: Reflex decrease of histamine-induced bronchoconstriction after laryngeal stimulation in asthmatic patients. *Am Rev Respir Dis* (1988) **138**: 1548–1552.

115. Barnes PJ, Dixon CMS: The effect of inhaled vasoactive intestinal peptide on bronchial reactivity to histamine in humans. *Am Rev Respir Dis* (1984) **130**: 162–166.

116. Ind PW, Barnes PJ, Brown MJ, Causon R, Dollery CT: Measurement of plasma histamine in asthma. *Cli Allergy* (1983) **13**: 61–67.

117. Skoner DP, Page R, Asman B, Gillen L, Fireman P: Plasma elevations of histamine and a prostaglandin metabolite in acute asthma. *Am Rev Respir Dis* (1988) **137**: 1009–1014.

118. Barnes PJ, Brown MJ: Plasma venous histamine in exercise and hyperventilation-induced asthma in man. *Clin Sci* (1981) **61**: 159–162.

119. Barnes PJ, Ind PW, Brown MJ: Plasma histamine and catecholamines in stable asthmatic subjects. *Clin Sci* (1982) **62**: 661–665.

120. McFadden ER, Soter NA: A search for chemical mediators of immediate hypersensitivity and hormonal factors in the pathogenesis of exercise-induced asthma. In Lichtenstein LM, Austin KF (eds) *Asthma—Physiology Immunopathology and Treatment.* New York, Academic Press, 1980, pp. 351–364.

121. Wang JY, Hsieh KH: The effect of immunotherapy on the *in vitro* productions of histamine, prostaglandin E2 and leukotriene C4 in asthmatic children. *Asian Pac J Allergy Immunol* (1989) **7**: 119–124.

122. Brown MJ, Ind PW, Causon R, Lee TH: A novel double isotope technique for the enzymatic assay of plasma histamine; application to estimation of mast cell activation assessed by antigen challenge in asthmatics. *J Allergy Clin Immunol* (1982) **69**: 20–24.

123. Durham SR, Lee TH, Cromwell O, *et al.*: Immunologic studies in allergen-induced late-phase asthmatic reactions. *J Allergy Clin Immunol* (1984) **74**: 49–60.

124. Howeth PH, Durham SR, Lee TH, Kay AB, Church MK, Holgate ST: Influence of albuterol, cromolyn sodium and ipratropium bromide on the airway and circulating mediator response to allergen bronchial provocation in asthma. *Am Rev Respir Dis* (1985) **132**: 986–992.

125. Phillips GD, Ng WH, Church MK, Holgate ST: The response of plasma histamine to bronchoprovocation with methacholine, adenosine 5'-monophosphate and allergen in atopic non-asthmatic subjects. *Am Rev Respir Dis* (1990) **141**: 9–13.

126. Busse WW, Swenson CA: The relationship between plasma histamine concentrations and bronchial obstruction to antigen challenge in allergic rhinitics. *J Allergy Clin Immunol* (1989) **84**: 658–666.

127. Lee TH, Nagakura T, Cromwell O, Brown MJ, Causon R, Kay AB: Neutrophil chemotactic activity (NCA) and histamine in atopic and nonatopic individuals after exercise-induced asthma. *Am Rev Respir Dis* (1984) **129**: 409–412.

128. Belcher NG, Murdoch RD, Dalton N, Clark TJH, Rees PJ, Lee TH: A comparison of mediator and catecholamine release between exercise- and hypertonic saline-induced asthma. *Am Rev Respir Dis* (1988) **137**: 1026–1032.

129. O'Hickey SP, Belcher NG, Rees PJ, Lee TH: Role of histamine release in hypertonic saline induced bronchoconstriction. *Thorax* (1989) **44**: 650–653.

130. Wenzel SA, Fowler AA, Schwartz LB: Activation of pulmonary mast cells by bronchoalveolar allergen challenge. *Am Rev Resp Dis* (1988) **137**: 1002–1008.

131. Rankin JA, Kaliner M, Reynolds HY: Histamine levels in bronchoalveolar lavage from patients with asthma, sarcoidosis and ideopathic pulmonary fibrosis. *J Allergy Clin Immunol* (1987) **79**: 371–377.

132. Flint KC, Leung KB, Hudspith BN, Brostoff J, Pearce FL, Johnson NMc: Bronchoalveolar mast cells in extrinsic asthma; a mechanism for the initiation of antigen specific bronchoconstriction. *Brit J Med* (1985) **291**: 923–926.

133. Casale TB, Wood D, Richerson HB, *et al.*: Elevated bronchoalveolar lavage fluid histamine levels in allergic asthmatics are associated with methacholine bronchial hyperresponsiveness. *J Clin Invest* (1987) **79**: 1197–1203.

134. Lui MC, Bleecker ER, Lichtenstein LM, *et al.*: Evidence for elevated levels of histamine, prostaglandin D2 and other bronchoconstricting prostaglandins in the airways of subjects with mild asthma. *Am Rev Respir Dis* (1990) **142**: 126–132.

135. Diaz P, Gonzalez C, Galleguillos FR, *et al.*: Leukocytes and mediators in bronchoalveolar lavage during allergen-induced late-phase asthmatic reactions. *Am Rev Respir Dis* (1989) **139**: 1383–1389.

136. Gittlin SD, MacDonald SM, Bleecker ER, Lui MC, Kagey-Sobotka A, Lichtenstein LM: An IgE-dependent histamine releasing factor (HRF) in human bronchoalveolar lavage (BAL) fluid. *FASEB J* (1988) **2**: A1232.

137. Alam R, Welter J, Forsythe PA, Lett-Brown MA, Rankin JA, Boyars M, Grant JA: Detection of histamine release inhibitory factor and histamine releasing factor-like activities in bronchoalveolar lavage fluids. *Am Rev Respir Dis* (1990) **141**: 666–671.

138. Alam R, Rozniecki J, Selmaj K: A mononuclear cell-derived histamine releasing factor in asthmatic patients. Histamine release from basophils *in vitro*. *Ann Allergy* (1984) **53**: 66–69.

139. Alam R, Rozniecki J, Kuzminska B: A mononuclear cell-derived histamine releasing factor (HRF) in asthmatic children. III. Further studies. *Ann Allergy* (1985) **55**: 825–829.

140. Alam R, Kuna P, Rozniecki J, Kuzminska B: The magnitude of spontaneous production of histamine releasing factor (HRF) by lymphocytes *in vitro* correlates with state of bronchial hyperreactivity in patients with asthma. *J Allergy Clin Immunol* (1987) **79**: 103–108.

141. Kuna P, Alam R, Kuzminska B, Rozniecki J: The effect of preseasonal immunotherapy on the production of histamine releasing factor (HRF) by mononuclear cells from patients with seasonal asthma. Results of a double blind placebo controlled randomised study. *J Allergy Clin Immunol* (1988) **83**: 816–824.

142. Popa VT: Bronchodilating activity of an H1-blocker chlorpheniramine. *J Allergy Clin Immunol* (1977) **59**: 54–63.

143. Nogrady SG, Hartley JPR, Handslip PDJ, Hurst NP: Bronchodilatation after inhalation of the antihistamine clemastine. *Thorax* (1978) **33**: 479–482.

144. Monie RD, White JP, Handslip PDJ, Hartley JPR, Nogrady SG: Bronchodilator properties of inhaled clemastine. *Brit J Dis Chest* (1980) **74**: 420.

145. MacFarlane PI, Heaf DP: Selective histamine blockade in childhood asthma; the effect of terfenadine on resting bronchial tone and exercise induced bronchoconstriction. *Resp Med* (1989) **83**: 19–24.

146. Cookson WOCM: Bronchodilator action of the anti-histaminic terfenadine. *Brit J Clin Pharmac* (1987) **24**: 120–121.

147. Hodges IGC, Milner AD, Stokes GM: Bronchodilator effect of two inhaled H1-receptor antagonists, clemastine and chlorpheniramine. *Brit J Dis Chest* (1983) **77**: 270–275.

148. Phillips MJ, Ollier S, Gould CAL, Davies RJ: Effect of antihistamines and antiallergic drugs on responses to allergen and histamine provocation tests in asthma. *Thorax* (1984) **39**: 345–351.

149. Partridge MR, Saunders KB: Effect of inhaled antihistamine (clemastine) as a bronchodilator and as maintenance treatment in asthma. *Thorax* (1979) **34**: 771–776.

150. Patel KR: Terfenadine in exercise induced asthma. *Brit J Med* (1984) **288**: 1496–1497.

151. Cheng HC, Woodward JK: A kinetic study of the antihistaminic effects of terfenadine. *Arzneim-Forsch Drug Res* (1982) **32**: 1160–1166.

152. Weich NL, Martin JS: Absence of the effect of terfenadine on guinea pig brain histamine H1-receptors *in vivo* determined by receptor binding techniques. *Arzneim-Forsch Drug Res* (1982) **32**: 1167–1170.

153. Cartier A, Malo JL, Begin P, Sestier M, Martin RR: Time course of the bronchoconstriction produced by histamine and methacholine. *J Appl Physiol* (1983) **54**: 821–826.

154. Malo JL, Gauthier R, Lemire L, Cartier A, Ghezzo H, Martin RR: Kinetics of recovery of airway response caused by inhaled histamine. *Am Rev Respir Dis* (1985) **132**: 848–852.

155. Weiss JW, Drazen JM, McFadden ER Jr, *et al.*: Airways constriction in normal humans produced by inhalation of leukotriene D. *JAMA* (1983) **249**: 2814–2817.
156. Griffin M, Weiss WJ, Leich AG, *et al.*: Effects of leukotriene D on the airways in asthma. *N Eng J Med* (1983) **308**: 436–439.
157. Barnes NC, Piper PJ, Costello JF: Comparative effects of inhaled leukotriene C4, leukotriene D4 and histamine in normal human subjects. *Thorax* (1984) **39**: 500–505.
158. O'Hickey SP, Arm JP, Rees PJ, Spur BW, Lee TH: The relative responsiveness to inhaled leukotriene E4, methacholine and histamine in normal and asthmatic subjects. *Eur Resp J* (1988) **1**: 913–917.
159. Arm JP, O'Hickey SP, Spur BW, Lee TH: Airway responsiveness to histamine and leukotriene E4 in subjects with aspirin-induced asthma. *Am Rev Respir Dis* (1989) **140**: 148–153.
160. Bisgaard H, Groth S, Madson F: Bronchial hyperreactivity to leukotriene D4 and histamine in exogenous asthma. *Brit J Med* (1985) **290**: 1468–1471.
161. Walters EH, Parrish RW, Bevan C, Smith AP: Induction of bronchial hypersensitivity: evidence for a role for prostaglandins. *Thorax* (1981) **36**: 571–574.
162. Heaton RW, Henderson AF, Dunlop LS, Costello JF: The influence of pretreatment with prostaglandin $F2_\alpha$ on bronchial sensitivity to inhaled histamine and methacholine in normal subjects. *Brit J Dis Chest* (1984) **78**: 168–174.
163. Walters EH, Bevan C, Parrish RW, Davies BH, Smith AP: Time-dependent effect of prostaglandin E2 inhalation on airway responses to bronchoconstrictor agents in normal subjects. *Thorax* (1982) **37**: 437–442.
164. Fuller RW, Dixon CMS, Dollery CT, Barnes PJ: Prostaglandin D2 potentiates airway responsiveness to histamine and methacholine. *Am Rev Respir Dis* (1986) **133**: 252–254.
165. Black PN, Fuller RW, Taylor GW, Barnes PJ, Dollery CT: Effect of inhaled leukotriene B4 alone and in combination with prostaglandin D2 on bronchial responsiveness to histamine in normal subjects. *Thorax* (1989) **44**: 491–495.
166. Arm JP, Spur BW, Lee TH: The effects of inhaled leukotriene E4 on the histamine airway responsiveness in asthmatic and normal subjects. *J Allergy Clin Immunol* (1988) **82**: 654–660.
167. O'Hickey SP, Hawsworth RJ, Arm JP, Crea AEG, Spur BW, Lee TH: Effect of inhalation of sulphidopeptide leukotrienes on airway responsiveness to histamine in asthmatic and normal subjects. *Thorax* (1990) **45**: 790.
168. Herxheimer H: Antihistamines in bronchial asthma. *Brit J Med* (1949) **2**: 901–904.
169. Popa VT: Effect of an H1-blocker, chlorpheniramine, on inhalation tests with histamine and allergen in allergic asthma. *Chest* (1980) **78**: 442–451.
170. Holgate ST, Emanuel MB, Howeth PH: Astemazole and other antihistaminic drug treatment of asthma. *J Allergy Clin Immunol* (1985) **76**: 375–380.
171. Rafferty P, Beasley R, Holgate ST: The contribution of histamine to immediate bronchoconstriction provoked by inhaled allergen and adenosine 5′ monophosphate in atopic asthma. *Am Rev Respir Dis* (1987) **136**: 369–373.
172. Curzen N, Rafferty P, Holgate ST: Effects of a cyclo-oxygenase inhibitor, flurbiprofen, and an H1-receptor antagonist, terfenadine, alone and in combination on allergen induced immediate bronchoconstriction in man. *Thorax* (1987) **42**: 946–952.
173. Eiser NM, Hayhurst M, Denman W: The contribution of histamine and leukotriene release to the production of early and late asthmatic responses to antigen. *Am Rev Respir Dis* (1989) **139**: A462.
174. Lai CKW, Beasley R, Holgate ST: The effect of an increase in inhaled allergen dose after terfenadine on the occurrence and magnitude of the late asthmatic response. *Clin Exp Allergy* (1989) **19**: 209–216.
175. Eiser NM: Effect of a β_2-adrenergic agonist and a histamine H_1-receptor antagonist on the late asthmatic response to inhaled antigen. *Resp Med* (1991) **85**: 393–399.
176. Hartley JPR, Nogrady SG: Effect of an inhaled antihistamine on exercise-induced asthma. *Thorax* (1980) **35**: 675–679.
177. Eiser NM: The role of histamine in bronchospasm in man, MD Thesis, London University (1983).

178. Finnerty JP, Holgate ST: Evidence for the roles of histamine and prostaglandins as mediators in exercise-induced asthma: the inhibitory effect of terfenadine and flurbiprofen alone and in combination. *Eur Respir J* (1990) **3**: 540–547.

179. Badier M, Beaumont D, Orehek J: Attenuation of hyperventilation-induced bronchospasm by terfenadine: a new antihistamine. *J Allergy Clin Immunol* (1988) **81**: 437–440.

180. Bewtra AK, Hopp RJ, Nair NM, Townley RG: Effect of terfenadine on cold air-induced bronchospasm. *Ann Allergy* (1989) **62**: 299–301.

181. Finnerty JP, Wilmot C, Holgate ST: Inhibition of hypertonic saline-induced bronchoconstriction by terfenadine and flurbiprofen. *Am Rev Respir Dis* (1989) **140**: 593–597.

182. Finney MJB, Anderson SD, Black JL: Terfenadine modifies airway narrowing induced by the inhalation of nonisotonic aerosols in subjects with asthma. *Am Rev Respir Dis* (1990) **141**: 1151–1157.

183. Eiser NM: Histamine antagonists and asthma. *Pharmac Ther* (1982) **17**: 239–250.

184. Eiser NM, Shelton DM: Effect of an H1-receptor antagonist, terfenadine, on nocturnal asthma. *Am Rev Respir Dis* (1989) **139**: A141.

185. Teale C, Morrison JFJ, Pearson SB: Terfenadine in nocturnal asthma. *Thorax* (1990) **45**: 795.

186. Kubo N, Shirakawa O, Kuno T, Tanaka C: Antimuscarinic effects of antihistamines: quantitative evaluation by receptor binding assay. *Japan J Pharmacol* (1987) **43**: 277–282.

187. Bousquet J, Lebel B, Chanal I, Morel Z, Michel F-B: Antiallergic activity of H1-receptor antagonists assessed by nasal challenge. *J Allergy Clin Immunol* (1988) **82**: 881–887.

17

Kinins

DAVID PROUD

INTRODUCTION

Kinins are potent vasoactive peptides that are generated during inflammatory events *in vivo*. Although the history of the kallikrein–kinin system can be traced back to the observation of Abelous and Bardier in 1909 that intravenous injection into the dog of an alcohol-insoluble fraction of human urine caused a pronounced, but reversible, fall in systolic blood pressure,[1] it was not until almost two decades later that Frey[2] established that the substance responsible for this effect was non-dialysable and thermolabile. Further studies, in collaboration with Werle and Kraut, showed that a similar activity was present in blood and in the pancreas.[3,4] On the incorrect assumption that the active substance, in each case, was identical and was derived from the pancreas, it was named kallikrein (from the Greek 'kallikreas', meaning pancreas). Werle subsequently demonstrated that kallikrein enzymatically released a substance from plasma that was capable of contracting smooth muscle.[5] This generated material was later named 'kallidin'. Working independently, Rocha e Silva and colleagues, coined the name 'bradykinin' for a similar smooth muscle spasmogen liberated from plasma by the action of either trypsin or the venom of the snake, *Bothrops jararaca*.[6]

In the years since these pioneering studies, major progress has been made in delineating the pharmacologic properties of kinins and in understanding the biochemical pathways by which these peptides are formed and metabolized in humans. Moreover, evidence has accumulated to suggest that kinins may be important mediators during inflammatory diseases of the airways, such as asthma. The present chapter will review our current knowledge of the potential role of kinins in airway inflammation.

ASTHMA: BASIC MECHANISMS AND CLINICAL MANAGEMENT (2nd Edn)
ISBN 0-12-079026-2

STRUCTURE, FORMATION AND METABOLISM

Kinins are generated from α_2-globulin precursor proteins, called kininogens. The two precursors found in humans, high molecular weight (HMW) kininogen and low molecular weight (LMW) kininogen, are derived from a single gene as a consequence of alternative RNA splicing.[7] Kininogens are synthesized in the liver. HMW kininogen represents approximately one-third of the kininogen in blood, while LMW kininogen constitutes the remaining two-thirds. Both kininogens gain access to the interstitium and the lymph and extravascular LMW kininogen has also been detected in the distal nephron.[8]

Three kinins have been reported to exist in humans: bradykinin, lysyslbradykinin (kallidin), amd methionyllysylbradykinin. All three peptides contain the C-terminal nonapeptide sequence of bradykinin (Fig.17.1). It is now accepted, however, that methionyllysylbradykinin is a laboratory artefact that is found only under conditions of acidification when it is produced, by the action of pepsin, from kininogen that has already undergone limited hydrolysis.[9] Thus, bradykinin and lysylbradykinin are the physiologically relevant kinins in humans.

Enzymes that release kinins from kininogens are generally referred to as kininogenases. Although plasmin, trypsin and mast cell tryptase[10] are capable of generating bradykinin *in vitro*, these enzymes are likely to play little role in kinin generation *in vivo*. The historical name, kallikrein, is still used to refer to the most physiologically important kininogenases from blood (plasma kallikrein) and from the major exocrine organs (tissue, or glandular, kallikrein). This shared nomenclature is unfortunate, since the plasma and tissue enzymes are derived from different genes and are biochemically and immunologically distinct from each other. Plasma kallikrein is synthesized in the liver

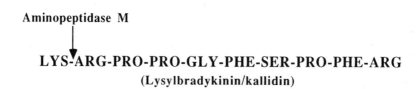

Aminopeptidase M

LYS-ARG-PRO-PRO-GLY-PHE-SER-PRO-PHE-ARG
(Lysylbradykinin/kallidin)

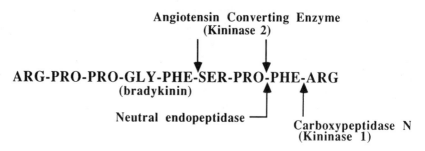

Angiotensin Converting Enzyme
(Kininase 2)

ARG-PRO-PRO-GLY-PHE-SER-PRO-PHE-ARG
(bradykinin)

Neutral endopeptidase ———

Carboxypeptidase N
(Kininase 1)

Fig. 17.1 Structure of bradykinin and lysylbradykinin and the sites of hydrolysis of these peptides by some of the major kininases.

and exists in the blood as a single chain, γ-globulin zymogen, prekallikrein, that circulates in a complex with HMW kininogen.[11] Activation of prekallikrein to kallikrein *in vivo* occurs principally as a result of the factor XII-dependent process, referred to as contact activation.[12] When kallikrein is generated by the interaction of prekallikrein, HMW kininogen and factor XII with certain negatively charged surfaces, this enzyme acts on its preferred substrate, HMW kininogen, to release bradykinin.[13] The kallikrein is then rapidly inactivated by the plasma protease inhibitors, C1-inactivator and α_2-macroglobulin. While plasma kallikrein generates bradykinin, tissue kallikreins are unique in that they hydrolyse two dissimilar bonds within either HMW or LMW kininogen to release lysylbradykinin. Although originally believed to be present only in the major exocrine organs, tissue kallikreins are acidic glycoproteins that are now known to enjoy a widespread distribution in exocrine and endocrine tissues.[12] Tissue kallikrein has also been reported to be present in both the upper and lower airways in humans.[14,15] There are no effective, naturally occurring inhibitors of tissue kallikreins in humans. The ability of tissue kallikrein to generate kinins from both HMW and LMW kininogens provides it with more available substrate than plasma kallikrein. This, together with its resistance to inhibition, suggests that tissue kallikreins may be of particular importance in kinin generation in inflammatory events.

Once bradykinin and lysylbradykinin are generated *in vivo*, metabolic destruction is a major mechanism for regulating their actions. Virtually all tissues and biological fluids contain enzymes (kininases) that are capable of degrading kinins.[16] Hydrolysis of any of the peptide bonds within the bradykinin moiety leads to a loss of biological activity. Although peptidases derived from all of the major classes of proteolytic enzymes can degrade kinins, those kininases that are believed to be the most important regulators of these peptides during airway inflammation in humans are shown in Fig.17.1. These peptidases are either derived from plasma and enter the airway mucosa by transudation during inflammatory events or are present on the surface of epithelial or endothelial cells. Hydrolysis of kinins by plasma peptidases has been reasonably well delineated but the full profile of peptidases on cells in the airways remains to be determined. An aminopeptidase M-like enzyme has been detected in airway secretions during allergic inflammation.[17] This enzyme does not result in the loss of biological activity of kinins but converts lysylbradykinin to bradykinin by removal of the N-terminal lysine residue. Aminopeptidase M in the airway originates, in part, from plasma but a similar activity is also present on the surface of respiratory epithelial cells (Proud D, Ward PE, unpublished observations). The major plasma enzymes that would contribute to kinin degradation are carboxypeptidase N (Kininase 1) and angiotensin-converting enzyme (ACE; Kininase 2). Carboxypeptidase N-like activity has been shown to enter airway secretions from plasma during allergic inflammation[17] and degrades kinins by removal of the C-terminal arginine residue to produce the B_1 kinin receptor agonists, des(Arg^9)-bradykinin and des(Arg^{10})lysylbradykinin (see below). Lower levels of ACE also enter the nasal mucosa from plasma,[17] although the major source of this enzyme is the endothelial cell surface. ACE degrades kinins by sequential removal of C-terminal dipeptides and will also degrade des(Arg) kinins by removal of the C-terminal tripeptide. Finally, a lot of attention has focused on the potential role of neutral endopeptidase in peptide hydrolysis during airway inflammation. This peptidase is present on the surface of the respiratory epithelial cell and hydrolyses kinins at the same site as ACE to release the C-terminal dipeptide.[18]

GENERAL PHARMACOLOGICAL PROPERTIES

Bradykinin and lysylbradykinin display essentially the same pharmacological properties. Some minor differences in the potencies of these two peptides are seen in intact
tissue preparations but this probably reflects minor variations in their rates of metabolism. Our knowledge of the receptor subtypes by which kinins act is still developing. In
1980, however, Regoli and Barabé[19] defined two types of receptors. On the B_1 kinin
receptor the kinin metabolites des(Arg⁹)bradykinin and des(Arg¹⁰lysylbradykinin are
more potent than the parent peptides and their actions can be antagonized by Leu⁸-
des(Arg⁹)bradykinin. On the B_2-receptor, these metabolites are essentially inactive. The
development and use of the first competitive antagonists of the actions of bradykinin at
the B_2-receptor[20] have led several investigators to suggest that other receptor subtypes
may remain to be defined.[21] To date, it appears as though the B_1 receptor does not play
a prominent role in the actions of kinins in humans.

In general, the pharmacological properties of kinins would suggest that they are ideal
mediators of inflammation.[21] Bradykinin and lysylbradykinin contract most types of
intestinal smooth muscle and either contract or have no effect on isolated airway smooth
muscle, depending on the species from which the tissue is derived (see below). Kinins
may contract or relax isolated vascular smooth muscle depending on the vessel being
examined. *In vivo,* however, the net effect of kinins is to cause peripheral vasodilation and
hypotension. In addition to being vasodilators, bradykinin and lysylbradykinin are
approximately 100-fold more potent than histamine in increasing the permeability of
postcapillary venules and, as a direct consequence of this, they are potent inducers of
oedema. Kinins are also potent stimulators of epithelial ion transport and can stimulate
sensory Aδ and C-fibres to cause pain and hyperalgesia. Moreover, they are clearly
capable of stimulating the release of biologically active lipids, such as prostaglandins
and platelet-activating factor, from a variety of cell types.[21]

KININ FORMATION IN AIRWAY INFLAMMATION

The first direct evidence that kinins could be generated during airway inflammation in
humans was provided using a model of nasal provocation with allergen in which
inflammatory mediators could be measured in secretions recovered by lavage. Insuffla-
tion of an appropriate allergen into the nasal cavity of allergic subjects resulted in the
immediate manifestation of sneezing, nasal congestion and rhinorrhoea. Concomitant
with this symptomatic response, strikingly increased levels of kinins could be measured
in recovered lavages.[22] Increased kinin generation correlated with symptoms and with
increases in other inflammatory mediators, including histamine. Kinin generation was
not observed following allergen challenge of non-allergic subjects nor when allergic
subjects were challenged with a non-relevant allergen. HPLC analysis showed that both
bradykinin and lysylbradykinin were produced. Following these initial observations,
kinin generation has now been documented in a variety of inflammatory conditions of
the upper airways, including the late-phase allergic response,[23] and both experimental
and naturally occurring viral infections.[24,25] Although the more limited accessibility of

the lower airways has made studies of kinin generation more difficult than in the upper airways, there is now also good evidence that increased kinin formation occurs during asthmatic reactions. Kinin levels were first shown to be elevated in bronchoalveolar lavage fluids from asthmatics who either had active symptoms of asthma or were responding to aerosolized allergen challenge when compared to lavage samples from normal subjects. The increased concentrations of free kinins correlated with the presence of increased levels of tissue kallikrein in lavages from asthmatics.[15] The identity of the enzyme in lavages as authentic tissue kallikrein was established by immunological criteria and by its ability to generate lysylbradykinin from kininogen (Fig. 17.2). More recently, segmental challenge has been used to demonstrate that allergen challenge of asthmatic subjects results in increased kinin generation compared to saline challenge of the same subjects,[26,27] and to show that increased levels of kinins are also detected 19 h after allergen challenge of asthmatics.[27]

EFFECTS OF KININS ON AIRWAYS

The effect of bradykinin on isolated airway smooth muscle varies depending on the species being examined. Kinins constrict isolated guinea-pig tracheal rings via a prostaglandin-dependent pathway but have no effect on airways from rabbits, rat or dogs.[28,29] At best, bradykinin is a weak constrictor of isolated human airways,[29–31] although Simonsson et al.[31] reported an enhanced sensitivity of bronchial strips taken from patients with chronic airflow obstruction.

The effects of bradykinin on human airway function in vivo depend upon the route of administration. When given intravenously, bradykinin causes a modest, transient fall in airway function that has been suggested to be due to alveolar duct constriction.[30] When given by inhalation, however, several investigators have now shown that bradykinin is a potent bronchoconstrictor in asthmatic, but not in normal, subjects.[31–35] The aerosolized peptide also induces retrosternal discomfort and cough in all subjects.[34] The bronchoconstrictor action of kinins in asthmatics is, apparently, mediated via B_2 kinin receptors, since bradykinin and lysylbradykinin are potent bronchoconstrictors, while the B_1-agonist, des(Arg^9)bradykinin, is inactive.[36] Bradykinin-induced bronchoconstriction is not inhibited by administration of cyclooxygenase inhibitors[34,35] or an antihistamine.[35] This latter observation is consistent with observations in the upper airways, where bradykinin induces increased vascular permeability, symptoms of rhinitis and a sore throat, regardless of atopic status, but does not induce histamine release.[37] Although the exact mechanism by which bradykinin induces bronchoconstriction remains to be elucidated, several pieces of evidence imply that neural reflexes are involved. The lack of a pronounced direct effect of bradykinin on isolated smooth muscle suggest the involvement of indirect pathways and the ability of bradykinin to evoke cough indicates that sensory nerves can be stimulated. Following bradykinin evoked bronchoconstriction there is a decreased sensitivity to subsequent challenges with either bradykinin or histamine,[34] suggesting a common, tachyphylactic pathway for these two mediators. Moreover, the ability of sodium cromoglycate and nedocromil sodium[38] to inhibit bradykinin-induced bronchoconstriction has been interpreted as supporting a role for sensory nerve stimulation, while the inhibitory effect of ipratroprium bromide[34] indicates that bradykinin's effects are mediated in part by a cholinergic reflex. These data, together with the observation that bradykinin causes bronchoconstriction in dogs by vagal reflex following stimulation of sensory C-fibres,[39] suggest that the bronchoconstrictor actions of bradykinin in humans may also involve C-fibre stimulation and the concomitant release of neuropeptides.

In addition to affecting bronchial tone, increased kinin generation during asthmatic reactions could lead to: (a) an increase in ciliary beat frequency via a prostaglandin

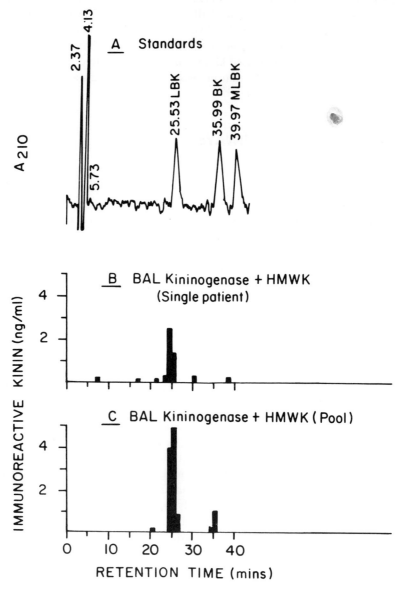

Fig. 17.2 Demonstration that bronchial tissue kallikrein generates lysylbradykinin upon incubation with highly purified human high molecular weight kininogen. The elution of standard lysylbradykinin (LBK), bradykinin (BK) and methionyllysylbradykinin (MLBK) are shown on the upper panel. (Reproduced from ref. 15, with permission.)

dependent pathway,[40] and (b) an increase in the volume of airway secretions. Lysyl-bradykinin has been shown to increase the production of respiratory mucus macromolecules in canine tracheal explants,[41] while bradykinin has been shown to increase canine tracheal gland secretion *in vivo* by a reflex mechanism after stimulation of bronchial C-fibres.[42] Moreover, since bradykinin can stimulate chloride secretion across the respiratory epithelium,[43,44] transepithelial water transport could also contribute to increased airway secretions. Kinins could also increase the volume of secretions as a result of increased vascular permeability and transudation of plasma. Although there have been no studies confirming that this occurs following kinin challenge of the lower airways *in vivo* in humans, there is clear evidence to support this concept in the upper airways.[37]

SUMMARY

In the last decade, there has been a renewed interest in the role of kinins in human airway inflammation. Our increased understanding of the biochemistry of the human kallikrein–kinin system has permitted the development of improved methods for the measurement of its components. With these improved methodologies, important evidence has been obtained documenting that kinin generation occurs in a variety of inflammatory reactions of the human airways, including asthma. Moreover, it has proven possible to delineate, to some degree, the mechanisms regulating kinin formation and destruction during inflammatory reactions *in vivo*.[12] The correlation between kinin generation and symptoms of inflammation, together with the demonstration that administration of kinins to the airway mucosa can induce relevant symptoms, provides strong circumstantial support for a role of kinins in the pathogenesis of diseases such as asthma. To establish definitively the contribution of kinins to asthma, however, it will clearly be necessary to be able to use specific pharmacological interventions to block their actions and demonstrate a concomitant effect on symptoms. The development of the first competitive kinin antagonists[20] appeared to provide an exciting opportunity to perform such interventive studies. Initial observations in the sheep were encouraging, in that a bradykinin antagonist inhibited both antigen-induced hyperreactivity and the late phase response.[45,46] Administration of the same compound to the upper airways of humans, however, failed to block the effects of a challenge with bradykinin.[47] This early compound suffered from a relatively low affinity for the kinin receptor and was, in addition, readily susceptible to hydrolysis by peptidases. The results obtained with these first generation antagonists, however, have led several laboratories to generate compounds with higher affinities and improved metabolic stabilities. It seems likely, therefore, that the next few years will provide exciting opportunities to delineate the role of kinins in the pathogenesis of asthma and other inflammatory diseases of the human airways.

ACKNOWLEDGEMENTS

Dr Proud acknowledges support from grant number HL 32272 from the National Institutes of Health. This is publication number 70 from the Johns Hopkins Asthma and Allergy Center.

REFERENCES

1. Abelous JE, Bardier E: Les substance hypotensives de l'urine humaine normale. *Compt Rend Soc Biol* (1909) **66**: 511–512.
2. Frey EK: Zusammenhange zwischen herzarbeit und nierentatigheit. *Arch Klin Chir* (1926) **142**: 663–669.
3. Frey EK, Kraut H: Ein neues kreislaufhormon und seine wirkung. *Arch Exp Path Pharm* (1928) **133**: 1–56.
4. Kraut H, Frey EK, Werle E: Der nachweis eines kreislaufhormons in der pankreasdrüse. *Hoppe-Seyler's Z Physiol Chem* (1930) **189**: 97–106.
5. Werle E, Götze W, Keppler A: Über die wirkung des kallikreins auf den isolierten darm und uber eine neue darmkontrahierende substanz. *Biochem Z* (1937) **281**: 217–233.
6. Roche e Silva M, Beraldo WT, Rosenfeld G: Bradykinin, a hypotensive and smooth muscle stimulating factor released for plasma globulin by snake venoms and by trypsin. *Am J Physiol* (1949) **156**: 261–273.
7. Kitamura N, Kitagawa H, Fukushima D, Takagaki Y, Miyata T, Nakanishi S: Structural organization of the human kininogen gene and a model for its evolution. *J Biol Chem* (1985) **260**: 8610–8617.
8. Proud D, Perkins M, Pierce JV, *et al.*: Characterization and localization of human renal kininogen. *J Biol Chem* (1981) **256**: 16034–16039.
9. Guimaraes JA, Pierce JV, Hial V, Pisano JJ: Methionyl-lysylbradykinin: the kinin released by pepsin from human kininogens. *Adv Exp Med Biol* (1976) **70**: 265–269.
10. Proud D, Siekierski ES, Bailey GS: Identification of human lung mast cell kininogenase as tryptase and relevance of tryptase kininogenase activity. *Biochem Pharmacol* (1987) **37**: 1473–1480.
11. Mandle RJ, Jr, Colman RW, Kaplan AP: Identification of prekallikrein and HMW-kininogen as a circulating complex in human plasma. *Proc Natl Acad Sci USA* (1976) **73**: 4179–4183.
12. Proud D, Kaplan AP: Kinin formation: Mechanisms and role in inflammatory disorders. *Annu Rev Immunol* (1988) **6**: 49–83.
13. Pierce JV, Guimaraes JA: Further characterization of highly purified human plasma kininogens. In Pisano JJ, Austen KF (eds) *Chemistry and Biology of the Kallikrien–Kinin System in Health and Disease.* Washington DC, DHEW Publ. No.(NIH)76-791, 1976, pp 121–127.
14. Baumgarten CR, Nichols RC, Naclerio RM, Proud D: Concentrations of glandular kallikrein in human nasal secretions increase during experimentally-induced allergic rhinitis. *J Immunol* (1986) **137**: 1323–1328.
15. Christiansen SC, Proud D, Cochrane CG: Detection of tissue kallikrein in the bronchoalveolar lavage fluids of asthmatic subjects. *J Clin Invest* (1987) **79**: 188–197.
16. Erdos EG: Kininases. In Erdos EG (ed) *Handbook of Experimental Pharmacology. Bradykinin, Kallidin and Kallikrein.* Vol. 25 (Suppl), New York, Springer-Verlag, 1979, pp 427–487.
17. Proud D, Baumgarten CR, Naclerio RM, Ward PE: Kinin metabolism in nasal secretions during experimentally-induced allergic rhinitis. *J Immunol* (1987) **138**: 428–434.
18. Erdos EG, Skidgel RA: Neutral endopeptidase 24.11 (enkephalinase) and related regulators of peptide hormones. *FASEB J* (1989) **3**: 145–151.
19. Regoli D, Barabé J: Pharmacology of bradykinin and related peptides. *Pharmacol Rev* (1980) **32**: 1–46.
20. Vavrek RJ, Stewart JM: Competitive antagonists of bradykinin. *Peptides* (1985) **6**: 161–164.
21. Bathon JM, Proud D: Bradykinin antagonists. *Annu Rev Pharmacol Toxicol* (1991) **31**: 129–162.
22. Proud D, Togias A, Naclerio RM, Crush SA, Norman PS, Lichtenstein LM: Kinins are generated *in vivo* following nasal airway challenge of allergic individuals with allergen. *J Clin Invest* (1983) **72**: 1678–1685.
23. Naclerio RM, Proud D, Togias AG, *et al.*: Inflammatory mediators in late antigen-induced rhinitis. *N Engl J Med* (1985) **313**: 65–70.
24. Naclerio RM, Proud D, Lichtenstein LM, *et al.*: Kinins are generated during experimental rhinovirus colds. *J Infect Dis* (1987) **157**: 133–142.
25. Proud D, Naclerio RM, Gwaltney JM, Jr, Hendley JO: Kinins are generated in nasal secretions during natural rhinovirus colds. *J Infect Dis* (1990) **161**: 120–123.

26. Christiansen SC, Proud D, Sarnoff RB, Cochrane CG, Zuraw BL: Human bronchial kallikrein (HBK) in bronchoalveolar lavage (BAL) fluid following local allergen challenge. *J Allergy Clin Immunol* (1989) **83**: 285 (Abstract).

27. Liu M, Hubbard WC, Proud D, *et al.*: Immediate and late inflammatory responses to ragweed antigen challenge of the peripheral airways in allergic asthmatics: Cellular, mediator, and permeability changes. *Am Rev Respir Dis* (1991) **144**: 51–58.

28. Collier HOJ: The action and antagonism of kinins on bronchioles. *Ann NY Acad Sci* (1963) **104**: 290–298.

29. Bhoola KD, Collier HOJ, Schachter M, Shorley PG: Actions of some peptides on bronchial muscle. *Br J Pharmacol* (1962) **19**: 190–197.

30. Newball HH, Keiser HR, Webster ME, Pisano JJ: Effects of bradykinin on human airways. In Pisano JJ, Austen KF (eds) *Chemistry and Biology of the Kallikrein–Kinin System in Health and Disease*. Washington DC, DHEW Publ. No. (NIH)76-791, 1976, pp 505–511.

31. Simonsson BG, Skoogh B-E, Bergh NP, Andersson R, Svedmyr N: *In vivo* and *in vitro* effects of bradykinin on bronchial motor tone in normal subjects and patients with airway obstruction. *Respiration* (1973) **30**: 378–388.

32. Herxheimer H, Stresemann E: The effects of bradykinin aerosol in guinea pigs and man. *J Physiol (Lond)* (1961) **158**: 38–39.

33. Varonier HS, Panzani R: The effect of inhalation of bradykinin on healthy and atopic (asthmatic) children. *Int Arch Allergy* (1968) **34**: 293–296.

34. Fuller RW, Dixon CMS, Cuss FMC, Barnes PJ: Bradykinin-induced bronchoconstriction in humans. Mode of action. *Am Rev Respir Dis* (1987) **135**: 176–180.

35. Polosa R, Phillips GD, Lai CKW, Holgate ST: Contribution of histamine and prostanoids to bronchoconstriction provoked by inhaled bradykinin in atopic asthma. *Allergy* (1990) **45**: 174–182.

36. Polosa R, Holgate ST: Comparative airway response to inhaled bradykinin, kallidin, and [des-Arg⁹]bradykinin in normal and asthmatic subjects. *Am Rev Respir Dis* (1990) **142**: 1367–1371.

37. Proud D, Reynolds CJ, LaCapra S, Kagey-Sobotka A, Lichtenstein LM, Naclerio RM: Nasal provocation with bradykinin induces symptoms of rhinitis and a sore throat. *Am Rev Respir Dis* (1988) **137**: 613–616.

38. Dixon CMS, Barnes PJ: Bradykinin-induced bronchoconstriction: inhibition by nedocromil sodium and sodium cromoglycate. *Br J Clin Pharmacol* (1989) **27**: 831–836.

39. Kaufman MP, Coleridge HM, Coleridge JCG, Baker DG: Bradykinin stimulates afferent vagal C-fibers in intrapulmonary airways of dogs. *J Appl Physiol* (1980) **48**: 511–517.

40. Tamaoki J, Kobayashi K, Saki N, Chiyotani A, Kanemura T, Takizawa T: Effect of bradykinin on airway ciliary motility and its modulation by neutral endopeptidase. *Am Rev Respir Dis* (1989) **140**: 430–435.

41. Baker AP, Hillegass LM, Holden DA, Smith WJ: Effect of kallidin, substance P, and other basic polypeptides on the production of respiratory macromolecules. *Am Rev Respir Dis* (1977) **115**: 811–817.

42. Davis B, Roberts AM, Coleridge HM, Coleridge JCG: Reflex tracheal gland secretion evoked by stimulation of bronchial C-fibers in dogs. *J Appl Physiol* (1982) **53**: 985–991.

43. Leikauf GD, Ueki IF, Nadel JA, Widdicombe JH: Bradykinin stimulates Cl secretion and prostaglandin E_2 release by canine tracheal epithelium. *Am J Physiol* (1986) **248**: F48–F55.

44. Widdicombe JH, Coleman DL, Finkbeiner WE, Tuet IK: Electrical properties of monolayers cultured from cells of human tracheal mucosa. *J Appl Physiol* (1985) **58**: 1729–1735.

45. Soler M, Sielczak M, Abraham WM: A bradykinin-antagonist blocks antigen-induced airway hyperresponsiveness and inflammation in sheep. *Pulmonary Pharmacol* (1990) **3**: 9–15.

46. Abraham WM, Burch RM, Farmer SG, Sielczak MW, Ahmed A, Cortes A: Effects of a bradykinin antagonist in allergen-induced pulmonary late responses and inflammation. *Am Rev Respir Dis* (1990) **141**: A116 (Abstract).

47. Pongracic JA, Naclerio RM, Reynolds CJ, Proud D: A competitive kinin receptor antagonist, [DArg,⁰Hyp³, DPhe⁷]-bradykinin, does not affect the response to nasal provocation with bradykinin. *Br J Clin Pharmacol* (1991) **31**: 287–294.

Adenosine, a Positive Modulator of the Asthmatic Response

RICCARDO POLOSA, WAI H. NG, AND MARTIN K. CHURCH

INTRODUCTION

Asthma is a complex disease which defies a clear definition let alone a good understanding of its mechanisms. Today much attention is being focused on the inflammatory events that underly the disease. However, we must also remember that it is the sudden exacerbation of symptoms which characterizes an asthma attack and which is the potentially life-threatening aspect of the disease. In order to investigate the mechanisms of bronchoconstriction in asthma it is necessary to use a variety of provocation approaches in addition to allergen.

One such form of bronchoconstriction is that induced by adenosine which was first described by Cushley et al. in 1983.[1] The observation that adenosine and its parent nucleotide, adenosine 5' monophosphate (AMP) produce a strong bronchoconstriction in asthmatic subjects, may produce a similar response in atopic subjects who are not asthmatic but not in subjects who show neither atopy nor asthma has led to its use in investigating the mechanisms of asthma and its association with allergic disease.

THE BIOCHEMICAL PHARMACOLOGY OF ADENOSINE

Adenosine is a naturally occurring purine nucleoside which promotes both intra- and extra-cellular physiological functions in a wide variety of different cell systems, the latter being effected through interaction with specific cell surface receptors (or purinoceptors).[2] Adenosine production is greatly increased under conditions of energy deficit,[3]

ASTHMA: BASIC MECHANISMS AND CLINICAL MANAGEMENT (2nd Edn)
ISBN 0-12-079026-2

tissue hypoxia[4] and following immunological activation.[5] Evidence that adenosine release may be increased under conditions that may prevail in areas of inflammation and in the asthmatic lung has been obtained from studies in allergic asthmatic subjects which have demonstrated significantly raised levels of plasma adenosine within minutes of challenge with allergen.[6,7]

Adenosine at extracellular sites behaves as an autocoid since it produces its pharmacological effects by stimulating cell surface P_1 purinoceptors to either decrease (A_1) or increase (A_2) intracellular levels of cyclic $3',5'$-AMP.[2] A_1- and A_2-receptors are defined by a unique agonist potency series of adenosine analogues to inhibit or stimulate adenylate cyclase, A_1-purinoceptors being stimulated by L-N^6-phenylisopropyladenosine (L-PIA) > adenosine > $5'$-N-ethylcarboxamidoadenosine (NECA) whilst the A_2-purinoceptors have a potency series of NECA > adenosine > L-PIA.[8] A third adenosine receptor subtype (A_3) controlling the function of calcium-related mechanisms has also been proposed.[9] In addition to cell surface receptors, there is also an intracellular P-site that is activated by adenosine analogues with an intact purine moiety such as $2'$-deoxyadenosine, $2',5'$-dideoxyadenosine, and 9-β-D-arabinofuranosyladenine.

THE EFFECT OF ADENOSINE ON HUMAN AIRWAYS

A possible modulatory effect of adenosine on airways tone was initially suggested by Coleman[10] and Fredholm et al.[11] when they demonstrated that this nucleoside caused a transient contraction followed by a more powerful and sustained relaxation in guinea-pig tracheal smooth muscle in vitro. Prompted by these findings, adenosine was investigated for its in vivo effects on human airways. Whilst inhalation of adenosine aerosols in concentrations up to 6.7 mg/ml was shown to have no detectable effect on airway calibre in normal subjects, when administered to patients with asthma it resulted in concentration-related bronchoconstriction rather than the expected bronchodilation.[1] A degree of selectivity for the adenine moiety was suggested by the finding that the purine nucleoside guanosine had no measurable effect on airways function in either normal or asthmatic subjects when inhaled over the same concentration range. However, inhalation of the adenosine nucleotides, AMP and adenosine diphosphate (ADP), in equivalent molar concentrations as adenosine, produced almost identical effects on the airways whereas the adenosine deamination product, inosine, was without effect.[7] Further evidence that adenosine-induced bronchoconstriction is a specific effect and not due to non-specific irritation of the airways is provided by the demonstration that theophylline, an antagonist at extracellular adenosine receptors at therapeutic concentrations, had a significant protective effect against adenosine and histamine challenge in asthmatic subjects, being two to three times more effective against adenosine than histamine.[12,13] Moreover, the adenosine uptake blocker dipyridamole, when administered by inhalation, also protected against adenosine challenge suggesting that adenosine does exert its effects by a cell surface receptor-mediated mechanism.[14]

When administered as an inhaled aerosol to allergic[1] or non-allergic[15] asthmatic subjects, adenosine provokes bronchoconstriction of rapid onset reaching maximum 2–5 min after challenge and then gradually recovering over the subsequent 45–60 min. Following AMP and ADP, the time course of bronchoconstriction is almost identical to that following adenosine inhalation. Since both nucleotides are rapidly dephosphory-lated to yield adenosine,[3] the airway effects of AMP and ADP are likely to be mediated following their hydrolysis to the purine nucleoside.[16] Because AMP is more soluble than adenosine in aqueous solvents, many of the ensuing *in vivo* studies in humans have utilized this nucleotide as the bronchoprovocative agent rather than adenosine itself.

THE MECHANISM OF ACTION OF ADENOSINE-INDUCED BRONCHOCONSTRICTION

Direct effects of adenosine on airway smooth muscle

Despite much research over the past decade, the mechanism by which adenosine mediates bronchoconstriction in asthmatic subjects is still not clear. Although initial studies with isolated guinea-pig tracheal tissue suggested that adenosine produced only relaxation in this tissue *in vitro*, subsequent studies by many groups have demonstrated that under certain conditions adenosine and its analogues can produce contraction. For example, several groups have reported a biphasic response to adenosine which was dependent on concentration: guinea-pig isolated airways preparations contracting in response to submicromolar concentrations and relaxing at higher concentrations.[17–20] In contrast, in guinea-pig whole isolated perfused lung, adenosine was reported to produce consistent bronchoconstriction,[21,22] the response being enhanced by prior sensitization of the animal to ovalbumin.[22] Similarly, in asthmatic or non-asthmatic human airways tissue, adenosine is reported to produce contraction, albeit only weakly.[23–25] The relative potency order of adenosine analogues in producing this response was NECA > adenosine > L-PIA suggesting an A_2-receptor mediated action.[26] Of great interest, however, is the recent finding by Bjorck *et al.* that bronchi from asthmatic subjects were more sensitive to adenosine than those prepared from non-asthmatic subjects in terms of both a lower threshold and a larger maximal amplitude of response, whereas the concentration–response lines for histamine and leukotriene (LT) C_4 were identical in these two groups.[27] The authors speculated that the increased sensitivity to adenosine in bronchi from asthmatics was specifically related to bronchial hyperrespon-siveness *in vivo*.

However, although adenosine is a weak contractile agonist on human airways tissue *in vitro*, it is unlikely that adenosine acts directly on smooth muscle cells, but indirectly through activation of specific receptors on intermediary inflammatory cells such as mast cells and basophils, or on afferent nerve endings.

Evidence for the involvement of mast cell mediators

That other inflammatory cells and their mediators are involved in the adenosine response is clearly demonstrated by clinical studies that have shown that premedication with histamine H_1 receptor antagonists such as terfenadine and astemizole inhibit by over 80% the bronchoconstriction response to AMP inhalation in asthmatic and atopic subjects.[15,28] Similarly, sodium cromoglycate and nedocromil sodium, both considered as inflammatory cell 'stabilizers',[29] also attenuate the response to AMP challenge,[30–32] although one recent study has reported that sodium cromoglycate competes with NECA for binding sites on plasma membranes prepared from normal human lung suggesting that the former may also act by adenosine receptor inhibition.[33] Furthermore, studies by Daxun et al.[34] have shown tachyphylaxis to repeated AMP challenge that could not be accounted for by a reduced sensitivity to histamine. These results strongly suggest either a depletion of preformed mast cell mediators or the downregulation of adenosine receptors whose stimulation initiates the response. This has also been found in exercise-induced asthma where repeated exercise challenge resulted in a refractoriness to the stimulus. Moreover, Finnerty and Holgate[35] reported that exercise was cross-tachyphylactic with AMP challenge suggesting that both stimuli share at least a common pathway within their mechanism. More recently, we have demonstrated a small, but significant increase in plasma histamine levels in atopic non-asthmatic subjects which was concomitant with the onset of AMP-induced bronchoconstriction.[36] All these studies would suggest that mast cell derived histamine is the major secondary mediator of adenosine-induced bronchoconstriction.

In addition to histamine, it is apparent from studies using cyclooxygenase inhibitors that newly formed mediators such as the prostaglandins may also contribute to the response to adenosine in the lung. Thus pretreatment with indomethacin and flurbiprofen also protected against the effect of AMP bronchoprovocation.[37,38] Interestingly, terfenadine and flurbiprofen are not additive in their effects on adenosine-induced bronchoconstriction, suggesting that prostanoids may modulate the release or action of histamine in some way or vice versa.[38] More direct evidence that newly generated mediators may indeed play a role in adenosine-induced bronchoconstriction comes from the recent study by Narushima et al.[39] who reported a significant increase in plasma levels of thromboxane B_2, but not LTB_4 or LTC_4, 15 min after adenosine challenge.

However, although it is clear from these clinical studies that various mast cell mediators play a role in the response to adenosine, exactly how the purine nucleoside promotes mediator release from mast cells remains to be elucidated. The first indication that adenosine could modulate mediator release from mast cells in vitro was reported by Marquardt et al. in 1978.[40] They found that although adenosine by itself had no effect on mediator release, preincubation with adenosine markedly enhanced histamine release elicited from rat peritoneal mast cells by stimuli as diverse as anti-IgE, concanavalin A, 48/80, and calcium ionophore A23187. Subsequently, these findings have been confirmed by other groups,[41–45] and have been extended to other tissues including guinea-pig lung fragments,[46,47] mouse cultured bone marrow-derived mast cells,[48] and human lung mast cells.[49]

The receptor mediating this enhancement of mediator release from human lung mast cells is thought to be of the A_2 subtype since NECA was more potent than R-PIA at reproducing this effect,[49,50] whereas in rat peritoneal mast cells, Burt and Stanworth[43] reported that PIA was more potent than NECA implying an A_1-receptor mediated action. However, it is becoming increasingly evident that the receptor(s) involved in this augmentation of mediator release may not be of the classical A_1 and A_2 subtypes since there appears to be no linkage with adenylate cyclase activity. For example, we have found in rat peritoneal mast cells that although the prolongation of the cyclic AMP peak, which is observed concomitantly with mediator release, could be inhibited by the potent

P_1-purinoceptor antagonist 8-phenyltheophylline (8-PT), the enhancement of mediator release by adenosine was not affected by this drug.[51] Similarly, in purified human lung mast cells, enhancement of mediator release by adenosine has been demonstrated to occur in the absence of any changes in intracellular cAMP content (Peachell, Lichtenstein, Schleimer, personal communication). These findings therefore suggest that these cellular actions of adenosine are not mediated by adenylate cyclase but by another second messenger system possibly linked to another hitherto undefined adenosine receptor. It has recently been recognized that the actions of adenosine may be mediated by a number of different second messenger mechanisms other that adenylate cyclase. These include activation of potassium conductance,[52] stimulation of guanylate cyclase,[53] modulation of phosphatidylinositol turnover,[54] and modulation of calcium currents.[55] Indeed, the existence of an A_3-purinoceptor linked to calcium currents has recently been proposed in the rat brain.[55]

Apart from a direct enhancement of mediator release elicited by other stimuli, adenosine may also increase the net amount of histamine released indirectly by reversing the inhibition of mediator release by β-adrenergic stimulation. Activation of β-adrenoceptors *in vitro* inhibits mast cell mediator release[56] and in an *in vivo* study with asthmatic subjects, circadian changes in circulating levels of adrenaline have been positively correlated with peak expiratory flow but inversely with plasma histamine.[57] Since adenosine has been reported to have anti-adrenergic effects in many tissues,[58] it is possible that adenosine itself may attenuate the inhibitory effects of adrenaline on mast cells to increase the net histamine released. That this may be the case has been confirmed by a preliminary study performed in our laboratory. We found that preincubation of tonsillar mast cells with adenosine or its stable analogues, NECA and L-PIA, reversed the effects of inhibition produced by adrenaline on immunologically stimulated histamine release.[59] This may therefore represent a further mechanism of action of adenosine.

Evidence for involvement of neuronal reflexes

Enhancement of mast cell mediator release may not be the only mechanism for adenosine within the airways in asthma. There is some evidence that local neural reflexes may also contribute to the bronchoconstrictor action of inhaled adenosine and AMP. Such an action of adenosine in the lung is conceivable since it is now widely acknowledged that purines have modulatory effects on synaptic transmission in both central and peripheral neurone arcs.

In isolated bronchial smooth muscle preparations from rabbits, adenosine has been shown to potentiate the constrictor response to transmural nerve stimulation via an A_2-receptor mechanism,[61] and in an *in vivo* rat model, the changes in airway response provoked by intravenous adenosine has been demonstrated to have an atropine-sensitive component.[62] Furthermore, although we have previously been unable to influence greatly the airway response to adenosine in asthmatics by prior muscarinic receptor blockade,[63] Okayama *et al.*[64] reported inhibition of adenosine bronchoconstriction by atropine and the local anaesthetic, lignocaine. More recently, we have also observed that premedication with the anticholinergic drug ipratropium bromide in a dose that caused profound reduction of the airway response to methacholine, is able to afford a significant protection to the airways against the bronchoconstrictor effect of AMP.[65] This therefore suggests that cholinergic pathways mediate a component of AMP-induced bronchoconstriction.

It is also possible that at least some of the reported protection afforded against the airways effect of AMP and adenosine by sodium cromoglycate and nedocromil sodium is due to the ability of these drugs to inhibit peptidergic neural reflexes in addition to their effect on mast cells.[66] Indeed, recent findings by Pauwels *et al.* suggest that adenosine may be synergistic with the neuropeptide, neurokinin A, in provoking bronchoconstriction in their *in vivo* rat model.[67] Moreover, Manzini and Ballati[68] have reported that the 2-chloroadenosine-induced bronchoconstriction in their *in vivo* guinea-pig model had a capsaicin-sensitive component. Capsaicin is thought to stimulate the release and subsequent depletion of sensory neuropeptides from sensory nerves, thus their findings also implicate the involvement of neuropeptides in the bronchoconstrictory response in the guinea-pig. Similarly, we have recently found that in asthmatic subjects, AMP shows some degree of tachyphylaxis with bradykinin, which is thought to stimulate the release of contractile neuropeptides from sensory nerve endings.[69] Interaction with cholinergic or peptidergic reflexes may therefore play an important role in the mechanism of adenosine-induced asthma.

CONCLUSIONS

In conclusion, the mechanism of action of adenosine-induced bronchoconstriction in atopic and asthmatic subjects, and the relevance of this in asthma is still far from understood. It is clear from clinical studies using selective histamine antagonists that histamine release plays an important role in the response although we were only able to detect a small, but significant, increase in plasma histamine following AMP challenge in asthmatic subjects.[36] It is therefore likely that other mechanisms are involved, of which direct contraction of airway smooth muscle and modulation of pulmonary neuronal reflexes are possibilities. Whether adenosine has a role in asthma, however, is still unclear. The observation by Persson[70] that enprofylline, a methylxanthine reportedly without adenosine antagonist properties,[71] is as effective in asthma as theophylline argues against the original postulate by Fredholm and Sydbom[41] that the mechanism of action of the latter methylxanthine is due to adenosine receptor blockade. Moreover, another observation by Larsson and Sollevi[72] showed that elevation of adenosine levels in asthmatic subjects by intravenous infusion failed to provoke any changes in lung function although it was acknowledged by these authors that higher concentrations of adenosine might have been required to trigger pulmonary effects. However, these findings have to be examined in the light of other recent evidence which do suggest a role for adenosine in asthma. For example, Eagle and Boucher[73] showed that infusion of dipyridamole, a drug that inhibits the facilitated uptake of adenosine, can precipitate severe asthma in susceptible individuals. Additionally, Rosati *et al.*[74] demonstrated that inhalation of AMP increased airway reactivity to methacholine in asthmatic subjects suggesting for the first time that, in addition to its immediate bronchonconstrictory effects when administered by inhalation, adenosine may also be involved in the pathogenesis of bronchial hyperreactivity. The precise role of adenosine in asthma can not be determined however, until potent and specific purinoceptor antagonists become available for study in man. Until then it may only be used as a unique exogenous agent with which to probe the mechanisms of asthma.

REFERENCES

1. Cushley MJ, Tattersfield AE, Holgate ST: Inhaled adenosine and guanosine on airway resistance in normal and asthmatic subjects. *Br J Clin Pharmacol* (1983) **15**: 161–165.
2. Wolff J, Londos C, Cooper DMF: Adenosine receptors and the regulation of adenylate cyclase. *Adv Cyclic Nucleotide Res* (1981) **14**: 199–214.
3. Fain JN, Malbon CC: Regulation of adenylate cyclase by adenosine. *Mol Cell Biochem* (1979) **25**: 143–169.
4. Mentzer RM, Rubio R, Berne RM: Release of adenosine from hypoxic canine lung tissue and its possible role in the pulmonary circulation. *Am J Physiol* (1975) **229**: 1625–1631.
5. Fredholm BB: The release of adenosine from rat lung by antigen and compound 48/80. *Acta Physiol Scand* (1981) **111**: 507–508.
6. Mann JS, Renwick AG, Holgate ST: Antigen bronchial provocation causes an increase in plasma adenosine levels in asthma (Abstract). *Clin Sci* (1983) **65**: 22P.
7. Mann JS, Holgate ST, Renwick AG, Cushley MJ: Airway effects of purine nucleosides and nucleotides and release with bronchial provocation in asthma. *J Appl Physiol* (1986) **61**: 1667–1676.
8. Daly JW: Adenosine receptors: targets for drugs. *J Med Chem* (1982) **25**: 197–207.
9. Ribeiro JA, Sebastiao AM: Adenosine receptor and calcium: basis for proposing a third (A3) adenosine receptor. *Prog Neurobiol* (1986) **26**: 179–209.
10. Coleman RA: Effects of some purine derivatives on the guinea pig trachea and their interaction with drugs that block adenosine uptake. *Br J Pharmacol* (1976) **57**: 51–57.
11. Fredholm BB, Brodin K, Strandberg K: On the mechanism of relaxation of tracheal muscle by theophylline and other cyclic nucleotide phosphodiesterase inhibitors. *Acta Pharmacol Toxicol (Copenh)* (1979) **45**: 336–344.
12. Cushley MJ, Tattersfield AE, Holgate ST: Adenosine induced bronchoconstriction in asthma: antagonism by inhaled theophylline. *Am Rev Respir Dis* (1984) **129**: 380–384.
13. Mann JS, Holgate ST: Specific antagonism of adenosine induced bronchoconstriction in asthma by oral theophylline. *Br J Clin Pharmacol* (1985) **19**: 685–692.
14. Crimi N, Palermo F, Oliveri R, et al.: Enhancing effect of dipyridamole inhalation on adenosine-induced bronchospasm in asthmatic patients. *Allergy* (1988) **43**: 179–183.
15. Phillips GD, Rafferty P, Beasley CRW, Holgate ST: The effect of oral terfenadine on the bronchoconstrictor response to inhaled histamine and adenosine 5'-monophosphate in non-atopic asthma. *Thorax* (1987) **42**: 939–945.
16. Arch JRS, Newsholme EA: The control of the metabolism and the hormonal role of adenosine. In Campbell PW, Aldridge WN (eds) *Essays in Biochemistry*, Vol 14. New York, Academic Press, 1978, pp 82–123.
17. Caparrotta L, Cillo F, Fassina G, Gaion RM: Dual effect of (-)-N6-phenylisopropyladenosine on guinea-pig trachea. *Br J Pharmacol* (1984) **83**: 23–29.
18. Farmer SG, Canning BJ, Wilkins DE: Adenosine-mediated contraction and relaxation of guinea-pig isolated tracheal smooth muscle: effects of adenosine antagonists. *Br J Pharmacol* (1988) **95**: 371–378.
19. Lundblad KAL, Persson CGA: The epithelium and the pharmacology of guinea-pig tracheal tone *in vitro*. *Br J Pharmacol* (1988) **93**: 909–917.
20. Le Gall G, Ukena D, Frossard N. Epithelium-independent contraction to adenosine is mediated through A1-receptor activation in guinea-pig airways. *Am Rev Respir Dis* (1989) **139**: A465.
21. Kroll F, Karlsson JA, Persson CGA, Ryrfeldt A: Interactions between xanthines, mepyramine and adenosine in the guinea-pig lung. In Andersson KE, Persson CGA (eds) *Anti-asthma Xanthines and Adenosine*. Current Clinical Practice Series No.19. Amsterdam, Excerpta Medicine (1985) pp 193–196.

22. Thorne J, Broadley KJ: A bronchoconstrictor response to adenosine of guinea-pig perfused lungs (Abstract). *Br J Pharmacol* (1988) **93** (Proceedings Suppl): 278P.

23. Finney MJB, Karlsson JA, Persson CGA: Effect of bronchoconstrictors and bronchodilators on a novel human small airway preparation. *Br J Pharmacol* (1985) **85**: 29–36.

24. Napier FE, Temple DM: Theophylline's inhibition of antigen-induced contraction of human parenchymal strips is independent of adenosine antagonism. *Eur J Pharmacol* (1987) **142**: 253–260.

25. Dahlen SE, Hansson G, Hedqvist P, Bjorck T, Granstrom E, Dahlen B: Allergen challenge of lung tissue from asthmatics elicits bronchial contraction that correlates with the release of leukotrienes C4, D4, and E4. *Proc Natl Acad Sci USA* (1983) **80**: 1712–1716.

26. Holgate ST, Cushley MJ, Mann JS, Hughes PJ, Church MK. The action of purines on human airways. *Arch Int Pharmacodyn Ther* (1986) **280**(Suppl): 240–252.

27. Bjorck T, Gustafsson LE, Wikstrom E, Dahlen B, Zetterstrom O, Dahlen SE: *In vitro* hyperresponsiveness to adenosine in bronchi from asthmatics. In: Piper PJ and Krell RD (eds). *Advances in the understanding and treatment of asthma*. Vol. 629: 458–59.

28. Rafferty P, Beasley R, Southgate P, Holgate S: The role of histamine in allergen and adenosine-induced bronchoconstriction. *Int Archs Allergy Appl Immunol* (1987) **82**: 292–294.

29. Kay AB, Walsh GM, Moqbel R, *et al.*: Disodium cromoglycate inhibits activation of human inflammatory cells *in vitro*. *J Allergy Clin Immunol* (1987) **80**: 1–8.

30. Cushley MJ, Holgate ST: Adenosine induced bronchoconstriction in asthma: role of mast cell mediator release. *J Allergy Clin Immunol* (1985) **75**: 272–278.

31. Crimi N, Brusasco V, Brancatisano M, Losurdo E, Crimi P: Adenosine-induced bronchoconstriction: premedication with chlorpheniramine and nedocromil sodium. *Eur J Respir Dis* (1986) **69**(Suppl 147): 255–257.

32. Altounyan REC, Lee TB, Rocchiccioli KMS, Shaw CL: A comparison of the inhibitory effects of nedocromil sodium and sodium cromoglycate on adenosine monophosphate-induced bronchoconstriction in atopic subjects. *Eur J Respir Dis* (1986) **69**(Suppl 147): 277–279.

33. Joad JP: Characterization of the human peripheral lung adenosine receptor. *Am J Respir Cell Mol Biol* (1990) **2**: 193–198.

34. Daxum Z, Rafferty P, Richards R, Summerel S, Holgate ST: Airway refractoriness to adenosine 5' monophosphate after repeated inhalation by atopic non-asthmatic subjects. *J Allergy Clin Immunol* (1989) **83**: 152–158.

35. Finnerty JP, Holgate ST: Effect of repeated bronchial challenges with adenosine monophosphate (AMP) on excercise induced bronchoconstriction in asthma (Abstract). *Thorax* (1989) **44**: 865P–866P.

36. Phillips GD, Ng WH, Church MK, Holgate ST: The response of plasma histamine to bronchocoprovocation with methacholine, adenosine 5'-monophosphate, and allergen in atopic non-asthmatic subjects. *Am Rev Respir Dis* (1990) **141**: 9–13.

37. Crimi N, Palermo F, Polosa R, *et al.*: Effect of indomethacin on adenosine-induced bronchoconstriction. *J Allergy Clin Immunol* (1989) **83**: 921–925.

38. Phillips GD, Holgate ST: The effect of oral terfenadine alone and in combination with flurbiprofen on the bronchoconstrictor response induced by inhaled adenosine 5'-monophosphate in non-atopic asthma. *Am Rev Respir Dis* (1989) **139**: 463–469.

39. Narushima M, Akisawa T, Tanaka K, Nakagami K, Suzuki H, Noguchi E: Studies of adenosine inhalation in asthmatic patients. *Arerugi* (1990) **39**: 322–329.

40. Marquardt DL, Parker CW, Sullivan TJ: Potentiation of mast cell mediator release by adenosine. *J Immunol* (1978) **120**: 871–878.

41. Fredholm BB, Sydbom A: Are the anti-allergic actions of theophylline due to antagonism at the adenosine receptor? *Agents Actions* (1980) **10**: 145–147.

42. Nishibori M, Shimamura K, Yokoyama H, Tsutsumi K, Saeki K: Differential effects of adenosine on histamine secretion induced by antigen and chemical stimuli. *Arch Int Pharmacodyn Ther* (1983) **265**: 17–28.

43. Burt DS, Stanworth DR: The effect of ribose and purine modified adenosine analogues on secretion of histamine from rat mast cells induced by ionophore A23187. *Biochem Pharmacol* (1983) **32**: 2729–2732.

44. Church MK, Hughes PJ: Adenosine potentiates immunological histamine release from rat mast cells by a novel cyclic-AMP independent cell surface action. *Br J Pharmacol* (1985) **85**: 3–5.

45. Leoutsakos A, Pearce FL: The effect of adenosine and its analogues on cyclic AMP changes and histamine secretion from rat peritoneal mast cells stimulated by various ligands. *Biochem Pharmacol* (1986) **35**: 1373–1379.

46. Welton AF, Simko BA: Regulatory role of adenosine in antigen-induced histamine release from the lung tissue of actively sensitized guinea pigs. *Biochem Pharmacol* (1980) **29**: 1085–1092.

47. Napier FE, Temple DM: The relation between the effects of adenosine, theophylline and enprofylline on the contractility of sensitized guinea-pig lung strips. *J Pharm Pharmacol* (1986) **39**: 432–438.

48. Marquardt DL, Gruber HE, Wasserman SI: Adenosine release from stimulated mast cells. *Proc Natl Acad Sci USA* (1984) **81**: 6192–6196.

49. Peachell PT, Columbo M, Kagey Sobotka A, Lichtenstein LM, Marone G: Adenosine potentiates mediator release from human lung mast cells. *Am Rev Respir Dis* (1988) **138**: 1143–1151.

50. Hughes PJ, Holgate ST, Church MK: Adenosine inhibits and potentiates IgE-dependent histamine release from human lung mast cells by an A2-purinoceptor mediated mechanism. *Biochem Pharmacol* (1984) **33**: 3847–3852.

51. Church MK, Featherstone RL, Cushley MJ, Mann JS, Holgate ST: Relationship between adenosine, cyclic nucleotides and xanthines in asthma. *J Allergy Clin Immunol* (1986) **78**: 670–676.

52. Zgombick JM, Beck SG, Mahle CD, Craddock Royal B, Masyani S: Pertussis toxin sensitive guanini nucleotide binding protein(s) couple adenosine A1 and 5-hydroxytryptamine 1A receptors to the same effector system in rat hippocampus: biochemical and electrophysiological studies. *Mol Pharmacol* (1989) **35**: 484–494.

53. Kurtz A: Adenosine stimulates guanylate cyclase activity in vascular smooth muscle. *J Biol Chem* (1987) **262**: 6296–6300.

54. Rubio R, Bencherif M: Adenosine: Sites of release in the nervous system and control of phosphatidylinositol turnover. In (eds) *Cardiac Electrophysiology and Pharmacology of Adenosine and ATP: Basic and Clinical Aspects*. Location Alan R. Liss 1987, pp 77–93.

55. Chin JH, De Lorenzo RJ: A new class of adenosine receptors in brain. Characterization by 2-chloro [3H] adenosine binding. *Biochem Pharmacol* (1986) **35**: 847–856.

56. Subramanian N: Inhibition of immunological and non-immunological histamine release from human basophils and lung mast cells by formoterol. *Arzneim Forsch* (1986) **36**: 502–505.

57. Barnes PJ, Fitzgerald GA, Brown M, Dollery CT: Nocturnal asthma and changes in circulating epinephrine, histamine and cortisol. *N Engl J Med* (1980) **303**: 263–267.

58. Braun S, Levitzki A: The attenuation of epinephrine-dependent adenylate cyclase and the characteristics of the adenosine stimulating and inhibitory sites. *Mol Pharmacol* (1979) **16**: 737–748

59. Ng WH, Polosa R, Church MK: Adenosine bronchoconstriction in asthma: investigations into its possible mechanism of action. *Br J Pharmacol* (1990) **30**: 89s–98s.

60. Snyder SH: Adenosine as a neuromodulator. *Ann Rev Neurosci* (1985) **8**: 103–124.

61. Gustafsson LE, Wiklund NP, Cederqvist B: Apparent enhancement of cholinergic transmission in rabbit bronchi via adenosine A2 receptors. *Eur J Pharmacol* (1986) **120**: 179–185.

62. Pauwels R, van der Straeten M: An animal model for adenosine-induced bronchoconstriction. *Am Rev Respir Dis* (1987) **136**: 374–378.

63. Mann JS, Cushley MJ, Holgate ST: Adenosine-induced bronchoconstriction in asthma: role of parasympathetic stimulation and adrenergic inhibition. *Am Rev Respir Dis* (1985) **132**: 1–6.

64. Okayama M, Ma JY, Hataoka I, *et al.*: Role of vagal nerve activity on adenosine-induced bronchoconstriction in asthma (Abstract). *Am Rev Dis* (1986) **133**(Suppl): A93.

65. Polosa R, Phillips GD, Rajakulasingam K, Holgate ST: The effect of inhaled ipratropium bromide alone and in combination with oral terfenadine on bronchoconstriction provoked by adenosine 5' monophosphate and histamine in asthma. *J Allergy Clin Immunol* (1991) **87**: 939–947.

66. Dixon M, Jackson DM, Richards IM: The action of sodium cromoglycate on 'C' fibre endings in the dog lung. *Br J Pharmacol* (1980) **70**: 11–13.
67. Pauwels R, Joos G, Kips J, Van der Straeten M: Synergistic mechanisms in the adenosine- and neuropeptide-induced bronchoconstriction. *Arch Int Pharmacodyn* (1990) **303**: 113–121.
68. Manzini S, Ballati L: 2-Chloroadenosine induction of vagally-mediated and atropine-resistant bronchomotor responses in anaesthetised guinea-pigs. *Br J Pharmacol* (1990) **100**: 251–256.
69. Polosa R, Rajakulasingam K, Holgate ST: Adenosine 5'-monophosphate (AMP) induced bronchospasm in asthma: effect of repeated challenges with bradykinin. *Thorax* (1991) **46**: 292.
70. Persson CGA: Experimental lung actions of xanthines. In Andersson KE, Persson CGA (eds) *Anti-asthma Xanthines and Adenosine.* Current Clinical Practice Series No. 19. Amsterdam: Excerpta Medica (1985) 61–83.
71. Persson CGA, Karlsson JA, Erjefalt J: Differentiation between bronchodilation and universal adenosine antagonism amongst xanthine derivatives. *Life Sci* (1982) **30**: 2181–2189.
72. Larsson K, Sollevi A: Influence of infused adenosine on bronchial tone and bronchial reactivity in asthma. *Chest* (1988) **93**: 280–284.
73. Eagle KA, Boucher CA: Intravenous dipyridamole infusion causes severe bronchospasm in asthmatic patients. *Chest* (1989) **95**: 258–259.
74. Rosati G, Hargreave FE, Ramsdale EH: Inhalation of adenosine 5'-monophosphate increases methacholine airway responsiveness. *J Appl Physiol* (1989) **67**: 792–796.

19

Platelet-activating Factor

CLIVE P. PAGE AND PETER J. BARNES

HISTORICAL BACKGROUND

In 1966, Barbaro and Zweifler demonstrated the release of histamine into rabbit plasma during the acute allergic reaction.[1] In this species, it had already been established that, among the blood elements, platelets provided the major source of histamine,[2] hence it was unclear whether release of histamine in an allergic reaction represented a direct or an indirect consequence of the recognition of allergen by antibody. It was subsequently demonstrated that histamine release in the rabbit was a consequence of IgE-dependent activation of basophils and that these cells responded to allergen stimulation by releasing a material that was capable of activating platelets.[3]

In 1972, Benveniste *et al.* described a method for preparing this basophil product, which was referred to as platelet-activating factor (PAF).[3] Benveniste *et al.* showed that PAF was released by IgE-activated basophils and initiated characterization of the biologically active constituent responsible for platelet activation.[4] On the basis of physicochemical characteristics, they concluded that the active material was a phospholipid, and the chemical structure of PAF was identified in 1979 by three independent groups as 1-*o*-alkyl-2-acetyl-sn-glyceryl-3-phosphorylcholine (Fig. 19.1).[5–7]

Partial synthesis of PAF was reported in 1979 by Benveniste *et al.*[8] and later total synthesis of this molecule was achieved.[9] To date, no properties of the synthetic material have been identified that are not established by PAF preparations of biological origin.

SYNTHESIS

Cell damage or disruption does not yield substantial amounts of PAF, suggesting that this material is neither preformed nor stored.[10] In several cell types, there is coincident

ASTHMA: BASIC MECHANISMS AND CLINICAL MANAGEMENT (2nd Edn)
ISBN 0-12-079026-2

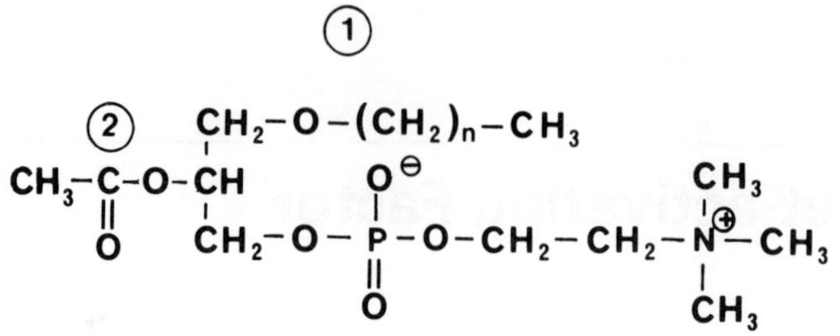

Fig. 19.1 Diagrammatic representation of platelet-activating factor (PAF), illustrating the location of the ether bond (position 1) and the acetyl side chain (position 2). Modification of the molecule at either of these carbon atoms results in reduction or loss of biological activity.

formation of PAF and a non-acetylated compound termed lyso-PAF.[11,12] Lyso-PAF has similar physicochemical properties to PAF, but is essentially devoid of biological activity. Lyso-PAF has been shown to be released *in vitro* by macrophages,[11] neutrophils[13] and platelets[12] in response to activation by a variety of agents, and the formation of lyso-PAF can be abolished by inhibitors of phospholipase A_2, indicating the involvement of this enzyme in the synthesis of PAF.[14]

A number of observations have lent support to the concept that lyso-PAF is a precursor of PAF; it can be shown that addition of synthetic lyso-PAF and acetyl-CoA to rat macrophages yields PAF.[15] This observation is consistent with the proposition that PAF is formed as a consequence of acetylation of lyso-PAF, and is further substantiated by the observation that platelets incorporate radiolabelled acetate into PAF.[16] It is now recognized that acetylation of lyso-PAF can be achieved by an acetyltransferase enzyme that has been described in a number of cell types;[17–19] this enzyme acts as a rate limiting enzyme for PAF synthesis (Fig. 19.2).[20] This pathway is sometimes referred to as the 'remodelling' pathway.

More recently, a second pathway sometimes called the '*de novo*' pathway, has been described for PAF synthesis involving the transfer of phosphorylcholine from ether-linked phospholipids (plasmalogens).[21,22] This is a single step reaction catalysed by the enzyme choline phosphotransferase.[20,21] The extent to which these enzymes participate in the production of PAF *in vivo* is not fully understood, but it appears that in inflammatory cells the two-step synthetic pathway involving the rate-limiting acetyl transferase enzyme predominates,[22] whereas in cell types such as renal cells, where PAF may be produced continuously and serve as a physiological hormone, the phosphocholine transferase enzyme appears active.[22] However, it is now recognized that certain cell types such as neurones may possess the ability to synthesize PAF by both pathways, although the precise role for each pathway in nerves remains to be established.[23]

METABOLISM

The lability of PAF *in vivo* is due to the widespread distribution of a cytosolic acetyl hydrolase enzyme[24] (phosphatide-2-acetyl-hydrolase) which is able to cleave the acetate moiety at the Sn-2 position to leave lyso-PAF. Recent evidence has suggested that a group of Japanese asthmatic children are genetically deficient of this enzyme and that

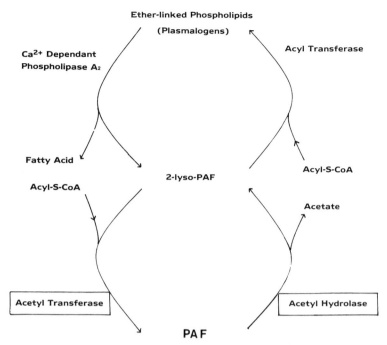

Fig. 19.2   PAF is generated from ether-linked phospholipids by a two step enzymatic process. The first step involves removal of a fatty acid to leave lyso-PAF, a biologically inactive precursor of PAF. Formation of PAF requires acetylation of lyso-PAF by a rate-limiting acetyl transferase enzyme. PAF is rapidly metabolized in plasma by an acetyl hydrolase to leave the inactive lyso-PAF. Lyso-PAF has been shown in some cell types to be reincorporated into ether-linked phospholipids.

this deficiency correlates with the severity of their asthma.[25] In experimental animals acetyl hydrolase will rapidly degrade ^{3}H-PAF to lyso-PAF such that 1 min following a bolus i.v. injection of PAF, 70% is present as lyso-PAF.[26] An acetylhydrolase enzyme has also been identified on the surface of platelets.[27] Furthermore, ^{3}H-PAF instilled into airways is very rapidly metabolized to ^{3}H-lyso-PAF suggesting the presence of a related enzyme within pulmonary tissue[28] although the precise cellular location of the enzyme in the lung has not been investigated. Lyso-PAF is further metabolized by removal of the o-alkyl group by an enzyme that is similar to, or identical with, the well-characterized tetrahydropteridine-dependent alkyl monooxygenase enzyme isolated from rat liver.[29] This process generates a fatty aldehyde and the hydrosoluble glyceryl-3-phosphoryl-choline.

The total synthesis of PAF has led to the synthesis of a wide range of analogues of PAF, permitting structure–activity relationships to determine the optimal requirements for the biological activity of PAF. This has been extensively reviewed elsewhere,[30] but in particular it is known that the presence of the ether linkage and the length of the alkyl side chain are critical determinants for biological activity, whereas the alkyl side chain at position 2 of the molecule is less critical. PAF derived from biological origin including human skin, is a mixture of mainly C_{16} and C_{18} types (31), and the biological activities of C_{16} PAF and C_{18}PAF do not appear to be qualitatively or quantitatively different.[32] Structure–activity studies have also allowed a putative structure of the binding site for PAF to be put forward (Fig. 19.3).[33]

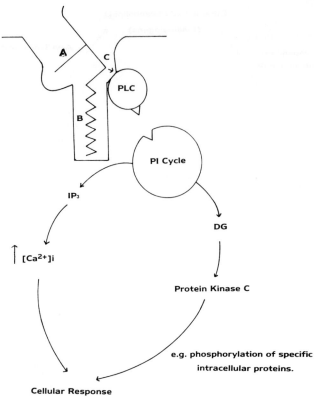

Fig. 19.3 Interaction of PAF with its putative receptor site results in activation of membrane-associated phospholipase C, leading to stimulation of the phosphotidylinositol (PI) cycle. Inositol triphosphate (IP_3) and diacylglycerol (DG) are generated from the PI cycle and act as second messages resulting in an increase in intracellular Ca^{2+} and activation of protein kinase C. PAF is suggested to interact with the putative receptor at three distinct points in the molecule: A, acetyl group at position 2; B, C_{16}–C_{18} backbone; C, ether link.

RECEPTORS

A number of groups have reported that high affinity binding sites exist for PAF and these have been demonstrated on platelets,[34–37] neutrophils,[37,38] eosinophils,[39] macrophages,[37,40] and lung tissue.[41,42] Recently, Honda *et al.* have cloned and expressed a PAF receptor from guinea-pig lung,[43] although whether this receptor is identical to the protein isolated as the PAF receptor from human platelets remains to be established.[44] The receptor protein fraction has seven transmembrane α-helices, typical of the structure of a G-protein linked surface receptor. With the availability of PAF antagonists, there have been preliminary suggestions that there may actually be more than one PAF receptor, although such evidence is still far from convincing,[40,45,46] and no selective antagonists for receptor subtypes have yet been described.

Following binding of PAF to its receptor, there is subsequent internalization of the PAF–receptor complex,[34] which probably explains the rapid desensitization of PAF-induced responses in a variety of tissues.[47,48] Several biochemical changes are also known to accompany the occupation of PAF receptors by PAF (Fig. 19.3). PAF is linked to intracellular events via a G protein, but there is some debate about the nature of the G proteins involved.[49] There is an activation of phospholipase C, triggering the hydrolysis of phosphoinositide (4,5)bisphosphate to inosine triphosphate (IP_3) and diacylglycerol (DG) (both substances known to be able to act as second messengers in bringing about a variety of intracellular events).[50–52] For instance, DG is able to activate protein kinase C, leading to the phosphorylation of specific intracellular proteins involved in physiological processes such as secretion or contraction.[53] IP_3 is able to release intracellular Ca^{2+} from internal stores which may in turn regulate other intracellular events such as Ca^{2+}-dependent K^+ channels.[54] In eosinophils PAF-receptor activation results in a rapid rise in intracellular $[Ca^{2+}]$ which is due to intracellular release and activation of Ca^{2+} via receptor-operated Ca^{2+} channels.[49] In some cell types, such as the human platelet, PAF activation will inhibit the formation of cyclic AMP induced by other endogenous agents such as prostaglandins.[55]

CELLULAR ORIGINS

PAF was originally described as a product of IgE-sensitized basophils in the rabbit.[3] However, it is unclear whether PAF is a product of human basophils, since a number of investigators have failed to demonstrate the formation of PAF from human basophil leukaemia cell lines.[56,57] There is also species variation in the ability of mast cells to form PAF. Bone-marrow derived mast cells from the mouse[58] and dog[59] mastocytoma cell lines have been shown to release PAF, but PAF appears not to be released by human lung mast cells in response to either antigenic or non-antigenic stimulation.[60]

On the other hand, a number of other cell types have been shown to release PAF, including neutrophils,[13] platelets,[12] nerves,[23] alveolar macrophages,[61] eosinophils[18] and vascular endothelial cells,[62] which have all been suggested to play a role in the pathogenesis of asthma. Eosinophils obtained from patients with eosinophilia (including asthmatics) have a much enhanced capacity to generate PAF which seems to reflect an underlying defect in the normally rate-limiting acetyl transferase enzyme controlling the 'remodelling' pathway of PAF synthesis.[18,20] Platelets, eosinophils and alveolar macrophages also possess IgE-binding sites, and antigen stimulation of these cell types leads to PAF release.[18,61,63] These latter observations are of particular interest as IgE-dependent activation of alveolar macrophages[64] and platelets[65–67] can be inhibited by anti-allergic drugs such as DSCG, nedocromil sodium and cetirizine.

All cell types capable of releasing PAF can be activated by non-antigenic stimuli specific to the particular cell type but not in response to non-specific cell damage. For instance, neutrophils can readily release PAF in response to phagocytosis of foreign particles,[13] and alveolar macrophages synthesize PAF following stimulation with foreign materials such as endotoxin.[68] However it is becoming increasingly apparent that many cells capable of synthesizing PAF retain the bulk of this mediator intracellularly (reviewed in ref. 69). Whilst the precise role of this cell-associated PAF is unknown, this has been suggested to be involved in phagocytosis in neutrophils[69] and possibly to act as a second messenger in macrophages.[70]

PROPERTIES RELEVANT TO ASTHMA

Bronchoconstriction

PAF induces an acute reversible bronchoconstriction in all species examined except the rat (reviewed in ref. 30). This includes man where, following inhalation by healthy volunteers, there is both bronchoconstriction that is rapidly reversed and that which exhibits tachyphylaxis.[71-73]

Pharmacological studies in man have suggested that PAF-induced bronchospasm is related in part to the generation of peptidoleukotrienes[73,74] but not histamine or cyclooxygenase products of arachidonic acid metabolism.[72] Since PAF does not contract airway smooth muscle directly[75] (except in rare cases),[76] it remains of interest to determine the cellular source of the peptidoleukotrienes responsible for this acute bronchospasm. Evidence in experimental animals suggests that treatment with anti-platelet antiserum reduces PAF-induced bronchoconstriction which, coupled with the inability of PAF to induce bronchospasm in rats—a species whose platelets do not possess PAF receptors, suggests that platelets may be involved in PAF-induced broncho-constriction (reviewed in ref. 30). However, whilst intratracheal administration of large doses of PAF to people with brainstem death results in acute reversible thrombocyto-paenia,[77] no thrombocytopaenia has been reported in healthy subjects undergoing bronchospasm following inhalation of PAF.[78] None the less, platelet activation has been shown to accompany PAF-induced bronchospasm in man detected as an increased expression of platelet-associated von Willebrand factor.[79] Perhaps not surprisingly PAF antagonists have been shown to inhibit bronchospasm induced by PAF in man.[78]

Increased vascular permeability

PAF appears to be one of the most potent agents for inducing increased vascular permeability and is able to induce oedema formation in all species tested, including man (reviewed in ref. 80). PAF is some 1000 times more potent than classical mediators such as histamine in inducing increased vascular permeability in human skin.[81] Unlike bronchoconstriction, this biological property of PAF is independent of platelet or neutrophil[82] activation and is most likely the result of a direct effect of PAF on vascular endothelial cells.[83] Thus, depletion of platelets or neutrophils is without effect on the ability of PAF to induce vascular permeability in the skin of experimental animals.[82] In human skin PAF will induce an acute wheal and flare response that can be potentiated by concomitant administration of vasodilator prostaglandins such as PGE_1, and ana-logues of PGI_2 (e.g. ZK 36374), known to be inhibitors of platelet function.[84] This suggests that in man, PAF-induced vascular permeability is probably platelet indepen-dent as well. Oedema formation in response to local administration of PAF seems to be independent of cyclooxygenase products of arachidonic acid metabolism or histamine, as it cannot be reduced by indomethacin or the histamine H_1 antagonist mepyramine.[81]

PAF is also able to elicit oedema formation in the bronchial circulation,[85] a process which is independent of platelet activation and of the generation of several mediators such as histamine, peptidoleukotrienes and cyclooxygenase products of arachidonic acid metabolism. However, it can be abolished by PAF receptor antagonists and as has been reported in other tissues, e.g. the skin, PAF is thought to increase vascular permeability via contraction of endothelial cells presumably as a result of interaction with high-affinity PAF receptors on the endothelial cells. The role of PAF in inducing oedema after allergen or other mediators is still not clear. PAF antagonists do not inhibit plasma extravasation after acute allergen exposure,[86] but partially inhibit the extravasation induced by bradykinin.[87] The role of PAF in chronic inflammation of the airways is not yet clear.

Inflammatory cell activation and recruitment

PAF is able to activate a wide range of inflammatory cells *in vitro*, including platelets, neutrophils, macrophages, monocytes (reviewed in ref. 30) and eosinophils.[88–93] In particular, it is a most potent inducer of chemotaxis of neutrophils and eosinophils,[88] and induces eosinophil degranulation.[89,90] Additionally, PAF will elicit the release of a variety of other mediators from these inflammatory cells, such as lipoxygenase products of arachidonic acid and oxygen free radicals from neutrophils,[30] macrophages[31] and eosinophils.[91,92] Interestingly, eosinophils from asthmatic subjects release higher amounts of certain mediators following activation with PAF when compared to eosinophils from normals or subjects with rhinitis.[91] PAF has also been demonstrated to stimulate the adherence of eosinophils to vascular endothelium[93] which could facilitate the migration of leucocytes through the vessel wall.

In vivo, PAF-induced cellular activation is reflected by the recruitment of various inflammatory cells into tissues following PAF administration. PAF is able to induce a sustained inflammatory response in rabbit lungs following local administration, a response that can last for up to 1 month and is associated with accumulation of inflammatory cells, fibroblasts and epithelial cell damage.[94] It is of particular interest that other investigators have noted that PAF elicits an eosinophil-rich infiltrate into the lungs following both local[95–97] and systemic administration[98] to experimental animals, although following inhalation by normal man, PAF elicits only neutrophil accumulation into the airway lumen.[99]

Following local administration of PAF to the skin of normal volunteers, an infiltration of neutrophils has also been described, 4–6 h after treatment, followed by a mixed cellular infiltrate comprising neutrophils and mononuclear cells at 24 h.[100] In contrast, local administration of PAF to the skin of atopic volunteers results in a selective eosinophil infiltration very reminiscent of antigen-induced eosinophil infiltration in the same subjects.[101] This is of interest because this PAF-induced eosinophil infiltration is susceptible to inhibition by anti-allergic drugs such as cetirizine.[102] The mechanisms of PAF-induced eosinophil infiltration are of interest because at least in some,[99,103] but not all studies[104] in experimental animals, this infiltration of eosinophils is dependent on platelet activation suggesting that it may be more complicated than mere chemotaxis.

PAF has been observed to elicit an extravascular recruitment of platelets into the lung of experimental animals which is followed by the close apposition of these platelets to bronchial smooth muscle.[105] Platelet-derived mitogens such as platelet-derived growth factor (PGDF) and transforming growth factor beta (TGF-ß) are thought to contribute to smooth muscle hyperplasia[106] and fibroblast proliferation[107] respectively, following tissue injury. Since bronchial smooth muscle hyperplasia and subepithelial fibrosis are now recognized histopathological features of even mild asthma,[108,109] the observation that chronic administration of PAF to guinea-pigs is able to induce airway smooth muscle thickening[110] and that a single administration of PAF to the lungs of rabbits induces fibrosis[94] in the airway may implicate this molecule in the pathogenesis of the long-term architectural changes found in the lungs of asthmatic subjects. The platelet dependence of these changes, however, remains to be established.

Effects on the mucocilliary escalator

PAF has not been studied extensively with regard to its effects on the mucocilliary escalator. However, PAF has been shown to increase mucus output and alter the physical properties of the mucus produced.[111] PAF also increases ion transport within the airway epithelium, and increases intracellular spaces as judged by mannitol flux.[112] Furthermore, topical administration of PAF to the lungs of experimental animals has been observed to cause loss of areas of the respiratory epithelium.[94] *In vitro* PAF-activated eosinophils release as yet undefined materials that cause epithelial shedding,[113] whereas PAF itself has no effect. Although the function of the mucocilliary escalator was not assessed in this study, it might be anticipated that mucocilliary clearance may well be impaired following PAF release if the respiratory epithelium is disrupted. Recently, inhaled PAF has also been shown to impair mucocilliary clearance in man, possibly via the release of LTB_4.[114]

Induction of bronchial hyperresponsiveness

One of the central features of asthma is non-specific bronchial hyperresponsiveness. One of the most interesting properties of PAF is the ability of this phospholipid to induce a non-selective increase in bronchial hyperresponsiveness in both experimental animals and man,[71,96,97,115] reviewed in ref. 80 (Fig. 19.4). However, this finding is not found universally[116,117] and at least in experimental animals is affected by the immunological status of the animals.[118] Thus rabbits that have been actively immunized from birth using a protocol designed to elicit the preferential production of IgE are consistently made hyperresponsive following exposure to PAF[118] whereas not all normal rabbits became hyperresponsive.[103,119] Whether this difference relates to the well-described ability of PAF to act as a 'priming' agent is not yet known.[30]

In normal subjects, increased responsiveness to methacholine has been observed up to 14 days following a single inhalation of PAF.[71] The time course and magnitude of PAF-induced bronchial hyperresponsiveness are very similar to that of antigen-induced changes in airway responsiveness observed in allergic asthmatics. None the less several other investigators have not found such changes in airway responsiveness in normal subjects following exposure to concentrations of PAF clearly capable of inducing bronchospasm.[116,117] However, other investigators have confirmed the original findings of Cuss *et al.*[120] and still others have reported that some, but not all, healthy subjects become hyperresponsive to exogenous spasmogens following exposure to aerosolized PAF.[121]

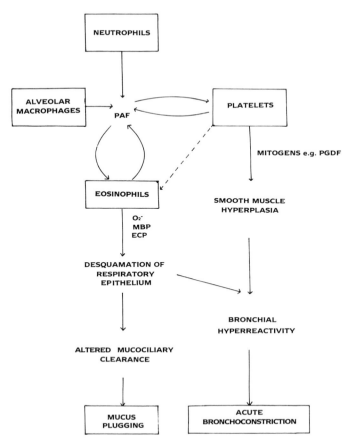

Fig. 19.4 A schematic representation of the possible relationship between PAF release from inflammatory cell populations within the lung and the subsequent pathological sequelae of asthma.

The mechanisms underlying PAF-induced bronchial hyperresponsiveness in man are not understood but in rabbits and guinea-pigs,[103,80] PAF-induced bronchial hyper-responsiveness is a platelet-dependent phenomenon. Furthermore, PAF has recently been reported to release a factor from human platelets capable of inducing bronchial hyperresponsiveness.[122] Furthermore, animals rendered hyperresponsive to exogenous spasmogens by prior treatment with systemic PAF have a reduced sensitivity to ß-adrenergic agonists such as isoprenaline, which cannot be attributed to loss of ß-receptor numbers or function in the lung.[115] Such observations are indirect evidence for a non-spasmogenic component contributing to the induction of bronchial hyperresponsiveness following PAF treatment which may involve oedema formation, cellular infiltration or epithelial cell damage. However, other studies have shown that PAF-induced hyper-responsiveness is not related to the extent of oedema formation[123] but in the rabbit can be inhibited by pretreatment with capsaicin, implying the involvement of sensory C-fibres in the expression of this phenomenon.[119]

Recent clinical studies have suggested that neither ß-agonists,[124] theophylline,[125] nor ketotifen[126] inhibit PAF-induced bronchial hyperresponsiveness in man although studies with other antiasthma drugs have yet to be carried out.

Release of PAF in asthma

A major factor hindering further investigation of PAF in the clinical arena is the lack of a convenient assay system for detecting this phospholipid in biological fluids. In 1977 Henson and Pinckard described the phenomenon of self-tachyphylaxis of platelets following exposure to PAF.[127] They utilized this phenomenon as the basis of a technique to detect PAF in the blood of rabbits undergoing IgE anaphylaxis. This technique is cumbersome but none the less has provided indirect data for PAF release in a variety of situations which have been verified by more sophisticated chemical procedures. This bioassay has been utilized for the detection of PAF in peripheral blood of asthmatics undergoing antigen provocation.[128] The bioassay has recently been modified to improve sensitivity, and the modified procedure has been utilized to confirm PAF release in allergic asthmatics undergoing bronchial provocation with antigens[129] and in aspirin-sensitive asthmatics undergoing provocation with aspirin.[130] Recent studies using this assay have also obtained a PAF-like material in the BAL fluid of some, but not all asthmatics.[131]

Recently, a radioimmunoassay procedure[132] for detection of this phospholipid in biological fluids has been described which should help the detection of PAF in the future, particularly with respect to looking for the release of PAF in clinical situations.

PAF ANTAGONISTS—FUTURE PROSPECTS

There is now a wide range of selective synthetic and naturally occurring PAF antagonists available as experimental tools to help unravel the physiological and pathophysiological roles of PAF (reviewed in ref. 133).

All of the PAF antagonists described are capable of inhibiting the wide array of PAF-induced pathological effects both *in vitro* and *in vivo* to varying extents (reviewed in ref. 133). This includes the ability of some of the PAF antagonists to inhibit PAF-induced bronchial hyperresponsiveness and eosinophil infiltration[96,97] in experimental animals. Several of the PAF antagonists have also been observed to inhibit allergic bronchocon-striction in experimental animals resulting from active or passive sensitization.[134,135] Furthermore, a number of PAF antagonists have been reported to inhibit allergen-induced late-onset responses in various animal models, including the rabbit[136,137] and sheep.[138] Furthermore, there have now been many investigations into the ability of PAF antagonists to inhibit allergen-induced cell infiltration and bronchial hyperresponsive-ness in a range of animal models.[96,97,137,138] Such studies have revealed that PAF antagonists can in certain circumstances inhibit the recruitment of inflammatory cells such as eosinophils and neutrophils into airway tissues and the bronchial hyperresponsi-veness, associated with this airway infiltration. However, not all investigators have found such inhibitory effects and the basis of these discrepancies is likely to in part reflect the wide array of sensitization methods utilized by investigators and the differences in route of administration of the drugs and/or antigen.[104]

Gingkolides have PAF-antagonistic activity and oral pretreatment of healthy volun-teers with a gingkolide mixture (BN 52063) selectively inhibits PAF-induced wheal and flare responses in the skin and PAF-induced aggregation of platelets removed from these individuals,[139] but has no significant effect on histamine-induced wheal and flare responses or ADP-induced platelet aggregation. However oral BN 52063 has only modest effects on PAF-induced bronchoconstriction or neutropaenia in normal volunteers, suggesting that it is not potent enough for use in asthma.[140] Oral BN 52063 also reduces allergen-induced late responses in the skin of allergic volunteers,[141] indicating that PAF may be involved in the late response in the skin, where there is a similar pathology to the late response in the airways. However, clinical studies in the airways with more potent PAF antagonists, such as WEB 2086 and MK-571, have failed to inhibit allergen-induced early and late responses in the airways of allergic asthmatics.[142,143] None the less, other potent, orally active antagonists are under development such as UK 74,505 which gives a prolonged inhibition against bronchoconstriction and neutropaenic responses induced by inhaled PAF.[144] It is possible that even the most potent PAF antagonists may not be effective in asthma, however, since it may be difficult to achieve a high enough local concentration of antagonist at sites of PAF release in the airways and the inhaled route may be a preferable route of delivery for PAF antagonists. Theoretically it may be better to develop inhibitors of PAF synthesis, particularly if it is shown that intracellular PAF has effects on cell function via mechanisms other than activation of the cell-surface receptor for PAF, which all of the existing PAF antagonists have been screened against. Ultimately, however, only double blind studies in chronic asthma will decide the precise role of PAF in the pathogenesis of chronic asthma.

REFERENCES

1. Barbero JF, Zweifler NJ: Antigen-induced histamine release from platelets in rabbits producing homologous PCA antibody. *Proc Soc Exp Biol Med* (1966) **122**: 1245–1247.
2. Humphrey JH, Jacques R: The histamine and serotonin content of platelets and polymorphonuclear leukocytes of various species. *J Physiol* (1954) **124**: 305–310.
3. Benveniste J, Henson PM, Cochrane CG: Leukocyte dependent histamine release from rabbit platelets: The role of IgE, basophils and platelet activating factor. *J Exp Med* (1972) **136**: 1356–1377.
4. Benveniste J, Le Couedic JP, Polonsky J, Tence M: Structural analysis of purified platelet activating factor by lipases. *Nature* (1977) **269**: 170–171.
5. Benveniste J: Platelet activating factor, a new mediator of anaphylaxis and immune complex deposition from rabbit and human basophils. *Nature* (1974) **249**: 581–582.
6. Demopolous CA, Pinckard RN, Hanahan DJ: Platelet activating factor: Evidence for 1-*o*-alkyl-2-acetyl-sn-glyceryl-3-phosphorylcholine as the active component of platelet activating factor (a new class of lipid chemical mediators). *J Biol Chem* (1979) **254**: 9355–9358.
7. Blank ML, Snyder F, Byers LW, Brooks B, Muirhead EE: Antihypertensive activity of an alkyl ether analog of phosphatidylcholine. *Biochem Biophys Res Commun* (1979) **90**: 1194–1200.
8. Benveniste J, Tence M, Varenne P, Bidault J, Boullet C, Polonsky J: Semi-synthese et structure. Proposee du facteur activant les plaquettes (PAF): Paf-acether, un alkyl ether analogue de la phosphatidylcholine. *C R Acad Sci (Paris)* (1979) **289**: 1037–1040.
9. Godfroid JJ, Heymans F, Michel E, Redenilh C, Steiner E, Benveniste J: Platelet activating factor (Paf-acether): total synthesis of 1-*o*-octadecyl-2-*o*-acetyl-sn-glyceryl-3-phosphorylcholine. *FEBS Lett* (1980) **116**: 161–164.
10. Tence M, Polonsky J, Le Couedic J-P, Benveniste J: Release, purification, and characterisation of platelet activating factor (PAF). *Biochimie* (1980) **62**: 251–259.
11. Mencia-Huerta JM, Ninio E, Roubin R, Benveniste J: Is platelet activating factor (PAF-acether) synthesis by murine peritoneal cells (Pc) a two step process? *Agents Actions* (1981) **11**: 556–558.

12. Benveniste J, Chignard M, Le Couedic JP, Vargaftig BB: Biosynthesis of platelet activating factor (PAF-acether). II. Involvement of phospholipase A2 in the formation of PAF-acether and lyso-PAF-acether from rabbit platelets. *Thromb Res* (1982) **25**: 375–385.

13. Jouvin-Marche E, Cerrina J, Coeffier E, Duroux P, Benveniste J: Effect of the calcium antagonist on the release of platelet activating factor (Paf-acether), and slow reacting substances SRS and beta-glucuronidase from human neutrophils. *Eur J Pharmacol* (1983) **89**: 19–26.

14. Vargaftig BB, Chignard M, Benveniste J: Present concepts on the mechanisms of platelet aggregation. *Biochem Pharmacol* (1981) **30**: 263–271.

15. Ninio EW, Mencia-Huerta JM, Heymans F, Benveniste J: Biosynthesis of platelet activating factor: Evidence for acetyl-transferase activity in murine macrophages. *Biochim Biophys Acta* (1982) **710**: 23–31.

16. Chap H, Mauco G, Simon MF, Benveniste J, Douste-Blazy L: Biosynthetic labelling of platelet activating factor (Paf-acether) from radioactive acetate by stimulated platelets. *Nature* (1981) **289**: 312–314.

17. Mencia-Huerta JM, Benveniste J: Platelet activating factor (PAF-acether) and macrophages. II. Phagocytosis-associated release of PAF-acether from rat peritoneal macrophages. *Cell Immunol* (1981) **57**: 281–292.

18. Lee T-C, Lenihan DJ, Malone B, Roddy LL, Wasserman SI: Increased biosynthesis of platelet activating factor in activated human eosinophils. *J Biol Chem* (1984) **259**: 5526–5530.

19. Pirotzky E, Ninio E, Bidault J, Pfister A, Benveniste J: Biosynthesis of platelet activating factor. VI. Precursor of platelet activating factor and acetyl-transferase activity in isolated rat kidney cells. *Lab Invest* (1984) **51**: 567–572.

20. Snyder F: Chemical and biochemical aspects of platelet activating factor: A novel class of acetylated ether-linked choline phospholipids. *Med Res Rev* (1985) **5**: 107–140.

21. Renooij W, Snyder FF: Biosynthesis of 1-alkyl-2-acetyl-sn-glycero-3-phosphorylcholine (platelet activating factor and a hypotensive lipid) by choline phosphotransferase in various rat tissues. *Biochim Biophys Acta* (1981) **663**: 545–556.

22. Snyder F: The significance of dual pathways for the biosynthesis of platelet activating factor: 1-alkyl-2-lyso-sn-glycero-3-phosphate as a branch point. In Winslow CM, Lee ML (eds) *New Horizons in Platelet Activating Research.* New York, John Wiley, 1987, pp 13–26.

23. Goracci G, Francascangeli E: Properties of PAF synthesising phosphocholine transferase and evidence for lyso-PAF acetyltransferase activity in rat brain. *Lipids* (1991) in press.

24. Farr RS, Cox CP, Wardlow ML, Jorgensen R: Preliminary studies of an acid-labile factor (ALF) in human sera that inactivates platelet activating factor (PAF). *Clin Immunol Pathol* (1980) **15**: 318–330.

25. Miwa M, Miyake T, Yamamaka T, *et al.*: Characterisation of serum platelet activating factor (PAF) acetylhydrolase: Correlation between deficiency of serum PAF-acetylhydrolase and respiratory symptoms in asthmatic children. *J Clin Invest* (1988) **82**: 1983–1991.

26. Lartigue-Mattei C, Godeneche D, Chabard JL, Petit J, Berger JA: Pharmacokinetic study of 3H-labelled PAF-acether II. Comparison with 3H-labelled lyso-PAF acether after intravenous administration in the rabbit and protein binding. *Agents Actions* (1984) **15**: 643–648.

27. Suzuki Y, Miwa M, Harada M, Matsumoto M: Acetylhydrolase released from platelets following aggregation with PAF. *Eur J Biochem* (1988) **172**: 1117–1120.

28. Haroldsen PE, Voelkel NF, Henson JE, Henson PM, Murphy RC: Metabolism of platelet-activating factor in isolated perfused lung. *J Clin Invest* (1987) **79**: 1860–1867.

29. Lee TC, Blank ML, Fitzgerald V, Snyder F: Substrate specificity in the biocleavage of the 1-alkyl-2-acetyl-sn-glyceryl-3-phosphorylcholine (a hypotensive and platelet activating lipid) and its metabolites. *Arch Biochem Biophys* (1981) **208**: 353–357.

30. Braquet P, Touqui L, Shen TY, Vargaftig BB: Perspectives in platelet activating factor research. *Pharmacol Rev* (1987) **39**: 97–145.

31. Mallet AJ, Cunningham FM, Daniel F: Rapid isocratic high performance liquid chromatographic purification of platelet activating factor (PAF) and lyso-PAF from human skin. *J Chromatogr* (1985) **309**: 160–164.

32. Archer CB, Cunningham FM, Greaves MW: Comparison of the inflammatory action of C18 isomers and C16 isomers of platelet activating factor. *Br J Dermatol* (1986) **113**: 779–780.

33. Braquet P, Godfroid JJ: Platelet activating factor (PAF-acether) specific binding sites: 2. design of specific antagonists. *Trends Pharmacol Sci* (1986) **7**: 397–403.

34. Valone FH, Coles E, Reinhold VR, Goetzl EJ. Specific binding of phospholipid platelet-activating factor by human platelets. *J Immunol* (1982) **129**: 1637–1641.

35. Kloprogge E, Akkerman JWN: Binding kinetics of Paf-acether (1-*o*-alkyl-2-acetyl-sn-glycero-3-phosphorylcholine) to intact human platelets. *Biochem J* (1984) **220**: 901–909.

36. Ukena D, Dent G, Birke FW, Robaut C, Sybrecht GW, Barnes PJ: Radioligand binding of antagonists of platelet activating factor to intact human platelets. *FEBS Lett* (1988) **228**: 285–289.

37. Stewart AG, Dusting GJ: Characterisation of receptors for platelet activating factor on platelets, polymorphonuclear leukocytes and macrophages. *Br J Pharmacol* (1988) **98**: 141–148.

38. Dent G, Ukena D, Chanez P, Sybrecht GW, Barnes PJ: Characterisation of PAF receptors on human neutrophils using the specific antagonist, WEB 2086: correlation between receptor binding and function. *FEBS Lett* (1989) **244**: 365–368.

39. Ukena D, Kroegel C, Yukawa T, Sybrecht G, Barnes PJ: PAF receptors on eosinophils: identification with a novel ligand [3H] WEB 2086. *Biochem Pharmacol* (1989) **38**: 1702–1705.

40. Lambrecht G, Parnham MJ: Kadsurenone distinguishes between different platelet activating factor receptor subtypes on macrophages and polymorphonuclear leukocytes. *Br J Pharmacol* (1986) **87**: 287–289.

41. Hwang S-B, Lam M-H, Biftu T, Beattie TR, Shen T-Y: *trans*-2-5-bis-(3,4,5-trimethoxyphenyl)tetrahydrofuran. An orally active specific and competitive receptor antagonist of platelet activating factor. *J Biol Chem* (1985) **260**: 15639–15645.

42. Dent G, Ukena D, Sybrecht GW, Barnes PJ: [3H] WEB 2086 labels platelet activating factor receptors in guinea pig and human lung. *Eur J Pharmacol* (1989) **169**: 313–316.

43. Honda Z, Nakamura M, Miki I, *et al.*: Cloning by functional expression of platelet-activating factor receptor from guinea-pig lung. *Nature* (1991) **349**: 342–345.

44. Valone FH: Isolation of a platelet membrane protein which binds platelet activating factor. *Immunology* (1984) **52**: 169–174.

45. Kroegel C, Yukawa T, Westwick J, Barnes PJ: Evidence for two platelet activating factor receptors on eosinophils: dissociation between PAF induced intracellular calcium mobilization, degranulation and superoxide anion generation. *Biochem Biophys Res Commun* (1989) **162**: 1265–1270.

46. Hwang SB: Specific receptors of platelet activating factor, receptor heterogenicity and signal transduction mechanisms. *J Lipid Med* (1990) **2**: 123–158.

47. Henson PM: Activation of rabbit platelets by platelet activating factor derived from IgE sensitized basophils: Characteristics of the aggregation and its dissociation from secretion. *J Clin Invest* (1977) **60**: 481–490.

48. Page CP, Paul W, Morley J: *In vivo* aggregation of guinea-pig platelets in response to synthetic platelet activating factor (Paf-acether). *Agents Actions* (1983) **13**: 506–507.

49. Kroegel C, Chilvers ER, Giembycz MA, Challiss RA, Barnes PJ: Platelet activating factor stimulates a rapid accumulation of inositol (1,4,5)-triphosphate in guinea pig eosinophils: relationship to calcium mobilization and degranulation. *J Allergy Clin Immunol* (1991) **88**: 114–124.

50. Lapetina EG: Platelet activating factor stimulates the phosphatidyl choline cycle. *J Biol Chem* (1982) **257**: 7314–7317.

51. Shukla SD, Hanahan DJ: An early transient decrease in phosphatidylinositol 4,5-bisphosphate upon stimulation of rabbit platelets with acetylglycerylether phosphorylcholine (platelet activating factor). *Arch Biochem Biophys* (1983) **227**: 626–629.

52. Kroegel C, Pleass R, Yukawa T, Chung KF, Westwick J, Barnes PJ: Characterization of platelet activating factor induced elevation of cytosolic free calcium concentration in eosinophils. *FEBS Lett* (1989) **243**: 41–46.

53. Ieyasu H, Takai Y, Kaibuchi K, Savamura M, Nishizuka Y: A role of calcium activated, phospholipid-dependent protein kinase in platelet activating factor induced serotonin release from rabbit platelets. *Biochem Biophys Res Commun* (1982) **108**: 1701–1708.

54. Garay R, Braquet P: Involvement of K^+ movements in the membrane signal induced by PAF-acether. *Biochem Pharmacol* (1986) **35**: 2811–2815.

55. Haslam RJ, Vanderwel M: Inhibition of platelet adenylate cyclase by 1-*o*-alkyl-2-acetyl-sn-glyceryl-3-phosphorylcholine (platelet activating factor). *J Biol Chem* (1982) **157**: 6879–6885.

56. Betz SJ, Lotner GZ, Henson PM: Generation and release of platelet activating factor (PAF) from enriched preparations of rabbit basophils, failure of human basophils to release PAF. *J Immunol* (1980) **125**: 2749–2755.

57. Sanchez-Crespo M, Alonso F, Egido J: Platelet activating factor in anaphylaxis and phagocytosis. I. Release from human peripheral polymorphonuclears and monocytes during the stimulation by ionophore A23187 and phagocytosis but not from degranulating basophils. *Immunology* (1980) **40**: 645–655.

58. Mencia-Huerta JM, Lewis RA, Razin E, Austen KF: Antigen-initiated release of platelet activating factor (Paf-acether) from mouse bone marrow derived mast cells sensitized with monoclonal IgE. *J Immunol* (1983) **131**: 2958–2964.

59. Elias DJ, Lazarus SC, Valone FH, Gold WM: Production of platelet activating factor by mastocytoma cells. *Fed Proc* (1985) **44**: 984.

60. Lichtenstein LM, Schleimer RP, MacGlaskin DW, *et al.*: In vitro and in vivo studies of mediators released from human mast cells. In Lichtenstein LM, Austen KF, Kay AB (eds) *Asthma: Physiology, Immunophysiology and Treatment.* Academic Press, London, 1984, pp 1–15.

61. Arnoux B, Grimfield A, Duroux P, Denjean A: Alveolar macrophages/Paf-acether. A new association in the pathogenesis of human asthma. In Benveniste J, Arnoux J (eds) *Platelet Activating Factor and Structurally Related Ether Phospholipids. INSERM Symposium No. 23.* Elsevier Science Publications, 1983, pp 335–341.

62. Prescott SM, Zimmerman GA, MacIntyre TM: Human endothelial cells in culture produce platelet activating factor (1-alkyl-2-acetyl-sn-glycero-3-phosphocholine) when stimulated by thrombin. *Proc Natl Acad Sci (USA)* (1984) **81**: 3534–3538.

63. Joseph M: The involvement of platelets in the allergic response. In Page CP (ed) *Platelets in Health and Disease.* Blackwell Scientific Publications, 1991, pp 120–131.

64. Joseph M, Tonnel AB, Capron A, Dessaint JP: The interaction of IgE antibody and human alveolar macrophages and its participation in the inflammatory processes of lung allergy. In Russo-Marie F, Vargaftig BB, Benveniste J (eds) *Pharmacology of Inflammation and Allergy. Colloques de l'INSERM, Vol 100.* 1981, pp 311–318.

65. Thorel T, Joseph M, Tsicopolous A, Tonnel AB, Capron A: Inhibition by nedocromil sodium of IgE mediated activation of human polymorphonuclear phagocytes and platelets in allergy. *Int Arch Allergy Appl Immunol* (1988) **85**: 232–237.

66. Tsicopolous A, Lasalle P, Joseph M, *et al.*: Effect of disodium cromoglycate on inflammatory cells bearing the Fc epsilon receptor type II [Fec RII]. *Int J Immunopharmacol* (1988) **10**: 227–236.

67. De Vos C, Joseph M, Leprevost C, *et al*: Inhibition of human eosinophil chemotaxis and of the IgE-dependent stimulation of human blood platelets by cetirizine. *Int Arch Allergy Appl Immunol* (1989) **88**: 212–215.

68. Rylander R, Beijer L: Inhalation of endotoxin stimulates alveolar macrophage production of platelet activating factor. *Am Rev Resp Dis* (1987) **135**: 83–86.

69. Bratton D, Henson PM: Cellular origins of PAF. In Barnes PJ, Page CP, Henson PM (eds) *Platelet Activating Factor and Human Disease.* Blackwell Scientific Publications, 1989, pp 23–57.

70. Stewart AG, Phillips WA: Intracellular platelet activating factor regulates eicosanoid generation in guinea pig resident peritoneal macrophages. *Br J Pharmacol* (1989) **98**: 141–148.

71. Cuss FM, Dixon CM, Barnes PJ: Inhaled platelet activating factor in man: effects on pulmonary function and bronchial responsiveness. *Lancet* (1986) **ii**: 189–191.

72. Smith HJ, Rubin AE, Patterson R: Mechanism of platelet activating factor-induced bronchoconstriction in humans. *Am Rev Resp Dis* (1988) **137**: 1015–1019.

73. Spencer DA, Evans JM, Green SE, Piper PJ, Costello JF: Bronchospasm induced by platelet activating factor is reduced by a selective cysteinyl-leukotriene antagonist in normal man. *Am Rev Resp Dis* (1990) **141**: A218.

74. Kidney JC, Ridge S, Chung KF, Barnes PJ: Inhibition of PAF-induced bronchoconstriction by the oral leukotriene antagonist ICI 204,219 in normal subjects. *Am Rev Resp Dis* (1991) **143**: A811.

75. Schellenberg RR, Walker B, Snyder F: Platelet dependent contraction of human bronchus by platelet activating factor. *J Allergy Clin Immunol* (1983) **71**: 145 (Abstract).

76. Johnson PRA, Armour CL, Black JL: The action of platelet activating factor on human isolated airways and its antagonism by WEB 2086. *Eur Resp J* (1990) **3**: 55–60.

77. Gateau O, Arnoux B, Deriaz H, Viars P, Benveniste J: Acute effects of intratracheal administration of Paf-acether (platelet activating factor) in humans. *Am Rev Resp Dis* (1984) **129**: A23.

78. Roberts NM, McCusker M, Chung KF, Barnes PJ: Effect of a PAF antagonist BN 52063, on PAF-induced bronchoconstriction in human subjects. *Br J Clin Pharmacol* (1988) **26**: 65–72.

79. Wilson JW, Lai C, Djukanovic R, Howarth PH, Holgate ST: The influence of inhaled platelet activating factor (PAF) on bronchoalveolar lavage (BAL) and peripheral blood leukocytes (PBL) and platelets. *J Allergy Clin Immunol* (1990) **85**: 1897 (Abstract).

80. Page CP: The role of platelet activating factor in asthma. *J Allergy Clin Immunol* (1988) **81**: 144–152.

81. Archer CB, Page CP, Paul W, Morley J, MacDonald DM: Inflammatory characteristics of platelet activating factor (Paf-acether) in human skin. *Br J Dermatol* (1984) **110**: 45–50.

82. Pirotzky E, Page CP, Roubin R, *et al.*: Paf-acether induced plasma exudation is independent of platelets and neutrophils in rat skin. *Microcirc Endothelium and Lymphatics* (1984) **1**: 107–122.

83. Humphrey DM, McManus LM, Hanahan DJ, Pinckard RN: Morphological basis of increased vascular permeability induced by acetyl glyceryl ether phosphorylcholine. *Lab Invest* (1984) **50**: 16–22.

84. Archer CB, Frohlich W, Page CP, Paul W, Morley J, MacDonald DM: Synergistic interactions between prostaglandins and Paf-acether in experimental animals and man. *Prostaglandins* (1984) **27**: 495–501.

85. Evans TW, Chung KF, Rogers DF, Barnes PJ: Effect of platelet-activating factor on airway vascular permeability: possible mechanisms. *J Appl Physiol* (1987) **63**: 479.

86. Evans TW, Rogers DF, Aursudkij B, Chung KF, Barnes PJ: Inflammatory mediators involved in antigen-induced microvascular leakage in guinea pigs. *Am Rev Respir Dis* (1988) **138**: 395–399.

87. Rogers DF, Dijk S, Barnes PJ: Bradykinin-induced plasma exudation in guinea pig airways: involvement of platelet activating factor. *Br J Pharmacol* (1990) **101**: 739–745.

88. Wardlaw AJ, Moqbel R, Cromwell O, Kay AB: Platelet activating factor. A potent chemotactic and chemokinetic factor for human eosinophils. *J Clin Invest* (1986) **78**: 1701–1706.

89. Kroegel C, Yukawa T, Dent G, Chanez P, Chung KF, Barnes PJ: Platelet activating factor induces eosinophil peroxidase release from human eosinophils. *Immunology* (1988) **64**: 559–562.

90. Kroegel C, Yukawa T, Dent G, Venge P, Chung KF, Barnes PJ: Stimulation of degranulation from human eosinophils by platelet activating factor. *J Immunol* (1989) **142**: 3518–3526.

91. Chanez P, Dent G, Yukawa T, Barnes PJ, Chung KF: Generation of oxygen free radicals from blood eosinophils from asthma patients after stimulation with PAF or phorbol ester. *Eur Respir J* (1990) **3**: 1002–1007.

92. Bruijnzeel Ph B, Kok PMT, Hamelink ML, Kijne AM, Verhagen J: Platelet activating factor induces leukotriene C_4 synthesis by purified human eosinophils. *Prostaglandins* (1987) **34**: 205–214.

93. Kimani G, Tonnesen G, Henson PM: Stimulation of eosinophil adherence to human vascular endothelial cells *in-vitro* by platelet activating factor. *J Immunol* (1988) **140**: 3161–3166.

94. Camussi G, Pawlowski I, Tetta C, *et al.*: Acute lung inflammation induced in rabbit by local instillation of 1-o-octadecyl-2-acetyl-sn-glyceryl-phosphorylcholine or of native platelet activating factor. *Am J Pathol* (1983) **112**: 78–88.

95. Arnoux B, Duval D, Benveniste J, *et al.*: Accumulation of platelets and eosinophils in a primate are inhibited by ketotifen. *Am Rev Resp Dis* (1988) **148**: 855–860.

96. Coyle AJ, Urwin S, Touvey C, Villain B, Page CP, Braquet P: The effect of the selective PAF antagonist BN 52021 on antigen-induced eosinophil infiltration and bronchial hyperreactivity. *Eur J Pharmacol* (1988) **148**: 51–58.

97. Seeds EAM, Coyle AJ, Page CP: The effect of the selective PAF antagonist WEB 2170 on PAF and antigen-induced airway hyperresponsiveness and eosinophil infiltration. *J Lipid Med* (1991) **4**: 111–112.

98. Wardlaw AJ, Chung KF, Moqbel R, *et al.*: Cellular changes in blood and bronchoalveolar lavage (BAL) fluid after inhaled PAF I in man. *Am Rev Resp Dis* (1988) **139**: A283.

99. Lellouch-Tubiana A, Lefort J, Simon MT, Pfister A, Vargaftig BB: Eosinophil recruitment into guinea pig lungs after Paf-acether and allergen administration. Modulation by prostaglandins, platelet depletion and selective antagonists. *Am Rev Resp Dis* (1988) **137**: 948–955.

100. Archer CB, Page CP, Morley J, MacDonald DM. Accumulation of inflammatory cells in response to intracutaneous platelet activating factor (Paf-acether) in man. *Br J Dermatol* (1985) **112**: 285–290.

101. Henocq E, Vargaftig BB: Skin eosinophilia in atopic patients. *J Allergy Clin Immunol* (1988) **81**: 691–695.

102. Fadel R, David B, Herpin-Richard N, Borgnon A, Rassermont R, Rioux JP: *In vivo* effects of cetirizine on cutaneous reactions and eosinophil migration by platelet activating factor (Paf-acether) (1990) **86**: 314–320.

103. Coyle AJ, Spina D, Page CP: The contribution of platelets and airway smooth muscle to PAF-induced bronchial hyperresponsiveness in the rabbit. *Br J Pharmacol* (1990) **101**: 31–38.

104. Sanjar S, Aoki S, Boubecker K, *et al.*: Eosinophil accumulation in pulmonary airways of guinea-pigs induced by exposure to an aerosol of platelet activating factor: effect of anti-asthma drugs. *Br J Pharmacol* (1990) **99**: 267–272.

105. Lellouch-Tubiana A, Lefort J, Pirotzky E, Vargaftig BB, Pfister A: Ultrastructural evidence for extra-vascular platelet recruitment in the lung upon intravenous injection of platelet activating factor (Paf-acether) to guinea pigs. *Br J Exp Pathol* (1985) **66**: 345–355.

106. Ross R, Raines EW, Bowen-Pope, DF: The biology of platelet derived growth factor. *Cell* (1986) **46**: 155–169.

107. Wahl SM, Hurst DA, Wakefield LM, McCartney-Francis LM, Roberts AB, Sporn MB: Transforming growth factor beta induces monocyte chemotaxis and growth factor production. *Proc Natl Acad Sci* (1987) **84**: 5788–5792.

108. Roche WR, Beasley R, Williams JH, Holgate ST: Sub-epithelial fibrosis in the bronchi of asthmatics. *Lancet* (1989) **i**: 520–528.

109. Brewster EP, Howarth PH, Djukanovic R, Wilson J, Holgate ST, Roche WR: Myofibroblasts and sub-epithelial fibrosis in bronchial asthma. *Am J Resp Cell Mol Biol* (1990) **3**: 507–511.

110. Touvey C, Pfister A, Villain B, *et al.*: Effect of long term infusion of platelet activating factor on pulmonary responses in the guinea pig. *Pulm Pharmacol* (1991) **4**: 43–51.

111. Lang M, Hansen D, Hahn HL: Effect of the PAF antagonist CV-3988 on PAF-induced changes in mucus secretion and in respiratory and circulatory variables in the ferret. In Schmitz-Schuman M, Menz G, Page CP (eds) *Platelets PAF and Asthma*. Birkhauser Verlag, Basle, 1987, pp 245–252.

112. Rogers DF, Alton EWFW, Aursudkij B, *et al.*: Effect of platelet activating factor on formation and composition of airway fluid in the guinea-pig trachea. *J Physiol* (1991) **431**: 643–658.

113. Yukawa T, Read RC, Kroegel C, *et al.*: The effect of activated eosinophils and neutrophils on guinea-pig airway epithelium *in vitro*. *Am J Resp Cell Mol Biol* (1980) **2**: 341–354.

114. Neiminen MM, Moilanen EK, Nyholm JEJ, *et al.*: Platelet activating factor impairs mucocilliary transport and modifies plasma leukotriene B$_4$ in man. *Eur Resp J* (1991) **4**: 551–560.

115. Barnes PJ, Grandordy B, Page CP, Rhoden KJ, Robertson DN: The effect of PAF-induced bronchial hyperreactivity on beta-adrenoceptor function. *Br J Pharmacol* (1987) **90**: 709–15.

116. Lai LKW, Jenkins JR, Polosa R, Holgate ST: Inhaled PAF fails to induce airway hyperresponsiveness in normal human subjects. *J Appl Physiol* (1990) **68**: 919–926.

117. Spencer DA, Green GE, Evans JM, Piper PJ, Costello JF: Platelet activating factor does not cause a reproducible increase in bronchial responsiveness in normal man. *Clin Exp Allergy* (1990) **20**: 525–532.

118. Herd CM, Shoupe TS, Page CP: Effect of PF 5901 on PAF-induced airway responses in neonatally immunized rabbits. *Br J Pharmacol* (1991) **104**: 170 P.

119. Spina D, McKenniff MG, Coyle AJ, *et al.*: Effect of capsaicin on PAF-induced bronchial hyperresponsiveness and pulmonary cell accumulation in the rabbit. *Br J Pharmacol* (1991) **103**: 1268–1274.

120. Di Maria GV, Bellafoe S, Inglese P, Ricciardolo FLM, Privitera S, Mistretta A: Platelet activating factor does not affect maximal airway narrowing to methacholine in normal subjects. *Am Rev Resp Dis* (1990) **141**: A174.

121. Kaye MG, Smith LS: Effects of inhaled leukotriene D$_4$ and platelet activating factor of airway reactivity in normal subjects. *Am Rev Resp Dis* (1990) **141**: 993–997.

122. Sanjar S, Smith D, Kristersson A: Incubation of platelets with PAF produces a factor which causes airway hyperreactivity in guinea pigs. *Br J Pharmacol* (1989) **96**: 76 (Abstract).

123. Roberts NM, Barnes PJ: Relationship between bronchoconstriction, bronchial hyper-responsiveness and microvascular leakage induced by inhaled PAF and antigen. *Am Rev Resp Dis* (1989) **139**: A463.

124. Chung KF, Dent G, Barnes PJ: Effects of salbutamol on bronchoconstriction, bronchial hyperresponsiveness and leukocyte responses induced by platelet activating factor in man. *Thorax* (1989) **44**: 102–107.

125. Chung KF, Lammers J-W, *et al.*: Effect of theophylline on airway responses to inhaled platelet activating factor. *Eur J Resp Dis* (1991) **2**: 763–768.

126. Chung KF, Minette P, McCusker M, Barnes PJ: Ketotifen inhibits the cutaneous but not the airway response to platelet activating factor in man. *J Allergy Clin Immunol* (1988) **81**: 1192–1198.

127. Henson PM, Pinckard RN: Basophil-derived platelet-activating factor (PAF) as an *in vivo* mediator of acute allergic reactions: demonstration of specific desensitization of platelets to PAF during IgE-induced anaphylaxis in the rabbit. *J Immunol* (1977) **119**: 2179–2184.

128. Thompson JM, Hanson H, Bilani M, Turner-Warwick M, Morley J: Platelets, platelet activating factor and asthma. *Am Rev Resp Dis* (1984) **129**: A3 (Abstract).

129. Beer HJ: Wirkungen des 'Platelet activating factor' (PAF) auf die Thrombozyten des Menschen. MD Thesis, University of Zurich (1984).

130. Page CP, Schmitz-Schumann M, Morley J: Pathophysiology and pharmacology of asthma. In Velo GP, Rainsford KD (eds) *Side Effects of Antiinflammatory Drugs. CRC Handbook of Anti-Rheumatic and Anti-Inflammatory Drugs, Vol. IV*, MTP Press, Lancaster, 1987, pp 331–342.

131. Stenton SC, Kingston WP, Court EN, *et al.*: Platelet activating factor in bronchoalveolar lavage fluid from asthmatic subjects. *Eur Resp J* (1990) **3**: 408–413.

132. Nishihira J, Ishibashi J, Imai Y: Production and characterisation of specific antibodies against 1-o-alkyl-2-acetyl-sn-glycero-3-phosphorylcholine (a potent hypotensive and platelet activating ether linked phospholipid). *J Biochem* (1984) **95**: 1247–1251.

133. Hosford D, Page CP, Barnes PJ, Braquet P: PAF receptor antagonists. In Barnes PJ, Page CP, Henson PM (eds) *Platelet Activating Factor in Human Disease*. Blackwell Scientific Publications, Oxford, pp 82–116.

134. Braquet P, Spinnewyn B, Braquet M, *et al.*: BN 52021 and related compounds: a new series of highly specific Paf-acether receptor antagonists isolated from Gingko biloba. *Blood and Vessels* (1985) **16**: 559–572.

135. Casals-Stenzel J: Effects of WEB 2086, a novel antagonist of platelet activating factor in active and passive anaphylaxis. *Immunopharmacol* (1987) **3**: 7–24.

136. Coyle AJ, Sjoerdsma K, Tuovey C, Page CP, Metzger WJ: Modification of the late asthmatic response and bronchial hyperreactivity by BN 52021, a platelet activating factor antagonist. *J Allergy Clin Immunol* (1988) **84**: 960–967.

137. Smith HR, Hennson PM, Clay KL, Larsen GL: Effect of the PAF antagonist L-659,989 on the late asthmatic response and increased airway reactivity in the rabbit. *Am Rev Resp Dis* (1988) **137**: A283.

138. Stevenson JS, Tallent M, Blinder L, Abraham WM: The effect of the PAF antagonist WEB 2086 on the early and late response in allergic sheep. *Fed Proc* (1987) **46**: 6683.
139. Chung KF, Dent G, McCusker M, Guinot PH, Page CP, Barnes PJ: Effect of a gingkolide mixture (BN 52063) in antagonising skin and platelet responses to platelet activating factor in man. *Lancet* (1987) **i**: 248–250.
140. Roberts NM, McCusker M, Chung KF, Barnes PJ: Effect of a PAF antagonist BN52063, on PAF-induced bronchoconstriction in normal subjects. *Br J Clin Pharmacol* (1988) **26**: 65–72.
141. Roberts NM, Page CP, Chung KF, Barnes PJ: Effects of BN 52063 on antigen-induced early and late cutaneous responses in volunteers. *J Allergy Clin Immunol* (1988) **81**: 236–242.
142. Freitag A, Watson RM, Matsos G, Eastwood C, O'Byrne PM: The effect of treatment with a oral platelet activating factor antagonist (WEB 2086) in allergen induced asthmatic responses in human subjects. *Am Rev Resp Dis* (1991) **143**: A157.
143. Bel EH, De Smut M, Rossing TH, Timrus MC, Dijkman JH, Sterzk PJ: The effect of a specific oral PAF antagonist, MK-287, on antigen-induced early and late asthmatic reactions. *Am Rev Resp Dis* (1991) **143**: A811.
144. O'Connor BJ, Ridge SM, Chen-Worsdell YM, Barnes PJ, Chung KF: Complete inhibition of airway and neutrophil responses to inhaled platelet activating factor by an oral PAF antagonist UK 74,505. *Am Rev Resp Dis* (1991) **143**: A156.

20

Cytokines

MARC CLUZEL AND TAK H. LEE

INTRODUCTION

Cytokines are cell-free soluble proteins of low molecular weight (less than 80 kDa) produced by immunologically competent cells. They are distinguished from other mediators by their ability to maintain the physiology of the immune system. Recent work has indicated that cytokines also modulate, *in vitro* and *in vivo*, the behaviour of a large number of target cells and play a role in inflammatory processes. In asthma the dual capacity of cytokines to both downregulate and promote inflammation has attracted increasing interest. Studies performed during the last 5 years have shown that cytokines have the ability to affect at least two major features of asthma, i.e. specific IgE production and eosinophilic accumulation in the bronchi.

The facts that cytokines are pluripotential, that there is a relative lack of characterization of their effects *in vivo*, and that there are possible antagonistic and synergistic effects between different cytokines make it difficult to define precisely an unequivocal role for one cytokine in asthma. We have therefore elected to describe first the major cytokines which might be involved in asthma. We will then discuss the potential role of cytokines for each of the major biological events which may contribute to the asthmatic process. Finally, we will develop a hypothesis about the role of the cytokine network in asthma, based on our present knowledge.

CHARACTERISTICS OF CYTOKINES

Interferon-γ

Interferon-γ (IFN-γ) is an antiviral and antiproliferative protein which has also potent immunoregulatory effects on a variety of cells. It induces class I and II major

ASTHMA: BASIC MECHANISMS AND CLINICAL MANAGEMENT (2nd Edn)
ISBN 0-12-079026-2

histocompatibility complex (MHC) on both macrophages and other cells of non haema-topoietic origin, and release of other cytokines such as IL-2 or TNF.

It is produced by T-lymphocytes upon stimulation with specific antigens, mitogens or alloantigens. CD4$^+$ and CD8$^+$ can produce IFN-γ although the former are considered to be the major cellular source in response to antigen.[1]

IFN-γ gene is located on chromosome 12. The human cDNA codes for 166 amino acids of which the first 23 are mostly hydrophobic. The secreted protein consists of 143 amino acids and has a structure unrelated to that of IFN-α or -β, suggesting that it has independent evolutionary origins. The extent of protein glycosylation of IFN-γ is variable but does not affect biological activity.

A specific receptor for IFN-γ has been characterized which is distinct from the receptor for IFN-α and IFN-β.[2] This receptor is sensitive to protease and is internalized when complexed with IFN-γ, resulting in the induction of protein synthesis. This is presumed to occur via a second message which acts on the interferon-responsive sequence of the genes leading to their transcription.[3]

Interleukin-1

Interleukin-1 (IL-1) is a polypeptide which was initially described as a comitogen for murine thymocytes incubated with a suboptimal concentration of a T-cell stimulant. It is produced mainly by monocytes and macrophages but it may be produced by other cell types, including endothelial cells. Upon stimulation by a broad range of agents including endotoxin and phorbol myristate acetate (PMA), basal low levels of IL-1 message rises after 2 h and the protein becomes detectable outside the cells after 3 h.[4]

IL-1 comprises two gene products, IL-1α and IL-1β. Human macrophages produce predominantly IL-1β. These proteins are derived from a 33 kDa protein precursor. The breakdown of the precursor is not fully understood but occurs at a membrane or an extracellular level. IL-1α and β have close biological activities and are bound to the same membrane receptor which is present on many cell types, including B and T lymphocytes and fibroblasts.

IL-1 regulates maturation of thymic T- and B-cell precursors and the induction of proteins, such as lymphokines IL-6 and TNF, or adhesion molecules. A key feature of IL-1 pro-inflammatory effects is the stimulation of arachidonic acid metabolism and the secretion of inflammatory proteins such as collagenases.

One signal transduction pathway has been described and this involves the activation of adenylate cyclase and a transient increase of cAMP.

Interleukin-2

Interleukin-2 (IL-2) is produced by T-cells and is a polypeptide characterized mainly by its property of promoting division of T-cell and other cells of the immune system, such as natural killer and B cells. IL-2 is a glycoprotein of 15.5 kDa where the first 20 amino acids of the amino-terminal end are hydrophobic and are cleaved off to give the mature protein. This latter may be glycosylated at the threonine residue at position 3. The gene is located on chromosome 4 in humans. A disulphide bond exists between residue 58 and 105 which is critical for biological activity.

A high- and low-affinity binding site for IL-2 have been described with a Kd of 1×10^{-11} and 1×10^{-8} M respectively, the former mediating the physiological response of T-cells to IL-2. Cells synthesize two different binding proteins of 55 and 75 kDa, which associate to give the high-affinity receptor. The 55-kDa binding protein alone corresponds to the low-affinity receptor and the 75-kDa protein has an intermediary binding capacity.[5] The 75-kDa protein is expressed on resting T-lymphocytes. Upon stimulation, synthesis of 55-kDa binding protein is induced to give rise to the high-affinity receptor. Binding of IL-2 to 75-kDa protein induces synthesis of the 55 kDa binding protein, thereby explaining T-cell proliferation in the presence of IL-2 alone.

IL-2 not only promotes division of T-cells but favours the formation of lymphokine-activated killer cells. The role of IL-2 on B-cells is less clear. Activated normal B-cells express IL-2 receptors. IL-2 is certainly not necessary in most B-cell lines for immunoglobin production but could regulate or potentiate B-cell proliferation and differentiation. Recently it has been shown that IL-2 stimulates certain B-cell activated subpopulations.[6]

Studies on signal transduction pathways suggest that IL-2 may stimulate T-cell proliferation via the activation of protein kinase C (PKC). A GTP-binding protein intermediate could also have been involved.

Interleukin-3

Interleukin-3 (IL-3) is a 28-kDa glycoprotein produced mainly by T-cells. It supports the growth and differentiation of pluripotent stem cells leading particularly to myeloid cells. IL-3 may also induce 20α-hydroxysteroid dehydrogenase in cultures of spleen cells from young athymic mice, proliferation of mast cells and macrophages, as well as the synthesis of histamine in mast cells. The human gene for IL-3 is located on long arm of chromosome 5 in the region of the gene for GM-CSF. IL-3 consists of 152 amino acids with a signal sequence of 19 amino acids.[7] It has two potential glycosylation sites and two cysteine residues involved in one disulphide bond.

IL-3-dependent cell lines express a single class of high affinity receptors of approximately 140 kDa which may possess tyrosine kinase activity. The binding of IL-3 with its receptor appears also to trigger the activation of PKC.

IL-3 in picomolar concentrations supports the colony formation of eosinophils, macrophages, basophils and other cell types. It seems that IL-3 preferentially acts on earlier progenitor cells while the final stage of development is supported by lineage-specific factors. IL-3 is also a potent activator for the end cells of the lineages whose development they support: IL-3 stimulates phagocytosis and cytoxicity by eosinophils[8] and IL-3 has been described to induce histamine release by basophils.[9]

Granulocyte-macrophage-colony stimulating factor

Granulocyte-macrophage-colony stimulating factor (GM-CSF) is an acidic glycoprotein of 23 kDa. It stimulates the formation of granulocytes and macrophages from pluripotent haematopoietic stem cells. It is produced by activated lymphocytes and by a number of other cell types, including monocytes and endothelial cells. Human GM-CSF precursor is composed of 144 amino acids. Seventeen amino acids are then cleaved from the amino-terminal end during secretion to give a 127 amino-acid protein. The protein is coded by a single gene on chromosome 5 in human. There are two potential N-glycosylation sites and four cysteine residue. The disulphide bond between the cysteine residue is critical for biological activity. Receptors for GM-CSF have been shown to be possessed by neutrophils, eosinophils and macrophages but are missing on lymphocytes.

GM-CSF is also able to stimulate the functional activity of neutrophils, eosinophils, and macrophages. GM-CSF is able to induce or enhance the production of other protein mediators including TNF.[10]

Granulocyte-colony stimulating factor

Granulocyte-colony stimulating factor (G-CSF) is mainly released by macrophages and stimulates granulocyte formation. It is composed of 207 amino acids, of which the first 30 have been determined as the probable active sequence. Five cysteine residues form disulphide bonds. Receptors are presents on neutrophils.

Macrophage colony-stimulating factor

Macrophage colony-stimulating factor (M-CSF) is produced by fibroblasts and stimulates macrophage colonies formation from pluripotent haematopoietic cell. Two natural forms of M-CSF comprising approximately 223 and 145 amino acids have been described. Receptors have been found expressed on macrophages.

Interleukin-4

Interleukin-4 (IL-4), a T-cell derived glycoprotein of 20 kDa, causes activation, proliferation and differentiation of B cells and enhances the expression of class II major histocompatibility complex on the same cell type. The gene for IL-4, located in humans on chromosome 5, codes for a 153 amino acids protein of which the first 22 amino acids are the signal sequence. It has two potential N-glycosylation sites and six cysteine residues. Receptors for IL-4 are found on B- and T-cells, macrophages, mast cells and myeloid cells and correspond to a single class of high-affinity receptors.

IL-4 plays a key role in the isotype switching in murine and human B-cells antibody responses. The stimulating effect of IL-4 on different cell types generally depends on the presence of another signal. IL-4 effects on B-cells may be potentiated by IL-1 but several actions are inhibited by IFN-γ. IL-4 is probably one of the principal cytokines involved in asthma pathogenesis due to its ability to induce IgE isotype switching. However IL-4 also possesses anti-inflammatory activities and inhibits IL-1, TNF-α and PGE$_2$ production by macrophages.[11] It inhibits IL-8 gene expression from stimulated monocytes.[12] Therefore IL-4 may regulate monocyte-macrophage cytokine expression.

Interleukin-5

Human interleukin-5 (IL-5) is a 45-kDa glycoprotein which enhances eosinophil differentiation. However IL-5 acts on precursor cells which were already directed to the eosinophil lineage by other cytokines such as IL-3. It also stimulates the production of superoxide anion by eosinophils and promotes their morphologic changes. B-cell activation (enhancing *in vitro* synthesis of IgM, IgG1 and IgA) has also been described in murine but remains controversial in humans.[13] The human IL-5 gene is located at 5q31, as one GM-CSF and IL-3. This gene codes for a 134 amino acid protein of which the first 29 are the signal sequence. It has two potential glycosylation sites and two cysteine residues. A high- and a low-affinity receptor have been described in B-cell lines.

Interleukin-6

Interleukin-6 (IL-6) is a 23–30-kDa glycoprotein that is produced by a large variety of cells including activated T-cells, B-cells, endothelial cells and monocytes/macrophages. It was originally identified as a B-cell activation factor which induces antibody production. It is now recognized to have a synergistic effect with IL-1 and TNFα on the induction of acute-phase proteins by hepatocytes. IL-6 seems responsible for most of the effects described during the acute-phase response, IL-1 and TNFα being mainly responsible for the production of IL-6. IL-6 has also been involved in human myeloma pathogenesis. IL-6 is composed of 212 amino acids of which the first 28 form a hydrophobic signal sequence. The protein has two glycosylation sites, and four cysteine residues which may be involved in disulphide bonds. The IL-6 receptor is expressed in IL-6 responsive cells, hepatocytes, and B- and T-cells.[14] The IL-6 signal is mediated through a membrane glycoprotein, gp130, which becomes associated with a ligand-binding 80-kDa IL-6 receptor at its extracellular portion.

Interleukin-8

Interleukin-8 (IL-8) is also called neutrophil attractant/ activation protein-1 (NAP) and is expressed as a 99 residue protein. Twenty of the first residues are hydrophobic and could be a signal peptide. The secreted form (79 residues, NAP-1α) is obtained after cleavage at position 20. Other cleavages occur and give 77 and 72 residues (NAP-1β and NAP-1γ respectively). There are four half-cysteine residues in the molecule. The gene for IL-8 maps to chromosome 4.[15]

IL-8 was initially described as being produced by monocytes/macrophages but can also be released by activated lymphocytes, virus-infected fibroblasts, endothelial and epithelial cells. Two other cytokines, IL-1 and TNF have been reported to induce IL-8 gene expression and release.[16,17]

A high-affinity receptor for IL-8 is present on neutrophils. This receptor is internalized after complexing with IL-8. IL-8 is a very potent neutrophil chemoattractant, with little or no activity on monocytes or eosinophils. IL-8 stimulates respiratory burst from neutrophils and promotes the release of azurophilic granules from neutrophils.

Tumour necrosis factor

Tumour necrosis factor (TNF or TNFα), a 17-kDa non-glycosylated protein, is coded by a gene on the short arm of chromosome 6. Recent evidence[18] suggests that TNFα exists as a membrane associated form of 26 kDa and as an extracellular form of 17 kDa after cleavage. Lymphotoxin (LT or TNFβ) is also coded by a gene present on chromosome 6.

TNFα is mainly produced by monocytes/macrophages and when appropriately stimulated may represent 1% of their total secretory product. LT is produced by lymphocytes. A high- and low-affinity site have been described on monocytes for TNFα,[19] but only one affinity site has been described on other cell type.

Both TNFα and LT induce synthesis of other cytokines which share the same related biological effects such as IL-1, GM-CSF and IL-6 and TNFα stimulates class I MHC expression.

CYTOKINES AND ASTHMA PATHOGENESIS

Antigen presentation

A large numbers of cells, including monocytes/macrophages, B-cells, dendritic cells and fibroblasts, may play a role in antigen presentation (Fig. 20.1). The alveolar macrophage has been shown to be a poor effector antigen-presenting cell. Indeed it has been

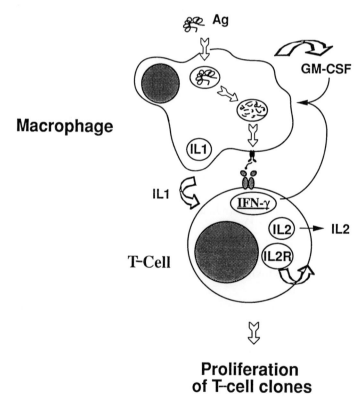

Fig. 20.1 Antigen presentation by macrophages. Antigen is processed and presented in association with the major histocompatibility complex on macrophages. This leads to differentiation and proliferation of T-helper lymphocytes. IL-1 increases IL-2 receptor expression which potentiates IL-2 effects. IFN-γ and GM-CSF may also enhance antigen presentation.

suggested that it might suppress antigen presentation.[20] One interpretation is that bronchi and lung are heavily exposed to antigen and that the poor antigenic presentation by alveolar macrophages is a way to avoid chronic lung inflammation.

Recent work has shown that cytokines may modulate antigen presentation. Falk et al.[21] showed that GM-CSF was more potent than IFN-γ in increasing the ability of bone-marrow derived macrophages to present antigen, and less potent than IFN-γ to induce the de novo synthesis of Ia molecules on bone-marrow derived macrophages. This observation was confirmed by Fischer et al.[22] GM-CSF was also able to induce morphological changes in murine alveolar macrophages.[23,24] Alveolar macrophages incubated with GM-CSF become small and round, whereas co-incubation with M-CSF results in stretched macrophages.

Cytokines might also affect T-cells during antigen presentation. In mice subsets of CD4$^+$ cells (Th1-Th2) differ for their responses to antigen presentation, and IL-1 is an important co-stimulator for the expansion of the Th2 subset after antigenic presentation[25,26] while the Th1 subset responds to IL-2 and IL-4.[27]

It is not known whether the capacity of alveolar macrophages to present antigen in asthma is enhanced. It has been reported that alveolar macrophages from asthmatic subjects are less able to suppress mitogen-driven T-cell proliferation.[28]

Lymphocytes and IgE regulation

Antigen presentation results in stimulation of specific T-cell clones. In allergic asthma these specific T-cell clones stimulate B-cells to produce specific IgE against defined airborne allergen. IgE, once fixed on mast cells and basophils, can trigger mediator release following cross-linking by allergen.

One mechanism for IgE production was clarified when it was shown that addition of IL-4, at a determined period of culture[29] was able to induce, in a dose-dependent manner, the production of IgE and IgG1 by B-cells.[30,31] Anti-IL-4 inhibits IgE- but not IgG1-production stimulated by IL-4, suggesting that other factors may interfere with IgG1 production. Other factors which favour IgE production, include cognate T/B-cell recognition and the presence of CD 23 soluble fragments.

IFN-γ antagonizes IL-4 effects on B-cells and inhibits IgE production.[32,33] As IL-4 decreases the expression of IFN-γ transcript,[34] these two factors probably interact in vivo to regulate IgE biosynthesis.

In the mouse, two types of T-cells, Th1 and Th2, have been described. The former secretes IL2, IFN-γ and lymphotoxin but not IL-4, IL-5 or IL-6. The latter secretes IL-4, IL-5 and IL-6 but not IL-2 or IFN-γ. Other cytokine such as IL-3 or GM-CSF are expressed by both sets of T-cells. An attractive hypothesis is that, in humans, specific IgE production occurs because of a defect in a Th1 clone of cells or via stimulation of Th2 clones. This hypothesis is supported by the fact that in humans an enhancement of IgE level is observed after total lymphoid irradiation and bone marrow transplantation[35,36] which in mouse favours Th2 proliferation over Th1. In this situation, even non-allergic patients are able to synthesize specific IgE antibodies to allergens that usually do not elicit IgE responses.[37]

However investigators have failed to clone Th1- and Th2-cells in humans. Furthermore, a small number of T-cells expressed IL-4 mRNA in normal subjects.[38] There are some indirect arguments to support the possibility of an imbalance between IFN-γ and IL-4 in humans. Thus T-cell clones from atopic patients produce more IL-4 than those of non-atopic patients.

Recent publications have reinforced the hypothesis that specific T-cell clone may regulate IgE production in humans. *Dermatophagoides pteronyssinus*-specific T-cell clones from an atopic individual were able to support IgE synthesis by autologous B-cells via an IL-4-dependent process, when the same specific clones from a non-atopic subject failed to support IgE production.[39] In another study, T-cell clones specific to *D. pteronyssinus* were isolated in allergic patients and these clones produced a larger amount of IL-4 than IFN-γ.[40] In non-atopic patients these clones produced more IFN-γ than IL-4. This specificity of T-cell clones to produce IL-4 is reinforced by the fact that T-cell clones from the same individual, directed against an allergen not responsible for sensitization, i.e. tetanus toxoid, produced high amounts of IFN-γ. A possible scenario is shown in Fig. 20.2.

Fcε RII/CD 23

Two different types of receptors for the Fc part of IgE have been described. Fcε RI is a receptor of high affinity (Kd 10^{-10} M) which is present on basophils and mast cells. Fcε RII is a receptor of low affinity, at least for monomeric IgE (Kd 10^{-7} M) which is present on B-cells, T-cells, monocytes, macrophages, platelets and possibly eosinophils. Fcε RII corresponds to CD23. CD23 which was already known as a 45-kDa glycoprotein is expressed on the cell surface. It is cleaved into soluble fragments and these are still recognized by anti-CD23 mAb.

Fcε RII/CD 23 and IgE production

Fcε RII plays a role in IgE production by B-cells and is regulated by cytokines. Fcε RII is poorly expressed on normal B-cells but its expression is enhanced by IL-4.[41] The expression occurs transiently while the B-cells are still expressing IgM and IgD, just prior to the Ig class switch to IgE.

IFNγ inhibits the effects of IL-4 on CD23 expression.[42] IgE production and CD23 expression on B-cells are therefore two closely related events. The chronological expression of CD23 before the switch for IgE supported the role of CD23 in IgE production. Supernatant fluid from Fcε RII-positive lymphoblastoid cell lines enhances IgE production by B-cells derived from atopic individuals[43] suggesting that soluble CD23 (sCD23) enhances IgE production. The central role of CD23 expression in IgE production was definitively established when F(ab') fragments of mAb25 (an anti-CD23 antibody) blocked IgE production.[44]

Although CD23 expression is necessary on B-cells for IgE production, the presence of CD23 on B-cells is not always associated with IgE synthesis. In highly purified splenic B-cells, IL-4 stimulates CD23 expression and sCD23 release, without IgE synthesis. IgE production is only restored by addition of autologous CD4$^+$ T-cells.[29] IL-4 also decreases IgG-mediated eosinophil degranulation, but not IgE-mediated secretion, through a reduction of IgG Fc but not IgE Fc receptor.[45] However, T-cell receptor-mediated and lymphokine-mediated signals show that IL-4 and IL-5 genes are differentially regulated.[46]

Fcε RII/CD23 on monocytes/macrophages, eosinophils and platelets

An active role for monocytes/macrophages, eosinophils and platelets in allergic reactions was suggested after the discovery of low-affinity Fcε RII/CD23 receptors on these cells. Following allergen provocation in the airways, the amount of β-glucuronidase in bronchoalveolar lavage (BAL) fluid was increased in asthmatic patients and this

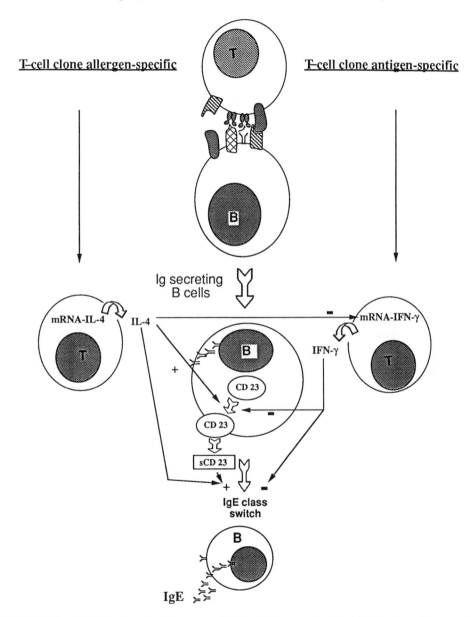

Fig. 20.2 Specific IgE production. Allergen-specific T-cell clones produce IL-4. IL-4 induces the expression of CD23 and the release of soluble CD23 fragments. These fragments with IL-4 induce IgE class switching by B lymphocytes. IFN-γ, produced by antigen specific T-cell clone can inhibit IL-4 effects on B cells. IL-4 decreases IFN-γ mRNA in T-lymphocytes.

enhancement correlated with the depletion of β-glucuronidase in BAL macrophages.[47] It suggests that macrophages have been activated by allergen, via an IgE-dependent mechanism, to release their granule products. Monocytes from atopics expressed more Fcε RII than non-atopic subjects. Sequence analysis of the cloned cDNAs for Fcε RII[48] indicated there were different subsets of Fcε RII. Fcε RIIa is constitutively expressed only in normal B cells, whereas Fcε RIIb is normally undetectable in B cells and monocytes, but can be induced by IL-4 and is expressed on peripheral blood monocytes in atopic individuals. Functional differences also exist between Fcε RII expressed on B-cells and monocytes: IFN-γ enhances Fcε RII expression on monocytes and inhibits it on B-cells.

Cytokines and mast cells/basophils

Upon IgE cross-linking, mast cells release a broad range of inflammatory mediators, including histamine, platelet-activating factor (PAF), LTB$_4$, LTC$_4$ and prostaglandins which may play a role in the mechanisms of airways inflammation in asthma. However, β_2-antagonists which prevent mast cells degranulation are not efficient against the allergen-induced late-phase reaction. This observation suggested that mast cells were not involved in the inflammatory process in asthma. The recent finding that mast cells secrete cytokines requires a re-appraisal of the mast cells in the allergic inflammation.

In 1987, Brown et al.[49] showed that mouse mast cells expressed mRNA for IL-4, and the latter was detected in medium of transformed mast cells. This study was further extended and it was shown that IgE cross-linking was able to induce both mRNA and secretion of IL-3, IL-4, IL-5, IL-6 and GM-CSF.[50,51] These factors have the capacity to recruit, to prime and to activate a large number of cells, including eosinophils. Thus mast cells continuously stimulated upon allergenic exposure might initiate bronchi inflammation by releasing cytokines. It is not established yet whether human mast cells secrete cytokines.

Cytokines and macrophages/monocytes in asthma

Macrophages/monocytes also produce cytokines. The release of cytokines, such as IL-1, GM-CSF and IL-8, may result in chronic bronchial inflammation. Thus IL-1 induces proliferation and activation of lymphocytes. IL-1 stimulates adhesion proteins for granulocytes on endothelial cells. It might play a role in antigen presentation leading to amplification of the lymphocytic reaction. Lung macrophages from asthmatic patients have an enhanced capacity to release GM-CSF. Macrophages/monocytes also release IL-8 which is a potent neutrophil chemoattractant. It also induces oxygen free-radical production and exocytosis of granular content from neutrophils. This novel protein is induced in monocytes by IL-1.[52]

Cytokines and adhesion molecules

The method by which leucocytes, especially eosinophils, accumulate in airways of asthmatic subjects is still not known. Cytokines have the potential to direct or to modulate the characteristic eosinophilic infiltration in asthma. IL-3, GM-CSF and IL-5 stimulate development of eosinophils from bone-marrow receptors. Cytokines may enhance the adherence of leucocytes to endothelial cells; IL-3 augments adhesiveness of human basophils, but not neutrophils, for endothelium;[53] IL-4, synergistically with IL-1β, promotes lymphocyte adhesion[54] and GM-CSF increases human monocyte adherence.[55] It has been suggested that IL-5 may preferentially cause adherence of eosinophils but not neutrophils. IL-3, IL-5 and GM-CSF have been shown to increase eosinophil viability in tissue culture *in vitro*, with no effect on the neutrophil.[56]

Cytokines and eosinophils

Eosinophils, at the site of inflammation, secrete major basic protein (MBP), eosinophilic cationic protein (ECP) and eosinophil-derived neurotoxin which induce desquamation of the respiratory epithelium. Eosinophils may also release LTC_4, a potent bronchoconstrictor and PAF.

IL-3, GM-CSF and IL-5 seem critical for the differentiation, proliferation, chemotaxis, survival and degranulation of eosinophils. IL-3 and GM-CSF induce eosinophil-colony formation from progenitor cells[57–59] and render eosinophil-forming units IL-5 responsive.[60] After this early stage, parasitic models have shown that IL-5 is necessary for the maturation and proliferation of eosinophils. Injection of monoclonal antibody to IL-5 suppresses completely the blood eosinophilia currently observed in these models. Indirect evidence in favour of a role of IL-5 in eosinophilia was the discovery that the majority of T-lymphocyte clones from patients with idiopathic hypereosinophilic syndrome were producing IL-5 and differed markedly from T-lymphocyte clones from healthy subjects.[61]

IL-5 induces expression of adherence-associated molecules LFA1 and Mol[62] and is believed to be selectively chemoattractant for eosinophils. GM-CSF is chemoattractant for both eosinophils and neutrophils[63] but contradictory reports exist.[64] Cytokines may also be indirectly involved in chemoattraction by potentiating activity of other molecules such as LTB_4.[65]

The action of cytokines on eosinophil infiltration may be amplified *in vivo*. Addition of GM-CSF to human eosinophils in the presence of 3T3 fibroblasts increases eosinophil viability in a dose-dependent manner.[56] The presence of GM-CSF in culture medium also modifies the morphology of eosinophils which become hypodense. This morphological change is correlated with an increasing capacity of eosinophils to kill *Schistosoma mansoni* larvae and a 2.5-fold increase in LTC_4 production after ionophore stimulation.[56] GM-CSF increases receptors for IL-5 in eosinophils.[66]

Cytokines may enhance eosinophil degranulation. Preincubation of eosinophils with cytokines increased the release of eosinophil-derived neurotoxin induced by IgA and IgG. IL-5 was the most potent but GM-CSF and IL-3 also had some activity.[67]

These observations demonstrate that IL-5 in association with IL-3 and GM-CSF support eosinophilia in humans and may play a role in augmenting the inflammatory potential of these cells. Factors that could lead to an increase of IL-5 production in asthma remain largely obscure.

Cytokines can also suppress eosinophil proliferation. IL-4 decreases the number of eosinophil colonies supported by both IL-5 and GM-CSF.[68] A possible scheme of cytokine effects on eosinophils is shown in Fig. 20.3.

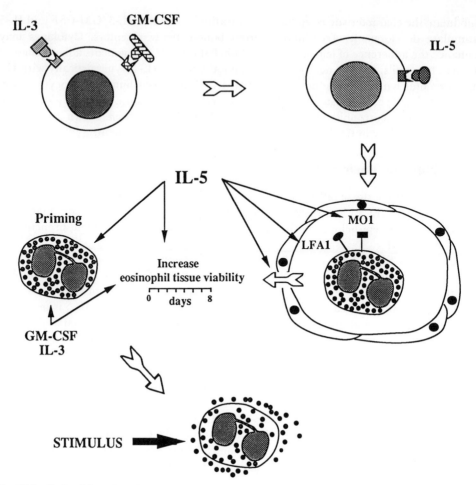

Fig. 20.3 Eosinophils and cytokines. IL-3 and GM-CSF induce eosinophil colony formation from progenitor cells and promote the formation of eosinophil-forming units which are IL-5 responsive. IL-5 leads to the maturation and proliferation of eosinophils and increases the expression of adhesion molecules Mo1 and LFA1. GM-CSF, IL-3 and IL-5 increase eosinophil viability in tissue and these cytokines prime eosinophils for enhanced function.

Cytokines and 'priming effects'

Preincubation of different cell types with cytokines, at concentrations that are not capable of causing release of mediators *per se*, potentiate mediator release in response to a second stimulus. This is called priming. Preincubation of basophils with IFN-γ or rIL-3 increases basophil releasability of arachidonic acid, LTB$_4$ and PAF.[71,72] IL-6 primes respiratory burst from neutrophils and monocytes. The phenomenon of priming also occurs between cytokines. Successive challenges with IL-3 and IL-8 cause release of histamine and sulphidopeptide leukotrienes without an IgE-mediated event.[73]

CYTOKINES AND ASTHMA

The biological activities of cytokines support the view that they may contribute to asthmatic bronchial inflammation. They may increase antigen presentation by monocytes/macrophages; induce and increase the production of specific IgE; favour the eosinophilic infiltration in bronchi and induce and/or increase the release of inflammatory mediators from primed cells.

A reasoned hypothesis which encompasses the known activities of cytokines and their enhanced secretion by cells in asthmatic airways, might be as shown in Fig. 20.4.

A genetic and/or environmental factor favours the growth of specific T-cell clones which produce and release IL-4. IL-4 production downregulates IFN-γ production and induces production of specific IgE. Cross-linking of IgE on mast cells and/or basophils leads to the release of inflammatory mediators and cytokines. As a result, eosinophil production increases and eosinophilic tissue infiltration appears. Monocytes/macrophages, directly stimulated by IgE cross-linking (in presence of IL-4) or indirectly stimulated by inflammatory mediators and/or phagocytosis of eosinophilic granules, secrete cytokines such as IL-1 and GM-CSF. Lymphocytes stimulated directly by inflammatory mediators or via monocyte/macrophage interaction would elaborate their own plethora of cytokine molecules. The end result is an airway in asthma that is

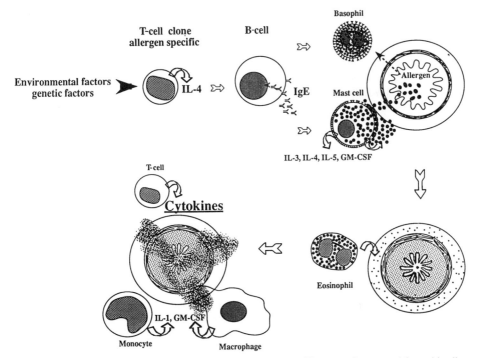

Fig. 20.4 Cytokines and asthma: a hypothesis. Upon a genetic and/or an environmental factor(s), allergen-specific T-cell clones proliferate and produce IL-4. T-cells and IL-4 favour IgE class switching and the production of specific IgE. Cross-linking of IgE on mast cell/basophil surfaces leads to the release of cytokines, which results in eosinophilic tissue infiltration. The concomitant release of inflammatory mediators stimulates monocytes/macrophages which produce IL-1 and GM-CSF and promotes further release of cytokines by T-cells. The end result is a chronic immune response with eosinophilia.

characterized by a chronic immune response with both reversible and irreversible inflammatory changes.

REFERENCES

1. Trinchieri G, Perussia B: Immune interferon: a pleiotropic lymphokine with multiple effects. *Immunology Today* (1985) **6**: 131–136.
2. Celada A, Gray PW, Rinderknecht E, *et al.*: Evidence for a gamma-interferon receptor that regulates macrophage tumoricidal activity. *J Exp Med* (1984) **160**: 55–72.
3. Friedman RL, Stark GR: Alpha-interferon-induced transcription of HLA and metallothionein genes containing homologous upstream sequences. *Nature* (1985) **314**: 637–639.
4. Windle JJ, Shin HS, Morrow JF: Induction of interleukin 1 messenger RNA and translation in oocytes. *J Immunol* (1984) **132**: 1317–1322.
5. Wang HM, Smith KA: The interleukin 2 receptor. Functional consequences of its bimolecular structure. *J Exp Med* (1987) **166**: 1055–1069.
6. Nakagawa T, Nagakawa N, Ambrus JL Jr, *et al.*: Differential effects of interleukin 2 vs B cell growth factor on human B cells. *J Immunol* (1988) **14**: 465–469.
7. Yang YC, Ciarletta AB, Temple PA, *et al.*: Human IL-3 (multi-CSF): identification by expression cloning of a novel hematopoietic growth factor related to murine IL-3. *Cell* (1986) **47**: 3–10.
8. Lopez AF, Dyson PG, To LB, *et al.*: Recombinant human interleukin-3 stimulation of responsiveness with differentiation in the neutrophilic myeloid series. *Blood* (1988) **72**: 1797–1804.
9. Haak-Frendcho M, Arai N, Arai K, *et al.*: Human recombinant granulocyte-macrophage colony-stimulating factor and IL-3 cause basophil histamine release. *J Clin Invest* (1988) **83**: 17–20.
10. Cannistra SA, Rambaldi A, Spriggs DR, *et al.*: Human granulocyte-macrophage colony-stimulating factor induces expression of the tumor necrosis factor gene by the U937 cell line and by normal human monocytes. *J Clin Invest* (1987) **79**: 1720–1728.
11. Essner R, Rhoades K, McBride WH, *et al.*: IL-4 down-regulates IL-1 and TNF gene expression in human monocytes. *J Immunol* (1989) **142**: 3857–3861.
12. Standford TJ, Strieter RM, Chensue SW, *et al.*: IL-4 inhibits the expression of IL-8 from stimulated human monocytes. *J Immunol* (1990) **145**: 1435–1439.
13. Sanderson CJ, Campbell HD, Young IG: Molecular and cellular biology of eosinophil differentiation factor (interleukin-5) and its effects on human and mouse B cells. *Immunol Rev* (1988) **102**: 29–50.
14. Taga T, Kawanishi Y, Hardy RR, *et al.*: Receptors for B cell stimulatory factor 2. Quantitation, specificity distribution, and regulation of their expression. *J Exp Med* (1987) **166**: 967–981.
15. Leonard EJ, Yoshimura T: Neutrophil attractant/activator protein-1 (NAP-1 [interleukin-8]). *Am J Respir Cell Mol Biol* (1990) **2**: 479–486.
16. Sica A, Matshushima K, Van Damme J, *et al.*: IL-1 transcriptionally activates the neutrophil chemotactic factor/IL-8 gene in endothelial cells. *Immunology* (1990) **69**: 548–553.
17. Strieter RM, Chensue SW, Basha MA, *et al.*: Human alveolar macrophage gene expression of interleukin-8 by tumour necrosis factor-alpha, lipopolysaccharide, and interleukin-1 beta. *Am J Respir Cell Mol Biol* (1990) **2**: 321–326.
18. Kriegler M, Perez C, DeFay K, *et al.*: A novel form of TNF/catechin is a cell surface cytotoxic transmembrane protein: ramifications of the complex physiology of TNF. *Cell* (1988) **53**: 45–53.
19. Imamura K, Spriggs D, Kufe D: Expression of tumour necrosis factor receptors on human monocytes and internalization of receptor bound ligand. *J Immunol* (1987) **139**: 2989–2992.
20. Toews GB, Vial WC, Dunn MM, *et al.*: The accessory cell function of human alveolar macrophages in specific T cell proliferation. *J Immunol* (1984) **132**: 181–186.

21. Falk LA, Wahl LM, Vogel SN: Analysis of Ia antigen expression in macrophages derived from bone marrow cells cultured in granulocyte-macrophage colony-stimulating factor or macrophage-colony stimulating factor. (Published erratum appears in *J Immunol* (1988) **141**: 709.)

22. Fischer HG, Frosch S, Reske K, *et al.*: Granulocyte-macrophage colony-stimulating factor activates macrophages derived from bone marrow cultures to synthesis of MHC class II molecules and to augmented antigen presentation function. *J Immunol* (1988) **141**: 3882–3888.

23. Chen BD, Mueller M, Chou TH: Role of granulocyte/macrophage colony-stimulating factor in the regulation of murine alveolar macrophage proliferation and differentiation. *J Immunol* (1988) **141**: 139.

24. Akagawa KS, Kamoshita K, Tokunaga T: Effects of granulocyte-macrophage colony-stimulating factor and colony-stimulating factor-1 on the proliferation and differentiation of murine alveolar macrophages. *J Immunol* (1988) **141**: 3383–3390.

25. Lichtman AH, Chin J, Schmidt JA, *et al.*: Role of interleukin 1 in the activation of T lymphocytes. *Proc Natl Acad Sci* (1988) **85**: 9699–9703.

26. Chang TL, Shea C, Urioste S, *et al.*: Heterogeneity of Helper/inducer T/lymphocytes: Responses of IL-2 and IL-4 producing (Th1 and Th2) clones to antigen presented by different accessory cells. *J Immunol* (1990) **145**: 2803–2808.

27. Kurt-Jones EA, Hamberg S, Ohara J, *et al.*: Heterogeneity of Helper/inducer T lymphocytes: lymphokine production and lymphokine responsiveness. *J Exp Med* (1987) **166**: 1774–1787.

28. Aubas P, Cosso B, Godard P, *et al.*: Decreased suppressor cell activity of alveolar macrophages in bronchial asthma. *Am Rev Respir Dis* (1984) **130**: 875–878.

29. Chretien I, Pene J, Briere F, *et al.*: Regulation of human IgE synthesis. I. Human IgE synthesis *in vitro* is determined by the reciprocal antagonistic effects of interleukin 4 and interferon-gamma. *Eur J Immunol* (1990) **20**: 243–251.

30. Coffman RL, Ohara J, Bond MW, *et al.*: B cell stimulatory factor-1 enhances the IgE response of lipopolysaccharide-activated B cells. *J Immunol* (1986) **136**: 4538–4541.

31. Finkelman FD, Katona IM, Urban JF Jr, *et al.*: Suppression of *in vivo* polyclonal IgE responses by monoclonal antibody to the lymphokine B-cell stimulatory factor 1. *Proc Natl Acad Sci USA* (1986) **83**: 9675–9678.

32. Snapper CM, Paul WE: Interferon-gamma and B cell stimulatory factor-1 reciprocally regulate Ig isotype production. *Science* (1987) **236**: 944–947.

33. Maggi E, Del Prete GF, Tiri A, *et al.*: Role of interleukin-4 in the induction of human IgE synthesis and its suppression by interferon-gamma. *Ric Clin Lab* (1987) **17**: 363–367.

34. Vercelli D, Jabara HH, Lauener RP, *et al.*: IL-4 inhibits the synthesis of IFN-gamma and induces the synthesis of IgE in human mixed lymphocyte cultures. *J Immunol* (1990) **144**: 570–573.

35. Heyd J, Donnenberg AD, Burns WH, *et al.*: Immunoglobulin E levels following allogenic, autologous, and syngeneic bone marrow transplantation: an indirect association between hyperproduction and acute graft-v-host disease in allogeneic BMT. *Blood* (1988) **72**: 442–446.

36. Abedi MR, Backman L, Persson U, *et al.*: Serum IgE levels after bone marrow transplantation. *Bone Marrow Transplant* (1989) **4**: 255–260.

37. Lakin JD, Strong DM, Sell KW: Polymixin B reactions, IgE antibody and T-cell deficiency. *Ann Int Med* (1975) **83**: 204–207.

38. Lewis DB, Prickett KS, Larsen A, *et al.*: Restricted production of interleukin 4 by activated human T cells. *Proc Natl Acad Sci* (1988) **85**: 9743–9749.

39. O'Hehir RE, Bal V, Quint D, *et al.*: An *in vitro* model of allergen-dependet IgE synthesis by human B lymphocytes: comparison of the response of an atopic and a non-atopic individual to *Dermatophagoides* spp. (house dust mite). *Immunology* (1989) **66**: 499–504.

40. Wierenga EA, Snoek M, de Groot C, *et al.*: Evidence for compartmentalization of functional subsets of CD2$^+$ T lymphocytes in atopic patients. *J Immunol* (1990) **144**: 4651–4656.

41. Defrance T, Aubry JP, Rousset F, *et al.*: Human recombinant interleukin 4 induces Fc epsilon receptors (CD23) on normal human B lymphocytes. *J Exp Med* (1987) **165**: 1459–1467.

42. Roussett F, Malefijt RW, Slierendregt B, *et al.*: Regulation of Fc receptor for IgE (CD23) and class II MHC antigen expression on Burkitt's lymphoma cell lines by human IL-4 and IFN-gamma. *J Immunol* (1988) **140**: 2625–2632.

43. Sarfati M, Rector E, Rubio-Trujillo M, *et al.*: *In vitro* synthesis of IgE by human lymphocytes. III. IgE-potentiating activity of culture supernatants from Epstein-Barr virus (EBV) transformed B cells. *Immunology* (1984) **53**: 207–214.

44. Pene J, Rousset F, Briere F, *et al.*: IgE production by normal human lymphocytes is induced by interleukin 4 and suppressed by interferons gamma and alpha and prostaglandin E2. *Proc Natl Acad Sci USA* (1988) **85**: 6880–6884.

45. Baskar P, Silberstein DS, Pincus SH: Inhibition of IgG-triggered human eosinophil function by IL-4. *J Immunol* (1990) **144**: 2321–2326.

46. Bohjanen PR, Okalima M, Hodes RJ: Differential regulation of interleukin 4 and interleukin 5 gene expression: a comparison of T-cell gene induction by anti-CD3 antibody or by exogenous lymphokines. *Proc Natl Acad Sci* (1990) **87**: 5283–5287.

47. Tonnel AB, Gosset P, Joseph M, *et al.*: Stimulation of alveolar macrophages in asthmatic patients after provocation test. *Lancet* (1983) (**i**)833983: 1406–1408.

48. Yokota A, Kikutani H, Tanaka T, *et al.*: Two species of human Fc epsilon receptor II (Fc epsilon RII/CD23): tissue-specific and IL-4-specific regulation of gene expression. *Cell* (1988) **55**: 611–618.

49. Brown MA, Pierce JH, Watson CJ, *et al.*: B cell stimulatory factor-1/interleukin-4 mRNA is expressed by normal and transformed mast cells. *Cell* (1987) **50**: 809–818.

50. Plaut M, Pierce JH, Watson CJ, *et al.*: Mast cell lines produce lymphokines in response to cross-linkage of Fc epsilon RI or to calcium ionophores. *Nature* (1989) **339**: 64–67.

51. Wodnar-Filipowicz A, Heusser CH, Moroni C: Production of the haemopoietic growth factors GM-CSF and interleukin-3 by mast cells in response to IgE receptor-mediated activation. *Nature* (1989) **339**: 150–152.

52. Matsushima K, Marishita K, Yoshimura T, *et al.*: Molecular cloning of a human monocyte-derived neutrophil chemotactic factor (MDNCF) and the induction of MDNCF mRNA by interleukin 1 and tumour necrosis factor. *J Exp Med* (1988) **167**: 1883–1893.

53. Bochner BS, McKelvey AA, Sterkinsky SA, *et al.*: IL-3 augments adhesiveness for endothelium and CD11b expression in human basophils but not neutrophils. *J Immunol* (1990) **145**: 1832–1837.

54. Masinovsky B, Urdal D, Gallatin WM: IL-4 acts synergistically with IL-1β to promote lymphocyte adhesion to microvascular endothelium by induction of cell adhesion molecule-1. *J Immunol* (1990) **145**: 2886–2895.

55. Elliott MJ, Vadas MA, Cleland LG, *et al.*: IL-3 and granulocyte-macrophage colony-stimulating factor stimulate two distinct phases of adhesion in human monocytes. *J Immunol* (1990) **145**: 167–176.

56. Owen WF Jr, Rothenberg ME, Silberstein DS, *et al.*: Regulation of human eosinophil viability, density, and function by granulocytes/macrophage colony-stimulating factor in the presence of 3T3 fibroblasts. *J Exp Med* (1987) **166**: 129–141.

57. Warren DJ, Moore MA: Synergism among interleukin 1, interleukin 3, and interleukin 5 in the production of eosinophilia from primitive haemopoeitic stem cells. *J Immunol* (1988) **140**: 94–99.

58. Clutterbuck EJ, Hirst EM, Sanderson EJ: Human interleukin-5 (IL-5) regulates the production of eosinophils in human bone marrow cultures: comparison and interaction with IL-1, IL-3, IL-6, and GMCSF. *Blood* (1989) **73**: 1504–1512.

59. Sonoda Y, Arai N, Ogawa M: Humoral regulation of eosinophilopoiesis *in vitro*: analysis of the targets of interleukin-3, granulocyte/macrophage colony-stimulating factor (GM-CSF), and interleukin-5. *Leukocyte* (1989) **3**: 14–18.

60. Clutterbuck EJ, Sanderson CJ: Regulation of human eosinophil precursor production by cytokines: a comparison of recombinant human interleukin-1 (rhIL-1), rhIL-3, rhIL-5, rhIL-6, and rh granulocyte-macrophage colony stimulating factor. *Blood* (1990) **75**: 1774–1779.

61. Raghavachar A, Fleischer S, Frickhofen N, *et al.*: T lymphocyte control of human eosinophilic granulopoiesis. Clonal analysis in an idiopathic hypereosinophilic syndrome. *J Immunol* (1987) **139**: 3753–3758.

62. Lopez AF, Williamson DJ, Gamble JR, *et al.*: Recombinant human granulocyte-macrophage colony-stimulating factor stimulates *in vitro* mature human neutrophil and eosinophil function, surface receptor expression, and survival. *J Clin Invest* (1986) **78**: 1220–1228.

63. Wang JM, Chen ZG, Cianciolo GJ, *et al.*: Production of a retroviral P15E-related chemotaxis inhibitor by Il-1-treated endothelial cells. A possible negative feedback in the regulation of the vascular response to monokines. *J Immunol* (1989) **142**: 2012–2017.
64. Arnaout MA, Wang EA, Clark SC, *et al.*: Human recombinant granulocyte-macrophage colony-stimulating factor increases cell-to-cell adhesion and surface expression of adhesion-promoting surface glycoproteins on mature granulocytes. *J Clin Invest* (1986) **78**: 597–601.
65. Wardlaw AJ, Moqbel R, Cromwell O, *et al.*: Platelet-activating factor. A potent chemotactic and chemokinetic factor for human eosinophils. *J Clin Invest* (1986) **78**: 1701–1706.
66. Chichara J, Plumas J, Gruart V, *et al.*: Characterization of a receptor for IL-5 on human eosinophils: variable expression and induction by granulocyte/macrophage colony-stimulating factor. *J Exp Med* (1990) **172**: 1347–1351.
67. Fujisawa R, Abu-Ghazaleh R, Kita H, *et al.*: Regulatory effect of cytokines on eosinophil degranulation. *J Immunol* (1990) **144**: 642–646.
68. Kajitan H, Enokihara H, Tsunogake S, *et al.*: Effect of human recombinant interleukin 4 on *in vitro* granulopoiesis of human bone marrow cells. *Growth Factors* (1989) **1**: 283–286.
69. Schleimer RP, Derse CP, Friedman B, *et al.*: Regulation of human basophil mediator release by cytokines. I. Interaction with antiinflammatory steroids. *J Immunol* (1989) **143**: 1310–1317.
70. Kurimoto Y, de Weck AL, Dahinden CA: Interleukin 3-dependent mediator release in basophils triggered by C5a. *J Exp Med* (1989) **170**: 467–479.
71. DiPersio JF, Billing P, Williams R, *et al.*: Human granulocyte-macrophage colony-stimulating factor and other cytokines prime human neutrophils for enhanced arachidonic acid release and leukotriene B4 synthesis. *J Immunol* (1988) **140**: 4315–4322.
72. Dahinden CA, Zingg J, Maly FE, *et al.*: Leukotriene production in human neutrophils primed by recombinant human granulocyte/macrophage colony stimulating-factor and stimulated with the complement component C5A and FMLP as second signals. *J Exp Med* (1988) **167**: 1281–1295.
73. Kurimoto Y, de Weck AL, Dahinden CA: Interleukin 3-dependent mediator release in basophils triggered by C5a. *J Exp Med* (1989) **170**: 467–479.

21

Other Mediators in Asthma

K.F. CHUNG AND P.J. BARNES

INTRODUCTION

Apart from the mediators such as histamine, adenosine, leukotrienes, prostaglandins and platelet-activating factor, which have been discussed in previous chapters, others have been implicated in asthma. In this chapter, several such mediators will be briefly considered, including the newly-discovered endothelin. Although it is unlikely that each of these mediators alone can explain all the features of asthma, they may as a whole contribute to the complex pathophysiological mechanisms observed in asthma.

OXYGEN RADICALS

The oxygen-derived molecules include superoxide anion (O_2^-), and hydroxyl radical (OH^-) and are characterized by their reactivity towards proteins, lipids and nucleic acids. This may result in damage to membranes, receptors or enzymes, which may lead to alterations in cell function. These molecules are generated as part of the inflammatory response and may therefore be involved in the pathophysiology of asthma. Activation of various inflammatory cells, including macrophages, neutrophils, eosinophils and mast cells, generate O_2^- and H_2O_2, with OH^- being secondarily formed.

Oxygen-radical species can act as initiators of lipid peroxidation for which arachidonic acid is an important substrate, with the synthesis of prostaglandins and leukotrienes. Thus, thromboxane generation has been shown to be stimulated by increased lung concentrations of reactive oxygen species in the isolated perfused rabbit lung.[1] In addition, hydrogen peroxide can induce arachidonic acid metabolism in rat alveolar macrophages.[2] Hydrogen peroxide may also induce the release of histamine from isolated rat peritoneal mast cells.[3]

ASTHMA: BASIC MECHANISMS AND CLINICAL MANAGEMENT (2nd Edn)
ISBN 0-12-079026-2

Effects on airways

Airway smooth muscle

Hydrogen peroxide is the oxygen radical which appears to have the major effect on airway tone and causes contraction both in bovine and guinea-pig airways.[4,5] In the guinea-pig, the contractile effect of H_2O_2 is greatly enhanced by removal of epithelium, suggesting that oxygen radicals release a relaxant factor from the epithelium. The bronchoconstriction is also reduced by indomethacin, suggesting that H_2O_2 also releases constrictor cyclooxygenase products.[5] Inhalation of xanthine and xanthine oxidase aerosols to generate oxygen radicals has been shown to cause bronchoconstriction in anaesthetized cats, an effect inhibited by superoxide dismutase, suggesting the involvement of superoxide anions.[6]

β-Receptor function

Oxygen-radical species may interfere with the sulphydryl groups of β-adrenoceptors in the lung, leading to dysfunction of the β-receptor. Pulmonary macrophages cause a specific deterioration of tracheal β-adrenergic responsiveness in the guinea-pig trachea, an effect inhibited by catalase and thiourea, indicating the oxygen species may be involved.[7] However, direct incubation of oxygen radicals with guinea-pig airways failed to alter β-receptor function.[5]

Bronchial hyperresponsiveness

Exposure of cats to xanthine and xanthine oxidase aerosols led to increased bronchial responsiveness to acetylcholine that lasted up to 1 h.[6] Ozone, which is a potent free-radical generator, is known to induce bronchial hyperresponsiveness and neutrophil influx into the airways of dogs and of normal volunteers. Arachidonic acid metabolites are increased in lungs of rats exposed to ozone,[8] and these may be metabolized by airway epithelial cells into lipoxygenase products such as leukotriene B_4 which has a potent chemotactic activity for neutrophils.[9] The involvement of oxygen-radical species in ozone-induced hyperresponsiveness is supported by the observation that this effect is inhibited by anti-oxidants.[10] Histamine hyperresponsiveness of guinea-pig trachea induced by leukotriene D_4 *in vitro* has been shown to be inhibited by pretreatment with superoxide dismutase, indicating the involvement of superoxide anions.[11]

Epithelial damage

Although oxygen-derived molecules such as H_2O_2 do not appear to be cytotoxic to respiratory epithelium, they markedly potentiate the cytotoxic effects of eosinophil-derived enzymes such as eosinophil peroxidase.[12] Epithelial damage induced by eosinophils activated by platelet-activating factor in guinea-pig tracheal rings *in vitro* is inhibited by catalase, supporting a role for H_2O_2.[13] Exposure of cultured epithelial cells to H_2O_2 may also increase paracellular permeability leading to increased penetration of exogenous substances.[14]

Possible role in asthma

Several studies suggest an association between the release of reactive oxygen species and asthma. Alveolar macrophages obtained from patients with asthma release larger quantities of reactive oxygen species than did those from normal subjects;[15,16] the amount of release of reactive oxygen species correlated with the severity of asthma.[15] In addition, significant correlations have been found between non-specific airway hyperresponsiveness to histamine aerosol and superoxide production by polymorphonuclear leucocytes in patients with chronic obstructive pulmonary disease.[17] Eosinophils obtained from venous blood of symptomatic asthmatic patients also show enhanced release of superoxide anions when stimulated by platelet-activating factor or a phorbol ester.[18]

Measuring oxygen-derived free radicals in the circulation is difficult because of their rapid degradation and neutralization by efficient local scavenger mechanisms. Glutathione peroxide, which removes H_2O_2 by oxidization of reduced glutathione to oxidized glutathione, has been reported to be lower in the blood of asthmatics with food and aspirin intolerance.[19] In addition, there is a reduction in whole blood glutathione peroxidase and selenium concentrations in asthmatic patients compared to controls,[20] selenium being required as a co-factor for glutathione oxidase. However blood levels of a specific non-peroxide product of free-radical attack on polyunsaturated lipids, used as a marker of lipid peroxidation, were not raised in patients with acute asthma.[21]

There have been very few studies of antioxidants or free-radical scavengers in asthma. Ascorbic acid is an effective antioxidant and reduces methacholine-induced bronchoconstriction in asthmatic subjects, although this could be mediated through an alternative mechanism.[22] In one study antioxidant supplementation with selenium and vitamins C and E did not improve bronchial hyperresponsiveness in asthmatic subjects, but the amount of supplementation may have been inadequate.[23] Further studies will be necessary in this area to determine the role of reactive oxygen species in asthma.

COMPLEMENT

The activation sequence and generation of various components of the complement cascade are complex and the reader is referred to other reviews for a thorough description.[24,25] A series of plasma proteins is generated during the complement cascade, and these may play an important role in host defence and in the pathophysiology of various disorders. In relation to asthma, we will focus specifically on two components of the complement cascade system for which there is documentation of airway effects, namely C3a and C5a.

Origin and metabolism

C3a, C4a and C5a are active fragments of the complement cascade which once formed do not participate in the cascade itself and are collectively known as anaphylatoxins. C3a and C5a are generated by the activation of the complement pathway by both the classical and alternative pathways. C5a has 74 amino acids and contains an oligosaccharide attached at position 64 with the active side being the carboxy-terminal pentapeptide

Met-Glu-Leu-Gly-Arg. The remainder of the molecule is required for functional binding to the C5a receptor, which is not so with C3a, although the carboxy-terminal of this molecule is again the active site. C3a has 77 aminoacids with the carboxy-terminal pentapeptide Leu-Gly-Leu-Ala-Arg.

The anaphylatoxins C3a and C5a are rapidly inactivated in plasma to the des-Arg form by the removal of the C-terminal arginine by serum carboxypeptidase N. Much of the biological activity of C3a and C5a is removed, although chemotactic activity is retained. The measurement of plasma levels of anaphylatoxins has been made possible with the development of carboxypeptidase N inhibitors.

Effects of C3a and C5a on airways

Airway smooth muscle

Intravenous injection of C5a into guinea-pigs causes bronchoconstriction by mechanisms which may involve direct effect on airway smooth muscle, as can be demonstrated *in vitro*.[26,27] However, C5a and C5a des-Arg can induce the release of other mediators such as histamine, prostaglandins, and leukotrienes from guinea-pig lung.[28,29] Both cyclooxygenase and lipoxygenase products appear to be important in C5a-induced contraction of airway smooth muscle preparations. C3a is a less potent inducer of airway smooth muscle contraction than C5a in the guinea-pig. This effect appears to be mediated predominantly by a cyclooxygenase product, despite the release of histamine.[30] Both C3a and C5a induce marked tachyphylaxis in airway smooth muscle preparations, although there is no cross-desensitization between them, indicating that they are likely to activate discrete receptors.[27]

Vascular effects

C5a and C3a induce vascular permeability in the skin through neutrophil activation, although the role of the neutrophil has not been fully elucidated.[31] Antagonists of platelet-activating factor do not inhibit C5a-induced oedema formation in rabbit skin, despite the observation that C5a can release platelet-activating factor from neutrophils.[32] In man, C5a produces immediate wheal and flare reactions in the skin; and H_1-antihistamine reduces the flare response but not the wheal.[33] Skin biopsies showed the presence of neutrophil infiltration, endothelial cell oedema, and mast cell degranulation.

Mucus secretion

Little is known about the effects of the anaphylatoxins on airway secretion or mucociliary clearance. C3a stimulates mucus glycoprotein secretion from human airways *in vitro*, probably via a direct effect on secretory cells.[34]

Chemotaxis and cell activation

C5a and C5a des-Arg possess chemotactic activity for neutrophils with a potency even greater than that of LTB_4.[35] C5a also has chemotactic activity of macrophages, basophils and eosinophils. By contrast, C3a is devoid of chemotactic activity. Both C5a and

C5a-des-Arg also stimulate the adhesion of inflammatory cells and elicit the release of other mediators including lysosomal enzymes, oxygen free radicals, both lipoxygenase and cyclooxygenase products of arachidonic acid metabolism, and platelet-activating factor from both neutrophils and eosinophils.[36-38]

Possible role in asthma

The role of anaphylatoxins in asthma is uncertain. Several clinical investigators have reported the activation of the complement cascade during asthma. Plasma C4 concentrations have been found to be elevated in childhood asthma and depressed in non-atopic adult asthmatics.[39] Other investigators have not confirmed this observation. No changes in circulating complement components have been detected in allergic asthmatics following either the early- or late-phase reactions after allergen provocation.[40,41] A few patients develop reduced haemolytic-component activity or C4 in arterial or venous blood following allergen provocation,[42] whereas others have reported an increase.[43] However, complement deposition has been found in the bronchial mucosa of asthmatic patients.[44] The alternative pathway can be activated in normal human serum by agents which may induce asthma such as cotton dust, plicatic acid and house dust mite extract.[45,46] The possibility that there may be local complement activation within the asthmatic airway cannot be excluded.

Exposure of guinea-pigs to an aerosol of C5a des-Arg causes an increase in airway responsiveness to histamine, in association with neutrophil infiltration into the airways. The increased airway responsiveness is reduced in animals rendered neutropenic, suggesting that neutrophils contribute to the induction of bronchial hyperresponsiveness by C5a.[47]

There is little experimental data on the effect of the anaphylatoxins on human lung and one cannot extrapolate the observations from various animal species to man. The effect of inhibitors of complement activation or of a specific antagonist of the anaphylatoxins in asthma has not yet been reported. Overall, more information is needed before the role of complement in asthma can be more clearly defined.

SEROTONIN

Serotonin is formed by decarboxylation of tryptophan in the diet and stored in secretory granules. In man, apart from the central nervous system, serotonin is localized in neuroendocrine cells of the gastrointestinal and respiratory tracts, in certain nerves and in secretory granules in platelets. Several types of serotonin receptors have been recognized, with the development of specific antagonists for the receptor subtypes. Of these subtypes, $5HT_2$-receptors are present on tracheal smooth muscle of the guinea-pig, mediating contraction.[48] In addition, $5HT_2$-receptors may also be located on postganglionic nerves to increase cholinergic neurotransmission in guinea-pig airways.[48] $5HT_3$-receptors are also present on nerves and stimulate neurotransmitter release from certain peripheral nerves.[50]

In several species including guinea-pig, cat, rat, dog and monkey, serotonin induces bronchoconstriction, but there is some doubt as to its effect in human airways. Serotonin may even relax human airways *in vitro*.[51] No consistent bronchoconstrictor response has been observed in either normal or asthmatic subjects.[52,53] Serotonin may facilitate acetylcholine release from airway nerves in dogs.[54] Serotonin induces airway microvascular leakage in the guinea-pig.[55]

Few studies have been performed with antagonists of serotonin in asthma. Ketanserin, a $5HT_2$-antagonist, has no protective action against exercise-induced asthma.[56] The use of more specific antagonists and agonists of serotonin-receptor subtypes may help to delineate the contribution of serotonin to the pathophysiology of asthma.

EOSINOPHIL PROTEINS

The human eosinophil is characterized by the presence of eosin-staining granules, the contents of which are mainly made up of four proteins: eosinophil cationic protein (ECP), eosinophil peroxidase (EPO), eosinophil-derived neurotoxin (EDN) and major basic protein (MBP).[57] These proteins have been purified and possess high isoelectric points. The cytotoxic potential of the eosinophil is mediated through the release of its granular constituents. Small amounts of MBP and ECP cause extensive damage to the epithelium, producing a histological picture similar to that seen in bronchial asthma; in addition, MBP slows ciliary beat frequency. The cytotoxic effects of eosinophil proteins on airway epithelium are potentiated by the presence of halide ions and reactive oxygen species.[59] Such damage to the airway epithelium may represent a mechanism by which bronchial hyperresponsiveness is triggered. However, potentiation of the contractile response of airway tissues *in vitro* may be observed with MBP, at concentrations that cause no histological evidence of epithelial damage.[60] MBP, but not EPO or ECP, induces bronchial hyperresponsiveness *in vivo* in primates.[61]

Both ECP and MBP have been demonstrated by immunohistochemical techniques in the lung tissue of patients who have died from asthma[62] with the extracellular deposition of ECP and MBP associated with damaged epithelium. During the late asthmatic reactions to allergen, elevated levels of ECP were measured in bronchoalveolar lavage fluid.[63] Large concentrations of MBP have been reported in sputum from asthmatic patients.[64] In addition, serum ECP levels rise significantly during the pollen season in atopic individuals with seasonal allergic symptoms, and these correlated significantly with the increase in histamine reactivity.[65]

The eosinophil proteins are therefore likely to be a major cause of epithelial damage in asthma. Eosinophils can also generate lipid mediators such as PAF and sulphidopeptide leukotrienes and must therefore be regarded as an important cellular source of mediators which can reproduce many of the pathophysiological features of asthma.

ENDOTHELIN

The endothelin family of peptides consists of three structurally related peptides (endothelin 1, 2 and 3). Endothelin-1 was first isolated from porcine aortic and human endothelial cell cultures.[66,67] These peptides are synthesized as separate precursors which are cleaved to yield a 38-amino-acid intermediate form called 'big' endothelin from which the 17C-terminal acids are removed to leave the mature peptide. Endothelins can be synthesized from a whole range of cells apart from the endothelium, including central nervous system nerves, renal and respiratory epithelia. Endothelins can also be released from canine, porcine and human tracheobronchial epithelial cell cultures.

Binding sites for endothelin-1 are present on the smooth muscle of animal and human airways.[68,69] Endothelin-1 can induce airway smooth muscle contraction *in vitro*[68] and causes bronchoconstriction when administered by inhalation to guinea-pigs.[70] In addition, endothelin-1 stimulates 15-lipoxygenase activity and increases 15-hydroxyeicosatetraenoic acid concentration in bronchoalveolar lavage fluid.[71] Endothelin-1 is also a potent mitogenic factor for fibroblasts[72] and may be involved in the subepithelial fibrosis seen in asthma.

In endobronchial biopsy specimens taken from patients with asthma, immunoreactivity for endothelin-1 was present in the glandular epithelium and the vascular endothelium at a significantly greater level than in atopic and non-atopic healthy control subjects.[73] Endothelin-like immunoreactivity has been detected in bronchoalveolar lavage fluid obtained from a patient with asthma.[74] These observations suggest that the synthesis of endothelin-1 may be increased in asthmatic tissues and that endothelin-1 may be involved in the pathophysiology of asthma.

REFERENCES

1. Tate RM, Morns HG, Schroeder WR, Repine JE: Oxygen metabolites stimulate thromboxane production and vasoconstriction in isolated saline-perfused rabbit lung. *J Clin Invest* (1984) **74**: 608–613.
2. Sporn PH, Peters-Golden M, Simon RH: Hydrogen peroxide-induced arachidonic acid metabolism in the rat alveolar macrophage. *Am Rev Respir Dis* (1988) **137**: 49–56.
3. Ohmori H, Komoriya K, Azuma A, Kurozumi S, Oto YH: Xanthine oxidase-induced histamine release from isolated rat peritoneal mast cells: involvement of hydrogen peroxide. *Biochem Pharmacol* (1978) **28**: 333–334.
4. Stewart RM, Weir EK, Montgomery MR, Niewoehner DE: Hydrogen peroxide contracts airway smooth muscle: a possible endogenous mechanism. *Respir Physiol* (1985) **45**: 333–342.
5. Rhoden KJ, Barnes PJ: Effect of hydrogen peroxide on guinea-pig tracheal smooth muscle *in vitro*: role of cyclo-oxygenase and airway epithelium. *Br J Pharmacol* (1989) **98**: 325–330.
6. Katsumata U, Miura M, Ichinose M, *et al.*: Oxygen radicals produce airway constriction and hyperresponsiveness in anesthetized cats. *Am Rev Respir Dis* (1990) **141**: 1158–1161.
7. Engels F, Oosting RS, Nijkamp F: Pulmonary macrophages induce deterioration of guinea pig tracheal β-adrenergic function through release of oxygen radicals. *Eur J Pharmacol* (1985) **111**: 143–144.
8. Shimasaki H, Takatori T, Anderson WR, Horten HL, Privett OS: Alteration of lung lipids in ozone exposed rats. *Biochem Biophys Res Commun* (1976) **68**: 1256–1262.
9. Holtzman MJ, Aizawa H, Nadel JA, Goetzel EJ: Selective generation of leukotriene B$_4$ by tracheal epithelial cells from dogs. *Biochem Biophys Res Commun* (1983) **114**: 1071–1076.
10. Matsui S, Jones GL, Lane CG, Wolley M, Gantovnick L, O'Byrne PM: The effect of antioxidants on ozone-induced airway hyperresponsiveness in dogs. *Amer Rev Respir Dis* (1991) **143**: A740.
11. Weiss EB: Leukotriene-associated toxic oxygen metabolites induce airway hyperreactivity. *Chest* (1986) **5**: 709–716.
12. Motojima S, Frigas E, Loegering DA, Gleich GJ: Toxicity of eosinophil cationic proteins for guinea pig tracheal epithelium *in vitro*. *Am Rev Respir Dis* (1989) **139**: 801–805.

13. Yukawa T, Read RC, Kroegel C, *et al.*: The effect of activated eosinophils and neutrophils on guinea pig airway epithelium *in vitro. Am Rev Respir Cell Mol Biol* (1990) **2**: 341–354.
14. Welsh MJ, Shasby DM, Russell MH: Oxidants increase paracellular permeability in a cultured epithelial cell line. *J Clin Invest* (1985) **76**: 1155–1168.
15. Cluzel M, Damon M, Chanez P, *et al.*: Enhanced alveolar cell luminol-dependent chemiluminescence in asthma. *J Allergy Clin Immunol* (1987) **80**: 195–201.
16. Kelly CJ, Stenton CS, Bird E, Hendrick DJ, Walters EH: Number and activity of inflammatory cells in bronchoalveolar lavage fluid in asthma and their relation to airway responsiveness. *Thorax* (1988) **43**: 684–692.
17. Postma DS, Renkema TEJ, Noordhoek JA, Faber H, Shuiter HJ, Kauffman H: Association between nonspecific bronchial hyperreactivity and superoxide anion production by polymorphonuclear leukocytes in chronic airflow obstruction. *Am Rev Respir Dis* (1988) **137**: 57–61.
18. Chanez P, Yukawa T, Dent G, Barnes PJ, Chung KF: Generation of oxygen free radicals from blood eosinophils from asthma patients after stimulation with platelet-activating factor and phorbol ester. *Eur Respir J* (1990) **3**: 1002–1007.
19. Malmgren R, Unge G, Zetterstrom O, Theovell H, de Wahl K: Lowered glutathione peroxidase activity in asthmatic patients with food and aspirin intolerance. *Allergy* (1986) **41**: 43–45.
20. Stone J, Hinks LJ, Beasley R, Holgate ST, Clayton BE: Selenium status of patients with asthma. *Clin Sci* (1989) **77**: 495–500.
21. Chilvers ER, Garratt H, Whyte MKB, Fink R, Ind PW: Absence of circulating products of oxygen derived free radicals in acute severe asthma. *Eur Respir J* (1988) **2**: 950–954.
22. Mohsenin V, Dubois AB, Douglas JS: Effect of ascorbic acid on responses to methacholine challenge in asthmatic subjects. *Am Rev Respir Dis* (1983) **127**: 143–147.
23. Owen S, Church S, Suarez-Mendez VJ, Pearson DJ, Woodcock A: Oral anti-oxidant therapy and bronchial hyperreactivity. *Am Rev Respir Dis* (1990) **141**: A832.
24. Muller-Eberhard HJ: Complement. *Ann Rev Biochem* (1975) **44**: 697–724.
25. Lachmann PJ, Peters DK: Complement. In *Clinical Aspects of Immunology*, 4th edn. Oxford, Blackwell Scientific, 1982, pp 18–49.
26. Bodammer G, Vogt, W: Actions of anaphyletoxins on circulation and respiration in the guinea-pig. *Int Arch Allergy Appl Immunol* (1967) **32**: 417–428.
27. Regal JF, Eastman AJ, Pickering RJ: C5a-induced tracheal contraction. A histamine independent mechanism. *J Immunol* (1980) **124**: 2876–2878.
28. Rocha E, Silva M, Bier O, Aronson M: Histamine release by anaphylatoxins. *Nature* (1951) **168**: 465–466.
29. Stimler NP, Bach MK, Blour CM, Hugli TE: Release of leukotrienes from guinea-pig lung stimulated by C5a des arg anaphylatoxin. *J Immunol* (1982) **128**: 2247–2252.
30. Stimler NP, Blour CM, Hugli TE: C3a-induced contraction of guinea-pig parenchyma. Role of cyclo-oxygenase metabolite. *Immunopharmacology* (1983) **5**: 251–257.
31. Wedmore CV, Williams TJ: Control of vascular permeability by polymorphonuclear leucocytes in inflammation. *Nature* (1981) **289**: 646–650.
32. Hellewell PG, Williams TJ: A specific antagonist of platelet-activating factor suppresses oedema formation in an Arthus reaction but not oedema induced by leukocyte chemoattractants in rabbit skin. *J Immunol* (1986) **137**: 302–307.
33. Yancey KB, Hammer CH, Harvalth L, Renfer L, Frank MM, Lawley TJ: Studies of human C5a as a mediator of inflammation in normal human skin. *J Clin Invest* (1985) **75**: 486–495.
34. Marom Z, Shelhamer J, Berger M, Frank M, Kaliner M: Anaphylatoxin C3a enhances mucous glycoprotein release from human airways *in vitro. J Exp Med* (1985) **16**: 657–668.
35. Movat HZ, Rettl C, Burrows CE, Johnston MG: The *in vivo* effect of leukotriene B₄ on polymorphonuclear leukocytes and microcirculation. Comparison with activated complement (C5a des Arg) and enhancement of prostaglandin E2. *Am J Pathol* (1984) **115**: 233–244.
36. Clancy RM, Dahinden CA, Hugli TE: Arachidonate metabolism of human polymorphonuclear leukocytes stimulated by *N*-formyl-Met-Leu-Phe or complement component C5a is independent of phosphodipose activation. *Proc Natl Acad Sci USA* (1983) **80**: 7200–7204.
37. Lee TC, Lenihan OJ, Malone B, Roddy L, Wasserman SI: Increased biosynthesis of platelet-activating factor in activated human eosinophils. *J Biol Chem* (1984) **259**: 5526–5530.

38. McCarthy K, Henson PH: Induction of lysosomal enzyme secretion by alveolar macrophages in response to the purified complement fragments C5a and C5a des arg. *J Immunol* (1979) **123**: 2511–2517.

39. Kay AB, Bacon GD, Mercer BA, Simpson H, Grafton JN: Complement components and IgE in bronchial asthma. *Lancet* (1974) **ii**: 916–920.

40. Kaufman HF, Van der Heide S, Demonchy JGR, De Vries K: Plasma histamine concentrations and complement activation during house dust mite-provoked bronchial obstructive reactions. *Clin Allergy* (1983) **13**: 219–228.

41. Durham SR, Lee TH, Cromwell O, *et al.*: Immunologic studies in allergen-induced late phase asthmatic reactions. *J Allergy Clin Immunol* (1984) **74**: 49–60.

42. Arroyave CM, Stevenson DD, Vaughan JH, Tan FM: Plasma component changes during bronchospasm provoked in asthmatic patients. *Clin Allergy* (1977) **7**: 173–182.

43. Baur X, Dorsch W, Becker T: Levels of complement factors in human serum during immediate and late asthmatic reactions and during acute hypersensitivity pneumants. *Allergy* (1980) **35**: 383–390.

44. Callerame ML, Condemi JJ, Milton G, Bohrod MG, Vaughan JH: Immunologic reactions of bronchial tissues in asthma. *N Engl J Med* (1971) **284**: 459–464.

45. Chan-Yeung M, Gidas PC, Henson PM: Activation of complement of plicatic acid, the chemical compound responsible for asthma due to western red cedar (*Thuja plicata*). *J Allergy Clin Immunol* (1980) **65**: 333–337.

46. Srivastava N, Gupta SP, Srivastava LM: Effect of house dust mite on serum complement activation and total haemophylic activity *in vitro* in normal subjects and in patients with bronchial asthma. *Clin Allergy* (1983) **13**: 43–50.

47. Irvin CG, Berend N, Henson PM: Airways hyperreactivity and inflammation produced by aerosolisation of human C5a des arg. *Am Rev Respir Dis* (1986) **134**: 777–783.

48. Cohen ML, Schenck KW, Colbert W, Wittenauer L: Role of 5-HT$_2$ receptors in serotonin-induced contractions of non-vascular smooth muscle. *J Pharmacol Exp Ther* (1985) **232**: 770–774.

49. Macquin-Mavier I, Jarreau PH, Istin N, Harf A: 5-hydroxytryptamine-induced bronchoconstriction in the guinea-pig: effect of 5-HT$_2$ receptor activation on acetylcholine release. *Br J Pharmacol* (1991) **102**: 1003–1007.

50. Richardson BP, Engel G: The pharmacology and function of 5-HT$_3$ receptors. *Trends Neurol Sci* (1986) **2**: 1986.

51. Raffestin B, Creeina J, Baullet C, Labat C, Benveniste J, Brink C: Response and sensitivity of isolated human pulmonary muscle preparations to pharmacological agents. *J Pharmacol Exp Ther* (1985) **233**: 186–194.

52. Tonnesen P: Bronchial challenge with serotonin in asthmatics. *Allergy* (1985) **40**: 136–140.

53. Cushley MJ, Wee LH, Holgate ST: The effect of inhaled 5-hydroxytryptamine (5-HT serotonin) on airway calibre in man. *Br J Clin Pharmacol* (1986) **22**: 487–490.

54. Hahn HL, Wilson AG, Graf PD, Fischer SP, Nadel JA: Interaction between serotonin and efferent vagus nerves in dog lungs. *J Appl Physiol* (1978) **44**: 144–149.

55. Tokuyama K, Lotvall J, Barnes PJ, Chung KF: Mechanism of airway narrowing caused by inhaled platelet-activating factor: role of airway microvascular leakage and edema. *Am Rev Respir Dis* (1991) **143**: 1345–1349.

56. So SY, Lam NK, Kuens S: Selective 5-HT$_2$ receptor blockade in exercise induced asthma. *Clin Allergy* (1985) **15**: 371–376.

57. Gleich GH, Adolphson CR: The eosinophilic leukocyte: structure and function. *Adv Immunol* (1986) **39**: 177–253.

58. Frigas E, Gleich GJ: The eosinophil and the pathophysiology of asthma. *J Allergy Clin Immunol* (1986) **77**: 527–537.

59. Gleich GJ, Flavahan NA, Fujisaura T, Vanhoutte PM: The eosinophil as a mediator of damage of respiratory epithelium: a model for bronchial hyperreactivity. *J Allergy Clin Immunol* (1988) **81**: 776–781.

60. Flavahan NA, Slifman NR, Gleich GJ, Vanhoutte PM: Human eosinophil major basic protein causes hyperreactivity of respiratory smooth muscle: role of the epithelium. *Am Rev Respir Dis* (1988) **138**: 685–688.

61. Grundel RH, Letts LG, Gleich GJ: Human eosinophil major basic protein induces airway constriction and airway hyperresponsiveness in primates. *J Clin Invest* (1991) **87**: 1470–1473.

62. Filley WV, Holley KE, Kephart GM, Gleich GJ: Identification by immunofluoresence of eosinophil granule major basic protein in lung tissues of patients with bronchial asthma. *Lancet* (1982) **2**: 11–16.

63. De Monchy JGR, Kauffman HF, Venge P, *et al.*: Bronchoalveolar eosinophilia during allergen-induced late asthmatic reactions. *Am Rev Respir Dis* (1985) **131**: 373–376.

64. Dor PJ, Ackerman SJ, Gleich GJ: Charcot–Leyden crystal protein and eosinophil major protein in sputum of patients with respiratory disease. *Am Rev Respir Dis* (1984) **130**: 1072–1077.

65. Rak S, Lowhagen O, Verger P: The effect of immunotherapy on bronchial hyperresponsiveness and eosinophil cationic protein in pollen allergic patients. *J Allergy Clin Immunol* (1988) **82**: 470–480.

66. Yanagisawa M, Kurichara H, Kimura S, *et al.*: A novel potent vasoconstrictor peptide produced by vascular endothelial cells. *Nature* (1988) **332**: 411–415.

67. Inoue A, Yanagisaura M, Kimura S, *et al.*: The human endothelin family: three structurally and pharmacologically distinct isopeptides predicted by three separate genes. *Proc Natl Acad Sci USA* (1989) **86**: 2863–2867.

68. Turner NC, Power RF, Polak JM, Bloom SR, Dollery CT: Endothelin-induced contractions of tracheal smooth muscle and identification of specific endothelin binding sites in the trachea of the rat. *Br J Pharmacol* (1989) **98**: 361–366.

69. Matolli S, Mezzetti M, Riva G, Allegra L, Fasoli A: Specific binding of endothelin on human bronchial smooth muscle cells in culture and secretion of endothelin-like material from bronchial epithelial cells. *J Resp Cell Mol Biol* (1990) **3**: 145–151.

70. Lagente V, Chabrier PE, Mencia-Huerta JM, Braquet P: Pharmacological modulation of the bronchopulmonary action of the vasoactive peptide, endothelin, administered by aerosol in the guinea-pig. *Biochem Biophys Res Commun* (1989) **158**: 625–632.

71. Nagase T, Fukuchi Y, Jo C, *et al.*: Endothelin-1 stimulates arachidonic 15-lipoxygenase activity and oxygen radical formation in the rat distal lung. *Biochem Biophys Res Commun* (1990) **168**: 485–489.

72. Takuwa N, Takuwa Y, Yanagisawa M, Yamashita K, Masaki T: A novel vasoactive peptide endothelin stimulates mitogenesis through inositol lipid turnover in Swiss 3T3 fibroblasts. *J Biol Chem* (1989) **264**: 7856–7861.

73. Springall DR, Howarth PH, Counihan H, Djukanovic R, Holgate ST, Polak JM: Endothelin immunoreactivity of airway epithelium in asthmatic patients. *Lancet* (1991) **337**: 697–701.

74. Nomura A, Uchida Y, Kameyama M, Saotome M, Oki K, Hasegawa S: Endothelin and bronchial asthma. *Lancet* (1989) **ii**: 747–748.

22

Neural and Humoral Control

PETER J. BARNES AND NEIL C. THOMSON

INTRODUCTION

There is now considerable evidence that neural control of the airways may be abnormal in asthma, and the neurogenic mechanisms may contribute to the pathophysiology of asthma. Indeed there is a complex interaction between inflammation and neural control of airways (Fig. 22.1). Autonomic nerves regulate many aspects of airway function and influence the tone of airway smooth muscle, airway secretions, blood flow, microvascular permeability and the migration and release of inflammatory cells.[1,2] In inflammatory diseases of the airways neural mechanisms may augment or modulate the inflammatory response.

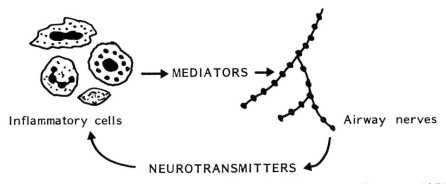

Fig. 22.1 Interaction between nerves and inflammatory cells. Inflammatory mediators may inhibit or facilitate the release of neurotransmitters from airway nerves, and in turn neurotransmitters may modulate or enhance the inflammatory response.

ASTHMA: BASIC MECHANISMS AND CLINICAL MANAGEMENT (2nd Edn)
ISBN 0-12-079026-2

Neural control of human airways is complex and the contribution of neurogenic mechanisms to the pathophysiology of airway disease is still debated. Because changes in bronchomotor tone in asthma occur rapidly, it was suggested many years ago that there might be an abnormality in autonomic neural control in asthma, with an imbalance between excitatory and inhibitory pathways, resulting in excessively reactive airways. Several types of autonomic defect have been proposed in asthma, including enhanced cholinergic, α-adrenergic, and excitatory non-adrenergic non-cholinergic (e-NANC) mechanisms, or reduced β-adrenergic and inhibitory NANC (i-NANC) mechanisms. Various abnormalities in airway control have been described in asthma, although it seems unlikely that these are primary defects but are secondary to the disease or its treatment.[1] Nevertheless, it is likely that neural mechanisms contribute to the symptoms and pathophysiology of asthma.

Airway function is also influenced by circulating hormones, which include adrenaline secreted from the adrenal medulla, and atrial natriuretic peptide released from the atria and, in some species, from pulmonary veins. Cortisol secreted from the adrenal cortex may also play an important role in regulating inflammation, and the circadian fall in plasma cortisol and adrenaline may play an important role in nocturnal asthma.[3]

The recognition that airway inflammation is critical in asthma raises the possibility that there may be interaction between neurohumoral and inflammatory mechanisms (Fig. 22.1). Inflammatory mediators may modulate or facilitate the release of neurotransmitters from airway nerves by acting at prejunctional receptors,[4] or may act on autonomic receptors on target cells of the airway. Similarly, neural mechanisms may contribute to the inflammatory reaction in the airway wall, and the concept of neurogenic inflammation, which is well established in skin and gut may also apply to the airways.[5,6]

In this chapter we review some of the possible neural and humoral mechanisms which may be relevant to asthma. The area of NANC neural mechanisms and the many neuropeptides which have potent effects on airway function[7] are reviewed in detail in Chapter 23.

NEURAL CONTROL

Cholinergic mechanisms

Cholinergic nerves are the dominant neural bronchoconstrictor pathway in animal and human airways,[8] and there has been considerable interest in whether cholinergic mechanisms are exaggerated in asthma or chronic obstructive airway disease (COAD). This is supported by the observation that many triggers which induce bronchospasm (such as sulphur dioxide, prostaglandins, histamine and cold air) also stimulate afferent receptors and may therefore lead to reflex cholinergic bronchconstriction. Anticholinergic drugs are the most effective bronchodilators in COAD. While they are effective in acute asthma, they are usually less effective in chronic asthma, suggesting that cholinergic mechanisms may become more important during exacerbations of asthma. There are several mechanisms which might contribute to cholinergic bronchoconstriction in asthma.[9]

Increased vagal tone

There may be an increase in central vagal drive, although there is no direct evidence for this in asthma. Indirect evidence which may suggest such an increase in vagal tone is the enhanced vagal cardiac tone (as determined by the Valsalva manoeuvre and sinus arrhythmia gap) which has been demonstrated in asthma,[10] and the increase in sinus arrhythmia gap at night, which corresponds with nocturnal bronchoconstriction.[11]

Reflex bronchoconstriction

There may be increased cholinergic reflex bronchoconstriction due to stimulation of sensory receptors in the airway (irritant receptors and C-fibre endings) by inflammatory mediators. Several mediators, such as histamine, prostaglandins and bradykinin, stimulate sensory receptors in the airways,[12] and it is possible that these receptors may be more easily triggered in asthma, since airway epithelium may be damaged, or sensory endings 'sensitized' by inflammatory mediators such as bradykinin, prostaglandins or cytokines.

Reflex bronchoconstriction may also be initiated from sensory receptors in the larynx, nose and oesophagus. Whether rhinitis exacerbates asthma through enhanced cholinergic reflex bronchoconstriction is not certain. However, there is evidence that gastro-esophageal acid reflux may exacerbate asthma through cholinergic mechanisms, since anticholinergic drugs inhibit the bronchoconstrictor associated with reflux ('the reflux reflex').

Increased acetylcholine release

There may be enhanced neurotransmission in cholinergic ganglia, perhaps because of release of other neurotransmitters or mediators, or facilitation of acetylcholine (ACh) release from postganglionic nerve terminals.[4] For example thromboxane, PGD_2 and tachykinins facilitate acetylcholine release from postganglionic nerves in the airways. Facilitation may also occur at parasympathetic ganglia in the airways; these structures are surrounded by inflammatory cells and have an afferent nerve input. There is evidence for facilitated transmission in sensitized animals exposed to allergen, although the mediators are not yet identified.[13] Histamine, surprisingly, has an inhibitory effect on ganglionic neurotransmission and on postganglionic nerves in guinea pig and human airways, which is mediated through H_3-receptors.[14,15] These receptors are activated by low concentrations of histamine and may represent a safety device to inhibit reflex bronchoconstriction, whereas larger concentrations of histamine may override this mechanism and cause bronchoconstriction directly by acting on H_1-receptors on airway smooth muscle.

Muscarinic receptors

There may be an increased effect of cholinergic stimulation of airway smooth muscle due to an increase in muscarinic receptor density or affinity, or due to increased efficacy of signal transduction. Asthmatic patients show an exaggerated bronchoconstrictor response to cholinergic agonists, but this is not specific, since a similar increased responsiveness is observed with other spasmogens, such as histamine, leukotrienes or prostaglandins, suggesting that a specific enhancement of muscarinic receptors is unlikely.

There are conflicting reports about the response to asthmatic airways *in vitro* to cholinergic agonists and other spasmogens, but in most studies neither an increased sensitivity nor an increased maximal response to cholinergic agonists has been reported.[16-18] In guinea-pigs, which become hyperresponsive to ACh *in vivo* after intravenous or inhaled platelet-activating factor (PAF), there is no increase in response of airways *in vitro* to ACh, no change in muscarinic receptors as determined by direct receptor binding, nor any change in coupling or biochemical consequences of receptor activation as measured by cholinergic stimulation of phosphoinositide turnover.[19] This indicates that the increased cholinergic responsiveness cannot be explained by enhancement of muscarinic receptors or their coupling in airway smooth muscle, and perhaps is more likely to be explained by mechanical factors such as airway oedema induced by PAF.

Muscarinic receptor subtypes. At least three subtypes of muscarinic receptor have been recognized pharmacologically and five distinct receptor subtypes have now been cloned. Muscarinic receptor subtypes have now also been recognized in airways,[20] and autoradiographic mapping shows that they are differentially distributed in human airways.[21]

M_1-receptors, which are excitatory, are present in airway parasympathetic ganglia of animals and may be inhibited by the M_1-selective blocker pirenzepine. The function of these M_1-receptors in regulation of airway tone is not yet certain, but they may play an important role in controlling the amount of filtering that occurs in parasympathetic ganglia, since these receptors appear to be important in the chronic regulation of ganglionic transmission, whereas the classical nicotinic receptors may be more important in rapid neurotransmission, as in reflexes. Similar receptors are also likely to be present in human parasympathetic ganglia, since pirenzepine inhibits reflex bronchoconstriction at doses that do not inhibit the direct effect of cholinergic agonists in airway tone.[22] M_1-receptors could be important in asthma if they facilitate cholinergic reflexes and they may play a role in nocturnal asthma in which increased vagal tone at night is important.

Inhibitory muscarinic receptors (autoreceptors) have been demonstrated on cholinergic nerves of airways in animals *in vivo*, and in human bronchi *in vitro*.[23] These prejunctional receptors inhibit ACh release and therefore may serve to limit vagal bronchoconstriction. Autoreceptors are of the M_2-receptor subtype and clearly different pharmacologically from M_3-receptors on airway smooth muscle (Fig. 22.2). Drugs such as atropine and ipratropium bromide, which block both prejunctional receptors and those on smooth muscle with equal efficacy, therefore increase ACh release which may then overcome the postjunctional blockade. This means that such drugs will not be as effective against vagal bronchoconstriction as against cholinergic agonists, so it may be necessary to re-evaluate the contribution of cholinergic nerves when drugs that are selective for the muscarinic receptors on airway smooth muscle (M_3-antagonists) are developed. Indeed, in animals low doses of ipratropium bromide increase vagally mediated bronchoconstriction.[24] It is possible that the *paradoxical* bronchoconstriction which is occasionally seen with inhaled anticholinergics may be due to this effect.

The presence of muscarinic autoreceptors has been demonstrated in human subjects *in vivo*. A cholinergic agonist, pilocarpine, which selectively activates M_2-receptors, inhibits cholinergic reflex bronchoconstriction induced by sulphur dioxide in normal subjects, but such an inhibitory mechanism does not appear to operate in asthmatic

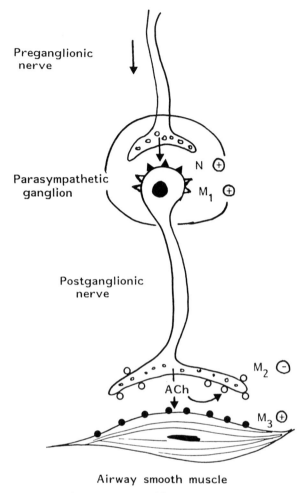

Preganglionic
nerve

Parasympathetic
ganglion

N ⊕

M₁ ⊕

Postganglionic
nerve

M₂ ⊖

ACh

M₃ ⊕

Airway smooth muscle

Fig. 22.2   Muscarinic receptor subtypes in airways. M_1-receptors in parasympathetic ganglia may *facilitate* neurotransmission which is mediated via nicotinic receptors (N), whereas M_2-receptors on postganglionic nerve terminals may *inhibit* the release of acetylcholine (ACh), thus reducing the stimulation of postjunctional M_3-receptors which constrict airway smooth muscle.

subjects, suggesting that there may be dysfunction of these autoreceptors.[25] Such a defect in muscarinic autoreceptors may then result in exaggerated cholinergic reflexes in asthma, since the normal feedback inhibition of acetylcholine release may be lost. This might also explain the sometimes catastrophic bronchoconstriction which occurs with β-blockers in asthma which, at least in mild asthmatics, appears to be mediated by cholinergic pathways.[26] Antagonism of inhibitory β-receptors on cholinergic nerves would result in increased release of acetylcholine which could be switched off in the asthmatic patient (Fig. 22.3).[27]

The mechanisms that lead to dysfunction of prejunctional M_2-receptors in asthmatic airways are not certain, but it is possible that M_2-receptors may be more susceptible to damage by oxidants or other products of the inflammatory response in the airways. Recent experimental studies have demonstrated that influenza virus infection in guinea-

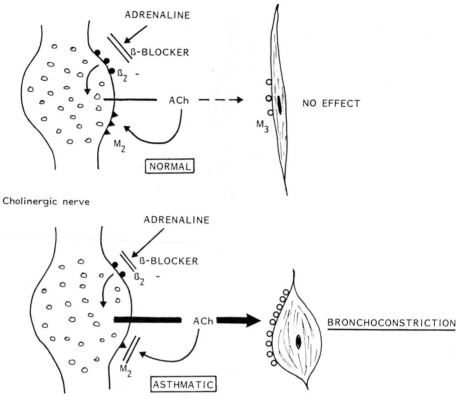

Fig. 22.3 A possible mechanism of β-blocker induced bronchoconstriction. β-Blockers may inhibit the modulatory effect of circulating adrenaline on β_2-receptors of cholinergic nerves, thus increasing acetylcholine (ACh) release. In normal subjects this may act at M_2-autoreceptors to inhibit further ACh release, so no effect on airway smooth muscle is seen. In asthmatic patients, if there is a defect in M_2 autoreceptors the increased ACh cannot switch itself off. Released ACh also has a greater effect on airway smooth muscle because of non-specific airway hyperresponsiveness in asthma.

pigs may result in a selective loss of M_2-receptors compared with M_3-receptors, due to the action of viral neuraminidase on the sialic acid residues on M_2-receptors which are necessary for their function. This results in a loss of autoreceptor function and enhanced cholinergic bronchoconstriction.[28] This may be a mechanism contributing to airway hyperresponsiveness after upper respiratory tract virus infections.

The development of more selective muscarinic drugs and the application of molecular biology techniques with cDNA probes for muscarinic subtypes will help to elucidate the role of muscarinic receptor subtypes in asthma.

Adrenergic mechanisms

Since β-agonists have a dramatic effect in relieving asthmatic bronchoconstriction, it was logical to suggest that there might be a defect in β-adrenoceptor function in asthma. Adrenergic mechanisms involve sympathetic nerves, circulating catecholamines and α- and β-adrenoceptors. Several possible abnormalities in adrenergic control have been proposed in asthma.[29]

Adrenergic innervation

Adrenergic nerves do not control human airway smooth muscle directly but could influence cholinergic neurotransmission via prejunctional α- or β-receptors.[1] There is no evidence to suggest that sympathetic neurotransmission may be abnormal in asthma, but it is theoretically possible that inflammatory mediators, such as histamine, might impair the release of noradrenaline from adrenergic nerves. Adrenergic neural control of the bronchial vasculature may also be important in asthma, particularly during exercise and cold air challenge, when conditioning of inspired air may be important.

β-Adrenoceptors

The possibility that β-receptors are abnormal in asthma has been extensively investigated. The suggestion that there is a primary defect in β-receptor function in asthma has not been substantiated and any defect in β-receptors is likely to be secondary to the disease, perhaps as a result of inflammation or as a consequence of adrenergic therapy. Some studies have demonstrated that airways from asthmatic patients fail to relax normally to isoprenaline, suggesting a possible defect in β-receptor function in airway smooth muscle.[16,17] Whether this is due to a reduction in β-receptors, a defect in receptor coupling, or some abnormality in the biochemical pathways leading to relaxation, is not yet known, although in a single asthmatic patient the density of β-receptors in airway smooth muscle appeared to be normal.[30] However, the fact that asthmatic airways may relax normally to theophylline suggests the defect may be specific for β-receptors.[16] β-Receptors are very widely distributed in the lungs and airways[31] and using labelled cDNA probes it has been possible to visualize sites of β_2-receptor gene transcription in human lung.[32] This may provide a new approach to the study of β-receptor regulation in airway disease and to the study of how inflammation may affect β-receptor expression and coupling.

α-Adrenoceptors

α-Receptors which mediate bronchoconstriction have been demonstrated in airways of several species, and may only be demonstrated under certain experimental conditions. There is now considerable doubt about the role of α-receptors in the regulation of tone in human airways, however, since it has proved difficult to demonstrate their presence functionally or by autoradiography,[33] and α-blocking drugs do not appear to be effective as bronchodilators. It is possible that α-receptors may play an important role in regulating airway blood flow, which may indirectly influence airway responsiveness, and there is some evidence that α-agonists may *reduce* airway narrowing in exercise-induced asthma.[34]

HUMORAL FACTORS

Circulating catecholamines

Since adrenergic nerves do not directly control airway smooth muscle, it seems probable that circulating catecholamines may play a more important role in regulation of bronchomotor tone.[35] Although the catecholamines, noradrenaline, adrenaline and dopamine, are present in the circulation, only adrenaline has effects on airway calibre at physiological concentrations.[36–43] Since β-blockers cause bronchoconstriction in asthmatic patients, but not in normal subjects this suggests that adrenergic drive to the airways is important in defending against bronchoconstriction, and in the absence of adrenergic innervation this drive might be provided by circulating adrenaline (see Chapter 30). Basal adrenaline concentrations, however, are not elevated in stable asthmatic patients,[44] even in those who bronchoconstrict with intravenous propranolol.[45] The circadian variation in adrenaline concentrations in asthmatic patients is similar to that found in normal subjects.[46] Furthermore, correction of the nocturnal fall in plasma adrenaline does not alter the peak flow values of patients with nocturnal asthma.[47] These findings taken together with the report of nocturnal asthma occurring in a patient after adrenalectomy[48] suggest that a fall in plasma adrenaline at night is not the only factor in nocturnal asthma. Nevertheless basal circulating adrenaline concentrations may have a role in the maintenance of airway calibre in some asthmatic patients particularly when airway calibre is reduced.

Bronchoconstriction *per se* is not a stimulus to adrenaline release.[42,49,50] Even during acute exacerbations of asthma there may be no elevation in plasma adrenaline level,[51] although very high adrenaline concentrations have been found in some patients with acute severe asthma.[52] Although a blunted catecholamine response to exercise in asthmatic patients has been reported by some investigators,[49,53] other studies have found no significant difference in either peak plasma catecholamine level between normal and asthmatic subjects nor in response to increasing levels of exercise.[54–57] All these reports confirm that the workload is of paramount importance in determining the sympatho-adrenal response to exercise and this might explain the apparent conflict between studies. Taking these studies together it seems unlikely that a reduced sympatho-adrenal response to exercise is an important mechanism in the pathogenesis of exercise-induced asthma.

Cortisol

The pharmacological effects of corticosteroids in the airways are thought to include anti-inflammatory actions on individual inflammatory cells such as eosinophils, associated with a reduction in vascular and airway permeability. Other possible actions of corticosteroids relevant to airway function include a reduction in mucus production and the potentiation of catecholamine effects (see Chapter 36). Treatment with inhaled or oral corticosteroids results in improved symptom control and reversal of airflow obstruction.

It is unclear whether physiological concentrations of cortisol have similar actions on the airways. The nadir in the circadian variation in plasma cortisol occurs 4 h before maximal bronchoconstriction,[46,58,59] although the delayed action of cortisol means that it could still have an influence on airway calibre. Although Kallenbach et al.[60] found a reduced nadir of plasma cortisol in patients with nocturnal asthma compared to patients without nocturnal asthma or non-asthmatic subjects, these authors could not exclude that their findings were not related to previous corticosteroid therapy. Furthermore, infused hydrocortisone has no effect on the nocturnal fall in PFR[52] suggesting that the circulating corticol level is not an important factor in determining nocturnal asthma.

The late asthmatic response following allergen challenge is associated with inflammatory reaction within the airways, but this response is not a result of an alteration in circulating cortisol levels.[61]

Corticosteroid resistant asthma

A subgroup of asthmatic patients responds well to bronchodilators but is unresponsive to corticosteroids ('corticosteroid resistant' asthma).[62] The cause of corticosteroid resistance in these patients remains unclear. Corticosteroid-resistant asthmatic patients show no evidence of reduced glucocorticoid receptor numbers and anti-lipocortin antibodies are no commoner when compared to corticosteroid-sensitive patients.[63–65] One report has suggested that corticosteroid-resistant patients may respond better to betamethasone than prednisolone.[66] Corticosteroid-resistant asthma may be explained by a relative insensitivity of the mononuclear and T-lymphocytes of these patients to the inhibitory effects of corticosteroids.[63,67,68] The defect in corticosteroid responsiveness may be more generalized since corticosteroid-resistant patients demonstrate a reduced skin vasoconstrictor response to topically applied beclomethasone diproprionate.[69]

Atrial natriuretic peptide

Atrial natriuretic peptide (ANP) is produced in the cardiac atria and released in response to stretch. It circulates in man as a 28 amino-acid peptide and affects volume homeostasis via a number of neuroendocrine mechanisms.[70] It is also known to have a direct relaxant effect on vascular smooth muscle.[71,72] Whilst the primary source of ANP is the cardiac atria, the biologically active hormone is also secreted from isolated perfused lung.[73] Specific ANP receptors have been localized to lung including airway smooth muscle.[74–76] These results suggest that ANP of pulmonary origin may contribute to circulating plasma levels and may also exert a local autocrine effect.

A dose-dependent relaxant effect of various atriopeptins and ANP has been demonstrated on airway smooth muscle in a number of animal studies and varying degrees of protection against induced tone have also been shown.[77–81] In bovine and guinea-pig trachea the relaxant effect of ANP appears to be mediated via the same mechanisms as in vascular tissue, namely by stimulation of particulate guanylate cyclase and subsequent generation of cGMP.[79,81] Previous studies have suggested that ANP does not cause significant relaxation of isolated human bronchial smooth muscle.[82,83] However, in a recent preliminary study in which higher concentrations of ANP (10^{-9}–10^{-5} M) were used, ANP had a direct relaxant effect in human bronchial smooth muscle against methacholine-induced tone.[84]

An intravenous infusion of exogenous ANP produces a very significant bronchodilator response in both normal and asthmatic subjects (Fig. 22.4)[85–87] and reduces the bronchoconstrictor response to inhaled histamine[88] and to fog challenge.[89] The rise in plasma ANP levels during exercise[57,90] is similar to these obtained during the lowest rates of ANP infusion[85] and these results suggest that these elevations may lead to attenuation of bronchospasm. Elevated plasma ANP levels are found in patients with cardiac failure[91] and cor pulmonale[92] and under these circumstances ANP may also play a protective role on the airways.

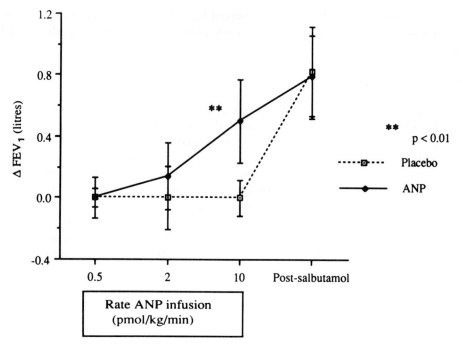

Fig. 22.4 Mean (95% confidence intervals) change in FEV_1 with varying rates of intravenous infusion of atrial natriuretic peptide compared with placebo (n = 8). Nebulized salbutamol was given after final infusion (adapted from ref. 85).

Thyroxine

The development of hyperthyroidism can be associated with deterioration in asthma control, with subsequent improvement in asthma after treatment of the thyrotoxicosis.[93–95] Conversely the occurrence of hypothyroidism has been reported to be associated with improvement in asthma control, which relapses following treatment with thyroxine replacement.[96] Several possible mechanisms have been suggested to account for the relationship between asthma and thyroid disease. Firstly β-adrenergic airway responsiveness has been reported to be inversely related to thyroxine levels both *in vitro*, in guinea-pig trachea specimens[97] and *in vivo*, in non-asthmatic subjects.[95] Following treatment of hyperthyroidism or hypothyroidism, airway β-adrenergic responses return to euthyroid level.[98] The alteration in β-adrenergic activity seems unlikely to be secondary to an alteration in circulating catecholamine levels[99] or to a reduction in β-adrenergic receptor numbers.[100,101] Possibly thyroxine is acting as a postreceptor site within the smooth muscle.[98,102] Secondly, Cockcroft *et al.*[103] reported a decrease in non-specific bronchial reactivity in an asthmatic patient after treatment of hyperthyroidism. Studies examining the effects of different circulating thyroid hormone levels on non-specific reactivity in non-asthmatic individuals, however, have produced conflicting results.[104–108] Possibly the effects of thyroid hormones on airway reactivity may differ between asthmatic and non-asthmatic individuals. The administration of triiodothronine to normal subjects was found not to increase airway reactivity[104] and two recent studies were unable to find any change in bronchial reactivity in groups of non-asthmatic patients after correction of hyperthyroidism.[105,106] In contrast, Israel *et al.*[107] reported that thyrotoxicosis was associated with reduced carbachol bronchial reactivity and Wieshammer *et al.*[108] found that acute hypothyroidism caused an increase in non-specific reactivity. Thirdly, although hydrocortisone metabolism is increased in hyperthyroidism, circulating corticosteroid levels are not elevated.[109] Fourthly, the metabolism of arachidonic acid is altered *in vitro* by the lungs of rats made hyperthyroid.[110] In particular, there is a reduction in the breakdown of the prostaglandins PGE_2 and $PGE_{2\alpha}$. Possibly the effects of elevated thyroxine levels in man may result in a potentiation of the effects of prostaglandins on the airways. Finally, respiratory muscle weakness which may occur in hyperthyroidism[105] could contribute to the dyspnoea that commonly accompanies thyrotoxicosis and this action may heighten the degree of breathlessness experienced by a patient with pre-existing airway disease. In conclusion it seems likely that more than one mechanism accounts for the effects of thyroid disease on co-existent asthma.

REFERENCES

1. Barnes PJ: Neural control of human airways in health and disease. *Am Rev Respir Dis* (1986) **134**: 1289–1314.
2. Barnes PJ: Neural control of airway function: new perspectives. *Molec Aspects Med* (1990) **11**: 351–423.
3. Barnes PJ: Inflammatory mechanisms and nocturnal asthma. *Am J Med* (1988) **85**(Suppl 1B): 64–70.
4. Barnes PJ: Neuromodulation in the airways. *Physiol Rev* (1992) in press.
5. Barnes PJ: Asthma as an axon reflex. *Lancet* (1986) **i**: 242–245.
6. Barnes PJ: Neurogenic inflammation in airways and its modulation. *Arch Int Pharmacodyn* (1990) **303**: 67–82.
7. Barnes PJ, Baraniuk J, Belvisi MG: Neuropeptides in the respiratory tract. *Am Rev Respir Dis* (1991) **144**: 1187–1198.
8. Barnes PJ: Cholinergic control of airway smooth muscle. *Am Rev Respir Dis* (1987) **136**: S42–S45.
9. Widdicombe JG, Karlsson J-A, Barnes PJ: Cholinergic mechanisms in bronchial hyperresponsiveness and asthma. In Kaliner MA, Barnes PJ, Persson CGA (eds) In *Asthma Its Pathology and Treatment*, 49th edn. New York, Marcel Dekker, 1991, pp 327–356.
10. Kallenbach JM, Webster T, Dowdeswell R, Reinach SG, Scott Millar RN, Zwi S: Reflex heart rate control in asthma. *Chest* (1985) **87**: 644–648.
11. Postma DS, Keyzer JJ, Koeter GA, Sluiter HJ, De Vries K: Influence of the parasympathetic and sympathetic nervous systems on nocturnal bronchial obstruction. *Clin Sci* (1985) **69**: 251–258.
12. Nadel JA, Barnes PJ, Holtzman MJ: Autonomic factors in the hyperreactivity of airway smooth muscle. In *Handbook of Physiology: The Respiratory System III*. Bethesda, MD, American Physiological Society, 1986, pp 693–702.
13. McCaig DJ: Comparison of autonomic responses in the trachea isolated from normal and albumin sensitive guinea-pigs. *Br J Pharmacol* (1987) **92**: 809–816.
14. Ichinose M, Stretton CD, Schwartz J-C, Barnes PJ: Histamine H_3-receptors inhibit cholinergic neurotransmission in guinea-pig airways. *Br J Pharmacol* (1989) **97**: 13–15.
15. Ichinose M, Barnes PJ: Inhibitory histamine M_3-receptors on cholinergic nerves in human airways. *Eur J Pharmacol* (1989) **163**: 383–386.
16. Goldie RG, Spina D, Henry PJ, Lulich KM, Paterson JW: *In vitro* responsiveness of human asthmatic bronchus to carbachol, histamine, β-adrenoceptor agonists and theophylline. *Br J Clin Pharmacol* (1986) **22**: 669–676.

17. Cerrina J, Ladurie ML, Labat C, Raffestin B, Bayol A, Brink C: Comparison of human bronchial muscle response to histamine *in vivo* with histamine and isoproterenol agonists *in vitro*. *Am Rev Respir Dis* (1986) **134**: 57–61.

18. Whicker SD, Armour CL, Black JL: Responsiveness of bronchial smooth muscle from asthmatic patients to relaxant and contractile agonists. *Pulm Pharmacol* (1988) **1**: 25–31.

19. Robertson DN, Rhoden KJ, Grandordy B, Page CP, Barnes PJ: The effect of platelet activating factor on histamine and muscarinic receptor function in guinea-pig airways. *Am Rev Respir Dis* (1988) **137**: 1317–1322.

20. Barnes PJ: Muscarinic receptors in airways: recent developments. *J Appl Physiol* (1990) **68**: 1777–1785.

21. Mak JCW, Barnes PJ: Autoradiographic visualization of muscarinic receptor subtypes in human and guinea pig lung. *Am Rev Respir Dis* (1990) **141**: 1559–1568.

22. Lammers J-WJ, Minette P, McCusker M, Barnes PJ: The role of pirenzepine-sensitive (M_1) muscarinic receptors in vagally mediated bronchoconstriction in humans. *Am Rev Respir Dis* (1989) **139**: 446–449.

23. Minette PA, Barnes PJ: Prejunctional inhibitory muscarinic receptors on cholinergic nerves in human and guinea-pig airways. *J Appl Physiol* (1988) **64**: 2532–2537.

24. Fryer AD, Maclagan J: Ipratropium bromide potentiates bronchoconstriction induced by vagal nerve stimulation in the guinea-pig. *Eur J Pharmacol* (1987) **139**: 187–191.

25. Minette PAH, Lammers J, Dixon CMS, McCusker MT, Barnes PJ: A muscarinic agonist inhibits reflex bronchoconstriction in normal but not in asthmatic subjects. *J Appl Physiol* (1989) **67**: 2461–2465.

26. Ind PW, Dixon CMS, Fuller RW, Barnes PJ: Anticholinergic blockade of beta-blocker induced bronchoconstriction. *Am Rev Respir Dis* (1989) **139**: 1390–1394.

27. Barnes PJ: Muscarinic receptor subtypes: implications for lung disease. *Thorax* (1989) **44**: 161–167.

28. Fryer AD, Jacoby DB: Parainfluenza virus infection damages inhibitory M_2-muscarinic receptors on pulmonary parasympathetic nerves in the guinea pig. *Br J Pharmacol* (1991) **102**: 267–271.

29. Barnes PJ: Adrenergic regulation of airway function. In Kaliner MA, Barnes PJ (eds) *The Airways: Neural Control in Health and Disease.* New York, Dekker, 1988, pp 57–85.

30. Spina D, Rigby PJ, Paterson JW, Goldie RG: Autoradiographic localization of beta-adrenoceptors in asthmatic human lung. *Am Rev Respir Dis* (1989) **140**: 1410–1415.

31. Carstairs JR, Nimmo AJ, Barnes PJ: Autoradiographic visualization of beta-adrenoceptor subtype in human lung. *Am Rev Respir Dis* (1985) **1332**: 541–547.

32. Hamid QA, Mak JC, Sheppard MN, Corrin B, Venter JC, Barnes PJ: Localization of β_2-adrenoceptor messenger RNA in human and rat lung using *in situ* hybridization: correlation with receptor autoradiography. *Eur J Pharmacol Mol Pharmacol* (1991) **206**: 133–138.

33. Spina D, Rigby PJ, Paterson JW, Goldie RG: α_1-Adrenoceptor function and autoradiographic distribution in human asthmatic lung *Br J Pharmacol* (1989) **97**: 701–708.

34. Dinh-Xuan AT, Chaussain M, Regnard J, Lockart A: Pretreatment with an inhaled α_1-adrenergic agonist, methoxamine, reduces exercise-induced asthma. *Eur Respir J* (1989) **2**: 409–414.

35. Barnes PJ: Endogeneous catecholamines and asthma. *J Allergy Clin Immunol* (1986) **77**: 791–795.

36. Berkin KE, Inglis GC, Ball SG, Thomson NC: Airway responses to low concentrations of adrenaline and noradrenaline in normal subjects. *Q J Exp Physiol* (1985) **70**: 203–209.

37. Thomson NC, Patel KR: Effect of dopamine on airways conductance in normals and extrinsic asthmatics. *Br J Clin Pharmac* (1978) **5**: 421–424.

38. Michoud MC, Amyot R, Jennertet-Grosjean A: Dopamine effect on bronchomotor tone *in vivo*. *Am Rev Respir Dis* 1984) **130**: 755–758.

39. Warren JB, Dalton N: A comparison of the bronchodilator and vasopressor effects of exercise levels of adrenaline in man. *Clin Sci* (1983) **64**: 475–479.

40. Warren JB, Dalton N, Turner C, Clark TJH: Protective effect of circulating epinephrine within the physiological range on the airway response to inhaled histamine in non-asthmatic subjects. *J Allergy Clin Immunol* (1984) **74**: 683–686.
41. Barnes PJ, FitzGerald GA, Dollery CT: Circadian variation in adrenergic responses in asthmatic subjects. *Clin Sci* (1982) **62**: 349–354.
42. Larssen K, Grunneberg R, Hjemdahl P: Bronchodilation and inhibition of allergen-induced bronchoconstriction by circulating epinephrine in asthmatic subjects. *J Allergy Clin Immunol* (1985) **75**: 586–593.
43. Berkin KE, Inglis GC, Ball SG, Thomson NC: Effect of low dose adrenaline and noradrenaline infusions on airway calibre in asthmatic patients. *Clin Sci* (1986) **70**: 347–352.
44. Barnes PJ, Ind PW, Brown MJ: Plasma histamine and catecholamines in stable asthmatic subjects. *Clin Sci* (1982) **62**: 661–665.
45. Ind PW, Barnes PJ, Durham SR, Kay AB: Propranolol-induced bronchoconstriction in asthma: beta-receptor blockage and mediator release. *Am Rev Respir Dis* (1984) **129**:10.
46. Barnes PJ, Fitzgerald G, Brown M, Dollery C: Nocturnal asthma and changes in circulating epinephrine, histamine and cortisol. *N Engl J Med* (1980) **303**: 263–267.
47. Morrison JFJ, Teale C, Pearson SB, *et al.*: Adrenaline and nocturnal asthma. *Br Med J* (1990) **301**: 473–476.
48. Morice A, Sever P, Ind PW: Adrenaline, bronchoconstriction and asthma. *Br Med J* (1986) **293**: 539–540.
49. Barnes PJ, Brown MJ, Silverman M, Dollery CT: Circulating catecholamines in exercise and hyperventilation induced asthma. *Thorax* (1981) **36**: 435–440.
50. Sands MF, Douglas FL, Green J, Banner AS, Robertson GL, Laff AR: Homeostatic regulation of bronchomotor tone by sympathetic activation during bronchoconstriction in normal and asthmatic humans. *Am Rev Respir Dis* (1985) **132**: 993–998.
51. Ind PW, Causson RC, Brown MJ, Barnes PJ: Circulating catecholamines in acute asthma. *Br Med J* (1985) **290**: 267–279.
52. Clarke B, Ind PW, Causson R, Barnes PJ: Bronchodilation and catecholamine responses to induced hypoglycaemia in acute asthma. *Clin Sci* (1985) **69**: 35P.
53. Warren JB, Keynes RJ, Brown MJ, Jenner DA, McNicol NW: Blunted sympathoadrenal response to exercise in asthmatic subjects. *Br J Dis Chest* (1982) **76**: 147–150.
54. Larsson K, Hjemdahl P, Martinsson A: Sympathoadrenal activity in exercise-induced asthma. *Chest* (1982) **82**: 560–567.
55. Berkin KE, Walker G, Inglis GC, Ball SG, Thomson NC: Circulating adrenaline and noradrenaline concentrations during exercise in patients with exercise induced asthma and normal subjects. *Thorax* (1988) **43**: 295–299.
56. Gilbert IA, Lennen KA, McFadden ER: Sympathoadrenal response to repetitive exercise in normal and asthmatic subjects. *J Appl Physiol* (1988) **64**: 2667–2674.
57. Hulks G, Mohammed AF, Jardine AG, Connell JMC, Thomson NC: Circulating plasma levels of atrial natriuretic peptide and catecholamines in response to maximal exercise in normal and asthmatic subjects. *Thorax* (1991) **46**: 824–828.
58. Reinberg A, Ghata J, Sidi E: Nocturnal asthma attacks: their relationship to the circadian adrenal cycle. *J Allergy* (1963) **34**: 323–330.
59. Soutar CA, Costello J, Ijaduola O, Turner-Warwick M: Nocturnal and morning asthma: relationship to plasma corticosteroid and response to cortisol infusion. *Thorax* (1975) **30**: 436–440.
60. Kallenbach JM, Panz VR, Joffe BI, *et al.*: Nocturnal events related to 'morning dipping' in bronchial asthma. *Chest* (1988) **93**: 751–757.
61. Durham SR, Keenan J, Cookson WOCM, Craddock CF, Benson MK: Diurnal variation in serum cortisol concentrations in asthmatics after allergen inhalation challenge. *Thorax* (1989) **44**: 582–585.
62. Carmichael J, Paterson IC, Diaz P, Crompton GK, Kay AB, Grant IWB: Corticosteroid resistance in chronic asthma. *Br Med J* (1981) **282**: 1419–1422.
63. Corrigan CJ, Brown PH, Barnes NC, *et al.*: Corticosteroid resistance in chronic asthma: glucocorticoid pharmacokinetics, glucocorticoid receptor characteristics and inhibition of peripheral blood T cell proliferation by corticosteroids *in vitro*. *Am Rev Respir Dis* (1991) **144**: 1016–1025.

64. Wilkinson JRW, Podgorski MR, Godolphin JL, Goulding NJ, Lee TH: Bronchial asthma is not associated with autoantibodies to lipocortin-1. *Clin Exp Allergy* (1990) **20**: 189–190.
65. Chung KF, Podgorski MR, Goulding NJ, *et al.*: Circulating autoantibodies to lipocortin in asthma. *Resp Med* (1991) **85**: 37–44.
66. Grandordy B, Belmatoug N, Morelle A, De Lauture D, Marsac J: Effect of betamethasone on airway obstruction and bronchial response to salbutamol in prednisolone resistant asthma. *Thorax* (1987) **42**: 65–71.
67. Pozansksy MC, Gordon ACH, Douglas JG, Krajewski AS, Wyllie AH, Grant IWB: Resistance to methylprednisolone in cultures of blood mononuclear cells from glucocorticoid-resistant asthmatic patients. *Clin Sci* (1984) **67**: 639–645.
68. Wilkinson JRW, Crea AEG, Clark TJH, Lee TH: Identification and characterisation of a monocyte-derived neutrophil activating factor in corticosteroid-resistant bronchial asthma. *J Clin Invest* (1989) **84**: 1930–1941.
69. Brown PH, Teelucksingh S, Matusiewicz SP, Greening AP, Crompton GK, Edwards CRW: Cutaneous vasoconstrictor response to glucocorticoids in asthma. *Lancet* (1991) **337**: 576–580.
70. Goetz KL: Physiology and pathophysiology of atrial peptides. *Am J Physiol* (1988) **254**: E1–E15.
71. Winquist RJ: The relaxant effects of atrial natriuretic factor on vascular smooth muscle. *Life Sci* (1985) **37**: 1081–1087.
72. Thibault G, Garcia R, Carrier F, *et al.*: Structure-activity relationships of atrial natriuretic factor (ANF). I Natriuretic activity and relaxation of intestinal smooth muscle. *Biochem Biophys Res Commun* (1984) **125**: 938–946.
73. Gutkowska J, Nemer M: Structure, expression and function of atrial natriuretic factor in extraatrial tissues. *Endocrine Rev* (1989) **10**: 519–536.
74. Olins GM, Patton DR, Tjoeng FS, Blehm DJ: Specific receptors for atriopeptin III in rabbit lung. *Biophys Biochem Res Commun* (1986) **140**: 302–307.
75. Von Schroeder HP, Nishimura E, McIntosh CHS, Buchan AMJ, Wilson N, Laidsome JR: Autoradiographic localisation of binding sites for atrial natriuretic factor. *Can J Physiol Pharmacol* (1985) **63**: 1373–1377.
76. Ishii Y, Watanabe T, Watanabe M, Hasegawa S, Uchiyama Y: Effects of atrial natriuretic peptide on type II alveolar epithelial cells of the rat lung. *J Anat* (1989) **166**: 89–95.
77. O'Donnell M, Garippa R, Welton AF: Relaxant activity of atriopeptins in isolated guinea-pig airway and vascular smooth muscle. *Peptides* (1985) **6**: 597–601.
78. Hamel R, Ford-Hutchinson AW: Relaxant profile of synthetic atrial natriuretic factor on guinea-pig pulmonary tissues. *Eur J Pharmacol* (1986) **121**: 151–155.
79. Ishii K, Murad F: ANP relaxes bovine tracheal smooth muscle and increases cGMP. *Am J Physiol* (1989) **256** (*Cell Physiol* **25**): C495–500.
80. Amyot T, Lesiège D, Michoud MC, Larochelle P, Hamet P: Effect of atrial natriuretic factor on airway sensitivity to histamine in anaesthetized dogs. *Eur Resp J* (1989) **2** (Suppl 5): 301s.
81. Watanabe H, Suzuki K, Takagui K, Sataki T: Mechanism of atrial natriuretic polypeptide and sodium nitroprusside-induced relaxation in guinea pig tracheal smooth muscle. *Arzneim-Forsch* (1990) **40**: 771–776.
82. Labat C, Norel Y, Benveniste J, Brink C: Vasorelaxant effects of atrial peptide II on isolated human pulmonary muscle preparations. *Eur J Pharmacol* (1988) **150**: 387–400.
83. Candenas ML, Naline E, Puybasset L, Devillier P, Advenier C: Effect of atrial natriuretic peptide and of atriopeptins on the human isolated bronchus. Comparison with the reactivity of the guinea-pig isolated trachea. *Pulm Pharmacol* (1991) **4**: 120–125.
84. Hulks G, Crabb K, McGrath JC, Thomson NC: *In vitro* effects of atrial natriuretic factor and sodium nitroprusside on bronchomotor tone in human bronchial smooth muscle. *Am Rev Respir Dis* (1991) **143**: A344.
85. Hulks G, Jardine A, Connell JMC, Thomson NC: Bronchodilator effect of atrial natriuretic peptide. *Brit Med J* (1989) **299**: 1081–1082.
86. Chanez P, Mann C, Bousquet J *et al.*: Atrial natriuretic factor (ANF) is a potent bronchodilator in asthma. *J Allergy Clin Immunol* (1990) **86**: 321–324.
87. Hulks G, Jardine A, Connell JMC, Thomson NC: The effect of atrial natriuretic factor on bronchomotor tone in the normal human airway. *Clin Sci* (1990) **79**: 51–55.

88. Hulks G, Jardine A, Connell JMC, Thomson NC: The influence of elevated plasma levels of atrial natriuretic factor on bronchial reactivity in asthma. *Am Rev Respir Dis* (1991) **143**: 778–782.

89. McAlpine LG, Hulks G, Thomson NC: The effect of an intravenous infusion of atrial natriuretic factor on fog-induced bronchoconstriction in patients with asthma. *Am Rev Respir Dis* (1991) **143**: A424.

90. Rubinstein I, Reiss TF, Gardner DG, Liu J, Bigby BG, Boushey HA: Effect of exercise hyperpnea, and bronchoconstriction on plasma atrial natriuretic peptide. *J Appl Physiol* (1989) **67**: 2565–2570.

91. Raine AEG, Erne P, Burgisser E, *et al.*: Atrial natriuretic peptide and atrial pressure in patients with congestive cardiac failure. *N Engl J Med* (1986) **315**: 533–537.

92. Burghuber OC, Harterr E, Punzengruber C, Weissel M, Woloszczuk W: Human atrial natriuretic peptide secretions in precapillary pulmonary hypertension. *Chest* (1988) **92**: 31–37.

93. Elliott CA: Occurrence of asthma in patients manifesting evidence of thyroid dysfunction. *Am J Surg* (1929) **7**: 333–337.

94. Ayres J, Clark TJH: Asthma and the thyroid. *Lancet* (1981) **ii**: 1110–1111.

95. Lipworth BJ, Dhillon DP, Clark RA, Newton RW: Problems with asthma following treatment of thyrotoxicosis. *Br J Dis Chest* (1988) **82**: 310–314.

96. Bush RK, Ehrlick EN, Reed CE: Thyroid disease and asthma *J Allergy Clin Immunol* (1977) **59**: 398–401.

97. Taylor SE: Additional evidence against universal modulation of β-adrenoceptor responses by excessive thyroxine. *Br J Pharmacol* (1983) **78**: 639–644.

98. Harrison RN, Tattersfield AE: Airway response to inhaled salbutamol in hyperthyroid and hypothyroid patients before and after treatment. *Thorax* (1984) **39**: 34–39.

90. Coulombe P, Dussault JH, Walker P: Plasma catecholamine concentrations in hyperthyroidism and hypothyroidism. *Metabolism* (1976) **25**: 973–979.

100. Williams RS, Guthrow CE, Lefkowitz, RJ: Beta-adrenergic receptors of human lymphocytes are unaltered by hyperthyroidism. *J Clin Endocrinal Metab* (1979) **48**: 503–505.

101. Scarpace PJ, Abrass IB: Thyroid hormone regulation of rat heart, lymphocyte and lung beta-adrenergic receptors. *Endocrinology* (1981) **108**: 1007–1011.

102. Guarnieri T, Filburn CR, Beard ES, Lakatta EG: Enhanced contractile response and protein kinase activation to threshold levels of beta-adrenergic stimulation in hyperthyroid rat heart. *J Clin Invest* (1980) **65**: 861–868.

103. Cockcroft DW, Silverberg JDH, Dosman JA: Decrease in nonspecific bronchial reactivity in an asthmatic patient following treatment of hyperthyroidism. *Ann Allergy* (1978) **41**: 160–163.

104. Irwin RS, Pratter MR, Stivers DH, Braverman LE: Airway reactivity and lung function in triiodothyronine-induced thyrotoxicosis. *J Appl Physiol* (1985) **58**: 1485–1488.

105. Kendrick AH, O'Reilly JF, Laslo G: Lung function and exercise performance in hyperthyroidism before and after treatment. *Q J Med* (1988) **68**: 615–627.

106. Roberts JA, McLellan AR, Alexander WD, Thomson NC: Effect of hyperthyroidism on bronchial reactivity in non-asthmatic patients. *Thorax* (1989) **44**: 603–604.

107. Israel RH, Poe RH, Cave WT, Greenblatt DW, DePapp Z: Hyperthyroidism protects against carbechol-induced bronchospasm. *Chest* (1987) **91**: 242–245.

108. Wieshammer S, Keck FS, Shäuffelen AC, Von Beauvais H, Seibold H, Hombach V: Effects of hypothyroidism on bronchial reactivity in non-asthmatic subjects. *Thorax* (1990) **45**: 947–950.

109. Hellman L, Bradlow HL, Zumoff B, Gallagher TF: The influence of thyroid hormone on hydrocortisone production and metabolism. *J Clin Endocrinol Metab* (1961) **21**: 1231–1247.

110. Hoult JRS, Moore P: Thyroid disease, asthma, and prostaglandins. *Br Med J* (1978) **i**: 366.

Airway NANC Nerves and Neuropeptides

PETER J. BARNES

INTRODUCTION

Many neuropeptides are localized to sensory, parasympathetic, and sympathetic neurons in the airways (Table 23.1).[1-3] These peptides have potent effects on bronchomotor tone, airway secretions, the bronchial circulation and on inflammatory and immune cells. The precise physiological roles of each peptide is still not known, but some clues

Table 23.1 Neuropeptides in the respiratory tract.

Peptide	Localization
Vasoactive intestinal peptide Peptide histidine isoleucine/methionine Peptide histidine valine-42 Helodermin PACAP-27 Galanin	Parasympathetic
Substance P Neurokinin A Neuropeptide K Calcitonin-gene related peptide Gastrin-releasing peptide	Afferent
Neuropeptide Y	Sympathetic
Somatostatin Enkephalin Cholecystokinin octapeptide	Afferent/uncertain

ASTHMA: BASIC MECHANISMS AND CLINICAL MANAGEMENT (2nd Edn)
ISBN 0-12-079026-2

are provided by their localization and functional effects. This chapter reviews what is known of these peptides, particularly in the human respiratory tract, and discusses their possible pathophysiological role in asthma.

NON-ADRENERGIC NON-CHOLINERGIC NERVES

In addition to classical cholinergic and adrenergic innervation of airways, there are neural mechanisms that are not blocked by cholinergic or adrenergic antagonists.[4] Non-adrenergic non-cholinergic (NANC) nerves were first described in the gut and therefore their existence in the respiratory tract is to be expected. NANC nerves were initially conceived as a 'third' nervous system in the lungs, but it rapidly became apparent that several distinct neural mechanisms are included. NANC mechanisms result in both bronchodilatation and bronchoconstriction, vasodilation and vasoconstriction, and mucus secretion, indicating that several neurotransmitters are likely to be involved.

Inhibitory NANC nerves

Inhibitory NANC (i-NANC) nerves relax airway smooth muscle. They have been demonstrated *in vitro* by electrical field stimulation after adrenergic and cholinergic blockade in several species, including humans.[4] In human airway smooth muscle the i-NANC mechanism is the only neural bronchodilator pathway, since there is no functional sympathetic innervation to airway smooth muscle and there has been considerable research into the identity of the neurotransmitter(s).

i-NANC nerves have also been demonstrated *in vivo* in some species by electrical stimulation of the vagus after adrenergic and cholinergic blockade. Stimulation of this pathway produces pronounced and long-lasting bronchodilatation, which may be inhibited by ganglion blockers. This pathway may be activated reflexly by mechanical or chemical stimulation of the larynx. In human subjects *in vivo* mechanical stimulation of the larynx or chemical stimulation with capsaicin in the presence of adrenergic and cholinergic blockers have also demonstrated reflex reversal of induced tone (Fig. 23.1).[5]

Purines

At first it was believed that purines may be the neurotransmitters in i-NANC nerves in airways, but the evidence does not support this view. Although exogenous ATP may relax airway smooth muscle, an antagonist quinidine fails to block NANC relaxation *in vitro* and *in vivo* and the purine uptake inhibitor, dipyridamole, does not enhance i-NANC responses.[6] Similarly, adenosine fails to mimic NANC relaxation and antagonists, such as theophylline, have no blocking effect.[6,7]

Nitric oxide

Recent evidence has demonstrated that nitric oxide (NO) may be a neurotransmitter of some NANC responses. The enzyme nitric oxide synthase, which produces NO from the

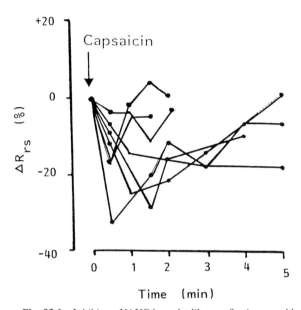

Normal human subjects   (n=7)

 ● Cholinergic blockade (inhaled ipratropium br)
 ● Adrenergic blockade (oral propranolol)
 ● Bronchoconstriction   (inhaled LTD_4)

Fig. 23.1   Inhibitory NANC bronchodilator reflex in normal human subjects.

precursor L-arginine, is localized to several peripheral nerves. Inhibition of NO synthase by L-N^Gnitroarginine markedly reduces i-NANC responses in guinea-pig trachea *in vitro*.[8] In human trachea another NO synthase inhibitor, L-N^Gmonomethyl arginine, also reduces i-NANC responses, producing approximately 50% inhibition at low frequencies of stimulation,[9] whereas L-N^Gnitroarginine methyl ester gives even greater inhibition, indicating that NO may be the *major* transmitter of i-NANC responses in human airways.

Neuropeptides

Evidence also favours a neuropeptide as a neurotransmitter of i-NANC nerves. Of the several neuropeptides identified in airways, only vasoactive intestinal peptide (VIP) and the related family of peptides (see below) relax airway smooth muscle and are, therefore, the only identified peptide candidates. In guinea-pig trachea there is compelling evidence that VIP contributes to the i-NANC response, since this is partially reduced by α-chymotrypsin, which degrades VIP[10] and by preincubation with a specific antiserum to VIP.[11] It now seems likely that both NO and VIP may contribute to the i-NANC response in airways and it is possible that they may be differentially released from airway nerves under different conditions of nerve stimulation. Thus VIP may only be released at high frequencies of stimulation, whereas NO may be released at all frequencies.

Excitatory NANC nerves

Electrical stimulation of guinea-pig bronchi, and occasionally trachea *in vitro*, and vagus nerve *in vivo* produces a component of bronchoconstriction that is not inhibited by atropine.[12] This bronchoconstrictor response has been termed the excitatory NANC (e-NANC) response and there is convincing evidence that it is mediated by the retrograde release of tachykinins from a certain population of sensory nerves. A similar e-NANC response has occasionally been reported in human airways *in vitro*, but this is not consistent.[13]

Other NANC responses

Other NANC responses in addition to effects on airway smooth muscle have been described in airways. NANC-mediated secretion of mucus has been demonstrated in cats *in vivo* using vagal nerve stimulation, and in ferret airways *in vitro* using electrical field stimulation.[14] NANC regulation of airway blood flow has been demonstrated in several species, with both vasodilator and vasoconstrictor effects.[15] NANC neurally mediated plasma extravasation has also been demonstrated in some species. These NANC secretory and vascular effects are likely to be mediated by a variety of neuropeptides, and in some instances by purines and NO.

Co-transmission

Although NANC nerves were originally envisaged as an anatomically separate nervous system, it is now more likely that NANC neural effects are mediated by the release of neurotransmitters from classical autonomic nerves (Table 23.1). Thus the i-NANC responses in airway smooth muscle are likely to be mediated by the release of co-transmitters such as NO and VIP from cholinergic nerves. NANC vasoconstrictor responses are mediated by the release of neuropeptide Y (NPY) from adrenergic nerves. e-NANC bronchoconstrictor responses are mediated by the release of tachykinins from unmyelinated sensory nerves. The physiological relevance of co-transmission is likely to be related to the 'fine tuning' of classical autonomic nerves, but the role of the co-transmitters may become more apparent in disease.

Co-existence of several peptides within the same nerve is commonly described in the peripheral nervous system, and multiple combinations are possible, giving rise to the concept of 'chemical coding' of nerve fibres. VIP and peptide histidine isoleucine (PHI) usually co-exist since they are derived from the same precursor peptide coded by a single gene. Galanin is often present with VIP in cholinergic neurons. In sensory nerves substance P (SP), neurokinin A (NKA) and calcitonin-gene related peptide (CGRP) often co-exist, but some sensory nerves may also contain galanin and VIP.[1] Similarly adrenergic nerves which contain NPY may also contain somatostatin, galanin, VIP and enkephalin. Thus there is a complex distribution of neuropeptides in the innervation of the airways, with the same peptides occurring in different types of nerve (Fig. 23.2). The physiological significance of this complexity is not yet clear, but it seems likely that there may be functional interactions between the multiple neuropeptides released and the classical transmitters which allow complex integration and regulation of functions in the airway.

Neuropeptides are often released by high-frequency firing and therefore may only be co-released with classical neurotransmitters with certain patterns of neural activation. Little is known about the optimal conditions for neuropeptide release, but it seems likely that release may be favoured by certain physiological and pathophysiological conditions. Furthermore little is known about the effect of repeated neural activation on the synthesis and release of neuropeptides, but it is possible that in certain diseases, when chronic nerve irritation may occur, that there may be increased neuropeptide gene expression, synthesis and release.

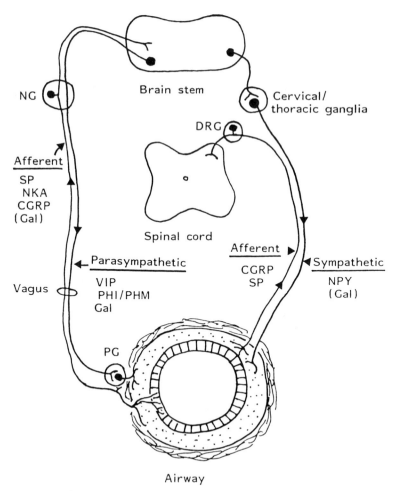

Fig. 23.2 Innervation of lower respiratory tract, showing neuropeptide co-localization in autonomic nerves. DRG, dorsal root ganglion; PG, parasympathetic ganglion; NG, nodose ganglion.

VASOACTIVE INTESTINAL PEPTIDE

VIP is a 28 amino-acid peptide that is localized to several types of nerve in the respiratory tract of several species, including humans. VIP has potent effects on airway and pulmonary vascular tone and on airway secretion, which suggests that it may have an important regulatory role.

Localization

VIP has been isolated from lung extracts of several species, including humans and is one of the most abundant of the neuropeptides found in lung. VIP-like immunoreactivity is localized to nerves and ganglia in airways.[1,16] VIP-immunoreactivity is present in ganglion cells in the posterior trachea and around intrapulmonary bronchi, diminishing in frequency as the airways become smaller. Usually VIP-immunoreactive neurones occur in parasympathetic ganglia, but isolated ganglion cells are also seen.

VIP-immunoreactive nerves are widely distributed throughout the respiratory tract. There is a rich VIP-ergic innervation in the proximal airways, but the density of innervation diminishes peripherally so that few VIP-ergic fibres are found in bronchioles. The pattern of distribution largely follows that of cholinergic nerves in airways consistent with the co-localization of VIP and acetylcholine (ACh) in human airways.[17] VIP-ergic nerves are found within airway smooth muscle, around bronchial vessels and surrounding submucosal glands. VIP may also be localized to some sensory nerves, including subepithelial nerves in the airways, which may arise in the jugular and nodose ganglia.[16] VIP, at least in some species, may also be localized to sympathetic nerves.

VIP receptors

VIP receptors have been identified in the lung of several species by receptor-binding techniques using [^{125}I]VIP.[18] Binding of VIP to its receptor activates adenylyl cyclase, and VIP stimulates cyclic AMP formation. The actions of VIP are, therefore, similar to those of β-adrenoceptor agonists and any differences in response of different tissues to VIP or β-agonists depends on the relative densities or coupling of their respective receptors. Autoradiographic mapping of VIP receptors demonstrates a high density in airway smooth muscle of large, but not small, airways.[19] VIP receptors are also found in high density in airway epithelium and submucosal glands.

Effect on airway smooth muscle

VIP is a potent relaxant of airway smooth muscle *in vitro* and is more potent than isoprenaline in relaxing human bronchi, making it one of the most potent endogenous bronchodilators.[20] Since there is a rich VIP-ergic innervation of human bronchi, this suggests that VIP may be an important regulator of bronchial tone and may be involved in counteracting the bronchoconstriction of asthma. In human airways, bronchi are potently relaxed by VIP, while bronchioles are unaffected. In contrast, both relax to an equal degree with isoprenaline.[20] This response of human airways is consistent with the distribution of VIP-receptors, since receptors are to be seen in bronchial smooth muscle, but not in bronchiolar smooth muscle.[19] This peripheral diminution of VIP-receptors is also consistent with the distribution of VIP-immunoreactive nerves which diminish markedly as airways become smaller.[16] These studies suggest that VIP, while regulating the calibre of large airways, is unlikely to influence small airways.

Intravenous VIP causes bronchodilatation *in vivo* in cat airways.[21] In asthmatic patients, however, inhaled VIP has no bronchodilator effect, and only a small protective effect against inhaled histamine, although a β-adrenergic agonist in the same subjects is markedly effective.[22] This lack of potency of inhaled VIP may be explained by the epithelium since this possesses proteolytic enzymes and may present a barrier to diffusion. Infused VIP has no bronchodilator effect in normal subjects who readily bronchodilate with isoprenaline.[23] However, infusion of VIP produces flushing, marked hypotension and reflex tachycardia. These effects limit the dose that can be given by infusion and, as VIP has a more potent relaxant effect on vessels than on airway smooth muscle, thus prevent administration of a sufficient bronchodilating dose. Infused VIP causes bronchodilation in asthmatic subjects, but the effect is trivial,[24] and might be explained by the reflex sympathoadrenal activation secondary to the profound cardiovascular effects. VIP therefore has little therapeutic potential in asthma.

Effects on airway secretion

VIP-immunoreactive nerves are closely associated with airway submucosal glands and form a dense network around the gland acini. VIP potently stimulates mucus secretion, measured by ^{35}S-labelled glycoprotein secretion, in ferret airway *in vitro*, being significantly more potent than isoprenaline.[25] VIP receptors have been localized to human submucosal glands, suggesting that VIP-ergic nerves may regulate mucus secretion in human airways.[19] VIP has an inhibitory effect on glycoprotein secretion from human tracheal explants,[26] which is surprising since agonists that stimulate cyclic AMP formation would be expected to stimulate secretion. More recently the effects of VIP on mucus secretion have been found to be more complex and may depend on the drive to gland secretion. Mucus secretion stimulated by cholinergic agonists is inhibited in ferret trachea but stimulated in cat trachea, whereas secretion stimulated with the α-adrenergic agonist phenylephrine is augmented.[14]

VIP is a potent stimulant of chloride ion transport and therefore water secretion of dog tracheal epithelium,[27] suggesting that VIP may be a regulator of airway water secretion and therefore mucociliary clearance. The high density of VIP receptors on epithelial cells of human airways, suggests that VIP may regulate ion transport and other epithelial functions in human airways.[19]

Vascular effects

VIP is a potent vasodilator in systemic vessels. It increases airways blood flow in dogs and pigs, and is more potent on tracheal than on bronchial vessels.[15] There is convincing evidence that VIP is a mediator of NANC vasodilatation in trachea, whereas in more peripheral airways other neuropeptides are involved.[28] Since VIP is likely to have a greater effect on bronchial vessels than on airway smooth muscle, it may provide a mechanism for increasing blood flow to contracted smooth muscle. Thus, if VIP is released from cholinergic nerves, it may improve muscular perfusion during cholinergic contraction. Perhaps the apparent protective effect of inhaled VIP against histamine-induced bronchoconstriction in human subjects,[29] despite a lack of effect on broncho-motor tone, may be explained by an increase in bronchial blood flow which would more rapidly remove inhaled histamine from sites of deposition in the airways.

Neuromodulatory effects

VIP is localized to nerves which surround airway ganglia, suggesting a possible neuro-modulatory effect on cholinergic neurotransmission. VIP appears to modulate cholin-ergic neurotransmission in guinea-pig parasympathetic ganglia[30] and postganglionic nerves,[31] since it has a greater inhibitory effect on neurally induced bronchoconstriction than on an equivalent contractile response induced by exogenous acetylcholine. VIP also modulates the release of peptides from sensory nerves in guinea-pig bronchi *in vitro*.[31]

Anti-inflammatory actions

VIP inhibits release of mediators from pulmonary mast cells,[32] and may have several other anti-inflammatory actions in airways. VIP may interact with T-lymphocytes and has the potential to act as a local immunomodulator in airways.[33]

VIP as an i-NANC transmitter

Several lines of evidence implicate VIP as a neurotransmitter of i-NANC nerves in airways:

(1) VIP produces prolonged relaxation of airway smooth muscle which is unaffected by adrenergic or neural blockade, and which has a time-course similar to that of i-NANC responses both *in vitro* and *in vivo* in several species. VIP also mimics the electrophysiological changes in airway smooth muscle produced by NANC nerve stimulation.[7]

(2) Electrical field stimulation of tracheobronchial preparations releases VIP into the bathing medium and this release is blocked by tetrodotoxin, proving that it is derived from nerve stimulation.[34]

(3) In the absence of potent specific blockers of VIP-receptors other strategies have been adopted. Incubation of cat and guinea-pig trachea with high concentrations of VIP induces tachyphylaxis and also reduces the magnitude of NANC nerve relaxation, while responses to sympathetic nerve stimulation and isoprenaline are unaffected.[7,34]

(4) VIP relaxes airway smooth muscle by increasing intracellular cyclic AMP and its effects are therefore potentiated by a selective inhibitor of cyclic AMP phosphodiesterase, which normally degrades intracellular cyclic AMP.[35] Under the same experimental conditions, this phosphodiesterase also potentiates i-NANC responses in guinea-pig trachea.

(5) Perhaps the most convincing evidence that VIP is a transmitter of i-NANC nerves in airways are studies with enzymes which degrade this peptide. VIP is rapidly broken down into inactive fragments by trypsin and α-chymotrypsin and also by mast cell tryptase.[36] Incubation of guinea-pig trachea with α-chymotrypsin, under conditions which completely block responses to exogenous VIP, results is a significant reduction in i-NANC response.[10] However inhibition is incomplete indicating that some other transmitter (now known to be NO) is involved. In human airways the i-NANC response is unaffected by α-chymotrypsin, but it is possible that the enzyme does not have good access to the sites where VIP is released.[9]

(6) The close association between responses to VIP and NANC relaxation in different sizes of human airways[20] provides supportive evidence for VIP as a neurotransmitter.

Some evidence argues *against* VIP as a neurotransmitter of i-NANC in airways. After pretreatment of guinea-pig trachea with maximally effective concentrations of VIP, there is no diminution of i-NANC relaxation, which would be expected if all VIP-receptors were occupied.[6] However, exogenous VIP may not have ready access to the VIP receptors related to VIP-ergic nerves. Removal of the epithelium potentiates the bronchodilator action of VIP *in vitro*, but has no enhancing effect on i-NANC responses.[37] This might be because VIP is released from cholinergic nerves distant from airway epithelium. In addition, there is convincing evidence from guinea-pig and human airways that NO contributes to bronchodilator i-NANC responses.[8,9] The precise role of VIP as an i-NANC transmitter can only be resolved when potent and specific VIP-antagonists become available.

Co-transmission with acetylcholine

VIP co-exists with ACh in airway cholinergic nerves. VIP may be released from cholinergic nerves only with high-frequency firing and may serve to increase the blood flow to exocrine glands under conditions of excessive stimulation. VIP also appears to co-exist with ACh in airways,[17] and it seems likely that there is a functional relationship between VIP and cholinergic neural control.

It is possible that excessive stimulation of cholinergic nerves and certain patterns of firing result in VIP release. In bovine tracheal smooth muscle, VIP has an inhibitory effect on cholinergic nerve-induced contraction only with high frequency firing, and also reduces the contractile effect of exogenous ACh.[38] This does not involve any change in muscarinic receptor density or affinity, and may be due to functional antagonism. VIP also has in inhibitory effect on the release of ACH from airway cholinergic nerves.[30,31] Conversely, α-chymotrypsin, which degrades VIP, potentiates cholinergic-nerve induced contractions in guinea-pig airways.[39] VIP and NO seem to counteract the bronchoconstrictor effect of cholinergic bronchoconstriction and thus may function as

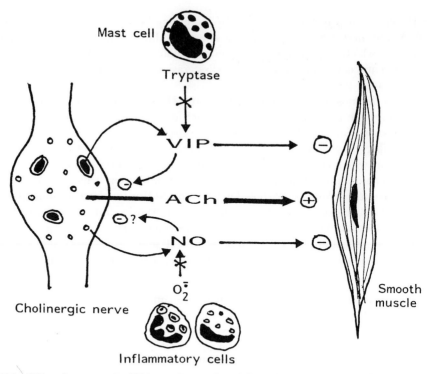

Fig. 23.3 VIP and nitric oxide (NO) may be co-released from cholinergic nerves and act as functional antagonists of cholinergic bronchoconstriction. In addition they may act prejunctionally to inhibit ACh release. In asthma enzymes such as tryptase released from airway mast cells may rapidly degrade VIP, and oxygen free radials, such as superoxide anions (O_2^-) from inflammatory cells may inactivate NO, thus leading to exaggerated cholinergic neural bronchoconstriction.

the 'braking' mechanism for airway cholinergic nerves (Fig. 23.3). If this mechanism were to be deficient with either reduced release or increased breakdown of VIP, then an exaggerated bronchoconstrictor response may result.

Possible abnormalities in asthma

Whether dysfunction of VIP-ergic innervation contributes to airway disease is uncertain. A striking absence of VIP-immunoreactive nerves has been described in the lungs of patients with asthma in tissues largely obtained at post-mortem.[40] The loss of VIP-immunoreactivity from all tissues including pulmonary vessels is so complete that it seems unlikely to represent a fundamental absence of VIP-immunoreactive nerves in asthma. More likely is the possibility that enzymes, such as mast cell tryptase, are released from inflammatory cells in asthma and that these rapidly degrade VIP when sections are cut.[41] Biopsies taken from patients with mild asthma suggest that VIP-immunoreactive nerves appear normal in asthma.[42] VIP antibodies, which would neutralize the effects of VIP, have also been described in the plasma of asthmatic patients.[43] They are found with the same prevalence in non-asthmatic patients, so that their significance is doubtful. While it seems unlikely that there would be any primary abnormality in VIP innervation in the airways of patients with asthma, it is possible that a secondary abnormality may arise as a result of the inflammatory process in the airway.

Mast cell tryptase is particularly active in degrading VIP.[36] Tryptase released from mast cells in the asthmatic airway may then more rapidly degrade VIP and related peptides released from airway cholinergic nerves. This would remove a 'brake' from cholinergic nerves and lead to exaggerated cholinergic reflex bronchoconstriction (Fig. 23.3). This may also have the effect of increasing inflammatory responses in the airway, since VIP has anti-inflammatory actions. In addition NO may also be more rapidly degraded by oxidants, such as superoxide anion released from activated inflammatory cells, further adding to the increase in cholinergic tone and inflammatory effects.

Whether i-NANC responses are impaired in asthma is not yet certain. In patients with mild asthma no evidence for an impaired NANC bronchodilator reflex has been observed.[5] However this does not preclude a defect in more severe asthmatics, in whom the degree of airway inflammation may be greater. In sensitized guinea-pigs exposed to allergen, a reduction in i-NANC responses has been reported.[44] This is presumably due to the release of enzymes or oxygen free radicals from inflammatory cells in the airways. However, as discussed above, the contribution of VIP to i-NANC responses in human airways is not yet established, and increased degradation of this peptide in asthma may have a relatively minor effect on airway tone.

VIP-RELATED PEPTIDES

Several other peptides that are similar in structure and effect to VIP have now been identified in the mammalian nervous system.

Peptide histidine isoleucine

Peptide histidine isoleucine (PHI) and its human equivalent peptide histidine methionine (PHM) have a marked structural similarity to VIP, with 50% amino-acid sequence homology. PHI and PHM are encoded by the same gene as VIP and both peptides are synthesized in the same prohormone. It is therefore not surprising to find that PHI has a similar immunocytochemical distribution in lung to VIP, and that PHI-immunoreactive nerves supply airway smooth muscle (especially larger airways), bronchial and pulmonary vessels, submucosal glands and airway ganglia.[16] PHI stimulates adenylyl cyclase and appears to activate the same receptor as VIP.[18] In human bronchi *in vitro* PHM is a potent relaxant, and is equipotent to VIP.[20] It is likely that PHI/PHM is released with VIP from airway nerves and may also be a contributory neurotransmitter in i-NANC nerves.

Peptide histidine valine

Peptide histidine valine (PHV-42) is an N-terminally extended precursor of VIP. PHV is a potent bronchodilator of guinea-pig airways *in vitro*,[45] but when infused in asthmatic patients has no demonstrable bronchodilator effect.[46] It is not yet clear whether this peptide is released from airway nerves.

Helodermin

Helodermin is a 35 amino-acid peptide of similar structure to VIP which has been isolated from the salivary gland venom of the Gila monster lizard. Helodermin-like immunoreactivity has been localized to airway nerves and has similar effects to VIP, but has a longer duration of action. Helodermin is a potent relaxant of airway smooth muscle *in vitro*, and heliodermin-like immunoreactivity has been found in trachea.[47] Helodermin appears to activate a high affinity form of the VIP receptor.[18]

Pituitary adenylate cyclase activating peptide (PACAP)

PACAP, a 38 amino-acid peptide isolated from sheep hypothalamus, and PACAP-27, a truncated fragment, have marked sequence homology with VIP and have been demonstrated in the peripheral nervous system. PACAP-like immunoreactivity has a similar distribution to VIP in airways of several species, and may be localized to cholinergic and also to capsaicin-sensitive afferent nerves.[48] The effects of PACAP-27 are likely to be similar to those of VIP.

TACHYKININS

Tachykinins are a family of peptides with the common C-terminal sequence Phe-X-Gly-Leu-Met-NH$_2$. NKA and SP are coded by the same preprotachykinin (PPT) gene, which encodes three mRNAs: α-PPT produces SP alone, β-PPT codes for SP, NKA and its N-terminally extended form neuropeptide K (NPK), and Y-PPT produces SP, NKA and a novel N-terminally extended form of NKA termed NP$_Y$.[49]

Localization

SP is localized to sensory nerves in the airways of several species, including humans,[1,50] although there has been debate about whether SP can be demonstrated in human airways. Rapid enzymatic degradation of SP in airways, and the fact that SP concentrations may decrease with age and possibly after cigarette smoking, could explain the difficulty in demonstrating this peptide in some studies. SP-immunoreactive nerves in the airway are found beneath and within the airway epithelium, around blood vessels and, to a lesser extent, within airway smooth muscle. SP-immunoreactive nerves fibres innervate parasympathetic ganglia, suggesting a sensory input which may modulate ganglionic transmission and so result in ganglionic reflexes.

SP appears to be localized predominantly to capsaicin-sensitive unmyelinated nerves in the airways. SP is predominantly synthesized in the nodose ganglion of the vagus nerve and then transported down the vagus to peripheral branches in the lung, although some SP-immunoreactive nerves also arise in dorsal root ganglia.[13] Treatment of animals with capsaicin, bradykinin, histamine, the nicotinic agonist dimethylphenyl piperazinium and electric nerve stimulation causes acute SP, NKA and CGRP release from sensory nerves in the lung.[13,51] Chronic administration of capsaicin only partially depletes the lung of tachykinins and CGRP indicating the presence of a population of capsaicin-resistant SP-immunoreactive nerves, as in the gastrointestinal tract.[13] Similar capsaicin denervation studies are not possible in human airways, but after extrinsic denervation by heart–lung transplantation there appears to be a loss of SP-immunoreactive nerves in the submucosa.[52] NKA-like immunoreactivity has been demonstrated in human airways, and appears to be co-localized with SP.[53] Neuropeptide K is also present in the airways. Neurokinin B (NKB) does not appear to be present in airways,[53] and it is not certain whether neuropeptides NP-Y or NP-δ are present.

Tachykinin receptors

Tachykinin effects on target cells are mediated via specific receptors and each tachykinin appears to activate selectively a distinct subtype of receptor: NK_1-receptors are activated preferentially by SP, NK_2-receptors by NKA, and NK_3 receptors by NKB (Fig. 23.4).[54] Three distinct tachykinin receptors have now been cloned.[55] With the development of selective agonists and antagonists it has now been possible to differentiate subtypes of NK_2-receptors; thus the NK_2-receptor in tracheal smooth muscle appears to differ from that in urinary bladder and pulmonary artery.[56]

Autoradiographic studies have mapped the widespread distribution of SP-receptors in guinea-pig and human lung.[57] SP-receptors are found in high density in airway smooth muscle from trachea down to small bronchioles and vascular endothelium, whereas pulmonary vascular smooth muscle and epithelian cells are less densely labelled. Submucosal glands in human airways are also labelled.

TACHYKININ RECEPTORS

● NK-1 (SP-P): SP > NKB > E > NKA

● NK-2 (SP-E): NKA > E > NKB > SP

● NK-3 (SP-N): NKB > NKA > SP

Substance P	SP	Arg-Pro-Lys-Pro-Gln-Gln-Phe-Phe-Gly-Leu-Met-NH₂
Physalaemin	PHY	Glp-Ala-Asp-Pro-Asn-Lys-Phe-Tyr-Gly-Leu-Met-NH₂
Eledoisin	E	Glp-Pro-Ser-Lys-Asp-Ala-Phe-Ile-Gly-Leu-Met-NH₂
Kassinin	KAS	Asp-Val-Pro-Lys-Ser-Asp-Gln-Phe-Val-Gly-Leu-Met-NH₂
Neurokinin A	NKA	His-Lys-Thr-Asp-Ser-Phe-Val-Gly-Leu-Met-NH₂
Neurokinin B	NKB	Asp-Met-His-Asp-Phe-Phe-Val-Gly-Leu-Met-NH₂

Fig. 23.4 Tachykinins and their receptors. At least three types of tachykinin receptor are now recognized, based on the relative potencies of naturally occurring tachykinins. Originally called SP-P, SP-E and SP-N receptors they are now known as NK_1-, NK_2- and NK_3-receptors respectively.

Metabolism

Tachykinins are subject to degradation by at least two enzymes, angiotensin converting enzyme (ACE, EC 3.4.15.1, kininase II) and neutral endopeptidase (NEP, EC 3.4.24.11, enkephalinase).[58] ACE is predominantly localized to vascular endothelial cells and therefore breaks down intravascular peptides. ACE inhibitors, such as captopril, enhance bronchoconstriction due to intravenous SP,[59] but not inhaled SP.[60] NKA is not a good substrate for ACE, however. NEP appears to be the most important enzyme for the breakdown of tachykinins in tissues. Inhibition of NEP by phosphoramidon or thiorphan markedly potentiates bronchoconstriction *in vitro*[61] and after inhalation *in vivo*.[60] NEP inhibition also potentiates mucus secretion in response to tachykinins.[62,63] NEP inhibition enhances e-NANC and capsaicin-induced bronchoconstriction, due to the release of tachykinins from airways sensory nerves.[64] The activity of NEP in the airways appears to be an important factor in determining the effects of tachykinins; any factors which inhibit the enzyme or its expression may be associated with enhanced tachykinin effects (see later).

Another endopeptidase (EC 3.4.24.15) which effectively degrades tachykinins, has also been described in rat airway epithelium and nerves.[65] This enzyme is not inhibited by drugs that inhibit NEP and its role in regulating tachykinin effects in the airway is not yet clear.

Effects on airway smooth muscle

While SP contracts airway smooth muscle of several species, including humans,[13] NKA is considerably more potent,[53] indicating that an NK_2-receptor is likely to be involved. This is confirmed by the use of selective synthetic agonists that are resistant to enzymatic degradation. The NK_2-selective agonist $[Nle^{10}]$-NKA^{4-10} is a potent constrictor of human bronchi *in vitro*, whereas NK_1- and NK_3-selective agonists are ineffective[66] Furthermore, an NK_2-selective antagonist L659,877 also has a high potency.[66] The NK_2-selective competitive antagonist R-396 appears to be 100 times more potent in hamster tracheal smooth muscle than MEN 10207, whereas the reverse is true in rabbit pulmonary artery, demonstrating that different subtypes of NK_2-receptor must exist.[56] The contractile response to NKA is significantly greater in smaller human bronchi than in more proximal airways, indicating that tachykinins may have a more important constrictor effect on more peripheral airways,[67] whereas cholinergic constriction tends to be more pronounced in proximal airways. *In vivo* SP does not cause bronchoconstriction either by intravenous infusion[68,69] or by inhalation,[68,70] whereas NKA causes bronchoconstriction after intravenous administration[69] and after inhalation in asthmatic subjects.[70] Surprisingly the bronchoconstrictor effect of nebulized NKA in asthmatic patients is inhibited by prior treatment with sodium cromoglycate, indicating that it is mediated indirectly, rather than via a direct effect on airway smooth muscle.[71]

Interactions with epithelium

Airway epithelium modulates the bronchoconstrictor effect of many spasmogens, possibly via the release of a relaxant substance termed epithelium-derived relaxant factor

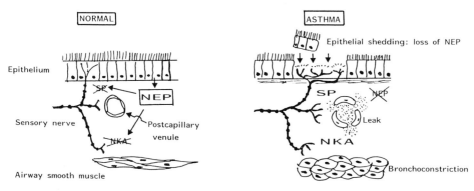

Fig. 23.5 Interaction of tachykinins with airway epithelium. When epithelium is intact neutral endopeptidase (NEP) degrades substance P (SP) and neurokinin A (NKA) released from sensory nerves (left panel). In asthmatic airways when epithelium is shed or NEP downregulated any tachykinins released will have an exaggerated effect (right panel).

(EpDRF), which may be similar but not identical to endothelium-derived relaxant factor. This may be of functional relevance in asthma since airway epithelium is often shed, even in patients with relatively mild asthma. Mechanical removal of epithelium markedly potentiates the bronchoconstrictor effect of tachykinins.[64,72] For NKA, the effect of epithelium removal can be mimicked by inhibiting NEP with phosphoramidon. Since NEP is localized to airway epithelium, mechanical denudation may remove the major site of tachykinin metabolism.[64] The situation for SP is more complex, since in addition SP may interact with NK_1-receptors on epithelial cells to release the putative EpDRF and other bronchodilators such as PGE_2. Epithelium removal also potentiates the effects of capsaicin, indicating that endogenous tachykinin effects are also enhanced.[64] If epithelium is shed in asthmatic airways any effects of tachykinins may be more pronounced, not only on airway smooth muscle, but also inflammatory effects of tachykinins in the mucosa and submucosa. (Fig. 23.5).

Airway secretion

SP stimulates mucus secretion from submucosal glands in animal and human airways *in vitro*.[62,63] In canine trachea, SP is one of the most potent stimulants of mucus secretion described, and at low concentrations appears to stimulate secretion without morphological effects on secretory cells. This suggests that SP may cause the myoepithelial cells which surround submucosal glands to contract and expel mucus from the glands and ducts rather like toothpaste is squeezed from a tube.[73] Direct measurement gland duct secretion in cats confirms this suggestion.[74] This is confirmed by functional studies that demonstrate an increased output of lysozyme, a serous cell marker.[14] SP is much more potent than NKA in stimulating airway mucus secretion, indicating that NK_1-receptors are involved,[14,63] and these have been localized by autoradiography to submucosal glands in human bronchi.[57]

Stimulation of the vagus nerve causes discharge from goblet cells in guinea-pig trachea, as measured by a morphometric technique.[75] This response is almost completely abolished by capsaicin pretreatment, indicating that the release of sensory neuropeptides is involved. Of the sensory neuropeptides, SP is by far the most potent in stimulating goblet cell secretion,[76] indicating that NK_1-receptor is involved. Since goblet cells are the only source of mucus in peripheral airways, it is possible that SP may play an important role in mucus secretion in peripheral airways in asthma and in cigarette smokers. Indeed cigarette smoking in guinea-pigs results in marked goblet cell discharge, which is partly mediated by the vapour phase which activates capsaicin-sensitive nerves.[77]

Tachykinins also stimulate ion transport in airway epithelium, with SP more potent than NKA,[78] indicating that NK_1-receptors are involved. SP also releases PGE_2 and possibly EpDRF from airway epithelial cells.[64] Tachykinins also increase mucociliary clearance in airways,[79] but this response may be secondary to an increase in airway secretions.

Vascular effects

Stimulation of the vagus nerve in rodents causes microvascular leakage, which is prevented by prior treatment with capsaicin or by a tachykinin antagonist, indicating that release of tachykinins from sensory nerves mediates this effect.[13] Amongst the tachykinins, SP is most potent at causing leakage in guinea-pig airways.[80] Inhaled SP also causes microvascular leakage in guinea-pigs and its effect on the microvasculature is more marked than its effect on airway smooth muscle;[81] inhaled SP causes an increase in airways resistance in anaesthetized guinea pigs, but unlike the increased resistance seen after a cholinergic agonist, this is not reversed by a full inflation. Whether tachykinins cause microvascular leakage in human airways is not yet certain, since no direct measurements have been made.

Tachykinins have potent effects on airway blood flow. Indeed the effect of tachykinins on airway blood flow may be the most important physiological and pathophysiological role of tachykinins in airways. In canine and porcine trachea both SP and NKA cause a marked increase in blood flow.[15] Tachykinins also dilate canine bronchial vessels *in vitro*, probably via an endothelium-dependent mechanism.[82] Tachykinins also regulate bronchial blood flow in pig; stimulation of the vagus nerve causes a vasodilatation mediated by the release of sensory neuropeptides, and it is likely that CGRP as well as tachykinins are involved.[28]

Effects on inflammatory cells

Tachykinins may also interact with inflammatory and immune cells, although whether this is of pathophysiologic significance remains to be determined. SP degranulates human skin mast cells and this response is not mediated by a classical tachykinin receptor, since it is dependent on the N-terminal sequence of the peptide,[83] whereas receptor binding is determined by the C-terminal sequence. However, human lung mast cells do not degranulate in response to SP.[84]

SP has a degranulating effect on eosinophils;[85] again the degranulation is related to high concentrations of peptide and is dependent on the N-terminal sequence. Tachykinins have effects on macrophage function *in vitro* and an NK_2-receptor appears to be involved.[86] Tachykinins may activate monocytes to release inflammatory cytokines, such as IL-6[87] and cause transient vascular adhesion of neutrophils in the airway circulation.[88]

Effects on nerves

In rabbit and ferret, the bronchoconstrictor effect of tachykinins is partly mediated by the release of ACh from postganglionic cholinergic nerves, since atropine reduces this response.[89] In guinea-pig trachea tachykinins also potentiate cholinergic neurotransmission at postganglionic nerve terminals, and an NK_2-receptor appears to be involved.[90] The potentiation is more marked at subthreshold voltages, suggesting that tachykinins may facilitate the *spread* of cholinergic transmission through postganglionic terminals. Endogenous tachykinins may also facilitate cholinergic neurotransmission since capsaicin pretreatment results in a significant reduction in cholinergic neural responses both *in vitro* and *in vivo*.[91,92] Interestingly capsaicin pretreatment also enhances i-NANC responses in airways, indicating that endogenous tachykinins may inhibit i-NANC mediated bronchodilatation.[93] SP-immunoreactive nerves appear to innervate parasympathetic ganglia in airways, suggesting that endogenous tachykinins may also have a facilitatory effect on cholinergic neurotransmission at a ganglionic level. Indeed SP and capsaicin appear to enhance ganglionic neurotransmission.[94] The interaction between tachykinins and human airway nerves is less certain. Although tachykinins do not facilitate cholinergic nerve-induced contraction of human bronchi under resting conditions, NKA has a facilitatory effect in the presence of potassium channel blockers.[95]

CALCITONIN-GENE RELATED PEPTIDE (CGRP)

CGRP is a 39 amino-acid peptide formed by the alternative splicing of the precursor mRNA coded by the calcitonin gene. There are two forms of CGRP which differ by three amino acids. Both α-CGRP and β-CGRP are expressed in sensory neurones[96] and both are potent vasodilators.

Localization

CGRP-immunoreactive nerves are abundant in the respiratory tract of several species. CGRP is co-stored and co-localized with SP in afferent nerves.[97] CGRP has been extracted from and is localized to human airways.[98] CGRP is found in trigeminal, nodose-jugular and dorsal root ganglia.[1] Unlike SP it has also been detected in neuroendocrine cells of the lower airways.

Receptors

CRGP binds to specific surface receptors which activate adenylyl cyclase, thus increasing intracellular cyclic AMP concentrations. CGRP receptors have been detected in lung by direct binding studies and localized by autoradiographic mapping.[99] At least two subtypes of receptor have been suggested on the basis of structure activity studies with CGRP analogues.[100]

Vascular effects

CGRP is a potent vasodilator, which has long lasting effects. CGRP potently dilates canine bronchial vessels *in vitro*[101] and produces a marked and long-lasting increase in airway blood flow in anaesthetized dogs.[102] Receptor mapping studies have demonstrated that CGRP receptors are localized predominantly to bronchial vessels rather than to smooth muscle or epithelium in human airways.[99] It is possible that CGRP may be the predominant mediator of arterial vasodilatation and increased blood flow in response to sensory nerve stimulation in the bronchi.[28] CGRP may be an important mediator of airway hyperaemia in asthma.

By contrast, CGRP has no direct effect of airway microvascular leak.[80] It is possible that potentiation of leak may occur when the two peptides are released together from sensory nerves.

Effect on airway smooth muscle

CGRP causes constriction of human bronchi *in vitro*.[98] This is surprising since CGRP normally activates adenylyl cyclase, which is usually associated with bronchodilatation. Receptor mapping studies suggest few, if any, CGRP receptors over airway smooth muscle in human or guinea-pig airways and this suggests that the paradoxical broncho-constrictor response reported in human airways may be mediated indirectly. In guinea-pig airways, CGRP has no consistent effect on tone.[103]

Other airway effects

CGRP has a weak inhibitory effect on cholinergically stimulated mucus secretion in ferret trachea[104] and on goblet cell discharge in guinea-pig airways.[76] This is probably related to the low density of CGRP receptors on mucus secretory cells, but does not preclude the possibility that CGRP might increase mucus secretion *in vivo* by increasing blood flow to submucosal glands.

NEUROGENIC INFLAMMATION

Pain, heat, redness and swelling are the cardinal signs of inflammation. Sensory nerves may be involved in the generation of each of these signs. There is now considerable evidence that sensory nerves participate in inflammatory responses. This 'neurogenic inflammation' is due to the antidromic release of neuropeptides from nociceptive nerves or C-fibres via an axon reflex. The phenomenon is well documented in several organs, including skin, eye, gastrointestinal tract and bladder.[105] There is also increasing evidence that neurogenic inflammation occurs in the respiratory tract,[106] and that it is possible that it may contribute to the inflammatory response in asthma.[107]

Neurogenic inflammation in asthma

There are several lines of evidence that neurogenic inflammation may be important in asthma.

Sensory neuropeptide effects

Sensory neuropeptides mimic many of the pathophysiological features of asthma. NKA is a very potent constrictor of human airways and enhances cholinergic neurotransmission; SP is a vasodilator, causes microvascular leakage and stimulates mucus secretion from submucosal glands and goblet cells; CGRP is a potent and long-lasting vasodilator (Fig. 23.6). In addition these peptides may have effects on regulation of local mucosal immunity.

Sensory nerve activation

Sensory nerves may be activated in airway disease. In asthmatic airways the epithelium is often shed, thereby exposing sensory nerve endings. Sensory nerves in asthmatic airways may be 'hyperalgesic' as a result of exposure to inflammatory mediators such as prostaglandins and certain cytokines. Hyperalgesic nerves may then be activated more readily by other mediators, such as kinins.

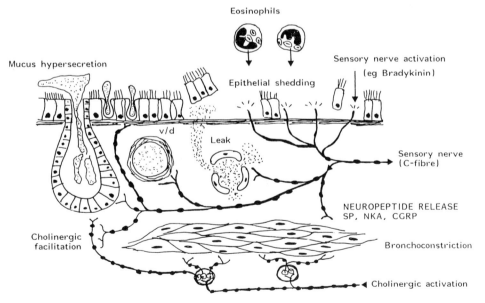

Fig. 23.6 Possible neurogenic inflammation in asthmatic airways via retrograde release of peptides from sensory nerves via an axon reflex. Substance P (SP) causes vasodilatation, plasma exudation and mucus secretion, whereas neurokinin A (NKA) causes bronchoconstriction and enhanced cholinergic reflexes and calcitonin-gene related peptide (CGRP) vasodilatation.

Bradykinin is a potent bronchoconstrictor in asthmatic patients and also induces coughing and a sensation of chest tightness, which closely mimics a naturally occurring asthma attack.[108] Yet it is a weak constrictor of human airways *in vitro*, suggesting that its potent constrictor effect is mediated indirectly. Bradykinin is a potent activator of bronchial C-fibres in dogs,[109] and releases sensory neuropeptides from perfused rodent lungs.[51] In guinea-pigs bradykinin instilled into the airways causes bronchoconstriction which is reduced significantly by a cholinergic antagonist (as in asthmatic patients),[108] and also by capsaicin pretreatment.[110] This indicates that bradykinin activates sensory nerves in the airways and that part of the bronchoconstrictor response is mediated by release of constrictor peptides from capsaicin-sensitive nerves. Whether the bronchoconstrictor response to bradykinin seen in asthmatic patients is also due to sensory peptide release is not certain, since specific tachykinin antagonists have not yet been studied in this situation. The inhibitory effects of sodium cromoglycate and nedocromil sodium on bradykinin-induced bronchoconstriction provides supportive evidence.[108,111]

Pattern of innervation

Chronic inflammation may lead to changes in the pattern of innervation, through the release of neurotrophic factors from inflammatory cells. Thus in chronic arthritis and inflammatory bowel disease there is an increase in the density of SP-immunoreactive nerves.[105] A striking increase in SP-like immunoreactive nerves has been reported in the airway of patients with fatal asthma.[112] This increased density of nerves is particularly noticeable in the submucosa. Whether this increase is due to proliferation of sensory nerves or is due to increased synthesis of tachykinins has not yet been established. Cultured sensory neurons are stimulated by nerve growth factor (NGF), which markedly increases the gene transcription of β-PPT, the major precursor peptide for tachykinins.[113] Since NGF may be released from several types of inflammatory cell, it is possible that this could lead to increased tachykinin synthesis and increased nerve growth. Several other neurotrophic factors have also recently been identified. However, bronchial biopsies of mild asthmatic patients have not revealed any evidence of increased SP-immunoreactive nerves. This may indicate that the increased innervation[112] may be a feature of either prolonged or severe asthma.

Neuropeptide metabolism

The metabolism of sensory neuropeptides may be impaired in asthmatic airways. The activity of NEP may be an important determinant of the extent of neurogenic inflammation in airways. Certain virus infections enhance e-NANC responses in guinea-pigs and mycoplasma infection enhances neurogenic microvascular leakage in rats,[114] an effect that is mediated by inhibition of NEP activity. Influenza virus infection of ferret trachea *in vitro* and of guinea-pigs *in vivo* inhibits the activity of epithelial NEP and markedly enhances the bronchoconstrictor responses to tachykinins.[115] This may explain why respiratory tract virus infections are so deleterious to patients with asthma. Hypertonic saline also impairs epithelial NEP function, leading to exaggerated tachykinin responses,[116] and cigarette smoke exposure has a similar effect which can be explained by an oxidizing effect on the enzyme.[117] Toluene diisocyanate, albeit at rather unrealistic doses, also reduces NEP activity and this may be a mechanism contributing to the airway hyperresponsiveness that may follow exposure to this chemical.[118] Thus many of the agents which lead to exacerbations of asthma appear to reduce the activity of NEP at the airway surface, thus leading to exaggerated responses to tachykinins (and other peptides) and so to increased airway inflammation. The role of NEP in human airway disease remains to be investigated.

Sensory nerve depletion

In several animal models of asthma, the role of neurogenic inflammation has been explored by selectively depleting sensory neuropeptides with capsaicin. In rat trachea capsaicin pretreatment inhibits the microvascular leakage induced by irritant gases, such as cigarette smoke[13] and inhibits goblet cell discharge and microvascular leak induced by cigarette smoke in guinea-pigs.[119] Capsaicin pretreatment also reduces the vasodilator response to allergen in pig bronchi[120] and to toluene diisocyanate in rat airways.[121] Capsaicin-sensitive nerves may also contribute to the bronchoconstrictor response to hypocapnia in rodents,[122] but not to the acute bronchoconstrictor response to allergen.[123] However more prolonged exposure of sensitized guinea-pigs to aerosolized antigen results in a pronounced increase in airway responsiveness, which is completely abolished by capsaicin pretreatment.[124] This suggests that capsaicin-sensitive nerves may play an important role in chronic inflammatory responses to allergen. It is probably not possible to apply capsaicin in high concentrations to human lower airways in order to study the role of capsaicin-sensitive nerves in asthma, but preliminary studies in which capsaicin has been topically applied to the nasal mucosa under local anaesthesia indicate that this treatment may be effective in controlling vasomotor rhinitis.[125]

Modulation of neurogenic inflammation

There are several ways in which neurogenic inflammation may be modulated,[126] and these may provide novel approaches to anti-inflammatory therapy in the future. These are discussed in more detail in Chapter 42.

OTHER NEUROPEPTIDES

Neuropeptide Y (NPY)

NPY is a 36 amino-acid peptide which is a co-transmitter with noradrenaline in adrenergic nerves and usually amplifies its effects.

The distribution of NPY follows the distribution of adrenergic nerves and is predominantly to nasal vessels, and bronchial vessels and glands, with less marked innervation of airway smooth muscle.[1] After extrinsic denervation in heart–lung transplantation recipients, there is an apparent increase in NPY-like immunoreactive nerves, suggesting that there may normally be some descending inhibitory neural influence on the expression of this peptide.[52] In rodents, depletion of sensory neuropeptides with capsaicin is associated with an increase in adrenergic nerves, indicating that there may be a reciprocal interaction between sensory and adrenergic innervation in lung.[127] NPY may also be found within parasympathetic ganglia, where it co-exists with VIP since sympathectomy does not completely deplete NPY. This suggests that there is a small population of NPY-immunoreactive fibres in the respiratory tract that are not sympathetic in origin.

NPY has no direct effect on airway smooth muscle of guinea-pig, but has a modulatory effect on cholinergic transmission of postganglionic cholinergic nerves.[128] This appears to be a direct effect on prejunctional NPY-receptors, rather than secondary to any effect on α-adrenoceptors. NPY also has a modulatory effect on e-NANC bronchoconstriction both *in vitro* and *in vivo*, and this effect is surprisingly long lasting.[128]

NPY is a potent vasoconstrictor in some vascular beds, acting predominantly on the resistance arterioles. NPY causes a long-lasting reduction in tracheal blood flow in anaesthetized dogs,[102] but has no direct effect on canine bronchial vessels *in vitro*,[82] suggesting a preferential effect on resistance vessels in the airways.

In ferret NPY enhances both cholinergic and adrenergic stimulation of airway mucus secretion, but inhibits stimulated serous cell secretion.[14]

Gastrin-releasing peptide (GRP)

GRP is a 27 amino-acid peptide, and is the mammalian form of the amphibian peptide bombesin. Other shorter peptides which share the common C-terminal sequence have also been described[129] and these peptides interact with specific receptors.

GRP/bombesin-like immunoreactivity is localized to neuroendocrine cells in human and animal lower airways.[1] GRP-containing nerve fibres have been demonstrated around blood vessels and submucosal glands in the airways of several species.

GRP and bombesin-like peptides may play important roles in lung maturation. GRP mRNA production in lungs is increased on the day prior to birth and then declines[130] and bombesin-like immunoreactivity decreases with maturation. Bombesin has a trophic effect on several cell types and may be important in epithelial growth.[131]

Bombesin is a potent bronchoconstrictor in guinea-pigs *in vivo*.[132,133] However *in vitro* it has no effect on either proximal airways or on lung strips, indicating that it produces bronchoconstriction indirectly. The bronchoconstrictor response is not blocked by an antihistamine, cyclooxygenase inhibitor, lipoxygenase inhibitor, platelet-activating factor antagonist or serotonin antagonist, indicating that mediator release is unlikely, nor is it inhibited by capsaicin pretreatment or by cholinergic antagonists, suggesting that neural reflex mechanisms are not involved. The bronchoconstrictor response is inhibited by a bombesin receptor antagonist, BIM 26159, indicating that bombesin/ GRP receptors are involved.[133] Bombesin reduces tracheal blood flow in dogs, indicating a vasoconstrictor action.[102] GRP and bombesin are potent stimulants of airway mucus secretion in human and cat airways *in vitro*.[134]

Cholecystokinin

Cholecystokinin octapeptide (CCK_8) has been identified in low concentration in lungs and airways of several species and may be localized to sensory nerves. CCK_8 is a potent constrictor of guinea-pig and human airways *in vitro*.[135] The bronchoconstrictor response is potentiated by epithelial removal and by phosphoramidon, suggesting that it is degraded by epithelial NEP. The bronchoconstrictor effect of CCK_8 is also potentiated in guinea-pigs sensitized and exposed to inhaled allergen, possibly because allergen exposure reduces epithelial NEP function. CCK_8 acts directly on airway smooth muscle and is potently inhibited by the specific CCK antagonist L363,851, indicating that CCK_A-receptors (peripheral type) are involved. CCK_8 has no apparent effect on cholinergic neurotransmission either at the level of parasympathetic ganglia, or at postganglionic nerve terminals. While few CCK-immunoreactive nerves are present in airways, it may still have a significant effect on airway tone if these particular neural fibres are activated selectively.

Somatostatin

Somatostatin has been localized to some afferent nerves,[105] but the concentration detectable in lung is low. Somatostatin has no direct action on airway smooth muscle *in vitro*, but appears to potentiate cholinergic neurotransmission in ferret airway.[136] While somatostatin has a modulatory effect on neurogenic inflammation in the rat foot pad,[137] no modulation of e-NANC nerves in airways is apparent (Stretton CD, Barnes PJ, unpublished observations).

Galanin

Galanin is a 29 amino-acid peptide named after its N-terminal glycine and C-terminal *alanine*.[138] Galanin is widely distributed in the respiratory tract innervation of several species. It is co-localized with VIP in cholinergic nerves of airways and is present in parasympathetic ganglia.[1] It is also co-localized with SP/CGRP in sensory nerves and dorsal root, nodose and trigeminal ganglia. Galanin has no direct effect on airway tone in guinea-pigs, but modulates e-NANC neurotransmission.[139] It has no effect on airway blood flow in dogs,[102] and its physiological role in airways remains a mystery.

Enkephalins

Leucine-enkephalin has been localized to neuroendocrine cells in airways and [Met]enkephalin-Arg^6-Gly^7-Leu^8 immunoreactive nerves have been described in guinea-pig and rat lungs, with a similar distribution to VIP.[140] The anatomical origins and functional roles of the endogenous opioids is not clear since the opioid antagonist naloxone has no effect on neurally mediated airway effects.[141,142] However it is possible that these opioid pathways may be selectively activated from brainstem centres under certain conditions. Exogenous opioids potently modulate neuropeptide release from sensory nerves in airways[141,142] via μ-opioid receptors.

ROLE OF NEUROPEPTIDES IN ASTHMA

The presence of so many neuropeptides in the respiratory tract raises questions about their physiological role. Neuropeptides appear to be co-transmitters in classical autonomic nerves and may be regarded as modulators of autonomic effects, perhaps acting to 'fine tune' airway functions, and to modulate the release of other neurotransmitters. Although much of the research on neuropeptides in the airways previously concentrated on their effects on airway smooth muscle, it is now clear that the most potent effect of many of the relevant peptides are on airway vasculature and secretions, and that neuropeptides may have an important role in regulating the mucosal surface of the airways. The lack of understanding of the physiological role of individual peptides is largely due to the lack of specific antagonists which can be given safely to man, but rapid advances in peptide chemistry are making the discovery of such antagonists possible, and there are now indications that non-peptide antagonists may be developed.[143]

Whether neuropeptides contribute to the pathophysiology of asthma has not yet been elucidated, although there are indications that increased effects of some peptides or defective function of other peptides may have effects on the inflammatory process and symptoms.

VIP appears to act as an anti-inflammatory peptide in general, as it inhibits mucus glycoprotein secretion from human airways[26] and inhibits mediator release from mast cells.[32] VIP is also a potent bronchodilator of proximal airways and may mediate part of the i-NANC response. Thus if VIP is more rapidly degraded in asthma by the action of enzymes such as tryptase released from mast cells, then inflammatory effects and bronchoconstriction may be exaggerated. Indeed a complete absence of VIP-immunoreactive nerves in lungs of severe asthmatic patients supports this possibility,[40] although it is likely that this reflects breakdown of VIP in the histological sections by the action of mast cell tryptase.[41] Although VIP is an effective bronchodilator *in vitro*, it has little or no effect on airway calibre in humans, probably because of degradation by the action of NEP and in asthmatic patients by tryptase in the airways. It is therefore unlikely that VIP, or even more stable analogues would have any therapeutic value in asthma.

There has been considerable interest in the possibility that sensory neuropeptides may contribute to the inflammatory response in asthmatic airways, but to date there is little direct evidence for this. Tachykinin-immunoreactive nerves are rather sparse in human airways, although it is possible that these nerves may be proliferated, sensitized or show increased neuropeptide expression in patients with severe asthma. It is also possible that the degradation of tachykinins may be impaired in asthma due to functional defects in NEP or other degradative enzymes. An understanding of the role of sensory neuropeptides in asthma may depend on the development of specific receptor antagonists or strategies to inhibit peptide release from these nerves.[126] It is possible that neurogenic inflammation may only be relevant in certain types of asthma, or in asthma of a certain degree of severity. This does point towards a need for more research on the distribution and effects of endogenous neuropeptides in the asthmatic patient, rather than reliance on animal models in which the importance of these neural mechanisms may be overemphasized.

REFERENCES

1. Uddman R, Sundler F: Neuropeptides in the airways: A review. *Am Rev Respir Dis* (1987) **136**: S3–S8.

2. Barnes PJ: Neuropeptides in the lung: localization, function and pathophysiological implications. *J Allergy Clin Immunol* (1987) **79**: 285–295.
3. Barnes PJ, Baraniuk J, Belvisi MG: Neuropeptides in the respiratory tract. *Am Rev Respir Dis* (1991) **144**: 1187–1198.
4. Barnes PJ: Neural control of human airways in health and disease. *Am Rev Respir Dis* (1986) **134**: 1289–1314.
5. Lammers J-WJ, Minette P, McCusker M, Chung KF, Barnes PJ: Capsaicin-induced bronchodilatation in mild asthmatic subjects: possible role of nonadrenergic inhibitory system. *J Appl Physiol* (1989) **67**: 856–861.
6. Karlsson JA, Persson CGA: Neither vasoactive intestinal peptide (VIP) nor purine derivatives may mediate nonadrenergic tracheal inhibition. *Acta Physiol Scand* (1984) **122**: 589–598.
7. Ito Y, Takeda K: Nonadrenergic inhibitory nerves and putative transmitters in the smooth muscle of cat trachea. *J Physiol (Lond)* (1982) **330**: 497–511.
8. Tucker JF, Brave SR, Charalambous L, Hobbs AJ, Gison A: L-N^G-nitro arginine inhibits nonadrenergic, noncholinergic relaxations of guinea-pig isolated tracheal smooth muscle. *Br J Pharmacol* (1990) **100**: 663–664.
9. Belvisi MG, Stretton CD, Barnes PJ: Evidence that nitric oxide is the neurotransmitter of inhibitory NANC nerves in human airways. *Eur J Pharmacol* (1992) in press.
10. Ellis JL, Framer SG: Effects of peptides on nonadrenergic noncholinergic inhibitory responses of tracheal smooth muscle; A comparison with effects on VIP- and PHI-induced relaxation. *Br J Pharmacol* (1989) **96**: 521–526.
11. Ellis JL, Farmer SG: The effects of vasoactive intestinal peptide (VIP) antagonists, and VIP and peptide histidine isoleucine antisera on nonadrenergic, noncholinergic relaxations of tracheal smooth muscle. *Br J Pharmacol* (1989) **96**: 513–520.
12. Andersson RG, Grundstrom N: The excitatory noncholinergic, nonadrenergic nervous system of the guinea-pig airways. *Eur J Respir Dis* (1983) **131** (Suppl): 141–157.
13. Lundberg JM, Saria A, Lundblad L, *et al*.: Bioactive peptides in capsaicin-sensitive C-fiber afferents of the airways: functional and pathophysiological implications. In Kaliner M and Barnes PJ (eds) The airways: neurol control in health and disease. New York, Marcel Decker, 1987, pp 417–445.
14. Webber SE: Non-adrenergic non-cholinergic control of mucus secretion in airways. *Arch Int Pharmacodyn* (1990) **303**: 100–102.
15. Widdicombe JG: The NANC system and airway vasculature. *Arch Int Pharmacodyn* (1990) **303**: 83–90.
16. Lundberg JM, Fahrenkrug J, Hökflet T, *et al*.: Coexistence of peptide histidine isoleucine (PHI) and VIP in nerves regulating blood flow and bronchial smooth muscle tone in various mammals including man. *Peptides* (1984) **5**: 593–606.
17. Laitinen A, Partanen M, Hervonen A, Peto-Juikko M, Laitinen LA: VIP-like immunoreactive nerves in human respiratory tract. Light and electron microscopic study. *Histochemistry* (1985) **82**: 313–319.
18. Robberecht P, Waelbroeck M, de Neef P, Camus JC, Coy DH, Christophe J: Pharmacological characterization of VIP receptors in human lung membranes. *Peptides* (1988) **9**: 339–345.
19. Carstairs JR, Barnes PJ: Visualization of vasoactive intestinal peptide receptors in human and guinea pig lung. *J Pharmacol Exp Ther* (1986) **239**: 249–255.
20. Palmer JBD, Cuss FMC, Barnes PJ: VIP and PHM and their role in nonadrenergic inhibitory responses in isolated human airways. *J Appl Physiol* (1986) **61**: 1322–1328.
21. Diamond L, Szarek JL, Gillespie MN, Altiere RJ: *In vivo* bronchodilatory activity of vasoactive intestinal peptide in the cat. *Am Rev Respir Dis* (1991) **128**: 827–832.
22. Barnes PJ, Dixon CMS: The effect of inhaled vasoactive intestinal peptide on bronchial reactivity to histamine in man. *Am Rev Respir Dis* (1984) **130**: 162–166.
23. Palmer JBD, Cuss FMC, Warren JB, Barnes PJ: The effect of infused vasoactive intestinal peptide on airway function in normal subjects. *Thorax* (1986) **41**: 663–666.
24. Morice A, Unwin RJ, Sever PS: Vasoactive intestinal peptide causes bronchodilation and protects against histamine-induced bronchoconstriction in asthmatic subjects. *Lancet* (1983) **ii**: 1225–1226.

25. Peatfield AC, Barnes PJ, Bratcher C, Nadel JA, Davis B: Vasoactive intestinal peptide stimulates tracheal submucosal gland secretion in ferret. *Am Rev Respir Dis* (1983) **128**: 89–93.

26. Coles SJ, Said SI, Reid LM: Inhibition by vasoactive intestinal peptide of glycoconjugate and lysozyme secretion by human airways *in vitro*. *Am Rev Respir Dis* (1981) **124**: 531–536.

27. Nathanson I, Widdicombe JH, Barnes PJ: Effect of vasoactive intestinal peptide on ion transport across dog tracheal epithelium. *J Appl Physiol* (1983) **55**: 1844–1848.

28. Matran R, Alving K, Martling CR, Lacroix JS, Lundberg JM: Effects of neuropeptides and capsaicin on tracheobronchial blood flow in the pig. *Acta Physiol Scand* (1989) **135**: 335–342.

29. Barnes PJ, Dixon CMS: The effect of inhaled vasoactive intestinal peptide on bronchial hyperreactivity in man. *Am Rev Respir Dis* (1984) **130**: 162–166.

30. Martin JG, Wang A, Zacour M, Biggs DF: The effect of vasoactive intestinal polypeptide on cholinergic neurotransmission in isolated innervated guinea pig tracheal preparations. *Respir Physiol* (1990) **79**: 111–122.

31. Stretton CD, Belvisi MG, Barnes PJ: Modulation of neural bronchoconstrictor responses in the guinea pig respiratory tract by vasoactive intestinal peptide. *Neuropeptides* (1991) **18**: 149–157.

32. Undem BJ, Dick EC, Buckner CK: Inhibition by vasoactive intestinal peptide of antigen-induced histamine release from guinea pig minced lung. *Eur J Pharmacol* (1983) **88**: 247–250.

33. O'Dorisio MS, Shannaon BT, Fleshman DJ, Campolito LB: Identification of high affinity receptors for vasoactive intestinal peptide on human lymphocytes of B cell lineage. *Immunol* (1989) **142**: 3533–3536.

34. Matsuzaki Y, Hamasaki Y, Said SI: Vasoactive intestinal peptide: a possible transmitter of nonadrenergic relaxation of guinea pig airways. *Science* (1980) **210**: 1252–1253.

35. Rhoden KJ, Barnes PJ: Potentiation of non-adrenergic non-cholinergic relaxation in guinea pig airways by a cAMP phosphodiesterase inhibitor. *J Pharmacol Exp Ther* (1990) **282**: 396–402.

36. Caughy GH, Leidig F, Viro NF, Nadel JA: Substance P and vasoactive intestinal peptide degradation by mast cell tryptase and chymase. *J Pharmacol Exp Ther* (1988) **244**: 133–137.

37. Rhoden K, Barnes PJ: Epithelial modulation of NANC and VIP-induced responses: role of neutral endopeptidase. *Eur J Pharmacol* (1989) **171**: 247–250.

38. Palmer JBD, Barnes PJ: Neuropeptides and airway smooth muscle function. *Am Rev Respir Dis* (1987) **136**: S50–S54.

39. Belvisi MG, Miura M, Stretton D, Barnes PJ: Nitric oxide (NO) modulates cholinergic neurotransmission in guinea pig tracheal smooth muscle. *Eur J Pharmacol* (1991) **198**: 219–221.

40. Ollerenshaw S, Jarvis D, Woolcock A, Sullivan C, Scheibner T: Absence of immunoreactive vasoactive intestinal polypeptide in tissue from the lungs of patients with asthma. *N Engl J Med* (1989) **320**: 1244–1248.

41. Barnes PJ: Vasoactive intestinal peptide and asthma. *New Engl J Med* (1989) **321**: 1128–1129.

42. Howarth PH, Britten KM, Djukanovic RJ, *et al.*: Neuropeptide containing nerves in human airways *in vivo*: a comparative study of atopic asthma, atopic non-asthma and non-atopic non-asthma (Abstract). *Thorax* (1990) **45**: 786–787.

43. Paul S, Said SI, Thompson AB, *et al.*: Characterization of autoantibodies to vasoactive intestinal peptide in asthma. *J Neuroimmunol* (1989) **23**: 133–142.

44. Miura M, Noue H, Ichinose M, Kimura K, Katsumata U, Takishima T: Effect of nonadrenergic, noncholinergic inhibitory nerve stimulation on the allergic reaction in cat airways. *Am Rev Respir Dis* (1990) **141**: 29–32.

45. Yiangou Y, DiMarzo V, Spokes RA, Panico M, Morris HR, Bloom SR: Isolation, characterization, and pharmacological actions of peptide histidine valine 42, a novel prepro-vasoactive intestinal peptide derived peptide. *J Biol Chem* (1987) **262**: 14010–14013.

46. Chilvers ER, Dixon CMS, Yiangou Y, Bloom SR, Ind PW: Effect of peptide histidine valine on cardiovascular and respiratory function in normal subjects. *Thorax* (1988) **43**: 750–755.

47. Foda HD, Higuchi J, Said SI: Helodermin, a VIP-like peptide is a potent long-acting pulmonary vasodilator. *Am Rev Respir Dis* (1990) **141**: A486.

48. Luts A, Uddman R, Arimura A, Sundler F: PACAP, a new VIP-like peptide in the respiratory tract. *Cell Tissue Res* (1991) in press.
49. Takeda Y, Takeda J, Smart BM, Krause JE: Regional distribution of neuropeptide gamma and other tachykinin peptides derived from the substance P gene in the rat. *Regulatory Peptides* (1990) **28**: 323–333.
50. Lundberg JM, Hökfelt T, Martling CR, Saria A, Cuello C: Substance P-immunoreactive sensory nerves in the lower respiratory tract of various mammals including man. *Cell Tissue Res* (1984) **235**: 251–261.
51. Saria A, Martling CR, Yan Z, Theodorsson-Norheim E, Gamse R, Lundberg JM: Release of multiple tachykinins from capsaicin-sensitive nerves in the lung by bradykinin, histamine, dimethylphenylpiperainium, and vagal nerve stimulation. *Am Rev Respir Dis* (1988) **137**: 1330–1335.
52. Springall DR, Polak JM, Howard L, *et al.*: Persistence of intrinsic neurones and possible phenotypic changes after extrinsic denervation of human respiratory tract by heart–lung transplantation. *Am Rev Respir Dis* (1990) **141**: 1538–1546.
53. Martling CR, Theodorsson-Norheim E, Lundberg JM: Occurrence and effects of multiple tachykinins: substance P, neurokinin A, and neuropeptide K in human lower airways. *Life Sci* (1987) **40**: 1633–1643.
54. Regoli D: Pharmacological receptors for substance P and neurokinins. *Life Sci* (1987) **403**: 66.
55. Shigemoto R, Yokota Y, Tsuchida K, Nakanishi S: Cloning and expression of a rat neuromedin K receptor cDNA. *J Biol Chem* (1990) **265**: 623–628.
56. Maggi CA, Patacchinin R, Guiliani S, *et al.*: Competitive antagonists discriminate between NK$_2$ tachykinin receptor subtypes. *Br J Pharmacol* (1990) **100**: 588–592.
57. Carstairs JR, Barnes PJ: Autoradiographic mapping of substance P receptors in lung. *Eur J Pharmacol* (1986) **127**: 295–296.
58. Skidgel RA, Engelbrecht A, Johnson AR, Erdos EG: Hydrolysis of substance P and neurotensin by converting enzyme and neutral endopeptidase. *Peptides* (1989) **5**: 767–776.
59. Martins MA, Shore SA, Gerard NP, Gerald C, Drazen JM: Peptidase modulation of the pulmonary effects of tachykinins in tracheal superfused guinea pig lungs. *J Clin Invest* (1990) **85**: 170–176.
60. Lötvall JO, Skoogh B-E, Barnes PJ, Chung KF: Effects of aerosolized substance P on lung resistance in guinea pigs: a comparison between inhibition of neutral endopeptidase and angiotensin-converting enzyme. *Br J Pharmacol* (1990) **100**: 69–72.
61. Black JL, Johnson PRA, Armour CL: Potentiation of the contractile effects of neuropeptides in human bronchus by an enkephalinase inhibitor. *Pulm Pharmacol* (1988) **1**: 21–23.
62. Borson DB, Corrales R, Varsano S, *et al.*: Enkephalinase inhibitors potentiate substance P-induced secretion of ^{35}S-macromolecules from ferret trachea. *Exp Lung Res* (1987) **12**: 21–36.
63. Rogers DF, Aursudkij B, Barnes PJ: Effects of tachykinins on mucus secretion on human bronchi *in vitro*. *Eur J Pharmacol* (1989) **174**: 283–286.
64. Frossard N, Rhoden KJ, Barnes PJ: Influence of epithelium on guinea pig airway responses to tachykinins: role of endopeptidase and cyclooxygenase. *J Pharmacol Exp Ther* (1989) **248**: 292–298.
65. Choi H-SH, Lesser M, Cardozo C, Orlowski M: Immunohistological localization of endopeptidase 24.15 in rat trachea, lung tissue and alveolar macrophages. *Am J Resp Cell Mol Biol* (1990) **3**: 619–624.
66. Rhoden KJ, Barnes PJ: Classification of tachykinin receptors on guinea pig and human airway smooth muscle. *Am Rev Respir Dis* (1990) **141**: A726.
67. Frossard N, Barnes PJ: Effects of tachykinins on small human airways. *Neuropeptides* (1991) **19**: 157–162.
68. Fuller RW, Maxwell DL, Dixon CMS, *et al.*: The effects of substance P on cardiovascular and respiratory function in human subjects. *J Appl. Physiol* (1987) **62**: 1473–1479.
69. Evans TW, Dixon CM, Clarke B, Conradson TB, Barnes PJ: Comparison of neurokinin A and substance P on cardiovascular and airway function in man. *Br J Pharmacol* (1988) **25**: 273–275.

70. Joos G, Pauwels R, van der Straeten ME: Effect of inhaled substance P and neurokinin A in the airways of normal and asthmatic subjects. *Thorax* (1987) **42**: 779–783.

71. Joos GF, Pauwels RA, van der Straeten ME: The effect of nedocromil sodium on the bronchoconstrictor effect of neurokinin A in subjects with asthma. *J Allergy Clin Immunol* (1989) **83**: 663–668.

72. Grandordy BM, Frossard N, Rhoden KJ, Barnes PJ: Tachykinin-induced phosphoinositide breakdown in airway smooth muscle and epithelium: relationship to contraction. *Mol Pharmacol* (1988) **33**: 515–519.

73. Coles SJ, Neill KH, Reid LM: Potent stimulation of glycoprotein secretion in canine trachea by substance P. *J Appl Physiol* (1984) **57**: 1323–1327.

74. Shimura S, Sasaki T, Okayama H, Sasaki H, Takishima T: Effect of substance P on mucus secretion of isolated submucosal glands from feline trachea. *J Appl Physiol* (1987) **63**: 646–653.

75. Tokuyama K, Kuo H-P, Rohde JAL, Barnes PJ, Rogers DF: Neural control of goblet cell secretion in guinea pig airways. *Am J Physiol* (1990) **259**: L108–L115.

76. Kuo H-P, Rhode JAL, Tokuyama K, Barnes PJ, Rogers DF: Capsaicin and sensory neuropeptide stimulation of goblet cell secretion in guinea pig trachea. *J Physiol* (1990) **431**: 629–641.

77. Kuo H-P, Rohde JAL, Barnes PJ, Rogers DF: Cigarette smoke induced goblet cell secretion: neural involvement in guinea pig trachea. *Eur Respir J* (1990) **3**: 189S.

78. Rangachari PK, McWade D: Effects of tachykinins on the electrical activity of isolated canine tracheal epithelium: an exploratory study. *Regulatory Peptides* (1985) **12**: 9–19.

79. Wong LB, Miller IF, Yeates DB: Stimulation of tracheal ciliary beat frequency by capsaicin. *J Appl Physiol* (1990) **68**: 2574–2580.

80. Rogers DF, Belvisi MG, Aursudkij B, Evans TW, Barnes PJ: Effects and interactions of sensory neuropeptides on airway microvascular leakage in guinea pigs. *Br J Pharmacol* (1988) **95**: 1109–1116.

81. Lötvall JO, Lemen RJ, Hui KP, Barnes PJ, Chung KF: Airflow obstruction after substance P aerosol: contribution of airway and pulmonary edema. *J Appl Physiol* (1990) **69**: 1473–1478.

82. McCormack DG, Salonen RO, Barnes PJ: Effect of sensory neuropeptides on canine bronchial and pulmonary vessels *in vitro*. *Life Sci* (1988) **45**: 2405–2412.

83. Lowman MA, Benyon RC, Church MK: Characterization of neuropeptide-induced histamine release from human dispersed skin mast cells. *Br J Pharmacol* (1988) **95**: 121–130.

84. Ali H, Leung KBI, Pearce FL, Hayes NA, Foreman JC: Comparison of histamine releasing activity of substance P on mast cells and basophils from different species and tissues. *Int Arch Allergy* (1986) **79**: 121–124.

85. Kroegel C, Giembycz MA, Barnes PJ: Characterization of eosinophil activation by peptides. Differential effects of substance P, melittin, and f-met-leu-phe. *J Immunol* (1990) **145**: 2581–2587.

86. Brunelleschi S, Vanni L, Ledda F, Giotti A, Maggi CA, Fantozzi R: Tachykinins activate guinea pig alveolar macrophages: involvement of NK_2 and NK_1 receptors. *Br J Pharmacol* (1990) **100**: 417–420.

87. Lotz M, Vaughn JH, Carson DM: Effect of neuropeptides on production of inflammatory cytokines by human monocytes. *Science* (1988) **241**: 1218–1221.

88. Umeno E, Nadel JA, Huang HT, McDonald DM: Inhibition of neutral endopeptides potentiates neurogenic inflammation in the rat trachea. *J Appl Physiol* (1989) **66**: 2647–2652.

89. Sekizawa K, Tamaoki J, Nadel JA, Borson DB: Enkephalinase inhibitor potentiates substance P and electrically induced contraction in ferret trachea. *J Appl Physiol* (1987) **63**: 1401–1405.

90. Hall AK, Barnes PJ, Meldrum LA, Maclagan J: Facilitation of tachykinins of neurotransmission in guinea-pig pulmonary parasympathetic nerves. *Br J Pharmacol* (1989) **97**: 274–280.

91. Martling C, Saria A, Andersson P, Lundberg JM: Capsaicin pretreatment inhibits vagal cholinergic and noncholinergic control of pulmonary mechanisms in guinea pig. *Naunyn Schmiedeberg Arch Pharm* (1984) **325**: 343–348.

92. Stretton CD, Belvisi MG, Barnes PJ: The effect of sensory nerve depletion on cholinergic neurotransmission in guinea pig airways. *Br J Pharmacol* (1989) **98**: 782P.

93. Stretton CD, Belvisi MG, Barnes PJ: Sensory nerve depletion potentiates inhibitory NANC nerves in guinea pig airways. *Eur J Pharmacol* (1990) **184**: 333–337.

94. Undem BJ, Myers AC, Barthlow H, Weinreich D: Vagal innervation of guinea pig bronchial smooth muscle. J Appl Physiol (1991) **69**: 1336–1346.

95. Black JL, Johnson PR, Alouvan L, Armour CL: Neurokinin A with K^+ channel blockade potentiates contraction to electrical stimulation in human bronchus. *Eur J Pharmacol* (1990) **180**: 311–317.

96. Noguchi K, Senba E, Morita Y, Sato M, Tohyama M: Coexistence of α-CGRP and β-CGRP mRNAs in rat dorsal root ganglion cells. *Neurosci Lett* (1990) **108**: 1–5.

97. Martling CR: Sensory nerves containing tachykinins and CGRP in the lower airways: functional implications for bronchoconstriction, vasodilation, and protein extravasation. *Acta Physiol Scand* (1987) **Suppl 563**: 1–57.

98. Palmer JBD, Cuss FMC, Mulderry PK, *et al.*: Calcitonin gene-related peptide is localized to human airway nerves and potently constricts human airway smooth muscle. *Br J Pharmacol* (1987) **91**: 95–101.

99. Mak JCM, Barnes PJ: Autoradiographic localization of calcitonin gene-related peptide binding sites in human and guinea pig lung. *Peptides* (1988) **9**: 957–964.

100. Dennis T, Fournier A, StPierre S, Quirion R: Structure activity profile of calcitonin gene-related peptide in peripheral and brain tissues. Evidence for receptor multiplicity. *J Pharm Exp Ther* (1989) **251**: 718–725.

101. McCormack DG, Mak JC, Coupe MO, Barnes PJ: Calcitonin gene-related peptide vasodilation of human pulmonary vessels: receptor mapping and functional studies. *J Appl Physiol* (1989) **67**: 1265–1270.

102. Salonen RO, Webber SE, Widdicombe JG: Effects of neuropeptides and capsaicin on the canine tracheal vasculature *in vivo*. *Br J Pharmacol* (1988) **95**: 1262–1270.

103. Martling CR, Saria A, Fischer JA, Hokfelt T, Lundberg JM: Calcitonin gene related peptide and the lung: neuronal coexistence and vasodilatory effect. *Regulatory Peptides* (1988) **20**: 125–139.

104. Webber SG, Lim JCS, Widdicombe JG: The effects of calcitonin gene related peptide on submucosal gland secretion and epithelial albumin transport on ferret trachea *in vivo*. *Br J Pharmacol* (1991) **102**: 79–84.

105. Maggi CA, Meli A: The sensory efferent function of capsaicin sensitive nerves. *Gen Pharmacol* (1988) **19**: 1–43.

106. Barnes PJ: Neurogenic inflammation in airways and its modulation. *Arch Int Pharmacodyn* (1990) **303**: 67–82.

107. Barnes PJ: Asthma as an axon reflex. *Lancet* (1986) **i**: 242–245.

108. Fuller RW, Dixon CMS, Cuss FMC, Barnes PJ: Bradykinin-induced bronchoconstriction in man: mode of action. *Am Rev Respir Dis* (1987) **135**: 176–180.

109. Kaufman MP, Coleridge HM, Coleridge JCG, Baker DG: Bradykinin stimulates afferent vagal C-fibres in intrapulmonary airways of dogs. *J Appl Physiol* (1980) **48**: 511–517.

110. Ichinose M, Belvisi MG, Barnes PJ: Bradykinin-induced bronchoconstriction in guinea-pig *in vivo*: role of neural mechanisms. *J Pharmacol Exp Ther* (1990) **253**: 1207–1212.

111. Dixon CMS, Barnes PJ: Bradykinin induced bronchoconstriction: inhibition by nedocromil sodium and sodium cromoglycate. *Br J Clin Pharmacol* (1989) **270**: 8310–8360.

112. Ollerenshaw SL, Jarvis DL, Woolcock AJ, Scheibner T, Sullivan CE: Substance P immuno-reactive nerve fibres in airways from patients with and without asthma. *Am Rev Respir Dis* (1989) **139**: A237.

113. Lindsay RM, Harmar AJ: Nerve growth factor regulates expression of neuropeptide genes in sensory neurons. *Nature* (1989) **337**: 362–364.

114. McDonald DM: Neurogenic inflammation in the respiratory tract: actions of sensory nerve mediators on blood vessels and epithelium of the airway mucosa. *Am Rev Respir Dis* (1987) **136**: S65–S72.

115. Jacoby DB, Tamaoki J, Borson DB, Nadel JA: Influenza infection increases airway smooth muscle responsiveness to substance P in ferrets by decreasing enkephalinase. *J Appl Physiol* (1988) **64**: 2653–2658.

116. Umeno E, McDonald DM, Nadel JA: Hypertonic saline increases vascular permeability in the rat trachea by producing neurogenic inflammation. *J Clin Invest* (1990) **85**: 1905–1908.

117. Dusser DJ, Djocic TD, Borson DB, Nadel JA: Cigarette smoke induces bronchoconstrictor hyperresponsiveness to substance P and inactivates airway neutral endopeptides in the guinea pig. *J Clin Invest* (1989) **84**: 900–906.

118. Sheppard D, Thompson JE, Scypinski L, Dusser DJ, Nadel JA, Borson DB: Toluene diisocyanate increases airway responsiveness to substance P and decreases airway and neutral endopeptidase. *J Clin Invest* (1988) **81**: 1111–1115.

119. Kuo HP, Rohde JAL, Barnes PJ, Rogers DF: Morphine inhibition of cigarette smoke induced goblet cell secretion in guinea pig trachea *in vivo*. *Respir Med* (1990) **84**: 425.

120. Alving K, Matran R, Lacroix JS, Lundberg JM: Allergen challenge induces vasodilation in pig bronchial circulation via a capsaicin sensitive mechanism. *Act Physiol Scand* (1988) **134**: 571–572.

121. Thompson JE, Scypinski LA, Gordon T, Sheppard D: Tachykinins mediate the acute increase in airway responsiveness by toluene diisocyanate in guinea-pigs. *Am Rev Respir Dis* (1987) **136**: 43–49.

122. Reynolds AM, McEvoy RD: Tachykinins mediate hypocapnia-induced bronchoconstriction in guinea pigs. *J Appl Physiol* (1989) **67**: 2454–2460.

123. Lötvall JO, Hui KP, Lofdahl C-G, Barnes PJ, Chung KF: Capsaicin pretreatment does not inhibit allergen-induced airway microvascular leakage in guinea pis. *Allergy* (1991) **46**: 105–108.

124. Matsuse T, Thomson RJ, Chen X-R, Salari H, Schellenberg RR: Capsaicin inhibits airway hyperresponsiveness, but not airway lipoxygenase activity nor eosinophilia following repeated aerosilized antigen in guinea pigs. *Am Rev Respir Dis* (1991) **144**: 368–372.

125. Wolfe G: Neue aspekte zur pathogenese und therapie der hyperflektorischen rhinopathie. *Laryngol Rhinol Otol* (1988) **67**: 438–445.

126. Barnes PJ, Belvisi MG, Rogers DF: Modulation of neurogenic inflammation: novel approaches to inflammatory diseases. *Trends Pharmacol Sci* (1990) **11**: 185–189.

127. van Ranst L, Lauweryns JM: Effects of long-term sensory vs sympathetic denervation of the distribution of calcitonin gene-related peptide and tyrosine hydroxylase immunoreactivity in the rat lung. *J Neuroimmunol* (1990) **29**: 131–138.

128. Stretton D, Barnes PJ: Modulation of cholinergic neurotransmission in guinea pig trachea by neuropeptide Y. *Br J Pharmacol* (1988) **93**: 672–678.

129. Cuittitta F, Fedorko J, Gu J, Labacq-Verheyden AM, Linnoila RI, Battey JF: Gastrin releasing peptide gene associated peptides are expressed in normal fetal lung and small cell lung cancer: a novel peptide family in man. *J Clin Endocrinol Metab* (1988) **67**: 576–583.

130. Sunday ME, Kaplan LM, Motoyama E, Chin WW, Spindel ER: Gastrin releasing peptide (mammalian bombesin) gene expression in health and disease. *Lab Invest* (1988) **59**: 5–24.

131. Woll PJ, Rozengurt E: Neuropeptides as growth regulators. *Br Med Bull* (1989) **45**: 492–505.

132. Impicciatore M, Bertaccini G: The bronchoconstrictor action of the tetradecapeptide bombesin in the guinea pig. *J Pharm Pharmacol* (1073) **25**: 812–815.

133. Belvisi MG, Stretton CD, Barnes PJ: Bombesin-induced bronchoconstriction in the guinea pig: mode of action. *J Pharmacol Exp Ther* (1991) **258**: 36–41.

134. Lundgren JD, Ostrowski N, Baraniuk JN, Shelhamer JH, Kaliner MA: Gastrin releasing peptide stimulates glycoconjugate release from feline tracheal explants. *Am J Physiol* (1990) **258**: L68–L74.

135. Stretton CD, Barnes PJ: Cholecystokinin octapeptide constricts guinea-pig and human airways. *Br J Pharmacol* (1989) **97**: 675–682.

136. Sekizawa K, Graf PD, Nadel JA: Somatostatin potentiates cholinergic neurotransmission in ferret trachea. *J Appl Physiol* (1989) **67**: 2397–2400.

137. Lembeck F, Donnerer J, Bartho L: Inhibition of neurogenic vasodilation and plasma extravasation by substance P antagonists, somatostatin and [D-Met^2, Pro^5]-enkephalinamide. *Eur J Pharmacol* (1982) **85**: 171–176.

138. Rökaeus Å: Galanin: a newly isolated biologically active peptide. *Trends Neurol Sci* (1987) **10**: 158–164.

139. Guiliani S, Amann R, Papini AM, Maggi CA, Meli A: Modulatory action of galanin on responses due to antidromic activation of peripheral terminals of capsaicin sensitive sensory nerves. *Eur J Pharmacol* (1989) **163**: 91–96.

140. Shimosegawa T, Foda HD, Said SI: [Met]enkephalin-Arg^6-Gly^7-Leu^8-immunoreactive nerves in guinea pig and rat lungs: distribution, origin, and coexistence with vasoactive intestinal polypeptide immunoreactivity. *Neuroscience* (1990) **36**: 737–750.

141. Belvisi MG, Rogers DF, Barnes PJ: Neurogenic plasma extravasation: inhibition by morphine in guinea pig airways *in vivo*. *J Appl Physiol* (1989) **66**: 268–272.

142. Belvisi MG, Chung KF, Jackson DM, Barnes PJ: Opioid modulation of non-cholinergic neural bronchoconstriction in guinea-pig in *in vivo*. *Br J Pharmacol* (1988) **95**: 413–418.

143. Snider RM, Constantine JW, Lowe JA, *et al.*: A potent nonpeptide antagonist of the substance P (NK$_1$) receptor. *Science* (1991) **251**: 435–437.

Pathogenesis of Asthma

PETER J. BARNES, IAN W. RODGER AND NEIL C. THOMSON

INTRODUCTION

Considerable progress has been made in our understanding of the pathophysiology of asthma. It is now clear that asthma is a special type of chronic inflammation of the airways and substantial progress has been made in understanding the nature of this inflammatory response, the cellular components and the inflammatory mediators involved. Yet we still have little understanding about the initiating stimuli that lead to this chronic and usually irreversible inflammatory response. Recent advances in pharmacology, immunology and molecular biology are now revealing much more about the components of the chronic inflammatory response which may lead to a greater understanding of the pathophysiology of asthma and airway hyperresponsiveness (AHR) and this may lead not only to more rational therapy, but in the future to the development of more specific treatments.

ASTHMA AS AN INFLAMMATORY DISEASE

An inflammatory response is concerned with defence against invasion by outside organisms and with tissue repair, and is thus a beneficial response. However in asthma the inflammatory response appears to have been mounted inappropriately, leading to adverse effects. Inflammation is a general process, but the type of inflammatory response may vary considerably from tissue to tissue and with different initiating stimuli. The cardinal signs of inflammation are *calor* and *rubor* (heat and redness from vasodilatation),

ASTHMA: BASIC MECHANISMS AND CLINICAL MANAGEMENT (2nd Edn)
ISBN 0-12-079026-2

tumor (swelling from plasma exudation and oedema) and *dolor* (pain from sensitization of sensory nerves). More recent research has highlighted the importance of migration of inflammatory cells from the circulation into the tissues. Recent studies have highlighted the fact that the inflammatory process in asthmatic airways appears to have common features from patient to patient, irrespective of whether asthma is allergic in origin ('extrinsic') or apparently non-allergic ('intrinsic').[1] Thus, although there may be several ways of initiating this inflammatory response, the type of inflammation that is characteristic of asthma is typified by infiltration with eosinophils and T-lymphocytes and by shedding of airway epithelial cells, as discussed in Chapter 3. These inflammatory changes may be seen even in the mildest of asthmatic patients.

It has long been recognized that patients who die from asthma attacks have grossly abnormal lungs. At post-mortem the lungs fail to deflate due to widespread occlusion of airways by tenacious mucus plugs, which have resulted in fatal hypoxia. Histological studies have demonstrated several common features, including occlusion of the airway lumen by plugs, comprised of exuded plasma proteins and mucus glucoproteins, which have trapped cellular debris, consisting of shed epithelial cells and inflammatory cells. The airway epithelium shows widespread shedding and there is thickening of the subepithelial layer.[2] The airway smooth muscle layer is invariably thickened, due to hypertrophy of airway smooth muscle cells.[3,4] There is also mucus gland and goblet cell hyperplasia. The whole airway wall is thickened and oedematous, and is infiltrated with various inflammatory cells, but most notably eosinophils and lymphocytes. This inflammatory response is seen throughout the length of the airways, from trachea down to terminal bronchioles, although the intensity of inflammation may vary from area to area. The inflammation never appears to extend into the lung parenchyma, but occasionally there is inflammation in pulmonary vessels adjacent to peripheral airways.[4] The pathological appearance of fatal asthma is characteristic, particularly in the presence of activated eosinophils and extensive epithelial shedding.

Bronchoalveolar lavage

Recently the use of bronchoalveolar lavage (BAL) and bronchial biopsies has revealed that there is an active inflammatory process even in patients with very mild asthma, who have infrequent symptoms. BAL has provided evidence for an active inflammatory process in asthmatic airways, with some increase in numbers of mast cells, eosinophils and lymphocytes.[5–10] The major problem in interpreting lavage is the variable dilution which may change the composition of the fluid collected and there appears to be no satisfactory method for correcting for this dilutional factor.[11] The cellular composition of BAL may not accurately reflect the inflammatory state in the underlying mucosa, as has become evident with interstitial lung disease. There are likely to be even greater discrepancies in asthmatic airways, since many of the lavaged cells originate in the alveolar spaces and 'dilute' the inflammatory cells derived from airways. This may be overcome by selected lavage of airways using double lumen catheters with balloons to isolate a segment of a proximal airway. This provides a more accurate assessment of the inflammatory status of a proximal airway, but does not provide sufficient cells for detailed study. Premedication and the persistence of previous antiasthma therapies may affect cell function and give misleading information about cell activation and regulation in asthma. These questions will have to be increasingly addressed as research into the cell biology of asthma progresses.

Bronchial biopsy

Although the inflammatory nature of fatal asthma has long been recognized, it is now apparent that inflammation may be present even in patients with mild asthma. Bronchial biopsies have confirmed that similar, though less severe, changes are present in the mucosa of mild asthmatics.[12–18] These studies have revealed eosinophil infiltration, and a variable degree of epithelial disruption and subepithelial fibrosis. However biopsy studies have limitations. The airways from which biopsies may be taken are proximal and therefore no information is provided about inflammatory changes in more peripheral airways which are known to be involved in asthma.[2,4] The inflammatory changes have long been recognized to be patchy, and it is therefore difficult to make useful correlations with asthma severity. The biopsy procedure itself, particularly with fibreoptic bronchoscopy, may lead to artefacts and pressure distortion, making a detailed analysis of structure difficult. Finally histological studies do not give information about cell activity, although an increasing number of cell surface markers are now available, which may give insights into the state of activation, particularly in immune cells. The use of cDNA probes and the polymerase chain reaction may provide useful information about the synthesis of various proteins (e.g. cytokines, enzymes, receptors) by cells in the asthmatic airway.

Inflammation and symptoms

There is compelling evidence that inflammation underlies the phenomenon of airway hyperresponsiveness (AHR), which is the hallmark of asthma (Fig. 24.1).[19,20] The

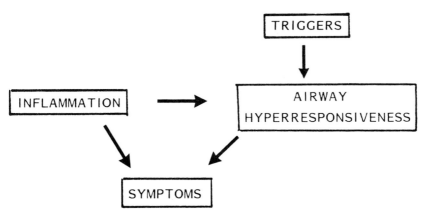

Fig. 24.1 Interrelationship between airway inflammation, airway hyperresponsiveness and symptoms in asthma.

precise relationship between airway inflammation, AHR and symptoms is still not certain and the commonly used tests of AHR, such as histamine or methacholine challenge, may not relate as closely to clinical symptoms in individual patients as had been suspected.[21,22] This may be because inflammation may directly lead to symptoms, perhaps by activating sensitized sensory nerve endings in the inflamed airway, and resulting in symptoms such as cough and chest tightness, which may be the equivalent of inflammatory pain in other organs. Anti-inflammatory treatments, such as inhaled steroids are often rapidly successful in the control of asthma symptoms, yet have a relatively small effect in reducing AHR.[23] This is presumably because the control of inflammation directly reduces some symptoms and there is some reduction in AHR which is due to active inflammation, but residual AHR may be due to structural changes in the airway that are not reversible by any known treatment.

Investigation of asthma mechanisms

Because of marked differences between species there has recently been increasing emphasis on studies in man. Thus human inflammatory cells may be obtained from peripheral blood and bronchoalveolar lavage, and human airways obtained at lung surgery. However normal cells and airways may not behave in the same way as asthmatic tissues, which may have been modified by chronic inflammation.

In vivo studies of asthmatic patients have proved to be very valuable in elucidating inflammatory mechanisms in asthma. Measurement of AHR is precise and can be measured repeatedly and after treatments or pharmacological interventions. Allergen challenge has proved particularly useful, as discussed in Chapter 25. The early response after allergen inhalation is completely inhibited and reversed by β-agonists and is likely to be due to airway smooth muscle contraction. A late phase response often follows 4–6 h after allergen challenge; the airway narrowing is slower in onset and associated with greater symptoms, which may include systemic symptoms.[20,24] This response is more difficult to reverse with β-agonists and may be due to infiltration of inflammatory cells and submucosal oedema.[20,25,26] The late response may be followed by a prolonged period of increased AHR, during which the patient experiences increased symptoms, such as exercise- and irritant-induced wheeze[27] and recurrent nocturnal asthma.[28] This period of increased AHR may last for 1–4 weeks, and is presumably due to increased inflammation in the airway resulting from allergen exposure. Although acute allergen exposure is a useful model of allergic asthma it is somewhat artificial, since asthmatic patients are rarely exposed over such a short time to such large doses of allergen. Usually the asthmatic is exposed to very small concentrations of allergen which may give rise to a 'grumbling' chronic inflammation that may differ in its nature and pharmacology from the acute and subacute inflammation provoked by the conventional allergen challenge.

A related question is how the inflammatory state of the airway should be assessed in asthmatic patients, particularly in the evaluation of new therapies. It is clearly impractical to consider repeated biopsy and BAL, although this may be indicated in exceptional circumstances for research purposes. Measurement of AHR by histamine or methacholine challenge may give some indication of the inflammatory state of the airways, although as noted above, there may be discrepancies between exacerbations of asthma and increases in AHR. Furthermore the effects of bronchodilator medications may interfere with these measurements. A more practical method of assessing inflammation may be the measurement of airway function during the day. Monitoring peak expiratory flow (PEF) in the morning and evening allows the measurement of diurnal variability of airway obstruction, which may be a reasonable assessment of airway inflammation. The need for β-agonist rescue medication may also give a similar indication. Further studies are needed on the relationship between symptoms, PEF variability, AHR and inflammation.

INFLAMMATORY CELLS

It is now clear that many different inflammatory cells are involved in asthma, although the precise role of each cell type is not yet certain (Fig. 24.2). These cells are discussed in some detail in Chapters 6–13. It is evident that no single inflammatory cell is able to account for the complex pathophysiology of asthma, but some cells are predominant in asthmatic inflammation.

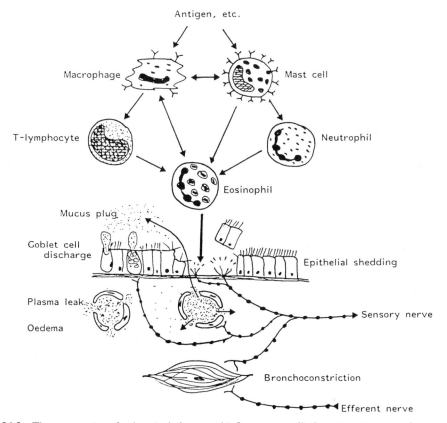

Fig. 24.2 The current view of asthma includes several inflammatory cells that interact in a complex manner and release multiple inflammatory mediators that act on various target cells of the airways to produce the characteristic pathophysiology of asthma.

Mast cells are clearly important in initiating the acute responses to allergen and probably to other indirect stimuli, such as exercise and hyperventilation (via osmolality or thermal changes) and fog. However there are questions about the role of mast cells in more chronic inflammatory events, and it seems more probable that other cells such as macrophages, eosinophils and T-lymphocytes are more important in the chronic inflammatory process, including airway hyperresponsiveness.

Macrophages, which are derived from blood monocytes, may traffic into the airways in asthma and may be activated by allergen via low affinity IgE receptors. The enormous repertoire of macrophages allows these cells to produce many different products, including a large variety of cytokines which may orchestrate the inflammatory response. Macrophages therefore have the capacity to initiate a particular type of inflammatory response via the release of a certain pattern of cytokines. Macrophages may both increase and decrease inflammation, depending on the stimulus. Alveolar macrophages normally have a suppressive effect on lymphocyte function, but this may be impaired in asthma after allergen exposure.[29,30] Macrophages may therefore play an important anti-inflammatory role, preventing the development of allergic inflammation. Macrophages, however, may also act as antigen-presenting cells which process allergen for presentation to T-lymphocytes, although alveolar macrophages are far less effective in this respect than macrophages from other sites, such as the peritoneum.[31] By contrast *dendritic* cells which are specialized macrophages in the airway epithelium, are very effective antigen-presenting cells,[32] and may therefore play a very important role in the initiation of allergen-induced responses.

Eosinophil infiltration is a characteristic feature of asthmatic airways and differentiates asthma from other inflammatory conditions of the airway. Indeed, asthma might more accurately be termed 'chronic eosinophilic bronchitis'. Allergen inhalation results in a marked increase in eosinophils in BAL fluid at the time of the late reaction[25,33] and there is a close relationship between eosinophil counts in peripheral blood or bronchial lavage and AHR.[9,34] Eosinophils were originally viewed as beneficial cells in asthma, as they have the capacity to inactivate histamine and leukotrienes, but it now seems more likely that they may play a damaging role, and may be linked to the development of AHR through the release of basic proteins and oxygen-derived free radicals.[35]

An important area of research is now concerned with the mechanisms involved in recruitment of eosinophils into asthmatic airways. Eosinophils are derived from bone marrow precursors. After allergen challenge eosinophils appear in BAL fluid during the late response,[25] and this is associated with a decrease in peripheral eosinophil counts and with the appearance of eosinophil progenitors in the circulation.[36] The signal for increased eosinophil production is presumable derived from the inflamed airway. Eosinophil recruitment initially involves adhesion of eosinophils to vascular endothelial cells in the airway circulation, their migration into the submucosa and their subsequent activation (Fig. 24.3). The role of individual cytokines and mediators in orchestrating these responses has yet to be clarified.

Adhesion of eosinophils involves the expression of specific glycoprotein molecules on the surface of eosinophils (integrins) and their expression of such molecules as intercellular adhesion molecular-1 (ICAM-1) on vascular endothelial cells (see below). An antibody directed at ICAM-1 markedly inhibits eosinophil accumulation in the airways after allergen exposure and also blocks the accompanying hyperresponsiveness.[37]

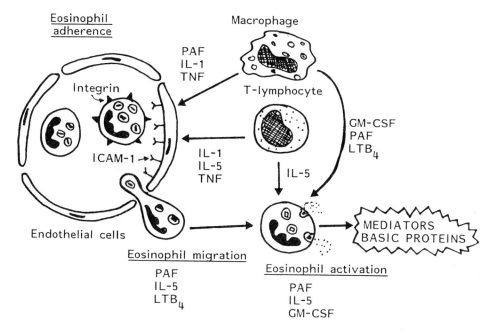

Fig. 24.3 Mechanisms of eosinophilic inflammation. Eosinophils firstly adhere to endothelial cells in the bronchial circulation, then migrate into the tissue where they survive and are activated to release mediators and granule products. Each step is directed by specific agents which may be released from macrophages and T-lymphocytes.

Eosinophil migration may be due to the effects of platelet-activating factor (PAF), which is selectively chemoattractant to eosinophils,[38] and to the effects of cytokines such as GM-CSF, IL-3 and IL-5.[39] These cytokines may be very important for the survival of eosinophils in the airways[40,41] and may 'prime' eosinophils to exhibit enhanced responsiveness. Eosinophils from asthmatic patients show greatly exaggerated responses to PAF and phorbol esters, than eosinophils from atopic non-asthmatic individuals,[42] suggesting that they may have been primed by exposure to cytokines in the circulation. Asthmatic patients characteristically have a high proportion of hypodense eosinophils in the circulation.[43] Hypodense eosinophils may arise from activation of these cells, and it is interesting that PAF and IL-5 are able to induce hypodense eosinophils *in vitro*.[44,45] There are several mechanisms that may lead to activation of eosinophils in the tissues.

The role of *neutrophils* in human asthma is now in doubt. Neutrophils are found in the airways of chronic bronchitics and patients with bronchiectasis who do not have the degree of AHR found in asthma.

Although the role of β-lymphocytes in the synthesis of IgE is well established, it is only recently that a role for *T-lymphocytes* in asthma has been recognized, as discussed in Chapter 9. Activated CD4[+] (helper) lymphocytes are prominent in asthmatic biopsies,[15,46,47] and it seems that these lymphocytes may be involved in orchestrating the chronic inflammatory response in asthma through the secretion of a specific pattern of lymphokines, such as IL-3, IL-4, IL-5 and GM-CSF, which may be important in

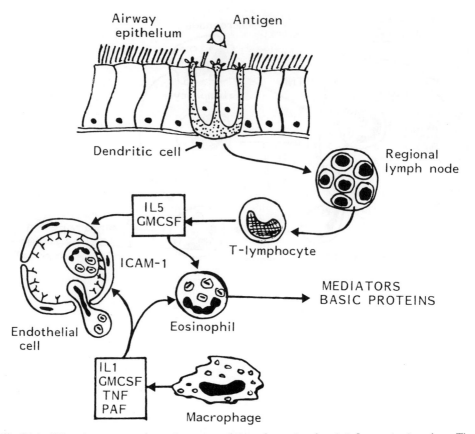

Fig. 24.4 T-lymphocytes may play an important role in orchestrating chronic inflammation in asthma. They may be programmed in regional lymph nodes by antigen-presenting cells, such as dendritic cells in the airway epithelium, which then migrate to regional lymph nodes.

recruitment and maintenance and differentiation of eosinophils and in the maintenance of mast cells in airway tissues. Presumably T-lymphocytes are coded to express a distinctive pattern of cytokines, which may be similar to that described in the murine Th2 type of T-lymphocyte,[48,49] which characteristically expresses IL-3, IL-4 and IL-5. This coding of T-lymphocytes is presumably due to antigen-presenting cells such as dendritic cells, which may migrate from the epithelium to regional lymph nodes (Fig 24.4).

Various abnormalities of *platelet* function have been described in asthma, and animal studies suggest that platelets may be implicated in certain types of AHR,[50] although their role in asthma has not yet been described.

Adhesion molecules

The movement of inflammatory cells from the circulation into the tissues depends on adhesion to endothelial cells. This adhesion is mediated by an interaction between specific adhesion glycoproteins expressed on the endothelial cell surface and on inflammatory cells. Several families of adhesion molecules have now been characterized.[51] The integrins are a large supergene family of adhesion molecules which include leucocyte adhesion molecules (LEUCAM) on lymphocytes, granulocytes and macrophages and intercellular adhesion molecules on endothelial (and epithelial) cells, such as ICAM-1. A monoclonal antibody to ICAM-1 inhibits eosinophil infiltration into primate airways after allergen challenge, emphasizing the importance of cell adhesion.[37] After allergen exposure there is increased expression of ICAM-1 bronchial endothelial and epithelial cells.[37] In other tissues various cytokines, such as IL-1 and TNFα have been shown to increase the expression of ICAM-1,[52] and this may be regulated in part by protein kinase C activation. ICAM-1 is also involved in the recruitment and activation of T-lymphocytes, and may play a critical role in cell immunity. Another integrin VCAM-1 may also be involved in leukocyte adhesion in inflammatory diseases and is induced by cytokines. The selectins are another large family of adhesion molecules involved in the adhesion between leucocytes and endothelial cells, and include ELAM-1. It is clear that further investigation of adhesion molecules and their regulation in asthma may lead to novel therapeutic approaches in the future.

INFLAMMATORY MEDIATORS

Many different mediators have been implicated in asthma and they may have a variety of effects on the airways which could account for the pathological features of asthma,[53] as discussed in Chapters 14–21. Mediators such as histamine, prostaglandins and leukotrienes contract airway smooth muscle, increase microvascular leakage, increase airway mucus secretion and attract other inflammatory cells (Table 24.1). It is therefore possible that interaction between inflammatory mediators might account for AHR. Because each mediator has many effects the role of individual mediators in the pathophysiology of asthma is not yet clear. Indeed the multiplicity of mediators makes it unlikely that antagonizing a single mediator will have a major impact in clinical asthma.

The sulphidopeptide leukotrienes LTC_4, LTD_4 and LTE_4 are potent constrictors of human airways and both LTD_4 and LTE_4 have been reported to increase AHR[54,55] and

Table 24.1 Inflammatory mediators implicated in asthma.

Mediator	Broncho-constriction	Airway secretion	Microvascular leakage	Chemotaxis	Airway hyper-responsiveness
Histamine	+	+	+	+	−
Prostaglandins D_2, $F_{2\alpha}$	+	+	−	?	+
Prostaglandin E_2	−	+	−	+	−
Thromboxane	+	?	−	?	+
Leukotriene B_4	−	−	−	+	?
Leukotrienes C_4, D_4, E_4	+	+	+	?	+
Platelet-activating factor	+	+	+	+	+
Adenosine	+	+	−	?	−
Bradykinin	+	+	+	−	−
Substance P	+	+	+	+	−

may play an important role in asthma.[56] The recent development of potent specific leukotriene antagonists has made it possible to evaluate the role of these mediators in asthma. Potent LTD_4 antagonists are remarkably effective against exercise-induced[57] allergen-induced responses,[58] suggesting that leukotrienes contribute to bronchoconstrictor responses. The role of leukotrienes in chronic asthma remains to be defined and several clinical trials with potent antagonists are currently underway.

A mediator that has attracted considerable attention recently is PAF, since it mimics many of the features of asthma, including AHR,[59] as discussed in Chapter 19. Although PAF appears to be produced by the inflammatory cells involved in asthmatic inflammation and mimics many of the pathophysiological features of asthma, its role in asthma will only become apparent with the use of potent and specific antagonists. Clinical trials of potent antagonists, such as WEB 2086, are currently underway.

Cytokines

Cytokines are increasingly recognized to be important in chronic inflammation and play a critical role in orchestrating the pattern of inflammation. Many inflammatory cells (macrophages, mast cells, eosinophils and lymphocytes) are capable of synthesizing and releasing these peptides, and it is now increasingly recognized that structural cells such as epithelial cells may also release a variety of cytokines and therefore may participate in the chronic inflammatory response. While inflammatory mediators like histamine, leukotrienes and PAF may be important in the acute and subacute inflammatory responses and in exacerbations of asthma, it is likely to be cytokines which play a dominant role in chronic inflammation. Multiple cytokines are now described in lungs[39] and almost every cell is capable of producing cytokines under certain conditions. Research in this area is hampered by the fact that there are no specific antagonists, although important observations have been made using specific neutralizing antibodies. Specific cytokines are discussed in detail in Chapter 20, and some of the cytokines that may be important in asthma are depicted in Fig. 24.6.

It is clear that no single mediator can be responsible for all the features of asthma, and it is likely that multiple mediators constitute an 'inflammatory soup' which may vary from patient to patient, depending on the relative state of activation of the different inflammatory cells (Fig. 24.5). There may be important interactions between the

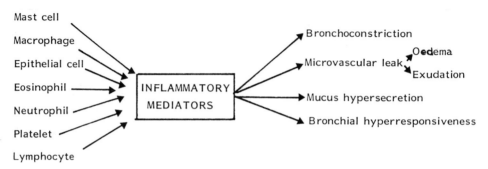

Fig. 24.5 Mediators may be released from a variety of inflammatory cells in asthma and make up a 'soup' of variable composition, which then leads to the characteristic pathology of asthma.

different mediators and the concept of 'priming' may be very important, since a combination of mediators may have a much greater effect than each mediator alone. This may be particularly important in the actions of cytokines, which may have no effect in isolation, but may have a very pronounced effect after a cell has been exposed to another cytokine.

EFFECTS OF INFLAMMATION ON TARGET CELLS

The chronic inflammatory response has several effects on the target cells of the airways, resulting in the characteristic pathophysiological changes associated with asthma (Fig. 24.1). Important advances have recently been made in understanding these changes, although their role in asthma symptoms is often not clear.

Acute vs chronic inflammation

Although much research has concerned the acute inflammatory events in asthma, it is apparent that asthma is a disease of chronic inflammation of the airways. This chronic inflammatory process may involve mediators such as cytokines, and may be perpetuated by chronic inflammatory cells such as T-lymphocytes. Chronic inflammation may lead to structural changes in the airways which involve proliferation of certain cell types (e.g. airway smooth muscle, sensory nerves) and may involve alterations in gene expression (e.g. increased expression of inflammatory receptor genes). In the future there will be increased emphasis on these chronic inflammatory processes, which may have different pharmacological control mechanisms from those involved in acute inflammatory events.

Airway epithelium

Airway epithelial damage may be a critical feature of AHR,[12,13] and may explain how several different mechanisms, such as ozone exposure, certain virus infections, chemical sensitizers and allergen exposure, can lead to its development, since all these stimuli may lead to epithelial disruption. Epithelium may be shed as a consequence of the action of inflammatory mediators, such as eosinophil basic proteins and oxygen-derived free radicals, together with various proteases released from inflammatory cells. Epithelial cells are commonly found in clumps in the BAL or sputum (Creola bodies) of asthmatics, suggesting that there has been a loss of attachment to the basal layer or basement membrane. Epithelium is not always shed in asthma,[16] but it is still possible that there may be abnormal functioning of airway epithelium. Epithelial damage may contribute to AHR in a number of ways, including loss of its barrier function to allow penetration of allergens, loss of enzymes that normally degrade inflammatory mediators, loss of relaxant factor (so called epithelial-derived relaxant factor), and exposure of sensory nerves which may lead to reflex neural effects on the airway. Epithelial cells also produce endothelin-1, and there is evidence for increased expression in asthma.[60]

Endothelin-1 may play a role in proliferation of airway smooth muscle cells and subepithelial fibrosis.

Subepithelial fibrosis

An apparent increase in the thickness of the basement membrane has been described in fatal asthma, although similar changes have been described in the airways in other conditions.[2] Electron microscopy of bronchial biopsies in asthmatic patients demonstrates that this thickening is due to subepithelial fibrosis.[14] Type III and V collagen appear to be laid down, and may be produced by myofibroblasts that are situated under the epithelium.[61] The mechanism of fibrosis is not yet clear but several cytokines, including transforming growth factor β may be produced by epithelial cells or macrophages in the inflamed airway.[39] The subepithelial fibrosis may be one of the factors which contributes to the irreversible airway obstruction, and the persisting AHR after steroid treatment, and is still present even after prolonged treatment with inhaled steroids.[62]

Airway smooth muscle

There is still considerable debate about the role and importance that abnormalities in airway smooth muscle play both in the pathogenesis of asthma and in the generation of AHR. Airway smooth muscle reactivity and function may be profoundly affected by the chemical milieu generated during the chronic inflammatory process. Several possible abnormalities in airway smooth muscle have been considered. The possibility that an electrical conduction defect may exist in asthmatic airway smooth muscle has been discussed in Chapter 5. Certain inflammatory mediators derived from arachidonic acid are capable of converting electrically quiescent airway smooth muscle cells into 'twitchy' cells that have a reduced threshold for excitability.[63] Any abnormality of contractile or relaxant mechanisms would necessarily involve abnormal control of calcium ion homeostasis in airway smooth muscle cells. This might arise in several ways: via an increased entry of Ca^{2+} through the cell membrane in response to spasmogens acting via their cell receptors; via increased release of Ca^{2+} from intercellular stores; via reduced efflux of Ca^{2+} from the cell via membrane processes; and via reduced sequestration of Ca^{2+} by intracellular organelles. *In vitro* and *in vivo* comparisons of airway responsiveness have been performed in relatively few asthmatic subjects.[64] While most of these studies failed to reveal enhanced sensitivity to mediators-induced contraction *in vitro*, as judged by EC_{50} values and maximal contractile responses, augmented maximal responses have occasionally been reported.[65,66] Relaxation may be defective, and reduced β-adrenoceptor responses have been reported in asthmatic airways *in vitro*.[67–70] Such abnormalities could be explained by phosphorylation of the stimulatory G-protein (G_s) that couples β-receptors to adenylyl cyclase.[71] Phosphorylation reactions may well be consequent upon the activation of protein kinase C by inflammatory mediators that are involved in the stimulation of airway smooth muscle cells.

In asthmatic airways there is also a characteristic hypertrophy and hyperplasia of airway smooth muscle,[3,72–74] which is presumably the result of stimulation of airway smooth muscle cells by various growth factors, such as platelet-derived growth factor, or endothelin[75] released from inflammatory cells. Even mediators such as histamine are able to stimulate growth in airway smooth muscle cells in measured by the increase in *c-fos* expression.[76] The functional significance of airway smooth muscle hypertrophy and hyperplasia is not yet certain, however. *In vitro* some studies have reported a correlation between maximal tension developed and the quantity of airway smooth muscle in the isolated strip,[77] but several studies have failed to show a relationship between airway responsiveness *in vivo* and the quantity of smooth muscle in bronchial specimens.[64] It is entirely conceivable that smooth muscle hypertrophy is a consequence rather than a cause of airway hyperresponsiveness.

Vascular responses

Vasodilatation occurs in inflammation, yet little is known about the role of the airway circulation in asthma, partly because of the difficulties involved in measuring airway blood flow. The bronchial circulation may play an important role in regulating airway calibre, since an increase in the vascular volume may contribute to airway narrowing. Passive venous congestion from left ventricular failure, results in increased

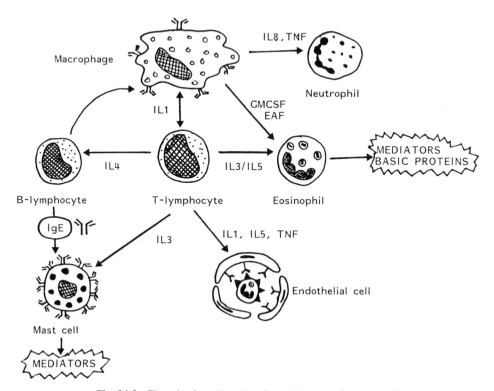

Fig. 24.6 The role of cytokines in asthma is increasingly recognized.

airway reactivity to methacholine challenge.[78] Increased venous congestion may also contribute to the increased AHR which occurs at night in association with the supine posture. Increased airway blood flow may be important in removing inflammatory apter mediators from the airway, and may play a role in the development of exercise-induced asthma.[79]

Plasma extravasation

Microvascular leakage is an essential component of the inflammatory response and many of the inflammatory mediators implicated in asthma produce this leakage.[53] There is good evidence for microvascular leakage in asthma, as discussed in Chapter 13, and it may have several consequences on airway function, including increased airway secretions, impaired mucociliary clearance, formation of new mediators from plasma precursors (such as kinins) and mucosal oedema which may contribute to airway narrowing and increased AHR.

Mucus hypersecretion

Mucus hypersecretion is a common inflammatory response in secretory tissues. Increased mucus secretion contributes to the viscid mucus plugs that occlude asthmatic airways, particularly in fatal asthma. There is evidence for hyperplasia of submucosal glands which are confined to large airways and of increased numbers of epithelial goblet cells (see Chapter 11). This increased secretory response may be due to inflammatory mediators acting on submucosal glands and due to stimulation of neural elements.[80] Little is understood about the control of goblet cells, which are the main source of mucus in peripheral airways, although recent studies investigating the control of goblet cells in guinea-pig airways suggest that cholinergic, adrenergic and sensory neuropeptides are important in stimulating secretion.[81,82]

Neural effects

There has recently been a renewal of interest in neural mechanisms in asthma. In the last century, asthma was explained by neural mechanisms. Autonomic nervous control of the airways is complex, for in addition to classical cholinergic and adrenergic mechanisms, non-adrenergic non-cholinergic (NANC) nerves and several neuropeptides have been identified in the respiratory tract.[83,84] Several studies have investigated the possibility that defects in autonomic control may contribute to AHR and asthma, and abnormalities of autonomic function, such as enhanced cholinergic and α-adrenergic responses or reduced β-adrenergic responses, have been proposed.[85] Current thinking suggests that these abnormalities are likely to be secondary to the disease, rather than primary defects.[86,87] It is possible that airway inflammation may interact with autonomic control by several mechanisms.[84]

Inflammatory mediators may act on various prejunctional receptors on airway nerves to modulate the release of neurotransmitters.[87] Thus thromboxane and PGD_2 facilitate the release of acetylcholine from cholinergic nerves in canine airways,[88,89] whereas histamine inhibits cholinergic neurotransmission at both parasympathetic ganglia and postganglionic nerves via H_3-receptors.[90] Inflammatory mediators may also activate sensory nerves, resulting in reflex cholinergic bronchoconstriction or release of inflammatory neuropeptides. Inflammatory products may also sensitize sensory nerve endings in the airway epithelium, so that the nerves become hyperalgesic. Hyperalgesia and pain (*dolor*) are cardinal signs of inflammation, and in the asthmatic airway may mediate cough and dyspnoea, which are such characteristic symptoms of asthma. The precise mechanisms of hyperalgesia are not yet certain, but mediators such as prostaglandins and certain cytokines (such as IL-1β) may be important.

Airway nerves may release neurotransmitters that are anti-inflammatory (such as VIP and nitric oxide), but may also release neurotransmitters that have inflammatory effects. Thus neuropeptides such as substance P, neurokinin A and calcitonin-gene related peptide may be released from sensitized inflammatory nerves in the airways which increase and extend the ongoing inflammatory response, as discussed in Chapter 23.

EFFECTS OF INFLAMMATION ON THE MECHANICS OF AIRWAY NARROWING

The influence on AHR of airway wall thickness, internal calibre and elastic loads on the airway smooth muscle has been discussed in Chapters 3 and 4. Alterations in these factors, due to the effects of airway inflammation, may be important in causing AHR in asthma.

Airway wall thickness

Airway wall thickness in asthma may be increased in size by mucosal oedema, smooth muscle hypertrophy, subepithelial fibrous and mucus gland and goblet hyperplasia. The variation between individuals in airway responsiveness to non-specific stimuli could be related principally to differences in airway wall thickness.[91,92] In support of this suggestion a recent study has shown that the wall area is markedly increased in the airways of asthmatic patients compared to normal controls.[93] The same reduction in airway radius will cause greater changes in airflow resistance in airways in which the wall thickness is increased (Fig. 24.7). Furthermore, a reduction in the internal dimensions of the airways due to increased secretions and smooth muscle contraction will also heighten the responsiveness of the airways to constrictor mediators, as a consequence of the inverse relationship of resistance to the fourth power of the radius.

Loss of the plateau of airway narrowing in asthma

Several workers have demonstrated that in normal subjects, but not in the majority of asthmatic patients, it is possible to produce maximum responses to inhaled histamine or

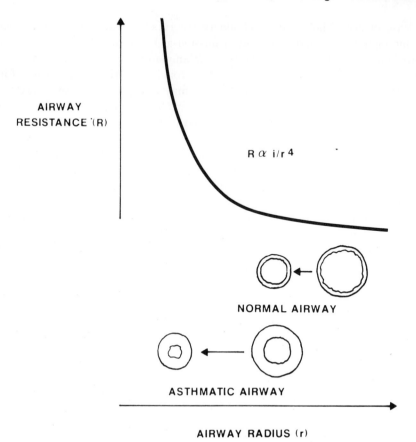

Fig. 24.7 Schematic representation of the response of a normal and an asthmatic airway of similar external diameter to a bronchoconstrictor stimulus. The same degree of smooth muscle contraction of each airway will produce little change in the airway resistance of the normal airway, but a marked increase in the resistance of the asthmatic airway. The wall:lumen ratio of the asthmatic airway is increased due to increased secretions, mucosal oedema and smooth muscle hypertrophy, and so a similar degree of smooth muscle contraction produces a greater reduction in the internal diameter of the asthmatic airway.

methacholine, i.e. a plateau response.[94,95] The results of pharmacological blocking studies using propranolol, hexamethonium and indomethacin would suggest that this response is not due to neural mechanism or to a product of the cyclooxygenase pathway.[96] The increased airway wall thickness found in asthmatic airway may result in early airway closure following smooth muscle contraction.[97] These authors have suggested that airway resistance will continue to increase because of airway closure, and this effect may explain the loss of a maximum response to inhaled bronchoconstrictor agents found in asthma.[97]

Elastic load on smooth muscle

Ding *et al.*[98] have postulated that the elastic load on smooth muscle is reduced in the airways of asthmatic patients as compared to the airways of normal subjects. Such an abnormality would produce increased maximum responses for a given concentration of an agonist. In support of this suggestion they showed that by changing the lung volume at which normal subjects inhaled methacholine, and thus altering the elastic load on the airways, the maximum response to mechacholine could be altered.[99] A reduction in lung volume, which is associated with a reduction in elastic recoil, produced an enhanced maximum response. Possible mechanisms by which the elastic load to airway smooth muscle shortening could be reduced in asthma include a loss of airway elastic recoil due, for example, to a softening of cartilage[99] or a loss of lung elastic recoil,[100] or an alteration in the relationship between airway and parenchymal function due, for example, to airway oedema. The inhibitory effects of the surrounding lung on smooth muscle contraction, however, may be important only after severe bronchoconstriction (see Chapter 4).

CONCLUSIONS

Many interacting mechanisms are involved in the pathophysiology of asthma, and many different inflammatory cells, mediators and inflammatory responses have been implicated. It is likely that different mechanisms may be operative in different patients and in the future it is likely that several pathophysiological variants of asthma may be recognized, as antagonists and inhibitors of specific pathways are used in a variety of asthmatic patients. In the future there will be more emphasis on the mechanisms of chronic inflammation, on the role of cytokines, and on the early events which sensitize the airways to allergens. Greater understanding of the pathophysiology of asthma should lead to more specific and possibly to more effective therapies in the future.

REFERENCES

1. Djukanovic R, Roche UR, Wilson JW, *et al.*: Mucosal inflammation in asthma. *Am Rev Respir Dis* (1990) **142**: 434–457.
2. Dunnill MS: the pathology of asthma, with special reference to the changes in the bronchial mucosa. *J Clin Pathol* (1960) **13**: 27–33.
3. Dunnill MS, Massarella GR, Anderson JA: A comparison of the quantitive anatomy on the bronchi in normal subjects, in status asthmaticus, in chronic bronchitis and emphysema. *Thorax* (1969) **24**: 176–179.
4. Saetta M, Di Stefano A, Rosina C, Thiene G, Fabbri LM: Quantitative structural analysis of peripheral airways and arteries in sudden fatal asthma. *Am Rev Respir Dis* (1991) **143**: 138–143.
5. Flint KC, Leung KBP, Hudspith BN, Brostoff J, Perce FL, Johnson NM: Bronchoalveolar mast cells in extrinsic asthma: a mechanism for the initiation of antigen specific bronchoconstriction. *Br Med J* (1985) **291**: 923–926.
6. Godard P, Chaintreuil J, Damon M, *et al.*: Functional assessment of alveolar macrophages: comparison of cells from asthmatics and normal subjects. *J Allergy Clin Immunol* (1982) **70**: 88–93.
7. Lam S, Leriche J, Phillips D, Chan-Yeung M: Cellular and protein changes in bronchial lavage fluid after late asthmatic reaction in patients with red cedar asthma. *J Allergy Clin Immunol* (1987) **80**: 44–50.

8. Kirby JG, Hargreave FE, Gleich GJ, O'Byrne PM: Bronchoalveolar lavage profiles of asthmatic and non asthmatic subjects. *Am Rev Respir Dis* (1987) **136**: 379–383.
9. Wardlaw AJ, Dunnette S, Gleich GJ, Collins JV, Kay AB: Eosinophils and mast cells in bronchoalveolar lavage in subjects with mild asthma. *Am Rev Respir Dis* (1988) **137**: 62–69.
10. Kelly CA, Ward C, Stenton SC, Bird G, Hendrick DJ, Walters EH: Numbers and activity of cells obtained at bronchoalveolar lavage in asthma, and their relationship to airway responsiveness. *Thorax* (1988) **43**: 684–692.
11. Walters EH, Duddridge M, Gardiner PV: Bronchoalveolar lavage: its place in diagnosis and research. *Resp Med* (1989) **83**: 457–458.
12. Laitinen LA, Heino M, Laitinen A, Kava T, Haahtela T: Damage of the airway epithelium and bronchial respiratory tract in patients with asthma. *Am Rev Respir Dis* (1985) **131**: 599–606.
13. Beasley R, Roche WR, Roberts JA, Holgate ST: Cellular events in the bronchi in mild asthma after bronchial provocation. *Am Rev Respir Dis* (1989) **139**: 806–817.
14. Roche WR, Beasley R, Williams JH, Holgate ST: Subepithelial fibrosis in the bronchi of asthmatics. *Lancet* (1989) **i**: 520–524.
15. Jeffrey PK, Wardlaw AJ, Nelson FC, Collins JV, Kay AB: Bronchial biopsies in asthma: an ultrastructural quantitative study and correlation with hyperreactivity. *Am Rev Respir Dis* (1989) **140**: 1745–1753.
16. Lozewicz S, Wells C, Gomez E, *et al.*: Morphological integrity of the bronchial epithelium in mild asthma. *Thorax* (1990) **45**: 12–15.
17. Bousquet J, Chanez P, Lacoste JY: Eosinophilic inflammation in asthma. *New Engl J Med* (1990) **323**: 1033–1039.
18. Poulter LW, Power C, Burke C: The relationship between bronchial immunopathology and hyperresponsiveness in asthma. *Eur J Respir Dis* (1990) **3**: 792–799.
19. Chung KF: Role of inflammation in the hyperreactivity of the airways in asthma. *Thorax* (1986) **41**: 657–662.
20. O'Byrne PM, Hargreave FE, Kirby JG: Airway inflammation and hyperresponsiveness. *Am Rev Respir Dis* (1987) **136**: S35–S37.
21. Josephs LK, Gregg I, Mullee MA, Holgate ST: Non-specific bronchial reactivity and its relationship to the clinical expression of asthma. *Am Rev Respir Dis* (1989) **140**: 350–357.
22. Britton JR, Burney PGJ, Chinn S, Papacosta AO, Tattersfield AE: The relation between changes in airway reactivity and change in respiratory symptoms and medication in a community survey. *Am Rev Respir Dis* (1988) **138**: 530–534.
23. Barnes PJ: Effect of corticosteroids on airway hyperresponsiveness. *Am Rev Respir Dis* (1990) **141**: S162–S165.
24. Pelikan Z, Pelikan-Filipek M: The late asthmatic response to allergen challenge—Part 1. *Ann Allergy* (1986) **56**: 414–420.
25. De Monchy JGR, Kauffman HP, Venge P, *et al.*: Bronchoalveolar eosinophilia during allergen-induced late asthmatic reactions. *Am Rev Respir Dis* (1985) **131**: 373–376.
26. Cockroft DW: Airway hyperresponsiveness: therapeutic implications. *Ann Allergy* (1987) **59**: 405–414.
27. Cockroft DW: Mechanisms of perennial allergic asthma. *Lancet* (1983) **ii**: 253–255.
28. Newman Taylor AJ, Davies RJ, Hendrick DJ, Pepys J: Recurrent nocturnal asthmatic reaction to bronchial-provocation tests. *Clin Allergy* (1979) **9**: 213–219.
29. Aubus P, Cosso B, Godard P, Miche FB, Clot J: Decreased suppressor cell activity of alveolar macrophages in bronchial asthma. *Am Rev Respir Dis* (1984) **130**: 875–878.
30. Spiteri MA, Knight RA, Wordsell M, Barnes PJ, Chung KF: Alveolar macrophage-induced suppression of T-cell hyperresponsiveness in asthma is reversed following allergen exposure *in vitro*. *Am Rev Respir Dis* (1991) **143**: A801.
31. Holt PG: Down-regulation of immune responses in the lower respiratory tract: the role of alveolar macrophages. *Clin Exp Immunol* (1986) **63**: 261–270.
32. Holt P, Schon-Hegrad MA, Phillips MJ: Ia positive dendritic cells form a tightly meshed network within human airway epithelium. *Clin Exp Allergy* (1989) **19**: 597–601.
33. Metzger WJ, Zavala D, Richerson HB, *et al.*: Local allergen challenge and bronchoalveolar lavage of allergic asthmatic lungs. *Am Rev Respir Dis* (1987) **135**: 433–440.

34. Taylor KJ, Luksza AR: Peripheral blood eosinophil counts and bronchial responsiveness. *Thorax* (1987) **42**: 452–456.

35. Gleich GJ, Flavahan NA, Fujisawa T, Vanhoutte PM: The eosinophil as a mediator of damage to respiratory epithelium: a model for bronchial hyperreactivity. *J Allergy Clin Immunol* (1988) **81**: 776–781.

36. Gibson PG, Manning PJ, O'Byrne PM, *et al.*: Allergen-induced asthmatic responses: relationship between increases in airway responsiveness and increases in circulating eosinophils, basophils and their progenitors. *Am Rev Respir Dis* (1991) **143**: 331–335.

37. Wegner CD, Gundel L, Reilly P, Haynes N, Letts LG, Rothlein R: Intracellular adhesion molecule-1 (ICAM-1) in the pathogenesis of asthma. *Science* (1990) **247**: 456–459.

38. Wardlaw AJ, Moqbel R, Cromwell O, Kay AB: Platelet activating factor. A potent chemotactic and chemokinetic factor from human eosinophils. *J Clin Invest* (1986) **78**: 1701–1706.

39. Kelley J: Cytokines of the lung. *Am Rev Respir Dis* (1990) **141**: 765–788.

40. Yamaguchi Y, Hayashi Y, Sugama Y, *et al.*: High purified murine interleukin 5 (IL-5) stimulates eosinophil function and prolongs *in vitro* survival. *J Exp Med* (1988) **167**: 1737–1742.

41. Owen WF, Rothenberg ME, Silberstein DS, *et al.*: Regulation of human eosinophil viability, density and function by granulocyte/macrophage colony stimulating factor in the presence of 3T3 fibroblasts. *J Exp Med* (1987) **166**: 129–141.

42. Chanez R, Dent G, Yukawa T, Barnes PJ, Chung KF: Generation of oxygen free radicals from blood eosinophils from asthma patients after stimulation with PAF or phorbol ester. *Eur Respir J* (1990) **3**: 1002–1007.

43. Fukuda T, Dunnette SL, Reed CE, Ackerman SJ, Peters MS, Gleich GJ: Increased numbers of hypodense eosinophils in the blood of patients with bronchial asthma. *Am Rev Respir Dis* (1985) **132**: 981–985.

44. Yukawa T, Kroegel C, Evans P, Fukuda T, Chung KF, Barnes PJ: Density heterogeneity of eosinophil leukocytes: induction of hypodense eosinophils by platelet activating factor. *Immunology* (1989) **68**: 140–143.

45. Rothenburg ME, Petersen J, Stevens RL, *et al.*: IL-5 dependent conversion of normodense human eosinophils to the hypodense phenotype uses 3T3 fibroblasts for enhanced viability, accelerated hypodensity and sustained antibody-dependent cytotoxicity. *J Immunol* (1989) **143**: 2311–2316.

46. Azzawi M, Bradley B, Jeffrey PK, *et al.*: Identification of activated T-lymphocytes and eosinophils in bronchial biopsies in stable atopic asthma. *Am Rev Respir Dis* (1990) **142**: 1407–1413.

47. Poulter LW, Power C, Burke C: The relationship between bronchial immunopathology and hyperresponsiveness in asthma. *Eur J Respir Dis* (1990) **3**: 792–799.

48. Mossman TR, Coffman RL: TH$_1$ and TH$_2$ cells: different patterns of lymphokine secretion lead to different functional properties. *Ann Rev Immunol* (1989) **7**: 145–173.

49. Wierenga EA, Snoek M, de Groot C, *et al.*: Evidence for compartmentalization of functional subjects of CD4$^+$ T-lymphocytes in atopic patients. *J Immunol* (1990) **144**: 4651–4656.

50. Coyle AJ, Spina D, Page CP: PAF-induced bronchial hyperresponsiveness in the rabbit: contribution of platelets and airway smooth muscle. *Br J Pharmacol* (1990) **101**: 31–38.

51. Albelda SM: Endothelial and epithelial cell adhesion molecules. *Am J Resp Cell Mol Biol* (1991) **4**: 195–203.

52. Rothlein R, Czaijkowski M, O'Neill M, Marlin SD, Nainolfi E, Merluzzi VJ: Induction of 1 Cam-1 on primary and continuous cell lines by proinflammatory cytokines. *J Immunol* (1988) **141**: 1665–1669.

53. Barnes PJ, Chung KF, Page CP: Inflammatory mediators and asthma. *Pharmacol Rev* (1988) **40**: 49–84.

54. Arm JP, Spur BW, Lee TH: The effects of inhaled leukotriene E4 on the airway responsiveness to histamine in subjects with asthma and normal subjects. *J Allergy Clin Immunol* (1988) **82**: 654–660.

55. Kaye MG, Smith LJ: Effects of inhaled leukotriene D$_4$ and platelet activating factor on airway reactivity in normal subjects. *Am Rev Respir Dis* (1990) **141**: 993–997.

56. Lewis RA, Austen KF, Soberman RJ; Leukotrienes and other products of the 5-lipoxygenase pathway. *New Engl J Med* (1990) **323**: 645–655.

57. Manning PJ, Watson RM, Margolskee DJ, Williams VC, Schwartz JI, O'Byrne PM: Inhibition of exercise-induced bronchoconstriction by MK-571, a potent leukotriene D$_4$-receptor antagonist. *New Engl J Med* (1990) **323**: 1736–1739.

58. Taylor IK, O'Shaughnessy KM, Fuller RW, Dollery CT: Effect of cysteinyl-leukotriene receptor antagonist ICI 204,219 on allergen-induced bronchoconstriction and airway hyper-reactivity in atopic subjects. *Lancet* (1991) **337**: 690–694.

59. Barnes PJ, Chung KF, Page CP: Platelet-activating factor as a mediator of allergic disease. *J Allergy Clin Immiunol* (1988) **81**: 919–934.

60. Springall DR, Howarth PH, Counihan H, Djukanovic R, Holgate ST, Polak JM: Endothelin immunoreactivity of airway epithelium in asthmatic patients. *Lancet* (1991) **337**: 697–701.

61. Brewster CEP, Howarth PH, Djukanovic R, Wilson J, Holgate ST, Roche WR: Myofibro-blasts and subepithelial fibrosis in bronchial asthma. *Am J Resp Cell Mol Biol* (1990) **3**: 507–511.

62. Lungren R, Soderberg M, Horstedt P, Stenling R: Morphological studies on bronchial mucosal biopsies from asthmatics before and after ten years' treatment with inhaled steroids. *Eur Resp J* (1988) **1**: 883–889.

63. Agrawal R, Daniel EE: Control of gap junction formation in canine trachea by arachidonic acid metabolites. *Am J Physiol* (1986) **250**: C495–C505.

64. Thomson NC: *In vivo* versus *in vitro* human airway responsiveness to different pharmacologic stimuli. *Am Rev Respir Dis* (1987) **136**: S58–S62.

65. Schellenberg RR, Foster A: *In vitro* responses of human asthmatic airway and pulmonary vascular smooth muscle. *Int Arch Allergy Appl Immunol* (1984) **75**: 237–241.

66. De Jongste JC, Mons H, Bonta IL, Kerrebijn KF: Human asthmatic airway responses *in vitro*: case report and literature review. *Eur J Respir Dis* (1987) **70**: 23–29.

67. Goldie RG, Spina D, Henry PJ, Lulich KM, Paterson JW: *In vitro* responsiveness of human asthmatic bronchus to carbachol, histamine, β-adrenoceptor agonists and theophylline. *Br J Clin Pharmacol* (1986) **22**: 669–676.

68. Cerrina J, Ladurie ML, Labat C, Raffestin B, Bayol A, Brink C: Comparison of human bronchial muscle response to histamine *in vivo* with histamine and isoproterenol agonists *in vitro*. *Am Rev Respir Dis* (1986) **134**: 57–61.

69. Beld AJ, Lammers JWJ, Mouris HG, *et al.*: Altered β-adrenoceptor characteristics in airway smooth muscle of a patient with atopic extrinsic asthma. *Br J Pharmacol* (1986) **89**: 477P.

70. Bai TR: Abnormalities in airway smooth muscle in fatal asthma: a comparison between trachea and bronchus. *Am Rev Respir Dis* (1991) **143**: 441–443.

71. Shehnaz D, Grady MW, Rodger IW, Pyne NJ: Muscarinic blockade of both isoprenaline and GTP-stimulated adenylate cyclase occurs via modification of G$_s$. *Br J Pharmacol* (1992) in press.

72. Heard BE, Hossain S: Hyperplasia of bronchial muscle in asthma. *J Pathol* (1973) **110**: 319.

73. Takizawa T, Thurlbeck WM: Muscle and mucus gland size in the major bronchi of patients with chronic bronchitis, asthma and asthmatic bronchitis. *Am Rev Respir Dis* (1971) **104**: 331–336.

74. Ebina M, Yaegashi H, Chiba R, Takahashi T, Motomiya M, Tanemura M: Hyperreactive site in the airway tree of asthmatic patients recoded by thickening of bronchial muscles: a morphometric study. *Am Rev Respir Dis* (1990) **141**: 1327–1332.

75. Komuro I, Kurimara H, Sugiyama T, Takaku F, Yazaki Y: Endothelin stimulates *c-fos* and *c-myc* expression and proliferation of vascular smooth muscle cells. *FEBS Lett* (1988) **238**: 249.

76. Panettieri RA, Yadish PA, Rubinstein VA, Kelly AM, Kotlikoff MI: Histamine induces proliferation and *c-fos* transcription in cultured airway smooth muscle. *Am J Physiol* (1990) **259**: L365–L371.

77. Armour CL, Black JL, Berend N, Woolcock AJ: The relationship between bronchial hyperresponsiveness to methacholine and airway smooth muscle structure and reactivity. *Respir Physiol* (1984) **58**: 223–233.

78. Cabanes LR, Weber SN, Matran R, *et al.*: Bronchial hyperresponsiveness to methacholine in patients with impaired left ventricular function. *N Engl J Med* (1989) **320**: 1317–1321.
79. McFadden ER: Hypothesis: exercise-induced asthma as a vascular phenomenon. *Lancet* (1990) **335**: 880–883.
80. Shelhamer J, Marom Z, Kaliner M: Immunologic and neuropharmacologic stimulation of mucous glycoprotein release from human airways *in vitro*. *J Clin Invest* (1980) **66**: 1400–1408.
81. Tokuyama K, Kuo H-P, Rohde JAL, Barnes PJ, Rogers DF: Neural control of goblet cell secretion in guinea pig airways. *Am J Physiol* (1990) **259**: L108–L115.
82. Kuo H-P, Rhode JAL, Tokuyama K, Barnes PJ, Rogers DF: Capsaicin and sensory neuropeptide stimulation of goblet cell secretion in guinea pig trachea. *J Physiol* (1990) **431**: 629–641.
83. Barnes PJ: Neural control of human airways in health and disease. *Am Rev Respir Dis* (1986) **134**: 1289–1314.
84. Barnes PJ: Airway inflammation and autonomic control. *Eur J Resp Dis* (1986) **69** (Suppl 147): 80–87.
85. Kaliner M, Shelhamer J, Davis PB, Smith LJ, Venter JC: Autonomic nervous system abnormalities and allergy. *Ann Intern Med* (1982) **82**: 349–357.
86. Barnes PJ: Neural control of airway function: new perspectives. *Molec Aspects Med* (1990) **11**: 351–423
87. Barnes PJ: Neuromodulation in the airways. *Physiol Rev* (1991) in press.
88. Chung KF, Evans TW, Graf PD, Nadel JA: Modulation of cholinergic neurotransmission in canine airways by thromboxane mimetic U46619. *Eur J Pharmacol* (1985) **117**: 373–375.
89. Tamaoki J, Sekizawa K, Graf PD, Nadel J: Cholinergic neuromodulation by prostaglandin D_2 in canine airway smooth muscle. *J Appl Physiol* (1987) **63**: 1396–1400.
90. Ichinose M, Stretton CD, Schwartz J-C, Barnes PJ: Histamine H_3-receptors inhibit cholinergic neurotransmission in guinea-pig airways. *Br J Pharmacol* (1989) **97**: 13–15.
91. Benson MK: Bronchial hyperreactivity. *Br J Dis Chest* (1975) **69**: 227–239.
92. Moreno RH, Hogg JC, Pare PD: Mechanisms of airway narrowing. *Am Rev Resp Dis* (1986) **133**: 1171–1180.
93. James AL, Pare PD, Hogg JC: The mechanisms of airway narrowing in asthma. *Am Rev Respir Dis* (1989) **139**: 242–246.
94. Woolcock AJ, Salome CM, Yan K: The shape of the dose–response curve to histamine in asthmatic and normal subjects. *Am Rev Respir Dis* (1984) **130**: 71–75.
95. Sterk PJ, Daniel EE, Zamel N, Hargreave FE: Limited bronchoconstriction to methacholine using partial flow-volume curves in non-asthmatic subjects. *Am Rev Respir Dis* (1985) **132**: 272–277.
96. Sterk PJ, Daniel EE, Zamel N, Hargreave FE: Limited maximal airway narrowing in non-asthmatic subjects. Role of neural control and prostaglandin release. *Am Rev Respir Dis* (1985) **132**: 865–870.
97. Wiggs BR, Moreno R, Hogg JC, Hilliam C, Paré PD: A model of the mechanics of airway narrowing. *J Appl Physiol* (1990) **69**: 849–860.
98. Ding DJ, Martin JG, Macklem PT: Effects of lung volume on maximal methacholine-induced bronchoconstriction in normal humans. *J Appl Physiol* (1987) **62**: 1324–1330.
99. Moreno RH, Dahlby R, Hogg JC, Pare PD: Increased airway responsiveness caused by airway calibre softening in rabbits. *Am Rev Respir Dis* (1985) **131**: 288.
100. Gold WM, Kaufman HS, Nadel JA: Elastic recoil of lungs in chronic asthmatic patients before and after therapy. *J Appl Physiol* (1967) **23**: 43.

25

Allergens

D.W. COCKCROFT

INTRODUCTION

Asthma is currently somewhat arbitrarily defined as symptoms associated with variable airflow obstruction.[1] Inhaled allergens producing IgE-mediated responses are amongst the many causes of airflow obstruction and symptoms in asthma.[1] The thinking regarding the importance of allergens in the pathogenesis of asthma is undergoing major revision. Allergens are more than just another trigger of bronchospasm along with exercise, cold air, smoke, irritants, etc. By inducing both inflammation[2,3] and airway hyperresponsiveness*,[4,5] allergens are now recognized as 'inducers' along with low molecular weight chemical sensitizers,[6-9] viral respiratory tract infections,[10] and occasionally extremely high levels of inhaled noxious gases or fumes.[11] Unlike simple triggers, inducers cause true asthma exacerbations and circumstantial evidence points to them as 'causes' of asthma. Evidence from several population studies points to inhalant atopic allergens as an important, perhaps *the* most important, cause of airway hyperresponsiveness and asthma. This shift in our thinking of the role of allergens in asthma, from that of one amongst many triggers of symptoms, to an important cause of the disease itself, has important therapeutic relevance.

In this chapter, naturally occurring complete allergens that trigger IgE-mediated Type I 'atopic' hypersensitivity, are discussed. Evidence implicating allergens, particularly inhaled allergens, as a cause of the disease itself is reviewed. IgE-mediated responses to haptenes (drugs, some occupational low molecular weight sensitizing

---

*The term 'airway (hyper) responsiveness' throughout this chapter, unless otherwise stated, refers to the non-allergic (hyper) responsiveness to histamine, cholinergic agonists, exercise, etc. which is a characteristic feature of symptomatic asthma.

ASTHMA: BASIC MECHANISMS AND CLINICAL MANAGEMENT (2nd Edn)
ISBN 0-12-079026-2

chemicals) and parasites will not be covered here, nor will asthma caused by other immune mechanisms, e.g. IgG_4.[12]

ATOPY

Atopy is the tendency to develop IgE antibodies to commonly encountered environmental allergens by natural exposure in which the route of entry of allergen is across intact mucosal surfaces.[13] The recognized familial nature of atopy is probably genetic; possibilities include either simple genetic inheritance with variable and low (<50%) penetrance or multiple gene inheritance.[14] Environmental factors are relevant also. The pathophysiologic basis of atopy remains unknown, although the likelihood appears to favour allergen handling perhaps at the mucosal surface rather than increased capacity to produce IgE.[15]

The prevalence of atopy in random populations, generally defined as the presence of positive(s) on prick skin tests with a small battery of indigenous allergens, ranges from 30 to almost 50%.[16–18] The peak period of sensitization is in the third decade; thereafter the prevalence falls.[13] Our experience with a random young population would suggest that about one-half of atopic subjects (or 15–17% of the population) will have some symptoms referrable to atopy, while about one-quarter of the atopics (or 7–8% of the population) will also have past or current 'allergic' asthma.[18] Thus, atopy is common, affecting about one in three, with about one in six having symptomatic atopy and an estimated one in 12 having historical evidence of atopic asthma.

INHALED ALLERGENS

Nature of allergens

Inhaled complete allergens that provoke asthma by IgE-mediated mechanisms are organic high molecular weight chemicals, most often protein or protein containing, which may be derived from virtually any of the phyla of both the plant and animal kingdoms (including bacteria).[19,20] However, in clinical, non-occupational settings the majority of inhaled allergens fall into four groups, namely pollen, fungal spores, animal danders, and house dust/mite.[21]

Pollen allergens that trigger asthma are predominantly from wind- (rather than insect-) pollenated plants, namely trees, grass, and weeds.[19,21] The relevant allergens and seasonal fluctuations will vary with locale and climatic conditions.[19] In general, tree pollens are prominent in spring months, grasses in the summer, and weeds in late summer and autumn.[19] Although whole pollen grains may have limited access to the lower respiratory tract,[22] the relationship of pollen to clinical asthma is convincing.[19]

Atmospheric fungal spores of many groups of fungi, much smaller and more respirable than pollen, are recognized as causing atopic sensitization, however, their role in triggering asthma is less certain than pollen.[19,21] Fungal spores are often associated with decaying vegetation. As for pollen, fungal spore types and seasons will vary with locale and climatic (temperature/humidity) conditions. Generally, there is a late summer and autumn peak for common fungal spores, *Alternaria, Cladosporium, Aspergillus, Sporobolomyces*, etc.[19] A spring peak for atmospheric fungal spores may be seen in some areas especially where late melting of snow cover leads to so-called 'snow mould'.[19] Thus atmospheric fungal spores may be responsible for autumn or spring/autumn asthma symptoms. Fungi may also be present inside living areas in moist basements, food storage areas, and waste receptacles.[19] *Aspergillus* may cause a distinct clinical syndrome, allergic bronchopulmonary aspergillosis, which will be covered separately.

Household animals,[20] particularly cats and dogs, but also small animals especially rodents (gerbils, hamsters, rabbits, etc.) and birds may release allergens in secretions (e.g. saliva) or excretions (e.g. urine, faeces). Large animals, particularly horses, may also provoke atopic sensitivity.

House dust, likely due to its content of mite antigens from various *Dermatophagoides* species, or insect antigens such as cockroach[23] is an important source of atopic sensitization. *Dermatophagoides* spp., in particular, are likely the most important cause of atopic sensitization worldwide. Again, climatic conditions are important, since areas of low (indoor) relative humidity do not favour growth of house dust mites.[20,24]

Other allergens are encountered less frequently, often in occupational settings, and include various plant parts (castor bean, cocoa bean, tobacco leaf, psyllium [laxative], vegetable gums, etc.), insect dusts, bacterial enzymes, and in the very highly sensitized even atmospheric molecular levels of foods (e.g. cooking fish).[20]

Patterns of allergen response

Bronchial responses to inhaled allergens have been assessed primarily by the somewhat artificial inhalation tests in the laboratory with aqueous allergen extracts.[4,5,25] Nevertheless, the results of such challenges, especially the late sequelae, appear to be clinically relevant,[26] and allergen inhalation tests allow study of both the pharmacology and pathophysiology of allergen-induced asthma. Bronchial responses to allergen can be divided into early and late sequelae.

The early or immediate asthmatic response is an episode of airflow obstruction which is maximal 10–20 min after allergen inhalation and resolves spontaneously in 1–2 h.[25,27] This response is predominantly bronchospastic.

The late sequelae include the late asthmatic response,[4,5,25,27–29] allergen-induced increase in airway responsiveness[4,5,26] and recurrent nocturnal asthma,[30,31] all of which are due, in whole or in part, to airway inflammation.

The late asthmatic response is an episode of airflow obstruction that develops after spontaneous resolution of the early response between 3 and 5 h after exposure, occasionally earlier, rarely later.[4,5,25,28,29] Resolution usually begins by 6–8 h but may require in excess of 12 h.[25,27] Modest late responses respond well to bronchodilators[32,33] but unpublished observations suggest this may be required often (e.g. up to 2 hourly). More severe late airway obstruction is not always completely reversible by bronchodilator.[27] Examples of early and late responses are shown in Fig. 25.1.

Allergen-induced increase in airway responsiveness (e.g. to histamine/methacholine) occurs following both experimental[4,5,26] and natural[26,34–36] allergen exposure. This is

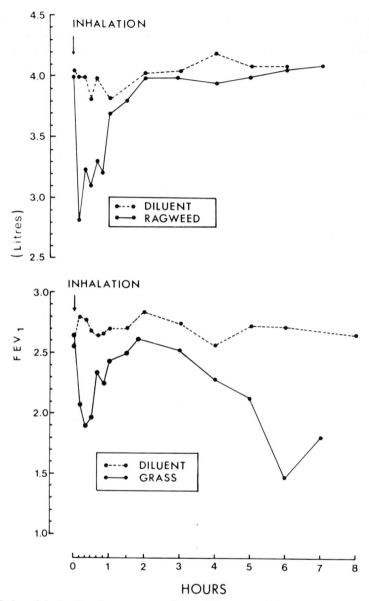

Fig. 25.1 Early and dual asthmatic responses to allergen. The top graph shows an isolated early asthmatic response following ragweed pollen inhalation and the bottom graph a dual asthmatic response (in another subject) following grass pollen inhalation.

correlated with the occurrence and severity of the late response, often appearing with small, previously ignored, late responses (5–15% FEV_1 autumn).[4,5] Airway responsiveness is not yet enhanced in most subjects 2 h after exposure,[37] appears to have developed at 3 h,[38–40] is present at 7–8 h[4,5] and may persist for days, occasionally worsening despite return of airway calibre to baseline[5] (Fig. 25.2). As expected,[41] the increased airway responsiveness is associated with symptoms of asthma.[4,5]

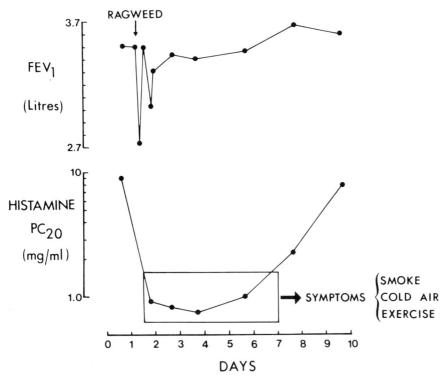

Fig. 25.2 Allergen-induced increase in non-allergic bronchial responsiveness to inhaled histamine. A dual asthmatic response, with spontaneous recovery, occurred after a single inhalation of ragweed pollen extract. Bronchial responsiveness to inhaled histamine, expressed as the provocation concentration causing a 20% FEV_1 fall (PC_{20}), increased after allergen exposure, and was associated with asthma symptoms on exposure to non-allergic stimuli. Reproduced from *Lancet* (1983) **2**: 253–256, with permission.

Recurrent nocturnal asthma following bronchoprovocation appears to be associated with late responses[30,31] and is secondary to the induced airway hyperresponsiveness.[31]

Pharmacology

Pharmacological inhibition of bronchial responses to inhaled allergen has been studied both for its potential therapeutic relevance and for further understanding of the pathophysiology of the responses.

Inhaled β_2 agonists

Inhaled β_2-agonists provide perhaps the most complete inhibition of the early asthmatic response.[29,42–45] This may be due to a direct effect on the bronchial smooth muscle and/ or to inhibition of mast cell mediator release as has been demonstrated both *in vitro*[46] and *in vivo*.[47] Despite inhibition of mast cell mediator release, however, several studies have demonstrated that there is no inhibition of the late asthmatic response when conventional inhaled β_2-agonists, e.g. salbutamol, fenoterol, etc. are administered prior to allergen exposure in a dose which will completely inhibit the early response.[29,42,43,45] Allergen-induced airway hyperresponsiveness is not inhibited by these short acting β-agonists.[45] By contrast, the new long-acting inhaled β-agonist, salmeterol, completely inhibited (or masked) both the early and late asthmatic responses; inhibition of the one dilution fall in PC_{20} at 32–34 h postallergen, however, suggested a mode of action different from salbutamol.[48] Further studies with these novel long-acting β-agonists, formoterol[49] and salmeterol, are clearly needed.

Anticholinegic agents

Anticholinegic agents cause variable and generally minor inhibition of early asthmatic responses[44,50–53] and no inhibition of late asthmatic responses.[50,53] Allergen-induced airway hyperresponsiveness appears uninfluenced by anticholinergics.[53] The enhanced bronchial responsiveness to histamine that develops following allergen inhalation is no more responsive to atropine than it was prior to allergen inhalation.[54]

Theophylline

Theophylline appears to offer minor protection against the early asthmatic response,[55–58] however, with therapeutic theophylline levels, there is a slight[58] to moderate[56,57] inhibition of the late asthmatic response. This probably represents a bronchodilator (smooth muscle) effect rather than true inhibition (reduced mediator release or anti-inflammatory effect) of the late response since the induced airway hyperresponsiveness is little influenced.[57,58]

Sodium cromoglycate

Sodium cromoglycate given prior to allergen exposure inhibits both the early and late asthmatic responses,[27,29,42,45,58,59] as well as the allergen-induced increased responsiveness to both histamine[45] and methacholine.[58] Nedocromil sodium appears to have similar effects on allergen-induced asthmatic responses.[60]

Corticosteroids

A single dose of inhaled corticosteroids, given prior to allergen, has no influence on the early asthmatic response but provides effective, often complete, inhibition of the late asthmatic response.[27,29,42,45,61–64] Longer treatment periods with inhaled corticosteroids will partially inhibit the early asthmatic response as well.[63,64] This might be secondary to the corticosteroid-induced improvement in airway responsiveness that is known to occur.[65,66] Airway responsiveness is recognized as an important determinant of the early asthmatic response.[67] Other mechanisms may be involved.

H_1-blockers

H_1-blockers have been shown to inhibit partially the early response, particularly the early portion thereof.[29,42,68–70] Newer H_1-blockers may also show some inhibition of the late response;[70] further studies are necessary.

Ketotifen

Ketotifen is an H_1-blocker that is reported to have some anti-allergic properties. Effects of short (≤4-day) courses of ketotifen on allergic responses have been conflicting. Reports have shown nil effect[71,72] to approximately a 25% reduction of the mean early asthmatic response measured by FEV_1.[73] Other reports show a variable proportion of individuals with 'significant' protection,[74–76] ranging from 47%[75] to 89%,[76] against the early response. The efficacy regarding the late response is also conflicting with studies showing no effect,[71,72] or improvement in 25%[75] to 75%.[76] We have shown minimal (non-significant) inhibition of the early response and no inhibition of the late response or postallergen methacholine hyperresponsiveness in six subjects.[77]

Other agents

Other agents have also been investigated. Non-steroidal anti-inflammatory agents, particularly indomethacin, appear to have no effect or perhaps enhance the early asthmatic response;[78] there is conflicting evidence regarding the late response.[79–81] Allergen-induced increase in airway responsiveness appears to be partially inhibited by indomethacin.[81] A thromboxane synthetase inhibitor had no effect on allergen-induced early or late responses or increased airway responsiveness.[82] Anti-seratonin agents have not been extensively studied, but appear to offer slight to no protection of early and late responses.[42]

Mechanisms

The mechanisms of allergen-induced asthmatic responses have been studied out of necessity in humans by indirect means. Animal studies, *in vitro* studies on excised human tracheobronchial smooth muscle, drug-inhibition studies and, more recently, bronchoalveolar lavage, have all been used to assess mechanisms.

The early asthmatic response appears to be almost purely bronchospastic in nature. Its complete inhibition and rapid reversal by β_2-agonists would support this. Histamine,[83] prostaglandin D_2[84] and leukotrienes[85] are released acutely from mast cells following allergen challenge. Failure of H_1-blockers to inhibit completely the early response suggests that histamine is only partially responsible. One *in vitro* study has shown that human tracheal smooth muscle contraction in response to anti-IgE can be inhibited only by the combination of H_1-blockers, cyclooxygenase inhibitors, and lipoxygenase inhibitors, implying that the early asthmatic response is caused by the combined release of histamine, prostaglandins and leukotrienes.[86]

Initially it was felt that the late asthmatic response might represent a Type III precipitin-mediated immune complex reaction.[27] This was based upon the time course, the steroid responsiveness and the presence of precipitins in some of the early patients who had allergic bronchopulmonary aspergillosis. Arguments were raised against this noting that there was no fever, no systemic symptoms, and no demonstrable precipitins to most common allergens which also produced late asthmatic responses.[29,42] More recently the analogous late allergic cutaneous response has been shown to be IgE dependent[87,88] and anti-human IgE inhalation, producing what is believed to be a pure

IgE-mediated response, has been shown to produce late asthmatic responses.[89] Thus, it is now felt that the late asthmatic response is part of the late (inflammatory) sequelae of the IgE-mediated allergic reaction.

The failure of bronchodilators to reverse completely late asthmatic responses led early to the speculation that oedema and/or inflammation as well as bronchospasm must be involved. With the development of animal models of late asthmatic responses to allergen,[90,91] and induced airways hyperresponsiveness to both non-allergic and allergic stimuli,[92–94] it is apparent that airways inflammation with eosinophils and/or neutrophils is an important requirement for both late responses and associated increased airway responsiveness. This has been well demonstrated in a rabbit allergic model where late responses and induced airway hyperresponsiveness were inhibited by polymorphonuclear leucocyte deletion.[94] Bronchoalveolar lavage data from human subjects during allergen-induced late asthmatic responses have shown that eosinophils[2,3] and to a lesser extent neutrophils[3] are increased; this supports the importance of inflammation in the pathogenesis of human late responses and increased responsiveness.

The nature of the mediator or mediators responsible for the late asthmatic inflammatory sequelae is uncertain. Attention has been focused on mediators with the potential to recruit inflammatory cells. Eosinophil chemotactic factor,[95] neutrophil chemotactic factor,[47,95] leukotrienes,[96] thromboxanes[97] and platelet-activating factor[98] have all been considered potential mediators of these sequelae. This list is neither intended to be complete nor exclusive.

A plausible diagrammatic scheme regarding the mechanism of early and late responses is shown in Fig. 25.3. The direct immediate effects of bronchoactive mediators lead to the bronchospastic early asthmatic response. The indirect effects requiring recruitment of inflammatory cells (neutrophils, eosinophils) lead to the late sequelae for which both bronchospasm and inflammation are felt to be important. The inflammation may further enhance the bronchial smooth muscle contraction by direct release of bronchoactive mediators from the recruited inflammatory cells by indirect release of mediators from the same or other effector cells within the airways and, of course, by the

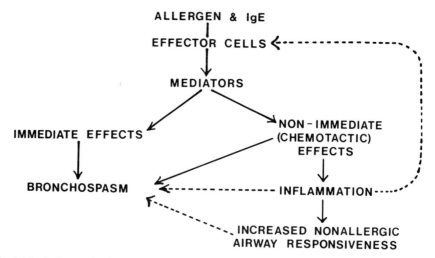

Fig. 25.3   Pathogenesis of early and late allergen-induced asthmatic sequelae. See text for explanation.

enhanced airway responsiveness which will increase the bronchial smooth muscle response to any stimulus.

Allergens as a cause of asthma

Increased airway responsiveness to non-allergic stimuli is a ubiquitous feature in bronchial asthma.[41] In the perennial atopic asthmatic, increased airway responsiveness appears to be of two types. Firstly, there is a chronic baseline level of airway hyperresponsiveness which appears to be non-reversible and non-responsive to environmental control and sodium cromoglycate, and incompletely responsive to corticosteroids. Secondly, there is superimposed transient hyperresponsiveness occurring as a result of allergen exposure. This latter is responsive to environmental avoidance,[99,100] steroid therapy,[35] sodium cromoglycate[36] and nedocromil.[101] This may explain the conflicting results obtained in investigations of these medications' inhibitory effects against histamine- and methacholine-induced airway responses. In subjects with only seasonal allergic asthma many,[102] if not most,[103] would appear to have only the transient seasonal increases in airway responsiveness with normal responsiveness out of season.

The clinical relevance of the allergen-induced asthmatic responses in the pathogenesis of asthma has been reviewed.[104] The late asthmatic (inflammatory) sequelae much more closely resemble, both clinically and pharmacologically, naturally occurring perennial and seasonal allergic asthma. A vicious circle hypothesis has been proposed (Fig. 25.4). Allergen exposure in sensitized individuals may lead to both early and late sequelae. The early responses may be missed either because they are mild, absent (as in occupational asthma), mistaken for non-allergic responses, or because they are completely inhibited by regular inhaled β_2-agonists. By contrast, the more important late sequelae may be difficult to associate with the exposure because of the delayed and prolonged nature of these responses. The enhanced airway responsiveness will lead to increased responses on further exposure to the allergen creating the vicious cycle. It will also lead to increased asthma symptoms on exposure to 'non-allergic' triggers such as smoke, dust, exercise and cold air; these latter often being more easily identified by the patient as triggering symptoms. The potential for erroneous diagnosis as intrinsic or mixed (extrinsic/intrinsic) asthma is obvious. Therapeutic relevance is discussed below.

The role of allergen exposure as a cause of the airway hyperresponsiveness of the perennial atopic asthmatic has been more speculative. The relationship between atopy and asthma is well recognized.[13] However, it has been difficult to demonstrate a relationship between atopy and airway hyperresponsiveness amongst asthmatics.[105] In atopics in a selected (clinic) population a low but significant correlation was seen between (log) histamine PC_{20} and the number of skin test positives from a panel of 16 allergens ($r=0.32$, $P<0.001$).[102] More recently, random population surveys in three countries (Canada, Australia, United Kingdom) have demonstrated a strong correlation between the degree of atopy and the prevalence of both airway hyperresponsiveness (Fig. 25.5) and asthma.[18,106–110] A longitudinal study has identified early onset atopy, in particular, as a risk factor for airway hyperresponsiveness.[111] The combined occurrence of airway hyperresponsiveness and atopy much more frequently than would be expected by chance strongly suggests the hypothesis that allergic asthma is more than just the coincidental occurrence of the two. Although some factors, be it congenital (genetic or

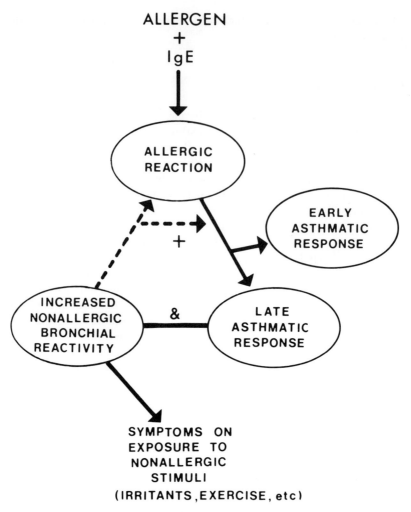

Fig. 25.4 Diagram of hypothesis explaining development and maintenance of perennial allergen-induced asthma. Reproduced from ref. 104, with permission.

otherwise) or acquired (e.g. airways inflammation at critical point(s) in life), could conceivably lead to both atopy and airway hyperresponsiveness, or alternatively airway hyperresponsiveness might predispose to atopy (a concept for which there is no scientific validity), it is speculated that atopy (allergic airway inflammation) causes airway hyperresponsiveness. Two unique and exciting observations support this. First, a striking increase in the prevalence of both atopy and asthma amongst the natives of Papua New Guinea has been documented in longitudinal studies.[112] This appears to be secondary to civilization; with modern ways came blankets and with blankets came mites leading to atopy leading to asthma. Second, neonatal induction of IgE sensitization to ragweed in dogs followed by repeated ragweed exposure leads to the development of chronic airway hyperresponsiveness.[113]

These observations in addition to the transient allergen-induced increases in airway responsiveness[4,5] and the apparent permanent airway hyperresponsiveness[114,115] caused

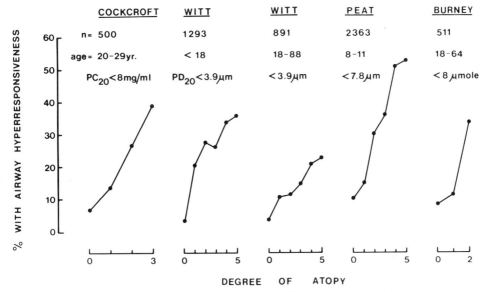

Fig. 25.5 Degree of atopy (various scales) from non-atopic (0) to highly atopic (highest number) on the horizontal axis vs prevalence of airway hyperresponsiveness (%) on the vertical axis from four population studies.[18,105–108] Reproduced from ref. 110, with permission.

by occupational exposures which also cause airway inflammation and transient increases in airway responsiveness,[6–9] make it attractive to speculate that the severity and/or duration of airways allergic reaction(s), particularly early in life, may lead to persistent hyperresponsiveness. The 'cumulative total of airways allergic reactions' should depend both upon environmental factors and the degree of atopy (recognizing that the latter may also be dependent to some extent upon the former).

Diagnosis

The diagnosis of allergic asthma rests predominantly with the history. Historical features that must be looked for include the allergens and potential allergens to which the patient might be exposed at home, at work, at school or during recreational activities. The temporal relationship between symptoms and exposure must be examined with regard to the above noted mechanisms (see particularly Fig. 25.4). Often low-grade sensitivity to an allergen may not be appreciated by the patient because of either the lack, the mildness, or the pharmacologic (especially β-agonist) inhibition of early responses. In such patients, immediate hypersensitivity is often better appreciated by the relationship of eye, nose, or cutaneous (following an animal scratch for example) symptoms immediately following exposure. The respiratory symptoms often lag behind and persist for several days after exposure. Seasonal variation in symptoms should give clues to sensitivity to atmospheric pollen and fungal spores; the precise seasonal variation and its relationship to various allergens will depend upon various climatic factors.

Following a good history, allergic skin testing, preferably by the prick technique, can be used to confirm suspected sensitivities.

Treatment

The treatment of allergen-induced asthma is the same as for asthma in general and is outlined in detail in the following chapters. The mechanisms outlined above, however, stress the importance of environmental control as well as the importance of the non-bronchodilator medications (sodium cromoglycate, inhaled corticosteroids) in the treatment of allergen-induced airway hyperresponsiveness, a particularly important aspect in the pathogenesis of allergic asthma. The likelihood that allergen exposure over the years can cause permanent airway hyperresponsiveness leads to the plausible speculation that early environmental control in subjects who are highly atopic, or at risk for being highly atopic, may have a role in the prophylaxis of asthma in addition to its above-noted role in the treatment of asthma. Likewise, early use of anti-inflammatory therapeutic strategies might also improve the prognosis of allergic asthma by reducing either the persistence of, or the future severity of, airway hyperresponsiveness.

ALLERGIC BRONCHOPULMONARY ASPERGILLOSIS

Introduction

A distinctive clinical syndrome occurs when atopic individuals have organisms, against which they have IgE antibodies, growing in their airways. The prototype and, by far the commonest of these 'allergic bronchopulmonary infestations', is allergic broncho-pulmonary aspergillosis.[116–119] Other fungi, including *Helminthosporium* species,[120,121] the closely related *Curvularia* and *Drechslera* species,[121,122] *Stemphylium*,[123] *Candida*,[124] and possibly even bacteria such as *Pseudomonas*,[125] may cause a similar syndrome. The syndrome that these organisms can produce involves complex immunologic and mechanical pathogenesis.

Pathogenesis

The pathogenesis of allergic bronchopulmonary aspergillosis initially involves acquisition of IgE-mediated Type I hypersensitivity to the fungus. Then, exposure to viable *Aspergillus* fungal spores released from decaying vegetation, particularly in the autumn and, in more temperate areas, in the winter months, will provoke Type I allergic reaction with reduced airway calibre and probably mucus hypersecretion. The spores then germinate and grow in the mucus within the lumen of the airways. The mucus will be held in place by the accompanying airway contraction allowing the developing of mucus plugs containing fungal hyphae and producing 'cast-like' outlines of the bronchial tree.

The presence in the airway of an allergen to which the subject is sensitive will lead to very high levels of both allergen-specific and total serum IgE as well as an intense peripheral and bronchial eosinophilia. The constant presence of a relatively large concentration of fungal antigen within the airways will also lead in most, but not all, individuals to the development of IgG-precipitating antibodies. Likewise, other immunologic responses including cell-mediated immunity may be stimulated.

The IgE-antigen reaction occurring continuously in the airways will lead to exacerbation of clinical asthma. The other immunologic reactions may be responsible for bronchial and parenchymal destruction with the development of (proximal) bronchiectasis and (upper lobe) interstitial pulmonary fibrosis. Fleeting or fixed pulmonary infiltrates may be produced either on the basis of immunologic reactions within the lung or by the mechanical effect of obstruction of major bronchi by mucus plugs.

Clinical features

Allergic bronchopulmonary aspergillosis is a fairly common condition in some areas; the precise prevalence is not certain. Amongst asthmatics the prevalence of Type I (IgE) sensitivity to *Aspergillus* is approximately 25%[126–128] and the prevalence of Type III (IgG) sensitivity to *Aspergillus* is approximately half this.[129,130] By contrast, on the dry Canadian prairies, *Aspergillus* skin sensitivity is uncommon and we have seen no new cases of allergic bronchopulmonary aspergillosis in over 10 years. Other organisms (e.g. *Helminthosporium*) are involved only rarely. The clinical picture is generally that of a subject with pre-existent atopy, and usually previous asthma, presenting with exacerbation of asthma accompanied by the expectoration of characteristic firm brown plugs.[116] Pulmonary infiltrates (with eosinophils) may be seen, occasionally but not always accompanied by febrile episodes. Chronic disease may manifest as bronchiectasis with chronic or recurrent pulmonary infection or pulmonary fibrosis with progressive dyspnea or both.[116,117]

Diagnosis (laboratory findings)

The two features that must be present in all subjects with allergic bronchopulmonary aspergillosis are Type I hypersensitivity to the *Aspergillus* and the presence of *Aspergillus* in the airways. However, it is not always possible to grow the organism.[131] Specific IgG precipitating antibodies are found in about 90% of cases.[118] Other features that are commonly seen include intense peripheral and bronchial eosinophilia,[131] marked elevations of total serum IgE,[132] and transient pulmonary infiltrates;[116–119] these all tend to correlate with activity of disease. Chronic changes in established or recurrent disease include radiographic demonstration of an unusual and essentially pathognomonic *proximal* bronchiectasis,[133] and in more severe cases progressive upper-lobe interstitial pulmonary fibrosis similar to tuberculosis and other upper-lobe scarring conditions.[117]

Allergic bronchopulmonary infestations with *Aspergillus* or other fungal organisms are not true infections; association with or progression to invasive fungal infections or mycetoma formation is rare. Treatment is thus directed against the asthma and the immunologic abnormalities. This generally means intensive asthma treatment with attention paid to the administration of systemic corticosteroids in doses sufficient to suppress clinical and laboratory features of the disease.[131,134,135] Total serum IgE may be useful to predict exacerbations.[135] With such treatment, the prognosis is favourable;

however, unlike other forms of allergic asthma, under-treatment can lead to substantial permanent bronchopulmonary damage.

INGESTED/INJECTED ALLERGENS

Isolated bronchial asthma induced by allergens that are introduced into the body via routes other than inhalation is uncommon but has been reported.[136,137] Both ingested allergens (foods)[137] and injected allergens (hyposensitization injections, insect bites and stings)[138] have the potential to produce Type-I mediated hypersensitivity. Such reactions are generally manifested by one or more of the following symptoms: angioedema, urticaria, anaphylactic shock, rhinitis, conjunctivitis, and bronchospasm.[136,138] Occasionally such reactions appear to be centred primarily within the lung.[137,139] It is likely that these most often represent systemic allergic reactions in asthmatics who have a pre-existing high level of airway hyperresponsiveness and, therefore, develop disproportionately severe bronchospasm. Although significant asthmatic responses to ingested and injected allergens are much less frequent than those to inhaled allergens, when they do occur, the rapidity and severity of the response may be striking. Often, a well-controlled asthmatic will experience sudden, at times apparently unexplained, life-threatening exacerbation of asthma such as is unlikely to occur secondary to inhaled allergens. We have seen patients in whom severe sudden life-threatening episodes of asthma appear to be due to ingestion of small amounts of a food to which they were very sensitive (nuts, shellfish), and two cases in whom circumstantial evidence pointed to unrecognized insect (black fly) bites as the cause of severe unexplained status asthmaticus.

Although uncommon, when confronted with a patient who has described sudden, otherwise unexplained, life-threatening episodes of asthma superimposed upon otherwise well-controlled asthma, severe IgE-mediated hypersensitivity to ingested foods (or drugs) or injected insect allergens (or allergen injections) must be considered. In addition, non-IgE mediated responses to non-steroidal anti-inflammatory agents, β-adrenergic blocking drugs, cholinesterase-inhibiting insecticides and certain food additives such as metabisulphites may cause sudden severe bronchospasm.

ACKNOWLEDGEMENTS

The author would like to thank Jacquie Bramley, Brenda Gore and Karen Murdock for their assistance in the preparation of this manuscript.

REFERENCES

1. Scadding JG: Definitions and clinical categories of asthma. In Clark TJH, Godfrey S (eds) *Asthma*. Chapman and Hall, London, 1983, pp 1–11.

2. de Monchy JGR, Kauffman HF, Venge P, *et al*.: Bronchoalveolar eosinophilia during allergen-induced late asthmatic reactions. *Am Rev Respir Dis* (1985) **131**: 373–376.
3. Metzger WJ, Richerson WB, Worden K, Monick M, Hunninghake GW: Bronchoalveolar lavage of allergic asthmatic patients following allergen bronchoprovocation. *Chest* (1986) **89**: 477–483.
4. Cockcroft DW, Ruffin RE, Dolovich J, Hargreave FE: Allergen-induced increase in nonallergic bronchial reactivity. *Clin Allergy* (1977) **7**: 503–513.
5. Cartier A, Thomson NC, Frith PA, Roberts R, Hargreave FE: Allergen-induced increase in bronchial responsiveness to histamine: Relationship to the late asthmatic response and change in airway caliber. *J Allergy Clin Immunol* (1982) **70**: 170–177.
6. Lam S, Wong R, Yeung M: Nonspecific bronchial reactivity in occupational asthma. *J Allergy Clin Immunol* (1979) **63**: 28–34.
7. Lam S, LeRiche J, Phillips D, Chan-Yeung M: Cellular and protein changes in bronchial lavage fluid after late asthmatic reaction in patients with red cedar asthma. *J Allergy Clin Immunol* (1987) **80**: 44–50.
8. Mapp CE, Polato R, Maestrelli P, Hendrick DJ, Fabbri LM: Time course of the increase in airway responsiveness associated with late asthmatic reactions to toluene diisocyanate in sensitized subjects. *J Allergy Clin Immunol* (1985) **75**: 568–572.
9. Fabbri LM, Boschetto P, Zocca E, *et al*.: Bronchoalveolar neutrophilia during late asthmatic reactions induced by toluene diisocyanate. *Am Rev Respir Dis* (1987) **136**: 36–42.
10. Empey DW, Laitinen LA, Jacobs L, Gold WM, Nadel JA: Mechanisms of bronchial hyperreactivity in normal subjects after upper respiratory tract infection. *Am Rev Respir Dis* (1976) **113**: 1331–139.
11. Brooks SM, Weiss MA, Bernstein IL: Reactive airways dysfunction syndrome (RADS). Persistent asthma syndrome after high level irritant exposures. *Chest* (1985) **88**: 376–384.
12. Gwynn CM, Smith JM, Leon GL, Stanworth DR: Role of IgG$_4$ subclass in childhood asthma. *Lancet* (1978) 910–911.
13. Pepys J: Atopy. In Gell PGH, Coombs RRA, Lachman PJ (eds) *Clinical Aspects of Immunology*. Blackwell Scientific Publications, Oxford, 1975, pp 877–902.
14. Marsh DG, Meyers DA, Bias WB: The epidemiology and genetics of atopic allergy. *N Engl Med J* (1981) **305**: 1555–1559.
15. Leskowitz S, Salvaggio JE, Schwartz HJ: An hypotheis for the development of atopic allergy in man. *Clin Allergy* (1972) **2**: 237–246.
16. Woolcock AJ, Colman MH, Jones MW: Atopy and bronchial reactivity in Australian and Melanesian populations. *Clin Allergy* (1978) **8**: 155–164.
17. Brown WG, Halonen MJ, Kaltenborn WT, Barbee RA: The relationship of respiratory allergy, skin test reactivity, and serum IgE in a community population sample. *J Allergy Clin Immunol* (1979) **63**: 328–335.
18. Cockcroft DW, Murdock KY, Berscheid BA: Relationship between atopy and bronchial responsiveness to histamine in a random population. *Ann Allergy* (1984) **53**: 26–29.
19. Solomon WR: Aerobiology and inhalant allergens. I Pollens & Fungi. In Middleton E Jr, Reed CE, Ellis EF (eds) *Allergy Principles and practice*. The CV Mosby Company, St Louis, 1978, pp 899–945.
20. Mathews KP: Aerobiology and inhalant allergens. II Other Inhaled Allergens. In Middleton E Jr, Reed CE, Ellis EF (eds) *Allergy Principles and Practice*. The CV Mosby Company, St Louis, 1978, pp 945–956.
21. Dolovich J, Zimmerman B, Hargreave FE: Allergy in asthma. In Clark TJH, Godfrey S (eds) *Asthma*. Chapman and Hall, London, 1983, pp 132–157.
22. Busse WW, Reed CE, Hoehne JH: Where is the allergic reaction in ragweed asthma? *J Allergy Clin Immunol* (1972) **50**: 289–293.
23. Pollart SM, Chapman MD, Fiocco GP, Rose G, Platts-Mills TAE: Epidemiology of acute asthma: IgE antibodies to common inhalant allergens as a risk factor for emergency room visits. *J Allergy Clin Immunol* (1989) **83**: 875–882.
24. Murray AB, Ferguson AC, Morrison B: The seasonal variation of allergic respiratory symptoms induced by house dust mites. *Ann Allergy* (1980) **45**: 347–350.

25. Robertson DG, Kerigan AT, Hargreave FE, Chalmers R, Dolovich J: Late asthmatic responses induced by ragweed pollen allergen. *J Allergy Clin Immunol* (1974) **54**: 244–254.
26. Boulet LP, Cartier A, Thomson NC, Roberts RS, Dolovich J, Hargreave FE: Asthma and increases in nonallergic bronchial responsiveness from seasonal pollen exposure. *J Allergy Clin Immunol* (1983) **71**: 399–406.
27. Pepys J: Immunopathology of allergic lung disease. *Clin Allergy* (1973) **3**: 1–22.
28. Herxheimer H: The late bronchial reaction in induced asthma. *Int Arch Allergy Appl Immunol* (1952) **3**: 323–333.
29. Booij-Noord H, deVries K, Sluiter HJ, Orie NGM: Late bronchial obstructive reaction to experimental inhalation of house dust extract. *Clin Allergy* (1972) **2**: 43–61.
30. Newman Taylor AJ, Davies RJ, Hendrick DJ, Pepys J: Recurrent nocturnal asthmatic reactions to bronchial provocation tests. *Clin Allergy* (1979) **9**: 213–219.
31. Cockcroft DW, Hoeppner VH, Werner GD: Recurrent nocturnal asthma after bronchoprovocation with Western Red Cedar sawdust: Association with acute increase in nonallergic bronchial responsiveness. *Clin Allergy* (1984) **14**: 61–68.
32. Cockcroft DW: Beta-adrenergic agonists. In Dorsch W (ed) *Late Phase Allergic Reactions*. CRC Press, Boca Raton, 1990, pp 270–275.
33. Dorsch W, Baur X, Emslander HP, Fruhmann G: Zur pathogenese und therapie der allergeninduzierten verzogerten bronchialostruktion. *Prax Klin Pneumol* (1980) **34**: 461–468.
34. Altounyan REC: Changes in histamine and atropine responsiveness as a guide to diagnosis and evaluation of therapy in obstructive airways disease. In Pepys J, Franklands AW (eds) *Disodium Cromoglycate in Allergic Airways Disease*. Butterworths, London, 1970, pp 47–53.
35. Sotomayor H, Badier M, Vervloet D, Orehek J: Seasonal increase of carbachol airway responsiveness in patients allergic to grass pollen. *Am Rev Respir Dis* (1984) **130**: 56–58.
36. Lowhagen O, Rak S. Modification of bronchial hyperreactivity after treatment with sodium cromoglycate during pollen season. *J Allergy Clin Immunol* (1985) **75**: 460–467.
37. Cockcroft DW, Murdock KY: Changes in bronchial responsiveness to histamine at intervals after allergen challenge. *Thorax* (1987) **42**: 302–308.
38. Millilo G: Discussion. In *International Conference on Bronchial Hyperreactivity*. The Medicine Publishing Foundation, Oxford, 1982, p 17.
39. Durham SR, Graneek BJ, Hawkins R, Newman Taylor AJ: The temporal relationship between increases in airway responsiveness to histamine and late asthmatic responses induced by occupational agents. *J Allergy Clin Immunol* (1987) **79**: 398–406.
40. Thorpe J, Steinberg D, Bernstein D, Bernstein IL, Murlas C: Bronchial hyperreactivity occurs soon after the immediate asthmatic response in dual responders. *Am Rev Respir Dis* (1986) **133**: A93.
41. Hargreave FE, Ryan G, Thomson NC, *et al.*: Bronchial responsiveness to histamine or methacholine in asthma: Measurement and clinical significance. *J Allergy Clin Immunol* (1981) **68**: 347–355.
42. Orie NGM, Van Lookeren Campagne JG, Knol K, Booij-Noord H, deVries K: Late reactions in bronchial asthma. In Pepys J, Yamamura I (eds) *Intal in Bronchial Asthma*. Proceedings of the 8th International Congress of Allergollogy, Tokyo, 1974, pp 17–29.
43. Hegardt B, Pauwels R, Van Der Straeten M: Inhibitory effect of KWD 2131, terbutaline, and DSCG on the immediate and late allergen-induced bronchoconstriction. *Allergy* (1981) **36**: 115–122.
44. Ruffin RE, Cockcroft DW, Hargreave FE: A Comparison of the protective effect of Sch1000 and fenoterol on allergen-induced asthma. *J Allergy Clin Immunol* (1978) **61**: 42–47.
45. Cockcroft DW, Murdock KY: Comparative effects of inhaled salbutamol, sodium cromoglycate and beclomethasone dipropionate on allergen-induced early asthmatic response, late asthmatic responses and increased bronchial responsiveness to histamine. *J Allergy Clin Immunol* (1987) **79**: 734–740.
46. Church MK, Young KD: The characteristics of inhibition of histamine release from human lung fragments by sodium cromoglycate, salbutamol, and chlorpromazine. *Br J Pharmacol* (1983) **78**: 671–679.

47. Howarth PH, Durham SR, Lee TH, Kay B, Church MK, Holgate ST: Influence on albuterol, cromolyn sodium, and ipratropium bromide on the airway and circulating mediator responses to allergen bronchial provocation in asthma. *Am Rev Respir Dis* (1985) **132**: 986–992.

48. Twentyman OP, Finnerty JP, Harris A, Palmer J, Holgate ST: Protection against allergen-induced asthma by salmeterol. *Lancet* (1990) **336**: 1338–1342.

49. Palmqvist M, Bolder B, Lohagen O, Melander B, Svedmyr N, Wahlander L: Late asthmatic reaction prevented by inhaled albuterol and formoterol. *J Allergy Clin Immunol* (1989) **83**: 244.

50. Yu DYC, Galant SP, Gold WM: Inhibition of antigen-induced bronchoconstriction by atropine in asthmatic patients. *J Appl Physiol* (1972) **32**: 823–828.

51. Orehek J, Gayrard P, Grimaud Ch, Charpin J: Bronchoconstriction provoquee par inhalation d'allergene dans l'asthme: Effet antagoniste d'un anticholinergique de synthese. *Bull Eur Physiopathol Respir* (1975) **11**: 193–201.

52. Fish JE, Rosenthal RR, Summer WR, Menkes H, Norman PS, Permutt S: The effect of atropine on acute antigen-medicated airway constriction in subjects with allergic asthma. *Am Rev Respir Dis* (1977) **115**: 371–379.

53. Cockcroft DW, Ruffin RE, Hargreave FE: Effect of Sch 1000 in allergen-induced asthma. *Clin Allergy* (1978) **8**: 361–372.

54. Boulet LP, Latimer KM, Roberts RS, *et al.*: The effect of atropine on allergen-induced increases in bronchial responsiveness to histamine. *Am Rev Respir Dis* (1984) **130**: 368–372.

55. Nissim JE, Bleecker ER, Norman PS, Menkes H, Permutt S, Rosenthal RR: Failure of aminophylline pretreatment to prevent antigen-induced bronchospasm. *J Allergy Clin Immunol* (1980) **65**: 180.

56. Pauwels R, van Renterghem D, Van Der Straeten M, Johannesson N, Persson GA: The effect of theophylline and enprofylline on allergen-induced bronchoconstriction. *J Allergy Clin Immunol* (1985) **76**: 583–590.

57. Crescioli S, Spinazzi A, Paleari D, Pozzan M, Mapp CE, Fabbri LM: Theophylline inhibits early and late asthmatic reactions induced by allergens in atopic subjects with asthma. *Am Rev Respir Dis* (1988) **137**(Suppl): 35(A).

58. Cockcroft DW, Murdock KY, Gore BP, O'Byrne PM, Manning P: Theophylline does not inhibit allergen-induced increase in airway responsiveness to methacholine. *J Allergy Clin Immunol* (1989) **83**: 913–920.

59. Pepys J, Chan M, Hargreave FE, McCarthy DS: Inhibitory effects of disodium cromoglycate on allergen-inhalation tests. *Lancet* (1968) **ii**: 134–137.

60. Dahl R, Pedersen B: Influence of nedocromil sodium on the dual asthmatic reaction after allergen challenge: A double-blind, placebo-controlled study. *Eur J Respir Dis* (1986) **69**(Suppl 147): 263–265.

61. Booij-Noord H, Orie NGM, deVries K: Immediate and late bronchial obstructive reactions to inhalation of house dust and protective effects of disodium cromoglycate and prednisolone. *J Allergy Clin Immunol* (1971) **48**: 344–354.

62. Pepys J, Davies RJ, Breslin ABX, Hendricks DJ, Hutchcroft BJ: The effects of inhaled beclomethasone dipropionate (Becotide®) and sodium cromoglycate on asthmatic reactions to provocation tests. *Clin Allergy* (1974) **4**: 13–24.

63. Van Der Star JG, Berg WC, Steenhuis EJ, deVries K: Invloed van beclometason-dipropionaat per aerosol op de obstructieve reactie in de bronchien na huisstofinhalatie. *Ned T Geneesk* (1976) **120**: 1928–1932.

64. Burge PS, Efthimiou J, Turner-Warwick M, Nelmes PTJ: Double-blind trials of inhaled beclomethasone dipropionate and fluocortin butyl ester in allergen-induced immediate and late reactions. *Clin Allergy* (1982) **12**: 523–531.

65. Du Toit JI, Salome CM, Woolcock AJ: Inhaled corticosteroids reduce the severity of bronchial hyperresponsiveness in asthma but oral theophylline does not. *Am Rev Respir Dis* (1987) **136**: 1174–1178.

66. Woolcock AJ, Yan K, Salome CM: Effect of therapy on bronchial hyperresponsiveness in the long-term management of asthma. *Clin Allergy* (1988) **18**: 165–176.

67. Cockcroft DW, Ruffin RE, Frith PA, *et al.*: Determinants of allergen-induced asthma: dose of allergen, circulating IgE antibody concentration and bronchial responsiveness to inhaled histamine. *Am Rev Respir Dis* (1979) **120**: 1053–1058.

68. Holgate ST, Emanuel MB, Howarth PH: Astemizole and other H_1-antihistaminic drug treatment of asthma. *J Allergy Clin Immunol* (1985) **76**: 375–380.

69. Rafferty P, Beasley R, Holgate S: The contribution of histamine to immediate bronchoconstriction provoked by inhaled allergen and adenosine 5' monophosphate in atopic asthma. *Am Rev Respir Dis* (1987) **136**: 369–373.

70. Hamid M, Rafferty P, Holgate ST: The inhibitory effect of terfenadine and flurbiprofen on early and late-phase bronchoconstriction following allergen challenge in atopic asthma. *Clin Exper Allergy* (1990) **20**: 261–267.

71. Wells A, Taylor B: A placebo-controlled trial of ketotifen (HC20-511, Sandoz) in allergen induced asthma and comparison with disodium cromoglycate. *Clin Allergy* (1979) **9**: 237–240.

72. Pelikan Z, Pelikan M: Early and late asthmatic response to allergen challenge and their pharmacologic modulation. *Ann Allergy* (1985) **55**: 318.

73. Pauwels R, Lamont H, Van Der Straeten M: Comparison between ketotifen and DSCG in bronchial challenge. *Clin Allergy* (1978) **8**: 289–293.

74. Craps L, Greenwood C, Radielovic P: Clinical investigation of agents with prophylactic antiallergic effects in bronchial asthma. *Clin Allergy* (1978) **8**: 373–382.

75. Klein G, Urbanek R, Matthys H: Long-term study of the protective effect of ketotifen in children with allergic bronchial asthma. The value of a provocation test in assessment of treatment. *Respiration* (1981) **41**: 128–132.

76. Adachi M, Kobayashi H, Aoki N, *et al.*: A comparison of the inhibitory effects of ketotifen and disodium cromoglycate on bronchial responses to house dust, with special reference to the late asthmatic response. *Pharmatherapeutics* (1984) **4**: 36–42.

77. Cockcroft DW, Keshmiri M, Murdock KY, Gore BP: Allergen-induced increase in airway responsiveness is not inhibited by ketotifen or clemastine. *Ann Allergy* (1992) in press.

78. Fish JE, Ankin MG, Adkinson NF, Jr, Peterman VI: Indomethacin modification of immediate-type immunologic airway responses in allergic asthmatic and nonasthmatic subjects. *Am Rev Respir Dis* (1981) **123**: 609–614.

79. Nakazawa T, Toyoda T, Furukawa M, Taya T, Kobayashi S: Inhibitory effects of various drugs on dual asthmatic responses in wheat flour-sensitive subjects. *J Allergy Clin Immunol* (1976) **58**: 1–9.

80. Fairfax AJ: Inhibition of the late asthmatic response to house dust mite by non-steroidal anti-inflammatory drugs. *Prostaglandins Leukotrienes Med* (1982) **8**: 239–248.

81. Kirby JG, Hargreave FE, Cockcroft, DW, O'Byrne PM: Indomethacin inhibits allergeninduced airway hyperresponsiveness but not allergen-induced asthmatic responses. *J Appl Physiol* (1989) **66**: 578–583.

82. Manning PJ, Stevens WH, Cockcroft DW, O'Byrne PM: The role of thromboxane in allergen-induced asthmatic responses. *Am Rev Respir Dis* (1990) **141**: A395.

83. Lee TH, Brown MJ, Nagy L, Causon R, Walport HJ, Kay AB: Exercise-induced release of histamine and neutrophil chemotactic factor in atopic asthmatics. *J Allergy Clin Immunol* (1982) **70**: 73–81.

84. Murray JJ, Tonnel AB, Brash AR, *et al.*: Release of prostaglandin D_2 into human airways during acute antigen challenge. *N Engl J Med* (1986) **315**: 800–804.

85. Lewis RA, Austen KF: The biologically active leukotrienes: biosynthesis, metabolism, receptors, functions and pharmacology. *J Clin Invest* (1984) **73**: 889–897.

86. Schellenberg RR, Duff MJ, Foster A: Human bronchial responses to anti-IgE *in vitro*. *Clin Invest Med* (1985) **8**: A41.

87. Dolovich J, Hargreave FE, Chalmers R, Shier KJ, Gauldie J, Bienenstock J: Late cutaneous allergic responses in isolated IgE-dependent reactions. *J Allergy Clin Immunol* (1973) **52**: 38–46.

88. Solley GO, Gleich GJ, Jordon RE, Schroeter AL: The late phase of the immediate wheal and flare skin reactions. *J Clin Invest* (1976) **58**: 408–420.

89. Kirby JG, Robertson DG, Hargreave FE, Dolovich J: Asthmatic responses to inhalation of anti-human IgE. *Clin Allergy* (1986) **16**: 191–194.

90. Schampain MP, Behrens BL, Larsen GL, Henson PM: An animal model of late pulmonary responses to *Alternaria* challenge. *Am Rev Respir Dis* (1982) **126**: 493–498.

91. Abraham WM, Delehunt JC, Yerger L, Marchette B: Characterization of a late phase pulmonary response after antigen challenge in allergic sheep. *Am Rev Respir Dis* (1983) **128**: 839–844.

92. Chung KF, Becker AB, Lazarus SC, Frick OL, Nadel JA, Gold WM: Antigen-induced hyperresponsiveness and pulmonary inflammation in allergic dogs. *J Appl Physiol* (1985) **58**: 1347–1353.

93. O'Byrne PM, Walters EH, Gold ED, *et al.*: Neutrophil depletion inhibits airway hyperresponsiveness induced by ozone exposure. *Am Rev Respir Dis* (1984) **130**: 214–219.

94. Murphy KR, Wilson MC, Irvin CG, *et al.*: The requirement for polymorphonuclear leukocytes in the late asthmatic response and heightened airways reactivity in an animal model. *Am Rev Respir Dis* (1986) **134**: 62–68.

95. Metzger WJ, Richerson HB, Wasserman SI: Generation and partial characterization of eosinophil chemotactic activity and neutrophil chemotactic activity during early and late phase asthmatic response. *J Allergy Clin Immunol* (1986) **78**: 282–290.

96. Lee TH, Shore S, Corey EJ, Austen KF, Drazen JM: Leukotriene E_4 (LTE_4)-induced airway hyperresponsiveness to histamine. *J Allergy Clin Immunol* (1985) **75**: 140(A).

97. Chung KF, Aizawa H, Becker AB, Frick O, Gold WM, Nadel JA: Inhibition of antigen-induced airway hyperresponsiveness by a thromboxane synthetase inhibitor (OKY-046) in allergic dogs. *Am Rev Respir Dis* (1986) **134**: 258–261.

98. Basran GS, Page CP, Paul W, Morley J: Platelet-activating factor: A possible mediator of the dual response to allergen? *Clin Allergen* (1984) **14**: 75–79.

99. Murray AB, Ferguson AC, Morrison B: The seasonal variation of allergic respiratory symptoms induced by house dust mites. *Ann Allergen* (1980) **45**: 347–350.

100. Platts-Mills TAE, Mitchell EB, Nock P, Tovey ER, Moszoro H, Wilkins SR: Reduction of bronchial hyperreactivity during prolonged allergen avoidance. *Lancet* (1982) **2**: 675–678.

101. Dorward AJ, Robers JA, Thomson NC: Effect of nedocromil sodium on histamine airway responsiveness in grass-pollen sensitive asthmatics during the pollen season. *Clin Allergy* (1986) **16**: 309–315.

102. Cockcroft DW, Killian DN, Mellon JJA, Hargreave FE: Bronchial reactivity to inhaled histamine: A method and clinical survey. *Clin Allergy* (1977) **7**: 235–243.

103. Cockcroft DW, Berscheid BA, Murdock KY, Gore BP: Sensitivity and specificity of histamine PC_{20} measurement in a random population. *J Allergy Clin Immunol* (1985) **75**: 142.

104. Cockcroft DW: Mechanism of perennial allergic asthma. *Lancet* (1983) **2**: 253–256.

105. Bryant DH, Burns MW: The relationship between bronchial histamine reactivity and atopic status. *Clin Allergy* (1976) **6**: 373–381.

106. Cookson WOCM, Musk AW, Ryan G: Association between asthma history, atopy, and non-specific bronchial responsiveness in young adults. *Clin Allergy* (1984) **16**: 425–432.

107. Witt C, Stuckey MS, Woolcock AJ, Dawkins RC: Positive allergy prick skin tests associated with bronchial histamine responsiveness in an unselected population. *J Allergy Clin Immunol* (1986) **77**: 698–702.

108. Peat JK, Britton WJ, Salome CM, Woolcock AJ: Bronchial hyperresponsiveness in two populations of Australian school children: III. Effect of exposure to environmental allergens. *Clin Allergy* (1987) **17**: 291–300.

109. Burney PFJ, Britton JR, Chinn S, *et al.*: Descriptive epidemiology of bronchial reactivity in an adult population: Results from a community study. *Thorax* (1987) **42**: 38–44.

110. Cockcroft DW, Hargreave FE: Relationship between atopy and airway responsiveness. In Sluiter HJ, van der Lende R (eds) *Bronchitis IV*. Royal Vangorcum, Assen, The Netherlands, 1988, pp 23–32.

111. Peat JK, Salome CM, Woolcock AJ: Longitudinal changes in atopy during a 4-year period: Relation to bronchial hyperresponsiveness and respiratory symptoms in a population sample of Australian schoolchildren. *J Allergy Clin Immunol* (1990) **85**: 65–74.

112. Dowse GK, Turner KJ, Stewart GA, Alpers MP, Woolcock AJ: The association between *Dermatophagoides* mites and the increasing prevalence of asthma in village communities within the Papua New Guinea highlands. *J Allergy Clin Immunol* (1985) **75**: 75–83.

113. Becker AB, Hershkovich J, Simons FER, Simons KJ, Lilley MK, Kepron MW: Development of chronic airway hyperresponsiveness in ragweed sensitized dogs. *JAP* (1989) **66**: 2691–2697.

114. Chan-Yeung M, Lam S, Koener S: Clinical features and natural history of occupational asthma due to Western Red Cedar (*Thuja plicata*). *Am J Med* (1982) **72**: 411–415.

115. Mapp CE, Corona PC, De Marzo N, Fabbri L: Persistent asthma due to isocyanates: A follow-up study of subjects with occupational asthma due to toluene diisocyanate (TDI). *Am Rev Respir Dis* (1988) **137**: 1326–1329.

116. Malo JL, Hawkins R, Pepys J: Studies in chronic allergic bronchopulmonary aspergillosis 1: Clinical and physiological findings. *Thorax* (1977) **32**: 254–261.

117. Malo JL, Pepys J, Simon G: Studies in chronic allergic bronchopulmonary aspergillosis 2: Radiological findings. *Thorax* (1977) **32**: 262–268.

118. Malo JL, Longbottom J, Mitchell J, Hawkins R, Pepys J: Studies in chronic allergic bronchopulmonary aspergillosis 3: Immunological findings. *Thorax* (1977) **32**: 269–274.

119. Malo JL, Inouye T, Hawkins R, Simon G, Turner-Warwick M, Pepys J: Studies in chronic allergic bronchopulmonary aspergillosis 4: Comparison with a group of asthmatics. *Thorax* (1977) **32**: 275–280.

120. Dolan CT, Weed LA, Dines DE: Bronchopulmonary helminthosporiosis. *Am J Clin Pathol* (1970) **53**: 235–242.

121. Matthiesson AM: Allergic bronchopulmonary disease caused by fungi other than *Aspergillus*. *Thorax* (1981) **36**: 719.

122. McAleer R, Kroenert DB, Elder JL, Froudist JH: Allergic bronchopulmonary disease caused by *Curvularia lunata* and *Drechslera hawaiiensis*. *Thorax* (1981) **36**: 338–344.

123. Benatar SR, Allan B, Hewitson RP, Don PA: Allergic bronchopulmonary stemphyliosis. *Thorax* (1980) **35**: 515–518.

124. Voisin C, Tonnel AB, Jacob M, Thermol P, Malin P, Lahoutte C: Infiltrats pulminaires avec grande eosinophilie sanguine associes a une candidose bronchique. *Rev Fr Allergie Immunol Clin* (1976) **16**: 279–281.

125. Gordon DS, Hunter RG, O'Reilly RJ, Conway BP: *Pseudomonas aeruginosa* allergy and humoral antibody-mediated hypersensitivity pneumonia. *Am Rev Respir Dis* (1973) **108**: 127–131.

126. Longbottom JL, Pepys J: Pulmonary aspergillosis: Diagnostic and immunologic significance of antigens and C-substance in *Aspergillus fumigatus*. *J Pathol Bacteriol* (1964) **88**: 141–151.

127. Hendrick DJ, Davies RJ, D'Souza MF, Pepys J: An analysis of prick skin test reactions in 656 asthmatic patients. *Thorax* (1975) **30**: 2–8.

128. Malo JL, Paquin R: Incidence of immediate sensitivity to *Aspergillus fumigatus* in a North American asthma population. *Clin Allergy* (1979) **9**: 377–384.

129. Hoehne JH, Reed CE, Dickie HA: Allergic bronchopulmonary aspergillosis is not rare. *Chest* (1973) **63**: 177–181.

130. Malo JL, Paquin R, Longbottom JL: Prevalence of precipitating antibodies to different extracts of *Aspergillus fumigatus* in a North American asthmatic population. *Clin Allergy* (1981) **11**: 333–341.

131. McCarthy DS, Pepys J: Allergic bronchopulmonary aspergillosis. *Clin Allergy* 1971) **1**: 261–286.

132. Patterson R, Fink JN, Pruzansky JJ, *et al.*: Serum immunoglobulin levels in pulmonary allergic aspergillosis and certain other lung disease, with special reference to immunoglobulin E. *Am J Med* (1973) **54**: 16–22.

133. Scadding JG: The bronchi in allergic bronchopulmonary aspergillosis. *Scand J Respir Dis* (1967) **48**: 372–377.

134. Safirstein BH, D'Souza MF, Simon G, Tai EHC, Pepys J: Five-year follow-up of allergic bronchopulmonary aspergillosis. *Am Rev Respir Dis* (1973) **108**: 450–459.

135. Wang JLF, Patterson R, Roberts M, Ghory AC: The management of allergic bronchopulmonary aspergillosis. *Am Rev Respir Dis* (1979) **120**: 87–92.

136. Metcalfe DD: The diagnosis of food allergy: Theory and practice. In Spector SL (ed) *Provocative Challenge Procedures: Bronchial, Oral, Nasal, and Exercise*. CRC Press, Boca Raton, 1983, pp 119–132.

137. Bock SA, Lee W-Y, Remigio LK, May CD: Studies of hypersensitivity reactions to foods in infants and children. *J Allergy Clin Immunol* (1978) **62**: 327–334.

138. Orange RP, Donsky GJ: Anaphylaxis. In Middleton E Jr, Reed CE, Ellis EF (ed) *Allergy Principles and Practice*. The CV Mosby Company, St Louis, 1978, pp 563–573.

139. Gluck JC, Pacin MP: Asthma from mosquito bites: A case report. *Annals of Allergy* (1986) **56**: 492–493.

Occupational Asthma

ANTHONY J. NEWMAN-TAYLOR

INTRODUCTION: INDUCERS AND INCITERS

Occupational asthma is asthma induced by an agent inhaled at work. Agents encountered at work that induce asthma should be distinguished from agents that incite asthma. *Inducers* of asthma can initiate asthma and when inhaled cause airway inflammation and airway hyperresponsiveness. *Inciters* of asthma provoke acute transient airway narrowing in individuals whose airways are hyperresponsive but do not initiate asthma or cause airway inflammation or increase airway responsiveness.

Inducers cause airway inflammation and initiate asthma either by causing toxic damage to the airway epithelium or as the outcome of an acquired specific hypersensitivity response. Toxic inducers include respiratory irritants such as chlorine and sulphur dioxide that cause airway inflammation by a direct toxic action. Viral respiratory tract infections may also initiate asthma by a similar mechanism. Hypersensitivity inducers include inhaled proteins (such as animal excreta, flour and enzymes), other complex biological molecules (such as wood-resin acids) and low molecular weight chemicals (such as isocyanates and acid anhydrides) which may bind covalently to body proteins to form haptens. Airway inflammation occurs as the outcome of a hypersensitivity (probably immunological) response. Inciters of acute airway narrowing may be physical, such as exercise and cold air inhalation, chemical such as sulphur dioxide inhaled in subtoxic concentrations or pharmacological such as histamine and methacholine. Avoiding exposure to an inducer can reduce the severity of asthma and airway responsiveness; avoiding an inciter will reduce the frequency of provoked attacks, but not the severity of asthma or of airway hyperresponsiveness.

Both inducers and inciters of asthma may be encountered at work. Cold air in storage rooms and outdoors, exertion and irritant chemicals may all provoke asthma in individuals with hyperresponsive airways. There is also increasing evidence that the effects

ASTHMA: BASIC MECHANISMS AND CLINICAL MANAGEMENT (2nd Edn)   ISBN 0-12-079026-2 of different inciters on the airways are additive. Asthma initiated by an irritant chemical inhaled in toxic concentrations has been described as 'reactive airways dysfunction syndrome' or RADS.[1] Although probably relatively uncommon, cases have been reported of patients without previous respiratory symptoms who, within hours of exposure to a toxic chemical in high concentration, develop respiratory symptoms and airway hyperresponsiveness which may resolve spontaneously but can persist indefinitely.

The great majority of cases of asthma induced by agents inhaled at work fulfil the criteria of an acquired hypersensitivity response and the term 'occupational asthma' is often reserved for cases of *asthma induced by sensitization to an agent inhaled at work*. Because hypersensitivity inducers are therefore considerably the more important causes of occupational asthma, the majority of this chapter will focus on them. However, it remains important to appreciate that asthma may also be initiated or provoked at work by chemicals directly irritant to the airways.

CAUSES OF OCCUPATIONAL ASTHMA

Many different agents encountered at work can stimulate a hypersensitivity response and cause asthma. Some of the more important are shown in Table 26.1. Proteins and other complex molecules of biological origin may be encountered in a wide variety of circumstances. These include agriculture, the storage and transport of crops, food production, forestry and carpentry, the use of laboratory animals and the commercial exploitation of microbes as sources of food, antibiotics and enzymes. Pinewood resin, colophony, widely used in the electronics industry as a soft solder flux, fumes at the temperature of soldering.

Table 26.1 Some causes of occupational asthma.

	Proteins	Low molecular weight chemicals
Animal	Excreta of rats, mice, etc; locusts, grain mites	
Vegetable	Grain/flour Castor bean Green coffee bean *Ispaghula*	Plicatic acid (Western Red Cedar) Colophony (pinewood resin)
Microbial	Harvest moulds *Bacillus subtilis* enzyme	Antibiotics, e.g. penicillins, cephalosporins
'Minerals'		Acid anhydrides Isocyanates Complex platinum salts Polyamines Reactive dyes

The synthetic chemicals that can cause asthma when inhaled are fewer in number, but exposure to them occurs in a wide variety of occupations. Isocyanates are probably the most important. They are bi- and tri-functional molecules that are used commercially to polymerize polyhydroxyl and polyglycol compounds to form polyurethanes. Isocyanates also react with water to form carbon dioxide, a reaction utilized in the production of flexible polyurethane foams. The polyurethane reaction is exothermic, and the heat generated is sufficient to evaporate isocyanates with high vapour pressures such as toluene (TDI) and hexamethylene (HDI). Diphenyl methane (MDI) and naphthalene (NDI) diisocyanates, whose vapour pressures are lower, evaporate when heat is applied. Polyurethanes are widely used and exposure to isocyanates occurs in many situations. These include the manufacture of rigid and flexible polyurethane foams, in inks and laminating adhesives used in flexible packaging and the use of two part polyurethane varnishes and paints, which when sprayed (e.g. on cars and aircraft) generate airborne isocyanates in high concentration both as vapour and droplets. Acid anhydrides such as phthalic anhydride (PA) are used as curing agents for epoxy and alkyd resins and in the manufacture of the plasticizer dioctyl phthalate. Complex platinum salts are essential intermediates in platinum refining. Reactive dyes are increasingly used to bind a colour (chromophore) covalently to textiles: asthma has been reported among both the manufacturers and users.

IMPORTANCE OF OCCUPATIONAL ASTHMA

The contribution of occupational causes to the prevalence of asthma in the community is not known. Estimates from different countries have varied between 2 and 15% but their basis is not secure. At present information in United Kingdom is limited to the numbers awarded compensation and the number of cases reported to voluntary surveillance schemes, both of which are likely to underestimate the true frequency of the disease.

At present statutory compensation in the UK is prescribed for 14 different groups of agents. The number of awards made in 1989 was 214.

A more promising source of information in the UK is the surveillance scheme for work related diseases (SWORD) started in January 1989 to which respiratory and occupational physicians voluntarily report *new cases* of occupational lung disease.

In 1989 2101 new cases were reported of which 554 (26%) were asthma. The annual incidence rate for the working population was calculated to be 22 per million. The rates in different occupational groups varied from less than 10 per million in professional management, clerical and selling occupations to 114 per million in industries processing metal and electrical materials and those engaged in painting assembly and packing. The agents most frequently reported to cause occupational asthma were isocyanates, which accounted for 22% of cases, and grain, wood dusts, and laboratory animals, which together accounted for 17% of cases.

The rates reported in this survey are lower than those reported in Finland, one of the few countries where occupational lung diseases are registered. The incidence in 1981 in Finland was estimated to be 71 per million (compared to the rate in the UK of 22 per million). However, within the UK considerable regional variation in reported rates occurred and the area of highest incidence, West Midlands Metropolitan County, had a rate of 63 per million, similar to the reported incidence in Finland. The authors of the report suggest that the differences in regional rates may at least in part be due to differences in ascertainment and reporting, and that the true incidence of occupational asthma in the UK is as much as three times the reported rate of 22 per million.[2]

OCCUPATIONAL ASTHMA AND ALLERGY

Occupational asthma fulfils the criteria for an acquired specific hypersensitivity response:

(1) It occurs in only a proportion—usually a minority—of those exposed to its cause.
(2) It develops only after an initial symptom-free period of exposure which is usually weeks or months but can be years.
(3) In those who develop asthma, airway responses (both reduction in calibre and in non-specific responsiveness) are provoked by inhalation of the specific agent in concentrations that were previously tolerable and that do not provoke similar responses in others equally exposed (i.e. is provoked by concentrations not toxic to mucosal surfaces).

These characteristics have stimulated a search for evidence of a specific immunological response to the causes of occupational asthma, both proteins and low molecular weight chemicals. Until recently, most attention has been directed towards the identification of specific IgE and IgG antibodies. In general, when demonstrated, IgE and IgG_4 have been found in exposed populations to be associated with disease and total specific IgG with exposure. Specific IgE was associated with asthma and IgG with exposure in those working with laboratory animals[3] and specific IgE and IgG_4 with asthma and IgG with exposure in acid anhydride workers.[4,5]

The central role of the T-lymphocyte (an allergic response equivalent to murine TH2) suggest that IgE and Ig_4 do not participate directly in the development of the eosinophilic bronchitis characteristic of asthma. Evidence of activation of T-lymphocytes and eosinophils in bronchial biopsy specimens from nine patients with isocyanate-induced asthma was reported recently.[6] None the less the IgE antibody–mast cell interaction is probably an important associated response and specific IgE remains a valuable marker of the immunological response associated with asthma caused by several agents inhaled at work.

Specific IgE antibody—inferred either from an immediate skin test response to a water-soluble extract of the specific protein or hapten protein conjugate, or its identification in serum by radioallergosorbent test (RAST)—has been identified in patients with occupational asthma caused by inhaled proteins of animal, vegetable or microbial origin. These include the excreta and secreta of laboratory animals, small mammals[7] and locusts,[8] wheat and rye flour[9] and proteolytic enzymes.[10] Specific IgE has also been identified in the sera of patients with asthma caused by some low molecular weight chemicals, particularly acid anhydrides[11–13] and reactive dyes.[14] In a study to examine the determinants of allergenicity of low molecular weight chemicals, the properties of two β lactam antibiotics were compared: clavulanic acid, which is not allergenic, and a carbapenam, MM2283, which can cause asthma and stimulate IgE antibody production in man. The characteristics relevant to allergenicity were (a) reactivity with body proteins (b) homogeneity with respect to the chemical hapten and (c) stability of the conjugate formed.[15]

Specific IgE antibody has been identified in only some 15% of cases of asthma induced by isocyanates. This may reflect the difficulties of working with reactive chemicals in *in vitro* systems or failure to prepare the relevant *in vivo* chemical–protein conjugate for the *in vitro* test. Reactants of the isocyanate water reaction are likely to form in the water-saturated respiratory tract and may bind to tissue proteins and form a number of different conjugates. Failure to find convincing evidence of a specific immunological response in cases of isocyanate-induced asthma has led to suggestions that it may be the outcome of a pharmacological rather than an immunological mechanism. In support of this, TDI was found to inhibit the *in vitro* stimulation of adenyl cyclase by isoprenaline in a dose-dependent fashion,[16] possibly by covalent binding of the isocyanate group to the membrane receptor, and provoke asthma by β-adrenoreceptor inhibition in those with pre-existing airway hyperresponsiveness. This however fails to explain the well-documented latent interval between exposure to TDI and the development of asthma and the failure of TDI to provoke asthma in patients with asthma and airway hyperresponsiveness from other causes.[17] Furthermore, inhalation of TDI induces an increase in non-specific airway responsiveness in sensitized individuals without pre-test airway hyperresponsiveness[18] and fails to inhibit isoprenaline-induced tracheal smooth muscle relaxation.[19]

The development of molecular biological techniques and their application in identifying specific mRNA in T-lymphocytes will provide a powerful tool to investigate further the immunological basis of these low molecular weight chemicals where evidence of associated IgE antibody, for whatever reason, is not obtainable.

DETERMINANTS OF OCCUPATIONAL ASTHMA

Three major factors been reported to contribute to the development of occupational asthma in populations exposed to its causes: intensity of exposure, atopy and tobacco smoking.

Exposure

Although exposure is the factor most directly amenable to control, to date it has received the least attention. No studies have reported the incidence of asthma in relation to measured exposure, although exposure response relationships have been reported for the incidence of skin test responses and in cross-sectional studies for asthma. Juniper *et al.* in a study of a cohort of enzyme detergent workers found the incidence of skin prick test responses to Alcalase was greatest in those most heavily exposed[20] and Coutts *et al.* found the prevalence of work-related nasal and lower respiratory symptoms increased with increasing frequency of exposure to cimetidine dust during the working week.[21] The prevalence of work-related respiratory symptoms and airway hyperresponsiveness in bakery workers was greater in those who had ever worked in dustier conditions[22] and a gradient of work-related respiratory symptoms in relation to measured concentration of airborne colophony was found in currently employed workers.[23]

Atopy

Atopy, defined in immunological terms as those who readily produce IgE antibodies on contact with environmental allergens encountered in everyday life, is commonly identified by the presence of one or more immediate skin prick test responses to common inhalant allergens (which in the UK would include grass pollen, *Dermatophagoides pteronyssinus* and cat fur). The prevalence in workforces of atopy, defined in this way, has been consistently reported to be between one quarter and one third. Asthma and IgE antibody induced by several causes of occupational asthma have been reported to occur more commonly among atopic individuals. This association is best described for asthma caused by laboratory animals, *Bacillus subtilis* enzymes and complex platinum salts. Several studies have shown asthma to be some four to five times more prevalent in atopic than non-atopic laboratory animal workers.[24,25] In a cohort study of enzyme detergent workers, Juniper *et al.* found the incidence of a skin test response to Alcalase was greater among atopics at each level of exposure.[20] The incidence of respiratory symptoms and skin prick test responses to ammonium hexachloroplatinate was greater among atopics in a platinum refinery workforce.[26] However, a subsequent study of the same population found smoking to be a more important risk factor.[27] On the other hand, for several causes of occupational asthma, such as isocyanates and plicatic acid, atopics seem at no greater risk of developing asthma than non-atopics.

Tobacco smoking

Tobacco smoking is associated with an increased risk of developing specific IgE and asthma caused by several different agents inhaled at work. Specific IgE antibody or an immediate skin test response has been found some four to five times more frequently in smokers than non-smokers exposed to the acid anhydride TCPA,[28] green coffee bean and ispaghula[29] and ammonium hexacholoroplatinate.[28] The risk of developing asthma is also increased, although less than for specific IgE: all seven cases of TCPA-induced asthma reported by Howe *et al.*[12] were cigarette smokers and the risk of asthma in platinum refinery workers[28] and snow crab processing workers was increased some two-fold.[30]

The mechanism of this 'adjuvant' effect of tobacco smoking is unknown, but may be a consequence of injury, whatever its cause, to the respiratory mucosa which is concurrent with the inhalation of novel antigens. Inhaled tobacco smoke was found to potentiate the IgE response in experimental animals to inhaled, but not subcutaneous, ovalbumin. Other respiratory irritants can exert a similar effect. The proportion of cynomolgus monkeys that developed asthma and a positive skin test after inhalation of complex platinum salts was increased in those animals who inhaled ozone concurrently.[32] Similarly, the frequency of IgE antibody production and airway responses provoked by inhaled ovalbumin were increased in a dose-dependent fashion in guinea-pigs that inhaled sulphur dioxide concurrently with the sensitizing dose of ovalbumin.[33]

DIAGNOSIS OF OCCUPATIONAL ASTHMA

Accurate and early diagnosis of cases of occupational asthma is important. Remission of respiratory symptoms and restoration of normal lung function, including non-specific airway responsiveness, can follow avoidance of exposure to the specific initiating cause. Furthermore, chronic asthma is more likely to develop in those who remain exposed to the initiating cause after the onset of symptoms. However, avoidance of exposure frequently requires a change of work which, particularly in the present economic climate, can mean loss of employment. Accurate diagnosis is therefore also essential if those whose asthma is not occupationally caused are to avoid being advised unnecessarily to change or leave their work.

The diagnosis of occupational asthma requires:

(1) Differentiation of asthma from other causes of respiratory symptoms, in particular chronic airflow limitation and hyperventilation.
(2) Differentiation of asthma of occupational cause from non-occupational asthma.
(3) Differentiation of asthma initiated by an agent inhaled at work from pre-existing or incident asthma provoked by non-specific irritants, such as sulphur dioxide and cold air, inhaled at work.

The diagnosis of occupational hypersensitivity asthma is usually suggested by the history. It usually occurs in an individual exposed at work to an agent recognized to cause occupational asthma and only develops after an initial symptom-free period when the patient has been exposed without symptoms to concentrations that later provoke his asthma. Symptoms from their onset are work related, occurring during the working week day by day when they may increase in severity, improving during absences from work, at weekends or during holidays. The patient may also be aware of others who have developed similar respiratory symptoms at his place of work.

Non-specific stimuli provoke asthmatic reactions that generally occur within minutes of exposure and usually resolve within 1–2 h of avoidance of exposure. Where work-related respiratory symptoms are due to the provocation of asthma by respiratory irritants encountered at work, the onset of asthma will often have preceded initial exposure to the irritant and the severity of the asthma does not improve when away from work. Non-specific irritants such as organic solvents, which can have a characteristic and unpleasant smell, may also provoke a hyperventilation response; breathing difficulties are associated with other symptoms suggestive of hyperventilation, such as tingling of the fingers, headaches and dizziness.

INVESTIGATION OF OCCUPATIONAL ASTHMA

In the majority of cases a confident diagnosis of occupational asthma can be made from knowledge of exposure at work to a recognized cause of occupational asthma and a characteristic history which, where possible, is supported by evidence from serial measurements of peak expiratory flow (PEF), or immunological tests or both. Inhalation testing is reserved for occasions when the results of these investigations do not provide an adequate basis for advice about future employment.

Serial peak expiratory flow (PEF) measurements

Asthma can be attributed with confidence to an agent inhaled at work where exposure to it in the workplace reproducibly provokes airway narrowing, particularly where this is increasingly severe during the working week. Repeated measurements of airway calibre, most conveniently made as peak expiratory flow rates (PEF), need to be made during a period long enough to allow observation of the consistency of any changes and their relationship to periods at work. Measurements need to be made repeatedly during each day for a period of several weeks; requiring the patient to make and record his own results. Such self-recording of PEF measurements is now widely used for both the diagnosis of occupational asthma and for examination of the effectiveness of intervention, such as relocation at work. Patients are lent a peak flow meter and asked to record the best of three measurements of PEF made every 2 h from waking to sleeping during a period of 1 month in the first instance. To allow sufficient time for lung function to recover from exposure to an agent at work, it is helpful if the month includes a period away from work longer than a weekend, ideally a 1–2-week holiday. Self-recording requires patient compliance and honesty. The measurements may be conveniently summarized to show the maximum, minimum and peak flow measurements for each day (Fig. 26.1); any differences between periods at work and periods away from work can be observed. This method of patient investigation has proved, in the hands of those experienced in its use, to be reliable and a relatively sensitive and specific index of occupational asthma.

Immunological investigations

The application of immunological tests in investigation of occupational asthma has widened because of:

(1) Identification of the nature and source of relevant allergens (e.g. the identification of laboratory animal urine as a major source of allergenic protein) allowing the preparation of immunologically relevant test extracts.
(2) Preparation of hapten protein conjugates suitable for immunological testing (e.g. acid anhydride–human serum albumin conjugates and reactive dye–human serum albumin conjugates).
(3) Development of reliable methods for identification of specific IgE antibody in serum.

Extracts of several of the causes of occupational asthma can be used to elicit skin test reactions and to identify specific IgE antibody in serum. These include the *B. subtilis* enzyme, Alcalase, urine proteins of laboratory animals, excreta of locusts, wheat and rye flour proteins, harvest moulds (e.g. *Alternaria tenius* and *Cladosporium herbarum*) and the

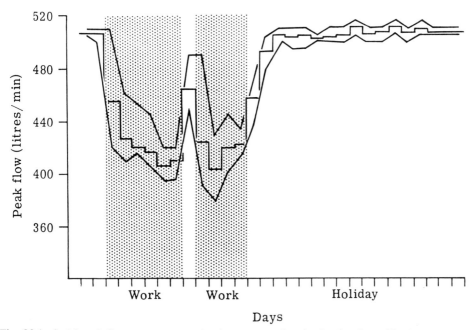

Fig. 26.1 Serial peak flow measurements showing pattern of work-related asthma. The best, worst and average peak flow results are plotted for each day. The shaded areas are periods at work, the unshaded areas periods away from work. Peak flow deteriorates at work and partially improves during 1-day absence from work. Complete improvement occurs within first 3 days of holiday and continues throughout this period.

grain mites (e.g. *Acaris siro* and *Leptidoglyphus destructor*). In addition, hapten protein conjugates, suitable for skin testing and identification of specific IgE antibody, have been prepared for acid anhydrides and reactive dyes. Complex platinum salts such as ammonium hexochloroplatinate can elicit immediate skin prick test responses without the need for conjugation to human serum albumin.

The value of such tests in the diagnosis of occupational asthma depends upon their sensitivity and specificity in populations exposed to the particular cause. Extracts of urine protein obtained from rats and mice have been shown in several studies to be a sensitive and relatively specific index of asthma, but not of rhinitis, conjunctivitis or urticaria.[24,25] Similarly, an immediate skin prick test response and specific IgE antibody, identified by RAST, to extracts of locust[8] and to conjugates of the acid anhydride, TCPA with human serum albumin[12] were associated with cases of asthma in exposed populations and not simply a reflection of exposure.

Inhalation tests

There are four major indications for inhalation testing in the diagnosis of occupational asthma.

(1) Where the agent thought to be responsible for causing asthma has not previously been reliably shown to do so.

(2) Where an individual with occupational asthma is exposed at work to more than one potential cause.
(3) Where asthma is of such severity that further uncontrolled exposure in the work environment is not justifiable.
(4) Where the diagnosis of occupational asthma remains in doubt after other investigations, including serial PEF and immunological tests, where appropriate, have been completed.

Inhalation tests undertaken solely for legal purposes are not justifiable.

The aim in an occupational-type inhalation test is to expose the individual under single blind conditions to the putative cause of his asthma in circumstances that resemble as closely as possible the conditions of his exposure at work. Wherever possible, atmospheric concentrations of the inhaled agent should be based on knowledge of the concentrations experienced at work and the physical conditions of exposure, e.g. the size of dust particles, whether vapour or aerosol and the temperatures to which the materials are heated, should be similar to the conditions encountered at work.

The different methods used in inhalation tests depend primarily on the physical state of the test material. Soluble allergens, such as urine proteins of laboratory animals, are inhaled as nebulized extracts in solution. Volatile organic liquids such as TDI may be painted onto a flat surface in increasing concentrations on different days; and the atmospheric concentration of vapour can be measured with an appropriate monitor. Exposure to dusts such as antibiotics, complex platinum salts and acid anhydrides can be made by tipping the test material, usually diluted in dried lactose, between two trays. The atmospheric concentration achieved is surprisingly reproducible and can be measured by use of a personal dust sampler.

Measurements of airway responses provoked by inhalation test should ideally include measurements of both changes in airway calibre and in non-specific airway responsiveness. Changes in airway calibre are most easily measured by regular measurements of FEV_1 and FVC or of PEF before and at regular intervals after the test, for at least 24 h. Changes in airway responsiveness can be made by estimating the concentration of inhaled histamine or methachlorine which provokes a 20% fall in FEV_1 (PC_{20}) before the test and at 3 h and 24 h after the test. The changes in airway calibre and non-specific responsiveness observed are compared to those following a control challenge test, each test being made on a separate day (Fig. 26.2).

The patterns of change in airway calibre provoked by inhalation testing are distinguished by their time of onset and duration. Immediate responses occur within minutes and resolve spontaneously within 1–2 h. Such reactions can be provoked by both allergic (e.g. grass pollen) and non-allergic (e.g. inhaled histamine or sulphur dioxide) stimuli. The response depends upon the concentration of the provoking agent and the degree of pre-existing non-specific airway responsiveness. Lone immediate responses are not usually associated with an increase in non-specific airway responsiveness. Late responses develop 1 h or more after the inhalation test, usually after some 3–4 h and may persist for 24–36 h. Unlike the immediate response, late responses are often associated with an increase in non-specific responsiveness which can be identified 3 h post-test prior to the onset of the late asthmatic response and, less reliably, at 24 h after the test (Fig. 26.2).[18]

A dual response is an immediate response followed by a late response. Recurrent

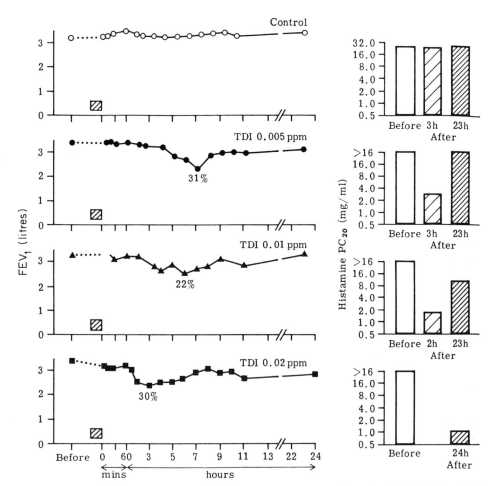

Fig. 26.2 Changes in airway calibre (FEV_1) and airway responsiveness (histamine PC_{20}) following inhalation test with control and increasing concentrations of TDI, FEV_1 and PC_{20} are stable during control day. Inhalation of TDI provokes a non-immediate asthmatic response with an increase in airway responsiveness at 3 h, but not 24 h at the lowest exposure concentration and at 24 h at the higher concentrations.

nocturnal responses may be provoked by a single inhalation test exposure with asthmatic responses occurring during several successive nights with partial or complete remission during the intervening days.[34] Such responses are almost certainly a manifestation of a provoked increase in non-specific airway responsiveness.

The question to be answered from the results of an inhalation test is whether or not the particular agent inhaled at work has induced asthma in the individual. The most satisfactory way to answer this question is to determine whether or not inhalation of the specific agents reproducibly provokes a non immediate asthmatic response and increases non-specific airway responsiveness. In such cases the specific agent can be regarded as the inducing cause in the particular individual. Non-specific irritants may provoke immediate responses in individuals with hyperresponsive airways but do not provoke either an increase in non-specific airway responsiveness or a late asthmatic reaction. Agents that induce specific IgE antibody, however, often provoke lone asthmatic responses; in these cases inferences from the inhalation test result should take the immunological test into account.

OUTCOME OF OCCUPATIONAL ASTHMA

Asthma induced by an agent inhaled at work may become chronic, and persist for several years, if not indefinitely, after avoidance of exposure to the initiating cause. This seems particularly, although not exclusively, to occur in patients with asthma caused by low molecular weight chemicals amongst whom asthma has been reported to persist in over a half. Six cases of asthma caused by the acid anhydride tetrachlorophthalic anhydride (TCPA) were followed up 4 years after avoidance of exposure: all had chronic respiratory symptoms consistent with persistent airway hyperresponsiveness and hista-mine PC_{20} was increased in the five in whom it was measured. The rate of decline of specific IgE to a TCPA-human serum albumin conjugate during the period of avoidance of exposure was exponential with a $t_{\frac{1}{2}}$ of 1 year, and parallel in all six subjects, making it very improbable their continuing asthma was caused by further inadvertent exposure.[35]

In another study, 31 snow-crab workers with occupational asthma, diagnosed by inhalation tests, were studied up to 5 years from their last exposure. All denied exposure to crabmeat by inhalation or ingestion. Respiratory symptoms persisted in all 31 of whom 26 had a measurable methacholine PC_{20}. Although FEV_1, FEV_1/FVC and PC_{20} improved during the initial period of avoidance of exposure, FEV_1 and FEV_1/FVC plateaued by 1 year and PC_{20} by 2 years.[36]

Continuing asthma in these patients seems likely to be a manifestation of chronic airway inflammation which, although initiated by an agent inhaled at work, persists in its absence. Ten patients with TDI-induced asthma, who had continuing respiratory symptoms and airway hyperresponsiveness, were investigated 4–40 months from their last exposure. Bronchial biopsies, obtained from eight, showed basement membrane thickening with infiltration of the mucosa by eosinophils, lymphocytes and neutrophils; in four patients, in whom airway responsiveness had not improved, the proportion of eosinophils in fluid recovered at bronchoalveolar lavage (BAL) was increased, whereas this was the case in only one of the five whose airway responsiveness had improved.[37]

The only important reported determinant of chronicity in occupationally induced asthma is duration of exposure to its initiating cause after the onset of respiratory symptoms. When examined, on average 4 years after avoidance of exposure, 60% of 136 cases of asthma caused by Western Red Cedar (*Thuja plicata*) continued to have asthma. The interval from onset of symptoms to diagnosis in those with continuing asthma was on average 2.5 years longer than in those whose symptoms had resolved.[38]

MANAGEMENT OF OCCUPATIONAL ASTHMA

Patients who develop occupational asthma and in whom the specific cause is identified should be advised to avoid further exposure to the cause of their asthma. This is

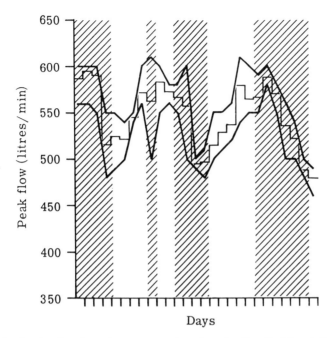

Fig. 26.3   Work related asthma in an isocyanate worker after relocation. Serial peak flow records demonstrate that despite avoidance of exposure to isocyanate (MDI) at work he has consistent deteriorations in PEF measurements while at work and is likely to be inadvertently continuing exposure to MDI.

particularly important if low molecular weight chemicals, such as isocyanates, plicatic acid or acid anhydrides, are the cause, as they are particularly associated with the development of chronic asthma and airway hyperresponsiveness.

Avoidance of further exposure can necessitate a change or loss of job which, for social or financial reasons, may not be possible. A change of occupation can be particularly difficult for highly trained individuals, such as experimental scientists, whose livelihood depends on their knowledge and experience of working with laboratory animals. Such individuals and others sensitized to biological dusts who are unable, at least in the short term, to change their job, should be advised to minimize their animal contact, and to wear respiratory protection, most conveniently laminar flow equipment, when in contact with animals. In addition background prophylaxis such as sodium cromoglycate will minimize the risk of the provocation of asthma by indirect allergen contact, as from dust on colleagues' clothing. None the less, it should be emphasized that such measures are temporary and in the long term, the means should be sought to avoid exposure to the cause of asthma.

When an individual does remain in employment where he is exposed to the cause of his asthma, either directly or indirectly, the effectiveness of relocation or of respiratory protection needs to be monitored. This can be conveniently done by serial self recordings of peak flow to determine whether or not asthma persists and if so if it is work related. (Fig. 26.3).

REFERENCES

1. Brookes SM, Weiss MA, Bernstein K: Reactive airways dysfunction syndrome (RADS): persistent asthma syndrome after high level irritant exposures. *Chest* (1985) **88**: 376–384.
2. Meredith SK, Taylor VM, McDonald JC: Occupational respiratory disease in the United Kingdom. *Brit J Indust Med* (1991) **48**: 292–298.
3. Platts Mills TAE, Longbottom J, Edwards J, Cockcroft A, Wilkins S: Occupational asthma and rhinitis related to laboratory animals: serum IgE and IgG antibodies to the rat urinary allergen. *J Allergy Clin Immunol* (1987) **79**: 505–515.
4. Howe W, Venables K, Topping M, *et al.*: Tetrachlorophthalic anhydride asthma: evidence for specific IgE antibody. *J Allergy Clin Immunol* (1983) **71**: 5–11.
5. Foster H, Topping M, Newman Taylor AJ: Specific IgG and IgG_4 antibody to tetra chlorophthalic anhydride. *Allergy Proc* (1988) **9**: 296.
6. Bentley AM, Maestrelli P, Fabri LM, *et al.*: Immunohistology of the bronchial mucosa in occupational, intrinsic and extrinsic asthma. *J Allergy Clin Immunol* (1991) 5246.
7. Newman Taylor AJ, Longbottom JL, Pepys J: Respiratory allergy to urine proteins of rats and mice. *Lancet* (1977) **2**: 847–849.
8. Tee RD, Gordon DJ, Hawkins ER, *et al.*: Occupational allergy to locusts: an investigation of the sources of the allergen. *J Allergy Clin Immunol* (1988) **81**: 517–525.
9. Bjorksten F, Backman A, Jarvinen AJ, Savilahti EK, Syvanen P, Karkkainen T: Immunoglobulin E specific to wheat and rye flour. *Clin Allergy* (1977) **7**: 473–483.
10. Pepys J, Wells ED, D'Souza M, Greenburg M: Clinical and immunological responses to enzymes of *Bacillus subtilis* in factory workers and consumers. *Clin Allergy* (1973) **3**: 143–160.
11. Maccia CA, Bernstein IL, Emmett EA, Brooks SM: *In vitro* demonstration of specific IgE in phthalic anhydride sensitivity. *Am Rev Resp Dis* (1976) **113**: 701–704.
12. Howe W, Venables KM, Topping MD, *et al.*: Tetrachlorophthalic acid anhydride asthma: evidence for specific IgE. *J Allergy Clin Immunol* (1983) **71**: 5–11.
13. Zeiss CR, Patterson R, Pruzansky JJ, Miller MM, Rosenburg M, Levitz D: Trimellitic anhydride induced airway syndromes. *J Allergy Clin Immunol* (1977) **60**: 96–103.
14. Luczynska CM, Topping MD: Specific IgE antibodies to reactive dye-albumin conjugates. *J Immunol Methods* (1986) **95**: 177–186.
15. Edwards RG, Dewdney JM, Dobrzanski RJ, Lee D: Immunogenicity and allergenicity studies on two beta lactam structures, a clavam, clavulancic acid and a carbapenam: structure activity relationships. *Int Arch Allergy Appl Immunol* (1988) **85**: 184–189.
16. Davies RJ, Butcher BT, O'Neil CE, Salvaggio JE: The *in vitro* effect of toluene di-isocyanate on lymphocyte cyclic adenosine monophosphate production by isoproterenol, prostaglandin and histamine. *J Allergy Clin Immunol* (1977) **60**: 223–229.
17. Lozewiz S, Assoufi BK, Hawkins R, Newman Taylor AJ: Outcome of asthma induced by isocyanates. *Br J Dis Chest* (1987) **81**: 14–22.
18. Durham SR, Graneek BJ, Hawkins R, Newman Taylor AJ: The temporal relationship between increases in airway responsiveness to histamine and late asthmatic responses induced by occupational agents. *J Allergy Clin Immunol* (1987) **79**: 398–406.
19. Mackay RT, Brooks SM: Effect of toluene diisocyanate on beta adrenergic receptor function. *Am Rev Resp Dis* (1983) **148**: 50–53.
20. Juniper CP, How MJ, Goodwin BFJ, Kinshott AJC: *Bascillus subtilis* enzymes: a 7 year clinical epidemiological and immunological study of an industrial allergen. *J Soc Occup Med* (1977) **27**: 3–12.
21. Coutts II, Lozewitcz S, Dally MD, Newman Taylor AJ, Burge PS, Rogers JD: Respiratory symptoms related to work in a factory manufacturing cimetidine tablets. *Brit Med J* (1984) **288**: 1418.
22. Musk AW, Venables KM, Crook B, Nunn AJ, *et al.*: Respiratory symptoms, lung function and sensitisation to flour in a British bakery. *Br J Ind Med* (1989) **46**: 636–642.
23. Burge PS, Edge G, Hawkins R, White V, Newman Taylor AJ: Occupational asthma in a factory making flux cored solder containing colophony. *Thorax* (1981) **36**: 828–834.
24. Slovak AMJ, Hill RN: Laboratory animal allergy: a clinical survey of an exposed population. *Br J Ind Med* (1981) **38**: 38–41.

25. Venables KM, Tee RD, Hawkins ER, *et al.*: Laboratory animal allergy in a pharmaceutical company. *Br J Ind Med* (1988) **45**: 660–666.

26. Dally MB, Hunter JV, Hughes EG, *et al.*: Hypersensitivity to platinum salts: a population study. *Am Rev Resp Dis* (1980) **4**: 120.

27. Venables KM, Dally MB, Nunn AJ, *et al.*: Smoking and occupational allergy in a platinum refinery. *Br Med J* (1989) **299**: 939–942.

28. Venables KM, Topping MD, Howe W, Luczynska CM, Hawkins R, Newman Taylor AJ: Interaction of smoking and atopy in producing specific IgE antibody against a hapten protein conjugate. *Br Med J* (1985) **290**: 201–204.

29. Zetterstrom O, Osterman K, Machado L, Johansson SGO: Another smoking hazard reused serum IgE concentrations and increased risk of occupational allergy. *Br Med J* (1981) **283**: 1215–1217.

30. Cartier A, Malo JL, Forest F, *et al.*: Occupational asthma in snow-crab processing workers. *J Allergy Clin Immunol* (1984) **74**: 261–269.

31. Zetterstrom O, Nordvall SL, Bjorksten B, Ahlstedt S, Stelander M: Increased IgE antibody responses to rats exposed to tobacco smoke. *J Allergy Clin Immunol* (1985) **75**: 594.

32. Biagini RE, Moorman WJ, Lewis TR, Bernstein IL: Ozone enhancement of platinum asthma in a primate model. *Ann Rev Respir Dis* (1986) **134**: 719–725.

33. Riedel F, Kramer M, Scheibenbogen C, Rieger CHC: Effects of SO_2 exposure on allergic sensitisation in the guinea pig. *J Allergy Clin Immunol* (1988) **82**: 527–534.

34. Newman Taylor AJ, Davies RJ, Hendrick DJ, Pepys J: Recurrent nocturnal asthmatic reactions to bronchial provocation tests. *Clin Allergy* (1979) **9**: 213–219.

35. Venables KM: Topping MD, Nunn AJ, Howe W, Newman Taylor AJ: Immunologic and functional consequences of chemical (tetrachlorophthalic anhydride) induced asthma after 4 years of avoidance of exposure. *J Allergy Clin Immunol* (1987) **80**: 212–218.

36. Malo JC, Cartier A, Ghezzo H, Lafrance M, Cante M, Lehrer SB: Patterns of improvement in spirometry, bronchial hyper responsiveness and specific IgE antibody levels after cessation of exposure in occupational asthma caused by snow-crab processing. *Am Rev Resp Dis* (1988) **138**: 807–812.

37. Paggiaro P, Bacci E, Paoetto P, *et al.*: Bronchoalveolar lavage and morphology of the airways after cessation of exposure in asthmatic subjects to toluene di-isocyanate. *Chest* (1990) **98**: 536–542.

38. Chan Yeung M, McLean L, Paggiaro PL: Follow up study of 232 patients with occupational asthma caused by Western Red Cedar (*Thuja plicata*). *J Allergy Clin Immunol* (1987) **79**: 792–796.

Infections

WILLIAM W. BUSSE AND WILLIAM J. CALHOUN

INTRODUCTION

Respiratory infections have a very important relationship to asthma and possibly the underlying mechanisms of airway hyperresponsiveness. For many patients with asthma, respiratory infections provoke wheezing. This relationship is especially evident in children. Furthermore, but less well established, is the possibility that respiratory infections actually are a pivotal event in the onset of asthma. Investigations into the relationship of respiratory infections and asthma have focused on two major issues: the epidemiology of respiratory infections and asthma and the mechanisms by which respiratory infections, particularly viral illnesses, affect the development of bronchial responsiveness and asthma. These areas will be the focus of this chapter.

EPIDEMIOLOGY OF RESPIRATORY INFECTIONS AND ASTHMA

Viral respiratory infections provoke asthma

For decades clinicians associated asthma exacerbations with respiratory infections. With prospective studies, it became apparent that viral, not bacterial, upper respiratory infections (URI) triggered these asthma attacks.

McIntosh et al.[1] prospectively studied 32 young children, aged 1–5 years, with severe asthma. The aetiology of each URI was carefully evaluated and confirmed by culture and serological tests for viral antibody titres. Further, each exacerbation of asthma was documented by physical examination and changes in bronchodilator medication. Over 2

ASTHMA: BASIC MECHANISMS AND CLINICAL MANAGEMENT (2nd Edn)
ISBN 0-12-079026-2

years, there were 102 confirmed viral respiratory infections and 139 episodes of wheezing. Fifty-eight episodes (42%) of wheezing occurred in relationship to viral respiratory infections of which respiratory syncytial virus (RSV) was the most prevalent and likely to provoke asthma. Respiratory bacteria, *Haemophilus influenza, Streptococcus pneumonia, β*-haemolytic streptococcus, and *Staphylococcus aureus,* were also cultured but their presence did not correlate with an asthma attack.

A prospective outpatient study from the University of Wisconsin evaluated 16 children, aged 3–11 years, with histories of four or more asthma attacks associated with respiratory illnesses during the previous year.[2] Detailed clinical records profiled each child's asthma severity, which was further substantiated with biweekly examinations. During an asthma exacerbation or apparent URI, additional bacteria and virus cultures were collected and asthma symptoms carefully quantitated.

The 16 children experienced 61 episodes of asthma; 42 occurred in conjunction with a symptomatic respiratory infection and 24 were confirmed to be of a viral aetiology by culture and/or serum haemagglutination titres. In this study, rhinovirus was the most frequently isolated virus in association with wheezing. Some patients had episodes of asymptomatic viral infection, but asthma was not worsened. Only one episode of wheezing coincided with a bacterial infection.

In contrast, the relationship between respiratory infections and episodes of wheezing is not as striking in adults. When both children and adults were evaluated, respiratory viruses were more frequently identified during episodes of asthma in children under 10 years of age than in adults.[3] Eight adult subjects evaluated by Minor *et al.*[3] had only three documented virus infections with increased wheezing. Although an explanation for such findings is not clear, it is likely that asthma flares are more difficult to delineate sharply, and the pattern of wheezing often appears chronic rather than episodic in adults. Similarly, when Hudgel *et al.*[4] evaluated 19 adult asthma patients over a 15-month period, 76 episodes of asthma were recorded but only eight could be documented with a viral URI. Although clinically apparent viral respiratory infections precipitate asthma in adults, the relative frequency appears less than in children.

Not all subjects are susceptible to wheezing with respiratory infections, nor are all respiratory viruses, or strains of one virus, capable of provoking asthma. Half of a normal adult volunteer population experimentally infected with rhinovirus by Halperin *et al.*[5] had positive cultures from their lower respiratory tract at bronchoscopy; neither spirometry nor bronchoprovocation with histamine changed during the respiratory illness. When the same investigators inoculated asthma volunteers with rhinovirus, only four of the 21 infected asthma patients had a 10% or greater decrease in FEV_1 and a concomitant increase in airway sensitivity to inhaled histamine.[6] Although the investigators interpreted their findings to show that experimental rhinovirus infections aggravate airway reactivity in a minority of adult asthma patients, and exacerbation of wheezing with other viral pathogens is more likely to play an important role in this relationship, this frequency of wheezing during URIs is not unusual for adults.[3,4] Moreover, it is important to recall that symptomatic respiratory infections, not merely the recovery of viruses from the airway, are more inclined to incite asthma in both children and adults.[2] Thus, the effect that a viral respiratory infection has on lung function will be dictated by many factors including the patient's age, underlying airway hyperreactivity, the particular respiratory virus, and the development of significant symptoms (rhinorrhoea, malaises, etc.).

Table 27.1 Disease characteristics before and after treatment for sinus disease in 48 children.

Characteristic	Before		After	
	No.	%	No.	%
Cough	48	100	14	29
Wheeze	48	100	7	15
Rhinorrhoea	30	63	10	21
Bronchodilator treatment	48	100	10	21
Normal pulmonary function tests	0/30	0	20/30	67
Normal sinus radiograph	0	0	38	79

Reproduced from ref. 9, with permission.

There is little evidence that bacterial respiratory infections, other than sinusitis, provoke asthma. Berman et al.[7] performed transtracheal aspirates on 27 adult asthma patients during an infectious exacerbation. Bacteria cultured from transtracheal aspirates was sparse, and more importantly, did not correlate with clinical illness. Moreover, transtracheal aspirates from normal subjects, without respiratory infections, yielded a similar degree of bacterial colonization.

Although the association between paranasal sinusitis and bronchial asthma has long been observed, it is conceivable that sinusitis and asthma co-exist as complications of the same respiratory infection. However, some feel that an aetiological relationship exists between sinusitis and asthma.[8] For example in 48 children with active sinusitis and asthma, Rachelefsky et al.[9] found that antibiotic treatment of sinusitis reduced asthma severity (Table 27.1). Although these observations are intriguing, additional insight is needed to understand how sinusitis exacerbates asthma.

Relationship of viral respiratory infections to the development of asthma

In comparison to the question as to whether viral respiratory infections exacerbate asthma, the issue becomes more complex when the role of respiratory illnesses is examined 'in the causation and perpetuation of airways hyperresponsiveness and, by implication, recurrent, chronic wheeze-associated respiratory illnesses including asthma'.[10] Although a significant body of information suggests an association between respiratory tract illness in early life and later development of airway dysfunction, this relationship cannot be definitively established but underscores the complexity of factors surrounding the development of bronchial reactivity and asthma.[11]

Eisen and Bacal[12] found that children hospitalized for bronchiolitis prior to age 2 had an increased risk for asthma. Rooney and Williams[13] also evaluated retrospectively the records of infants hospitalized for bronchiolitis at 18 months or younger; allergic manifestations and a family history of asthma were more frequent in children who eventually experienced one or more episodes of wheezing. Finally, McConnochie and Roghmann[14] identified 77 patients who had bronchiolitis at 25 months or younger and compared their outcome to children without a history of bronchiolitis. When these children were evaluated approximately 7 years later, only upper respiratory allergy, bronchiolitis and passive smoking exposure were found to be independent predictors of wheezing following bronchiolitis. Consequently it is apparent that final conclusions on the relationship between respiratory infections in infancy and later asthma must consider a host of influences, including parental smoking, air pollution, underlying airway reactivity and gender.

A more difficult issue to resolve is the relationship between respiratory infections and the genesis of airway hyperresponsiveness. To evaluate the effect of bronchiolitis on airway responsiveness, Sims et al.[15] identified 8-year-old children who had RSV respiratory infection and quantitated bronchial 'lability' by exercise tests. Compared to appropriate controls, the fall in the peak flow to exercise was greater in children who had bronchiolitis; however, airway reactivity to exercise was not different between children with or without subsequent episodes of wheezing. Since other variables confounded their study, Sims et al.[15] could not prove that respiratory infections led to the later development of asthma.

Other efforts have been made to ascertain if lower respiratory tract viral infections (LRI) in early life cause persistent pulmonary function abnormalities. Pullan and Hey[16] evaluated 130 children admitted to hospital during the first 5 years of life with RSV LRIs. Forty-two per cent of the hospitalized children had future episodes of wheezing, while only 19% of control subjects experienced similar airway symptoms. However, few patients (6.2% vs 4.5% of controls) had troublesome respiratory symptoms by 10 years of age. Furthermore, although a three-fold increase in bronchial reactivity was found in children with bronchiolitis, atopy was not increased. Analogous conclusions were reached by Weiss et al.[17] when they assessed the outcome of an antecedent acute respiratory illness on airway responsiveness and atopy in young adults. Airway responsiveness, evaluated by eucapnic hyperventilation to subfreezing air, was increased in children with a previous history of either croup or bronchiolitis, or greater than two acute lower respiratory illnesses but atopy was not greater.

The possibility has also been raised that a predisposition to wheezing in infancy depends more on intrinsic airway structure, or bronchial reactivity, than atopy.[18] This position is supported by the high degree of airway responsiveness found in infancy both in physiological evaluations[19–21] and incidence of wheezing with respiratory infections.[22]

To help clarify the relationship between premorbid lung function and wheezing with respiratory illnesses Martinez et al.[23] conducted a prospective study of respiratory illness in infancy and childhood. Lung function values were determined *prior* to any LRIs. Included in these measurements were patterns of tidal expiratory patterns, specifically the ratio of time to peak tidal expiratory flow (T_{me}) divided by total expiratory time (T_E), or the T_{me}/T_E ratio; Morris and Lane[24] had shown that decreasing T_{me}/T_E ratios correlated with lower lung function in patients with progressive chronic obstructive lung disease.

Thirty-six infants developed a lower respiratory infection and 24 wheezed with at least one of these infections. There was no difference in preinfection lung function between those infants who did not have an LRI and those with an infection but no wheezing (Table 27.2). However, infants who wheezed with the respiratory infection had diminished T_{me}/T_E values and reduced expiratory system conductance when measured *prior* to wheezing with the infection. These data suggest that alterations in lung function are compatible with reduced airway conductance or a slow respiratory system time constant precedes and predicts wheezing with respiratory infections in infants. Furthermore, it

Table 27.2   Pulmonary function and LRI outcome.

Index	No LRI	LRI (no wheeze)	(wheeze)	P value
T_{me}/T_E	31.2 ± 9.2 (88)	31.4 ± 8.5 (12)	$25.4 \pm 6.9^*$ (24)	0.01
G_{RS} (litre/s/cm H_2O)	0.035 ± 0.009 (30)	0.036 ± 0.010 (6)	$0.028 \pm 0.006^{**}$ (11)	0.04
FRC (ml)	103.2 ± 16.7 (71)	102.5 ± 15.6 (8)	97.1 ± 20.8 (15)	0.63
$\dot{V}_{max}$ (ml/s)	131.2 ± 47.9 (77)	119.1 ± 44.0 (11)	118.6 ± 51.2 (21)	0.5

Plus-minus values are means ± SD. The number of subjects are shown in parentheses. All values are age- or length-adjusted.

$^*P < 0.01$ for the comparison with the no LRI group.
$^{**}P < 0.05$ for the comparison with the no LRI group.

Reproduced from ref. 23, with permission.

Table 27.3   Mechanisms of virus-induced asthma.

Sensitization of rapidly adapting afferent vagus
   sensory fibres.

Damage to airway epithelium
   Loss of relaxing factor
   Inactivation of enkephalinase, substance-P
     degrading enzyme

β-adrenergic blockade

Production of virus-specific IgE antibody

Development of late asthmatic reactions to inhaled
   antigen

Enhanced leucocyte inflammatory function

appears that a given child's response to infection is determined not only by the infection but the pre-existing lung function.

Taussig et al.[25] also noted that lower levels of lung function predispose to wheezing with LRI, as opposed to the infection per se. The precise nature of this predisposition remains to be defined but may lie in airway geometry, airway–parenchymal interaction, or mucosal and smooth muscle response. Furthermore this pulmonary-structural predisposition may be enhanced by an exaggerated IgE response to viral infection,[26,27] resulting in more inflammation and severe wheezing with hospitalization. Since the majority of infants who develop wheezing with LRIs do not wheeze throughout life,[28] it is likely that pulmonary function abnormalities that favour wheezing with viral infections are modified with the growth and development of the lung. Long-term outcome then seems to be more closely linked to the persistence of ongoing airway damage or bronchospasm associated with the development of atopy and true clinical asthma.[18]

MECHANISMS OF VIRUS-INDUCED AIRWAY HYPERRESPONSIVENESS

A number of mechanisms have been identified to explain how viral respiratory infections enhance airway responsiveness or provoke an attack of asthma (Table 27.3). As each of these mechanisms is reviewed, it should become apparent that no single, unifying cause has yet to be established, but rather the virus-effects are multiple, interrelated and interactive.

The role of virus-specific IgE antibody responses

Welliver et al.[26] tested 79 children, all less than 12 months of age and with documented RSV infection, for the presence of IgE-specific antibody to the infecting virus (Fig. 27.1). The clinical patterns of illness were divided into four groups: (a) upper respiratory tract

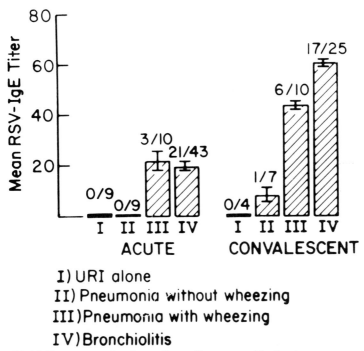

Fig. 27.1 The RSV-IgE response analysed according to illness group. The fractions represent the number of patients positive for RSV-IgE per number tested. Bars represent arithmetic mean for the RSV-IgE titre (± 1 SE). Group I had upper respiratory tract disease only, Group II pneumonia without wheezing, Group III pneumonia with wheezing, and Group IV bronchiolitis without pneumonia. The acute phase represents the first 7 days after the onset of illness, and the convalescent phase of the 14th through the 90th day after the onset of illness. Reproduced from ref. 26, with permission.

illness; (b) pneumonia without wheezing; (c) pneumonia and wheezing; and (d) wheezing (bronchiolitis). Nasal secretions from each patient were measured for IgE-specific antibody to RSV and histamine. When RSV-IgE antibody titres were compared with the patient's clinical illness, a striking and intriguing association appeared. IgE titres to RSV were highest in patients with evidence of airway obstruction, e.g. pneumonia/wheezing or bronchiolitis. Furthermore, patients with the highest RSV-IgE titres also had the lowest arterial pO_2 values. Similarly, parainfluenza virus (PV)-specific IgE responses were examined in individuals with upper respiratory illness alone or bronchiolitis by Welliver et al.[29] PV-specific IgE antibody were detected in eight of 12 with bronchiolitis but only one of 10 with upper respiratory disease alone. These studies indicate that respiratory viruses stimulate IgE-specific antibody responses and the degree to which this occurs is associated with the clinical manifestations of upper versus lower airway disease.

Generation of chemical mediators

A biological role for virus-specific IgE is strengthened by the presence of chemical mediators. The frequency and mean concentrations by which histamine was detected were greater in children with bronchiolitis (lower airway disease) than subjects not

Table 27.4 Histamine content of nasopharyngeal secretions following RSV
infection.

Illness group	No. with histamine/ No. tested (%)	Histamine content* (Mean ± SE)
Upper respiratory infection alone	1/2 (50)	1.1 ± 1.0
Pneumonia, no wheezing	2/10 (20)	0.6 ± 0.01
Bronchiolitis	27/37 (73)	2.8 ± 0.2

*Nanograms per milligram of protein in fluid.

Reproduced from ref. 26, with permission.

experiencing any wheezing (Table 27.4). Although these observations imply a role for
histamine in defining the type and severity of illness from RSV, the correlations were
weaker than those noted with IgE-specific antibody titres.

Leukotriene C_4 (LTC_4) was also measured in children with either bronchiolitis or
upper respiratory infection alone to RSV (Table 27.5).[30] LTC_4 was detected twice as
frequently in patients with bronchiolitis as those with upper airway disease alone;
furthermore, the concentration of LTC_4 was greater in those with bronchiolitis. Finally,
Skoner et al.[31] found elevated plasma histamine and prostaglandin metabolites in infants
with acute bronchiolitis (Table 27.6). A correlation was noted between plasma elevations of these mediators and disease severity. Since plasma measurements in a comparative control group indicated that the histamine and prostaglandin elevations were
not a mere reflection of general illness, a role for these mediators is suggested in the
clinical characteristics of bronchiolitis.

Virus-specific IgE concentrations predict future wheezing episodes

To further evaluate the significance of virus-specific IgE antibody, Welliver et al.[32]
prospectively monitored 38 infants for 48 months after an initial episode of bronchiolitis.
Only 20% of infants with undetectable titres of RSV IgE had subsequent episodes of
documented wheezing (Table 27.7). In contrast, 70% of those children with high RSV
IgE antibody titres experienced wheezing. To explain their observation, the authors

Table 27.5 LTC_4 release in nasopharyngeal secretions of infants and
children with RSV infection.

Diagnosis	No. with LTC_4/ No. tested (%)	Group mean LTC_4 concentration*
Upper respiratory infection alone	7/21 (33)	224 ± 114‡
Bronchiolitis	29/43 (67)†	1271 ± 239‡

*Picograms per 0.1 ml of fluid.
†$P < 0.025$.
‡$P < 0.02$.

Reproduced from ref. 30, with permission.

Table 27.6   Plasma histamine (pg/ml) and 13,14-dihydro-15-keto-PGF$_{2\alpha}$ (pg/ml) levels before and after initial therapy for acute bronchiolitis.

Mediator	Group I* (n = 9)	Group II (n = 14)	Group III (n = 12)	Group IV (n = 9)
Histamine	1923 ± 980	1035 ± 250†	9210 ± 5242	360 ± 125
PG metabolite	1033 ± 419‡	1613 ± 527‡	27 ± 7	68 ± 25

*Group I: acute bronchiolitis before therapy; Group II: acute bronchiolitis 15 min to 48 h after therapy; Group III: non-wheezing infants 6 months after bronchiolitis; Group IV: non-wheezing infants 18 months after bronchiolitis.

†$P < 0.05$ compared to 18-month value.
‡$P < 0.025$ compared to 6- and 18-month values.

Reproduced from ref. 31, with permission.

Table 27.7   Risk of subsequent wheezing after RSV bronchiolitis analysed by peak RSV-IgE titre in nasopharyngeal secretions.

RSV-IgE titre in secretions	Subjects with titre	Documented subsequent wheezing episode (No./%)	P*
Undetectable	15	3 (20)	—
1–6	13	6 (46)	<0.025
>6	10	7 (70)	<0.025

*Compared with undetectable.

Reproduced from ref. 32, with permission.

questioned whether RSV infection in early age identifies individuals with airways congenitally prone to obstruction. As a consequence, the investigators concluded that their 'results, which suggest that the number of wheezing episodes experienced after RSV bronchiolitis can be predicted on the basis of a genetically determined phenomenon (over production of IgE), are more consistent with the concept that the increased frequency of lower respiratory tract illnesses, airway hyperreactivity, and small airway dysfunction observed in children examined years after an episode of bronchiolitis are also genetically determined'.

The effect of viral respiratory infections on airway hyperresponsiveness and the development of late-phase asthmatic reactions

To evaluate the effects of respiratory infection on airway responsiveness, we experimentally infected subjects with rhinovirus and determined its action on a non-allergic stimulus of airway contraction, histamine, and an IgE-dependent activator, antigen.[33] The patients selected for study were evaluated on three separate occasions: at baseline, during acute infection, and recovery. Each study period was separated by approximately

4 weeks with the following determinations made at each testing. First, airway response to inhaled histamine was determined and provided an index of airway reactivity. In addition, both the *immediate* and *late-phase asthmatic responses* (LAR) to inhaled antigen were evaluated. Thus, we could determine the effect of a rhinovirus infection on non-specific airway responsiveness and compare this response to antigen. Airway responsiveness was determined by measuring the provocative dose of either histamine or antigen that was required to drop the forced expiratory volume in 1 s (FEV_1) by 20% (PD_{20}). These values were used as indices of bronchial reactivity and to determine virus effects.

Effect of rhinovirus infection on airway response to histamine and antigen

All 10 patients had a rhinovirus respiratory infection at time of study as ascertained by either virus recovery from nasal washings and/or a rise in hemagglutination titre, or both. During the acute rhinovirus respiratory infection, airway responsiveness to histamine significantly increased over baseline values (Fig. 27.2). Likewise, acute airway reactivity to inhaled antigen was increased. The change in airway responsiveness to histamine and antigen was similar, suggesting that the respiratory infection effects on responsiveness to antigen related to alterations in non-specific bronchial reactivity.

The airways' response to inhaled antigen is not necessarily limited to immediate bronchoconstriction. Many individuals experience bronchoconstriction and a recurrence of airway obstruction approximately 4–8 h after inhalation of antigen, the late-phase asthmatic response. Recognition that LARs follow antigen inhalation has been instrumental to better understanding of the pathogenesis, airway inflammation and bronchial hyperresponsiveness in asthma. For example, LARs are characterized by a number of important features:[34] diminished responsiveness to bronchodilator, increased airway reactivity, and the presence of bronchial inflammation. These particular features suggest that LARs resemble chronic asthma and are the component of an airway's response to inhaled antigen most likely to yield insight on the pathogenesis of asthma.

For these reasons, it was of interest to determine the effect of the viral respiratory illness on the late-phase asthmatic response to inhaled antigen. Prior to rhinovirus inoculation, only one of the 10 patients had an LAR to inhaled antigen (Fig. 27.3). However, during the acute respiratory infection, eight of 10 patients experienced late-phase airway obstruction. Furthermore, when evaluated during the recovery period (4 weeks after rhinovirus inoculation), five of the seven patients available for testing still had late asthmatic reactions to inhaled antigen. These observations indicate that rhinovirus respiratory infection not only increased airway responsiveness but also changed the pattern of the airway response to inhaled antigen.

The recovery pattern of airway responsiveness following the viral respiratory infection was also evaluated. Although increased airway responsiveness was still detected 4 weeks after rhinovirus inoculation, there was a trend towards recovery in both the reaction to inhaled histamine and the immediate response to antigen. However, as already discussed, the increased frequency of late-phase asthmatic reactions to antigen was still noted 4 weeks post-viral infection. These observations suggest that the viral respiratory infection has a greater, and possibly more lasting, effect on factors which participate in the development of LARs.

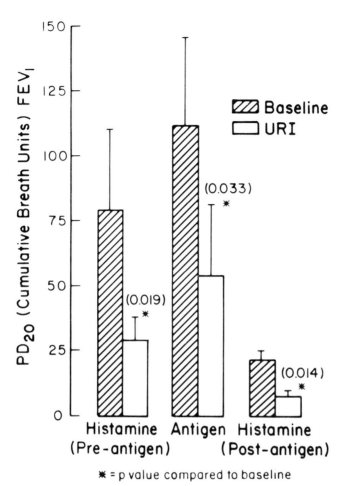

Fig. 27.2 The effect of an acute rhinovirus respiratory infection on airway reactivity to histamine and antigen along with reactivity to histamine following antigen challenge. Values are mean ± SEM, $n = 10$. Reproduced from ref. 33, with permission.

Possible mechanisms by which respiratory infections may influence the development of a late-phase asthmatic reaction

Virus-associated airway hyperresponsiveness is a multifactorial process involving a complex interplay of IgE-dependent reactions, epithelial damage, autonomic nervous system dysfunction, and enhanced inflammation.[35] In addition, individual patient features, such as inborn lung function and a family history of atopy, also contribute to the outcome in specific patients.[18]

To begin to unravel the mechanisms by which a respiratory viral infection increases the potential for late-phase asthma, it is helpful to examine those steps which determine the airway's response to inhaled antigen. From this analysis a number of sites emerge as being potentially susceptible to respiratory virus effects and eventually influence the development of late-phase asthma (Fig. 27.4). Of the identified influences, we have been

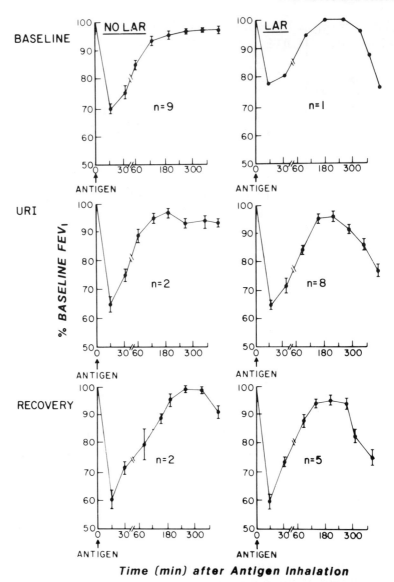

Fig. 27.3 The pattern of airway response to inhaled ragweed antigen in patients prior to, during and following an acute rhinovirus infection. Reproduced from ref. 33, with permission.

principally interested in factors that could cause, or accentuate, airway inflammation: mediator release and recruited inflammatory cells.

Effect of respiratory viruses on the inflammatory response and late-phase asthmatic responses

In IgE-mediated reactions, the tissue response, be it the skin, nose, or airway, is influenced by IgE sensitization of mast cells and basophils, release of bronchospastic

RELATIONSHIP OF RHINOVIRUS 16 RESPIRATORY
INFECTION TO LATE PHASE ASTHMA

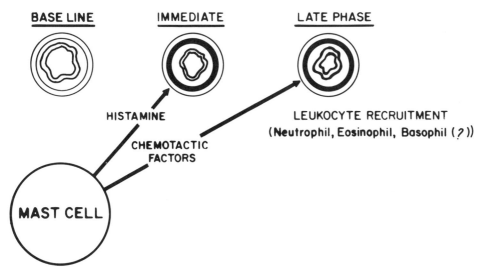

Fig. 27.4 Mechanisms by which rhinovirus infection promotes the development of late-phase asthma. During the 'baseline' period of the respiratory infection, airway reactivity is increased. Changes in mast cell mediator or the cells recruited to the airway may determine the likelihood of a late-phase reaction.

and inflammatory mediators from sensitized cells, and the response of the target organ, which, in asthma, is bronchial smooth muscle. Welliver et al.[26,27] have evidence that respiratory viruses stimulate the production of virus-specific IgE. However, there are no available data to suggest that the concentration of IgE antibody necessarily determines either the intensity or likelihood of a late reaction.[33,34]

To evaluate the effects of respiratory viruses on another facet of the immediate hypersensitivity response, mediator release, basophil histamine secretion was determined. For these studies, isolated human white cells were obtained, incubated *in vitro* with live respiratory virus, challenged with antigen and histamine release measured. We, and others, have found increased IgE-dependent basophil histamine release following an *in vitro* incubation with live respiratory viruses.[36,37] There is evidence that enhanced basophil histamine release occurs, in part, as interferon is produced during the virus–leucocyte incubation and then acts on sensitized basophils.[36,37] On the other hand, Chonmaitree et al.[38] incubated leucocytes from healthy, non-allergic donors with different strains of inactivated respiratory viruses and found that respiratory viruses could augment IgE-mediated histamine release *with* or *without* interferon present; they concluded that although interferon may play a role in virus-induced hypersensitivity reactions, other mechanisms were probably also involved.

In the studies that showed increased airway reactivity to histamine and the development of late-phase asthma during a rhinovirus infection,[33] basophil histamine release was also enhanced. Although this association does not indicate a 'cause-and-effect' relationship between enhanced leucocyte secretion and changes in airway reactivity and the development of an LAR, it does imply that the *in vivo* viral infection had effects upon human basophil function similar to that found with *in vitro* exposure to respiratory viruses.

Since the role of basophils in allergic disease and asthma is not fully established, it is difficult to ascertain the importance of *in vitro* and *in vivo* studies with basophils. None the less, recent investigations at Johns Hopkins Hospital may help clarify the contribution of basophils in allergic diseases. To evaluate nasal responses to inhaled antigen, Naclerio *et al.*[39] found that nasal histamine concentrations increased during both the immediate and late-phase nasal response to inhaled antigen. Prostaglandin D_2 (PGD_2) was also measured and found elevated only during the *acute*-phase reaction. Because histamine is found in *both* the mast cell and basophil whereas PGD_2 is limited to the mast cell, the rise in histamine during late phase nasal response was attributed to the basophil. Although the basophil has not been established as a participant in late-phase airway obstructive reaction, it is possible that the changes in basophil function during respiratory viral infections may be relevant to the development of a late asthmatic reaction.

Late-phase reactions also involve leucocyte recruitment. When Lett-Brown *et al.*[40] incubated leucocytes with a PV and then measured leucocyte chemotaxis to a C5 peptide component of complement or a leucocyte-derived chemotactic factor, only basophils demonstrated enhanced chemotaxis. Furthermore, if interferon was substituted for virus, basophil migration was likewise enhanced. Collectively, these observations are a further example that basophil function may be particularly susceptible to effects of respiratory viruses with an end result being the promotion of this cell's inflammatory potential and hence greater contribution to the allergic reaction.

Effect of respiratory viruses on polymorphonuclear leucocyte function

Since other cells, i.e. neutrophils and eosinophils, are also associated with airway inflammation and late-phase asthmatic reactions, we have begun to examine the effect of respiratory viruses on their function. Isolated neutrophils were incubated *in vitro* with influenza virus. Following a 30-min incubation, the cells were collected, activated by a chemotactic peptide, and the generation of superoxide measured. Superoxide generation was increased with neutrophils that had been incubated with influenza virus.[41] Since superoxide is a toxic substance for pulmonary tissue and may cause bronchial injury,[42] it is possible that respiratory virus enhancement of the inflammatory function of leucocytes promotes airway injury and the likelihood of obstruction.

To integrate these findings into understanding the development of late-phase asthma, we propose the following series of events. During initiation of the allergic response in the airway, inflammatory cells (neutrophils, eosinophils, and possibly basophils) are recruited to the airway and, when activated, release inflammatory mediators. The amount of inflammatory mediators released will determine the intensity of the response and possibly whether a late-phase reaction occurs. If this same allergic reaction occurs during a viral respiratory infection, leucocytes recruited to the airway are 'primed' and, when activated, produce a greater inflammatory response. Thus, because the cells recruited to the lung during the respiratory illness are activated leucocytes, the likelihood for airway injury and the development of a late asthmatic reaction increases (Fig. 27.4).

Other mechanisms by which viral respiratory infections can increase airway reactivity and possibly late-phase asthma

Alterations in autonomic nervous system function

Airway smooth muscle function is regulated by the autonomic nervous system. β-adrenergic receptors on the bronchial smooth muscle are activated by catecholamines and reduce bronchial smooth muscle tone. In addition, β-adrenergic receptors on leucocytes modulate their inflammatory response and mediator release. Nearly three decades ago, Szentivanyi[43] proposed that diminished β-adrenergic function was found in asthma and this autonomic nervous system imbalance contributed to the bronchial hyperresponsiveness and bronchoconstriction in asthma. He further suggested that viral infections exacerbate 'β-blockade' to further increase the underlying airway abnormalities in asthmas.

The existence of diminished β-adrenergic function has been proposed to explain airway hyperresponsiveness and the lack of complete bronchodilation with the administration of catecholamines in patients with asthma. Although evidence for 'β-blockade' exists in asthma, the precise role of altered autonomic nervous system function has yet to be fully established.

We have used isolated human leucocytes as an *in vitro* model to evaluate β-adrenergic function in asthma. In this model, β-adrenergic suppression of lysosomal enzyme release was used as the test response. Leucocytes isolated from patients during viral respiratory infection,[44] or following incubation with respiratory viruses,[45] had diminished β-adrenergic function. These observations indicated that respiratory viruses can alter β-adrenergic function of circulating human leucocytes. Even though airway smooth muscle β-adrenergic function may not be altered by respiratory viruses, the virus-associated autonomic nervous system dysfunction can affect regulation of leucocyte-dependent inflammation. Since catecholamines normally inhibit leucocyte inflammatory responses, virus alteration of β-adrenergic function may increase cellular secretion of inflammatory mediators. The consequence of virus-associated changes in leucocyte regulatory responses could translate to increased tissue inflammation.

Viral upper respiratory infections also enhance airway cholinergic sensitivity. In a study of 16 non-asthmatic patients, Empey *et al.*[46] documented significantly increased airway sensitivity to inhaled histamine. Since the enhanced response to inhaled histamine was blocked by pretreatment with atropine, the authors speculated that airway injury by respiratory viruses sensitized rapidly adapting sensory fibres of the vagus nerve to promote reflex bronchospasm. These observations indicate that respiratory viruses may not have to directly change the function of airway smooth muscle to promote bronchial hyperreactivity but can accomplish this alteration by 'indirect' methods.[47]

To localize and characterize the effect of a respiratory virus on cholinergic function further, Fryer and co-workers[48] evaluated parainfluenza action on cholinergic receptor binding. In membrane preparations from guinea-pig lung, PV incubation decreased cholinergic binding. Although not conclusive, these observations suggest that the virus effect is on the M_2-receptor of the lung. Because 'M_2-receptors modulate vagally induced bronchoconstriction in the lungs, the investigators[48] postulate that the virus-induced decrease in agonist affinity for M_2-receptors is responsible for the increase in vagally mediated bronchoconstriction observed in animals and man with viral respiratory infections'.

Damage to airway epithelium

Damage to airway epithelium can also contribute to airway hyperreactivity.[49] In addition to serving as a protective barrier to the diffusion of antigens and noxious substances, bronchial epithelium actively produces substances that modulate airway responsivity and smooth muscle tone.[50] Since some respiratory viruses directly injure airway epithelium, the consequences of this damage have been examined.

In studies with parainfluenza 3-infected guinea-pigs, Saban et al.[51] detected enhanced isolated airway contractility to the neuropeptide substance P. In addition, Jacoby et al.[52] found that isolated ferret trachea, which had been incubated with influenza virus, had epithelial desquamation, increased contractility to substance P, and reduced activity of enkephalinase, an epithelial-derived enzyme which degrades substance P. Based upon these findings, Jacoby et al.[52] proposed that the influenza virus infection altered enkephalinase activity such that the substance P-induced contraction was enhanced.

Moreover, damage to epithelium may lead to the loss of epithelium-derived relaxing factor(s).[53] These factor(s) include inhibitory cyclooxygenase metabolites of arachidonic acid[54] which may act by reducing cholinergic neurotransmitter release.[55] In this fashion, virus-associated damage to airway epithelium would further alter control of airway calibre and reactivity without directly affecting smooth-muscle physiology.

The role of neuropeptides in airway inflammation has been further elucidated by McDonald[56] who demonstrated that naturally occurring viral infections caused rat tracheas to become more susceptible to neurogenic inflammation which arose from direct stimulation of vagal sensory nerves or by injection of capsaicin or substance P. Interestingly, the enhanced susceptibility to inflammation occurred even in the absence of virus-induced changes in the airway such as increased vascular permeability, adherence of neutrophils to blood vessel walls or influx of neutrophils into tracheal mucosa. Moreover, the increased susceptibility to neurogenic inflammation outlasted the brief pathologic changes observed with acute infection. Collectively, the described changes in airway epithelium could result in increased airway responsiveness. Evidence that increased airway reactivity enhances the likelihood for late asthma reactions has yet to be established.

Effects on the cellular immune response

To appreciate the effects of a viral respiratory infection on airway function more fully, it is essential to consider the complex interaction of respiratory viruses with the cellular immune system. To initiate an immune response, viruses must first attach to a target cell. Evidence now indicates that this attachment occurs through specific cell surface receptors.[57] Following cellular processing, which may involve intracellular alteration of the virus, viral antigen(s) may be expressed on the surface of the target cell in conjunction with proteins of the HLA system. The newly expressed viral antigen–HLA complex is then recognized by T-lymphocytes and an immune response is triggered. Before this specific binding occurs, however, T-lymphocytes bind non-specifically to

CD4⁺ T–Lymphocyte

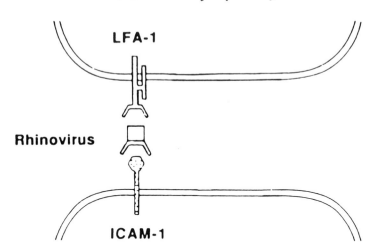

Fig. 27.5 Rhinovirus blocking adhesion of antigen-presenting cell to T-lymphocyte. Reproduced from ref. 58, with permission.

other cells by means of surface adhesion molecules.[58] Following this non-specific adhesion, antigen-specific recognition and T-cell activation occurs.

One non-specific T-cell adhesion molecule, lymphocyte function-associated antigen (LFA)-1, is found on almost all leucocytes.[59] During cell adhesion, LFA-1, or other T-cell adhesion molecules, binds to a ligand on the target cell. One such ligand for LFA-1 is intercellular adhesion molecule (ICAM)-1, a glycoprotein expressed on the surface of endothelial cells, fibroblasts, lymphocytes and monocytes.[60]

Interestingly, the major human rhinovirus receptor has recently been identified to be ICAM-1.[61] Thus, an early step in rhinovirus infection would involve virus attachment to ICAM-1 potentially blocking adhesion of the antigen-presenting cells to the T-lymphocyte (Fig. 27.5). Significantly, the surface expression of ICAM-1 is increased by cytokines, such as γ-interferon and tumour necrosis factor, which may be released by activated T-cells. Therefore, it has been suggested that an initial immune, or inflammatory, response to rhinovirus infection may actually enhance the spread of infection by generating factors to increase the number of ICAM-1 receptors for rhinovirus.[62] Although preliminary, these findings promise to have important implications for future study and understanding of the pathogenesis of virus-induced airway hyper-responsivity.

Viral infections may alter the regulation of IgE synthesis by modifying the combined actions of T-helper and T-suppressor lymphocytes.[63] To evaluate the effect of viral infection on IgE synthesis, Lin *et al.*[64] studied house-dust allergic children following a community-acquired influenza A illness. Twelve of their study patients experienced attacks of asthma in association with the influenza illness. When compared to subjects who did not wheeze during the influenza infection, those patients with increased asthma symptoms had alterations in their T-helper/T-suppressor lymphocyte ratio and increases in specific house-dust antibody. Thus, Lin *et al.*[64] postulated that virus infection-associated changes in the T-helper/T-suppressor cell ratio may result in an increased lymphoproliferative response to antigen which in turn can contribute to increased symptoms of asthma.

SUMMARY

The mechanisms involved in the development of airway hyperresponsiveness, airway obstruction, and recurrent wheezing with viral respiratory infections have yet to be fully appreciated. None the less, current evidence indicates that viruses, or products of virus-infected cells, influence the inflammatory property and potential of many cells. Precisely how these virus-effects translate into increased airway injury, responsiveness, and obstruction will require further work. As the mechanisms of these interactions are established, so will improved understanding of asthma pathogenesis and treatment.

ACKNOWLEDGEMENTS

Support for this chapter has come from grants from NIH HL 44098, AI-26609, K08-01828 and General Clinical Research Grant RR-03186.

REFERENCES

1. McIntosh K, Ellis EF, Hoffman LS, Lybass TG, Eller JJ, Fulginiti VA: The association of viral and bacterial respiratory infections with exacerbations of wheezing in young asthmatic children. *J Pediatr* (1973) **83**: 578–590.
2. Minor TE, Dick EC, DeMeo AN, Ouellette JJ, Cohen M, Reed CE: Viruses as precipitants of asthmatic attacks in children. *JAMA* (1974) **227**: 292–298.
3. Minor TE, Dick EC, Baker JW, Ouellette JJ, Cohen M, Reed CE: Rhinovirus and influenza A infections as precipitants of asthma. *Am Rev Respir Dis* (1976) **113**: 149–153.
4. Hudgel DW, Lanston E Jr, Selner JC, McIntosh K: Viral and bacterial infections in adults with chronic asthma. *Am Rev Respir Dis* (1979) **120**: 393–397.
5. Halperin SA, Eggleston PA, Hendley JO, Suratt PM, Gröschel DHM, Gwaltney JM Jr: Pathogenesis of lower respiratory tract symptoms in experimental rhinovirus infection. *Am Rev Respir Des* (1983) **128**: 806–810.
6. Halperin SA, Eggleston PA, Beasley P, *et al.*: Exacerbations of asthma in adults during experimental rhinovirus infection. *Am Rev Respir Dis* (1985) **132**: 976–980.
7. Berman SZ, Mathison DA, Stevenson DD, Tan EM, Vaughan JH: Transtracheal aspiration studies in asthmatic patients in relapse with 'infective' asthma and in subjects without respiratory disease. *J Allergy Clin Immunol* (1975) **56**: 206–214.
8. Slavin RG, Cannon RF, Friedman WH, Palitang E, Sundaram M: Sinusitis and bronchial asthma. *J Allergy Clin Immunol* (1980) **66**: 250–257.

9. Rachelefsky GS, Katz RM, Siegel SC: Chronic sinus disease associated with reactive airway disease in children. *Pediatr* (1984) **73**: 526–529.

10. Tager IB: Epidemiology of respiratory infections in the development of airway hyperreactivity. *Sem Respir Med* (1990) **11**: 297–305.

11. Samet JM, Tager IB, Speizer FE: The relationship between respiratory illness in childhood and chronic air-flow obstruction in adulthood. *Am Rev Respir Dis* (1983) **127**: 508–523.

12. Eisen AH, Bacal HL: The relationship of acute bronchiolitis to bronchial asthma — a 4-to-14 year follow-up. *Pediatr* (1963) **31**: 859–861.

13. Rooney JC, Williams HE: The relationship between proven viral bronchiolitis and subsequent wheezing. *J Pediatr* (1971) **79**: 744–747.

14. McConnochie KM, Roghmann KJ: Bronchiolitis as a possible cause of wheezing in childhood. *Pediatr* (1984) **74**: 1–10.

15. Sims DG, Downham MAPS, Gardner PS: Study of 8-year-old children with a history of respiratory syncytial virus bronchiolitis in infancy. *Br Med J* (1978) **1**: 11–14.

16. Pullan CR, Hey EN: Wheezing, asthma, and pulmonary dysfunction 10 years after infection with respiratory syncytial virus in infancy. *Br Med J* (1982) **284**: 1665–1669.

17. Weiss ST, Tager IB, Munoz A, Speizer FE: The relationship of respiratory infections in early childhood to the occurrence of increased levels of bronchial responsiveness and atopy. *Am Rev Respir Dis* (1985) **131**: 573–578.

18. Morgan WJ: Viral respiratory infection in infancy: Provocation or propagation? *Sem Respir Med* (1990) **11**: 306–313.

19. Tepper RS: Airway reactivity in infants: A positive response to methacholine and metaproterenol. *J Appl Physiol* (1987) **62**: 1155–1159.

20. Geller DE, Morgan WJ, Cota K: Airway response to cold, dry air in normal infants. *Pediatr Pulmonol* (1988) **4**: 90–97.

21. LeSouef PN, Geelhoed GC, Turner DJ, Morgan SEG, Landau LI: Response of normal infants to inhaled histamine. *Am Rev Respir Dis* (1989) **139**: 62–66.

22. Wright AL, Taussig LM, Ray CG, Harrison HR, Holberg CJ, The Group Health Medical Associates: The Tucson children's respiratory study. II. Lower respiratory tract illness in the first year of life. *Am J Epidemiol* (1989) **129**: 1232–1246.

23. Martinez FD, Morgan WJ, Wright AL, Holberg CJ, Taussig LM, Group health Medical Associates Personnel: Diminished lung function as a predisposing factor for wheezing respiratory illnesses in infants. *N Engl J Med* (1988) **319**: 1112–1117.

24. Morris MJ, Lane DJ: Tidal expiratory flow patterns in air-flow obstruction. *Thorax* (1981) **36**: 135–142.

25. Taussig LM, Harris TR, Lebowitz MD: Lung function in infants and young children: Functional residual capacity, tidal volume, and respiratory rate. *Am Rev Respir Dis* (1977) **116**: 233–239.

26. Welliver RC, Wong DT, Sun M, Middleton E Jr, Vaughan RS, Ogra PL: The development of respiratory syncytial virus specific IgE and the release of histamine in nasopharyngeal secretions after infection. *N Engl J Med* (1981) **305**: 841–846.

27. Welliver RC, Wong DT, Middleton E Jr, Sun M, McCarthy RN, Ogra PL: Role of parainfluenza virus-specific IgE in pathogenesis of croup and wheezing subsequent to infection. *J Pediatr* (1982) **101**: 889–896.

28. Voter KZ, Henry MM, Stewart PW, Henderson FW: Lower respiratory illness in early childhood and lung function and bronchial reactivity in adolescent males. *Am Rev Respir Dis* (1988) **137**: 302–307.

29. Welliver RC, Wong DT, Sun M, McCarthy N: Parainfluenza virus bronchiolitis. Epidemiology and pathogenesis. *AJDC* (1986) **140**: 34–40.

30. Volovitz B, Welliver RC, DeCastro G, Krystofik DA, Ogra PL: The release of leukotriene in the respiratory tract during infection with respiratory syncytial virus: Role in obstructive airway disease. *Pediatr Res* (1988) **24**: 504–507.

31. Skoner DP, Fireman P, Caliguiri L, Davis H: Plasma elevations of histamine and prostaglandin metabolite in acute bronchiolitis. Am Rev Respir Dis (1990) **142**: 359–364.

32. Welliver RC, Sun M, Rinaldo D, Ogra PL: Predictive value of respiratory syncytial virus-specific IgE response for recurrent wheezing following bronchiolitis. *J Pediatr* (1986) **109**: 776–780.

33. Lemanske RF Jr, Dick EC, Swenson CA, Vrtis RF, Busse WW: Rhinovirus upper respiratory infection increases airway reactivity in late asthmatic reactions. *J Clin Invest* (1989) **83**: 1–10.

34. Lemanske RF Jr, Kaliner MA: Late-phase allergic reactions. In Middleton E Jr, Reed CE, Ellis EF, Adkinson NF Jr, Yuninger JW (eds) *Allergy: Principles and Practice*. St Louis, MO, C V Mosby Co., 1988, pp 224–246.

35. Frick WE, Busse WW: Respiratory infections: their role in airway responsiveness and pathogenesis of asthma. *Clin Chest Med* (1988) **9**: 539–549.

36. Ida S, Hooks JJ, Siraganian RP, Notkens AL: Enhancement of IgE-mediated histamine release from human basophil by viruses: Role of interferon. *J Exp Med* (1979) **145**: 892–896.

37. Busse WW, Swenson CA, Borden EC, Treuhauft MW, Dick EC: The effect of influenza A virus on leukocyte histamine release. *J Allergy Clin Immunol* (1983) **71**: 382–388.

38. Chonmaitree T, Lett-Brown MA, Tsong Y, Goldman AS, Baron S: Role of interferon in leukocyte histamine release caused by common respiratory viruses. *J Inf Dis* (1988) **157**: 127–132.

39. Naclerio RM, Proud D, Togias AG, *et al.*: Inflammatory mediators in late antigen-induced rhinitis. *N Engl J Med* (1985) **313**: 65–70.

40. Lett-Brown MA, Aelvoet M, Hooks JJ, Georgiades JA, Thueson DO, Grant JA: Enhancement of basophil chemotaxis *in vitro* by virus-induced interferon. *J Clin Invest* (1981) **67**: 547–552.

41. Busse WW, Vrtis RF, Steiner R, Dick EC: *In vitro* incubation with influenza virus primes human polymorphonuclear leukocyte generation of superoxide. *Am J Respir Cell Mol Bio* (1991) **4**: 347–354.

42. Cross CE, Halliwell B, Borish ET, *et al.*: Oxygen radicals and human disease. *Ann Intern Med* (1987) **107**: 526–545.

43. Szentivanyi A: The beta-adrenergic theory of atopic abnormality in asthma. *J Allergy* (1968) **42**: 203–223.

44. Busse WW: Decreased granulocyte response to isoproterenol in asthma during upper respiratory infections. *Am Rev Respir Dis* (1977) **115**: 783–791.

45. Busse WW, Anderson CL, Dick EC, Warshauer D: Reduced granulocyte response to isoproterenol, histamine, prostaglandin E, after *in vitro* incubation with rhinovirus 16. *Am Rev Respir Dis* (1980) **122**: 641–646.

46. Empey DW, Laitinen LA, Jacobs L, Gold WM, Nadel JA: Mechanisms of bronchial hyperreactivity in normal subjects after upper respiratory tract infection. *Am Rev Respir Dis* (1976) **133**: 131–139.

47. deJongste JC, Kerrebijn, KF: Is bronchial hyperresponsiveness in humans a smooth muscle abnormality? *Prog Clin Biol Res* (1988) **263**: 255–265.

48. Fryer AD, El-Fakahany EE, Jacoby DB: Parainfluenza virus type 1 reduces the affinity of agonists for muscarinic receptors in guinea-pig lung and heart. *Eur J Pharmacol* (1990) **181**: 51–58.

49. Laitinen LA, Heino M, Laitinen A, Kava T, Haahtela T: Damage of the airway epithelium and bronchial reactivity in patients with asthma. *Am Rev Respir Dis* (1985) **131**: 599–606.

50. Nadel JA: Role of airway epithelial cells in the defense of airways. *Prog Clin Biol Res* (1988) **263**: 331–339.

51. Saban R, Dick EC, Fishleder RJ, Buckner CK: Enhancement by parainfluenza 3 infection of contractile responses to substance P and capsaicin in airway smooth muscle from the guinea pig. *Am Rev Respir Dis* (1987) **136**: 586–591.

52. Jacoby DB, Tamaoki J, Bornson BD, Nadel JA: Influenza infection causes airway hyperresponsiveness by decreasing enkephalinase. *J Apply Physiol* (1988) **64**: 2653–2658.

53. Vanhoutte PM: Epithelium-derived relaxing factor(s) and bronchial reactivity. *J Allergy Clin Immunol* (1989) **83**: 855–861.

54. Butler GB, Adler KB, Evans JN, Morgan DW, Szarek JL: Modulation of rabbit airway smooth muscle response by respiratory epithelium. *Am Rev Respir Dis* (1987) **135**: 1099–1104.

55. Barnett K, Jacoby DB, Nadel JA, Lazarus SC: The effects of epithelial cell supernatant on contraction of isolated canine tracheal smooth muscle. *Am Rev Respir Dis* (1988) **138**: 780–783.
56. McDonald DM: Respiratory tract infections increase susceptibility to neurogenic inflammation in the rat trachea. *Am Rev Respir Dis* (1988) **137**: 1432–1440.
57. White JM, Littman DR: Viral receptors of the immunoglobulin superfamily cell. *Cell* (1988) **56**: 725–728.
58. Bierer BE, Burakoff SJ: T cell adhesion molecules. *FASEB J* (1988) **2**: 2584–2590.
59. Krensky AM, Sanchez-Madrid F, Robbins E, Nagy JA, Springer TA, Burakoff SJ: The functional significance, distribution, and structure of LFA-1, LFA-2, and LFA-3: cell surface antigens associated with CTL-target interactions. *J Immunol* (1983) **131**: 611–616.
60. Makgoba MW, Sanders ME, Luce GEG, *et al.*: ICAM-1 a ligand for LFA-1 dependent adhesion of B, T and myeloid cells. *Nature (Lond.)* (1988) **331**: 86–88.
61. Greve JM, Davis G, Meyer AM, *et al.*: The major human rhinovirus receptor is ICAM-1. *Cell* (1989) **56**: 839–847.
62. Staunton DE, Merluzzi VJ, Rothlein R, Barton R, Marlin SC, Springer TA: A cell adhesion molecule, ICAM-1, is the major surface receptor for rhinoviruses. *Cell* (1989) **56**: 849–853.
63. Roitt IM, Brostoff J, Male DK: *Immunology*, 2nd edn. London, Gower, 1989, pp 19.3–19.6.
64. Lin CY, Kuo YC, Liu WT, Lin CC: Immunomodulation of influenza virus infection in the precipitating asthma attack. *Chest* (1988) **93**: 1234–1238.

Asthma Provoked by Exercise, Hyperventilation, and the Inhalation of Non-isotonic Aerosols

SANDRA D. ANDERSON

INTRODUCTION

Exercise-induced asthma (EIA) is the name used to describe the transitory increase in airway resistance which follows vigorous exercise in most patients with asthma. In addition to increasing airway resistance, exercise causes transient hyperinflation and arterial hypoxaemia.[1] It is the increase in ventilation rate, rather than exercise itself, that is the stimulus for provoking an attack of asthma.[2] For this reason voluntary isocapnic hyperventilation is often used instead of exercise to measure bronchial responsiveness to hyperpnoea and the asthma provoked by it is called hyperventilation-induced asthma (HIA). The similarity between the changes in lung function provoked by exercise and isocapnic hyperventilation has led to the suggestion that the stimulus, mechanism, and pathway by which these challenges provoke an attack of asthma are probably the same. However there are some differences in relation to the effect of drugs, particularly when air of subfreezing temperature is inhaled. Further there are differences between isocapnic hyperventilation and exercise in relation to the refractory period and the cardiovascular, metabolic and hormonal changes, all of which have the potential to modify responses during and possibly even after challenge.

The stimulus by which hyperpnoea induces an attack of asthma is the loss of water from the respiratory mucosa.[3,4] Evaporative water loss is thought to cause the airways to narrow when the increase in the concentration of ions leads to an increase in osmolarity of the airway surface liquid (ASL) of the respiratory tract,[5] often referred to as the periciliary fluid. Unfortunately there have been no direct measurements showing an increase in osmolarity of the ASL of the lower airways after exercise but hyperosmolar changes do occur in the nose in response to hyperpnoea,[6] and at rest when the upper

ASTHMA: BASIC MECHANISMS AND CLINICAL MANAGEMENT (2nd Edn)
ISBN 0-12-079026-2

airways are bypassed as occurs in laryngectomized subjects.[7] Studies that have compared the responses to exercise and hyperventilation with the inhalation of hyperosmolar aerosols have shown no inconsistencies with this hypothesis and have confirmed that hyperosmolarity is a potent stimulus for provoking airway narrowing in asthmatics.[8-13] These observations followed on the study of Allegra and Bianco[14] which showed that inhaling an aerosol of distilled water could also provoke an attack of asthma. This is often referred to as 'fog-induced' asthma. These observations have led to the use of non-isotonic aerosols to increase or decrease the osmolarity of the ASL and thus induce acute narrowing of the airways.[15,16]

It is estimated that the volume of fluid lining the large airways is small and less than 1 ml in the first 10 generations.[5,17] The osmolarity is approximately 359 mosmoles and the major ions contributing to this are chloride and sodium.[18] The small volume of the ASL creates the potential for a rapid change in its osmolarity. Only microlitres (equivalent to milligrams) of water need to be lost by evaporation and only microlitres of non-isotonic fluid need to be deposited on the ASL to cause a rapid and significant change in ion concentration.

Exercise, hyperventilation, and the inhalation of non-isotonic aerosols are thought to cause the release of chemical mediators from cells in the airway mucosa. The release of chemotactic factors suggests that cell activation is also a consequence of these challenges.[19-22] The release of endogenous mediators and chemotactic factors resembles the events that occur in response to inhaling naturally occurring aeroallergens. Thus these challenges are now considered as useful for diagnosing asthma in the pulmonary function laboratory. The airway response to all these challenges is prevented by the acute administration of β_2-adrenoceptor agonists, sodium cromoglycate and nedocromil sodium,[1,23,24] and modified by the chronic administration of aerosol steroids.[25-27] A refractory period has been observed in many patients following these challenges and this is prevented by pretreatment with indomethacin.[28-30] For these reasons these challenges are useful for identifying and for assessing the benefits, or otherwise, of asthma treatment.

The recognition that an attack of asthma can be provoked by a change in the osmolarity in the respiratory tract has advanced our understanding of non-immunologically mediated factors that can provoke an attack of asthma. It has also drawn to our attention the importance of maintaining a normal balance of water in the respiratory tract. This is particularly important as many events encountered in daily life have the potential to change the osmolarity of the airways. For example exercise, accidental aspiration of non-isotonic fluid whilst swimming or diving, infection, smoke, and inhalation of aerosol particles of therapeutic and non-therapeutic substances may all lead to an alteration in airway osmolarity.

RESPIRATORY WATER LOSS AND CONDITIONING OF THE INSPIRED AIR

Under most ambient conditions the air inspired is cooler and drier than alveolar air and it must be heated and humidified as it enters the body. At rest, air is conditioned as it passes over the nasal mucosa and is almost fully conditioned by the time it reaches the pharynx. The nasal mucosa has a surface area of around 160 cm^2 and acts not only to give heat and water vapour to the inspired air, but, because it cools during inspiration, it conserves heat and water during expiration.[31] As the rate of ventilation increases during exercise, the increase in inspiratory resistance causes a switch from nasal to mouth breathing. Therefore the burden to heat and humidify the inspired air is transferred to the intrathoracic airways.

Direct measurements of temperature flux occurring during hyperpnoea in human airways have demonstrated that the number of generations of airways required to condition the inspired air fully will vary depending upon the temperature and the humidity of the inspired air, and on the rate of ventilation.[32,33] Furthermore, these and other studies have demonstrated that the number of generations involved in conditioning inspired air increases with time. This implies that, during hyperpnoea, the rate of return of water to the respiratory mucosa is not sufficient to provide continuous humidification from the same generations of airways. This concept can be more easily understood when one considers the need to humidify air, even at low ventilations, when the upper airways are bypassed during mechanical ventilation.[34]

The amount of water required to humidify the inspired air will depend on its water content and the rate of ventilation. When dry air between 23 and 42°C is inhaled, the net loss of water during exercise[35,36] and isocapnic hyperventilation[8,37] is between 29 and 35 mg of H_2O per litre of air. A considerable proportion of this water will be provided by the intrathoracic airways which will be cooled as a result of the latent heat of vaporization of water. Because of this cooling process, most of the water will be returned to the mucosa on expiration and the net loss of water from the airways below the pharynx is small. It has been estimated to be only between 1 and 7 μl (mg) of water per litre during moderate exercise.[17,38] If the loss of water is accumulated over 1 min during exercise while ventilating at 80 litre/min, a loss of 80–560 μl of water loss would result. Considering even these small volumes in relation to available water (Table 28.1), it can easily be appreciated that a transient alteration in osmolarity could occur if replacement is not instantaneous.[17]

Changing the temperature of the inspired air has the potential to change the site of the osmotic stimulus. When the air is cool, and therefore dry, more generations of airways will need to be recruited in order to heat and humidify the air completely. In some asthmatic subjects there is an increase in severity of the airway response after exercise breathing cold air.[39] This may be due to a greater number of airways being recruited and made hyperosmolar by evaporative water loss breathing cold air compared with the number of recruited breathing dry air of temperate conditions. The fact that inspiring cold air does not enhance the airway response[37,40] in all subjects may reflect a limitation in the number of airways that can become hyperosmolar. Beyond the 14th generation it is unlikely that the osmolarity of the ASL changes as there is enough water available to humidify the air fully before it reaches the alveoli. Because of the substantial amount of water available in the small airways, there is no need for water to be replaced rapidly in the large airways. The potential for the osmolarity to increase in the large airways as a consequence is, however, of great physiological significance to the patient with asthma.

Several years ago there was some debate as to whether cooling of the airways or hyperosmolarity of the periciliary fluid was the primary stimulus to asthma provoked by hyperpnoea.[17,35,40,41] The results of recent studies now suggest that airway cooling is an inhibitory rather than excitatory stimulus.[9,42–44] This may account for the observation that inhaling hot dry air during exercise or hyperventilation is a potent stimulus to

Table 28.1 Surface area and volume of periciliary fluid available in the first 17 generations of human airways.

Airway generation No.	Surface area (cm²)	Periciliary fluid volume (μl) at depth of		Cumulative surface area (cm²)	Cumulative volume (μl) of periciliary fluid at a depth of	
		5 μm	10 μm		5 μm	10 μm
0	68	34	68	68	34	68
1	37	18	37	105	52	105
2	21	10	21	124	63	126
3	9	4	9	135	67	135
4	29	15	29	164	82	164
5	37	18	37	201	100	201
6	51	25	51	252	126	252
7	70	35	70	322	160	322
8	95	47	95	417	208	417
9	135	67	135	552	276	552
10	190	95	190	742	371	742
11	275	137	275	1015	507	1015
12	397	198	397	1412	706	1412
13	584	292	584	1996	998	1996
14	870	435	870	2866	1433	2866
15	1312	656	1312	4178	2089	4178
16	1905	950	1901	6183	3091	6183
17	3100	1550	3100	9283	4641	9283

Reproduced from ref. 17. The depth of the periciliary fluid (sol layer) has been taken to be uniform at 5 and 10 μm.

airway narrowing.[35,37,39] The effect of heating the inspired air may be to concentrate the osmotic stimulus in the larger airways.

Both duration and intensity of exercise are important determinants of the severity of the airway response[1] and the reason for this is likely to relate to the number of airways involved in the process of conditioning air.

ROLE OF THE BRONCHIAL CIRCULATION

Although it is now generally acknowledged that airway cooling, *per se*, is not the mechanism whereby hyperpnoea provokes asthma, it has been suggested that rapid rewarming of the airways may be important.[45] A hypothesis put forward recently suggests that 'rapid expansion of the blood volume in perivascular plexi may be an important cause of the airway narrowing after exercise and isocapnic hyperventilation'.[46] It is proposed that the bronchial circulation constricts in response to cooling of the airways during exercise, and that, on cessation of exercise, there is a reactive hyperaemia of the circulation and oedema within the airway wall.

There is no direct evidence in man to show that the bronchial circulation is reduced with exercise and studies in man at rest[47] and in animals show an increase in blood flow in response to inhaling dry air.[48,49]

The concept of vasoconstriction and a compromised bronchial circulation during exercise is of interest in that it is this circulation that provides the water to the airways. If this circulation is decreased rather than increased with exercise, it would allow a change in osmolarity to occur more rapidly and it would reduce the rate of clearance of released mediators. Further, oedema may occur as a response to an increase in osmolarity of the submocosa if dehydration was severe.

The concept of rapid expansion of this circulation accounting for the airway narrowing is difficult to justify on the basis of the responses to drugs such as sodium cromoglycate and nedocromil sodium, and the rapid reversal of EIA and HIA by the administration of β_2-agonists.[1] None of these drugs has profound effects on vascular smooth muscle. Further, EIA and HIA may occur when no abnormal cooling of the airways has occurred[35,50] or during exercise before rewarming takes place.[17,50,51] The inability of this hypothesis to account for many of the established facts about EIA and HIA has led to a vigorous debate on the topic.[52,53] It seems unlikely that vasoconstriction followed by reactive hyperemia could account for the airway narrowing observed with inhaling non-isotonic aerosols as the bronchial circulation is not affected by this challenge.[54]

These arguments do not detract from the importance of this circulation in the bronchial hyperresponsiveness observed in asthma, particularly as oedema of the airway wall can serve to amplify the airway narrowing produced by contraction of bronchial smooth muscle.[55] Further, this circulation is important for maintaining a steady osmotic environment and the balance of water within the airways[56] and it is likely to be the major source of ASL under conditions of thermal stress. Normally there would be a number of sources for replenishment of the ASL. For example, some water will be returned to the larger airways during expiration as warm humid air passes over the cooled mucosal surface. Other possible sources include the submocosal glands and the mucociliary escalator. Taking into account the length of the respiratory tract, considerable time would be required to replace the ASL from the mucociliary escalator as it moves at about 5 mm/min. The depth, and amount, of ASL is most likely controlled locally by the passage of water across the epithelial cells and through paracellular channels in response to the movement of sodium and chloride ions.[57] Because the volume of fluid moving up the mucociliary escalator is large, the epithelial cells are thought to absorb rather than secrete water by the movement of ions.[58,59] As sodium ions move from the lumen into the epithelial cells, chloride ions move passively and with these, water. Although water can move into the airway lumen by the active transport of chloride across the epithelium, there is some debate as to whether an abnormally high chloride ion concentration in the periciliary fluids is of itself a stimulus for water to cross the epithelial cells into the airway lumen. It is likely, under the conditions of continued osmotic stress, that adaptive processes will occur to improve water return to the mucosa and to the airway lumen.

GENERATION AND DEPOSITION OF NON-ISOTONIC AEROSOLS IN THE RESPIRATORY TRACT

Distilled water and 3.6–4.5% saline have been the most common non-isotonic solutions used for challenging patients with asthma.[11,14,15,24] Because of their high output (66–

100 μl/litre) of aerosol, ultrasonic nebulizers rather than jet nebulizers are used to generate the aerosol particles. The mass median aerodynamic diameter (MMAD) of the particles ranges from 2 to 10 μm for most ultrasonic nebulizers. When the MMAD is 3–5 μm, between 15% and 35% of the aerosol particles inhaled are predicted to deposit in the human respiratory tract.[60] A volume of 80–480 μl (0.08–0.48 ml)/min has been predicted to deposit in the lower airways under these conditions.[60] Even at the lower rate a significant change in osmolarity could occur in the ASL in less than 5 min.

The distribution of aerosol within the airways may vary according to the tonicity of the aerosol and the relative humidity of the airways.[61] Theoretically, water particles could shrink and hypertonic aerosol particles grow as they traverse the human airways. Thus there may be regional differences in the deposition of hypotonic and hypertonic aerosols which could account for the poor correlation in the airway responses to aerosols of different osmolarities.[10]

COMPARISON BETWEEN CHALLENGE WITH EXERCISE AND HYPERVENTILATION AND CHALLENGE WITH NON-ISOTONIC AEROSOLS

Because the volume of ASL is so small and distributed over a large surface area, no attempt has been made to measure osmolarity of ASL before, during, and after exercise or hyperventilation. Rather, the airway responses to exercise and hyperventilation have been compared with a known hyperosmolar stimulus. Some findings are illustrated in Fig. 28.1 and demonstrate that there is excellent concordance between responses to exercise, hyperventilation, and to the inhalation of hyperosmolar saline.[8–10,62] One study,[9] which compared the responses to multiple 1-min exposures of 4.5% saline aerosol and isocapnic hyperventilation, demonstrated a difference in the time-course of the maximal response (Fig. 28.2). During aerosol challenge 86% of the maximal reduction in FEV_1 occurred, whereas only 54% of the response was documented during challenge with isocapnic hyperventilation. This finding is in keeping with the suggestion that airway cooling may act to inhibit responses to hyperventilation.[42–44] Cross refractoriness has been demonstrated between exercise and hyperosmolar saline, suggesting that the mechanisms for the development of the refractoriness are the same (Fig. 28.3).[63]

Although asthmatics are sensitive to inhaling both water and hyperosmolar aerosols, the responses in some individuals are not well correlated[9] suggesting some differences in the development of the response.

There has been some attention given to comparing responses to isocapnic hyperventilation and exercise, and distilled water.[64–68]

THE MECHANISM BY WHICH CHANGE IN OSMOLARITY AND AIRWAY DRYING INDUCE AIRWAY NARROWING

There are a number of sites in the airways where a change in osmolarity could act as a stimulus to induce airway narrowing (Fig 28.4).[69] However it is likely that the broncho-constrictor response to hyperpnoea and to the deposition of particles of non-isotonic

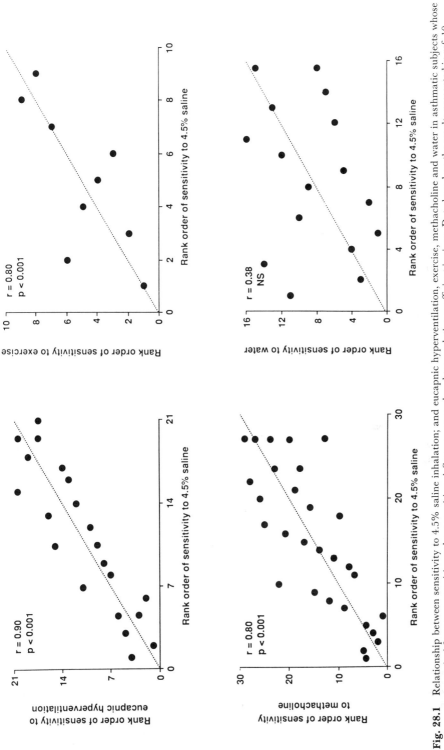

Fig. 28.1 Relationship between sensitivity to 4.5% saline inhalation; and eucapnic hyperventilation, exercise, methacholine and water in asthmatic subjects whose responses were ranked from most sensitive to least sensitive. A Spearmans rank order correlation coefficient is given. Data based on the results presented in ref. 10.

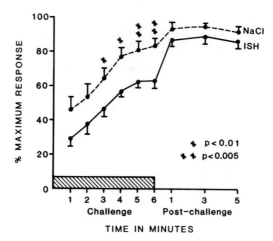

Fig. 28.2 A comparison of the percentage of the maximum response recorded for the reduction in FEV_1 during the last 6 min of challenge with 4.5% saline and isocapnic hyperventilation in nine asthmatic subjects. Data taken from ref. 9.

aerosols is initiated by events that occur in, or close to, the airway lumen.[3] This is based on the observation that both EIA and HIA are prevented by inhaling warm humid air during challenge and the prediction that small volumes of non-isotonic aerosols deposited in the respiratory tract are unlikely to alter osmolarity beyond the ASL or epithelial cells.

There is now considerable evidence in humans that mast cells are present in or on the airway epithelium and thus are in an ideal situation to respond to a change in the osmotic environment.[70] It is also known that human lung mast cells and basophils can degranulate and release mediators in response to either an increase or a decrease in osmolarity.[71–73] Flint et al.[73,74] demonstrated that the mast cells, recovered during bronchoalveolar lavage in patients with asthma, release histamine in response to a hyperosmolar stimulus and that this release is inhibited by sodium cromoglycate. These observations are in keeping with the *in vitro* findings of Eggleston et al.[71] who have shown that dispersed human lung mast cells release histamine in response to hyperosmolar solutions and that this release is dissociated from release of leukotrienes and prostaglandins.[75] Studies of the effect of changing temperature on the hyperosmolar release of

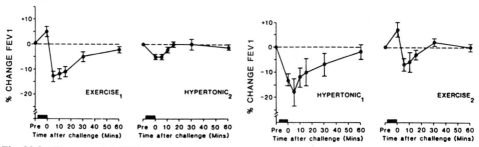

Fig. 28.3 The mean ± 1 SEM per cent change in FEV_1 from baseline following exercise (60% of maximal predicted oxygen consumption) and hypertonic challenge (3.6% saline) in four asthmatic subjects. The data demonstrate the cross refractoriness between these two challenge tests. Reproduced from ref. 63, with permission.

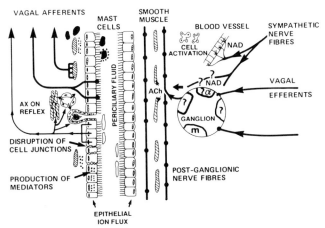

Fig. 28.4 Schematic diagram of the human airways illustrating the various sites which may be affected by an alteration of osmolarity. Modified from ref. 69.

histamine from mast cells and basophils have shown that release is greatest at 32°C,[71] a temperature that is easily achieved in the large airways during exercise.[32] Furthermore the optimum osmolarity for release of histamine was between 600–800 mosmoles.[71] This is a value similar to that which would be induced *in vivo* by either evaporative water loss or the inhalation of aerosols of hyperosmolar saline of around 4.5%.

In vivo mediator release studies do not correlate so well with these findings. An increase in plasma histamine is not a universal finding in patients after challenge with exercise and non-isotonic aerosols.[20,21,76] Studies of isolated segment lavage[77] and bronchoalveolar lavage[78] have been disappointing in their failure to demonstrate large changes in mediator levels in response to changes in osmolarity and to exercise. However the techniques are limited in their ability to sample adequately from the airways and bronchoconstriction can occur in response to minute quantities of mediators making changes difficult to detect. By contrast, studies of mediator release in the nose have shown hyperosmolarity as an important stimulus and that it is related to hyperpnoea.[6,79] Although histamine may not be the most potent mediator, it must contribute to airway narrowing after these challenges because antihistamines markedly reduce the changes in lung function caused by exercise, isocapnic hyperventilation, and non-isotonic aerosols.[16,80–82] As the only source of histamine is either mast cells or basophils, it is likely that mast cells are involved and release their mediators in response to evaporative water loss and a change in osmolarity of the ASL.

There are other cells which could also participate in events that lead to airway narrowing. For example human epithelial cells produce leukotrienes which have the potential to contract bronchial smooth muscle.[83] These cells may also produce prostaglandin E_2,[84] in response to an increase in osmolarity. This could be an important mode of protection against bronchoconstriction and would function best in those who have an intact epithelium. A change in osmolarity in the airway lumen could stimulate the release of other substances associated with the inflammatory response and this could change the permeability of the cells to water. Normally, epithelial cells defend the submocosa from environmental insults but a change in osmolarity may cause a loosening of the tight junctions between these cells. With a breakdown in integrity of the epithelium, substances in the airway lumen would have easier access to bronchial and vascular smooth muscle and surrounding tissue to cause contraction, extravasation, and mucosal oedema. There are contradictory findings from studies on human airways *in vitro*. Some investigators have found an osmolarity-dependent contraction of human isolated airways[85] while others have found relaxation.[86] It is possible that there is a direct osmotic effect on blood vessels or submucosal cells. A high osmolarity in the mucosa may lead to microvascular leakage of water in an attempt to regain normal osmolarity.

The possibility that a change in osmolarity can stimulate vagal afferent nerve activity has been considered[87–89] and there is recent evidence in animals that activation of sensory nerve endings is important in the bronchoconstriction induced by changes in osmolarity.[90]

Cells associated with inflammation, such as eosinophils and neutrophils, are not normally present in the respiratory mucosa but may be attracted to the airways by changes in airway osmolarity and subsequent release of mediators. Evidence to support a role for these cells in the bronchial responsiveness to osmolarity changes comes from the knowledge that chemotactic activity increases in serum in response to these challenges[20–22] and drugs that modify airway inflammation decrease airway responsiveness to these challenges.[24–27,91] It is unlikely, however, that the cell activation and inflammatory events that follow allergen challenge are exactly reproduced by osmotic challenge. The evidence to support this comes from studies showing only small, if any, change in non-specific bronchial hyperresponsiveness after these challenges compared with large changes after allergen challenge.[92–94]

THE EFFECT OF PHARMACOLOGICAL AGENTS

Most drugs that are commonly used to treat or prevent attacks of asthma will inhibit or modify the airway responses to these challenges.[23–27,91,95–97] The most effective drugs are the β_2-adrenoceptor agonists, sodium cromoglycate and nedocromil sodium. The anticholinergic agents are not as effective as the β_2-adrenoceptor agonists although, in some patients, they do inhibit the responses.[24,91,97,98]

Regular treatment with the inhaled steroid beclomethasone dipropionate has been shown to increase the threshold at which the stimulus provokes airway narrowing, i.e. sensitivity, and the rate at which the airways narrow, i.e. reactivity, to these challenges.[25–27] However, it should be noted that chronic treatment with aerosol beclomethasone does not necessarily reduce the capacity of the airways to narrow excessively in response to 4.5% saline aerosol.[27] Similar findings have been made with exercise,[99] and hyperventilation[100] where patients have severe responses even though they are receiving high doses of beclomethasone and have lung function within the normal range. The effect of the newer steroids has not been widely studied but there is a report that regular treatment with budesonide can markedly reduce severity of EIA.[25] Thus the particular steroid used in the treatment of bronchial hyperresponsivenss may be as important as the dose.

There has been a renewed interest in the role of antihistamines in these challenges because of the development of terfenadine and astemizole which are non-sedating drugs and do not have anticholinergic activity. Both agents are effective in inhibiting responses to these challenges.[16,80–82] Although antihistamines can be given as aerosols and do inhibit these challenges,[101–103] they are not commercially available in the aerosol formulation.

The cyclooxygenase inhibitor flurbiprofen, when given orally in a dose of 100 mg, has been shown to reduce the bronchoconstrictor response to both exercise[80] and hypertonic saline.[104] The reduction was less with flurbiprofen compared with terfenadine, suggesting that histamine was a more important mediator in these challenges. Further, when flurbiprofen was given before continuous challenge, rather than a progressive one, it afforded no protection against hypertonic saline. Leukotriene antagonists have also been investigated with limited success when delivered as an aerosol[105] but improved efficacy given in large doses intravenously before exercise.[106]

There are a number of drugs that are not used in the treatment of asthma but that have been investigated for their effectiveness in preventing the response to these challenges. The most interesting development has come from the work of Bianco et al. with the diuretic furosemide. They showed that this drug, when given as an aerosol in a dose of 28 mg, was effective in preventing EIA,[107] while it was ineffective when administered in the same dose as a tablet. Inhaled furosemide prevents airway responses to challenge with water,[108] hyperventilation,[109] hyperosmolar saline,[110] allergen,[111] metabisulphite,[112] and adenosine.[113] Inhaled furosemide reduces the frequency of cough to low chloride ion concentration but not capsaicin.[114] Furosemide has been shown in vitro to prevent the release of histamine and leukotrienes from human lung fragments.[115]

There have been many studies on the effect of calcium antagonists, α-adrenoceptor antagonists, and the sodium nitrates on these challenges.[24,91,116–120] The precise mode of action of these drugs in reducing the response is not known but for EIA and HIA it has been proposed that they act to prevent vasoconstriction of the bronchial circulation. Thus calcium antagonists and nitrates may have some beneficial effect by their direct vasodilator action. Vasodilatation of the bronchial circulation would permit more direct return of water and clearance of bronchoconstrictor mediators and reactive hyperaemia would be prevented from occurring after exercise. α-Adrenoceptor antagonists may also act in this way by preventing the vasoconstriction induced by the release of noradrenaline during exercise. Paradoxically the α_1-adrenergic agonist, methoxamine, has also been shown to modify EIA,[121] which makes some of these findings difficult to interpret.

The findings with these drugs have, on the whole, been variable and the benefits not sufficient to warrant inclusion in treatment. However the dose and route of administration may be important and there may be other sites of action for these drugs and they should not be excluded from further study.

There have been a number of studies using local anaesthetics to prevent airway narrowing to these challenges. It would appear that lignocaine prevents the cough but does not prevent the bronchoconstriction induced by these challenges.[89,91] More studies are required to exclude the possibility that sensory nerves are involved because of the recent finding that hyperosmolarity is a stimulus to neuropeptide release.[90]

The study of the effects of pharmacological agents, given both as aerosol and by tablet, has given us a better understanding of the possible mechanisms whereby these challenges provoke acute airway narrowing. The relative failure of orally administered drugs such as β_2-adrenoceptor agonists, methylxanthines, and anticholinergic agents to prevent the responses to these challenges at a time when bronchodilation is evident is of interest.[24,91] It suggests that the concentration of a drug at the smooth muscle receptor required to induce relaxation is less than that required to prevent contraction,[122] and that events other than contraction of bronchial smooth muscle contribute to airway narrowing. It is also likely that when drugs are administered as aerosols they reach the airways in higher concentrations and they have easy access to cells other than bronchial smooth muscle. For example β_2-adrenoceptor agonists are potent inhibitors of mediator release from mast cells[123] and have the potential to improve the delivery of water to the airways, by enhancing ion movement across epithelial cells[57] and by the mucociliary escalator. All these modes of action may contribute to their ability to prevent the airway narrowing induced by evaporative water loss and changes in osmolarity of ASL.

It is quite clear that a drug need not have a relaxing effect on smooth muscle to prevent the responses to these challenges. Sodium cromoglycate, nedocromil sodium, and furosemide are good examples of this. Their action in preventing mediator release from mast cells is likely to be the most important one and their effectiveness in doing so may relate to their ability to alter ion transport. There are sites other than the mast cell at which these drugs could act to prevent airway narrowing and their prevention of the release of neuropeptides from sensory nerves is of current interest.

The precise mechanism whereby aerosol steroids reduce the sensitivity and reactivity to these challenges is unknown but there are many possibilities. A decrease in sensitivity may reflect an improvement in the integrity of the airway epithelium resulting in an improved mechanical barrier. Thus nerve endings may be protected from the stimulus and less mediator may reach the smooth muscle. Steroids have the potential to reduce airway oedema and the amplifying effect that bronchial smooth muscle contraction has on airway calibre. Steroids may also improve water transport to the airway by their effect on the Na^+ K^+ ATPase pump. By reducing the numbers of mast cells steroids act to reduce the amount of bronchoconstricting mediators.[124] In addition, by reducing the number of other inflammatory cells, the smooth muscle may become less sensitive to contractile agents in the presence of steroids.[125]

The most effective of all agents in blocking EIA is water vapour.[3,4,39] Although it was originally considered that water prevented EIA by modifying the effects of heat loss,[39] it is now appreciated that water blocks EIA by preventing respiratory water loss and the subsequent changes in osmolarity of the periciliary fluid.[4] Although the inhalation of fully saturated air at body temperature (37°C, 44 mgH$_2$O/litre) usually prevents EIA, bronchoconstriction can still occur with these conditions.[4] As 33 mg/litre is normally lost during expiration, inhaling air with a water concentration greater than this may create a hypoosmolar environment and thus a stimulus to asthma. This observation highlights the importance of maintaining a normal balance of water and ions in the respiratory tract.

If the significant amount of water loss that occurs during exercise is from the first 14 generations of the airways, it may be that all that is required to prevent EIA is to ensure that sufficient water is given back to these airways during exercise. The small amounts lost may explain the benefits obtained from the respiratory heat exchangers, such as masks and filters, which permit a small amount of water vapour to be inhaled with each breath.[126] In the future drugs that act specifically to stimulate transport of water to these airways may be used to control EIA.

REFERENCES

1. Anderson SD, Silverman M, Godfrey S, Konig P: Exercise-induced asthma: A review. *Br J Dis Chest* (1975) **69**: 1–39.
2. Deal EC, McFadden ER, Ingram RH, Jaeger JJ: Hyperpnea and heat flux: initial reaction sequence in exercise-induced asthma. *J Appl Physiol* (1979) **46**: 476–483.
3. Chen WY, Horton DJ: Heat and water loss from the airways and exercise-induced asthma. *Respiration* (1977) **34**: 305–313.
4. Anderson SD, Schoeffel RE, Follet R, Perry CP, Daviskas E, Kendall M: Sensitivity to heat and water loss at rest and during exercise in asthmatic patients. *Eur J Respir Dis* (1982) **63**: 459–471.
5. Anderson SD: Is there a unifying hypothesis for exercise-induced asthma? *J Allergy Clin Immunol* (1984) **73**: 660–665.
6. Togias AG, Proud D, Lichtenstein LM, *et al.*: The osmolarity of nasal secretions increases when inflammatory mediators are released in response to inhalation of cold, dry air. *Am Rev Respir Dis* (1988) **137**: 625–629.
7. Potter JL, Matthews LW, Spector S, Lemm J: Studies on pulmonary secretions. II. Osmolarity of the ionic environment of pulmonary secretions from patients with cystic fibrosis, bronchiectasis and laryngectomy. *Am Rev Respir Dis* (1967) **96**: 83–87.
8. Smith CM, Anderson SD: Hyperosmolarity as the stimulus to asthma induced by hyperventilation? *J Allergy Clin Immunol* (1986) **77**: 729–736.
9. Smith CM, Anderson SD: A comparison between the airway response to isocapnic hyperventilation and hypertonic saline in subjects with asthma. *Eur Respir J* (1989) **2**: 36–43.
10. Smith CM, Anderson SD: Inhalational challenge using hypertonic saline in asthmatic subjects: a comparison with responses to hyperpnoea, methacholine and water. *Eur Respir J* (1990) **3**: 144–151.
11. Belcher NG, Lee TH, Rees PJ: Airway responses to hypertonic saline, exercise and histamine challenges in bronchial asthma. *Eur Respir J* (1989) **2**: 44–48.
12. Boulet LP, Legris C, Thibault L, Turcotte H: Comparative bronchial responses to hyperosmolar saline and methacholine in asthma. *Thorax* (1987) **42**: 953–958.
13. Magyar P, Dervaderics M, Toth A, Lantos A: Inhalation of hypertonic potassium chloride solution: A specific bronchial challenge for asthma. *Ital J Chest Dis* (1983) **37**: 29–34.
14. Allegra L, Bianco S: Non-specific bronchoreactivity obtained with an ultrasonic aerosol of distilled water. *Eur J Respir Dis* (1980) **61**: 41–49.
15. Smith CM, Anderson SD: Inhalation provocation tests using non-isotonic aerosols. *J Allergy Clin Immunol* (1989) **84**: 781–790.
16. O'Hickey SP, Belcher NG, Rees PJ, Lee TH: Role of histamine release in hypertonic saline induced bronchoconstriction. *Thorax* (1989) **44**: 650–653.
17. Anderson SD, Daviskas E, Smith CM: Exercise-induced asthma: a difference in opinion regarding the stimulus. *Allergy Proc* (1989) **10**: 215–226.
18. Boat TF, Matthews L-RW: Chemical composition of human tracheo-bronchial secretions. In: Dulfano MJ (ed) Fundamentals and Clinical Pathology of Sputum. Springfield, IL, Thomas, 1973, pp 243–273.
19. Lee TH, Brown MJ, Nagy L, Causon R, Walport MJ, Kay AB: Exercise-induced release of histamine and neutrophil chemotactic factor in atopic asthmatics. *J Allergy Clin Immunol* (1982) **70**: 73–81.
20. Shaw RJ, Murdoch SD, Durham SR, *et al.*: Mediators of hypersensivity and 'fog'-induced asthma. *Allergy* (1985) **40**: 48–57.
21. Belcher NG, Murdoch RD, Dalton N, *et al.*: A comparison of mediator and catecholamine release between exercise- and hypertonic saline-induced asthma. *Am Rev Respir Dis* (1988) **137**: 1026–1032.
22. Arm JP, Horton CE, House F, Clark TJH, Spur BW, Lee TH: Enhanced generation of leukotriene B_4 by neutrophils stimulated by unopsiinized zymosan and by calcium ionophore after exercise-induced asthma. *Am Rev Respir Dis* (1988) **138**: 47–53.

23. Latimer KM, O'Byrne PM, Morris MM: Bronchoconstriction stimulated by airway cooling. Better protection with combination of terbutaline sulphate and cromolyn sodium than either alone. *Am Rev Respir Dis* (1983) **128**: 440–443.

24. Anderson SD: Bronchial challenge by ultrasonically nebulized aerosols. *Clin Rev Allergy* (1985) **3**: 427–439.

25. Henriksen JM, Dahl R: Effects of inhaled budesonide alone and in combination with low-dose terbutaline in children with exercise-induced asthma. *Am Rev Respir Dis* (1983) **128**: 993–997.

26. Pomari C, Turco P, Trevisan F, Zoccatelli D, Dal Negro RW: Multiparametrical approach to fog-challenge-induced bronchial hyperreactivity in asthmatics—protective effects of salbutamol plus beclomethasone dipropionate. *Int J Clin Pharmacol Ther Toxicol* (1984) **22**: 515–518.

27. Rodwell LT, Anderson SD: Inhaled beclomethasone dipropionate (BDP) modifies airway sensitivity (PD_{20}) but does not reduce excessive airway narrowing to 4.5% saline in asthmatic subjects (Abstract). *Am Rev Respir Dis* (1991) **143**: A423.

28. O'Byrne PM, Jones GL: The effect of indomethacin on exercise-induced bronchoconstriction and refractoriness after exercise. *Am Rev Respir Dis* (1986) **134**: 69–72.

29. Mattoli S, Foresi A, Corbo GM, Valente S, Ciappi G: The effect of indomethacin on the refractory period occurring after the inhalation of ultrasonically nebulized distilled water. *J Allergy Clin Immunol* (1987) **79**: 678–683.

30. O'Hickey SP: Hypertonic saline challenge and refractory behaviour in asthmatic subjects. MD Thesis, University of London (1989).

31. Proctor DF: Physiology of the upper airway. In: Fenn WO, Rahn H (eds) *Handbook of Physiology, Section 3, Respiration.* Vol 1. Washington DC, American Physiological Society (1964) **1**: 309–345.

32. McFadden ER, Pichurko BM, Bowman HF, et al.: Thermal mapping of the airways in humans. *J Appl Physiol* (1985) **58**: 564–570.

33. McFadden ER, Pichurko BM: Intraairway thermal profiles during exercise and hyperventilation in normal man. *J Clin Invest* (1985) **76**: 1007–1010.

34. Chalon J, Loew DAY, Malebranche J: Effects of dry anesthetic gases on tracheobronchial ciliated epithelium. *Anesthesiology* (1972) **37**: 338–343.

35. Anderson SD, Schoeffel RE, Black JL, Daviskas E: Airway cooling as the stimulus to exercise-induced asthma. A re-evaluation. *Eur J Respir Dis* (1985) **67**: 20–30.

36. Tabka Z, Ben Jebria A, Guenard H: Effect of breathing dry warm air on respiratory water loss at rest and during exercise. *Respirat Physiol* (1987) **67**: 115–125.

37. Eschenbacher WL, Sheppard D: Respiratory heat loss is not the sole stimulus for bronchoconstriction induced by isocapnic hyperpnea with dry air. *Am Rev Respir Dis* (1985) **131**: 894–901.

38. Daviskas E, Gonda I, Anderson SD: Local airway heat and water vapour losses. *Respiration Physiology* (1991) in press.

39. Deal EC, McFadden ER, Ingram RH, Strauss RH, Jaeger JJ. Role of respiratory heat exchange in production of exercise-induced asthma. *J Appl Physiol: Respirat Environ Exercise Physiol* (1979) **46**: 467–475.

40. Hahn A, Anderson SD, Morton AR, Black JL, Fitch KD. A re-interpretation of the effect of temperature and water content of the inspired air in exercise-induced asthma. *Am Rev Respir Dis* (1984) **130**: 575–579.

41. McFadden ER. Exercise-induced asthma. Assessment of current etiologic concepts. *Chest* (1987) **91S**: 151S–157S.

42. Freed AN, Kelly LJ, Menkes HA: Airflow-induced bronchospasm: imbalance between airway cooling and airway drying? *Am Rev Respir Dis* (1987) **136**: 595–599.

43. Blackie SP, Hilliam C, Village R, Paré PD: The time course of bronchoconstriction in asthmatics during and after isocapnic hyperventilation. *Am Rev Respir Dis* (1990) **142**: 1133–1136.

44. Freed AN, Stream CE: Airway cooling: stimulus specific modulation of airway responsiveness in the canine lung periphery. *Eur Respir J* (1991) **4**: 568–574.

45. McFadden ER, Lenner KAM, Strohl KP: Postexertional airway rewarming and thermally induced asthma. New insights into pathophysiology and possible pathogenesis. *J Clin Invest* (1986) **78**: 18–25.

46. McFadden ER: Hypothesis: exercise-induced asthma as a vascular phenomenon. *Lancet* (1990) **335**: 880–882.

47. Agostini P, Arena V, Doria E, Susini G: Inspired gas relative humidity affects systemic to pulmonary bronchial blood flow in humans. *Chest* (1990) **97**: 1377–1380.

48. Baile EM, Dahlby RW, Wiggs BR, Parsons GH, Pare PD: Effect of cold and warm dry air hyperventilation on canine airway blood flow. *J Appl Physiol* (1987) **62**: 526–532.

49. Parsons GH, Paré PD, White DA, Baile EM: Airway blood flow response to eucapnic dry air hyperventilation in sheep. *J Appl Physiol* (1989) **66**: 1443–1447.

50. Zawadski DK, Lenner KA, McFadden ER: Comparison of intraairway temperatures in normal and asthmatic subjects after hyperpnea with hot, cold, and ambient air. *Am Rev Respir Dis* (1988) **138**: 1553–1558.

51. Smith CM, Anderson SD, Walsh S, McElrea MS: An investigation of the effects of heat and water exchange in the recovery period after exercise in children with asthma. *Am Rev Respir Dis* (1989) **140**: 598–605.

52. Letters: Exercise-induced asthma as a vascular phenomenon. *Lancet* (1990) **335**: 1410–1412.

53. Letters: The effects of heat and water exchange in the recovery period after exercise in children with asthma. *Am Rev Respir Dis* (1990) **141**: 801–803.

54. Godden DJ, Baile EM, Okazawa M, Paré PD: Hypertonic aerosol inhalation does not alter central airway blood flow in dogs. *J Appl Physiol* (1988) **65**: 1990–1994.

55. Moreno RG, Hogg JC, Paré PD: Mechanics of airway narrowing. *Am Rev Respir Dis* (1986) **133**: 1171–1180.

56. Deffebach ME, Charan NB, Lakshminarayan S, Butler J: The bronchial circulation. Small, but a vital attribute of the lung. State of the Art. *Am Rev Respir Dis* (1987) **135**:463–481.

57. Nadel JA, Widdicombe JH, Peatfield AC: Regulation of airway secretions, ion transport, and water movement. In Fishman AP (ed) *Handbook of Physiology, The Respiratory System 1.* Bethesda, MD, American Physiological Society, 1985, pp 419–445.

58. Kilburn KH: A hypothesis of pulmonary clearance and its implications. *Am Rev Respir Dis* (1968) **98**: 449–463.

59. Frizzell RA: Role of absorptive and secretory processes in hydration of the airway surface. *Am Rev Respir Dis* (1988) **138** (Suppl): S3–S6.

60. Anderson SD, Smith CM: The use of nonisotonic aerosols for evaluating bronchial hyper-responsiveness. In Spector S (ed) *Bronchial Provocation Tests.* Futura, New York, 1989, pp 227–252.

61. Ferron GA, Haider B, Kreyling WG: Inhalation of salt aerosol particles. 1. Estimation of the temperature and relative humidity of the air in the human upper airways. *J Aerosol Sci* (1988) **19**: 343–363.

62. Kivity S, Greif J, Reisner B, Fireman E, Topilsky M: Bronchial inhalation challenge with ultrasonically nebulized saline: comparison to exercise-induced asthma. *Ann Allergy* (1986) **57**: 355–358.

63. Belcher NG, Rees PJ, Clark TJM, Lee TH: A comparison of the refractory periods induced by hypertonic airway challenge and exercise in bronchial asthma. *Am Rev Respir Dis* (1987) **135**: 822–825.

64. Galdes-Sebalt M, McLaughton FJ, Levison H: Comparison of cold air, ultrasonic mist and methacholine inhalations as tests of bronchial reactivity in normal and asthmatic children. *J Pediatr* (1985) **107**: 526–530.

65. Foresi A, Mattoli S, Corbo GM, Polidori G, Ciappi G: Comparison of bronchial responses to ultrasonically nebulized distilled water, exercise, and methacholine in asthma. *Chest* (1986) **90**: 822–826.

66. Foresi A, Corbo GM, Valente S: Airway responsiveness to exercise and ultrasonically nebulized distilled water in children: relationship to clinical and functional characteristics. *Respiration* (1988) **53**: 205–213.

67. Lemire TS, Hopp RJ, Bewtra A, Nair NM, Townley RG: Comparison of ultrasonically nebulized distilled water and cold-air hyperventilation challenges in asthmatic patients. *Chest* (1989) **95**: 958–961.
68. Fourie PR, Joubert JR: Determination of airway hyper-reactivity in asthmatic children: a comparison among exercise, nebulized water, and histamine challenge. *Pediatr Pulmonol* (1988) **4**: 2–7.
69. Anderson SD: Issues in exercise-induced asthma. *J Allergy Clin Immunol* (1985) **76**: 763–772.
70. Tomioka M, Ida S, Shindoh Y, Ishihara T, Takishima T: Mast cells in bronchoalveolar lumen of patients with bronchial asthma. *Am Rev Respir Dis* (1984) **129**: 1000–1005.
71. Eggleston PA, Kagey-Sobotka A, Lichtenstein LM: A comparison of the osmotic activation of basophils and human lung mast cells. *Am Rev Respir Dis* (1987) **135**: 1043–1048.
72. Rimmer J, Bryant DH: Effect of hypo- and hyper-osmolarity on basophil histamine release. *Clin Allergy* (1986) **16**: 221–230.
73. Flint KC, Hudspith BN, Leung KBP, Pearce FL, Brostoff J, Johnson NMcI: The hyper-osmolar release of histamine from bronchoalveolar mast cells and its inhibition by sodium cromoglycate. *Thorax* (1985) **40**: 717.
74. Flint KC, Leung KBP, Pearce FL, Hudspith BN, Brostoff J, Johnson NMcI: Human mast cells recovered by bronchoalveolar lavage: their morphology, histamine release and the effects of sodium cromoglycate. *Clin Sci* (1985) **68**: 427–432.
75. Eggleston PA, Kagey-Sobotka A, Proud D, Adkinson NF, Lichtenstein LM: Disassociation of the release of histamine and arachidonic acid metabolites from osmolatically activated basophils and human lung mast cells. *Am Rev Respir Dis* (1990) **141**: 960–964.
76. Anderson SD, Bye PTP, Schoeffel RE, Seale JP, Taylor KM, Ferris L: Arterial plasma histamine levels at rest, during and after exercise in patients with asthma: Effects of terbutaline aerosol. *Thorax* (1981) **36**: 259–267.
77. Gravelyn TR, Pan PM, Eschenbacher WL: Mediator release in an isolated segment in subjects with asthma. *Am Rev Respir Dis* (1988) **137**: 641–646.
78. Broide DH, Eisman S, Ramsdell JW, Ferguson P, Schwartz, Wasserman SI: Airway levels of mast cell-derived mediators in exercise-induced asthma. *Am Rev Respir Dis* (1990) **141**: 563–568.
79. Silber G, Proud D, Warner J, *et al.*: *In vivo* release of inflammatory mediators by hyperosmolar solutions. *Am Rev Respir Dis* (1988) **137**: 606–612.
80. Finnerty JP, Holgate ST: Evidence for the roles of histamine and prostaglandins as mediators in exercise-induced asthma: the inhibitory effect of terfenadine and flurbiprofen alone and in combination. *Eur Respir J* (1990) **3**: 540–547.
81. Finney MJB, Anderson SD, Black JL: Terfenadine modifies airway narrowing induced by the inhalation of non-isotonic aerosols in subjects with asthma. *Am Rev Respir Dis* (1990) **141**: 1151–1157.
82. Townley RG, Hopp RJ, Bewtra A, Nabe M: Effect of terfenadine on pulmonary function, histamine release, and bronchial challenges with nebulized water and cold-air hyperventilation. *Ann Allergy* (1989) **63**: 455–460.
83. Hunter JA, Finkbeiner WE, Nadel JA, Goetzl EJ, Holtzman MJ: Predominant generation of 15-lipoxygenase metabolites of arachidonic acid by epithelial cells from human trachea. *Proc Natl Acad Sci, USA* (1985) **82**: 4633–4637.
84. Assouline G, Leibson V: Stimulation of prostaglandin output from rat stomach by hypertonic solutions. *Eur J Pharmacol* (1977) **44**: 271–273.
85. Jongejan RC, de Jongste JC, Raatgeep RC, Bonta IL, Kerrebijn KF: Effects of changes in osmolarity on isolated human airways. *J Appl Physiol* (1990) **68**: 1568–1575.
86. Finney MJB, Anderson SD, Black JL: Effect of non-isotonic solution on human isolated airway smooth muscle. *Respirat Physiol* (1987) **69**: 277–286.
87. Anderson SD, Schoeffel RE, Finney M: Evaluation of ultrasonically nebulised solutions as a provocation in patients with asthma. *Thorax* (1983) **38**: 284–291.
88. Sheppard D, Epstein J, Holtzman MJ, Nadel JA, Boushey HA: Dose-dependent inhibition of cold air-induced bronchoconstriction by atropine. *J Appl Physiol: Respirat Environ Exercise Physiol* (1982) **53**: 169–174.

89. Eschenbacher WL, Boushey HA, Sheppard D: Alterations in osmolarity of inhaled aerosols cause bronchoconstriction and cough, but absence of a permeant anion causes cough alone. *Am Rev Respir Dis* (1984) **129**: 211–215.

90. Umeno E, Nadel JA, McDonald DM: Neurogenic inflammation is evoked in the rat trachea by inhalation of hypertonic saline aerosols. *Am Rev Respir Dis* (1990) **141**: A182.

91. Anderson SD: Exercise-induced asthma. In Middleton E, Reed C, Ellis E, Adkinson NF, Yunginger JW (eds) *Allergy: Principles and Practice*, 3rd edn. Vol. 2. St Louis, CV Mosby, 1988, pp. 1156–1175.

92. Smith CM, Anderson SD,.Black JL: Methacholine responsiveness increases after ultrasonically nebulized water, but not after ultrasonically nebulized hypertonic saline in patients with asthma. *J Allergy Clin Immunol* (1987) **79**: 85–92.

93. Hahn AG, Nogrady SG, Tumilty DMcA, Lawrence SR, Morton AR: Histamine reactivity during the refractory period after exercise induced asthma. *Thorax* (1984) **39**: 919–923.

94. Malo JL, Cartier A, L'Acheveque J, Ghezzo H, Martin RR: Bronchoconstriction due to isocapnic cold air inhalation minimally influences bronchial hyperresponsiveness to methacholine in asthmatic subjects. *Bull Eur Physiopathol Respir* (1986) **22**: 473–477.

95. del Bufalo C, Fasano L, Patalano F, Gunella G: Inhibition of fog-induced bronchoconstriction by nedocromil sodium and sodium cromoglycate in intrinsic asthma: a double-blind, placebo-controlled study. *Respiration* (1989) **55**: 181–185.

96. Albazzaz MK, Neale MG, Patel KR: Dose-response study of nebulised nedocromil sodium in exercise induced asthma. *Thorax* (1989) **44**: 816–819.

97. Boulet L-P, Turcotte H, Tennina S: Comparative efficacy of salbutamol, ipratropium and cromoglycate in the prevention of bronchospasm induced by exercise and hyperosmolar challenges. *J Allergy Clin Immunol* (1989) **83**: 882–887.

98. Wilson NM, Barnes PJ, Vickers H, Silverman M: Hyperventilation-induced asthma: evidence for two mechanisms. *Thorax* (1982) **37**: 657–662.

99. Anderson SD, Rodwell LT, Du Toit J, Young IH: Duration of protection of inhaled salmeterol in exercise-induced asthma. *Chest* (1991) **100**: 1254–1260.

100. Smith CM, Anderson SD, Seale JP: The duration of the combination of fenoterol hydrobromide and iptratropium bromide in protecting against asthma provoked by hyperpnea. *Chest* (1988) **94**: 709–717.

101. Hartley JPR, Nogrady SG: Effect of an inhaled antihistamine on exercise-induced asthma. *Thorax* (1980) **35**: 675–679.

102. O'Byrne PM, Thomson NC, Morris M, Roberts RS, Daniel EE, Hargreave FE: The protective effect of inhaled chlorpheniramine and atropine on bronchoconstriction stimulated by airway cooling. *Am Rev Respir Dis* (1983) **128**: 611–617.

103. Rodwell LT, Anderson SD, Seale JP: Clemastine prevents airway narrowing caused by aerosols of hypertonic saline (HS) in asthmatic subjects. *Eur Respir J* (1990) **3**(Suppl 10): 129S.

104. Finnerty JP, Wilmot C, Holgate ST: Inhibition of hypertonic saline-induced bronchoconstriction by terfenadine and flurbiprofen. Evidence of the predominant role of histamine. *Am Rev Respir Dis* (1989) **140**: 593–597.

105. Mann JS, Robinson C, Sheriden AQ, Clement P, Bach MK, Holgate ST: Effect of inhaled Piriprost (U-60,257) a novel leukotriene inhibitor, on allergen and exercise induced bronchoconstriction in asthma. *Thorax* (1986) **41**: 746–752.

106. Manning PJ, Watson RM, Margolskee DJ, Schwartz JI, O'Byrne PM: The effect of a leukotriene D_4 receptor antagonist MK571 on exercise-induced bronchoconstriction. *Eur Resp J* (1990) **3**(Suppl 10): 203S.

107. Bianco S, Vaghi A, Robuschi M, Pasargiklian M: Prevention of exercise-induced bronchoconstriction by inhaled frusemide. *Lancet* (July 1988) **30**: 252–355.

108. Robuschi M, Gambaro G, Spagnotto S, Vaghi A, Bianco S: Inhaled frusemide is highly effective in preventing ultrasonically nebulised water bronchoconstriction. *Pulmonary Pharmacol* (1989) **1**: 187–191.

109. Grubbe RE, Hopp R, Dave NK, Brennan B, Bewtra A, Townley R: Effect of inhaled furosemide on the bronchial response to methacholine and cold-air hyperventilation challenges. *J Allergy Clin Immunol* (1990) **85**: 881–884.

110. Rodwell LT, Anderson SD, Du Toit J, Seale JP: A comparison between the inhibitory effects of furosemide and nedocromil sodium on hyperosmolar challenge in asthmatic subjects. Personal communication.

111. Bianco S, Pieroni MG, Refini RM, Rottli L, Sestini P: Protective effect of inhaled furosemide on allergen-induced early and late asthmatic reactions. *New Engl J Med* (1989) **321**: 1069–1073.

112. Nichol GM, Alton EWFW, Nix A, Geddes DM, Chung KF, Barnes PJ: Effect of inhaled furosemide on metabisulphite- and methacholine-induced bronchoconstriction and nasal potential differences in asthmatic subjects. *Am Rev Respir Dis* (1990) **142**: 576–580.

113. Polosa R, Lau LCK, Holgate ST: Inhibition of adenosine 5′-monophosphate- and methacholine-induced bronchoconstriction in asthma by inhaled frusemide. *Eur Respir J* (1990) **3**: 665–672.

114. Ventresca PG, Nichol GM, Barnes PJ, Chung KF: Inhaled furosemide inhibits cough induced by low chloride content solutions but not by capsaicin. *Am Rev Respir Dis* (1990) **142**: 1434–146.

115. Anderson SD, Wei He, Temple DM: Furosemide inhibits antigen-induced release of sulfidopeptide-leukotrienes and histamine from sensitized human lung fragments. *New Engl J Med* (1991) **324**: 131.

116. Patel KR, Peers E: Felopidine: A new calcium antagonist, modifies exercise-induced asthma. *Am Rev Respir Dis* (1988) **138**: 54–56.

117. Kivity S, Ganem R, Greif J, Topilsky M: The combined effect of nifedipine and sodium cromoglycate on the airway response to inhaled hypertonic saline in patients with bronchial asthma. *Eur Respir J* (1989) **2**: 513–516.

118. Patel KR, Kerr JW, MacDonald EB, Mackenzie AM: The effect of thymoxamine and cromolyn sodium on postexercise bronchoconstriction in asthma. *J Allergy Clin Immunol* (1976) **57**: 285–292.

119. Barnes PJ, Wilson NM, Vickers H: Prazosin, an alpha$_1$-adrenoceptor antagonist, partially inhibits exercise-induced asthma. *J Allergy Clin Immunol* (1981) **68**: 411–415.

120. Tullett WM, Patel KR: Isosorbide dinitrate and isoxsuprine in exercise induced asthma. *Br Med J* (1983) **286**: 1934–1935.

121. Dinh Xuan AT, Chaussain M, Regnard J, Lockhart A: Pretreatment with an inhaled alpha$_1$-adrenergic agonist, methoxamine, reduces exercise-induced asthma. *Eur Respir J* (1989) **2**: 409–414.

122. Jenne JW, Tashkin DP: Bronchodilators and bronchial provocation. In Spector SL (ed) *Provocative Challenge Procedures. Background and Methodology.* Mount Kisco, NY, Futura, 1989, pp. 451–517.

123. Morr H: Immunological release of histamine from human lung. 1. Studies on the beta$_2$ sympathomimetic stimulator fenoterol. *Respiration* (1979) **38**: 163–167.

124. Pipkorn U, Enerback L: Nasal mucosal mast cells and histamine in hay fever. Effect of topical glucocorticoid treatment. *Int Arch Allergy Appl Immunol* (1987) **84**: 123–128.

125. Hallahan AR, Armour CL, Black JL: Products of neutrophils and eosinophils increase the responsiveness of human isolated bronchial tissue. *Eur Respir J* (1990) **3**: 554–558.

126. Eiken O, Kaiser P, Holmer I, Baer R: Physiological effects of a mouth-borne heat exchanger during heavy exercise in a cold environment. *Ergonomics* (1989) **32**: 645–653.

29

Gases

DEAN SHEPPARD

INTRODUCTION

Inhalation of noxious gases is a well-recognized cause of exacerbations of asthma. Considerable anecdotal evidence suggests that acute inhalation of high concentrations of some noxious gases might also be capable of causing asthma in previously healthy individuals. This chapter will first focus on sulphur dioxide as an example of a gas that has clearly been shown to cause bronchospasm in patients with asthma, and will then consider the evidence suggesting that airway injury from noxious gases could be a cause of asthma.

EXACERBATIONS OF PRE-EXISTING ASTHMA

Non-specific airway hyperresponsiveness, a central feature of asthma, is characterized by exaggerated bronchomotor responses to a wide variety of bronchoconstrictor stimuli.[1] It is thus generally assumed that patients with asthma will develop symptomatic bronchoconstriction on exposure to any irritating gas. On the basis of this assumption, physicians often advise patients with asthma to avoid 'irritating vapours and fumes' and sometimes prevent these patients from working in industries in which such exposures might occur. However, there is little scientific basis for this approach. It is incorrect to equate 'irritancy' with bronchoconstrictor potency. For example, formaldehyde is highly 'irritating' to the mucous membranes of the eyes and throat in airborne concentrations of 1 p.p.m. or higher.[2] However, inhalation of up to 3 p.p.m. formaldehyde, even during heavy exercise, does not cause bronchoconstriction in most subjects with asthma.[3]

ASTHMA: BASIC MECHANISMS AND CLINICAL MANAGEMENT (2nd Edn)
ISBN 0-12-079026-2

Similarly, inhalation of an aerosol of an isotonic solution that lacks a permanent anion (e.g. solutions of dextrose or sodium gluconate) is quite 'irritating' and a potent stimulus to cough, but does not generally cause bronchoconstriction.[4] In contrast, inhalation of concentrations of sulphur dioxide gas that are generally not detected by normal subjects and do not cause cough or any other symptoms of mucosal 'irritation' can cause severe symptomatic bronchoconstriction in patients with asthma.[5–8]

SULPHUR DIOXIDE

Sulphur dioxide (SO_2) is one of the few noxious gases that has been carefully studied as a potential cause of bronchoconstriction. More than 20 years ago studies in guinea-pigs, cats and normal human subjects show that inhalation of SO_2 causes contraction of airway smooth muscle within minutes of the onset of exposure.[9–12] In normal humans, this effect occurs with exposure to concentrations of SO_2 that can be encountered in industrial settings (< 5 p.p.m.), but the resultant changes in airway resistance are small and not likely to be of clinical significance. However, several recent studies have shown that people with asthma are exquisitely sensitive to the bronchoconstrictor effects of SO_2 and can develop bronchoconstriction on exposure to concentrations of SO_2 at least an order of magnitude lower than the highest concentrations commonly encountered in the workplace: concentrations that can be encountered in polluted urban air.

Sources of exposure to SO₂

Sulphur dioxide is either used or generated in a wide variety of industries. Concentrations of SO_2 in excess of 5 p.p.m. can occur in metal smelters, paper pulp mills, petroleum refineries, wineries and food-processing plants. In the USA, the present standard set by the Occupational Safety and Health Administration allows exposure of workers up to 5 p.p.m. SO_2 calculated as a time-weighted average over an 8 h workshift. These industrial plants also serve as important point sources of SO_2 emissions into the atmosphere. As the major air pollutant produced by combustion of sulphur-containing fossil fuels, SO_2 is also an important emission from fuel-burning power plants, which account for approximately 70% of atmospheric emissions in the USA.[13] The concentrations of SO_2 in outdoor air is usually considerably lower than the concentrations found in the workplace, but short-term (3–6 min) peak concentrations of SO_2 in excess of 3 p.p.m. have been measured in the vicinity of point sources. In non-industrial setting, SO_2 has not generally been considered an important indoor air pollutant. However, kerosene space heaters, a form of household heating that has recently gained worldwide popularity, can produce large quantities of SO_2, leading to indoor concentrations of 1–2 p.p.m. or more.[14]

Effect of SO₂ on people with asthma

During resting tidal breathing, human subjects with mild asthma develop significant increases in specific airway resistance (SRaw) on inhaling 1 p.p.m. SO_2 for 5–10 min, and can develop symptomatic asthma attacks on inhaling 3 p.p.m. SO_2.[15] However, since SO_2 is highly soluble in water, during resting tidal breathing more than 95% of the SO_2 is removed from inspired air by the moist mucous membranes of the mouth and/or nose.[16] With increases in minute ventilation and inspiratory flow, a larger dose of SO_2 is delivered to the mouth and a higher percentage of inspired SO_2 actually reaches the airways.[16] Thus, increases in ventilation, such as the increases that occur during exercise, can greatly potentiate the bronchoconstrictor effect of a given concentration of SO_2. As a result, during moderate or heavy exercise, concentrations of SO_2 as low as 0.25 p.p.m. can cause statistically significant increases in SRaw,[17,18] and 0.4 p.p.m. can cause symptomatic asthma attacks after exposures as brief as 3 min in duration.[19,20] These effects are not merely due to exercise (or hyperventilation) alone, since they have repeatedly been shown to occur even when SO_2 is inhaled in warm, humidified air at exercise work rates and levels of ventilation that do not cause bronchoconstriction in the same subjects in the absence of SO_2.[5,6,18,20]

In most studies of the bronchoconstrictor effects of SO_2, investigators have administered the gas in warm, humid air to avoid the potentially confounding effects of airway drying and/or cooling on subjects with asthma. However, a few studies have examined the hypothesis that the effect of SO_2 would be potentiated by cold and/or dry air. In most such studies, dry air did appear to potentiate SO_2-induced bronchoconstriction,[20–22] an effect that was equally large at ambient and at subfreezing temperatures.[19] Again, this was not merely due to known bronchoconstrictor effects of dry air, since in two studies subjects inhaled SO_2 at a minute ventilation chosen to be below the ventilation at which dry air caused any detectable increase in SRaw.[20,21]

Thus, on the basis of available data, it is possible for physicians to predict reasonably accurately the likelihood that patients with asthma will develop symptomatic exacerbations from exposure to SO_2 if the anticipated SO_2 concentration, the patient's anticipated exercise work rate and the probable atmospheric conditions (e.g. inspired water content) are known. Consequently, for example, it is quite clear that patients with asthma should be advised to avoid employment in industries known to be associated with exposure to high SO_2 concentrations (i.e. smelters and pulp mills) and to avoid residence in buildings heated by kerosene space heaters. The same approach can be used to predict that concentrations of SO_2 in outdoor air that exceed 0.4 p.p.m. for periods of 3 min or more have the potential to cause symptomatic bronchoconstriction in exercising subject with asthma. Based on this knowledge, effective pollution control strategies need to be developed to prevent these concentrations from occurring, especially in populated areas.

BRONCHOCONSTRICTOR EFFECTS OF OTHER 'IRRITANTS'

Unfortunately, as alluded to above, little is known about the bronchoconstrictor potency of most noxious gases, especially on patients with asthma. Surprisingly, most of the 'irritants' that have been studied have not been found to be terribly potent stimuli to bronchoconstriction. For example, formaldehyde, ozone and nitrogen dioxide have all been reported to cause either clinically insignificant or no bronchoconstriction in irritating concentrations up to or exceeding presently allowable workplace exposure limits in the USA. Inhaled acid aerosols can cause bronchoconstriction in subjects with asthma. However, the concentration required to produce meaningful symptomatic effects is orders of magnitude higher than concentrations likely to be encountered in outdoor polluted air.[23]

Thus, on the basis of available data, it is not possible for physicians to predict accurately bronchoconstrictor responses to most noxious gases or aerosols, even known respiratory irritants. Therefore, it is not reasonable to prohibit patients with known asthma from working in industries or occupations that include exposure to irritant gases or aerosols. On the other hand, since such patients can clearly be exquisitely sensitive to bronchoconstrictor substances that might have little effect on normal co-workers, a history suggesting work-induced exacerbations of asthma by irritants must be taken seriously and usually requires either a change in work practices or a change in employment. As in patients suspected of having new asthma caused by work, frequent measurements of peak flow at and away from the workplace can help to clarify the relationship (if any) between bronchospasm and work exposures.

DIRECT INJURY BY INHALED GASES AS A POSSIBLE CAUSE OF ASTHMA

Sporadic cases of new-onset asthma following a single massive exposure to a noxious gas have appeared in the medical literature over at least the past 50 years.[24–26] Although all of these reports have been anecdotal, several have been sufficiently dramatic to suggest that such an effect can occur. There is considerable experimental evidence that a single exposure to a variety of noxious gases and particles including ozone,[27–31] cigarette smoke,[32] fire smoke[33] and toluene diisocyanate,[34,35] can acutely increase non-specific bronchoconstrictor responsiveness in both human subjects and in experimental animals.

MECHANISMS OF AIRWAY HYPERRESPONSIVENESS INDUCED BY NOXIOUS GASES

Each of the noxious agents listed above causes an increase in airway responsiveness in association with morphological evidence of airway mucosal injury and acute airway inflammation.[31,32,34] These findings suggest that the increased airway responsiveness may be a consequence of some aspect or aspects of the acute inflammatory response. Because polymorphonuclear leucocytes (PMN) are rapidly recruited into the airways of animals (and humans) exposed to these agents, it has been suggested that PMN themselves may play a mechanistic role in causing airway hyperresponsiveness. This hypothesis was supported by the finding that the increase in bronchomotor responsiveness to inhaled acetylcholine caused by exposure of dogs to ozone was abolished when the animals were depleted of circulating (and airway) PMN by treatment with the cytotoxic drug hydroxyurea.[36] However, PMN depletion by another cytotoxic drug, cyclophosphamide, failed to inhibit the increase in airway responsiveness caused by ozone exposure in guinea-pigs.[37] A study of the effects of cytotoxic drugs on the increase in airway responsiveness caused by exposure of guinea-pigs to toluene diisocyanate (TDI) may explain the apparent discrepancy in these results. In this study, PMN depletion with hydroxyurea inhibited the TDI-induced increase in airway responsiveness, whereas equivalent PMN depletion with cyclophosphamide (documented by circulating PMN counts less than $200/mm^3$ and an absence of PMN in airway sections) did not.[38] These results suggest that hydroxyurea may inhibit increases in airway responsiveness caused by noxious gases.

Several studies have examined the role of various humoral mediators of acute inflammation in the airway hyperresponsiveness that follows acute exposure to noxious gases. Thus far the results of these studies have not produced a unifying hypothesis to explain this phenomenon. The significance of specific mediators seems to vary considerably among mammalian species. For example, cyclooxygenase metabolites of arachidonic acid, especially thromboxanes, appear to be required in the increased airway responsiveness caused by ozone exposure in dogs, since this response to ozone is inhibited by indomethacin[39] and by the thromboxane synthetase inhibitor OKY-046.[40] However, indomethacin does not inhibit the increase in airway responsiveness caused by ozone in guinea-pigs[41] or in humans (unpublished observation). Furthermore, the role of specific mediators may be different in response to different noxious gases in the same species. For example, the increases in airway responsiveness caused by exposure of guinea-pigs to ozone[41] or to acrolein[42] can be inhibited by inhibitors and antagonists of sulphadopeptide leukotrienes, whereas the same drugs have no effect on the increased airway responsiveness caused by exposure of guinea-pigs to TDI.[43]

Treatment of guinea-pigs with repeated doses of capsaicin in a regimen shown to deplete animals of airway tachykinins has been found to inhibit the increase in airway responsiveness caused by exposure to TDI. Administration of the competitive tachykinin antagonist (D-Arg,[1] D-Pro,[2] D-Trp,[7-9] Leu[11]) substance P also inhibited this effect of TDI.[44] These observations suggest that, at least in the guinea-pig, tachykinins released from airway afferent nerves might play a role in the increase in airway responsiveness caused by some noxious gases. Interestingly, although TDI exposure also causes airway oedema, treatment with capsaicin did not prevent the production of oedema by TDI, suggesting that the presence of oedema itself is not sufficient to cause airway hyperresponsiveness in this model. The effects of tachykinins on the airways are strongly influenced by the local activity of neutral endopeptidase, an ectoenzyme that rapidly cleaves the two principal tachykinins in the airways substance P and neurokinin P, to inactive fragments. TDI exposure augments the effects of tachykinins by decreasing neutral endopeptidase activity.[45]

The experimental observations summarized above provide a useful opportunity to study how various aspects of airway injury and inflammation could contribute to the airway hyperresponsiveness that characterizes asthma. However, these experimental models differ from clinical asthma in that the alterations in airway responsiveness caused by noxious gases are usually short-lived and completely resolve over a period of hours to weeks. This transient increase in airway responsiveness probably helps to explain the prominent bronchoconstriction commonly seen in patients hospitalized after smoke or other gas inhalation. However, a major question that remains unanswered by these observations is why after acute injury occasional patients develop airway hyperresponsiveness that persists for months to years.

Elucidation of the factor or factors responsible for the persistence of airway hyperresponsiveness after acute injury could provide important clues to the mechanisms underlying clinical asthma.

REFERENCES

1. Boushey HA, Holtzman MJ, Sheller JR, Nadel JA: Bronchial hyperreactivity: state of the art. *Am Rev Respir Dis* (1980) **121**: 389–413.
2. Dally KA, Hanrahan LP, Woodbury MA, Kanarek MS: Formaldehyde exposure in nonoccupational environments. *Arch Environ Health* (1981) **36**: 277–284.
3. Sheppard D, Eschenbacher WL, Epstein J: Lack of bronchomotor response to up to 3 ppm formaldehyde in subjects with asthma. *Environ Res* (1984) **35**: 133–139.
4. Eschenbacher WL, Boushey HA, Sheppard D: Alterations in osmolarity of inhaled aerosols cause bronchoconstriction and cough but absence of a permeant anion causes cough alone. *Am Rev Respir Dis* (1984) **129**: 211–215.
5. Sheppard D, Saisho A, Nadel JA, Boushey HA: Exercise increases sulfur dioxide-induced bronchoconstriction in asthmatic subjects. *Am Rev Respir Dis* (1981) **123**: 486–491.
6. Bethel RA, Erle DJ, Epstein J, Sheppard D, Nadel J, Boushey HA: Effect of exercise rate and route of inhalation on sulfur dioxide induced bronchoconstriction in asthmatic subjects. *Am Rev Respir Dis* (1983) **128**: 592–596.
7. Bethel RA, Epstein J, Sheppard D, Nadel JA, Boushey HA: Sulfur dioxide induced bronchoconstriction in freely breathing exercising asthmatic subjects. *Am Rev Respir Dis* (1983) **128**: 987–990.
8. Koenig JQ, Pierson WE, Horike M, Frank NR: Effects of inhaled sulfur dioxide (SO_2) on pulmonary function in healthy adolescents. Exposure to SO_2 alone or SO_2 + sodium chloride droplet aerosol during rest and exercise. *Environ Res* (1982) **37**: 5–9.
9. Nadel JA, Salem H, Tamplin B, Tokjwa G: Mechanism of bronchoconstriction during inhalation of sulfur dioxide. *J Appl Physiol* (1965) **20**: 164–167.
10. Frank NR, Amdur MO, Whittenberger JH: Effects of acute controlled exposure to SO_2 on respiratory mechanics in healthy male adults. *J Appl Physiol* (1962) **17**: 252–258.
11. Frank NR, Speizer FE: SO_2 effects on the respiratory system in dogs: changes in mechanical behavior at different levels of the respiratory system during acute exposure to the gas. *Arch Environ Health* (1965) **11**: 624–634.
12. Amdur MO: Respiratory absorption data and SO_2 dose-response curves. *Arch Environ Health* (1966) **112**: 729–736.
13. Committee on Sulfur Oxides: Sulfur Oxides, Washington DC, National Academy of Sciences, 1978.
14. Leaderer BP: Air pollutant emission from kerosene heaters. *Science* (1982) **218**: 1113–1115.
15. Sheppard D, Wong SC, Uehara CF, Nadel JA, Boushey HA: Lower threshold and greater bronchomotor responsiveness of asthmatic subjects to sulfur dioxide. *Am Rev Respir Dis* (1980) **122**: 873–878.
16. Frank NR, Yoder RE, Brain JD, Yokoyama E: SO_2 (^{35}S-labeled) absorption by the nose and mouth under conditions of varying concentration and flow. *Arch Environ Health* (1969) **18**: 315–322.
17. Bethel RA, Sheppard D, Geffroy B, Tam E, Nadel JA, Boushey HA: Effect of 0.25 ppm sulfur dioxide on airway resistance in freely breathing, heavily exercising, asthmatic subjects. *Am Rev Respir Dis* (1985) **131**: 659–661.
18. Linn WS, Venet TG, Shamoo DA, *et al.*: Respiratory effects of sulfur dioxide in heavily exercising asthmatics: a dose-response study. *Am Rev Respir Dis* (1983) **127**: 278–283.
19. Sheppard D, Epstein J, Bethel RA, Nadel J, Boushey HA: Tolerance to sulfur dioxide-induced bronchoconstriction in subjects with asthma. *Environ Res* (1983) **30**: 412–419.
20. Sheppard D, Eschenbacher WL, Boushey HA, Bethel RA: Magnitude of the interaction between the bronchomotor effects of sulfur dioxide and those of dry (cold) air. *Am Rev Respir Dis* (1984) **130**: 52–55.

21. Bethel RA, Sheppard D, Epstein J, Tam E, Nadel JA, Boushey HA: Interaction of sulfur dioxide and airway cooling in causing bronchoconstriction in people who have asthma. *J Appl Physiol* (1984) **57**: 419–423.

22. Linn WS, Shamoo DA, Anderson KR, Whynot JD, Avol EL, Hackney JD: Effects of heat and humidity on the responses of exercising asthmatics to sulfur dioxide. *Am Rev Respir Dis* (1985) **13**: 222–225.

23. Fine JM, Gordon T, Thompson JE, Sheppard D: The role of titratable acidity in acid aerosol-induced bronchoconstriction. *Am Rev Respir Dis* (1987) **135**: 826–830.

24. Romanoff A: Sulfur dioxide poisoning as a cause of asthma. *J Allergy* (1938) 166–169.

25. Flury KE, Dines DE, Rodarte JR, Rodgers R: Airway obstruction due to inhalation of ammonia. *Mayo Clin Proc* (1983) **58**: 389–393.

26. Brooks SM, Weiss MA, Bernstein IH: Reactive airways dysfunction syndrome (RADS); Persistent asthma syndrome after high level irritant exposures. *Chest* (1985) **88**: 376–384.

27. Easton RE, Murphy SD: Experimental ozone preexposure and histamine. *Arch Environ Health* (1967) **15**: 160–166.

28. Lee L-Y, Bleecker EA, Nadel JA: Effect of ozone on bronchomotor response to inhaled histamine aerosol in dogs. *J Appl Physiol* (1977) **43**: 626–631.

29. Golden J, Nadel JA, Boushey HA: Bronchial hyperirritability in healthy subjects after exposure to ozone. *Am Rev Respir Dis* (1978) **118**: 287–294.

30. Gordon T, Amdur MO: Effect of ozone on respiratory response of guinea pigs to histamine. *J Toxicol Environ Health* (1980) **6**: 185–191.

31. Holtzman MJ. Fabbri LM, O'Byrne PM, *et al.*: Importance of airway inflammation for hyperresponsiveness induced by ozone. *Am Rev Respir Dis* (1983) **127**: 686–690.

32. Hulbert WM, Mclean T, Hogg JC: The effect of acute inflammation on bronchial reactivity in guinea pigs. *Am Rev Respir Dis* (1985) **132**: 7–11.

33. Sheppard D, Distefano S, Morse L, Becker C: Acute effects of routine firefighting on lung function. *Am J Ind Med* (1986) **9**: 333–340.

34. Gordon T, Sheppard D, McDonald D, Scypinski L, Distefano S: Airway hyperresponsiveness and inflammation induced by toluene diisocyanate in guinea pigs. *Am Rev Respir Dis* (1985) **132**: 1106–1112.

35. Cibulus W Jr, Murlas CG, Miller ML, *et al.*: Toluene diisocyanate-induced airway hyperreactivity and pathology in the guinea pig. *J Allergy Clin Immunol* (1986) **77**: 828–834.

36. O'Byrne PM, Walter E, Gold B, *et al.*: Neutrophil depletion inhibits airway hyperresponsiveness induced by ozone. *Am Rev Respir Dis* (1984) **130**: 214–219.

37. Murlas C, Roum J: Bronchial reactivity occurs in steroid-treated guinea pigs depleted of leukocytes by cyclophosphamide. *J Appl Physiol* (1985) **58**: 1630–1637.

38. Thompson JE, Scypinski L, Gordon T, Sheppard D: Hydroxyurea inhibits airway hyperresponsiveness in guinea pigs by a granulocyte-independent mechanism. *Am Rev Respir Dis* (1986) **134**: 1713–1718.

39. O'Byrne P, Walters EH, Aizawa H, Fabbri LM, Holtzman MJ, Nadel JA: Indomethacin inhibits the airway hyperresponsiveness, but not the neutrophil influx induced by ozone in dogs. *Am Rev Respir Dis* (1984) **130**: 220–224.

40. Aizawa H, Chung KF, Leikauf GD, *et al.*: Significance of thromboxane generation in ozone-induced airway hyperresponsiveness in dogs. *J Appl Physiol* (1985) **59**: 1918–1923.

41. Lee HK, Murlas C: Ozone-induced bronchial hyperreactivity in guinea pigs is abolished by BW755C or FPL55712 but not by indomethacin. *Am Rev Respir Dis* (1985) **132**: 1005–1009.

42. Leikauf GD, Doupnik CA, Leming LM, Wey HE: Sulfidopeptide leukotrienes mediate acrolein-induced bronchial hyperresponsiveness. *Am Phys Society* (1989): 1838.

43. Gordon T, Thompson JE, Sheppard D: Modulation by arachidonic acid metabolites of the toluene diisocyanate airway hyperresponsiveness in guinea pigs. *Prostaglandins* (1988) **35**: 699–706.

44. Thompson J, Gordon T, Scypinski L, Sheppard D: The role of tachykinins in TDI-induced airway hyperresponsiveness. *Am Rev Respir Dis* (1987) **136**: 43–49.

45. Sheppard D, Thompson JE, Scypinski L, Dusser D, Nadel JA, Borson DB: Toluene diisocyanate increases airway responsiveness to substance P and decreases airway neutral endopeptidase. *J Clin Invest* (1988) **81**: 1111–1115.

Drug-induced Asthma

PETER J. BARNES AND NEIL C. THOMSON

ASPIRIN-INDUCED ASTHMA

In the early part of this century it was first recognized that aspirin could precipitate asthma in susceptible individuals.[1] Similar asthmatic reactions were later shown to occur with other non-steroid anti-inflammatory drugs.[2–4] It was also demonstrated that patients with aspirin-induced asthma were sensitive to other cyclooxygenase inhibitors.[4] Various terms have been used to describe this asthmatic reaction including aspirin-induced asthma, aspirin-sensitive asthma or aspirin hypersensitivity, idiosyncratic reaction to aspirin, aspirin intolerance or aspirin allergy.

Clinical features

Aspirin-induced asthma is characterized by the development of bronchoconstriction within minutes to several hours after the ingestion of aspirin or other non-steroidal anti-inflammatory drugs.[2–4] The asthmatic reaction may be associated with other symptoms including rhinorrhoea, flushing, loss of consciousness, and very rarely the attack may be fatal.

In the typical case the patient has had symptoms of chronic rhinitis for many years before asthma develops. The rhinitis starts as intermittent watery rhinorrhoea which develops during the second or third decade of life. The rhinorrhoea becomes progressively more severe and is complicated by nasal polyp formation and sinusitis. In later years symptoms of asthma appear associated with the development of acute asthma after the ingestion of cyclooxygenase inhibitors. Although the latter drugs may precipitate asthma these patients continue to have nasal and asthmatic symptoms in the absence of

ASTHMA: BASIC MECHANISMS AND CLINICAL MANAGEMENT (2nd Edn)
ISBN 0-12-079026-2

ingesting aspirin or non-steroidal anti-inflammatory drugs. Respiratory symptoms tend to be chronic, severe, perennial and steroid dependent. Individuals with aspirin-induced asthma are more commonly female. Skin tests to common external allergens are usually negative but the eosinophil count is elevated. A small percentage of patients with aspirin-induced asthma also develop associated symptoms of urticaria and angioedema after ingestion of aspirin.[5,7]

Incidence

The true incidence of aspirin-induced asthma is unknown and estimates vary from 1.9 to 19% of asthmatic patients.[6,8-12] Many of these studies are undertaken in specialized allergy centres which may result in an over-estimate of the incidence of aspirin-induced asthma in the general population.[13] Incidence figures based on a history of aspirin-induced asthma only, are lower than surveys based on oral aspirin challenge. In adult asthmatic patients the incidence rises from 3 to 5% based on historical data only[9] to 8–19% based on the results of oral challenge.[6,10] Similarly, in children with asthma the incidence rises from 1.9% based on historical data[8] to 13% based on the results of oral challenge.[12]

Diagnosis

In most clinical circumstances the diagnosis is based on a history of bronchoconstriction following the ingestion of a cyclooxygenase inhibitor. It should be appreciated that a history of either the presence or absence of aspirin-induced asthma may result in both false positive and false negative diagnosis. For example after oral aspirin challenge the reported incidence is approximately 9% in adult asthmatic patients with no history of aspirin-induced asthma,[10] approximately 30% in patients with no history of aspirin-induced asthma but who do have chronic steroid-dependent asthma, chronic rhinitis and nasal polyps and 60–85% in patients with a history of aspirin-induced asthma.[10,11] The negative oral challenge results in some patients with a history of aspirin-induced asthma may be due to changing responsiveness to aspirin, a high threshold to aspirin or to a misleading history.[10]

Aspirin challenge is indicated in adult asthmatic patients who require treatment with a non-steroidal anti-inflammatory drug. The oral challenge procedure has been reported to be safe provided a standardized protocol is used.[10,11,13] The challenge should be undertaken in hospital, by experienced physicians, and when the patient's asthma is stable and the FEV_1 is 1.5 litres or greater. Bronchodilators such as β-adrenergic agonists, antihistamines,[14] sodium cromoglycate[15,16] and ketotifen[17] should be withheld for the duration of the action of the drug prior to challenge. Corticosteroids and theophylline can be continued.[13] Some investigators undertake the challenge by the double blind sequential administration of 15, 37.5, 75, 150, 325 mg of aspirin randomized with placebo on different days.[10] Others undertake the challenge over 2 days.[13] On one day increasing doses of aspirin are administered with at least 3 h elapsing between doses. On the other day a control placebo challenge is performed. A 20–25% fall in FEV_1 from baseline values is considered a positive test.[10,11] Very sensitive patients will bronchoconstrict to 30 mg of aspirin or less.

An alternative but less widely used method of detecting aspirin-induced asthma is undertaken by administering aspirin by inhalation.[18,19] An 18% solution of lysine acetylsalicylate which, unlike aspirin, is soluble in water, nebulized at hourly intervals for 30 s and then 2 min using a 1 in 3 dilution and then for 5 min using the undiluted solution. A control inhalation is performed on a separate day using a lysine solution. It is claimed that this method is safe and that compared to oral challenge the procedure is shorter and the reaction is localized to the respiratory tract.[19] Most patients with a positive reaction respond to the first 30-s inhalation of lysine acetylsalicylate.[19]

Until recently no *in vitro* test has been available to detect aspirin-induced asthma. Ameisen *et al.*[20] have identified an abnormality of platelet activation specific to patients with aspirin-induced asthma. Cyclooxygenase drugs induce *in vitro* activation of platelets as assessed by the release of cytocidal mediators measured by the percentage of killed *Schistosoma mansoni* parasites, and by the generation of oxygen metabolites measured by chemiluminescence in patients with aspirin-induced asthma but not in asthmatic controls. These findings could be developed into an *in vitro* diagnostic test for aspirin-induced asthma.[20]

Mechanisms

Abnormality of arachidonic acid metabolism

A characteristic feature of patients with aspirin-induced asthma is the occurrence of airway obstruction following the ingestion of drugs that inhibit cyclooxygenase, the enzyme that converts arachidonic acid into prostaglandins and thromboxanes. The severity of the asthmatic attack induced by aspirin or other non-steroid anti-inflammatory drugs such as indomethacin, flufenamic acid, mefanamic acid and naproxen is directly proportional to their ability to inhibit cyclooxygenase *in vitro*.[4] Based on these findings it has been proposed that inhibition of cyclooxygenase in the respiratory tract of patients with aspirin-induced asthma is central to the development of an asthma attack after the ingestion of non-steroidal anti-inflammatory drugs.[4,21] Although the site within the respiratory tract where this proposed biochemical event might take place is unknown, several different mechanisms have been postulated by which inhibition of cyclooxygenase might result in bronchoconstriction.[22]

Firstly, enhanced synthesis of products of the lipoxygenase pathway following inhibition of the cyclooxygenase pathway would result in the release of bronchoconstrictor mediators such as leukotrienes.[23] This reaction would either have to occur more readily in patients with aspirin-induced asthma or they would require to be more sensitive to the effects of the leukotrienes. In support of this hypothesis aspirin challenge causes the release of immunoreactive LTC_4 into nasal secretions of patients with aspirin-induced asthma, but not in controls or in patients after desensitization to aspirin.[24] Basal levels of LTE_4 are increased in the urine of aspirin-sensitive patients and there is a further increase in LTE_4 after challenge with aspirin.[25,26] Furthermore, aspirin-sensitive patients show a selective increased airway responsiveness to LTE_4 which is lost after desensitization.[27]

Secondly, the influence of prostaglandins and thromboxanes on airway cells may differ between asthmatic patients with and without aspirin-induced asthma.[4,21] The control of airway calibre in this latter group could be more dependent on a direct bronchodilator effect of prostaglandins such as PGE_2 or PGI_2 or these agents might normally suppress the release of bronchoconstrictor mediators such as histamine.[28] Recently Szczeklik[29] proposed that non-steroidal anti-inflammatory drugs block the inhibitory effect of PGE_2 on cytotoxic lymphocytes that have been produced against virus-infected respiratory cells. In the absence of PGE_2 the cytotoxic lymphocytes would release inflammatory mediators. Alternatively, it has been suggested that non-steroidal anti-inflammatory drugs could produce a greater inhibition in the synthesis of broncho-dilator prostaglandins than bronchoconstrictor substances such as PGD_2, PGF_α or the thromboxanes, and that these patients are more sensitive to one or more of these bronchoconstrictor mediators.

There is, however, no direct evidence to support a specific defect in arachidonic acid metabolism in the lung of patients with aspirin-induced asthma. Nevertheless, there are some unexplained differences between patients with and without aspirin-induced asthma that suggest there may be an abnormality of the cyclooxygenase pathway in the aspirin-induced asthma group, although the nature of such a defect is uncertain. Firstly patients with aspirin-induced asthma are more sensitive to inhaled PGE_2[30] and less sensitive to inhaled PGF_α[30,31] than other asthmatic patients. Secondly, specimens of nasal polyps removed from patients with aspirin-induced asthma have been reported to be more sensitive to the inhibition effects of aspirin on the cyclooxygenase pathway.[32] Thirdly, basal plasma levels of $PGF_{2\alpha}$ are significantly higher in patients with aspirin-induced asthma than in control subjects.[33] Fourthly, alveolar macrophages obtained by bronchoalveolar lavage release reduced amounts of PGE_2, PGF_α and thromboxane B_2 in aspirin-sensitive patients.[34]

Abnormality of platelet function

A specific abnormality of platelet function has been found in patients with aspirin-induced asthma.[20] Drugs that inhibit the cyclooxygenase pathway cause *in vitro* activation of platelets as demonstrated by increased platelet chemiluminescence and by an increased percentage of dead *S. mansoni* larvae after incubation of the platelets and parasites for 24 h.[20] These results were not found with platelets obtained from allergic asthmatics or healthy controls, nor from basophils or monocytes from patients with aspirin-induced asthma. The abnormality of platelet function can be inhibited by preincubation of the platelets with prostaglandin endoperoxides and sodium salicylate. These results have been interpreted as indicating that platelets may be involved in the pathogenesis of aspirin-induced asthma due perhaps to an abnormality in the control by prostaglandin endoperoxides of the activation processes in the platelet.[35] Pearson and Suarez-Mendez[36] confirmed an abnormality of platelet function in eight individuals out of a mixed group of 25 aspirin-sensitive patients. The proportion of patients with aspirin-sensitive asthma with this abnormality was, however, higher. The mean level of glutathione peroxidase, an important enzyme in the degradation of hydrogen peroxide, was significantly lower in the aspirin-sensitive group suggesting an abnormality in oxygen peroxide metabolism may be involved in aspirin-sensitive asthma.

Other mechanisms

Recently, a significant increase in HLA-DQW2 was reported in patients with aspirin-induced asthma suggesting this or an associated genetic factor may be involved in the pathogenesis of this disorder.[37] There is no convincing evidence that aspirin-induced asthma is due to IgE-mediated mechanisms.[38] For example specific anti-aspiryl IgE antibodies are generally absent[39] and skin tests to aspiryl-polylysine negative[40] in these patients. Skin-prick test reactivity to a non-immunological stimulus such as codeine phosphate is similar to control subjects.[33] Basal and post-aspirin challenge complement levels are not altered in patients with aspirin-induced asthma.[41,42]

Inflammatory mediators such as histamine[43] and neutrophil chemotactic factor[44,45] blood levels are raised after aspirin challenge in patients with aspirin-induced asthma although these changes are thought to be secondary to the primary biochemical events.

Desensitization

Following the administration of oral or inhaled aspirin to patients with aspirin-induced asthma there is a refractory period to further aspirin challenge which lasts for 2–5 days.[13,19,46,47] Continued administration of aspirin on a daily basis will maintain this refractory state, and this effect has been termed desensitization.[46,47] Patients are not only desensitized to aspirin but also to other non-steroidal anti-inflammatory drugs. Those patients who react to small doses of aspirin require several aspirin challenges before desensitization is accomplished whereas less aspirin-sensitive patients are more quickly desensitized.[47]

The processes by which aspirin ingestion might cause desensitization is unknown[38] although it is associated with reversal of the abnormal platelet function found in aspirin-induced asthmatic patients[20] and with LTE_4-induced airway hyperresponsiveness.[27]

Management

Patients with a history of acute bronchoconstrictor response after the ingestion of aspirin or a non-steroidal anti-inflammatory drug must be warned to avoid these drugs in the future. If they require a simple analgesic then non cyclooxygenase inhibiting agents such as paracetamol (acetaminophen) and sodium salicylate should not cross-react with aspirin. However, care should be exercised in prescribing these drugs since a small percentage of patients with aspirin-induced asthma can react to paracetamol.[48] If a patient with aspirin-induced asthma should require a non-steroidal anti-inflammatory drug for the treatment of another condition such as arthritis then the patient can be desensitized to aspirin. This procedure should be undertaken in hospital by doctors with experience in aspirin challenge.

These patients frequently have severe chronic asthma unrelated to the ingestion of non-steroidal anti-inflammatory drugs. Treatment of their asthma is along similar lines to non-aspirin-induced asthma patients, i.e. inhaled bronchodilators, inhaled steroids, oral steroids, etc. Pretreatment with a number of drugs including sodium cromoglycate,[15] the H_1 receptor antagonist clemastine,[14] and ketotifen[17] can inhibit the bronchoconstrictor response to aspirin ingestion in patients with aspirin-induced asthma. A small percentage of patients with aspirin-induced asthma develop bronchoconstriction after the intravenous injection of hydrocortisone[49] and occasionally the bronchospastic response can be severe.[50] These patients do not react adversely to other intravenous steroids such as methylprednisolone, dexamethasone or betamethasone[49] and it has been suggested that these steroids rather than hydrocortisone should be used in patients with aspirin-induced asthma.

Finally since chronic aspirin desensitization and sodium salicylate both inhibit the abnormal platelet response found in patients with aspirin-induced asthma it has been suggested that these forms of treatment might not only prevent the bronchoconstrictor response to aspirin ingestion but might also influence the long-term severity of the disease.[20,51]

β-BLOCKERS

Worsening or precipitation of asthma by β-adrenoceptor antagonists was observed shortly after their introduction into clinical practice.[52,53] Although this property of β-blockers is well recognized, occasional reports of fatal asthma precipitated by β-blockers still occur and severe asthma may be precipitated even in relatively mild asthmatics. The dose of β-blocker required to precipitate bronchoconstriction may be low and there are several reports of severe asthma precipitated by eye drops of timolol, a non-selective β-blocker used to treat glaucoma.[54,55] Propafenone is a new anti-arrythmic agent with a structure similar to propranolol that has been reported to cause bronchoconstriction in asthmatics.[56]

The severity of bronchoconstrictor response to a given β-antagonist is not predictable and does not appear to relate closely to the degree of airway hyperresponsiveness. The amount of bronchodilatation with a β-agonist may be an indication of sensitivity to β-blockers,[57] and patients with chronic obstructive airways disease are less likely to develop deterioration in lung function after a β-blocker.[58,59]

Non-selective β-blockers are more likely to precipitate bronchospasm than β_1-selective drugs. Thus, atenolol, acebutolol and metoprolol may give less fall in lung function than propranolol in asthmatic subjects.[60-64] Moreover, any fall in lung function found with β_1-selective antagonists is reversible by an inhaled β_2-agonist. This may be explained by the fact that there are no bronchodilator β_1-receptors in human airways.[65,66] Non-selective β-blockers with intrinsic sympathomimetic activity, such as pindolol, are also less likely to produce bronchoconstriction than those without,[60] although the bronchoconstriction with any non-selective β-blocker cannot be reversed by a β_2-agonist.

Since the severity of bronchoconstriction that will result from a β-blocker is not predictable, it is safest to avoid *all* β-blockers, even if β_1-selective, in all patients with airway obstruction. Safe alternative therapies exist for both hypertension (such as thiazides, calcium antagonists, ACE inhibitors, hydralazine, clonidine, prazosin and α-methyl dopa) and ischaemic heart disease (calcium antagonists, nitrates).

Possible mechanisms

Despite the fact that β-blocker-induced asthma has been recognized for over 20 years, the mechanism is still not certain. Normal subjects do not develop any deterioration in lung function after β-blockers,[67,68] and do not show an increase in sensitivity to bronchoconstricting agents such as histamine or methacholine.[69] This suggests that some endogenous activation of β-receptors may be important in asthmatic subjects to counteract bronchoconstrictor mechanisms (neural and inflammatory mediators).

Because most cases of bronchoconstriction were associated with propranolol, it was suggested that the mechanism was unrelated to β-blockade, and could be explained by some non-specific property of propranolol (such as membrane-stabilizing activity). In rodents it was found that D-propranolol, which has no significant β-blocking effect, was as potent as L-propranolol in causing bronchoconstriction,[70,71] and D-propranolol was as potent as L-propranolol in releasing histamine from guinea-pig lung.[72] In asthmatic subjects, however, while infused racemic DL-propranolol causes bronchoconstriction, D-propranolol does not, and the bronchoconstrictor response is related to the degree of β-blockade as assessed by isoprenaline dose-response curves.[73]

β-Blockers presumably antagonize some tonic adrenergic bronchodilator tone that is present in asthmatic patients, but not in normal subjects. Since human airway smooth muscle has no demonstrated adrenergic innervation,[74] this might suggest that circulating catecholamines might provide this drive.[75] Yet circulating catecholamines are not elevated in asthmatic subjects,[76] even in those subjects who have demonstrable bronchoconstriction after propranolol[77] (see Chapter 22). In any case, the concentrations of adrenaline in plasma (< 0.3 nmol/litre) are too low to have a direct effect on human airway smooth muscle tone. This has suggested that β-blockers may inhibit the action of catecholamines on some other target cell, such as airway mast cells or cholinergic nerves. Mediator release from human lung mast cells is potently inhibited by β-agonists.[78] The effect of β-blockers may, therefore, be an increase in mediator release, which may be more marked in the 'leaky' mast cells of asthmatics. This idea is supported by the observation that sodium cromoglycate, a mast cell 'stabilizer', prevents the bronchoconstriction produced by inhaled propranolol.[79] However, after intravenous propranolol, no increase in plasma histamine has been detected.[73]

A more likely explanation for β-blocker-induced asthma is that there is an increase in neural bronchoconstrictor mechanisms. β_2-Receptors on cholinergic nerves in human airways[80] may be tonically activated by adrenaline to modulate acetylcholine (ACh) release and therefore to dampen cholinergic tone. Blockade of these receptors would therefore increase the amount of ACh released tonically, but this would be compensated for by the increased stimulation of prejunctional M_2-autoreceptors which would act homeostatically to inhibit any increase in ACh release,[81] and therefore no increase in airway tone would occur, even with high doses of β-blocker. By contrast, in asthmatic patients β-blockers inhibit prejunctional β-receptors in the same way, increasing the release of ACh, but as discussed in Chapter 22, there may be a defect in M_2-receptor function in asthmatic airways, so that the increased release in ACh cannot be compensated. Thus increased ACh reaches M_3-receptors on airway smooth muscle. In addition bronchoconstrictor responses to ACh are exaggerated in asthma as part of airway hyperresponsiveness and thus two interacting amplifying mechanisms may lead to marked bronchoconstriction. Since the apparent defect in M_2-receptors may occur even in patients with mild asthma,[82,83] this explains why β-blockers may be dangerous even in patients with relatively mild asthma. Evidence to support this theory is provided by the inhibitory effect of an inhaled anticholinergic drug oxitropium bromide on β-blocker-induced asthma.[84]

In patients with more severe asthma there may be an additional neural mechanism by which β-blockers may cause bronchoconstriction. β_2-Receptors inhibit the release of tachykinins from airway sensory nerves,[84;85] and thus β-blockers may increase the release of these neuropeptides, thereby increasing bronchoconstriction and airway inflammation. While this mechanism may not be relevant in patients with mild asthma, in whom cholinergic mechanisms appear to account for the bronchoconstrictor response to β-blockers,[83] it may be relevant in more severe asthmatic patients in whom cholinergic mechanisms do not appear to be as important.

LOCAL ANAESTHETICS

Local anaesthetics inhibit different vagal sensory endings and postganglionic parasympathetic motor fibres in animals.[86,87] *In vitro* studies have shown that the local anaesthetic lignocaine can inhibit and reverse the contraction induced by histamine and acetylcholine in isolated guinea-pig trachealis muscle,[88] and also inhibit mediator release from passively sensitized guinea-pig lung tissue.[89] The inhibiting effect of lignocaine on smooth muscle contraction and mediator release from mast cells may be due to effects on calcium binding or flux.[89] These effects on neural reflexes, smooth muscle contraction and mediator release from mast cells in the lungs would suggest that local anaesthetics might be useful in the treatment of asthma.

In both normal subjects and asthmatic patients the cough reflex elicited by citric acid or capsaicin can be abolished following inhalation of the local anaesthetics bupivacaine or lignocaine.[90–92] Weiss and Patwardhan[93] reported that lignocaine had a protective effect against methacholine-induced bronchospasm in asthmatic patients. Pretreatment with inhaled local anaesthetics, however, does not inhibit exercise-induced asthma[94,95] or bronchoconstriction induced by inhaled distilled water aerosol in asthmatics,[96] or bronchospasm induced by histamine, methacholine, $PGF_{2\alpha}$ or capsaicin in normal subjects.[91,92]

Several studies have found that aerosols of the local anaesthetics bupivacaine and lignocaine produce a bronchoconstriction response in a proportion of asthmatic patients[90,91,93–95,97–99] but not in normal subjects.[90,91] The degree of histamine airway hyperresponsiveness does not predict the development or extent of bronchoconstriction following lignocaine inhalation.[99] The mechanism of local-anaesthetic-induced bronchoconstriction is unclear. Pretreatment with anticholinergic drugs partially attenuates the bronchoconstrictor response to aerosols of local anaesthetics suggesting that they may be acting partially via a vagal pathway.[91,93,97] Possibly inhaled local anaesthetics selectively inhibit non-adrenergic non-cholinergic bronchodilator nerves and allow unopposed vagal tone. Some evidence for this is provided by the demonstration that lignocaine inhalation blocks non-adrenergic non-cholinergic reflex bronchodilatation in human subjects, leading to a reflex bronchoconstrictor response.[100]

It is important to be aware that some asthmatic patients may develop bronchoconstriction with topical local anaesthetics during fibreoptic bronchoscopy. All asthmatic patients should receive premedication with a bronchodilator prior to bronchoscopy.

ADDITIVES

Several chemicals that are used as additives to drug preparations and food have been associated with worsening of asthma and should, where possible, be avoided.

Tartrazine

Tartrazine (E102), a yellow dye, is used as a colouring in many foods, beverages (such as orange squash) and pharmaceutical preparations. Tartrazine sensitivity is relatively common and may affect 4% of asthmatics, especially children.[101,102] Ingestion of tartrazine may result in urticarial rashes and bronchoconstriction. The mechanism may depend upon mediator release from mast cells. As previously discussed, there is no association between tartrazine sensitivity and aspirin-induced asthma.[101]

Benzalkonium chloride

Benzalkonium chloride is a bactericidal compound added to certain nebulizer solutions, such as ipratropium bromide nebulizer solution. Paradoxical bronchoconstriction with nebulized ipratropium bromide was reported in asthma and was initially ascribed to the hypotonicity of the nebulizer solution.[103] When this was corrected by the use of isotonic solutions, bronchoconstriction was still occasionally reported, which might be explained by the presence of the preservatives benzalkonium chloride and ethylene diamine tetraacetic acid (EDTA) in the nebulizer solution.[104] Nebulization of ipratropium bromide with preservatives causes significant bronchoconstriction in a proportion of asthmatic patients, whereas nebulization of ipratropium bromide alone gives the expected bronchodilator response.[104,105] Nebulization of the preservatives gave a bronchoconstrictor response. The presence of benzalkonium chloride in beclomethasone nebulizer solution may also explain the bronchoconstriction that has been reported with this solution.[106] The mechanism of bronchoconstriction may be due to release of mediators from mast cells, perhaps due to a non-specific effect on the cell membrane.

Metabisulphite

Bisulphites and metabisulphites (E220, 221, 222, 226 and 227) are anti-oxidants used as preservatives in several foods, including wines (especially sparkling wines), beer, fruit juices, salads and medications. Characteristically, they produce bronchoconstriction within 30 min of ingestion[107,108] and this may account for several cases of 'food allergy'. The mechanism of metabisulphite-induced asthma is probably explained by release of sulphur dioxide after ingestion which is then inhaled, since nebulized metabisulphite solutions generate SO_2 in sufficient quantities to provoke bronchoconstriction in asthmatic subjects.[109,110]

Monosodium glutamate

Monosodium glutamate (MSG, E621) is added to food as a flavour enhancer. It is found in soy sauce, spices, stock cubes, hamburgers and in Chinese restaurant food. Some people react with sweating, flushing and numbness of the chest; in patients with asthma this may be accompanied by wheezing, which may begin several hours after ingestion ('Chinese restaurant asthma syndrome').[111,112]

ACE INHIBITORS

There has recently been concern that drugs that inhibit angiotensin converting enzyme (ACE), such as captopril and enalapril, might lead to exacerbation of asthma, since ACE is an enzyme that degrades the bronchoconstrictor mediator bradykinin. Exacerbation of asthma has only very rarely been reported in patients with asthma after ACE inhibitors.

Administration of a potent ACE inhibitor (ramipril) to a group of mild asthmatics showed no change in lung function or bronchial reactivity to inhaled histamine, nor was there any increase in bronchoconstrictor response to inhaled bradykinin.[113] As many as 20% of hypertensive patients treated with ACE inhibitors may develop an irritant cough,[114] but this is unrelated to the presence of underlying airway disease or atopic status. Perhaps this might be related to inhibition of bradykinin metabolism, with resultant stimulation of unmyelinated C-fibres in the larynx. ACE-inhibitor cough is prevented by cyclooxygenase inhibitors,[115] and may be due to prostaglandin release by endogenous bradykinin, since PGE_2 and $PGF_{2\alpha}$ increase cough sensitivity.[116,117]

OTHER DRUGS

Many other drugs have been reported to lead to exacerbation of asthma in occasional patients. Bronchoconstriction may constitute part of an anaphylactic reaction to a drug, such as penicillin.[118] Other drugs, such as opiates, may cause direct degranulation of mast cells. Bronchoconstriction has also rarely been reported in association with a wide variety of drugs, including nitrofurantoin, pyrazone derivatives, ACTH, aminophylline, insulin, α-methyldopa, bleomycin, carbamazepine and tetracyclines.[119]

Bronchodilator aerosols may occasionally cause a paradoxical bronchoconstriction. This is presumed to be due to the propellant (freon) or other additives (such as oleic acid which is used as a surfactant).[120–122] The mechanism of bronchoconstriction may be via a cholinergic reflex.

REFERENCES

1. Cooke RA: Allergy in drug idiosyncrasy. *J Am Med A* (1919) **73**: 759–760.
2. Vanselow NA, Smith JR: Bronchial asthma induced by indomethacin. *Ann Inter med* (1967) **66**: 567–572.

3. Smith AP: Response of aspirin-allergic patients to challenge by some analgesics in common use. *Br Med J* (1971) **2**: 494–496.

4. Szczeklik A, Gryglewski PR, Czerniawaska MG: Relationship of inhibition of prostaglandin biosynthesis by analgesics to asthma attacks in aspirin sensitive patients. *Br Med J* (1975) **1**: 67–69.

5. Samter M, Beers RF: Intolerance to aspirin. Clinical studies and consideration of its pathogenesis. *Ann Intern Med* (1968) **68**: 975–983.

6. McDonald JR, Mathison DA, Stevenson DD: Aspirin intolerance in asthma. *J Allergy Clin Immunol* (1972) **50**: 198–207.

7. Szczeklik A, Gryglewski PR, Czerniawska MG: Clinical patterns of hypersensitivity to nonsteroidal anti-inflammatory drugs and their pathogenesis. *J Allergy Clin Immunol* (1977) **60**: 276–284.

8. Falliers CJ: Aspirin and subtypes of asthma: risk factors analysis. *J Allergy Clin Immunol* (1973) **53**: 141–147.

9. Giraldo B, Bumethal MN, Spink WW: Aspirin intolerance and asthma. Clinical and immunological study. *Ann Intern Med* (1969) **71**: 479–496.

10. Spector SL, Wangaard CH, Farr RS: Aspirin and concomitant idiosyncrasies in adult asthmatic patients. *J Allergy Clin Immunol* (1979) **64**: 500–506.

11. Pleskow WW, Stevenson DD, Mathison DA, Schatz M, Zeiger RS: Aspirin sensitive rhinosinusitis/asthma: spectrum of adverse reactions. *J Allergy Clin Immunol* (1983) **71**: 574–579.

12. Vedanthan PR, Menon MM, Bell TD, Bergin D: Aspirin and tartrazine oral challenge: incidence of adverse response in chronic childhood asthma. *J Allergy Clin Immunol* (1977) **60**: 8–13.

13. Stevenson DD: Adverse reactions to aspirin and nonsteroidal anti-inflammatory drugs. In Reed CE (ed) *Proceedings of the XII International Congress of Allergology and Clinical Immunology* 1985, pp 79–83.

14. Szczeklik A, Serwonska M: Inhibition of idiosyncratic reactions to aspirin in asthmatic patients with clemastine. *Thorax* (1979) **34**: 654–657.

15. Martelli NA, Usandivaras G: Inhibition of aspirin-induced bronchoconstriction by sodium cromoglycate inhalation. *Thorax* (1977) **32**: 684–690.

16. Martelli NA: Bronchial and intravenous provocation tests with indomethacin in aspirin-sensitive asthmatics. *Am Rev Respir Dis* (1979) **120**: 1073–1079.

17. Szczeklik A, Czerniawska MG, Serwonska M, Kuklinski P: Inhibition by ketotifen of idiosyncratic reactions to aspirin. *Allergy* (1980) **35**: 421–424.

18. Pasargiklian M, Bianco S, Allegra L, et al.: Aspects of bronchial reactivity to prostaglandins and aspirin in asthmatic patients. *Respiration* (1977) **34**: 78–91.

19. Bianco S, Robuschi M, Petrigni G: Aspirin sensitivity in asthmatics. *Br Med J* (1981) **282**: 146.

20. Ameison JC, Capron A, Joseph M, et al.: Aspirin-sensitive asthma: abnormal platelet response to drugs inducing asthmatic attacks. *Int Archs Allergy Appl Immunol* (1985) **78**: 438–448.

21. Szczeklik A: Aspirin-sensitive asthma and arachidonic acid transformation. In Reed CE (ed) *Proceedings of the XII International Congress of Allergology and Clinical Immunology* 1986, pp 504–508.

22. Szczeklik A: The cyclooxygenase theory of aspirin-induced asthma. *Eur Resp J* (1990) **3**: 588–593.

23. Undem BJ, Pickett WC, Lichtenstein LM, Adams GK: The effect of indomethacin on immunologic release of histamine and sulfidopeptide leukotrienes from human bronchus and lung parenchyma. *Am Rev Respir Dis* (1987) **136**: 1183–1187.

24. Ferreri NR, Howland WC, Stevenson DD, Spiegelberg HL: Release of leukotrienes, prostaglandins and histamine into nasal secretions of aspirin-sensitive asthmatics during reaction to aspirin. *Am Rev Respir Dis* (1988) **137**: 847–854.

25. Dahlen B, Kumlin M, Johansson H, et al.: Aspirin-sensitive asthmatics have elevated basal levels of leukotriene E_4 in the urine: and bronchial provocation with lysine-aspirin results in further release. *Am Rev Respir Dis* (1991) **143**; A599.

26. Christie PE, Togari P, Ford-Hutchison AW, *et al.*: Urinary leukotriene E_4 concentrations increase after aspirin challenge in aspirin sensitive asthmatic subjects. *Am Rev Respir Dis* (1991) **143**: 1025–1029.

27. Arm JP, O'Hickey SP, Spur BW, Lee TH: Airway responsiveness to histamine and leukotriene E_4 in subjects with aspirin-induced asthma. *Am Rev Respir Dis* (1989) **140**: 148–153.

28. Okazaki T, Llea VS, Rosario NA, *et al.*: Regulatory role of prostaglandin E in allergic histamine release with observations on the responsiveness of basophil leukocytes and the effect of acetylsalicytic acid. *J Allergy Clin Immunol* (1977) **60**: 360–366.

29. Szczeklik A: Aspirin-induced asthma as a viral disease. *Clin Allergy* (1988) **18**: 15–20.

30. Szczeklik A, Niazankowska E, Nizankowski R: Bronchial reactivity to prostaglandin $F_{2\alpha}$, E2 and histamine in different types of asthma. *Respiration* (1977) **34**: 323–331.

31. Thomson NC, Roberts R, Bandouvakis J, Newball H, Hargreave FE: Comparison of bronchial responses to prostaglandin $F_{2\alpha}$ and methacholine. *J Allergy Clin Immunol* (1981) **68**: 392–398.

32. Szczeklik A, Gryglewski RJ, Olszewski E, Dembinska-kiee A, Czerniawska-Mysik G: Aspirin sensitive asthma: the effect of aspirin on the release of prostaglandins from nasal polyps. *Pharmacol Res Commun* (1977) **9**: 415–425.

33. Asad SI, Kemeny DM, Youlten LJF, Frankland AW, Lessof MH: Effect of aspirin in 'aspirin sensitive' patients. *Br Med J* (1984) **288**: 745–748.

34. Godard P, Chaintreuil J, Damon M, *et al.*: Functional assessment of alveolar macrophages: comparison of cells from asthmatic and normal subjects. *J Allergy Clin Immunol* (1982) **70**: 88–93.

35. Ameisen JC, Capron A: Aspirin-sensitive asthma. *Clin Exp Allergy* (1990) **20**: 127–129.

36. Pearson DJ, Suarez-Mendez VJ: Abnormal platelet hydrogen metabolism in aspirin hypersensitivity. *Clin Exp Allergy* (1990) **20**: 157–163.

37. Mullarkey MF, Thomas PS, Hansen JA, Webb DR, Nisperos B: Association of aspirin-sensitive asthma with HLA-DQW2. *Am Rev Respir Dis* (1986) **133**: 261–263.

38. Slepian IK, Mathews KP, McLean JA: Aspirin-sensitive asthma. *Chest* (1985) **87**: 386–391.

39. Weltman JK, Szaro RP, SeHipane GA: An analysis of the role of IgE in intolerance to aspirin and tartrazine. *Allergy* (1978) **34**: 273–281.

40. Shumberger HD, Lobbecke EA, Kallos P: Acetylsalicylic acid intolerance. *Acta Med Scand* (1974) **196**: 451–458.

41. Delaney JC, Kay AB: Complement components and IgE in patients with asthma and aspirin idiosyncrasy. *Thorax* (1976) **31**: 425–427.

42. Pleskow WW, Chenoweth DE, Simon RA, Stevenson DD, Curd JG: The absence of detectable complement activation in aspirin-sensitive patients during aspirin challenge. *J Allergy Clin Immunol* (1983) **72**: 462–468.

43. Stevenson DD, Arroyave CM, Bhat KN, Tan EM: Oral aspirin challenges in asthmatic patients: a study of plasma histamine. *Clin Allergy* (1976) **6**: 493–505.

44. Hollingwoth HM, Downing ET, Braman SS, Glassroth J, Binder R, Center DM: Identification and characterization of neutrophil chemotactic activity in aspirin-induced asthma. *Am Rev Respir Dis* (1984) **130**: 373–379.

45. Zeiss CR, Lockey RF: Refractory period to aspirin in a patient with aspirin-induced asthma. *J Allergy Clin Immunol* (1976) **57**: 440–448.

46. Stevenson DD, Simon RA, Mathison DA: Aspirin-sensitive asthma: tolerance to aspirin after positive oral aspirin challenges. *J Allergy Clin Immunol* (1980) **66**: 82–88.

47. Pleskow WW, Stevenson DD, Mathison DA, Simon RA, Schatz M, Zeiger RS: Aspirin desensitization in aspirin-sensitive asthmatic patients: clinical manifestations and characterisation of the refractory period. *J Allergy Clin Immunol* (1982) **69**: 11–19.

48. Settipane RA, Stevenson DD: Cross sensitivity with acetaminophen in aspirin-sensitive patients with asthma. *J Allergy Clin Immunol* (1989) **84**: 26–33.

49. Szczeklik A, Niazankowska E, Czerniawska-Mysik G, Sek S: Hydrocortisone and airflow impairment in aspirin-induced asthma. *J Allergy Clin Immunol* (1985) **76**: 530–536.

50. Partridge MR, Gibson GJ: Adverse bronchial reactions to intravenous hydrocortisone in two aspirin-sensitive asthmatic patients. *Br Med J* (1978) **i**: 1521–1522.

51. Sweet JM, Stevenson DD, Simon RA, Mathison DA: Long term effects of aspirin desensitization-treatment for aspirin-sensitive rhinosinusitis-asthma. *J Allergy Clin Immunol* (1990) **85**: 59–65.

52. McNeill RS: Effect of β-adrenergic blocking agent, propranolol, on asthmatics. *Lancet* (1964) **ii**: 1101–1102.

53. McNeill RS, Ingram CG: Effect of propranolol on ventilatory function. *Am J Cardiol* (1966) **18**: 473–475.

54. Shoene RB: Timolol-induced bronchospasm in asthmatic bronchitis. *JAMA* (1981) **245**: 1460.

55. Dunn TL, Gerber MJ, Shen AS, Fernandez E, Iserman MD, Cherniak RM: The effect of topical opthalmic instillation of timolol and betexolol on lung function in asthmatic subjects. *Am Rev Respir Dis* (1986) **133**: 264–268.

56. Hill MR, Gotz VP, Harman E, McLeod I, Hendeles L: Evaluation of the asthmogenicity of propaferone, a new antiarrhythmic drug. *Chest* (1986) **90**: 698–702.

57. van Herwaarden CLA: β-Adrenoceptor blockade and pulmonary function in patients suffering from chronic obstructive lung disease. *J Cardiovasc Pharmacol* (1983) **5**: S46–50.

58. Perks W, Chatterjee S, Croxson R, Cruikshank J: Comparison of atenolol and oxprenolol in patients with angina or hypertension and coexistent chronic airways obstruction. *Br J Clin Pharmacol* (1978) **5**: 101–106.

59. Lammers JWJ, Folgering HTM, van Herwaarden CLA: Ventilatory effects of long-term treatment with pindolol and metoprolol in hypertensive patients with chronic obstructive lung disease. *Br J Clin Pharmacol* (1985) **20**: 205–210.

60. Benson MK, Berrill WT, Cruikshank JM, Sterling GS: A comparison of four β-adrenoceptor antagonists in patients with asthma. *Br J Clin Pharmacol* (1978) **5**: 415–419.

61. Greefhorst APM, van Herwaarden CLA: Comparative study of the ventilatory effects of three β_1-selective blocking drugs in asthmatic patients. *Eur J Clin Pharmacol* (1981) **20**: 417–421.

62. Ruffin RE, Frith MB, Anderton RC, Kumana CR, Newhouse MT, Hargreave FE: Selectivity of beta-adrenoceptor antagonist drugs assessed by histamine bronchial provocation. *Clin Pharmacol Ther* (1979) **25**: 536–540.

63. Lammers JWJ, Folgering HTM, van Herwaarden CLA: Ventilatory effects of beta$_1$-receptor selective blockade with bisoprolol and metoprolol in asthmatic patients. *Eur J Clin Pharmacol* (1984) **27**: 141–145.

64. Wilcox PG, Ahmad D, Darke AC, Parsons J, Carruthers SG: Respiratory and cardiac effects of metoprolol and bevantolol in patients with asthma. *Clin Pharmacol Ther* (1986) **39**: 29–34.

65. Zaagsma J, van der Heijden PJCM, van der Schaar MWG, Bank CMC: Comparison of functional β-adrenoceptor heterogeneity in central and peripheral airway smooth muscle of guinea pig and man. *J Recept Res* (1983) **3**: 89–106.

66. Carstairs JR, Nimmo AJ, Barnes PJ: Autoradiographic visualization of β-adrenoceptor subtypes in human lung. *Am Rev Respir Dis* (1985) **1332**: 541–547.

67. Tattersfield AE, Leaver DG, Pride NB: Effects of β-adrenergic blockade and stimulation on normal human airways. *J Appl Physiol* (1973) **35**: 613–619.

68. Zaid G, Beall GN: Bronchial response to beta-adrenergic blockade. *New Engl J Med* (1966) **275**: 580–584.

69. Townley RG, McGeady S, Bewtra A: The effect of beta-adrenergic blockade on bronchial sensitivity to acetyl-beta-methacholine in normal and allergic rhinitis subjects. *J Allergy Clin Immunol* (1976) **57**: 358–366.

70. Maclagan J, Ney UM: Investigation of the mechanisms of propranolol induced bronchoconstriction. *Br J Pharmacol* (1979) **66**: 409–418.

71. Ney UM: Propranolol-induced airway hyperreactivity in guinea-pigs. *Br J Pharmac* (1983) **79**: 1003–1009.

72. Terpstra GK, Raaijmakers JAM, Wassink GA: Propranolol-induced bronchoconstriction: a non-specific side-effect of β-adrenergic blocking therapy. *Eur J Pharmacol* (1981) **73**: 107–108.

73. Ind PW, Barnes PJ, Brown MJ, Dollery CT: Plasma histamine concentration during propranolol-induced bronchoconstriction. *Thorax* (1985) **40**: 903–909.

74. Barnes PJ: Neural control of human airways in health and disease. *Am Rev Respir Dis* (1986) **134**: 1289–1314.

75. Barnes PJ: Endogenous catecholamines and asthma. *J Allergy Clin Immunol* (1986) **77**: 791–795.

76. Barnes PJ, Ind PW, Brown MJ: Plasma histamine and catecholamines in stable asthmatic subjects. *Clin Sci* (1982) **62**: 661–665.

77. Church MK, Hiroi J: Inhibition of IgE-dependent histamine release from human dispersed lung mast cells by anti-allergic drugs and salbutamol. *Br J Pharmacol* (1987) **90**: 421–429.

78. Koeter GH, Meurs H, Kauffman HF, De Vries K: The role of the adrenergic systems in allergy and bronchial hyperreactivity. *Eur J Respir Dis* (1982) **63**: (Suppl 121): 72–78.

79. Rhoden KJ, Meldrum LA, Barnes PJ: Inhibition of cholinergic neurotransmission in human airways by β_2-adrenoceptors. *J Appl Physiol* (1988) **65**: 700–705.

80. Barnes PJ: Muscarinic receptor subtypes: implications for lung disease. *Thorax* (1989) **44**: 161–167.

81. Minette PAH, Lammers J, Dixon CMS, McCusker MT, Barnes PJ: A muscarinic agonist inhibits reflex bronchoconstriction in normal but not in asthmatic subjects. *J Appl Physiol* (1989) **67**: 2461–2465.

82. Ayala LE, Ahmed T: Is there a loss of a protective muscarinic receptor mechanism in asthma? *Chest* (1991) **96**: 1285–1291.

83. Ind PW, Dixon CMS, Fuller RW, Barnes PJ: Anticholinergic blockade of β-blocker induced bronchoconstriction. *Am Rev Respir Dis* (1989) **139**: 1390–1394.

84. Kamikawa Y, Shimo Y: Inhibitory effects of catecholamines on cholinergically and non-cholinergically mediated contractions of guinea-pig isolated bronchial muscle. *J Pharm Pharmacol* (1990) **42**: 131–134.

85. Verleden GM, Belvisi MG, Rabe K, Barnes PJ: Inhibition of nonadrenergic noncholinergic neural bronchoconstriction in guinea pig airways *in vitro* by β_2-adrenoceptors. *Am Rev Respir Dis* (1991) **143**: A347.

86. Jain SK, Trenchard D, Reynolds F, Noble MM, Guz A: The effect of local anaesthesia of the airway on respiratory reflexes in the rabbit. *Clin Sci* (1973) **44**: 519–538.

87. Dain DS, Boushey HA, Gold WM: Inhibition of respiratory reflexes by local anaesthetic aerosols in dogs and rabbits. *J Appl Physiol* (1975) **38**: 1045–1050.

88. Weiss EB, Anderson WH, O'Brien KP: The effect of a local anaesthetic, lidocaine on guinea pig trachealis muscle *in vitro*. *Am Rev Respir Dis* (1975) **112**: 393–400.

89. Weiss EB, Hargreaves WA, Viswaneth SG: The inhibitory action of lidocaine in anaphyl-axis. *Am Rev Respir Dis* (1978) **117**: 859–869.

90. Cross BA, Guz A, Jain SK, Archer S, Stevens J, Reynolds F: The effect of anaesthesia of the airway in dog and man: a study of respiratory reflexes, sensations and lung mechanics. *Clin Sci Molec Med* (1976) **50**: 439–454.

91. Thomson NC: The effect of different pharmacological agents on respiratory reflexes in normals and asthmatic subjects. *Clin Sci* (1979) **56**: 235–241.

92. Choudry NB, Fuller RW, Anderson N, Karisson J-A: Separation of cough and reflex bronchoconstriction by inhaled local anaesthetics. *Eur Respir J* (1990) **3**: 579–583.

93. Weiss EB, Patwardhan AV: The response to lidocaine in bronchial asthma. *Chest* (1977) **72**: 429–438.

94. Tullett WM, Patel KR, Berkin KE, Kerr JW: Effect of lignocaine, sodium cromoglycate and ipratropium bromide in exercise-induced asthma. *Thorax* (1982) **37**: 737–740.

95. Griffin MP, McFadden ER, Ingram RH, Pardee S: Controlled analysis of the effects of inhaled lignocaine in exercise-induced asthma. *Thorax* (1982) **37**: 741–745.

96. Sheppard D, Rizk NB, Boushey HA, Bethel RA: Mechanisms of cough and bronchoconstric-tion induced by distilled water aerosol. *Am Rev Respir Dis* (1983) **127**: 691–694.

97. Fish JE, Peterman VI: Effect of inhaled lidocaine on airway function in asthmatic subjects. *Respiration* (1979) **37**: 201–207.

98. Miller WC, Awe R: Effect of nebulized lidocaine on reactive airways. *Am Rev Respir Dis* (1975) **111**: 739–741.

99. McAlpine LG, Thomson NC: Lidocaine-induced bronchoconstriction in asthmatic patients. Relation to histamine airway responsiveness and effect of preservative. *Chest* (1989) **96**: 1012–1015.

100. Lammers J-W, Minette P, McCusker MT, Chung KF, Barnes PJ: Nonadrenergic broncho-dilator mechanisms in normal human subjects *in vivo. J Appl Physiol* (1988) **64**: 1817–1822.

101. Stevenson DD, Simon RA, Lumry WR, Mathison DA: Adverse reactions to tartrazine. *J Allergy Clin Immunol* (1986) **78**: 182–191.

102. Tarlo SM, Broder I: Tartrazine and benzoate challenge and dietary avoidance in chronic asthma. *Clin Allergy* (1982) **12**: 303–310.

103. Mann JS, Howarth PH, Holgate ST: Bronchoconstriction induced by ipratropium bromide in asthma: relation to hypotonicity. *Br Med J* (1984) **289**: 469.

104. Beasley CRW, Rafferty P, Holgate ST: Bronchoconstrictor properties of preservatives in ipratropium bromide (Atrovent®) nebuliser solution. *Br Med J* (1987) **294**: 1197–1198.

105. Rafferty P, Beasley R, Holgate ST: Comparison of the efficacy of preservative from ipratro-pium bromide and Atrovent® nebuliser solution. *Thorax* (1988) **43**: 446–450.

106. Clark RJ: Exacerbation of asthma after nebulised beclomethasone diproprionate. *Lancet* (1986) **1**: 574–575.

107. Stevenson DD, Simon RA: Sulfites and asthma. *J Allergy Clin Immunol* (1984) **74**: 469–472.

108. Stevenson DD, Simon RA: Sensitivity to ingested metabisulfites in asthmatic subjects. *J Allergy Clin Immunol* (1981) **68**: 26–32.

109. Schwartz HJ, Chester EH: Bronchospastic responses to aerosolised metabisulfite in asth-matic subjects: potential mechanisms and clinical implications. *J Allergy Clin Immunol* (1984) **74**: 511–513.

110. Nichol GM, Nix A, Chung KF, Barnes PJ: Characterisation of bronchoconstrictor responses to sodium metabisulphite aerosol in atopic asthmatic and non-asthmatic subjects. *Thorax* (1989) **44**: 1009–1014.

111. Allen DH, Baker GJ: Chinese restaurant asthma. *New Engl J Med* (1981) **305**: 1114–1115.

112. Allen DH, Delomery J, Baker G: Monosodium L-glutamate induced asthma. *J Allergy Clin Immunol* (1987) **80**: 530–537.

113. Dixon CMS, Fuller RW, Barnes PJ: The effect of an angiotensin converting enzyme inhibitor, ramipil, on bronchial responses to inhaled histamine and bradykinin in asthmatic subjects. *Br J Clin Pharmacol* (1987) **23**: 91–93.

114. Fuller RW: Cough associated with angiotensin converting enzyme inhibitors. *J Hum Hypert* (1989) **3**: 159–161.

115. McEwan JR, Choudry NB, Fuller RW: The effect of sulindac on the abnormal cough reflex associated with dry cough. *J Pharmacol Exp Ther* (1990) **255**: 161–164.

116. Chaudry NB, Fuller RW, Pride NB: Sensitivity of the human cough reflex: effect of inflammatory mediators prostaglandin E$_2$, bradykinin and histamine. *Am Rev Respir Dis* (1989) **40**: 137–141.

117. Nichol G, Nix A, Barnes PJ, Chung KF: Prostaglandin F$_{2\alpha}$ enhancement of capsaicin induced cough in man: modulation by beta$_2$-adrenergic and anticholinergic drugs. *Thorax* (1990) **45**: 694–698.

118. Sogn DD: Penicillin allergy. *J Allergy Clin Immunol* (1984) **74**: 589–593.

119. Israel-Biet D, Labrune S, Huchon GJ: Drug-induced lung disease: 1990 review. *Eur Resp J* (1991) **4**: 465–478.

120. Engel T, Heinig JH, Malling H-J, Scharing B, Nikander K, Masden F: Clinical comparison of inhaled budesonide delivered either by pressurized metered dose inhaler or Turbuhaler. *Allergy* (1989) **44**: 220–225.

121. Yarbrough J, Lyndon RN, Mansfield E, Ting S: Metered dose inhaler induced broncho-spasm in asthmatic patients. *Ann Allergy* (1985) **55**: 25–27.

122. Shim CS, Williams MH: Cough and wheezing from beclomethasone diproprionate aerosol are absent after triamcinolone acetronide. *Ann Intern Med* (1987) **106**: 700–703.

31

Allergen Avoidance

THOMAS A.E. PLATTS-MILLS, FREDERICK DE BLAY,

GEORGE W. WARD, JR AND MARY L. HAYDEN

INTRODUCTION

Over the last decade it has become increasingly clear that despite many new medicines for asthma the therapeutic problem has not been solved. Indeed progressive increases in hospital admissions, morbidity, and mortality suggest that a different direction is needed in the management of the disease. It has actually been suggested that some of the bronchodilators are harmful. This could occur either because a short-term beneficial effect masks an increase in bronchial reactivity or because bronchodilation allows the patient to inhale more allergen. Whatever the reasons for the increasing severity of the disease the logical approach is to try to control the primary causes of bronchial reactivity. In the last 5 years it has become clear that asthma is an inflammatory disease of the bronchi in which eosinophils, lymphocytes, mast cells and probably basophils play a role.[1-3] It also seems more and more likely that non-specific bronchial reactivity is a consequence of this inflammation. Given the fact that exposure to common inhaled allergens is the best established cause of this inflammation, reducing exposure is the logical first line of treatment. Indeed we would now recommend that any patient who requires more than occasional treatment for asthma should be evaluated for sensitivity and offered specific advice about allergen avoidance. Although dozens of different 'causes' of asthma have been described only a few are common. In many cases once the specific sensitivity is identified the relevant avoidance measures become obvious, e.g. occupational exposure to Western Red Cedar, isocyanate or solder fumes. Similarly with some domestic exposures, avoidance measures are obvious and not difficult, e.g. removing a guinea-pig, a room humidifier, a horse hair mattress or a feather pillow. Thus, the problem comes down to those sources of indoor allergens that are not obvious to the

ASTHMA: BASIC MECHANISMS AND CLINICAL MANAGEMENT (2nd Edn)
ISBN 0-12-079026-2

patient and/or not simple to avoid. Indeed the problem can be focused on dust mites, domestic animals and fungi.

Real progress has come with the ability to measure indoor allergens particularly dust mite and cat.[4,5] This has allowed the proposal of threshold values for exposure and progressive evidence about the quantitative reductions in exposure that are necessary to achieve clinical improvement.[6,7] In addition, it has been possible to start defining the levels of exposure that increase the risk of sensitization and the development of asthma.[8-11] This in turn suggests that allergen avoidance should be considered both as a treatment for established cases of asthma and also a possible method for reducing the prevalence of the disease.

DUST MITES

The evidence that dust mites are a major cause of asthma world wide has been reviewed by an international workshop.[6] Although sensitization is extremely common (in some studies up to 80% of asthmatics have positive skin tests to mite extracts), the association between exposure to dust and asthma is usually not obvious to the patients. Thus there is no such thing as a 'typical history of dust mite allergy'. This is probably because the real role of dust-mite exposure is progressive, chronic inflammation of the lungs, with maximum exposure occurring slowly while lying down or resting.[12] In addition, the form in which dust-mite allergens become airborne (i.e. mite faecal pellets) does not create a challenge to the lung which would be recognized by the patient.[13] Thus the history is not a useful guide as to who should be given advice on avoidance. All patients require skin tests or RAST to establish sensitivity; a wheal of 4×4 mm is generally considered positive, a wheal of 5×5 mm correlates well with a positive RAST.

Quantitation of exposure to mites

Originally mites were counted microscopically and it was suggested that 200 mites/gram of dust represented a significant level of exposure.[14] Subsequently it became possible to measure mite allergens, first by RAST inhibition then by specific assay of the major allergens; e.g. the Group I allergens which include *Der p* I, *Der f* I and *Der m* I.(4).[4] The assays for mite allergens have progressively improved and currently two site monoclonal antibody ELISA assays for Group I allergens are widely used.[15] Since 1981 it has been possible to measure airborne mite allergens, and several groups have recommended airborne measurements to evaluate exposure.[13,16,17] However, mite allergens only become airborne during disturbance and the allergen falls rapidly after disturbance.[13,16,18] At present no coherent plan has been offered for standardizing domestic disturbance during measurements of room air. Similarly no satisfactory system for personal monitoring has been developed. Thus the standard method for monitoring exposure is to collect samples from flooring, mattress or bedding, and upholstered furniture. Results are expressed as allergen in micrograms/gram of dust.[4,6] In 1987 threshold levels for mite allergen were first proposed.[16,19] These levels are not absolute but simply represent a guide to the levels above which the risk of sensitization and disease increases.

The threshold levels proposed, i.e. 2 µg and 10 µg Group I allergen/gram of dust have now been applied in several countries and have been related to mite counts.[8–11] Thus 2 µg/g has been recognized in Marseilles and Berlin as a level which is associated with increased risk of mite allergic asthma.[8,9] In Denmark and Australia 100 mites/gram of dust (which is equivalent of 2 µg Group I/g) has been reported as creating an increased risk for asthma.[10,11] Finally in England it has been found that exposure to ≥ 10 µg/g of dust in early childhood increases the risk of asthma and is associated with recurrent admissions to hospital.[20] Finally there is limited evidence about the quantitative reduction in exposure necessary to produce clinical benefit. Patients who were moved from houses with allergen levels of 13 µg/g of dust to hospital rooms with ~0.2 µg/g dust improved dramatically both in symptoms and bronchial reactivity.[7] In houses reductions as complete as that are very difficult to achieve, however reductions of 80–90% have been achieved and have been associated with significant improvement.[21–24]

Physical measures to reduce mite allergen exposure

The primary methods for reducing levels of dust mite allergens are physical measures designed to control the sites in which mites grow. The single most consistently effective measure is to cover mattresses and pillows with plastic or vapour-permeable fabric covers. Owen *et al.* reported that covering mattresses with a vapour-permeable cover reduced the mean concentration of mite allergen on the outside of the mattress from 20.3 to 0.3 µg *Der p* I/g dust.[25] This should be accompanied by covering the duvet or comforter *and/or* a regular regime of washing all bedding in hot water (130°F/55°C weekly or biweekly).

The second priority is the flooring and remainder of the bedroom. Whenever possible the carpet should be replaced by wood or vinyl flooring which can be polished. The carpet is not only a source of airborne allergen but is an important source for reinfesting bedding and clothing. Curtains should be washable (i.e. cotton or venetian blinds). It is important to remember that under humid conditions mites can grow in any fabric, including clothing such as sweaters, coats and trousers as well as in any upholstered furniture. The bedroom should be made as simple as possible.

In the rest of the house high levels of mite allergen can be found in sofas, chairs, carpets, curtains, and indeed any material. Reduction of exposure can be achieved by replacing these items with polished floors; wooden, vinyl or leather furniture; and washable curtains or blinds. However, these measures are expensive and it is these areas of the house that may best be managed by reducing overall humidity or treating with acaricides.[26–30] Reducing humidity in a house can be achieved in several ways. In some climates simply increasing ventilation e.g. from 0.2 air changes per hour (ACH) up to 1 ACH will be effective.[26] However, in more humid climates e.g. south eastern United States in the summer, Brazil, Hong Kong, Venezuela, etc., control can only be achieved by air conditioning and helped by simple dehumidifiers. The objective is to keep relative humidity below 50% and absolute humidity below 7 g/kg (Fig.31.1). Structural faults in a building which allow entry of rain water or ground water can create ideal growth conditions. Also some social groups artificially raise the humidity in their houses with water pans, boiling kettles, etc. A special problem is posed by carpets laid on unventilated floors e.g. basements or concrete slab houses. If these carpets become wet due to

Humidity, Temperature and Mite Growth

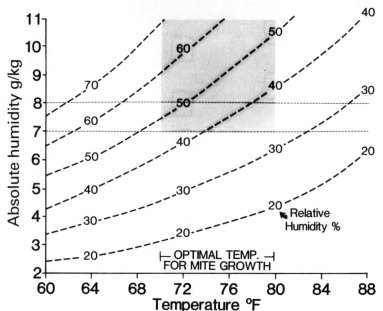

Fig. 31.1 Optimal conditions for mite growth are indicated by the grey square, i.e. 70–80°F and >7 g/kg absolute humidity. It is obvious that progressive increases in central heating and decreasing ventilation has created many houses with optimal conditions for mite growth.

leakage or condensation they dry very slowly and may become sites of very high mite growth.[19] It is essential that mite or fungal allergic patients do not live or work in basements. All unventilated floors should have primary polished flooring and carpets should be removed or at least lifted during hot/damp weather.

Acaricides and denaturing agents for mite allergens

Soon after mites were shown to be the major source of allergens in house dust, studies were started to evaluate methods of killing them.[27,29,30] Many different chemicals had already been identified as killing those mites that are pests in agriculture.[27] The next and more difficult question was whether these acaricides could successfully be applied to carpets or sofas. A carpet is a very dense object with multiple layers which becomes full of skin scales, food and other debris from the house. This creates a deep nest for mites, and extreme problems with getting an acaricide to penetrate. Various formulations have been tried, either as a liquid spray, a foam, or a powder. For example, a benzoate (acaricide) is marketed in Australia in a liquid form combined with 1% tannic acid (denaturing agent).[31] This product works *in vitro*, but recent experiments suggest it needs to be applied at higher rates than those recommended in order to get effective reductions.[32] Similarly the powder form of benzyl benzoate is very effective at killing mites in culture but is less effective in carpets. Application of the powder over 12–18 h with repeated brushing is more effective than applying the powder as recommended i.e.

Table 31.1 Carpet treatment to control dust mites and dust mite allergens.

Chemical	Trade name	Mechanism*	Form
Benzyl benzoate	Acarosan	Acaricide (used for scabies)	Powder (USA/Europe) Foam (Europe)
Pyrethroids	Actomite (Acardust)	Insecticide/acaricide	Pressurized canister (Europe only)
Pirimphos methyl	Actellic	Insecticide/acaricide (treating grain)	(not available)
Natamycin	Tymasil	Anti-fungal (treating food)	Powder (Europe)
Tannic acid (3%)	Allergy control solution	Protein denaturing	Fluid (USA)
Liquid nitrogen	—	Kills mites by freezing	—
Benzyl tannate	DMS spray	Acaricide and protein denaturing	Fluid (Australia)
Mixture of surface wetting agents and solvents	Allerex	Cleaning solution used with special vacuum cleaner	Europe

*Several of the available preparations are in use for other purposes: e.g. benzyl benzoate is a traditional treatment to kill scabies mites; pirimphos methyl is widely used for treating grain to prevent the growth of storage mites; natamycin, which controls mite reproduction is also used as a fungicide on cheeses and other foods.

for 4 h.[28] When brushed in repeatedly the white powder (which also acts as a cleaning agent) remains in the carpet producing increased recovery of 'dust' for several weeks. Other compounds have been recommended including natamycin (a fungicide that prevents mite reproduction) and second generation pyrethroids (Table 31.1). In each case the compound is effective at killing mites in culture but the evidence for a prolonged effect in carpets is less compelling. Mattresses and sofas are if anything more difficult to treat; natamycin, benzyl benzoate foam, or liquid mixtures of acaricide and tannic acid have each been found to be relatively ineffective. For those acaricides that have been demonstrated to be effective on carpets, the results of this treatment on airborne allergen have not been reported and this information is needed. Other acaricides are currently being tested for use in carpets, however it appears that the major problem will be the method of delivery not the ability of the agent to kill mites. In the final analysis leaving carpets down all year long creates a major cleaning problem to which we have only very limited answers.

Putting tea leaves on carpets has been recommended as a health measure in some parts of China for many years, and it is well known that tannic acid can denature proteins (this is the basis for tanning leather). Green *et al.* in Australia recommended tannic acid as a method of denaturing allergens in house dust.[31] Applied either as a 1% or a 3% solution, tannic acid has a very rapid effect on reducing the allergenicity of dust. This effect can be demonstrated either by assaying allergen using ELISA assays, or by extracting the treated dust and showing that the extract no longer produces positive skin tests.[31] Tannic acid is very effective on Group I mite allergen (>95% loss of activity) and slightly less effective on Group II allergens or the cat allergen *Fel d* I.[33] The acid has little effect on live mites, which can even survive being bathed in 3% tannic acid at pH 2.8, so the effect on carpets can only be temporary. However, this is certainly an effective method of producing rapid short term i.e. ~6 weeks' reductions in allergen.

Conclusions *re* mites

House dust mites can live in multiple sites in the house and no single physical measure can solve the problem. Similarly there is no acaricide that can be applied to treat the whole house. However, the evidence is steadily accumulating that specific measures can produce major reductions in mite allergen levels. In addition, a series of studies has now shown that treating the whole house with appropriate measures for each site can reduce symptoms of asthma.[21–24] Convincing patients to carry out avoidance measures requires demonstrating that they are specifically allergic, educating them about mites and providing a specific set of instructions which indicate the priorities and the long-term objectives (Table 31.2). Two groups have reported marked benefit including reduction in non-specific bronchial reactivity from treating the bedroom only.[21,22] However, this must reflect local housing conditions since in many areas the highest levels of mite allergen exposure occur outside the bedroom. There is still need for further information on methods of applying acaricides and the design of furniture to control the growth of mites.

CAT ALLERGEN

Assessing random patients who presented to emergency rooms in the United States 30/188 asthmatics had high levels of IgE antibody to cat dander. The comparable figure for controls was 1/202. This gives an odds ratio of 38 and supports the well-established view that exposure to cat allergens is a major risk factor for both acute and chronic asthma. Dust from houses with a cat (or cats) in them will contain between 10 μg and 1500 μg of the cat allergen *Fel d* I.[5,34,35] The primary method of reducing exposure to cat allergen is to remove the cat from the house. Removing the cat will produce some effects rapidly because the cat itself gives off significant quantities of airborne allergen.[36,37] However, a house in which a cat has been living will contain large quantities of allergen in carpets, sofas, bedding, etc. Even with continued routine cleaning of a house, cat allergen levels will take 12–16 weeks to fall below the levels associated with disease i.e. below 1 μg *Fel d* I/g dust.[38] Aggressive cleaning measures (i.e. removing carpets and furniture combined with washing down walls) can remove cat allergen from a house rapidly. Cat allergen becomes airborne on a wide range of particle sizes including particles ≤2.0 mm in diameter.[16,39] In keeping with their size these particles remain airborne for hours and are always measurable even when the cat is not present and the room is undisturbed.[36,39] For these small particles it is possible to make a direct comparison with bronchial provocation. In some houses during domestic disturbance the level of allergen

Table 31.2 University of Virginia allergy clinic instructions for reducing exposure to house dust mites.

House dust mites require humidity (>50% relative humidity) and warmth (>70°F) to grow. Because mites avoid the light and because surfaces dry out rapidly, mites flourish in mattresses, bedding, upholstered furniture, carpets, pillows, and quilts. Under really humid conditions mites will also grow in clothing, curtains (drapes) and any material.

Procedures to reduce dust mites should focus first on the bedroom because more time is spent there than any other room and it is generally easiest to change. However, in the long run it is best to modify much of the house and this should certainly be considered when moving.

Priority objectives

Mattresses and pillows should be enclosed in a zippered, plastic cover or a special vapour-permeable, allergen-proof fabric. Damp wipe the mattress cover every 2 weeks.

Wash all bedding including mattress pad, pillow cases, and blankets in hot cycle (~130°F) *weekly*. Comforters (or duvets) should be replaced with dacron or orlon which can be washed with the bedding or covered with vapour-permeable covers.

Small objects that accumulate dust such as knick-knacks, books, stuffed animals and records should be placed in drawers or closed cabinets. Clothing should be stored in closed cupboards or closet. Unused clothing should be stored away from the bedroom.

Carpets should be vacuum cleaned weekly using a vacuum cleaner with an effective filter. The patient should either avoid vacuum cleaning or wear a mask during cleaning. In general, dust mite allergens will take about 20 min to fall after vacuum cleaning.

Medium-term objectives

Removing carpets from bedrooms makes it much easier to control mites. This is because carpets are very difficult to clean and will tend not only to grow mites (in humid seasons) but also to act as a source to reinfest bedding, clothing, etc.

Replace curtains/drapes with washable cotton curtains or venetian/slat blinds.

Control humidity in the house; this can be achieved by increasing ventilation if the outdoor conditions are cold and/or dry; alternatively, reducing humidity can be achieved with central air conditioning. Dehumidifiers are helpful in basements. The objective is to keep relative humidity below 50%.

Treat carpets with acaricides (e.g. acarosan) or tannic acid (e.g. allergy control solution).

Choice of houses/apartments

Basements are not recommended for any allergic patients (in some cases moving out of a basement may be urgent because it is so difficult to control mite and/or fungal growth in a basement). Bedrooms should be upstairs.

Carpets fitted to a concrete slab either in a basement or on the ground floor tend to become damp and remain damp. We recommend that all floors should have a primary polished floor (vinyl or wood) and carpets should be movable.

Upholstered sofas and chairs should be avoided.

Air filters on central air conditioning should be cleaned regularly. Good quality, e.g. electrostatic, filters may be helpful but are no substitute for reducing available mite nests in the house.

---

on small particles can be as high as 100 ng/m^3 of allergen. Since it takes ~10 ng to achieve a positive bronchial provocation, at these levels it would take only 6 min to inhale sufficient cat allergen to produce a measurable fall in FEV_1. Thus a decrease in the level of airborne small particles could be expressed as the length of time to inhale a

Table 31.3   Proposed procedures for reducing airborne
cat allergen levels

Remove cat either completely or keep outdoors*

If the cat 'cannot' be removed:
  Polish flooring, no carpeting
  Minimize upholstered furniture
  Vacuum clean with high efficiency filter
  Air filtration**
  Wash cat weekly

*Cat allergen will still take up to 16 weeks to remove.
**Room air cleaners with a HEPA filter are only effective if the carpet has been removed.

provocation dose, i.e. after a reduction of the airborne level to 5 ng/m^3 it would take as long as 120 min to inhale 10 ng.

Despite continued symptoms and education many allergic patients insist on keeping a cat in the house; possibly as many as 2 million patients in the USA. Recent evidence has suggested that even if the cat remains in the house it is possible to reduce airborne cat allergen levels.[36] The primary observation was that when cats are washed repeatedly the quantity of allergen recovered progressively decreases.[40,41] If washing cats is combined with washable furniture, a high efficiency (e.g. HEPA) room air cleaner, and removing carpets, airborne levels of allergen can be reduced 90% or more (Table 31.3). The feasibility of this approach with patients or the long-term effectiveness of washing cats remains to be demonstrated. However, it is normal practice to wash dogs or to keep them outside and this may explain why there is much less asthma associated with dog allergy. Because airborne cat allergen is associated with small particles, ventilation may also play a role in controlling exposure.[36,39] Particles < 2 mm in diameter will remain suspended for hours and increasing ventilation rates (e.g. from 0.2 ACH to 1.0 ACH) may be effective in physically removing small particles.

FUNGAL ALLERGENS

There is no question that moulds grow in domestic houses and that many patients with asthma give positive immediate skin tests to fungal extracts.[42,43] In addition, there is striking evidence that exposure to outdoor fungi may play an important role in severe asthma.[44] However, information about the role of indoor fungal allergens in asthma is very incomplete. Thus there is little epidemiological evidence connecting sensitization (with or without exposure) to indoor fungi with asthma. Indeed there are no simple assays for indoor fungal allergens, and we do not even know whether fungal spores or some other part of the organism are the major form in which these allergens become airborne. Thus most advice given about reducing fungal allergens in houses is based on basic knowledge about their growth conditions rather than any objective measurements of the relationship between exposure and disease. Fungal growth can occur on any surface and is primarily dependent on humidity plus a source of organic matter. Fungi can grow under much colder conditions than mites and are a common contaminant of unheated basements. These organisms commonly grow on food, stored wood, wicker baskets and household plants, as well as kitchen or bathroom surfaces. Normal recommendations include reducing organic matter in the house to the minimum and controlling humidity by structural maintenance, and ventilation *or* dehumidification. In addition, surfaces which tend to grow moulds particularly in the kitchen or bathrooms should be cleaned with chemicals designed to kill moulds e.g. chlorine bleach. In common usage 4 or 6 parts of water to 1 part chlorine bleach is effective at cleaning surfaces. The use of room (or house) humidifiers presents a special hazard for mould growth, and if used, they should be washed with chlorine solution at least twice weekly.

OTHER ALLERGENS

Almost any foreign protein that accumulates in a house can give rise to sensitization and asthma. Circumstantial evidence has been provided for cockroaches, guinea-pigs, rabbits, rodent urine, and others.[16,35,45] In each case once the cause of sensitization is established avoidance advice is obvious, although in most cases the details have not been confirmed by accurate measurements. In addition, outdoor allergens including pollens and moulds can become part of the indoor environment. During the season, grass pollen may become the dominant source of foreign protein in house dust.[46] Reducing the quantities of pollen that enter the house is important. Ultimately closing a house and using full air conditioning may be the most effective measure. It is essential not to use window fans blowing into a bedroom and wiser to have some form of filter over bedrooms windows if they must be kept open. There is a large literature on exterminating both insects and rodents in houses, however there is little published data on the effectiveness of these measures in reducing allergen exposure.

CONCLUSIONS

The logical first treatment for extrinsic asthma is to reduce exposure to the causative allergen. There is now good evidence that levels of mite allergen can be reduced and that these reductions can produce symptomatic improvement and reduced requirement for medications.[21-24] Furthermore the proposed threshold levels do provide a guide to the levels of exposure that are associated with disease and also the quantitive reductions necessary to achieve benefit.[6,7] Mite allergens become airborne in large particles which fall rapidly so that reducing reservoirs (or breeding grounds) is the primary method to control exposure and air filters have little role.

The primary steps to reduce mite exposure are physical: (a) covering mattresses, pillows and duvets; (b) removing carpets where possible; (c) reducing humidity. Acaricides or tannic acid may play a role particularly on fitted carpets but further work is needed on the best methods for application.

Cat allergen becomes airborne on small particles which remain airborne for prolonged periods. In keeping with this, measures to filter the air or increase air exchange may be effective. However, as with all allergens it is essential to reduce the source as well. This can be achieved either by removing the cat permanently *or* by washing the cat and removing furnishings which can act as a reservoir. For cat allergen the quantitative data is less clear than for mites but it already seems clear that 8 μg *Fel d* I/g dust is a level associated with symptoms and that 1 μg *Fel d* I/g dust can increase the risk of sensitization.

Many other allergens can be important in house dust including fungi, cockroaches, pollen, mouse urine, etc. There is little quantitative data about these allergens and so most advice is based simply on a knowledge of the biology of the source. None the less, specific advice about avoidance is appropriate to reduce mould growth, exterminate cockroaches, reduce pollen entry into the house, etc.

Air exchange rates as low as 0.3 ACH without air conditioning can create problems with indoor air because humidity, chemical air pollutants (such as tobacco smoke), and the smaller airborne particles carrying allergens (e.g. cat) will all accumulate without adequate ventilation.

Allergen avoidance has become progressively more specific and more detailed, and it can be expensive (in fact the expenses of allergen avoidance measures are modest by comparison with the long-term cost of asthma medications particularly the inhaled medicines). It is therefore essential to establish that the patient is specifically allergic. This can be achieved most simply by skin tests but also by RAST assays. For any patient whose asthma requires more than occasional treatment, establishing sensitivities and offering detailed advice about avoiding relevant allergens should be a routine part of management.

ACKNOWLEDGEMENTS

This work was supported by NIH Grant No. A1-20565 and a grant from the American Lung Association of Virginia.

REFERENCES

1. Kirby JG, Hargreave FE, Gleich GJ, O'Byrne PM: Bronchoalveolar cell profiles of asthmatic and nonasthmatic subjects. *Am Rev Respir Dis* (1987) **136**: 379–383.
2. Djukanovic R, Roche WR, Wilson JW, *et al.*: Mucosal inflammation in asthma. *Am Rev Respir Dis* (1990) **142**: 434–457.
3. Bousquet J, Chanez P, Lacoste JY, *et al.*: Eosinophilic inflammation in asthma. *N Eng J Med* (1990) **323**: 1033–1039.
4. Platts-Mills TAE, Chapman MD: Dust mites: immunology, allergic disease, and environmental control [published erratum appears in *J Allergy Clin Immunol* (1988 Nov) **82**(5 Pt 1): 841] [Review]. *J Allergy Clin Immunol* (1987) **80**: 755–775.
5. Chapman MD, Aalberse RC, Brown MJ, Platts-Mills TAE: Monoclonal antibodies to the major feline allergen *Fel d* I. II. Single step affinity purification of *Fel d* I, N-terminal sequence analysis, and development of a sensitive two-side immunoassay to assess *Fel d* I exposure. *J Immunol* (1988) **140**: 812–818.
6. Platts-Mills TAE, de Weck AL: Dust mite allergens and asthma—A world-wide problem. *J. Allergy Clin Immunol* (1989) **83**: 416–427.

7. Platts-Mills TAE, Tovey ER, Mitchell EB, Moszoro H, Nock P, Wilkins SR: Reduction of bronchial hyperreactivity during prolonged allergen avoidance. *Lancet* (1982) **2**: 675–678.
8. Lau S, Rusche A, Weber A, Bischoff E, Wahn U: Short term efficacy of benzyl benzoate on mite allergen concentrations in house dust. *J Allergy Clin Immunol* (1989) **83**: 1–263.
9. Charpin D, Birnbaum J, Haddi E, Genard G, Toumi M, Vervloet D: Attitude and allergy to house dust mites: an epidemiological study in primary school children. *J Allergy Clin Immunol* (1990) **85**: 185.
10. Peat JK, Britton WJ, Salome CM, Woolcock AJ: Bronchial hyperresponsiveness in two populations of Australian schoolchildren. III. Effect of exposure to environmental allergens. *Clin Allergy* (1987) **17**: 297–300.
11. Korsgaard J: Mite asthma and residency. A case-control study on the impact of exposure to house-dust mites in dwellings. *Am Rev Resp Dis* (1983) **128**: 231–235.
12. Platts-Mills TAE, Pollart S, Chapman MD, Luczynska CM: The role of allergens in asthma and airway hyperresponsiveness. Relevance to immunotherapy and allergen avoidance. In Kaliner M, Barnes P, Persson C (eds) *Pharmacology and Pathophysiology of Airway Hyperresponsiveness*. New York, Marcel Dekker, 1991, pp 595–631.
13. Tovey ER, Chapman MD, Wells CW, Platts-Mills TAE: The distribution of dust mite allergen in the houses of patients with asthma. *Am Rev Resp Dis* (1981) **124**: 630–635.
14. Voorhorst R, Spieksma FThM, Varekamp N: House dust atopy and the house dust mite *Dermatophagoides pteronyssinus* (Troussart, 1897). In Leiden (ed) Leiden, Stafleu's Scientific Publishing Co., 1969.
15. Luczynska CM, Arruda LK, Platts-Mills TAE, Miller JD, Lopez M, Chapman MD: A two-site monoclonal antibody ELIZA for the quantitation of the major *Dermatophagoides* spp. allergens, *Der p* I and *Der f* I. *J. Immunol Meth* (1989) **118**: 227–235.
16. Swanson MC, Agarwal MK, Reed CR: An immunochemical approach to indoor aeroallergen quantitation with a new volumetric air sampler: Studies with mite, roach, cat, mouse, and guinea pig antigens. *J Allergy Clin Immunol* (1987) **76**: 724–729.
17. Price JA, Pollock J, Little SA, Longbottom JL, Warner JO: Measurements of airborne mite allergen in houses of asthmatic children. *Lancet* (1990) **336**: 895–897.
18. De Blay F, Heymann PW, Chapman MD, Platts-Mills TAE: Airborne dust mite allergens: Comparison of airborne concentrations and particle size distribution of Group II mite allergen with Group I and cat. *J All Clin Immunol* **88**: 919–926.
19. Platts-Mills TA, Hayden ML, Chapman MD, Wilkins SR: Seasonal variation in dust mite and grass-pollen allergens in dust from the houses of patients with asthma. *J Allergy Clin Immunol* (1987) **79**: 781–791.
20. Sporik R, Holgate ST, Platts-Mills TAE, Cogswell J: Exposure to house dust mite allergen (*Der p* I) and the development of asthma in childhood: A prospective study. *N Eng J Med* (1990) **323**: 502–507.
21. Murray AB, Ferguson AC: Dust-free bedrooms in the treatment of asthmatic children with house dust or house dust mite allergy: a controlled trial. *Pediatrics* (1983) **71**: 418–422.
22. Ehnert B, Lau S, Weber A, Wahn U: Reduction of mite allergen exposure and bronchial hyper-reactivity. *J Allergy Clin Immunol* (1991) **87**: 320.
23. Walshaw MJ, Evans CC: Allergen avoidance in house dust mite sensitive adult asthma. *Q J Med* (1986) **58**: 199–215.
24. Dorward AJ, Colloff MJ, MacKay NS, McSharry C, Thomson NC: Effect of house dust mite avoidance measures on adult atopic asthma. *Thorax* (1988) **43**: 98–105.
25. Owen S, Morganstern M, Hepworth J, Woolcock A: Control of house dust mite antigen in bedding. *Lancet* (1990) **335**: 396–397.
26. Korsgaard J: House dust mites and absolute indoor humidity. *Allergy* (1983) **38**: 85–92.
27. Heller-Haupt A, Busvine JR: Tests of acaricides against house dust mites. *J Med Entomol* (1974) **11**: 551–558.
28. Hayden ML, Rose G, Diduch KB, *et al.*: Reduction of dust mite allergens in carpets using benzyl benzoate in the form of a wet powder. *J All Clin Immunol* (1991) in press.
29. Bischoff E, Krause-Michel B, Nolte D: Zur bekampfung von houstaubmilben in haushalten von patienten mit milbenasthma. *Allergologie* (1987) **10**: 473–478.

30. Colloff MJ: Use of liquid nitrogen in the control of house dust mite populations. *Clin Allergy* (1986) **16**: 41–47. See also *Pesticide Outlook* (1989) **1.1**: 17–18 and (1990) **1.2**: 3–8.
31. Green WF, Nicholas NR. Salome CM, Woolcock AJ: Reduction of house dust mites and mite allergens: effects of spraying carpets and blankets with Allersearch DMS, an acaricide combined with an allergen reducing agent. *Clin Exp Allergy* (1989) **19**: 203–207.
32. Tovey ER: Paper presented at the 2nd International Workshop on Dust Mite Allergens and Asthma, 1990.
33. Miller JD, Miller A, Luczynska CM, Rose G, Platts-Mills TAE: Effect of tannic acid spray on dust-mite antigen levels in carpets (Abstract). *J Allergy Clin Immunol* (1989) **83**: 1: 262.
34. Ohman JL Jr, Lorusso JR, Lewis S: Cat allergen content of commercial house dust extracts: comparison with dust extracts from cat-containing environment. *J. Allergy Clin Immunol* (1987) **79**: 955–959.
35. Gelber L, Pollart S, Chapman MD, Platts-Mills TAE: Serum IgE antibodies and allergen exposure as a risk factor for acute asthma (Abstract). *J Allergy Clin Immunol* (1990).
36. De Blay F, Chapman MD, Platts-Mills TAE: Airborne cat allergen (*Fel d* I): Environmental control with the cat *in situ*. *Am Rev Resp Dis* (1991) **143**: 1334–1339.
37. Swanson MC, Campbell AR, Klauck MJ, Reed CE: Correlations between levels of mite and cat allergens in settled and airborne dust. *J Allergy Clin Immunol* (1989) **83**: 776–783.
38. Wood RA, Chapman MD, Adkinson NF Jr, Eggleston PA: The effect of cat removal on allergen content in household-dust samples. *J Allergy Clin Immunol* (1989) **83**: 730–734.
39. Luczynska CM, Li Y, Chapman MD, Platts-Mills TAE: Airborne concentrations and particle size distribution of allergen derived from domestic cats (*Felis domesticus*): Measurements using cascade impactor, liquid impinger and a two site monoclonal antibody assay for *Fel d* I. *Am Rev Resp Dis* (1990) **141**: 361–367.
40. Glinert R, Wilson P, Wedner HJ: *Fel d* I is markedly reduced following sequential washing of cats (Abstract). *J Allergy Clin Immunol* (1990) **85**: 327.
41. Ohman JL, Baer H, Anderson MC, Leitermann K, Brown P: Surface washes of living cats: An improved method of obtaining clinically relevant allergen. *J Allergy Clin Immunol* (1983) **72**: 288–293.
42. Lehrer SR, Lopez M, Butcher BT, Olson J, Reed M, Salvaggio JE: Basidiomycete mycelia and spore-allergen extracts: skin test activity in adults with symptoms of respiratory allergy. *J Allergy Clin Immunol* (1986) **78**: 478–485.
43. Salvaggio J, Aukrust L: Postgraduate course presentations. Mold-induced asthma. *J Allergy Clin Immunol* (1981) **68**: 327–346.
44. O'Hallaren MT, Yunginger J, Offord KP, *et al.*: Exposure to aeroallergen as a possible precipitating factor in respiratory arrest in young patients with asthma. *New Eng J Med* (1991) **324**: 359–363.
45. Pollart SM, Chapman MD, Fiocco GP, Rose G, Platts-Mills TAE: Epidemiology of acute asthma: IgE antibodies to common inhalant allergens as a risk factor for emergency room visits. *J Allergy Clin Immunol* (1989) **83**: 875–882.
46. Pollart SM, Reid MJ, Fling JA, Chapman MD, Platts-Mills TAE: Epidemiology of emergency room asthma in northern California: association with IgE antibody to rye grass pollen. *J Allergy Clin Immunol* (1988) **82**: 224–230.

β-Adrenoceptor Agonists

A.E. TATTERSFIELD AND J.R. BRITTON

CHEMISTRY

β-Adrenoceptor agonists are sympathomimetic amines, the parent basic structure consisting of a benzene ring attached to an amine group via two carbon atoms (Fig. 32.1). The distinctive features of the different β-agonists depend on the substitutions on this basic structure, and on the substituent on the amine group in particular.[1] The main features of the structure–activity relationships are summarized below:

(1) β-Adrenoceptor agonists consist of catecholamines and non-catecholamines. Catecholamines are characterized by hydroxyl groups in the 3 and 4 positions of the benzene ring—the catechol nucleus. Naturally occurring catecholamines include dopamine, noradrenaline and adrenaline; synthetic catecholamines include isoprenaline, isoetharine and rimiterol.

(2) Non-catecholamines have other substitutions or a repositioning of the hydroxyl groups on the benzene ring. These modifications tend to make the drug less potent than isoprenaline but resistant to breakdown by catechol-O-methyltransferase (COMT). Non-catecholamines include salbutamol, terbutaline, orciprenaline, fenoterol, salmeterol and formoterol.

(3) The larger the substitution on the amine head, the greater the β-agonist activity and the less the α-agonist activity. Although most substitutions reduce the potency (biological activity per unit weight of drug) of the agonist for β-adrenoceptors compared to isoprenaline this is not true for the new long-acting β_2-agonists salmeterol and formoterol (Fig. 32.2).

(4) Substitutions on the α-carbon atom and large substitutions on the amine head (e.g. salbutamol, terbutaline) block oxidation by monoamine oxidase (MAO).

ASTHMA: BASIC MECHANISMS AND CLINICAL MANAGEMENT (2nd Edn)
ISBN 0-12-079026-2

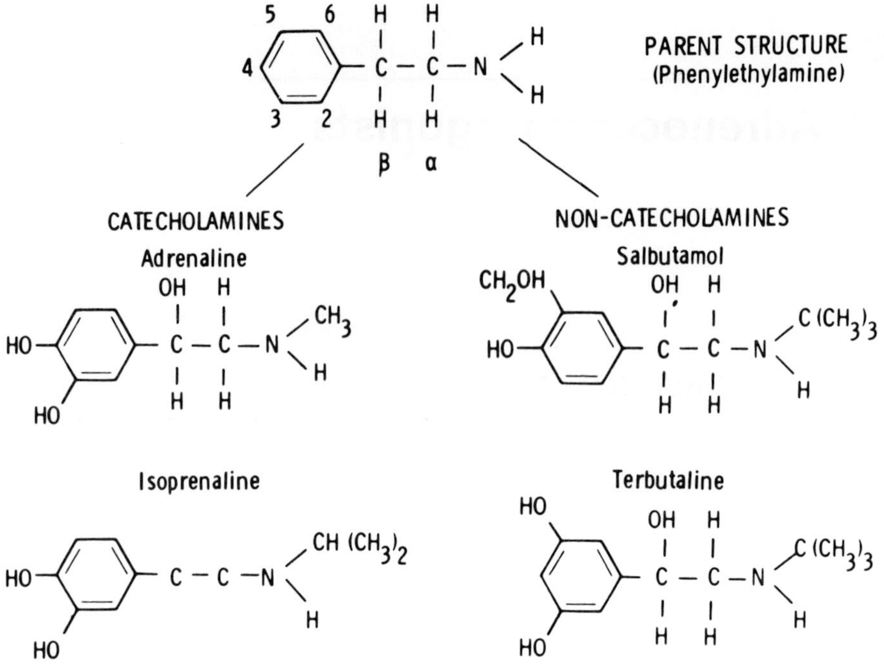

Fig. 32.1 Structure of some catechol and non-catechol sympathomimetic amines.

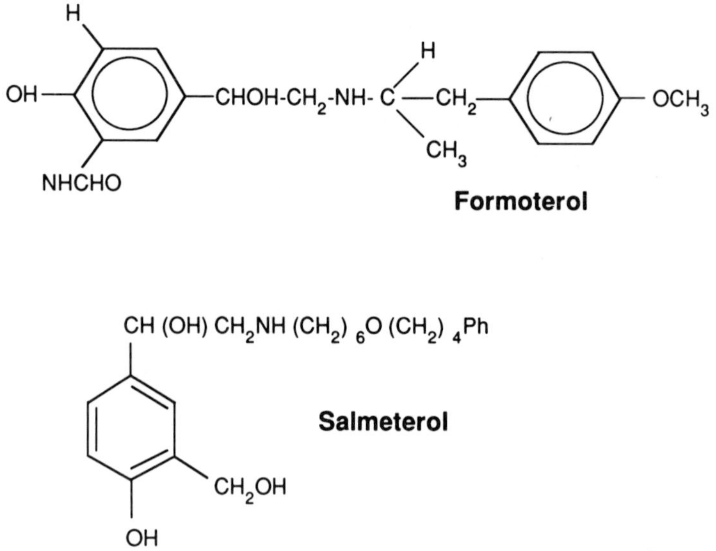

Fig. 32.2 Structure of two new long-acting sympathomimetic amines salmeterol and formoterol.

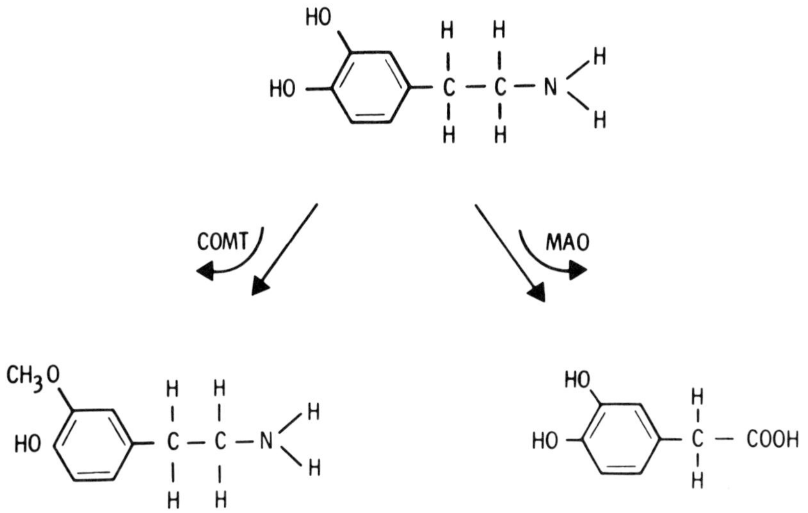

Fig. 32.3 Effect of metabolism by catechol-*O*-methyltransferase (COMT) and monoamine oxidase (MAO) on structure of sympathomimetic amines.

(5) Drugs with a lone benzene ring, such as amphetamine and ephedrine, show greater penetration of the central nervous system.

PHARMACOKINETICS

Catecholamines

Although well absorbed from the buccal mucosa and lung, catecholamines are almost completely conjugated and inactivated following ingestion. Catecholamines, whether exogenous or endogenous, are removed by active uptake mechanisms and metabolized by two widely distributed enzymes, COMT and MAO. Hence catecholamines have a relatively short half-life.

Uptake 1, the mechanism by which catecholamines are taken up into the sympathetic nerve terminal to be stored in granules, is an important method for terminating the action of adrenaline and noradrenaline but not isoprenaline. It is inhibited by amphetamine, cocaine and imipramine. Uptake 2 involves the uptake of catecholamines including isoprenaline into non-neuronal tissue such as smooth muscle cells, where metabolic degradation occurs.[2] It is inhibited by corticosteroids.

The main metabolic pathway for catecholamines is 3-*O*-methylation of the catechol nucleus by COMT and cleavage of the sympathomimetic amine between the α-carbon atom and the amine group by monoamine oxidase (Fig. 32.3). In general, 3-*O*-methylation by COMT is the more important. MAO is clearly making a significant contribution, however, since dangerous hypertension can occur in patients on monoamine oxidase inhibitors following ingestion of food containing tyramine or drugs such as ephedrine which release noradrenaline from sympathetic nerve endings. The metabolic products of catecholamines are excreted in urine.

Non-catecholamines

Non-catecholamines are well absorbed from the buccal mucosa and lung; following ingestion they are partially conjugated during first pass metabolism. Steady-state pharmacokinetic studies of oral salbutamol show that around 95% is absorbed, of which roughly half is unchanged and half converted to the sulphate conjugate.[3] Non-catecholamines have a longer half-life than catecholamines since they are not taken up by either uptake mechanism, and are resistant to degradation by COMT and usually resistant to deamination by MAO. The drugs are largely excreted in urine unchanged or as inactive conjugates.

The longer-acting β_2-agonists formoterol and salmeterol xinafoate are well absorbed from the lung and gut. Following oral administration formoterol is largely metabolized, mainly to the glucoronide, and about two thirds of the dose is excreted in urine. Salmeterol and hydroxynaphthoic acid dissociate in solution and are therefore absorbed, distributed and cleared independently. Following oral administration salmeterol is metabolized extensively by hydroxylation and eliminated predominantly in the faeces. Hydroxynaphthoic acid and conjugate are excreted in urine.

MODE OF ACTION

β-Agonists act through β-adrenoceptors, which belong to a family of G-protein linked receptors. The β_1 and β_2 receptors have been cloned and their sequences determined.[4,5] Like other G-protein linked receptors the β-receptor has seven hydrophobic segments that span the cell membrane with hydrophyllic extracellular and intracellular loops (Fig. 32.4). The native receptor differs from the cloned receptor in being glycosylated and hence has a higher molecular weight (around 60 kDa). Site-directed mutagenesis studies suggest that the ligand binding domain of the β-receptor is within the membrane, in the second and third transmembrane segments. The third intracellular loop appears to be important for coupling of the receptor to the Gs protein.[6]

The three components of the membrane–β-adrenoceptor complex, the β-adrenoceptor, Gs protein and adenylate cyclase, exist in an active and an inactive form. Stimulation of the receptor by an agonist causes a transient sequential change of each from the inactive to the active form, the agonist–adrenoceptor complex stimulating the Gs protein, which in turn activates adenylate cyclase.[7] Activation of adenylate cyclase catalyses the intracellular conversion of adenosine triphosphate (ATP) to cyclic 3,5-adenosine monophosphate (3,5-AMP). The concentration of cyclic 3,5-AMP is determined by the relative activity of adenylate cyclase and the phosphodiesterase enzymes which metabolize cyclic 3,5-AMP to adenosine monophosphate. Intracellular cyclic 3,5-AMP is capable of causing bronchodilatation through several different actions. These include reduction of intracellular calcium, inhibition of inositol phospholipid hydrolysis, activation of K^+ channels and Na^+/K^+ ATPase and activation of specific protein kinases, which, in the case of bronchial smooth muscle, reduces calcium-dependent coupling of actin and myosin (see ref. 8).

Tolerance, an attenuated response to chronic stimulation, is seen with high concentrations of β-agonists in vitro and in certain situations in vivo; it is associated with a reduced cyclic AMP response to β-agonist stimulation in vitro. Recent studies have identified several mechanisms at the level of the β-receptor whereby this can occur.[7,9]

Phosphorylation of the plasma membrane receptor by the enzyme β-adrenoceptor kinase (βARK) or protein kinase A causes uncoupling of the adrenoceptor from the Gs protein and rapid desensitization *in vitro*.[7] Alternatively, receptors may be reversibly sequestered within the cell where they can be recycled back to the cell surface. Finally, with prolonged exposure, receptors may be downregulated and degraded. This appears to be associated with a fall in β-adrenoceptor mRNA so that synthesis of new receptors is reduced.[10] The relative importance of any or all of these different processes in clinical practice is uncertain. Homologous or agonist-specific desensitization provides a feedback control mechanism to protect the cell from excessive agonist stimulation and provides increased sensitivity when agonist concentrations are low. β-Agonists could, however, be rendered less effective by this feedback mechanism though this will depend on the number of 'spare' receptors in the lung.

PHARMACOLOGICAL ACTION

The main actions of β-agonists are effected through β_1- and β_2-receptors, as shown in Table 32.1; the main pharmacological actions of relevance to patients with asthma are

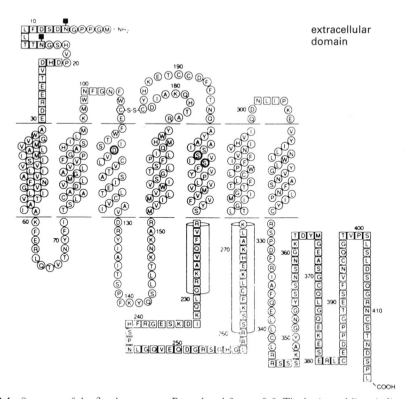

Fig. 32.4 Structure of the β_2-adrenoceptor. Reproduced from ref. 6. The horizontal lines indicate the cell membrane. There are seven transmembrane segments, an intracellular C terminal and three intracellular loops. The regions identified on the third intracellular loop are thought to be important for coupling to G proteins and the residues outlined in bold for ligand binding.

Table 32.1   β-Adrenoceptor sites and effects of stimulation.

Tissue	Receptors	Response
Airways	β_2	Smooth muscle relaxation, inhibition of mediator release by mast cells and basophils; diminution of mucosal oedema; increased mucociliary clearance; decreased airway reactivity
Heart	β_1, β_2 $\beta_1, ?\beta_2$	Tachycardia Inotropy
Blood vessels	β_2	Dilatation
Uterus	β_2	Relaxation
Muscle	β_2	Tremor
Metabolic	β_2/β_3	Increased serum concentrations of glucose, insulin lactate, pyruvate, non-esterified fatty acids, glycerol and ketone bodies; decreased concentrations of potassium, phosphate and calcium

discussed below. β_2-Adrenoceptor agonists vary in their selectivity for β_2-adrenoceptors, but none is β_2-specific, i.e. they all stimulate β_1-receptors to a lesser, but dose-dependent, extent. The pathophysiological relevance of atypical β-receptors on gastro-intestinal and cardiac tissue and the β_3-adrenoceptor subtype[11] in adipose cells is still under investigation and is not discussed further.

Airways

β-Receptors are widely distributed in human airways and alveoli. Their distribution has been studied by autoradiography carried out in the presence of selective adrenoceptor antagonists.[12] The greatest density of β-receptor labelling is seen on airway epithelium, alveolar walls and submucosal glands, with less dense labelling over airway and vascular smooth muscle. The receptors on airway and vascular smooth muscle, and on airway epithelium, appear to be entirely β_2-receptors, whereas β_1-receptors account for 10% and 30% of β-receptors on submucosal glands and alveolar walls respectively.

β-Adrenoceptor agonists have several pharmacological actions in the lung which directly or indirectly affect airway function.

Bronchial smooth muscle

The density of β_2-receptors on airway smooth muscle increases progressively from the trachea to small bronchioles.[12] The receptors have little if any innervation. *In vitro*, β-agonists have a direct relaxant effect on preconstricted or spontaneously contracting human bronchial smooth muscle, and this reponse is inhibited competitively by β-adrenoceptor antagonists.[13,14] Isoprenaline is a very potent relaxant of bronchial smooth muscle, with EC_{50} values ranging from 10^{-9} to 10^{-7} M;[14–16] β_2-agonists are in general, less potent, with EC_{50} values ranging from 10^{-7} to 10^{-3}M.[14,15] In some studies of human bronchial smooth muscle, salbutamol appears to be a partial agonist when compared with isoprenaline,[14,15] and this may be true for some other selective β-agonists.[15] The relaxation seen with β-agonists is due to functional antagonism, since it occurs whatever the contractile stimulus.

Cholinergic neurotransmission

β-Adrenoceptors are found on autonomic ganglia and postsynaptic nerve terminals and β_2-agonists are able to inhibit cholinergic neurotransmission in animals[17] and in human bronchi.[18] Loss of this protective effect may explain the bronchoconstriction induced by β-adrenoceptor antagonists in some asthmatic subjects.[19]

Inflammatory cells and mediator release

Adrenaline was shown to inhibit the release of histamine from guinea-pig lung by Schild in 1936,[20] and subsequent work has shown that β-agonists are potent inhibitors of histamine release from several tissues, including sensitized human lung,[21,22] blood from atopic subjects after incubation with allergen,[23] human basophils[24] and dispersed human mast cells.[25] The potency of β-agonists in inhibiting mediator release from human lung is greater than that seen for bronchial smooth muscle, with EC_{50} values being 10^{-9} M or less for isoprenaline[21,26] and of the order of 10^{-7} M or less for salbutamol and terbutaline.[24–26] The receptors on human mast cells are of the β_2-subtype,[26] as are the β-receptors on lymphocytes[27] and leucocytes[28] where β_2-agonists increase cyclic AMP production. β_2-Receptors have also been found on human eosinophils but do not appear to inhibit degranulation.[29] Salmeterol and formoterol are potent inhibitors of mediator release from sensitized human lung.[30,31] Other anti-inflammatory effects have been described[32] though the extent to which either drug differs qualitatively from shorter-acting β-agonists is not clear at present.

The shorter-acting β_2-agonists reduce the early response to inhaled allergen and the response to exercise in asthmatic subjects and they reduce the associated rise in plasma histamine,[33] neutrophil chemotactic factors,[33,34] platelet-derived factors[35] and eosinophil cationic protein.[36] Some of these changes are likely to be due to a direct effect of β-agonists on mediator-releasing cells, whereas others, such as platelet-derived factors, appear to be secondary effects. Early evidence suggested that the shorter acting β_2-agonists did not affect the late response to antigen[37] though recent studies have shown inhibition.[38] Salmeterol inhibited the early response to antigen in one study and although a late reponse occurred and was similar to that following placebo,[39] FEV_1 values were higher during the late response period as a result of the prolonged bronchodilatation.

How much of the airway response to β_2-agonists is due to smooth muscle relaxation and how much to inhibition of mediator release is not clear. In the nose, where there is no smooth muscle, β_2-agonists reduce the increase in nasal resistance in response to allergen to some extent,[40,41] suggesting that mediator inhibition may contribute to protection against allergen in the airways.

Vascular permeability and mucosal oedema

Airway oedema resulting from microvascular leakage and local mediator release is a prominent feature of the inflammatory response to allergen in animal models of asthma and is thought to make a large contribution to the airflow obstruction that occurs in severe asthma.[42] There is evidence that β-agonists can reduce oedema formation in some animal models but the extent to which physiological doses of β-agonists reduces vascular permeability and mucosal oedema in asthmatic airways is uncertain.[42,43]

Mucociliary clearance

The effect of β-agonists on mucociliary clearance in patients with asthma has been variable, some studies showing no effect,[44,45] and others showing an increase in clearance[46,47] attributed to increased ciliary beat frequency and increased production of periciliary cytosol. These mechanisms are difficult to study in man but β-agonists are known to stimulate mucus secretion from human airways mounted in an Ussing chamber,[48] and in animals they promote secretion of chloride ions into the airway lumen[49] and produce a small volume of viscous secretions with a high protein content.[50]

β-Agonists clearly have the potential to affect several aspects of airway function. It is difficult to determine the relative importance of the different actions to the overall therapeutic response. Measurements of airway calibre, such as the FEV_1 do not distinguish between them. The rapid time course of action of β-agonists in acute asthma suggests that they are probably acting predominantly on bronchial smooth muscle. Other actions may make a larger contribution in other situations.

Cardiovascular effects

Radioligand studies suggest that approximately a third of the β-receptors in human atria are β_2- and two-thirds β_1-receptors.[51–53] It is widely appreciated that β_1-selective agonists cause an increase in force and rate of myocardial contraction in the isolated heart, but β_2-inotropy has also been demonstrated in human atria *in vitro*.[54] β_2-agonists cause vasodilatation, a fall in systemic vascular resistance, tachycardia and increased cardiac output and the extent to which the tachycardia and increased cardiac output are due to reflex changes following peripheral vasodilatation[55,56] or to stimulation of cardiac β_2-adrenoceptors[57,58] is uncertain.

Radioligand-binding studies suggest that β-adrenoceptors on pulmonary vascular smooth muscle are exclusively β_2-receptors, a surprising finding since isoprenaline appears to be more effective than β_2-agonists in relaxing isolated human pulmonary arteries[59] and in reducing pulmonary vascular resistance in dogs.[60]

Metabolic effects

A wide range of metabolic and hormonal effects is modulated by β_2-receptor stimulation including glycogenolysis and lipolysis, and release of renin, insulin, glucagon, parathyroid and antidiuretic hormone. Studies in man, usually with an intravenous β-agonist, have demonstrated a large number of metabolic changes, including increased levels of glucose, insulin, non-esterified fatty acids, glycerol, lactate, pyruvate, ketone bodies and high-density lipoprotein cholesterol, and a fall in serum potassium phosphate, calcium and magnesium.[61-63] Patients with severe asthma show similar metabolic abnormalities prior to treatment, presumably due to release of endogenous catecholamines. The decrease in serum potassium concentrations appears to be due to stimulation of membrane-bound Na^+/K^+ ATPase on skeletal muscle, rather than to insulin release.[64,65]

Tremor

The β-receptors on skeletal muscle fibres and muscle spindles are mainly of the β_2-subtype and there is a close correlation between the EC_{50} values for relaxation of airway smooth muscle and skeletal muscle with different β-agonists.[66] β-Agonists increase physiological tremor,[67] particularly in subjects with a high basal tremor[68] by accelerating the relaxation phase of slowly contracting fibres and increasing the gain on the servomechanism (γ loop) which uses opposing muscle groups to control position.[69]

CLINICAL EFFECTS OF β_2-AGONISTS

Airways

Bronchodilatation

β_2-Agonists cause bronchodilatation in normal subjects and subjects with airflow obstruction, the greatest therapeutic benefit and largest increase in FEV_1 being seen in patients with asthma. Normal subjects will usually show a 30–100% increase in measurements which do not involve a maximum inspiration, such as specific airway conductance (sGaw) or flow rates from partial flow volume curves, but little or no change in the FEV_1. This inability to detect bronchodilatation in normal subjects by tests such as the FEV_1 is attributed to transient loss of normal resting bronchomotor tone following a maximal inspiratory manoeuvre, due to the fact that airway hysteresis is greater than parenchymal hysteresis in normal subjects.[70] Bronchodilatation can only be assessed in normal subjects by measurements which do not involve a full inflation.

Dose–response curves to inhaled β-agonists in subjects with mild asthma have been compared to those from normal subjects, and the curves are very similar, showing a similar maximum response and similar D_{max50} values (Fig. 32.5).[71] These data suggest that airway β-adrenoceptor responsiveness is normal in subjects with asthma, and provide no support for the suggestion that asthma is associated with partial β-adrenoceptor blockade of the airways. When patients with more severe asthma have been compared with normal subjects there have been small differences in responsiveness to β-agonists,[72] but interpretation is difficult in this situation due to differences in baseline airway calibre and in the patients' need for other therapy which could interfere with the response.

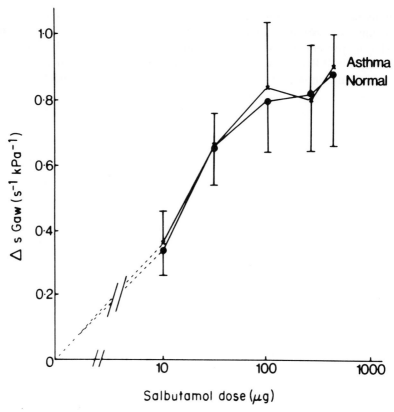

Fig. 32.5 Change in specific airways conductance (sGaw, s^{-1} kPa$^-$$^{-1}$) with increasing doses of inhaled salbutamol (10–400 μg) in six normal (●– – –●) and eight asthmatic (×– – –×) subjects.

Although some studies *in vitro* have suggested that some β_2-selective agonists may only be partial agonists with respect to isoprenaline,[14,15] there is no evidence *in vivo* of a reduced maximal bronchodilator response with β_2-agonists relative to isoprenaline. Dose–response studies with inhaled salbutamol and isoprenaline[72,73] and with salbutamol, terbutaline and fenoterol[74] have shown the same maximal airway response when carried out in the same subjects.

Bronchial reactivity

In subjects with asthma, β-agonists cause a marked reduction in non-specific bronchial reactivity to stimuli such as histamine, methacholine, eucapnic hyperventilation and exercise.[75–78] A single dose of inhaled β_2-agonist has usually caused a shift in the dose–response curve to histamine or methacholine of between two and four doubling doses, depending on the dose of β-agonist; the change is smaller when β_2-agonists have been given by the oral route.[75,78] The magnitude of this protection against non-specific stimuli is consistently greater with β-agonists than that seen with any other class of drug used to treat asthma. It does not appear to be due to bronchodilatation *per se* since ipratropium bromide does not provide similar protection for the same degree of bronchodilatation.[77] The time course of reduction in bronchial reactivity following a single dose of β-agonist is roughly similar to the time course of bronchodilatation.[76,79] The new long-acting β$_2$-agonists formoterol and salmeterol have been shown to reduce bronchial responsiveness for at least 12 h.[80,81]

The long-term effects of β-agonists on bronchial reactivity are however less straightforward and several studies now have shown a small rebound increase in bronchial reactivity following cessation of treatment with β-agonists for 2 weeks to 12 months.[79,82-85] This effect appears to be a function of prolonged treatment since terbutaline when administered in high doses over 12 h during the day did not cause a rebound increase in bronchial reactivity overnight.[79] The mechanism underlying these findings and their clinical relevance is uncertain and is discussed later.

Interaction with other therapies used in asthma

Corticosteroids. Corticosteroids are frequently said to restore airway responsiveness to β-agonists in patients with asthma. This is based on studies in animals,[86-88] in normal subjects[89] and in asthmatic patients who were unresponsive to β-agonists[90] and thus, by definition, an atypical group. When the interaction has been studied in conventional patients with stable asthma the response to the two drugs has been additive with no evidence of synergism.[91,92]

Theophylline. It was anticipated that β-agonists and theophylline might produce a synergistic effect on the airways, since theophylline causes phosphodiesterase inhibition *in vitro* and should therefore potentiate the cyclic-AMP mediated effects of β-agonists. The majority of clinical studies have been unable to demonstrate this.[93,94] Studies investigating the addition of oral theophylline to an inhaled β$_2$-agonist have usually found only a small further increase in FEV$_1$ or PEFR, of the order of a further 5–10% above the increase seen with the β-agonist alone. The addition of theophylline has sometimes caused an increase in side-effects, and this may occur when aminophylline is added to an inhaled β$_2$-agonist.[95]

Ipratropium bromide. The addition of ipratropium bromide to conventional doses of β$_2$-agonists has also usually produced slightly greater bronchodilatation than the β-agonist alone.[96-98] The magnitude of this additional response in patients with chronic asthma is variable, depending on the dose of β-agonist, but it has usually consisted of a further 5–10% increase in FEV$_1$ or PEFR above the increase seen with the β-agonist alone. In acute asthma the addition of ipratropium bromide to 10 mg nebulized salbutamol caused a greater increment improvement in peak flow rate after 1 h (77 litres/min), than salbutamol alone (31 litres/min).[99]

Thus there is no good clinical evidence of a synergistic action between β$_2$-agonists and either steroids or other bronchodilators. The benefit at best is likely to be additive. When a large dose of any bronchodilator is used, the effect of a second is invariably much less than additive, suggesting that there is a ceiling effect for response. The point at which the patient is better served by taking two drugs rather than by increasing the dose of the first drug depends on the benefit, side-effects and potential toxicity of the two drugs. Many physicians have a relatively low threshold for adding an inhaled steroid to a β$_2$-agonist, a higher threshold for adding ipratropium bromide and a higher threshold still for adding theophylline.

Development of tolerance

Tolerance, the tendency of a biological response to wane in the presence of a stimulus of constant intensity, is a common and widespread phenomenon. Following the epidemic of asthma deaths in the 1960s[100] it was suggested that tolerance may have developed in patients tending to overuse their isoprenaline inhalers who might then be expected to show a reduced bronchodilator response to an inhaled β-agonist and a subsequent inability to respond to endogenous catecholamines released during an acute attack of asthma.[101] The clinical phenomenon often referred to as tolerance or tachyphylaxis could result from desensitization of the β-adrenoceptor as discussed on page 530, although it could also occur through other mechanisms such as impaired drug access due to increased mucus production, altered drug pharmacokinetics or intracellular adaptation to increased receptor stimulation.

The development of tolerance with higher doses of β-agonists is well documented in man for certain responses such as tremor[102] and cyclic AMP production by lympho- cytes[103,104] and leucocytes,[105] but there are large differences in susceptibility between tissues.[62,102,104,106] Fortunately, the airways of asthmatic patients appear to be relatively resistant to the development of tolerance.[104,107] Bronchodilator responsiveness is fre- quently determined in clinical practice and responsiveness to β-agonists appears to be well maintained in most patients taking regular β-agonists. Two studies in the 1960s however showed that patients taking very high doses of isoprenaline improved when their isoprenaline was reduced or stopped.[108,109] Numerous prospective studies have been carried out since then looking at bronchodilator responsiveness before and after a period of treatment with recommended doses of β-agonists, and although the majority of studies have failed to show the development of tolerance[110] others have come to the opposite conclusion. The reasons for these differences are not obvious, though very few have included a control group and changes with time might occur, for example, if the selection criteria encouraged entry into the study when patients were either better or worse than average. Studies looking at the effect of higher doses of β-agonists given by nebulizer in patients with severe asthma have not shown clear evidence of tolerance[111] though these studies are difficult to carry out and interpret. Three studies have looked at bronchodilator responsiveness following salmeterol and formoterol and none has shown any reduction in bronchodilator responsiveness; however 37 of the 47 patients studied were taking an inhaled steroid and the studies were carried out a relatively short time after stopping treatment.[112-114]

The question of airway tolerance has also been approached by looking at the ability of β-agonists to protect against a bronchoconstrictor challenge. It has been suggested that the protection afforded by terbutaline against histamine challenge may be reduced following regular treatment with terbutaline for 2 weeks[79] though other studies have failed to show a significant effect.

Cardiovascular

Tachycardia and palpitations

Tachycardia and palpitations are infrequent problems when β_2-agonists are given by the inhaled route but they can occur with higher doses and are more marked with systemic therapy and with non-selective drugs. The cardiovascular changes appear to be due to direct stimulation of cardiac β_1- and β_2-receptors and to secondary compensatory effects following β_2-mediated vasodilatation. When autonomic dysfunction prevents compensatory changes, as in quadriplegic patients, β-agonist cause a large fall in system vascular resistance and blood pressure.[115] The increase in cardiac output and reduction in systemic vascular resistance with β_2-agonists has been made use of in cardiogenic shock and low cardiac output states.

Serious adverse cardiac effects

The question of whether β-agonists might cause more serious cardiac effects was first raised 25 years ago, when it was suggested that the use of isoprenaline metered-dose inhalers may have contributed to the epidemic of asthma deaths in the UK and elsewhere during the 1960s.[100,116] Cardiac dysrhythmias were suggested as the cause of death in an early anecdotal report.[117] This theory has proved difficult to substantiate because patients usually die at home and it is almost impossible to establish whether a dysrhythmia caused or contributed to death in these circumstances; the finding of widespread mucus plugging at autopsy does not exclude a fatal dysrhythmia. Evidence of myocardial damage has rarely been sought in autopsy studies of asthma, though in one such study four of 13 children who had died of asthma had histological evidence of myocardial contraction band necrosis (Fig. 32.6).[118] These lesions can be induced by catecholamine infusion[119] although only two of the four children described had been given catecholamines.[118] It may be relevant that both myocardial damage and dysrhythmias after subarachnoid haemorrhage are inhibited by β_1 blockade.[120]

The toxic effects of β-agonists on the heart are difficult to investigate in man, but studies in animals suggest that they can cause myocardial necrosis and dysrhythmias and that these effects occur with lower doses of β-agonists in the presence of theophylline. Both selective and non-selective β-agonists have caused myocardial necrosis and death from ventricular tachydysrhythmias when given alone in high doses[121–124] or, when combined with theophylline, in doses comparable to those given to man.[123–125] In animals subjected to hypoxia or in whom heart failure has been produced, isoprenaline has produced bradycardia and cardiac arrest at doses which in the unstressed heart produced tachycardia.[126,127] Isoprenaline appears to cause a 'coronary steal' in dogs with intramyocardial diversion of coronary blood flow away from the vulnerable subendocardium to cause ischaemia and subendocardial infarction.[128]

Evidence for cardiac toxicity in man has consisted to date of rather anecdotal case reports and a few prospective studies in small numbers of subjects. There are several reports of documented adverse cardiac effects during treatment with β-agonists, either alone or in combination with other drugs, including systemic steroids and methylxanthines (see Table 32.2).[128–137] It is not possible to separate the effects of the different drugs in these episodes nor the effect of the underlying disease in some instances, but the data suggest that β-agonists, usually in high doses, may have contributed to the development of dysrhythmias, pulmonary oedema, myocardial ischaemia and infarction. These patients had symptoms referable to the heart, but in a prospective study of 15 consecutive pregnant women receiving intravenous rimiterol, with no cardiac symptoms other than palpitations, 11 had ST segment depression and three of four patients studied by echocardiography had septal hypokinesia.[138]

A few prospective studies have looked at the incidence of cardiac toxicity with β-agonists given alone or in combination with methylxanthines. The results are conflicting,[125] with some showing no increase in cardiac dysrhythmias[138–142] and others a significant increase.[143–147] All the studies contained a small number of subjects, however, and many excluded patients with known cardiac problems. If dysrhythmia or myocardial ischaemia is a significant complication of β-agonists it is clearly very uncommon and the chance of a type II error in these studies is very high. If serious dysrhythmia occurred in one in a thousand patients on high-dose β-agonists it would be clinically important, but tens of thousands of patients would need to be studied prospectively to detect such an effect.

The possibility that fluorinated hydrocarbon propellants used in metered-dose inhalers might cause dysrhythmias has been investigated.[148] Cardiac toxicity only occurred in dogs when the most toxic propellant, freon 11, was taken in very high doses in conjunction with a β-agonist[149] (freon blood levels exceeded 20 μg/ml).[150] These compounds have a relatively short half-life, however, and freon 11 was undetectable in blood from patients overusing their inhalers.[151] When normal subjects deliberately

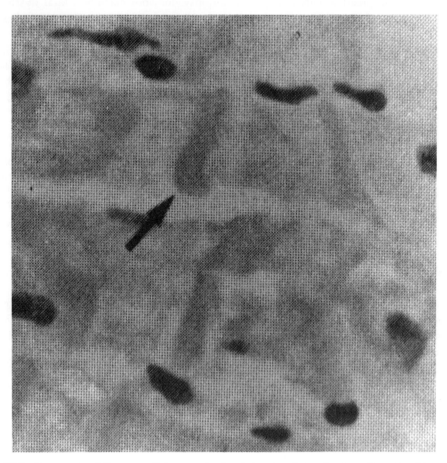

Fig. 32.6   Dense eosinophilic myocardial contraction bands in a boy dying of asthma. Reproduced from ref. 118, with permission.

Table 32.2 Summary of reports of adverse effects of β-agonists on the heart.

First author		
Winsor[128]	Isoprenaline (inhalation and IV)	ST depression in eight patients, most with coronary artery disease Myocardial infarction in one patient
Neville[129]	Salbutamol (nebulizer)	Increased angina in three patients with coronary heart disease
Lawyer[130]	Terbutaline (subcutaneous) aminophylline, prednisolone	Chest pain, tachycardia (160 b/min) and ST segment depression following terbutaline overdose in 67-year-old patient with asthma
Matson[131]	Isoprenaline (inhalation and IV), aminophylline, hydrocortisone	Chest pain and ST segment depression in 14-year-old boy with asthma
Szczeklik[132]	Salbutamol (IV), aminophylline, hydrocortisone	Myocardial infarction in 54-year-old patient with asthma
Kurland[133]	Isoprenaline (IV), aminophylline, hydrocortisone	Fatal myocardial infarction in 18-year-old patient with asthma
Elliott,[134] Tinga[135]	Rimiterol (IV), betamethasone	Pulmonary oedema in two patients with premature labour
Rogge[136]	Terbutaline (subcutaneous and oral), dexamethasone	Pulmonary oedema in three patients with premature labour
Tandon[137]	Fenoterol, salbutamol (inhaled)	Ventricular dysrhythmias after fenoterol

inhaled 10–30 puffs over 2 min from a metered-dose inhaler containing 80 μg of isoprenaline per puff, blood levels rarely exceeded 2 μg/ml.[152] These findings suggest that freons are unlikely to contribute significantly to cardiac toxicity.

Pulmonary artery pressure

β-Agonists cause pulmonary vasodilatation in patients with pulmonary hypertension,[153] and isoprenaline caused a small fall in pulmonary artery pressure in patients with asthma.[154] Vasodilatation of blood vessels constricted in response to hypoxia is the likely explanation for the fall in arterial oxygen tension (PaO_2) which sometimes occurs after β-agonist administration.

Arterial oxygen tension

Arterial oxygen tension may increase or decrease following administration of β-agonists, the response depending on the net effect of two separate actions of β-agonists. The increase in cardiac output and hence increase in mixed venous PO_2 will cause PaO_2 to increase, whereas the increased perfusion of poorly ventilated areas will cause PaO_2 to fall. Inert gas studies showed a doubling of blood flow to low V/Q areas following isoprenaline.[154] However, the fall in PaO_2 when it occurs is usually small, around 0.5 kPa (3–4 mmHg), although occasional patients show larger changes.[155,156] An increase in PaO_2 appears to be more common after higher doses of β-agonists given by nebulizer or intravenously,[157,158] situations in which a predominant effect on cardiac output might be expected.

Metabolic changes

Metabolic complications of β-agonist therapy are rarely recognized. With coventional single doses by metered-dose inhaler, nebulizer, subcutaneous or intravenous injection, the mean decrease in plasma potassium has ranged from 0.4 to 1.1 mmol/litre.[74,159–161] with falls up to 1.6 mmol/litre in individual patients. However, these acute changes may not be sustained with long-term treatment. The reduction in potassium and change in other metabolites seen with the acute administration of oral pirbuterol was not seen after treatment for 3 months, with the exception of fasting glucose and insulin.[162] β-Agonists can precipitate ketoacidosis in diabetic patients.[163]

Tremor and other side-effects

A fine tremor can be a nuisance with oral β-agonists or with high doses by nebulizer, though it tends to decrease with prolonged treatment as tolerance develops. It is rarely a problem with low-dose inhaled therapy. Cramp occurs relatively infrequently with β-agonists. Seizures have been reported following a high dose of an oral β-agonist in one child.[164]

CHOICE OF β-AGONIST

When selecting a β-agonist in clinical practice, the main points to consider are β-selectivity, dose equivalence, duration of action and formulation. There is no evidence that one β-agonist causes a greater maximal effect than another. Although some patients claim to respond better to one β-agonist than to another these preferences are inconsistent and are probably due to differences in dose or other factors at the time that the drug was taken.

β_2-Selectivity

When the bronchial selectivity of β-agonists is assessed in man it is always considerably less than would be expected from assessment of β_2-selectivity of the drug in isolated tissues.[73,165,166] This is because the β_2-adrenoceptor-mediated fall in peripheral vascular resistance causes a compensatory reflex tachycardia through vagal withdrawal, so the increase in heart rate is greater than would be expected from *in vitro* studies. The studies in man are relevant to clinical practice. They show a roughly 7–10-fold bronchial selectivity for salbutamol compared to isoprenaline.[73,165] Salbutamol and terbutaline appear to be similar in terms of bronchial selectivity, with orciprenaline being slightly less bronchial selective.[167] Fenoterol may be less β_2-selective than salbutamol and terbutaline[74,168–171] though the main reason that it causes more cardiovascular effects than the other two drugs is because it has been marketed at a relatively higher dose.[74,168,169] Formoterol showed similar β_2 selectivity to salbutamol in one study;[172] data on salmeterol are not available.

Dose equivalence

Differences in potency between different β-agonists (e.g. orciprenaline 20 mg = salbutamol 4 mg), are unimportant, since lower potency is easily compensated for by giving a larger dose of drug. Differences in dose equivalence between recommended doses of different β-agonists is more important. Salbutamol and terbutaline appear to have roughly similar effects on β_1 and β_2 receptors for each dose from a metered-dose inhaler (100 μg and 250 μg). Fenoterol (200 μg) has somewhere between two and four times the effect on both β_1 and β_2 receptors.[74,169,170] Formoterol (12 μg) appears to be roughly equivalent to salbutamol 100 μg;[172] salmeterol 50 μg is probably equivalent to rather more than 200 μg salbutamol.[81]

Duration of action

The duration of action of β-agonists, as with any bronchodilator, is very dependent on dose; the higher the dose the longer the half-life. When given in recommended doses by metered-dose inhaler the duration of action varies, the short-acting catecholamines lasting from 1 to 2 h with recommended doses, the intermediate acting drugs such as salbutamol and terbutaline lasting 3–6 h, and the new long-acting β-agonists such as formoterol and salmeterol lasting around 12 h.[79,80] Salbutamol, terbutaline and fenoterol have a slightly longer duration of action than orciprenaline.[173] The onset of action also varies considerably being more rapid with the catecholamines (near maximum within 5 min of inhalation) than with the intermediate acting drugs such as salbutamol, although 80% of the peak effect in the latter group is seen by 5 min and values close to maximum by 15 min. The onset of action with formoterol appears to be similar to that of salbutamol and terbutaline and more rapid than that seen with salmeterol (around 1 h).[32,80,81,174]

DRUGS AND ROUTE OF ADMINISTRATION

Whenever possible, β_2-agonists should be given by inhalation, since this allows bronchodilatation to be achieved with a smaller dose and fewer side-effects than either the oral or intravenous routes. The metered-dose inhaler is widely used and is usually convenient and effective, though care is needed to make sure that it is used correctly. For patients unable to use a metered-dose inhaler, other routes of administration should be tried. These include a dry powder inhaler, a metered-dose inhaler attached to a spacing device, or a nebulizer.

β_2-Selective non-catecholamines

Salbutamol and terbutaline combine β_2-selectivity with a reasonably long duration of action and are used most widely at present. Orciprenaline and possibly fenoterol are less β_2-selective and fenoterol has been marketed at a high dose relative to salbutamol and terbutaline.

β_2-Selective catecholamines

Rimiterol, apart from being β_2 selective, is similar to isoprenaline; isoetherine is conjugated to a lesser extent in the gut wall.

Isoprenaline

Isoprenaline, a non-selective β-agonist, was the first relatively pure β-agonist with little α-adrenoceptor activity to be used widely. It has a short duration of action, causes more tachycardia for a given degree of bronchodilatation than the β_2-agonists, and is ineffective when given orally, being conjugated in the gut wall to an inert sulphate. Although it has been the yardstick for the assessment of newer drugs, it has been superseded in clinical practice by the β_2-selective agonists.

Ephedrine

Ephedrine, a non-catecholamine, has no place in the modern treatment of asthma. It lacks β_2-selectivity and has more side-effects such as insomnia and retention of urine due to penetration of the central nervous system. Since it acts in part by release of noradrenaline from sympathetic nerve terminals, it is dangerous in the presence of MAO inhibitors.

Adrenaline

Adrenaline is still used for severe asthma in some countries. It appears to cause more adverse cardiac effects than β_2-agonists,[145,175] as would be expected from its α-adrenoceptor agonist activity and lack of β-selectivity.

ROLE OF β-AGONISTS IN THE MANAGEMENT OF ASTHMA

The role of β-agonists in the management of asthma is undergoing re-appraisal following the introduction of the long-acting β-agonists and the recent studies concerned with mortality and morbidity in relation to β-agonists in New Zealand and elsewhere. Unlike the epidemic of asthma deaths in the 1960s, New Zealand was the only country to experience a marked increase in asthma mortality in the late 1970s.[176] This increase in mortality coincided with the introduction of the inhaled β-agonist fenoterol in 1976, and the increase in prescriptions of this drug in New Zealand was greater than in any other country.[177] Three case-control studies from New Zealand have shown that patients who died from asthma were more likely to have been taking fenoterol than any other β-agonist, in effect salbutamol.[177–179] What cannot be determined from these studies is whether the association between fenoterol and mortality is due to a direct effect of fenoterol or to confounding by severity, the patients with more severe asthma being more likely to be given fenoterol. The fact that fenoterol has been marketed at a higher dose by metered-dose inhaler than salbutamol[74,169,170] and may be less $β_2$-selective [74,168–171] could mean that it was more likely to have caused adverse effects or that it was perceived as being more effective and hence was given to the more vulnerable patients with severe or brittle asthma.

To try to disentangle these effects Sears *et al.*[85] carried out a prospective study in patients with asthma comparing the effect of regular treatment with fenoterol (400 μg q.i.d.) with treatment with β-agonists taken as required. The patients receiving regular fenoterol did less well according to a variety of clinical measures of asthma control than patients taking β-agonists as required, suggesting that regular high doses of fenoterol can cause asthma to deteriorate. The mechanism whereby this deterioration might happen is not clear. Sears *et al.*[85] suggest that bronchodilatation with $β_2$-agonists may increase the antigen load to the airways. Such a feedback mechanism would mitigate against maintained benefit with β-agonists but does not easily explain why patients should deteriorate with regular treatment. If this mechanism is correct a similar effect would be expected with other bronchodilators, and there is some support for this.[180] An alternative hypothesis, that heparin released by mast cells is an important anti-inflammatory agent and that β-agonists, by suppressing mast cell mediator release, increase inflammation[181] is only tenable if the effects of heparin are more important than the combined effects of the pro-inflammatory mediators released by mast cells. The evidence for this is not strong. The mechanism for which there is most evidence *in vitro* is downregulation of β-receptors (see page 530). Sears *et al.*[85] argue against receptor downregulation because most of their patients were taking an inhaled steroid which would be expected to prevent it. Also van Schayck *et al.*[84] found no evidence of β-receptor downregulation on lymphocytes, but this is perhaps not surprising since the drugs were given by inhalation. On present evidence it is not possible to determine the underlying mechanism; these different hypotheses need to be tested in further studies.

SUMMARY

Regular short-acting β-agonists

There is confusion at present about the role of regular β-agonists in the treatment of asthma. There is circumstantial evidence to suggest that in high doses they can cause dysrhythmias and it seems likely that they will do so in some vulnerable patients.

Dysrhythmias cannot explain the deterioration seen in the study by Sears et al.[85] nor do they easily explain the increased mortality in young patients in New Zealand. The study by Sears et al.[85] and the studies showing increased bronchial responsiveness following cessation of treatment with β-agonists suggest that β-agonists can make asthma worse. To what extent this relates to drug (fenoterol) or dose (high doses only) is not clear and requires urgent investigation. The only important recognized difference in pharmacological activity between fenoterol and drugs such as salbutamol and terbutaline is that fenoterol has been used in higher doses and it may be less β_2-selective. It could well be the case that β-agonists are helpful for most patients with asthma and only cause problems when given in high doses; it is important to determine the extent to which, overall, β-agonists are helpful or unhelpful to patients and in what circumstances.

Role of long-acting β-agonists

The role of long-acting β-agonists in the management of asthma is still far from clear,[182] and there may be differences between salmeterol and formoterol since the mechanism underlying the longer duration of action of the two drugs may be different. The longer duration of action will be convenient for patients, should help nocturnal asthma and may be of benefit by providing continuous inhibition of mast-cell mediator release. It is also possible that the way in which the agonists interact with the receptor will protect the receptor against desensitization and some of the side-effects or shorter-acting β-agonists.[183] Data however are lacking and until further evidence is available to show that these drugs do not cause the changes seen with fenoterol, or the findings of Sears et al.[85] are refuted, they should be introduced cautiously. They are being recommended as an addition to inhaled steroids in patients not adequately controlled on the steroid alone, and, in the case of salmeterol, for twice-daily treatment only.

ACKNOWLEDGEMENTS

We thank Dr W. Richardson at Ciba Geigy and Dr J. Maconochie at Glaxo for information on the pharmacokinetics of formoterol and salmeterol respectively.

REFERENCES

1. Brittain RT, Dean CM, Jack D: Sympathomimetic bronchodilator drugs. In Widdicombe JG (ed) *Respiratory Pharmacology*. Oxford, Pergamon, 1981, pp 613–653.
2. Iverson LL: Role of transmitter uptake mechanisms in synaptic neurotransmission. *Br J Pharmac* (1971) **41**: 571–591.
3. Morgan DJ, Paull JD, Richmond BH, Wilson-Evered E, Ziccone SP: Pharmacokinetics of intravenous and oral salbutamol and its sulphate conjugate. *Br J Clin Pharmacol* (1986) **22**: 587–593.
4. Dixon RAF, Kobilka BK, Strader D, et al.: Cloning of the gene and cDNA for mammalian β-adrenergic receptor and homology with rhodopsin. *Nature* (1986) **321**: 75–79.
5. Barnes PJ: Molecular biology of receptors: implications for lung disease. *Thorax* (1990) **45**: 482–488.

6. Strader CD, Sigal IS, Dixon RAF: Mapping the functional domains of the β-adrenergic receptor. *Am J Respir Cell Mol Biol* (1989) **1**: 81–86.

7. Hausdorff WP, Caron MG, Lefkowitz RJ: Turning off the signal: desensitization of β-adrenergic receptor function. *FASEB J* (1990) **4**: 2881–2889.

8. Hall IP, Tattersfield AE: Beta agonists. In Clark TJH, Lee TH, Godfrey S (eds) *Asthma*. London, Chapman and Hall, 1991, pp 341–365.

9. Bouvier M, Collins S, O'Dowd BF, *et al.*: Two distinct pathways for cAMP-mediated down-regulation of the β₂-adrenergic receptor. *J. Biol Chem* (1989) **264**: 16786–16792.

10. Hadcock JR, Malbon CC: Down-regulation of β-adrenergic receptors: Agonist-induced reduction in receptor mRNA levels. *Proc Natl Acad Sci* (1988) **85**: 5021–5025.

11. Emorine LJ, Marullo S, Briend-Sutren M-M, *et al.*: Molecular characterisation of the human β₃-adrenergic receptor. *Science* (1989) **245**: 1118–1121.

12. Carstairs JR, Nimmo AJ, Barnes PJ: Autoradiographic visualization of beta-adrenoceptor subtypes in human lung. *Am Rev Respir Dis* (1985) **132**: 541–547.

13. Mathé AA, Astrom A, Persson N-A: Some bronchoconstriction and bronchodilating responses of human isolated bronchi: evidence for the existence of alpha-adrenoceptors. *J Pharm Pharmac* (1971) **23**: 905–910.

14. Davis C, Conolly ME, Greenacre JK: Beta-adrenoceptors in human lung, bronchus and lymphocytes. *Br J Clin Pharmac* (1980) **10**: 425–432.

15. Goldie RG, Spina D, Henry PJ, Lulich KM, Paterson JW: *In vitro* responsiveness of human asthmatic bronchus to carbachol, histamine, beta-adrenoceptor agonists and theophylline. *Br J Clin Pharmac* (1986) **22**: 669–676.

16. van Koppen CH, Rodrigues de Miranda JF, Beld AJ, van Ginneken CAM: β-Adrenoceptor binding and induced relaxation in airway smooth muscle from patients with chronic airflow obstruction. *Thorax* (1989) **44**: 28–35.

17. Skoogh BE: Transmission through airway ganglia: *Eur J Respir Dis* (1983) **64** (Suppl 131): 159–170.

18. Rhoden KJ, Meldrum LA, Barnes PJ: Inhibition of cholinergic neurotransmission in human airways by β₂-adrenoceptors. *J Appl Physiol* (1988) **65**: 700–705.

19. Ind PW, Dixon CMS, Fuller RW, Barnes PJ: Anticholinergic blockade of beta-blocker-induced bronchoconstriction. *Am Rev Respir Dis* (1989) **139**: 1390–1394.

20. Schild HO: Histamine release and anaphylactic shock in isolated lungs of guinea-pigs. *Quart J Experimental Physiol* (1936) **26**: 165–179.

21. Assem ESK, Schild HO: Inhibition by sympathomimetic amines of histamine release induced by antigen in passively sensitized human lung. *Nature* (1969) **224**: 1028–1029.

22. Butchers PR, Fullarton JR, Skidmore IF, Thompson LE, Vardeu CJ, Wheeldon A: A comparison of the anti-anaphylactic activities of salbutamol and disodium cromoglycate in the rat, the rat mast cell and in human lung tissue. *Br J Pharmac* (1979) **67**: 23–32.

23. Radermecker M, Guston M: An *in vivo* demonstration of the antianaphylactic effect of terbutaline. *Clin Allergy* (1981) **11**: 79–86.

24. Marone G, Kagey-Sobotka A, Lichtenstein LM: Effects of arachidonic acid and its metabolites on antigen-induced histamine release from human basophils *in vitro*. *J. Immunol* (1979) **123**: 1669–1677.

25. Peters SP, Schulman ES, Schleimer RP, Macglashan DW, Newball HH, Lichtenstein LM: Dispersed human lung mast cells. Pharmacological aspects and comparison with human lung tissue fragments. *Am Rev Respir Dis* (1982) **126**: 1034–1039.

26. Butchers PR, Skidmore IF, Vardey CJ, Wheeldon A: Characterization of the receptor mediating the anti-anaphylactic effects of beta-adrenoceptor agonists in human lung tissue *in vitro*. *Br J Pharmacol* (1980) **71**: 663–667.

27. Conolly ME, Greenacre JK: The beta-adrenoceptor of the human lymphocyte and human lung parenchyma. *Br J Pharmacol* (1977) **59**: 17–23.

28. Logsdon PJ, Middelton E, Coffey RG: Stimulation of leukocyte adenyl cyclase by hydrocortisone and isoproterenol in asthmatic and non-asthmatic subjects. *J Allergy Clin Immunol* (1972) **50**: 45–56.

29. Yukawa T, Ukena D, Kroegel C, *et al.*: β₂-Adrenergic receptors on eosinophils. *Am Rev Respir Dis* (1990) **141**: 1446–1452.

30. Mita H, Shida Takao: Anti-allergic activity of formoterol, a new β-adrenoceptor stimulant, and salbutamol in human leukocytes and human lung tissue. *Allergy* (1983) **38**: 547–552.

31. Butchers P, Cousins SA, Vardey CJ: Salmeterol: a potent and long-acting inhibitor of the release of inflammatory and spasmogenic mediators from human lung. *Br J Pharmacol* (1987) **92**: 745.

32. Lofdahl CG, Chung KF: Long-acting β_2-adrenoceptor agonists: a new perspective in the treatment of asthma. *Eur Respir J* (1991) **4**: 218–226.

33. Howarth PH, Durham SR, Lee TH, *et al*.: Influence of albuterol, cromolyn sodium and ipratropium bromide on the airway and circulating mediator responses to allergen bronchial provocation in asthma. *Am Rev Respir Dis* (1985) **132**: 986–992.

34. Martin GL, Atkins PC, Dunsky EH, Zweiman B: Effects of theophylline, terbutaline, and prednisone on antigen-induced bronchospasm and mediator release. *J Allergy Clin Immunol* (1980) **66**: 204–212.

35. Johnson CE, Belfield PW, Davis S, Cooke NJ, Spencer A, Davies JA: Platelet activation during exercise induced asthma: effect of prophylaxis with cromoglycate and salbutamol. *Thorax* (1986) **41**: 290–294.

36. Venge P, Dahl R, Peterson CGB: Eosinophil granule proteins in serum after allergen challenge of asthmatic patients and the effects of anti-asthmatic medication. *Int Arch Allergy Appl Immunol* (1988) **87**: 306–312.

37. Cockcroft DW, Murdock KY: Comparative effects of inhaled salbutamol, sodium cromoglycate and beclomethasone dipropionate on allergen-induced early asthmatic reponses, late asthmatic responses and increased bronchial responsiveness to histamine. *J. Allergy Clin Immunol* (1987) **79**: 734–740.

38. Twentyman OP, Finnerty JP, Holgate ST: The inhibitory effect of nebulised albuterol on the early and late asthmatic reactions and increase in airways responsiveness provided by inhaled allergen in asthma. *Am Rev Respir Dis* (1991) **144**: 782–787.

39. Twentyman OP, Finnerty JP, Harris A, Palmer J, Holgate ST: Protection against allergen-induced asthma by salmeterol. *Lancet* (1990) **336**: 1338–1342.

40. Schumacher MJ: Effect of a beta-adrenergic agonist, fenoterol, on nasal sensitivity to allergin. *J. Allergy Clin Immunol* (1980) **66**: 33–36.

41. Borum P, Mygind N: Inhibition of the immediate allergic reaction in the nose by the β_2-adrenostimulant fenoterol. *J Allergy Clin Immunol* (1980) **66**: 25–32.

42. Persson CGA: Role of plasma exudation in asthmatic airways. *Lancet* (1986) **ii**: 1126–1129.

43. Chung KF, Rogers DF, Barnes PJ, Evans TW: The role of increased airway microvascular permeability and plasma exudation in asthma. *Eur Respir J* (1990) **3**: 329–337.

44. Isawa T, Teshima T, Hirano T, *et al*.: Does a β_2-stimulator really facilitate mucociliary transport in the human lungs *in vivo*? *Am Rev Respir Dis* (1990) **141**: 715–720.

45. Bateman JRM, Pavia D, Sheahan NF, Newman SP, Clarke SW: Effects of terbutaline sulphate aerosol on bronchodilator response and lung mucociliary clearance in patients with mild stable asthma. *Br J Clin Pharmacol* (1983) **15**: 695–700.

46. Pavia D. Agnew JE, Sutton PP, *et al*.: Effect of terbutaline administered from metered dose inhaler (2 mg) and subcutaneously (0.25 mg) on tracheobronchial clearance in mild asthma. *Br J Dis Chest* (1987) **81**: 361–370.

47. Mossberg B, Strandberg K, Philipson K, Camner P: Tracheobronchial clearance in bronchial asthma: response to beta-adrenoceptor stimulation. *Scand J Respir Dis* (1976) **57**: 119–128.

48. Phipps RJ, Williams IP, Richardson PS, Pell J, Pack RJ, Wright N: Sympathomimetic drugs stimulate the output of secretory glycoproteins from human bronchi *in vitro*. *Clin Sci* (1982) **63**: 23–28.

49. Davis B, Marin MG, Yee JW, Nadel JA: Effect of terbutaline on movement of Cl and Na across the trachea of the dog *in vitro*. *Am Rev Respir Dis* (1979) **120**: 547–552.

50. Lopez-Vidriero MT: Lung secretions. In Clarke SW, Pavia D (eds) *Aerosols and the Lung. Clinical and Experimental Aspects*, 1st edn. London, Butterworths, 1984, pp 19–41.

51. Heitz A, Schwartz J, Velly J: Beta-Adrenoceptors of the human myocardium: determination of β_1 and β_2 subtypes by radioligand binding. *Br J Pharmacol* (1983) **80**: 711–717.

52. Robberecht P, Delhaye M, Taton G, *et al.*: The human heart beta-adrenergic receptors. *Mol Pharmacol* (1983) **24**: 169–173.

53. Stiles GL, Taylor S, Lefkowitz RJ: Human cardiac beta-adrenergic receptors: subtype heterogeneity delineated by direct radioligand binding. *Life Sci* (1983) **33**: 467–473.

54. Zerkowski H-R, Ikezono K, Rohm N, Reidemeister J Chr, Brodde O-E: Human myocardial beta-adrenoceptors: demonstration of both *β₁*- and *β₂*-adrenoceptors mediating contractile responses to *β*-agonists on the isolated right atrium. Naunyn-Schmiedeberg's *Arch Pharmacol* (1986) **332**: 142–147.

55. Bourdillon PDV, Dawson JR, Foale RA, Timmis AD, Poole-Wilson PA, Sutton GC: Salbutamol in treatment of heart failure. *Br Heart J* (1980) **43**: 206–210.

56. Arnold JMO, McDevitt DG: Contribution of the vagus to the haemodynamic responses following intravenous boluses of isoprenaline. *Br J Clin Pharmacol* (1983) **15**: 423–429.

57. McGibney D, Singleton W. Strike B, Taylor SH: Observations on the mechanisms underlying the differences in exercise and isoprenaline tachycardia after cardioselective and non-selective beta-adrenoceptor antagonists. *Br J Clin Pharmacol* (1983) **15**: 15–19.

58. Arnold JMO, O'Connor PC, Riddell JG, Harron DWG, Shanks RG, McDevitt DG: Effects of the *β₂*-adrenoceptor antagonists ICI 118 151 on exercise tachycardia and isoprenaline-induced beta-adrenoceptor responses in man. *Br J Clin Pharmacol* (1985) **19**: 619–630.

59. Boe J, Simonssen BG: Adrenergic receptors and sympathetic agents in isolated human pulmonary arteries. *Eur J Respir Dis* (1980) **61**: 195–202.

60. Rodriguez-Roisin R, Bencowitz HZ, Ziegler MG, Wagner PD: Gas exchange responses to bronchodilators following methacholine challenge in dogs. *Am Rev Respir Dis* (1984) **130**: 617–626.

61. Phillips PJ, Vedig AE, Jones PL, *et al.*: Metabolic and cardiovascular side effects of the beta adrenoceptor agonists, salbutamol and rimiterol. *Br J Clin Pharmacol* (1980) **9**: 483–491.

62. Harvey JE, Baldwin CJ, Wood PJ, Alberti KGMM, Tattersfield AE: Airway and metabolic responsiveness to intravenous salbutamol in asthma—effect of regular inhaled salbutamol. *Clin Sci* (1981) **60**: 579–585.

63. Hooper PH, Woo W, Visconti L, Pathak DR: Terbutaline raises high-density-lipoprotein-cholesterol levels. *N Engl J Med* (1981) **305**: 1455–1456.

64. Struthers AD, Reid JL: The role of adrenal medullary catecholamines in potassium homeostasis. *Clin Sci* (1984) **66**: 377–382.

65. Whyte KF, Addis GJ, Whitesmith R, Reid JL: The mechanism of salbutamol-induced hypokalaemic. *Br J Clin Pharmacol* (1987) **23**: 65–71.

66. Olsson OAT, Swanberg E, Svedinger I, Waldeck B: Effects of beta-adrenoceptor agonists on airway smooth muscle and on slow-contracting skeletal muscle: *In vitro* and *in vivo* results compared. *Acta Pharm Toxicol* (1979) **44**: 272–276.

67. Marsden CD, Foley TM, Owen DAL, McAllister RG: Peripheral beta-adrenergic receptors concerned with tremor. *Clin Sci* (1967) **33**: 53–65.

68. Jenne JW, Ridley DJ, Marcucci RA, Druz WS, Rook JC: Objective and subjective tremor responses to oral *β₂*-agents on first exposure. *Am Rev Respir Dis* (1982) **126**: 607–610.

69. Lippold OCJ: Oscillation in the stretch reflex arc and the origin of the rhythmical, 8-12 C/S component of physiological tremor. *J Physiol* (1970) **206**: 359–382.

70. Ingram RH: Site and mechanism of obstruction and hyperresponsiveness in asthma. *Am Rev Respir Dis* (1987) **136**: S62–S64.

71. Tattersfield AE, Holgate ST, Harvey JE, Gribbin HR: Is asthma due to partial beta-blockade of airways? *Agents Actions* (1983) **13**: 265–271.

72. Barnes PJ, Pride NB: Dose–response curves to inhaled beta-adrenoceptor agonists in normal and asthmatic subjects. *Br J Clin Pharmacol* (1983) **25**: 677–682.

73. Warrell DA, Robertson DG, Newton Howes J, *et al.*: Comparison of cardiorespiratory effects of isoprenaline and salbutamol in patients with bronchial asthma. *Br Med J* (1970) **i**: 65–70.

74. Wong CS, Pavord ID, Williams J, Britton JR, Tattersfield AE: Bronchodilator, cardiovascular, and hypokalaemic effects of fenoterol, salbutamol, and terbutaline in asthma. *Lancet* (1990) **336**: 1396–1399.

75. Salome CM, Schoeffel RE, Yan K, Woolcock AJ: Effect of aerosol and oral fenoterol on histamine and methacholine challenge in asthmatic subjects. *Thorax* (1981) **36**: 580–584.

76. Salome Cm, Schoeffel RE, Yan K, Woolcock AJ: Effect of aerosol fenoterol on the severity of bronchial hyperreactivity in patients with asthma. *Thorax* (1983) **38**: 854–858.
77. Britton JR, Hanley SP, Garrett HV, Hadfield JW, Tattersfield AE: Dose related effects of salbutamol and ipratropium bromide on airway calibre and reactivity in subjects with asthma. *Thorax* (1988) **43**: 300–305.
78. Tattersfield AE: Effect of beta agonists and anticholinergic drugs on bronchial reactivity. *Am Rev Respir Dis* (1987) **136**: S64–S68.
79. Vathenen AS, Knox AJ, Higgins BG, Britton JR, Tattersfield AE: Rebound increase in bronchial responsiveness after treatment with inhaled terbutaline. *Lancet* (1988) **i**: 554–558.
80. Becker AB, Simons FER, McMillan JL, Faridy T: Formoterol, a new long-acting selective β_2-adrenergic receptor agonist: Double-blind comparison with salbutamol and placebo in children with asthma. *J. Allergy Clin Immunol* (1989) **84**: 891–895.
81. Campos-Gongora H, Wisniewski AFZ, Tattersfield AE: A single dose comparison of inhaled albuterol and two formulations of salmeterol on airway reactivity in asthmatic subjects. *Am Rev Respir Dis* (1991) **144**: 626–629.
82. Kraan J, Keoter GH, van der Mark Th W, Sluiter H-, de Vries K: Changes in bronchial hyperreactivity induced by 4 weeks of treatment with antiasthmatic drugs in patients with allergic asthma: a comparison between budesonide and terbutaline. *J Allergy Clin Immunol* (1985) **76**: 628–636.
83. Kerrebijn KF, van Essen-Zandvliet EEM, Neijens HJ: Effect of long term treatment with inhaled corticosteroids and beta agonists on the bronchial responsiveness in children with asthma. *J Allergy Clin Immunol* (1987) **79**: 653–659.
84. van Schayck CP, Graafsma SJ, Visch MB, Dompeling E, van Weel C, van Herwaarden CLA: Increased bronchial hyperresponsiveness after inhaling salbutamol during 1 year is not caused by subsensitisation to salbutamol. *J Allergy Clin Immunol* (1990) **86**: 793–800.
85. Sears MR, Taylor DR, Print CG, *et al.*: Regular inhaled β-agonist treatment in bronchial asthma. *Lancet* (1990) **336**: 1391–1396.
86. Mano K, Akbarzedeh A, Townley RG: Effect of hydrocortisone on beta-adrenergic receptors in lung membranes. *Life Sci* (1979) **25**: 1925–1930.
87. Handslip PDJ, Ward JPT, Cameron IR: The effect of steroids on beta-adrenergic receptor density and affinity in rat lung membrane. *Clin Sci* (1981) **61**: 11.
88. Geddes BA, Jones TR, Dvorsky RJ, Lefcoe NH: Interaction of glucocorticoids and bronchodilators on isolated guinea-pig tracheal and human bronchial smooth muscle. *Am Rev Respir Dis* (1974) **110**: 420–427.
89. Holgate ST, Baldwin CJ, Tattersfield AE: Beta-adrenergic agonist resistance in normal human airways. *Lancet* (1977) **ii**: 375–377.
90. Ellul-Micallef R, French FF: Effect of intravenous prednisolone in asthmatics with diminished adrenergic responsiveness. *Lancet* (1975) **ii**: 1269–1271.
91. Dahl R, Johansson SA: Effect on lung function of budesonide by inhalation, terbutaline s.c. and placebo given simultaneously or as single treatments. *Eur J Respir Dis* (1982) **63**(Suppl 122): 132–137.
92. Grandordy B, Belmatoug N, Morelle A, De Lauture D, Marsac J: Effect of betamethasone on airway obstruction and bronchial response to salbutamol in prednisolone resistant asthma. *Thorax* (1987) **42**: 65–71.
93. Svedmyr K: β_2-Adrenoceptor stimulants and theophylline in asthma therapy. *Eur J Respir Dis* (1981) **62**(Suppl. 116): 1–48.
94. Handslip PDJ, Dar AM, Davies BH: Intravenous salbutamol and aminophylline in asthma. A search for synergy. *Thorax* (1981) **36**: 741–744.
95. Siegel D, Sheppard D, Gelb A, Weinburgh PF: Aminophylline increases the toxicity but not the efficacy of an inhaled beta-adrenergic agonist in the treatment of acute exacerbations of asthma. *Am Rev Respir Dis* (1985) **132**: 283–286.
96. Jenkins CR, Chow CM, Fisher BL, Marlin GE: Ipratropium bromide and fenoterol by aerosolized solution. *Br J Clin Pharmacol* (1982) **14**: 113–115.
97. Pierce RJ, Allen CJ, Campbell AH: A comparative study of atropine methonitrate, salbutamol, and their combination in airways obstruction. *Thorax* (1979) **34**: 45–50.

98. Ullah MI, Newman GB, Saunders KB: Influence of age on response to ipratropium and salbutamol in asthma. *Thorax* (1981) **36**: 523–529.

99. O'Driscoll BR, Taylor RJ, Horsley MG, Chambers DK, Bernstein A: Nebulised salbutamol with and without ipratropium bromide in acute airflow obstruction. *Lancet* (1989) **i**: 1418–1420.

100. Inman WHW, Adelstein AM: Rise and fall of asthma mortality in England and Wales in relation to use of pressurised aerosols. *Lancet* (1969) **ii**: 279–285.

101. Conolly ME, Davies DS, Dollery CT, George CF: Resistance to beta-adrenoceptor stimulants, a possible explanation of the rise in asthma deaths. *Br J Pharmacol* (1971) **43**: 389–402.

102. Larrson S, Svedmyr N, Thiringer G: Lack of bronchial beta adrenoceptor resistance in asthmatics during long-term treatment with terbutaline. *J Allergy Clin Immunol* (1977) **59**: 93–100.

103. Conolly ME, Greenacre JK: The beta adrenoreceptor of human lymphocyte and human lung parenchyma. *Br J Pharmacol* (1977) **59**: 17–23.

104. Tashkin DP, Conolly ME, Deutsch RI, *et al.*: Subsensitization of beta-adrenoceptors in airways and lymphocytes of healthy and asthmatic subjects. *Am Rev Respir Dis* (1982) **125**: 185–193.

105. Galant SP, Duriseti L, Underwood S, Allred S, Insel PA: Beta adrenergic receptors of polymorphonuclear particulates in bronchial asthma. *J Clin Invest* (1980) **65**: 577–585.

106. Eichler H-G, Blochl-Daum B, Eichler I, Wolzt M, Korn A, Gotz M: Normal responsiveness of superficial hand veins to alpha- and beta-adrenergic stimuli in allergic asthma: Effects of terbutaline and prednisolone on beta-adrenergic responsiveness. *J Allergy Clin Immunol* (1990) **86**: 714–725.

107. Harvey JE, Tattersfield AE: Airway response to salbutamol: effect of regular salbutamol inhalations in normal, atopic, and asthmatic subjects. *Thorax* (1982) **37**: 280–287.

108. Van Metre TE: Adverse effects of inhalation of excessive amounts of nebulised isoproterenol in status asthmaticus. *J Allergy* (1969) **43**: 101–113.

109. Reisman RE: Asthma induced by adrenergic aerosols. *J Allergy* (1970) **46**: 162–177.

110. Tattersfield AE: Tolerance to beta agonists. *Bull Eur Physiopathol Respir* (1985) **21**: 1S–5S.

111. McGivern DV, Ward M, Revill S, Sechiari A, Macfarlane J, Davies D: Home nebulisers in severe chronic asthma. *Br J Dis Chest* (1984) **78**: 376.

112. Wallin A, Melander B, Rosenhall L, Sandstrom T, Wahlander L: Formoterol, a new long acting β_2-agonist for inhalation twice daily, compared with salbutamol in the treatment of asthma. *Thorax* (1990) **45**: 259–261.

113. Arvidsson P, Larsson S, Lofdahl C-G, Melander B, Wahlander L, Svedmyr N: Formoterol, a new long-acting bronchodilator for inhalation. *Eur Respir J* (1989) **2**: 325–330.

114. Ullman A, Hedner J, Svedmyr N: Inhaled salmeterol and salbutamol in asthmatic patients. *Am Rev Respir Dis* (1990) **142**: 571–575.

115. Pingleton SK, Schwartz O, Szymanski D, Epstein M: Hypotension associated with terbutaline therapy in acute quadriplegia. *Am Rev Respir Dis* (1982) **126**: 723–725.

116. Stolley PD, Schinnar R: Association between asthma mortality and isoproterenol aerosols: A review. *Prev Med* (1978) **7**: 519–538.

117. Greenberg MJ: Isoprenaline in myocardial failure. *Lancet* (1965) **ii**: 442–443 (letter).

118. Drislane FW, Samuels MA, Kozakewich H, Schoen FJ, Strunk RC: Myocardial contraction band lesions in patients with fatal asthma: possible neurocardiologic mechanisms. *Am Rev Respir Dis* (1987) **135**: 498–501.

119. Karch ST, Billingham ME: Myocardial contraction bands revisited. *Hum Pathol* (1986) **17**: 9–13.

120. Cruickshank JM, Neil-Dwyer G, Degaute JP, *et al.*: Reduction of stress/catecholamine-induced cardiac necrosis by β_1-selective blockade. *Lancet* (1987) **ii**: 585–589.

121. Rona G, Chappel CI, Balazs T, Gaudry R: An infarct-like myocardial lesion and other toxic manifestations produced by isoproterenol in the rat. *Arch Pathol* (1959) **67**: 443–445.

122. Todd GL, Baroldi G, Pieper GM, Clayton FC, Eliot RS: Experimental catecholamine-induced myocardial necrosis. I. Morphology, quantification and regional distribution of acute contraction band lesions. *J Mol Cell Cardiol* (1985) **17**: 317–338.

123. Food and Drug Administration: Interactions between methylxanthines and beta adrenergic agonists. *FDA Drug Bull* (1981) **11**: 19–20.

124. Joseph X, Whiteburst VE, Bloom S, Balazs T: Enhancement of cardiotoxic effects of beta-adrenergic bronchodilators by aminophylline in experimental animals. *Fundam Appl Toxicol* (1981) **1**: 443–447.

125. Nicklas RA, Whitehurst VE, Donohoe RF, Balazs T: Concomitant use of beta adrenergic agonists and methylxanthines. *J Allergy Clin Immunol* (1984) **73**: 20–24.

126. Lockett MF: Dangerous effects of isoprenaline in myocardial failure. *Lancet* (1965) **ii**: 104–106.

127. Collins JM, McDevitt DG, Shanks RG, Swanton JG: The cardiotoxicity of isoprenaline during hypoxia. *Br J Pharmacol* (1969) **36**: 35–45.

128. Winsor T, Mills B, Winbury MM, Howe BB, Berger HJ: Intramyocardial diversion of coronary blood flow: effects of isoproterenol-induced subendocardial ischemia. *Microvasc Res* (1975) **9**: 261–278.

129. Neville E, Corris PA, Vivian J, Nariman S, Gibson GJ: Nebulized salbutamol and angina. *Br Med J* (1982) **285**: 796–797.

130. Lawyer C, Pond A: Problems with terbutaline. *N Engl J Med* (1977) **296**: 821.

131. Matson JR, Loughlin GM, Strunk RC: Myocardial ischemia complicating the use of isoproterenol in asthmatic children. *J Pediatr* (1978) **92**: 776–778.

132. Szczeklik A, Nizankowski R, Mruk J: Myocardial infarction in status asthmaticus. *Lancet* (1977) **i**: 658–659.

133. Kurland G, Williams J, Lewiston NF: Fatal myocardial toxicity during continuous infusion intravenous isoproterenol therapy of asthma. *J Allergy Clin Immunol* (1979) **63**: 407–411.

134. Elliott HR, Abdulla U, Hayes PJ: Pulmonary oedema associated with ritodrine infusion and betamethasone administration in premature labour. *Br Med J* (1978) **ii**: 799–800.

135. Tinga DJ, Aarnoudse JG: Post-partum pulmonary oedema associated with preventive therapy for premature labour. *Lancet* (1979) **i**: 1026.

136. Rogge P, Young S, Goodlin R: Post-partum pulmonary oedema associated with preventive therapy for premature labour. *Lancet* (1979) **i**: 1026–1027.

137. Tandon MK: Cardiopulmonary effects of fenoterol and salbutamol aerosols. *Chest* (1980) **77**: 429–431.

138. Ben-Shlomo T, Zohar S, Marmor A, Blondheim DS, Sharir T: Myocardial ischaemia during intravenous ritodrine treatment; is it so rare? *Lancet* (1986) **ii**: 917–918.

139. Gilmartin JJ, Veale D, Murray A, Adams PC, Gibson GJ: Cardiac effects of salbutamol given by air driven nebuliser at home. *Thorax* (1986) **41**: 331–332.

140. Coleman JJ, Vollmer JWM, Barker AF, Schultz GE, Buist AS: Cardiac arrhythmias during the combined use of beta-adrenergic agonist drugs and theophylline. *Chest* (1986) **90**: 45–51.

141. Kelly HW, Menendez R, Voyles W: Lack of significant arrhythmogenicity from chronic theophylline and beta-2-therapy in asthmatic subjects. *Ann Allergy* (1985) **54**: 405–410.

142. Kemp JP, Chervinsky P, Orgel HA, Meltzer EO, Noyes JH, Mingo TS: Concomitant bitolterol mesylate aerosol and theophylline for asthma therapy, with 24 h electrocardiographic monitoring. *J Allergy Clin Immunol* (1984) **73**: 32–43.

143. Al-Hillawi AH, Hayward R, Johnson NM: Incidence of cardiac arrhythmias in patients taking slow release salbutamol and slow release terbutaline for asthma. *Br Med J* (1984) **288**: 367.

144. Cookson WOCM, John S, McCarthy G, McCarthy S, Lane DJ: Nebuliser therapy and cardiac dysrhythmias in patients with COAD. *Thorax* (1985) **40**: 704–705.

145. Josephson GW, Kennedy HL, MacKenzie EJ, Gibson G: Cardiac dysrhythmias during the treatment of acute asthma. *Chest* (1980) **78**: 429–435.

146. Nicotra MB, Rivera M, Faber B, Clark PL, Crisp GO: Are high theophylline levels of benefit to stable patients with chronic airways obstruction (CAO) receiving beta-adrenergic agents or do they increase the risk of cardiac arrhythmias? *Am Rev Respir Dis* (1983) **127**: 137.

147. Conradson T-B, Eklundh G, Olofsson B, Pahlm O, Persson G: Cardiac arrhythmias in patients with mild-to-moderate obstructive lung disease. *Chest* (1985) **88**: 537–542.

148. Taylor GJ, Harris WS: Cardiac toxicity of aerosol propellants. *JAMA* (1979) **214**: 81–85.

149. Clark DG, Tinston DJ: Cardiac effects of isoproterenol, hypoxia, hypercapnia and fluorocarbon propellants and their use in asthma inhalers. *Ann Allergy* (1972) **30**: 536–541.
150. Jack D: Sniffing syndrome. *Br Med J* (1971) **2**: 708–709.
151. Paterson JW, Sudlow MF, Walker SR: Blood-levels of fluorinated hydrocarbons in asthmatic patients after inhalation of pressurised aerosols. *Lancet* (1971) **ii**: 565–568.
152. Dollery CT, Draffan GH, Davies DS, Williams FM, Conolly ME: Blood concentrations in man of fluorinated hydrocarbons after inhalation of pressurised aerosols. *Lancet* (1970) **ii**: 1164–1166.
153. Pietro DA, LaBresh KA, Shulman RM, Folland ED, Parisi AF, Sasahara AA: Sustained improvement in primary pulmonary hypertension during six years of treatment with sublingual isoproterenol. *N Engl J Med* (1984) **310**: 1032–1034.
154. Wagner PD, Dantzker DR, Iacovoni VE, Tomlin WC, West JB: Ventilation–perfusion inequality in asymptomatic asthma. *Am Rev Respir Dis* (1978) **118**: 511–525.
155. Ingram RH, Krumpe PE, Duffell GM, Maniscalco B: Ventilation–perfusion changes after aerosolised isoproterenol in asthma. *Am Rev Respir Dis* (1970) **101**: 364–370.
156. Pierson RN, Grieco MH: Isoproterenol aerosol in normal and asthmatic subjects. *Am Rev Respir Dis* (1969) **100**: 533–541.
157. Tribe AE, Wong RM, Robinson JS: A controlled trial of intravenous salbutamol and aminophylline in acute asthma. *Med J Aust* (1976) **2**: 749–752.
158. Bloomfield P, Carmichael J, Petrie GR, Jewell NP, Crompton GK: Comparison of salbutamol given intravenously and by intermittent positive-pressure breathing in life-threatening asthma. *Br Med J* (1979) **1**: 848–850.
159. Clifton GD, Hunt BA, Patel FC, Burki NK: Effects of sequential doses of parenteral terbutaline on plasma levels of potassium and related cardiopulmonary responses. *Am Rev Respir Dis* (1990) **141**: 575–579.
160. Smith SR, Ryder C, Kendall MJ, Holder R: Cardiovascular and biochemical responses to nebulised salbutamol in normal subjects. *Br J Clin Pharmacol* (1984) **18**: 641–644.
161. Haalboom JRE, Deenstra M, Struyvenberg A: Hypokalaemia induced by inhalation of fenoterol. *Lancet* (1985) **i**: 1125–1127.
162. Canepa-Anson R, Dawson JR, Kuan P, *et al.*: Differences between acute and long-term metabolic and endocrine effects of oral *β*-adrenoceptor agonist therapy with pirbuterol for cardiac failure. *Br J Clin Pharmacol* (1987) **23**: 173–181.
163. Leslie D, Coats PM: Salbutamol-induced diabetic ketoacidosis. *Br Med J* (1977) **2**: 768.
164. Friedman R, Zitelli B, Jardine D, Fireman P: Seizures in a patient receiving terbutaline. *Am J Dis Child* (1982) **136**: 1091–1092.
165. Cullum VA, Farmer JB, Jack D, Levy GP: Salbutamol: a new, selective beta adrenoceptive receptor stimulant. *Br J Pharmac* (1969) **35**: 141–151.
166. Rossing TH, Fanta CH, McFadden ER: A controlled trial of the use of single versus combined drug therapy in the treatment of acute episodes of asthma. *Am Rev Respir Dis* (1981) **123**: 190–194.
167. Kennedy MCS, Simpson WT: Human pharmacological and clinical studies on salbutamol: a specific *β*₁-adrenergic bronchodilator. *Br J Dis Chest* (1969) **63**: 165–174.
168. Gray BJ, Frame MH, Costello JF: A comparative double-blind study of the bronchodilator effects and side effects of inhaled fenoterol and terbutaline administered in equipotent doses. *Br J Dis Chest* (1982) **76**: 341–350.
169. Svedmyr N: Fenoterol: A *β*-adrenergic agonist for use in asthma. *Pharmacotherapy* (1985) **5**: 109–126.
170. Heel RC, Brogden RN, Speight TM, Avery GS: Fenoterol: A review of its pharmacological properties and therapeutic efficacy in asthma. *Drugs* (1978) **15**: 3–32.
171. Crane J, Burgess C, Beasley R: Cardiovascular and hypokalaemic effects of inhaled salbutamol, fenoterol, and isoprenaline. *Thorax* (1989) **44**: 136–140.
172. Lofdahl C-G, Svedmyr N: Formoterol fumarate, a new *β*₂-adrenoceptor agonist. *Allergy* (1989) **44**: 264–271.
173. Formgren H: Clinical comparison of inhaled terbutaline and orciprenaline in asthmatic patients. *Scand J Respir Dis* (1970) **51**: 203–211.

174. Ullman A, Svedmyr N: Salmeterol, a new long acting inhaled β_2-adrenoceptor agonist: comparison with salbutamol in adult asthmatic patients. *Thorax* (1988) **43**: 674–678.
175. Rossing TH, Fanta CH, McFadden ER, Medical House Staff of the Peter Bent Brigham Hospital: A controlled trial of the use of single versus combined drug therapy in the treatment of acute episodes of asthma. *Am Rev Respir Dis* (1981) **123**: 190–194.
176. Jackson RT, Beaglehole R, Rea HH, Sutherland DC: Mortality from asthma: a new epidemic in New Zealand. *Br Med J* (1982) **285**: 771–774.
177. Crane J, Pearce N, Flatt A, *et al.*: Prescribed fenoterol and death from asthma in New Zealand, 1981–83; case-control study. *Lancet* (1989) **i**: 917–922.
178. Pearce N, Grainger J, Atkinson M, *et al.*: Case-control study of prescribed fenoterol and death from asthma in New Zealand, 1977–81. *Thorax* (1990) **45**: 170–175.
179. Grainger J, Woodman K, Pearce N. *et al.*: Prescribed fenoterol and death from asthma in New Zealand, 1981–7: a further case-control study. *Thorax* (1991) **46**: 105–111.
180. van Schayck CP, Dompeling E, van Herwaarden CLA, *et al.*: Long term effects of continuous versus symptomatic bronchodilator treatment in asthma or COPD. *Am Rev Respir Dis* (1991) **143**: A653.
181. Page CP: On explanation of the asthma paradox: inhibition of natural anti-inflammatory mechanism by β_2-agonists. *Lancet* (1991) **337**: 717–720.
182. Editorial: β_2-agonists in asthma: relief, prevention, morbidity. *Lancet* (1990) **336**: 1411–1412.
183. Jack D: A way of looking at agonism and antagonism: Lessons from salbutamol, salmeterol and other β-adrenoceptor agonists. *Br J Clin Pharmacol* (1991) **31**: 501–514.

33

Anticholinergic Bronchodilators

NICHOLAS J. GROSS

INTRODUCTION

Anticholinergic alkaloids such as atropine exist in many plants and have consequently been used in herbal remedies for many centuries. They were introduced into Western medicine in the early 1800s and enjoyed enormous use as bronchodilators until well into the present century. When adrenaline was discovered in the 1920s, followed soon by ephedrine, other adrenergic drugs, and then methylxanthines, their use declined. The natural anticholinergic agents produced side-effects that resulted in poor acceptability by patients, besides being less effective bronchodilators then newer agents. Interest in their use has returned with better understanding of the role of cholinergic mechanisms in the control of airway tone, and the development of synthetic congeners of atropine and scopolamine that are topically active but much less prone to produce side-effects.[1]

RATIONALE FOR THE USE OF ANTICHOLINERGIC BRONCHODILATORS

Autonomic control of airway calibre

In normal human airways the bulk of efferent autonomic nerves are cholinergic.[2] Branches of the vagus nerve travel along the airways and synapse at peribronchial ganglia that are distributed predominantly among larger airways (Chapter 22). From ganglion cells, short postganglionic fibres travel to smooth muscle cells, pulmonary arterioles, mucus glands, and possibly ciliated epithelial cells. Acetylcholine is released

ASTHMA: BASIC MECHANISMS AND CLINICAL MANAGEMENT (2nd Edn)
ISBN 0-12-079026-2

from varicosities and terminals of the postganglionic nerves and activates muscarinic receptors on these structures. This results in smooth muscle contraction, liberation of mucus from mucus glands, and possibly, acceleration of ciliary beating. A low level of cholinergic vagal (bronchomotor) tone can be recorded in the normal, resting state in experimental animals, but can be considerably augmented in response to stimuli (see below).

Anticholinergic agents are competitive inhibitors of acetylcholine at muscarinic receptors. The rationale for their use as bronchodilators, then, is that they inhibit the cholinergic activity responsible for bronchomotor tone and this allows the airways to dilate. They do not inhibit other mechanisms or mediators that may cause airway smooth muscle contraction; nor, indeed, do they affect the numerous other mechanisms of airway obstruction in abnormal states such as asthma.

Vagal reflexes in airways

Reflex-mediated bronchoconstriction has been extensively studied in animal models.[3,4] Cholinergic, bronchomotor activity can be reflexly augmented by a number of stimuli (Fig. 33.1). The territory from which reflex bronchoconstriction can arise is wide and probably includes, in addition to the upper and lower airways, the oesophagus and the carotid bodies. Receptors through which the reflex acts include the rapidly adapting 'irritant receptors' and non-myelinated C-fibres, both of which are found in the airway epithelium. Stimuli to which they respond and which result in bronchoconstriction include mechanical irritation, a wide variety of irritant gases, aerosols, and particles of

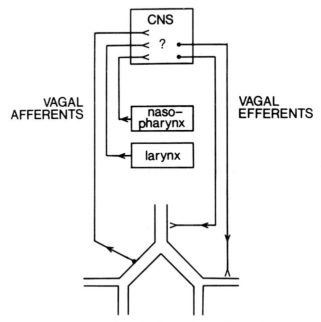

Fig. 33.1 Diagrammatic representation of vagal reflex pathways from irritant receptors through vagal afferents, central nervous system (CNS), and vagal efferents to effector cells in the airways. Reproduced from ref. 1, with permission.

many sorts, and to some extent the inhalation of cold dry air and specific mediators such as histamine. Impulses originating from the receptors travel in afferent vagal nerves to the central nervous system and back to the lungs in vagal efferents, resulting in rapid bronchoconstriction (<1 s).

A solid body of research derived from elegant physiologic studies, mostly in animals, indicates that bronchoconstriction can be mediated through such vagal reflex mechanisms. However, the extent to which such reflex mechanisms actually contribute to airflow limitation in patients with airway disease is not at all clear. As vagally mediated bronchoconstriction can be entirely ablated by anticholinergic agents, and as anticholinergic agents rarely entirely reverse airflow obstruction in any airway disease, one assumes that vagal activity rarely accounts for more than part of the pathophysiology of airflow limitation. This part may be the only reversible component in patients with emphysema where airflow obstruction is due mainly to structural damage,[5] but may be a trivial component in diseases such as asthma where airflow obstruction is largely due to inflammation. Inflammatory mechanisms can be mitigated by anti-inflammatory therapy and to some extent by β-adrenergic agents, but are not amenable to anticholinergic therapy, except to the extent (probably minor) that they are due to cholinergic activity. One might predict from this that anticholinergic agents would be less useful in airway inflammation, i.e. asthma, than in chronic bronchitis and emphysema, as is shown below.

Muscarinic receptor subtypes

A detailed discussion of muscarinic receptor subtypes, a topic that is rapidly expanding at present, is outside the scope of this chapter (see Chapter 22). Two points can be briefly made. One is that airway muscarinic receptors are distributed preferentially in larger airways,[6] a distribution that corresponds to that of vagal parasympathetic nerves. This implies that the bronchodilator action of anticholinergic agents will also be concentrated on the larger airways.

The second point is that molecular biology has revealed that there are possibly as many as nine muscarinic receptor genes, raising the possibility of this number of unique receptor subtypes, called M_1, M_2 ..., etc. Three muscarinic receptor subtypes have been identified in airway structures.[7] Inhibition of M_1 and M_3 receptors would tend to limit muscarinic bronchomotor activity; inhibition of M_2, an autoreceptor, might be expected to augment bronchomotor activity. None of the anticholinergic agents that are currently available for clinical use are selective for these subtypes—they inhibit all three subtypes. It is possible that inhibitors selective for M_1 and M_3, for example, may be developed with greater bronchodilator potential.

ACTION OF ANTICHOLINERGIC AGENTS

Cholinergic control of airway functions

In summary, cholinergic fibres mediate at least three functions in the airways. They promote airway smooth muscle contraction, promote the release of secretions from submucosal glands and, possibly, augment ciliary activity of epithelial cells. Perhaps the most important of these is their effect on airway smooth muscle (bronchomotor tone, as discussed above), inhibition of which is the principal rationale for administering anticholinergic agents as bronchodilators. They increase airflow even in normal subjects.[8] There is some evidence that basal cholinergic tone is increased in both asthma[9] and chronic obstructive pulmonary disease (COPD),[8] which, if correct, provides a practical reason for using anticholinergic agents in these conditions. Airway secretions are stimulated by cholinergic activity, as is (probably) ciliary clearance;[10] the therapeutic role of anticholinergic agents in inhibiting these latter two actions in airway disease, whether beneficial or not, is unclear.

Site of action of anticholinergic agents

When administered systemically, anticholinergic agents tend to have their principal physiological action on more central airways than do adrenergic bronchodilators.[1] This site conforms to the distribution of both cholinergic nerve terminals and muscarinic receptors in the airways (above). Current practice favours the aerosol administration of bronchodilators, by which route all bronchodilators tend to be preferentially delivered to the larger, central airways. Consequently, the site of action of inhaled anticholinergic and alternative bronchodilators is predominantly central, and not distinguishably different for these different classes of agents.

PHARMACOLOGY OF ANTICHOLINERGIC AGENTS

Naturally occurring anticholinergic agents such as atropine, scopolamine, hyoscine, etc. are all tertiary ammonium compounds, i.e. the nitrogen atom on the tropine ring is 3-valent (Fig. 33.2). Such compounds are freely water- and lipid-soluble and are well absorbed from mucosal surfaces. They are thus widely distributed in the body and cross the blood–brain barrier. They counteract parasympathetic, cholinergic activity in almost every system and consequently result in widespread systemic effects. In the dose that results in bronchodilatation, 1.0–2.5 mg in adults, they produce some dryness of the mouth, and possibly tachycardia and flushing of the skin. In only slightly higher doses these effects are accentuated, and they produce blurred vision and urinary retention. At doses above 5 mg central nervous system effects can occur—irritability, ataxia, hallucinations, delirium and coma. Their therapeutic margin is thus small.

Synthetic anticholinergic agents, e.g. ipratropium bromide (Fig. 33.2) have been developed to minimize such side-effects. The nitrogen atom in the tropine ring has been made 5-valent and carries a charge, making the molecule virtually incapable of absorption from mucosal surfaces. Such agents are fully anticholinergic at the site of deposition and will, for example, dilate the pupil if delivered to the eye, or dilate the bronchi if delivered to the airways. They are not sufficiently absorbed from these sites, however, to produce detectable effects on other organs. They can thus be regarded as topical forms of atropine.

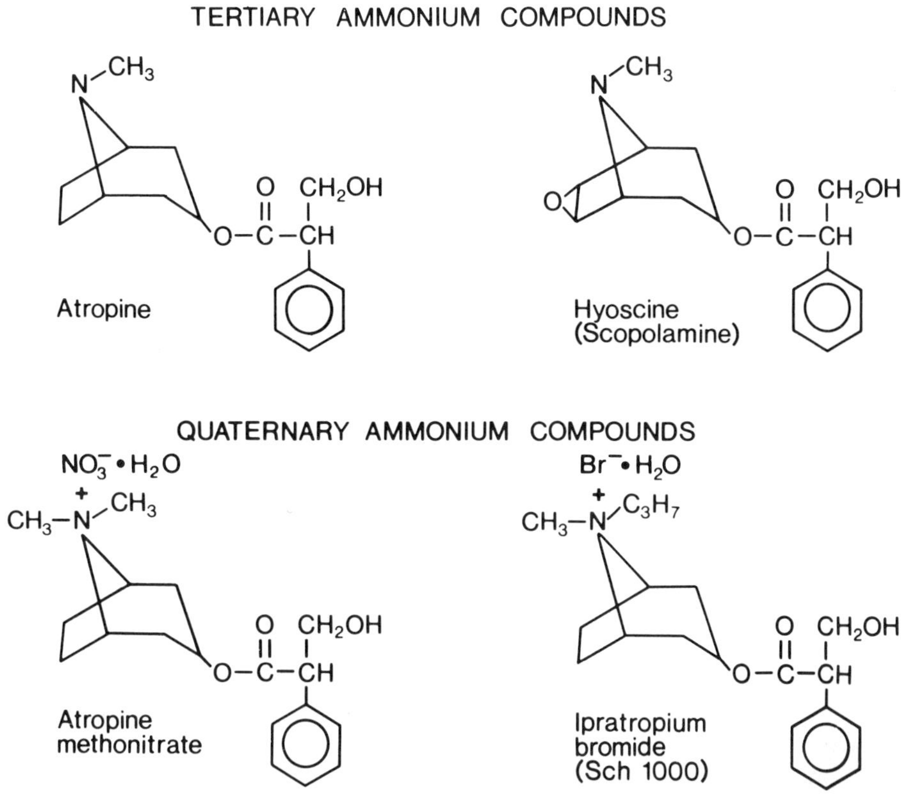

TERTIARY AMMONIUM COMPOUNDS

Atropine

Hyoscine
(Scopolamine)

QUATERNARY AMMONIUM COMPOUNDS

Atropine
methonitrate

Ipratropium
bromide
(Sch 1000)

Fig. 33.2 Structures of some anticholinergic bronchodilators. Reproduced from ref. 1, with permission.

In addition to ipratropium bromide (Atrovent®), which has been in use in Europe for about 15 years and in the United States for about 5 years, other synthetic quaternary anticholinergic agents include atropine methonitrate, oxitropium bromide (Oxivent®), and glycopyrrolate bromide (Robinul®).

Pharmacokinetics

Atropine and its naturally occurring congeners exist in two optical isomers, only one of which is physiologically active. Most synthetic agents, e.g. ipratropium, are synthesized in the active form, a fact that must be taken into account in dose–response studies.

Atropine sulphate administration results in peak blood levels in 1 h or less. It has a half-life of 3 h in the circulation in adults, but longer in children and the elderly.[11] Most of the drug is recovered unchanged in the urine within 24 h, traces occur in the faeces and in the breast milk of lactating women. Ipratropium administration by mouth or by inhalation results in very low blood levels peaking at about 1–2 h, declining with a half-life of up to 4 h. Its biological effect following inhalation is somewhat longer than that of atropine, probably because it is not removed by absorption. Over 90% of the orally administered dose is recovered in the faeces, some of the remainder is recovered in the urine as inactive metabolites. It is largely excluded from the central nervous system.

EFFICACY IN ASTHMA

Dose–response[11]

The optimal dose of nebulized atropine solution has been reported to be 0.025–0.4 mg/kg in adults, 0.05 mg/kg in children. For nebulized atropine methonitrate the optimal dose is somewhat less, 0.015–0.02 mg/kg. For nebulized ipratropium the optimal dose in adults is about 500 μg. For nebulized glycopyrrolate bromide the optimal dose is 0.02 mg/kg. These figures will vary according to severity of airway disease, and the equipment and technique used for nebulization. For metered-dose inhalers (MDI), the optimal dose of oxitropium bromide has been reported to be 500 μg. The optimal dose of ipratropium by MDI is unclear. In stable young asthmatics a dose of 40–80 μg may be optimal, in stable older patients with COPD the optimal dose may be as much as 160 μg.[12] It seems possible that patients with more severe airway obstruction may need higher doses because of reduced penetration of particles into the airway tree.

Against specific stimuli

Anticholinergic agents when given in advance of specific bronchospastic stimuli show varying degrees of protection. They protect more or less completely against the bronchospasm induced by cholinergic agonists such as methacholine. They are also prophylactic against bronchospasm induced in asthmatics by β-blocking agents and by psychogenic factors. They provide only partial protection against bronchospasm due to most other specific stimuli, e.g. histamine, prostaglandins, non-specific dusts and irritant aerosols, and exercise, hyperventilation and the inhalation of cold dry air (reviewed in ref. 1). In many of the later instances, adrenergic agents usually provide greater prophylaxis.

Stable asthma

A very large number of studies have compared the bronchodilator potential of anticholinergic agents with that of adrenergic agents. While many of these studies are flawed by the fact that they used recommended doses rather than optimal doses, they provide the clinician with useful information about the comparative actions of these bronchodilators. Figure 33.3[13] which is typical of most such studies, illustrates many of these points. Anticholinergic agents are slower to reach peak effect, typically 1–2 h, than adrenergic agents. At their peak effect they almost invariably result in less bronchodilatation. The quaternary forms may be slightly longer acting than agents such as salbutamol. Among asthmatics there is, however, substantial variation in responsiveness, some patients responding very little to anticholinergic agents, others responding almost as well to them as to adrenergic agents.

It has been difficult to identify subgroups of asthmatics who are likely to manifest the most responsiveness to anticholinergic agents. Older asthmatics (over 40 years of age) may respond better than younger ones,[14] although even children aged 10–18 years have

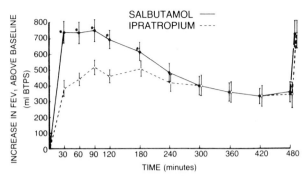

Fig. 33.3   Increase in FEV_1 in 25 patients with asthma after inhalation of 200 μg salbutamol by MDI, or 40 μg ipratropium by MDI on separate days. All patients received an additional dose of salbutamol at 480 min. Asterisks denote significant differences ($P < 0.05$). Reproduced from ref. 13, with permission.

been shown to benefit.[15] Intrinsic asthmatics and those with longer duration of asthma may also respond better than extrinsic asthmatics[16] although these too appear to be poor predictors.[13] An individual trial remains the best way to identify responsiveness.[17]

Acute severe asthma

Rebuck et al.[18] found that 500 μg nebulized ipratropium resulted in less bronchodilatation than 1.25 mg of nebulized fenoterol over the first 90 min of treatment of acute asthma. However the combination of both agents was significantly more effective than either alone. Moreover, patients with more severe airway obstruction obtained the greatest benefit from the combination. In a similar setting, however, Gilman et al. found no difference in the improvement in airflow between 2 mg nebulized glycopyrrolate and 15 mg nebulized metaproterenol.[19] They found fewer side-effects in the group that received the anticholinergic agent.

It seems appropriate to recommend that both classes of bronchodilators be given in acute severe asthma, particularly in the early hours of treatment and particularly in patients with more severe airflow obstruction.

CHRONIC BRONCHITIS AND EMPHYSEMA OR COPD

Stable COPD

A very large number of studies have compared anticholinergic agents with other bronchodilators in patients with COPD. In general, patients with COPD do not manifest as much absolute increase in airflow to any agent or combination of agents as do patients with asthma. However, almost all are capable of some. With very few exceptions, these studies show the anticholinergic agent to provide at least as great and prolonged an increase in airflow as other agents. Most, like the largest such study (Fig. 33.4),[20] show the anticholinergic agent to be a more potent bronchodilator. Even when large cumulative doses of each agent, rather than 'recommended' doses, are given the

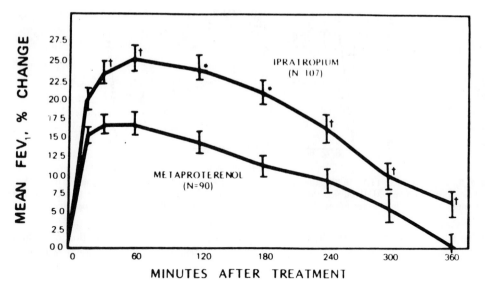

Fig. 33.4 Increase in FEV$_1$ in patients with COPD after inhalation of 40 µg ipratropium by MDI (107 patients), or 1.5 mg metaproterenol by MDI (90 patients). Symbols denote significant differences. Reproduced from ref. 20, with permission.

anticholinergic agent alone achieves all the available bronchodilatation in these patients.[5,21]

As this is clearly not the case in asthmatic patients there may thus be a systematic difference between asthmatic and COPD patients with respect to their responsiveness to bronchodilators. This point is brought out by about five studies in which patients with asthma and COPD who had similar baseline airflows have been studied side-by-side, e.g. Fig. 33.5.[22] This shows that the combination of fenoterol and theophylline results in

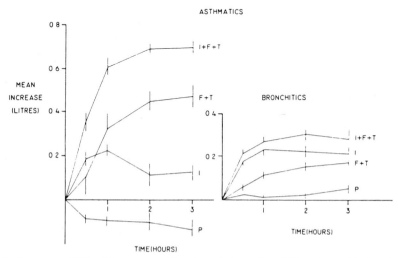

Fig. 33.5 Increase in FEV$_1$ of 15 patients with asthma (left panel) and 15 patients with chronic bronchitis (right panel). P, placebo; I, ipratropium 40 µg MDI; F + T, fenoterol 5 mg plus oxtriphylline 400 mg oral. Reproduced from ref. 22, with permission.

more bronchodilatation than did ipratopium in the asthmatic group; but that ipratropium resulted in more bronchodilatation in the bronchitic group. Reasons for the difference between these two groups of patients are not known but seem likely to include the fact that airflow obstruction in asthma is due to factors related to airway inflammation that are amenable at least in part to adrenergic agents but not amenable to anticholinergic agents. These factors are present to a lesser extent in patients with COPD whose major reversible component is bronchomotor tone, the latter being best reversed by anticholinergic agents.[5] Whatever the reason, COPD represents the group of patients in whom anticholinergic agents are the most useful bronchodilators.

Acute exacerbations of COPD

Three recent studies comparing the efficacy of bronchodilators in acute exacerbations of COPD found no significant differences between adrenergic and anticholinergic agents or their combination.[18,23,24]

Combination with other bronchodilators

Combinations of different classes of bronchodilators often provide more improvement in airflow than single agents, and this effect is seen in many of the studies cited above, e.g. Fig. 33.5. However, this is probably due to the fact that most clinical studies are performed with recommended rather than optimal doses of the bronchodilators. Consequently when two classes of agents are given together, both in recommended dosage, the effects may simply be additive rather than potentiating. As anticholinergic agents act through a different pathway from that of other bronchodilators it is not unreasonable to use them in combination with other agents, but the evidence that this is an advantage over using a larger dose of either agent alone is limited to acute asthma (above).

There is no physiological or pharmacological contraindication to the combination of anticholinergic agents with other agents used in the treatment of airway diseases. No unfavourable interactions between anticholinergic bronchodilators and other drugs have been reported. When patients are taking both adrenergic and anticholinergic agents by MDI, there is little evidence to suggest that it matters how and in what order they use these agents. One common practice is to use the adrenergic agent first to obtain an immediate effect, and to follow with the anticholinergic agent. This might improve penetration of the second aerosol into the respiratory tract.

OTHER EFFECTS

On lung mechanics

Anticholinergic agents, like adrenergic bronchodilators, reduce the hyperinflation associated with airflow obstruction.[5] They also improve effort tolerance.[25] The quaternary forms have negligible effects on haemodynamics[26] and the pulmonary circulation.

Consequently they do not carry the risk of increasing hypoxaemia, as do adrenergic agents,[23,27] an important consideration in exacerbations of asthma and COPD.

Side-effects

Atropine sulphate results in numerous side-effects related to the inhibition of physiological functions of the parasympathetic system. These effects occur in doses at or only slightly above the bronchodilator dose, and include skin flushing, dryness of the mouth and other mucosal secretions, tachycardia, blurred vision, and mental disturbances. Atropine is contraindicated in patients with glaucoma or prostatism. The principal advantage of quaternary anticholinergic agent is that they are so poorly absorbed from mucosae that the risk of such effects is insignificant. Even massive, inadvertent overdosage of one such agent resulted in trivial effects.[28] Ipratropium, the most widely studied quaternary anticholinergic, has been exonerated after extensive exploration for atropine-like side-effects.[29] It can, for example, be given to patients with glaucoma without affecting intra-ocular tension (provided it is not sprayed directly into the eye). It has been found not to affect urinary flow characteristics in older men. Nor has it been found to alter the viscosity and elasticity of respiratory mucus, or mucociliary clearance, as does atropine.[30]

In normal clinical usage the only side effect that the patient might experience with ipratropium MDI is a brief coughing spell which has been reported to occur in 5% of patients.[20] Rarely it can result in paradoxical bronchoconstriction. This has been variously attributed to hypotonicity of the nebulized solution, idiosyncrasy to the bromine radical, the benzalkonium preservative, and a selective effect on the M_2 muscarinic receptor. Paradoxical bronchoconstriction may also occur with other anticholinergic agents. Although rare, occurring in possibly 0.3% of patients, the possibility of paradoxical bronchoconstriction in a patient warrants withdrawal of the drug from that patient. Other than these two effects, very extensive investigation and the worldwide use of ipratropium for over a decade demonstrate a remarkably low incidence of untoward reactions.

CLINICAL RECOMMENDATIONS

The use of anticholinergic bronchodilators is best limited to the poorly absorbed quaternary forms, e.g. ipratropium, oxitropium, atropine methonitrate, glycopyrrolate, administered by inhalation. They are sometimes useful in stable asthma as adjuncts to other bronchodilator therapy, and have a demonstrated role in combination with adrenergic agents in the treatment of acute severe asthma. Their principal role is in the long-term management of stable COPD where they are probably the most efficacious bronchodilators. Because of their slow onset of action they are best used on a regular, maintenance basis, rather that p.r.n. The usual dose, two puffs of 20 μg each, is probably suboptimal for many patients with COPD and can safely be doubled or quadrupled.[31]

REFERENCES

1. Gross NJ, Skorodin MS: Anticholinergic, antimuscarinic bronchodilators. *Am Rev Respir Dis* (1984) **129**: 856–870.
2. Richardson JB: Innervation of the lung. *Eur J Respir Dis* (1982) **117**(Suppl): 13–31.
3. Widdicombe JG: The parasympathetic nervous system in airways disease. *Scand J Respir Dis* (1979) **103**(Suppl): 38–43.
4. Nadel JA: Autonomic regulation of airway smooth muscle. In Nadel JA (ed) *Physiology and Pharmacology of the Airways.* NY, Marcel Dekker, 1980, pp 217–257.
5. Gross NJ, Skorodin MS: Role of the parasympathetic system in airway obstruction due to emphysema. *N Engl J Med* (1984) **311**: 421–426.
6. Barnes PJ, Basbaum CB, Nadel JA: Autoradiographic localization of autonomic receptors in airway smooth muscle, marked differences between large and small airways. *Am Rev Respir Dis* (1983) **127**: 758–762.
7. Gross NJ, Barnes PJ: A short tour around the muscarinic receptor. *Am Rev Respir Dis* (1988) **138**: 765–767.
8. Gross NJ, Co E, Skorodin MS: Cholinergic bronchomotor tone in COPD, estimates of its amount in comparison to normal. *Chest* (1989) **96**: 984–987.
9. Shah PKD, Lakhotia M, Mehta S, Jain SK, Gupta GL: Clinical dysautonomia in patients with bronchial asthma, study with seven autonomic function tests. *Chest* (1990) **98**: 1408–1413.
10. Gross NJ: Cholinergic control. In Barnes PJ, Rodger IW, Thomson NC (eds) *Asthma, Basic Mechanisms and Clinical Management.* London, Academic Press, 1988, pp 381–393.
11. Gross NJ, Skorodin MS: Anticholinergic agents. In Jenne JW, Murphy S (eds) *Drug Therapy for Asthma, Lung Biology in Health and Disease,* Vol 31. NY, Marcel Dekker, 1987. pp 615–668.
12. Gross NJ, Petty TL, Friedman M, Skorodin MS, Silvers GW, Donohue JF: Dose–response to ipratropium nebulized solution in COPD, a 3-center study. *Am Rev Respir Dis* (1989) **139**: 1188–1191.
13. Ruffin RE, McIntyre E, Crockett AJ, Zeilonka K, Alpers JH: Combination bronchodilator therapy in asthma. *J Allergy Clin Immunol* (1982) **69**: 60–65.
14. Ullah MI, Newman GB, Saunders KB: Influence of age on response to ipratropium and salbutamol in asthma. *Thorax* (1981) **36**: 523–529.
15. Vichyanond P, Sladek WA, Syr S, Hill MR, Szefler SJ, Nelson HS: Efficacy of Atropine methylnitrate alone and in combination with albuterol in children with asthma. *Chest* (1990) **98**: 637–642.
16. Jolobe OMP: Asthma versus non-specific reversible airflow obstruction, clinical features and responsiveness to anticholinergic drugs. *Respiration* (1984) **45**: 237–242.
17. Brown IG, Chan CS, Kelley CA, Dent AG, Zimmerman PV: Assessment of the clinical usefulness of nebulised ipratropium bromide in patients with chronic airflow limitation. *Thorax* (1984) **39**: 272–276.
18. Rebuck AS, Chapman KR, Abboud R, *et al.*: Nebulized anticholinergic and sympathomimetic treatment of asthma and chronic obstructive airways disease in the emergency room. *Am J Med* (1987) **82**: 59–64.
19. Gilman MJ, Meyer L, Carter J, Slovis C: Comparison of aerosolized glycopyrrolate and metaproterenol in acute asthma. *Chest* (1990) **98**: 1095–1098.
20. Tashkin DP, Ashutosh K, Bleeker E, *et al.*: Comparison of the anticholinergic ipratropium bromide with metaproterenol in chronic obstructive pulmonary disease, a 90 day multicenter study. *Am J Med* (1986) **81**(Suppl 5A): 81–86.
21. Easton PA, Jadue C, Dhingra S, Anthonisen NR: A comparison of the bronchodilating effects of a beta-2 adrenergic agent (albuterol) and an anticholinergic agent (ipratropium bromide), given by aerosol alone or in sequence. *N Engl J Med* (1986) **315**: 735–739.
22. Lefcoe NM, Toogood JH, Blennerhassett G, Patterson NAM: The addition of an aerosol anticholinergic to an oral beta agonist plus theophylline in asthma and bronchitis. *Chest* (1982) **82**: 300–305.

23. Karpel JP, Pesin J, Greenberg D, Gentry E: A Comparison of the effects of ipratropium bromide and metaproterenol sulfate in acute exacerbations of COPD. *Chest* (1990) **98**: 835–839.
24. Patrick DM, Dales RE, Stark RM, Laliberte G, Dickinson G: Severe exacerbations of COPD and asthma, incremental benefit of adding irpratropium to usual therapy. *Chest* (1990) **98**: 295–297.
25. Leitch AG, Hopkin JM, Ellis DA, Merchant S, McHardy GJR: The effect of aerosol ipratropium bromide and salbutamol on exercise tolerance in chronic bronchitis. *Thorax* (1978) **33**: 711–713.
26. Chapman KR, Smith DL, Rebuck AS, Leenen FHH: Hemodynamic effects of inhaled ipratropium bromide alone and in combination with an inhaled beta2-agonist. *Am Rev Respir Dis* (1985) **132**: 845–847.
27. Gross NJ, Bankwala Z: Effects of an anticholinergic bronchodilator on arterial blood gases of hypoxemic patients with COPD. *Am Rev Respir Dis* (1987) **136**: 1091–1094.
28. Gross NJ, Skorodin MS: Massive overdose of atropine methonitrate with only slight untoward effects. *Lancet* (1985) **2**: 386.
29. Gross NJ: Ipratropium bromide. *N Engl J Med* (1988) **319**: 486–494.
30. Pavia D, Bateman JRM, Sheahan NF, Clarke SW: Effect of ipratropium bromide on mucociliary clearance and pulmonary function in reversible airways obstruction. *Thorax* (1979) **34**: 501–507.
31. Leak A, O'Connor T: High dose ipratropium—is it safe? *Practitioner* (1988) **232**: 9–10.

34

Xanthines

NILS SVEDMYR AND IAN W. RODGER

INTRODUCTION

During the last 15 years, slow-release theophylline preparations and reliable theophylline assays have increased the therapeutic efficacy of this drug in asthma therapy.[1,2] Although it is today the most frequently prescribed *oral* antiasthmatic drug for maintenance therapy worldwide, it is also widely used intravenously in the treatment of acute severe asthma and to treat premature infants with idiopathic apnoea.

In recent years the use of xanthines has been somewhat controversial, since the incidence of side-effects (occasionally fatal) has continued unabated. Furthermore, there are an increasing number of reports suggesting that inhaled bronchodilators and corticosteroids are substantially safer and that they provide a more efficacious therapy in the majority of patients.[3-8]

CELLULAR MECHANISM(S) OF ACTION

The precise mechanism of action of xanthine-like drugs has been the subject of considerable debate over the last 30 or so years. Since the early observations of Butcher and Sutherland,[9] that theophylline inhibited cyclic AMP phosphodiesterase (PDE), there have been numerous studies aimed at establishing that precisely such a mechanism underlies the airway smooth muscle relaxant action of xanthines. To date, however, there exists no single, universally acceptable explanation of how xanthines exert their clinical efficacy (see, for example, ref. 10).

ASTHMA: BASIC MECHANISMS AND CLINICAL MANAGEMENT (2nd Edn)
ISBN 0-12-079026-2

Several potential mechanisms of action have been proposed. These include:

(1) Inhibition of cyclic nucleotide phosphodiesterases;
(2) Interaction with guanine nucleotide regulatory proteins (G-proteins);
(3) Adenosine antagonism;
(4) Effects via catecholamine release;
(5) Effects on phospholipid metabolism;
(6) Effects on Ca^{2+} availability and utilization.

It is important to note that in this list all of the proposed effects of the xanthines may well be attributable to an action mediated via either cyclic AMP and/or cyclic GMP. Both of these cyclic nucleotides are known to be intimately involved in controlling airway smooth muscle relaxation[11,12] and regulating the activity of certain inflammatory cells.[13–17]

INHIBITION OF CYCLIC NUCLEOTIDE PHOSPHODIESTERASES (PDEs)

PDEs are a family of enzymes that perform a critical role in the catabolism of the two intracellular second messengers, cyclic AMP and cyclic GMP. It is now known that there are, at least, five main families of PDEs, some of which selectively metabolize cyclic AMP whilst others selectively metabolize cyclic GMP.[18] Within these five families 25 different phosphodiesterase isoenzymes have been identified.[18]

Cyclic AMP-phosphodiesterase inhibition

Theophylline and other xanthines have been shown to inhibit cyclic AMP-PDE derived from airway smooth muscle of several animal species including man.[19–28] Inhibition of the PDE is, however, observed at concentrations of xanthines that are substantially below those producing maximal relaxant effects on airway preparations *in vitro*.[22,23,29] Notwithstanding, there is a good correlation between the rank orders of potency of the xanthines in causing both relaxation and enzyme inhibition[10,23,26]

Whilst most authors agree that xanthines can inhibit cyclic AMP-PDE derived from homogenates of lung tissues there is less agreement with regard to the ability of xanthines to elevate cyclic AMP levels in airway preparations from a variety of species. Some studies show clear increases in cyclic AMP,[29,30] others report increases but only at maximally effective relaxant concentrations[31] whilst others observe no effect.[19] Such a diversity of observations has led to several re-appraisals, and questioning, of the role of cyclic AMP as the mediator underlying xanthine-induced bronchodilation.[26,30] Such re-appraisals have also been strengthened by the knowledge that theophylline is a very weak PDE inhibitor at therapeutically effective plasma concentrations.[22,25] Furthermore, there are numerous other inhibitors of cyclic AMP-PDE more potent than theophylline that are ineffective as bronchodilators.[32]

One possible explanation of these anomalies lies in the existence of several different isoenzymes of cyclic AMP-PDE.[18,33] The fact that nearly all these isoenzymes possess unique primary amino-acid sequences in their catalytic and regulatory domains and that they are often selectively expressed implies that selective inhibition of the PDEs should be possible. Selective inhibition, however, is not a property inherent in xanthine bronchodilators. Furthermore, the tissue distribution and subcellular localization of these PDE isoenzymes appears to be of critical importance in relation to the function that they subserve. For example, in airway smooth muscle the Type I isoenzyme accounts for the majority (c. 85–90%) of the total cyclic AMP hydrolytic activity of tissue homogenates.[34,35] There is, however, no evidence that this isoenzyme plays any role in regulating contractile events in intact tissue. In contrast, the Type III and Type IV isoenzymes, which account for approximately 5% and 10% respectively of the total cyclic AMP hydrolytic activity of tissue homogenates, are thought to be critically important regulators of both cyclic AMP content and contractile events.[34] This being the case, then in experiments involving measurements of total tissue cyclic AMP content, very small, xanthine-induced changes in the cellular levels of the nucleotide, occurring in a restricted cellular domain essential for inducing relaxation, might well go undetected. Consequently, there would appear little or no relationship between tissue relaxation and cyclic AMP accumulation.

Thus, the case for rejecting cyclic AMP-dependent PDE inhibition as a mechanism underlying xanthine-induced airway smooth muscle relaxation remains not proven. The case will only be sustained once it has been demonstrated that there is no correlation between a xanthine's potency as a bronchodilator and its potency as an inhibitor of the specific isoenzyme that regulates tissue contractility.

In relation to the differential tissue distribution of the Type IV isoenzyme there is a further point that is worthy of note. Recent observations suggest that cyclic AMP plays an important role in modulating the inflammatory activity of eosinophils and neutrophils.[14–17] In these cells the type IV isoenzyme is the sole means whereby cyclic AMP is degraded.[14–17] Thus, inhibitors of the Type IV isoenzyme may well possess anti-inflammatory activity of relevance to the therapy of asthma. Such an effect, however, is unlikely to contribute to the clinical efficacy of theophylline since it is a poor inhibitor of the Type IV isoenzyme at therapeutic plasma concentrations.

Cyclic GMP-phosphodiesterase inhibition

There are several reports of drugs that selectively increase cyclic GMP levels producing relaxation of airway smooth muscle.[31,36–38] Such circumstantial evidence does suggest, therefore, that cyclic GMP has a functional role to play in the relaxation process. Whether xanthine bronchodilators exert their effect via a cyclic GMP-dependent mechanism is an open question. There is little doubt that certain xanthines, such as theophylline and isobutylmethylxanthine, are capable of inhibiting cyclic GMP-PDE and elevating cyclic GMP levels in airway tissues.[31,36–38] Notwithstanding, a systematic examination of about 30 xanthine derivatives has demonstrated a wide variation in their efficacy as inhibitors of cyclic GMP-PDE. Critically, this activity is poorly correlated with smooth muscle relaxant activity.[26] Furthermore, the anti-allergic drug disodium cromoglycate is also a potent cyclic GMP-PDE inhibitor (of equal potency with theophylline) yet it is devoid of smooth muscle relaxant activity.[39]

These observations, therefore, pose similar questions, regarding the involvement of cyclic GMP as a mediator underlying xanthine-induced bronchodilator activity, as were raised above for cyclic AMP. Perhaps not surprisingly a similar 'isoenzyme/localization' defence can be mounted for cyclic GMP/cyclic GMP-PDE, as was the case for cyclic AMP. In this instance, the PDE isoenzymes involved are the Types I, II and V. Generally, it is the Type V PDE that is the principal isoenzyme involved in the breakdown of cyclic GMP. In keeping with the other PDE isoenzymes, the Type V enzyme has its own unique tissue distribution and subcellular localization. Just how important the Type V isoenzyme is with regard to lung function is not yet known. However, the observation that zaprinast (a potent inhibitor of the Type V isoenzyme) is both a bronchodilator and an inhibitor of histamine release from mast cells[13] may well signal an important functional role. As far as the xanthines are concerned there is insufficient evidence of their activity against Type I and IV isoenzymes to allow a definitive verdict to be reached.

INTERACTION WITH GUANINE NUCLEOTIDE REGULATORY PROTEINS (G-PROTEINS)

Heterotrimeric guanine nucleotide regulatory proteins (G-proteins) are now widely regarded as critical elements that couple hormone and neurotransmitter receptors to an array of cellular processes, via modulation of the concentrations of intracellular second messengers.[40] In the context of cyclic nucleotides, G-proteins are involved only in the control of cyclic AMP levels via interaction with adenylyl cyclase. The two G-proteins in question are either stimulatory (Gs) or inhibitory (Gi) on adenylyl cyclase activity. Thus, increases in cyclic AMP levels within cells can be achieved either via activation of Gs or inhibition of Gi.

Recently, it has been reported that certain inhibitors of cyclic nucleotide phosphodiesterase, including xanthines, have a capacity to inhibit the activity of Gi.[41] In so doing, these compounds disinhibit the influence of Gi on adenylyl cyclase. Thus, the enzyme activity is enhanced and cyclic AMP levels are increased. Whilst this interaction with G-proteins represents an attractive new possible mechanism of action for the xanthines, the concentrations at which the effect is manifest are substantially in excess of those achieved in the plasma of man. It is unlikely, therefore, that this evidence provides a satisfactory explanation for the therapeutic efficacy of the xanthines as bronchodilators.

ADENOSINE ANTAGONISM

Another mechanism that has been thoroughly investigated is adenosine antagonism.[42,43] Adenosine activates two types of membrane receptors both of which are coupled to adenylyl cyclase. The A_1 receptors exert an inhibitory influence on adenylyl cyclase whilst the A_2 receptors stimulate the enzyme. The plasma adenosine level is increased after an allergen provocation, and adenosine has been shown to cause bronchoconstriction when inhaled by asthmatic subjects. This bronchoconstrictor effect is mediated via the A_1 receptor, via a reduction in the intracellular levels of cyclic AMP. Xanthines, at therapeutic plasma concentrations, are potent inhibitors of the A_1 adenosine receptors. Theophylline, for example, antagonizes this action of adenosine more effectively than it does the bronchoconstriction induced by histamine.[44] Enprofylline, however, a xanthine derivative practically devoid of adenosine antagonistic activity and which has only weak PDE inhibitory activity, is three to four times more potent as a bronchodilator than theophylline in both animals[45] and asthmatic subjects.[46] Thus, it seems unlikely that adenosine antagonism is the principal cellular mechanism of action underlying the bronchodilator effects of the xanthines.

EFFECTS VIA CATECHOLAMINE RELEASE

Theophylline has been shown to increase the release of endogenous catecholamines in animals[46–49] but the resultant effect on airways was not blocked by β-adrenoceptor antagonists.[50] Studies in man have shown that xanthine treatment does not induce changes in the plasma catecholamine levels.[51] This observation, allied to the fact that asthmatic subjects are unable to elevate their plasma adrenaline levels even in an acute attack[52,53] would lead one to conclude safely that xanthines do not exert their therapeutic effects via adrenaline release from the adrenal medullae.

EFFECT ON PHOSPHOLIPID METABOLISM

It is now recognized that contraction of airway smooth muscle is associated with receptor/G-protein activated, phospholipase C-catalysed phosphatidyl-inositol bisphosphate hydrolysis. This results in the generation of an intracellular second messenger, inositol trisphosphate, which is responsible for the release of calcium ions from intracellular stores and contraction (see Chapter 4). Despite early observations to the contrary[54] recent studies have demonstrated that certain drugs (including xanthines) that elevate cyclic AMP (and in some instances cyclic GMP) levels in airway tissue inhibit the formation of inositol trisphosphate.[55,56] Precisely how this effect is mediated is not yet known. It is, however, likely to involve a cyclic AMP-dependent protein kinase-mediated phosphorylation of certain elements (G-protein and/or phospholipase C) of the membrane signalling pathway. As far as xanthines are concerned this is yet another mechanism of action that would be dependent upon their ability to increase cyclic nucleotide levels within airway tissues. The caveats pertaining to this possibility have already been elaborated above.

EFFECTS ON Ca^{2+} AVAILABILITY AND UTILIZATION

Xanthines are known to inhibit Ca^{2+} entry through voltage-operated calcium channels by virtue of their ability to hyperpolarize the cell membrane (for references see ref. 57). However, given the lack of involvement of these Ca^{2+} channels in the initiation or maintenance of bronchospasm (see Chapter 4), this mechanism is unlikely to play any significant role in the smooth muscle relaxation process.[57]

There is no evidence that xanthines exert any direct inhibitory effect upon the airway smooth muscle contractile apparatus.[31,58] However, an indirect effect, mediated by increases in either cyclic AMP or cyclic GMP, consequent upon PDE inhibition, would certainly alter the sensitivity of the contractile apparatus to the triggering effects of Ca^{2+}.[31]

Reductions in the intracellular concentration of Ca^{2+} would certainly bring about relaxation of airway smooth muscle. Such an effect has been proposed[30] although precisely how it is mediated is not yet known. It may well, again, be consequent upon the generation of cyclic nucleotides since both are known to facilitate uptake of Ca^{2+} by intracellular organelles.[59,60]

ANTIASTHMATIC EFFECTS

Several effects of theophylline have been proposed to be of therapeutic importance in asthma:

(1) Bronchial smooth muscle relaxation;
(2) Increase in mucociliary transport;
(3) Inhibition of release of mediators;
(4) Suppression of permeability oedema;
(5) Decrease of pulmonary hypertension and increase in right ventricular ejection fraction;
(6) Improved contractility of fatigued diaphragmatic muscle;
(7) Central stimulation of ventilation.

All but the last two effects are shared with β_2-adrenoceptor stimulants. The most important of these effects in the treatment of asthma is probably bronchial smooth muscle relaxation, but the other effects may contribute to the antiasthmatic effect, especially when the drugs are given regularly and prophylactically. At the present time, however, it is difficult to evaluate their clinical significance.

Bronchial smooth muscle relaxation

Different β-adrenoceptor stimulants and theophylline derivatives all had the same maximum relaxant effect on isolated human bronchial muscle contracted by a moderate dose of carbachol[61] the relative potency being proportional to the potencies found clinically. Thus theophylline is about 1000 times less potent than isoprenaline.

Experiments with isolated airway preparations from animal and man show that both theophylline and β_2-receptor stimulants relax smooth muscle in large and small airways, irrespective of whether they have been contracted by carbachol, histamine, serotonin, prostaglandins, leukotrienes or substance P.[62] These findings show that terbutaline, theophylline and enprofylline are effective *functional* antagonists of the bronchoconstrictory action of a large variety of potential chemical mediators of asthma. This functional antagonistic effect at the level of the smooth muscle in the whole respiratory tree is probably of importance for the substantial therapeutic effect of β_2-receptor agonists and xanthines. Their effects are usually superior to those of anticholinergics, which only block acetylcholine and consequently only reflex mediated constriction. However, when the concentration of carbachol was increased to a maximum, the degree of relaxation induced by isoprenaline relative to that caused by theophylline was gradually reduced.[63] The concentration of theophylline used in these studies was, however, far above the therapeutic one. The concentration of carbachol was also very high, and the significance of these differences is difficult to assess. In fact, they may have none, since clincal studies have not shown a better antiasthmatic effect of theophylline compared to the β_2-adrenoceptor stimulants in emergency treatment of asthma.

When given systemically, theophylline and β_2-receptor stimulants have a comparable bronchodilating effect. *Inhaled β_2-agonists* produce, however, a much more pronounced bronchodilation. In the treatment of acute severe asthma, theophylline may have additive effects in *some* patients not responding adequately to initial therapy with high dose inhaled β_2-receptor agonists.

Increase in mucociliary transport

Both β_2-receptor stimulants and theophylline have been shown to increase mucociliary transport, and this effect may contribute to their therapeutic efficacy in asthma.[64–68] Matthys *et al.*[69] have shown that β_2-receptor stimulants and theophylline have only an additive effect on this parameter.

Inhibition of mediator-release

One week of pretreatment with theophylline (final blood concentrations 8–22 μg/ml) (44–121 μmol/litre) has been shown to reduce the response to nasal challenge with antigen and inhibit the release of mediators from mast cells.[70] Both terbutaline and theophylline given orally to asthmatics protect against allergen provocation and at the same time partly inhibit the release of histamine.[71] Both theophylline and enprofylline partly inhibit 'late reactions' after antigen provocation in asthmatics.[72] (See also 'Effect of bronchial hyperreactivity' below.)

Suppression of permeability oedema

Theophylline and enprofylline have shown an ability to decrease permeability oedema induced by different asthma mediators in the microcirculation.[73] This property may also contribute to their therapeutic effects, but so far it has not been possible to evaluate this clinically.

Decrease of pulmonary hypertension and increase in right ventricular ejection fraction

Theophylline reduces pulmonary artery pressure and increases the right ventricular ejection fraction in acute tests in patients with emphysema.[74,75] These effects, however, can hardly be of importance in the normal treatment of asthma. In contrast, they might be of importance in patients with chronic obstructive pulmonary disease (COPD), where pulmonary hypertension and right ventricular failure carry a poor prognosis.[76]

Improved contractility of fatigued diaphragmatic muscle

Theophylline improves the contractility of fatigued diaphragmatic muscle.[77] The same effect has also been shown with β_2-receptor stimulants in animal studies, in which these two types of drugs appeared to have an additive effect.[78] This effect is probably without clinical relevance in normal asthma treatment, when pCO_2 is comparatively low. It might, however, be of importance when patients are no longer able to breath and pCO_2 starts to increase, i.e. when asthmatics need respirator treatment. This effect may also be of clinical importance in patients with chronic obstructive pulmonary disease.

Central stimulation of ventilation

Stimulation of ventilation may be of clinical importance. It seems to depend on the adenosine-blocking properties of theophylline, since the effect is not shared by enprofylline and since adenosine is a potent depressant of the respiratory centre.[79,80] The lack of this effect with enprofylline may be favourable in asthma therapy, but may be a disadvantage in patients with COPD, if this effect is of any clinical importance. Theophylline and caffeine are also currently used to treat premature infants with idiopathic apnoea.[81,82]

Effect on bronchial hyperreactivity

There is now increasing evidence that inflammation of the airways contributes to their hyperreactivity. The anti-inflammatory effect of theophylline is disputed. It has been argued that the clinical efficacy of xanthines may reflect their anti-inflammatory properties more than smooth muscle relaxation.[83] At therapeutic levels, xanthines produced only slight reduction of the immediate response in asthmatics challenged with allergen, while they markedly inhibited the late response occurring after several hours.[72] The antipermeability effect of theophylline may be important in preventing this late reaction. Theophylline had an acute protective effect on histamine and methacholine responsiveness in asthmatics[84] and also on exercise-induced bronchospasm.[85] There is, however, no evidence that these effects are attributable to mechanisms other than smooth muscle relaxation and theophylline did not inhibit allergen-induced increase in airway responsiveness to methacholine.[86] Several weeks of treatment with oral theophylline did not change the bronchial hyperreactivity in asthmatics in comparison to the marked attenuation achieved with inhaled steroids over the same time period.[87]

SIDE-EFFECTS

Theophylline's narrow therapeutic window and potentially lethal side-effects need to be recognized and monitored. In an excellent review, theophylline toxicity reported in the literature during the last decade is updated.[88] During this time 63 deaths were reported in the studies. The actual number of all theophylline-induced toxicities including death is obviously much higher than reported in the literature.

The most common side-effects of oral theophylline treatment are anorexia, nausea, vomiting and mild central nervous stimulation.[89] Nausea is probably both a central effect and a direct toxic effect on the gastric mucosa, as the problem seems to be greater if oral therapy is given. Actual abdominal pain, diarrhoea and, rarely, gastric bleeding may also occur. In maintenance therapy, initial dosage should be low to avoid these gastrointestinal side-effects, which seem to occur much more frequently if the initial oral dose is high. A few patients do not, however, tolerate theophylline at all because of this side-effect.

There are an increasing number of reports demonstrating that nausea and vomiting might not occur as presenting features of toxicity when theophylline is given by the intravenous route, and that some patients experience more severe complications as a first indication that theophylline in the blood has reached a toxic level.

Mild CNS stimulation is common, especially if the maintenance dose is increased too fast. Recently, theophylline has been found to induce both subtle and gross central nervous system side effects such as change in mood and personality, particularly in children, also school performance may be impaired.[90,91] The most serious toxicity is the risk of seizures, which have been associated with a mortality rate as high as 50%. Theophylline-induced seizures, however, appear to be rare under a concentration of 40 mg/litre (220 μmol/litre).

In theophylline-induced seizures, higher than normal doses of benzodiazepines should be used as theophylline antagonizes the effect of benzodiazepines on GABA-receptors in the brain.[93]

The cardiovascular side-effects are seen mainly with intravenous theophylline. Palpitations, tachycardia and arrhythmias may occur and are relatively common with serum levels in excess of 30 mg/litre (165 μmol/litre).[1,2] Headache, however, is quite common, especially when initiating theophylline therapy, and nausea and headache are normally the practical dose-limiting side-effects in maintenence therapy.

Children may have a relatively greater tolerance for theophylline therapy than adults, but reports of sudden deaths are common in the older paediatric literature. If modern kinetic principles are used, they should not occur.[2]

Drug interactions are also a major problem sometimes leading to theophylline toxicity due to delayed clearance (see Pharmacokinetics).

XANTHINE DRUGS

Theophylline (1,3-dimethylxanthine), caffeine (1,3,7-trimethylxanthine) and theobromine (3,7-dimethylxanthine) exemplify the fact that small changes in the chemical structure of alkylxanthines significantly alters pharmacodynamic properties. Several soluble salts of theophylline have been introduced, but no salt of theophylline will be present in the body. Theophylline itself will be produced as soon as the salt dissolves in body fluids. Theophylline as such is also sufficiently soluble to be completely and reliably absorbed after oral intake. The theophylline salts contain 50–85% water-free theophylline. They seem to offer no advantage over theophylline.

The solubility can also be increased by making true chemical derivatives of theophylline. Various substituents have been attached to the xanthine molecule, and it is important to realize that they are different molecules from theophylline and will not

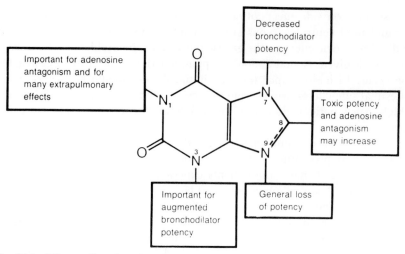

Fig. 34.1   Effect profiles of xanthine derivatives related to structure. Reproduced from ref. 94.

generate theophylline in the body. Figure 34.1 summarizes the structure–activity of xanthines with bronchodilating properties based on *in vitro* and *in vivo* data obtained with about 300 derivatives.[94] Various substituents have been attached at the 7-position in theophylline (e.g. dyphylline, etophylline, proxyphylline, acephylline). What seems to make these drugs of doubtful value is the finding that they are less active, some of them are poorly absorbed, and most importantly they are certainly less well documented than theophylline.

3-Propylxanthine (enprofylline) is three to four times as potent a bronchodilator as theophylline and is an interesting derivative because it is nearly devoid of adenosine-receptor antagonist properties and therefore also devoid of the following effects of theophylline.[194]

(1) CNS stimulation, including anxiety, restlessness, respiratory stimulation and life-threatening seizures;
(2) Increased release of free fatty acids;
(3) Increased gastric acid secretion;
(4) Vasoconstriction;
(5) Increased natriuretic and volume diuresis.

Enprofylline also has the advantage of being eliminated through the kidney unmetabolized, thus avoiding the large variation in elimination rate, provided that the kidney function is normal. Unfortunately, it produced (reversible) liver damages and has been withdrawn from the market.

PHARMACOKINETICS

The bronchodilating effect of theophylline is proportional to the log of the plasma concentration over a range of 5–30 mg/litre (30–165 μmol/litre).[95,97] The optimal concentration is 10–20 mg/litre (55–110 μmol/litre). During maintenance treatment of asthma, theophylline is very often combined with a β_2-adrenoceptor stimulant and then a concentration of 5–10 mg/litre (25–50 μmol/litre) is sometimes sufficient.[98] The therapeutic index for theophylline is very low, and cardiac side-effects may occur with theophylline at lower plasma concentrations when it is combined with systemically administered β_2-stimulants than when it is given alone. The bonchodilating effects of β_2-adrenoreceptor agonists and theophylline are additive[98–99] and the concentration-effect curve for theophylline will be shifted more to the left, the more intensive the simultaneous β_2-agonist therapy.[99] Between individuals there is a great variation in response to theophylline when related to similar steady-state concentrations.[99] Theophylline seems to be especially beneficial in a minor setup of severe asthmatics.[100] Slight nausea and mild gastrointestinal side-effects occur frequently at therapeutic plasma concentrations and appear to have little direct relationship to the plasma concentration. Risk for severe toxicity such as seizure and serious arrhythmias is high when serum theophylline concentrations exceed 30 mg/litre (165 μmol/litre).

The possibility for determination of serum theophylline concentration ('Therapeutic drug monitoring') is a main advantage in theophylline therapy and is mandatory when higher doses are used.

Absorption

Gastointestinal absorption from rapidly disintegrating tablets is complete and almost as rapid as from a solution. The absorption may be somewhat slower, but not less complete, when food is present. Poor absorption has been documented for some slow-release theophylline tablets and for suppositories. Rectal solutions, however, have good bioavailability.[2] The maintenance dose per 24 h for theophylline is therefore the same for intravenous, oral or rectal treatment.[1,2]

With some of the new sustained-release theophylline preparations absorption can be influenced by diet. Food increases the extent of absorption of some preparations, while decreasing absorption of others. The rate of absorption can increase to such an extent that clinical toxicity develops.[1,2]

Slow-release theophylline preparations with reliable and complete bioavailability intended for administration once or twice a day are to be preferred. They minimize fluctuations in serum concentrations and consequent variation in effect between doses. They also increase patients' compliance.

Distribution

The apparent volume of distribution varies very little between patients. It is around 0.45 litres/kg body weight in both adults and children. Therefore, a loading dose of theophylline always gives about the same increase of plasma concentration (e.g. a loading dose 6 mg/kg increases the concentration $6/0.45 = 13$ mg/litres $= 74\,\mu$mol/litre).[1,2]

Elimination

Theophylline is eliminated by metabolic degradation (N-demethylations and C-deoxidations) to around 90% and is renally excreted only around 10%. The most

Table 34.1   Non-genetic factors altering theophylline clearance.

Increased clearance	Decreased clearance
Enzyme-inducing drugs:	Enzyme-inhibiting drugs:
phenobarbitone	cimetidine
rifampicine	oral contraceptives
fenytoin	erythromycin
β-receptor agonists (high doses)	ciprofloxacine
Smoking (tobacco and marihuana)	quinolones
Barbecued meat	Methylxanthines (Michaelis-Menten kinetics)
Medical coal	Age
High protein, low carbohydrate diet	Liver cirrhosis
Youth	Congestive heart failure
	Respiratory insufficiency with *cor pulmonare*
	Fever

important source of variation in theophylline concentration is the variation in elimination rate. The individual variation is up to 20-fold and the single most important variable factor is the genetic one, with an approximately six-fold variation in clearance in the population. Other factors influencing theophylline elimination are summarized in Table 34.1.[1,2,101,102] All of these factors may be combined to cause the highly variable steady-state levels after a standard dose. The theophylline dose must therefore be individualized.

A considerable degree of knowledge concerning clinical pharmacology of theophylline is required to use it safely and effectively.

CLINICAL USE

Theophylline has been used in the treatment of reversible airflow obstruction associated with asthma or COPD due to chronic bronchitis and/or emphysema for more than 50 years. It is also used in premature infants with apnoea.[81,82] Over the years it has gained an increasing role in the therapy of these conditions, particularly since the introduction of sustained release formulations about 15 years ago.

Maintenance treatment

β_2-Receptor stimulants and theophylline have proved to have an acute prophylactic effect against bronchoconstriction triggered by exercise, allergen provocation and inhalation of irritants such as histamine, methacholine or cold.[103,104]

Table 34.2 compares β_2-receptor stimulants and theophylline in maintenance treatment of asthma. Given by the systemic route they seem to have the same antiasthmatic effect. However, only the β_2-receptor stimulants can be given by inhalation producing much better acute antiasthmatic effects. In many countries, inhaled β_2-receptor stimulants are therefore considered the drug of choice both for treating acute asthma attacks and in maintenance therapy. The duration of action of inhaled β_2-receptor stimulants

Table 34.2 Comparison of β_2-receptor stimulants and theophylline in asthma treatment.

	β_2-Receptor stimulants	Theophylline
Antiasthmatic effect (systemic)	+	+
Antiasthmatic effect (inhalation)	+++	−
Duration of action	Too short	Long (in slow-release form)
Therapeutic margin	Very wide	Narrow
Development of tolerance	Perhaps but probably without clinical importance	No

+, Moderate effect; +++, Pronounced effect.

available for the clinicians today is, however, too short except for the new long-acting drugs formoterol and salmeterol.

In the USA, theophylline in a 'high-dose' slow-release form is considered the drug of first choice by many specialists for maintenance treatment of asthma. No doubt this therapy is effective but it can produce life-threatening theophylline intoxication. With appropriate patient selection and education and a better understanding of theophylline kinetics and potential drugs interaction, the risk of inadvertent theophylline intoxication can be minimized.

Today asthma is regarded as primarily an inflammatory disease. Drug therapy of asthma is therefore increasingly focused on preventing and treating airway inflammation. Inhaled glucocorticosteroids and to a minor degree cromoglycate and nedocromil reduce airway inflammation and suppress bronchial hyperresponsiveness and can be used at a greatly reduced risk. For symptomatic treatment of airway obstruction inhaled β_2-agonists are now widely regarded as a bronchodilator treatment of choice. Inhaled β_2-agonists produce bronchodilation several times greater than that produced by theophylline and with fewer side-effects. Theophylline is therefore no longer the mainstay in the treatment of airway obstruction.[3-8] In chronic asthma, sustained-release theophylline preparations should be added to maintenance therapy only if adequate control is not achieved with inhaled glucocorticosteroids combined with inhaled β_2-sympathomimetics. The most common indication for sustained-release theophylline is control of nocturnal asthma and early morning wheezing. In this situation theophylline may be more effective if given as a single dose at night.[105] However, with the introduction of the new long-acting inhaled β_2-agonists, formoterol and salmeterol, this indication for theophylline is challenged.

Maintenance dosage

The dosage during oral maintenance treatment is preferably low and could slowly be increased to the following mean doses when combined with a β_2-adrenoceptor stimulant:

Under 9 years—12 mg/kg and 24 h
9–12 years—10 mg/kg and 24 h
12–16 years—9 mg/kg and 24 h
Over 16 years—7 mg/kg and 24 h

These dosages are related to the ideal body weight excluding the obesity and usually give a plasma concentration of 30–55 μmol/litre (5–10 mg/litre). This dosage is to be preferred if there is no possibility of estimation of plasma concentration.

If the schedule results in an insufficient response, careful increases in dose should be considered. If possible it should be guided by plasma theophylline monitoring. In the following situations theophylline assay in asthmatics is favourable:

(1) Optimizing drug therapy in the severely ill asthmatics;
(2) Insufficient response in spite of a high dose (>15 mg/kg/day) in adults and addition of other bronchodilating therapy (rapid metabolism? non-compliance?);
(3) Suspected side-effects in spite of a low or moderate (< 10 mg/kg/day) maintenance dose (slow metabolism?);
(4) High-risk patients (cardiac decompensation, liver cirrhosis, respiratory insuffi-ciency).

It is important that when oral theophylline is indicated, it should be given as a single drug and the dose should be individualized. Therefore, combination preparations should not be used. It is important to teach patients on maintenance theophylline therapy that they should not change the dosage of oral theophyllines even during exacerbations. An increased dose of theophylline might give life-threatening intoxication.

Intravenous treatment

The value of theophylline in the treatment of acute asthma attacks has been questioned, as several deaths have occurred due to acute theophylline intoxication.[3,7,8,106]

A recent 'meta-analysis'[107] carefully reviewed 347 clinical trials involving the use of aminophylline in acute severe asthma published between 1966 and 1986. Of these only 13 were judged to be eligible for analysis based on adequacy of study design and statistical validity. These studies compared aminophylline therapy with treatment with either salbutamol, adrenaline or other bronchodilators. The 13 reports did not agree. Seven reported no difference in spirometric values between aminophylline treatment and the control regimens. Three found aminophylline treatment superior, three favoured the control regimen. The results of the 13 trials were re-analysed and pooled. Overall there was no difference between the aminophylline-treated groups and the control groups. Several studies emphasized that side-effects such as nausea, anxiety, palpitation, occurred more often and at times exclusively in the aminophylline-treated patients. This important review suggests that in acute severe asthma repeated relatively high doses of nebulized β_2-adrenergic aerosols provide optimal bronchodilation. Recently, however, Connelly and Jenkins[108] indicated that intravenous theophylline had a significant beneficial effect above treatment with steroids and nebulized terbutaline. In this study the terbutaline dose was, however, not maximal.

In emergencey room treatment, the preferred initial treatment of acute severe asthma today is nebulized β_2-agonist in high dosage, salbutamol 0.10–0.15 mg/kg, repeated after 20–30 min if necessary (or terbutaline at double the dose), combined with

Table 34.3 Initial intravenous maintenance dosage of theophylline in asthma following the loading dose. Reproduced from ref. 2.

	Infusion rate (mg/kg/h)
Neonates	0.13
Infants 2–6 months	0.4
Infants 6–11 months	0.7
Children 1–9 years	0.8
Children over 9 and adults who smoke	0.6
Healthy non-smoking adults	0.4
Cardiac decompensation and liver dysfunction	0.2

intravenous glucocorticosteroids. Intravenous theophylline should be reserved for those patients who fail to respond to this treatment within 1 h.[109]

Kelly and Murphy[4] point out that studies of hospitalized patients after emergency treatment, in which the patients were monitored for at least 24 h, all demonstrate a positive therapeutic effect of theophylline and still recommend theophylline as continuous infusion for the management of hospitalized patients with *status asthmaticus*.

Intravenous dosage

The recommended bolus dose to all, independently of age and other diseases, is 6 mg theophylline per kilogram, if the patient has not been treated with oral theophylline. This dose usually increases the blood concentration about 12 mg/litre or 66 μmol/litre (depending on the distribution volume around 0.5 litres/kg). If the patient is on maintenance treatment with oral theophyllines, this bolus should be halved.

It is to be noted that the intravenous theophylline should always be given in a peripheral vein. Administration via a central venous catheter has probably induced fatal cardiac arrhythmias.

The initial intravenous maintenance dosage following this loading dose is shown in Table 34.3.[2]

CONCLUSIONS

Theophylline is a moderately potent bronchodilator and respiratory stimulant. The therapeutic index is very low and its pharmacokinetics are complicated. Benefits and risks of theophylline have been shown to relate directly to serum concentration, which is a function of dose, and the elimination characteristics of the drug in an individual patient.

In acute severe asthma, intravenous theophylline should be reserved for those patients who fail to respond to an initial treatment with high-dose nebulized β_2-agonists plus intravenous glucocorticosteroids and, if necessary, also an inhaled anticholinergic drug within the first hour.

In chronic asthma, slow-release theophyllines should be added to maintenance therapy if adequate control to asthma is not achieved with inhaled β_2-agonists combined with inhaled corticosteroids. The most frequent indication for slow-release theophylline is in the control of nocturnal asthma and early morning wheeze not controlled by inhaled corticosteroids in combination with inhaled β_2-receptor agonists. In this situation slow-release theophyllines may be more effective if given as a single dose at night.

The present drug treatment of asthma has undoubtedly increased the quality of life of asthmatic patients. Unfortunately, no good long-term studies of any antiasthmatic drugs are available to show which drug or drug combination is most beneficial for long-term treatment. Studies of this kind could perhaps explain why the number of acute asthma deaths has not decreased during the last 15 years.

REFERENCES

1. Hendeles L, Weinberger M: Theophylline: a 'state of the art' review. *Pharmacotherapy* (1983) **3**: 2–44.
2. Hendeles L, Iafrate R, Weinberger M: A clinical and pharmacokinetic basis for the selection and use of slow release theophylline products: *Clin Pharmacokinet* (1984) **9**: 95–135.
3. Self TH, Ellis RF, Abou-Shala N, Amarshi N: Is theophylline use justified in acute exacerbations of asthma? *Pharmacotherapy* (1989) **9**(4): 260–266.
4. Kelly HW, Murphy S: Should we stop using theophylline for the treatment of the hospitalized patient with status asthmaticus? *DICP, the Annals of Pharmacotherapy* (1989) **23**: 995–998.
5. Trigg CJ, Davies RJ: Use of slow-release theophylline in asthma—is it justified? *Respiratory Medicine* (1990) **84**: 1–3.
6. Ukena D, Sybrecht W: Management of chronic airway obstruction: Theophylline—is it still necessary? *Lung* (1990) (Suppl): 627–633.
7. Newhouse MT, Lam A: Management of asthma and chronic airflow limitation: Are methylxanthines obsolete? *Lung* (1990) (Suppl): 634–641.
8. Johnston IDA: Theophylline in the management of airflow obstruction. Difficult drug to use, few clinical indications. *Br Med J* (1990) **300**: 929–931.
9. Butcher RW, Sutherland EW: Adenosine 3',5',-phosphate in biological materials. I. Purification and properties of cyclic-3',5'-nucleotide phosphodiesterase and use of this enzyme to characterise adenosine 3',5'-phosphate in human urine. *J Biol Chem* (1963) **237**: 1244–1250.
10. Howell RE: Multiple mechanisms of xanthine actions on airway reactivity. *J Pharmac Exp Ther* (1990) **255**: 1008–1013.
11. Rodger IW: Calcium ions and contraction of airways smooth muscle. In Kay AB (ed) *Asthma: Clinical Pharmacology and Therapeutic Progress.* Oxford, Blackwell, 1986, pp 114–127.
12. Rodger IW: Excitation–contraction coupling mechanisms in airway smooth muscle: new targets in drug design. *Drug, Design & Delivery* (1990) **5**: 169–193.
13. Frossard N, Landry Y, Pauli G, Ruckstuhl M: Effects of cyclic AMP- and cyclic GMP-phosphodiesterase inhibitors on immunological release of histamine and on lung contraction. *Br J Pharmac* (1981) **73**: 933–938.
14. Giembycz MA, Rabe K, Dent G, Barnes PJ: Identification and partial characterisation of cyclic nucleotide-dependent phosphodiesterase activities in guinea-pig peritoneal eosinophils. *Br J Pharmac* (1991) **102** 29P.
15. Turner NC, Souness JE, Wood LJ, Diocee BK, Hassal GA, Scott L: Effects of phosphodiesterase inhibitors on granulocyte superoxide generation. *Br J Pharmac* (1991) **102** 39P.
16. Wright CD, Kuipers PJ, Kobylarz-Singer D, Devall LJ, Klinkefus BA, Weishaar RE: Differential inhibition of human neutrophil functions. Role of cyclic AMP specific, cyclic GMP-insensitive phosphodiesterase. *Biochem Pharmac* (1990) **40**: 699–707.

17. Nielson CP, Vestal RE, Sturm RJ, Heaslip R: Effects of selective phosphodiesterase inhibitors on the polymorphonuclear leukocyte respiratory burst. *J Allergy Clin Immunol* (1990) **86**: 801–808.

18. Beavo JA, Reifsnyder DH: Primary sequence of cyclic nucleotide phosphodiesterase isoenzymes and the design of selective inhibitors. *Trends Pharmacol Sci* (1990) **11**: 150–155.

19. Lohmann SM, Miech RP, Butcher FR: Effects of isoproterenol, theophylline and carbachol on cyclic nucleotide levels and relaxation of bovine tracheal smooth muscle. *Biochim Biophys Acta* (1977) **499**: 238–250.

20. Newman DJ, Colella DF, Spainhour CB. Brann EG, Zabko-Potapovich B, Wardell JR: cAMP-phosphodiesterase inhibitors and tracheal smooth muscle relaxation. *Biochem Pharmac* (1978) **27**: 729–732.

21. Polson JB, Krzanowski JJ, Goldman AL, Szentivanyi A: Inhibition of human phosphodiesterase by therapeutic levels of theophylline. *Clin Exp Pharmac Physiol* (1978) **5**: 535–539.

22. Polson JB, Krzanowski JJ, Anderson WH, Fitzpatrick DF, Hwang DPC, Szentivanyi A: Analysis of the relationship between pharmacological inhibition of cyclic nucleotide phosphodiesterase and relaxation of canine tracheal smooth muscle. *Biochem Pharmac* (1979) **28**: 1391–1395.

23. Polson JB, Krzanowski JJ, Szentivanyi A: Inhibition of a high affinity cyclic AMP phosphodiesterase and relaxation of canine tracheal smooth muscle. *Biochem Pharmac* (1982) **31**: 3403–3406.

24. Bergstrand H: Phosphodiesterase inhibition and theophylline. *Eur J Resp Dis* (1980) **61**(Suppl 109): 37–44.

25. Bergstrand H: Xanthines as phosphodiesterase inhibitors. In Andersson K-E, Persson CGA (eds) *Anti-asthma Xanthines and Adenosine*. Amsterdam, Excerpta Medica, 1985, pp 16–22.

26. Persson CGA: Experimental lung actions of xanthines. In Andersson K-E, Persson CGA (eds) *Anti-asthma Xanthines and Adenosine*. Amsterdam, Excerpta Medica, 1985, pp 61–83.

27. Small RC, Boyle JP, Duty S, Elliott KRF, Foster RW, Watt AJ: Analysis of the relaxant effects of AH 21-132 in guinea-pig isolated trachealis. *Br J Pharmac* (1989) **97**: 1165–1173.

28. Selvig K, Bjerve KS: Inhibition of human lung cyclic nucleotide phosphodiesterases by proxyphylline, theophylline and their metabolites. *Acta Pharmac Tox* (1982) **51**: 250–252.

29. Katsuki S, Murad F: Regulation of adenosine cyclic 3′,5′-monophosphate and guanosine cyclic 3′,5′-monophosphate levels and contractility in bovine tracheal smooth muscle. *Mol Pharmac* (1977) **13**: 330–341.

30. Kolbeck RC, Spier WA, Carrier GO, Bransome ED: Apparent irrelevance of cyclic nucleotides to relaxation of tracheal smooth muscle induced by theophylline. *Lung* (1979) **156**: 173–183.

31. Bryson SE, Rodger IW: Effects of phosphodiesterase inhibitors on normal and chemically-skinned isolated airway smooth muscle. *Br J Pharmac* (1987) **92**: 673–681.

32. Persson CGA: The profile of action of enprofylline, or why adenosine antagonism seems less desirable with xanthine antiasthmatics. In Morley J, Rainsford KD (eds) *Pharmacology of Asthma*. Basle, Birkhauser Verlag, 1983, pp 115–129.

33. Nicholson CD, Challiss RAJ, Shahid M: Differential modulation of tissue function and therapeutic potential of selective inhibitors of cyclic nucleotide phosphodiesterase isoenzymes. *Trends Pharmac Sci* (1991) **12**: 19–27.

34. Torphy TJ: Action of mediators on airway smooth muscle: Functional antagonism as a mechanism for bronchodilator drugs. In O'Donnell SR, Persson CGA (eds) *Directions for New Anti-Asthma Drugs*. Agents & Actions, Suppl 23, Basle, Birkhauser Verlag, 1988, pp 37–53.

35. Pyne NJ, Rodger IW: Selective phosphodiesterase inhibitors. *Eur Resp J* (1990) **3**(Suppl 10): 306S.

36. Jamieson DD, Taylor KM: Comparison of the bronchodilator and vasodilator activity of sodium azide and sodium nitroprusside in the guinea-pig. *Clin Exp Pharmac Physiol* (1979) **6**: 515–525.

37. Murad F: Effects of phosphodiesterase inhibitors and the role of cyclic nucleotides in smooth muscle relaxation. In Andersson K-E, Persson CGA (eds) *Anti-Asthma Xanthines and Adenosine*. Amsterdam, Excerpta Medica, 1985, pp 10–15.

38. Suzuki K, Takagi K, Satake T, Sugiyama S, Ozawa T: The relationship between tissue levels of cyclic GMP and tracheal smooth muscle relaxation in the guinea-pig. *Clin Exp Pharmac Physiol* (1986) **13**: 39–46.

39. Bergstrand H, Kristoffersson J, Lundquist B, Schurmann A: Effects of antiallergic agents, compound 48/80 and some reference inhibitors of the activity of partially purified human lung tissue adenosine cyclic 3′,5′-monophosphate and guanosine cyclic 3′,5′-monophosphate phosphodiesterase. *Mol Pharmac* (1977) **13**: 38–43.

40. Gilman AG: G proteins: transducers of receptor-generated signals. *Annu Rev Biochem* (1987) **56**: 615–649.

41. Parsons WJ, Ramkumar V, Stiles GL: Isobutylmethylxanthine stimulates adenylate cyclase by blocking the inhibitory regulatory protein, Gi. *Mol Pharmac* (1988) **34**: 37–41.

42. Fredholm BB: Are methylxanthine effects due to antagonism of endogenous adenosine? *Trends Pharmac Sci* (1980) **1**: 129–132.

43. Holgate ST, Cushley MJ, Church MK, Hughes P, Mann JS: Adenosine: A potential mediator of bronchial asthma and its antagonism by methylxanthines. In Andersson K-E, Persson CGA (eds) *Anti-Asthma Xanthines and Adenosine*. Amsterdam, Excerpta Medica, 1985, pp 84–93.

44. Mann JS, Cushley MJ, Holgate ST: Adenosine-induced bronchoconstriction in asthma and its antagonism by theophylline. In Herzog H, Perruchoud AP (eds) *Progress in Respiration Research*, Vol. 19, *Asthma and Bronchial Hyperreactivity*. Basel, Karger, 1985, pp 102–105.

45. Persson CGA, Kjellin G: Enprofylline, a principally new antiasthmatic xanthine. *Acta Pharmac Tox* (1981) **49**: 313–318.

46. Lunell E, Svedmyr N, Andersson K-E, Persson CGA: A novel bronchodilator xanthine apparently without adenosine receptor antagonism and tremorogenic effect. *Eur J Resp Dis* (1984) **64**: 333–339.

47. Higbee MD, Kumar M, Galant SP: Stimulation of endogenous catecholamine release by theophylline; A proposed additional mechanism of action for theophylline effects. *J Allergy Clin Immunol* (1982) **70**: 377–382.

48. Poisner AM: Direct stimulant effect of aminophylline on catecholamine release from the adrenal medulla: *Biochem Pharmac* (1973) **22**: 469–476.

49. Snider S, Waldeck B: Increased synthesis of adrenomedullary catecholamines induced by caffeine and theophylline. *Naunyn-Schmiedeberg's Arch Pharmac* (1974) **281**: 257–260.

50. Persson CGA, Ekman M, Erjefält I: Vascular anti-permeability effects of β-receptor agonists and theophylline in the lung. *Acta Pharmac Tox* (1979) **44**: 216–220.

51. Andersson K-E, Johannesson N, Karlberg B, Persson CGA: Xanthine induced increase of plasma free fatty acid and natriuresis in man may reflect adenosine antagonism. *Eur J Clin Pharmac* (1985) **26**: 33–38.

52. Barnes PJ, Brown MJ, Siverman M, Dollery CT: Circulating catecholamines in exercise- and hyperventilation-induced asthma. *Thorax* (1981) **36**: 435–440.

53. Dahlöf C, Dahlöf P, Lundberg JM, Strömbom U: Elevated plasma concentration of neuropeptide Y and low level of circulating adrenaline in elderly asthmatics during rest and acute severe asthma. *Pulmonary Pharmacol* (1988) **1**: 3–6.

54. Grandordy BM, Cuss FM, Barnes PJ: Breakdown of phosphoinositides in airway smooth muscle: Lack of influence of antiasthma drugs. *Life Sci* (1987) **41**: 1621–1627.

55. Hall IP, Donaldson J, Hill SJ: Inhibition of histamine-stimulated inositol phospholipid hydrolysis by agents which increase cyclic AMP levels in bovine tracheal smooth muscle. *Br J Pharmac* (1989) **97**: 603–613.

56. Hall IP, Donaldson J, Hill SJ: Modulation of fluoroaluminate-induced inositol phosphate formation by increases in tissue cyclic AMP content in bovine tracheal smooth muscle. *Br J Pharmac* (1990) **100**: 646–650.

57. Rodger IW, Small RC: Pharmacology of airway smooth muscle. In Barnes PJ, Page CP (eds) *Pharmacology of Asthma: Handbook of Experimental Pharmacology*, Berlin, Springer-Verlag, 1991, Vol. 98, pp 107–141.

58. Allen SL, Cortijo J, Foster RW, Morgan GP, Small RC, Weston AH: Mechanical and electrical aspects of the relaxant action of aminophylline in guinea-pig isolated trachealis. *Br J Pharmac* (1986) **88**: 473–483.

59. Felbel J, Trockur B, Ecker T, Landgraf W, Hofman F: Regulation of cytosolic calcium by cAMP and cGMP in freshly isolated smooth muscle cells from bovine trachea. *J Biol Chem* (1988) **263**: 16764–16771.

60. Raeymaekers J, Hofmann F, Casteels R: Cyclic GMP-dependent protein kinase phosphory-lates phospholamban in isolated sarcoplasmic reticulum from cardiac and smooth muscle. *Biochem J* (1988) **252**: 269–273.

61. Svedmyr N: Treatment with β-adrenostimulants. *Scand J Respir Dis* (1977) **101**(Suppl): 59–68.

62. Persson CGA, Karlsson JA: *In vitro* responses to bronchodilator drugs. In Jenne JW, Murphy S (eds) *Drug Therapy for Asthma*. New York, Marcel Dekker, 1987, pp 129–176.

63. Karlsson J-A, Persson CGA: Influence of tracheal contraction on relaxant effects *in vitro* of theophylline and isoprenaline. *Br J Pharmacol* (1981) **74**: 73.

64. Mossberg B, Strandberg K, Philipson K, Camner P: Tracheobronchial clearance in bronchial asthma response to β-adrenoceptor stimulation. *Scand J Respir Dis* (1976) **57**: 119.

65. Matthys H, Köhler D: Effect of theophylline on mucociliary clearance in man. *Eur J Respir Dis* (1980) **61**(Suppl 109): 98.

66. Sutton PP, Pavia D, Bateman JRM, Clarke SW: The effect of oral aminophylline on lung mucociliary clearance in man: *Chest* (1981) **80**: 889.

67. Wanner A: Effects of methylxanthines on airway mucociliary function. *Am J Med* (1985) **20**(Suppl 79): 16–21.

68. Pavia D, Sutton PP, Lopez-Vidriero MD, Agnew JE, Clarks SW: Drug effects on mucocili-ary function. *Eur Respir Dis* (1983) (Suppl 28): 304–317.

69. Matthys H, Köhler D, Daikeler G: Additive actions of bronchodilators on mucous transport. *Respiration* (1984) **46**(Suppl): 34.

70. Naclerio RM, Bartenfelder D, Proud D, et al.: Theophylline reduces the response to nasal challenge with antigen. *Am J Med* (1985) **20**(Suppl 79): 43–47.

71. Martin GL, Atkins PC, Dynsky EG, Zweiman B: Effects of theophylline, terbutaline and prednisone on antigen-induced bronchospasm and mediator release. *J Allergy Clin Immunol* (1980) **66**: 204.

72. Pauwels R, Van Renterghem D, Van der Straeten M, et al.: The effect of theophylline and enprofylline on allergen-induced bronchoconstriction. *J Allergy Clin Immunol* (1985) **76**(4): 583–590.

73. Persson CGA, Svensjö E: Airway hyperreactivity and microvascular permeability to large molecules. *Eur J Respir Dis* (1986) **64**(Suppl 131): 183.

74. Parker JO, Ashekian PB, Di Georgi S, West RO: Hemodynamic effects of aminophylline in chronic obstructive pulmonary disease. *Circulation* (1976) **35**: 365.

75. Winter RJD, Langford JA, George RJD, et al.: The effect of theophylline and salbutamol on right and left ventricular function in chronic bronchitis and emphysema. *Br J Dis Chest* (1984) **78**: 358.

76. Wetzenblum E, Hirth C, Dulolone A, Mirhom R: Prognostic value of pulmonary artery pressure in chronic obstructive pulmonary disease. *Thorax* (1981) **36**: 752.

77. Aubier M: The clinical importance of methylxanthines for diaphragmatic contractility. In Andersson KE, Persson CGA (eds) *Anti-asthma Xanthines and Adenosine*. Amsterdam, Excerpta Medica, 1985, pp 110–120.

78. Howell S, Roussos C: Isoproterenol and aminophylline improve contractility of fatigued canine diaphragmae. *Am Rev Respir Dis* (1984) **129**: 118.

79. Hedner T, Hedner J, Wessberg P, Jonason J: Regulation of breathing in the rat: indications for a role of central adenosine mechanisms. *Neurosci Lett* (1982) **33**: 147.

80. Hedner J, Hedner T, Wessberg P, et al.: Central respiratory effects of adenosine analogues, theophylline and enprofylline. In Andersson KE, Persson CGA (eds) *Anti-asthma Xanthines and Adenosine*. Amsterdam, Excerpta Medica, 1985, pp 467–471.

81. Gerhardt T, McCarthy J, Bancalore E: Effect of aminophylline on respiratory centre activity and metabolic rate in premature infants with idiopathic apnoea. *Pediatrics* (1979) **63**: 537–542.

82. Lagercrantz H, Rane A, Tunell R: Plasma concentration-effect relationship of theophylline in treatment of apnoea in preterm infants. *Eur J Clin Pharmacol* (1980) **18**: 65–68.
83. Persson CGA: Xanthines: new developments. In Barnes PJ (ed) *New Drugs for Asthma*. London, IBC, 1989, pp 21–32.
84. Magnusson H, Reuss G, Jorres R: Theophylline has a dose-related effect on the airways response to inhaled histamine and metacholine in asthmatics. *Am Rev Respir Dis* (1987) **136**: 1163–1167.
85. Phillips MJ, Ollier S, Trembath PW, Boobis SW, Davies RJ: The effect of slow-release aminophylline on exercise-induced asthma. *Br J Dis Chest* (1981) **75**: 181–189.
86. Cockroft DW, Murdock KY, Gore BP, O'Byrne PM, Manning P: Theophylline does not inhibit allergen-induced increase in airway responsiveness to metacholine. *J Allergy Clin Immunol* (1989) **83**: 913–920.
87. Dutoit JE, Salome CM, Woolcock NJ: Inhaled corticosteroids reduce the severity of bronchial hyperresponsiveness in asthma but oral theophylline does not. *Am Rev Respir Dis* (1987) **136**: 1174–1178.
88. Tsiu SJ, Self TH, Burns R: Theophylline toxicity: update. *Ann Allergy* (1990) **64**: 241–257.
89. Ellis EF: Theophylline toxicity. In Andersson KE, Persson CGA (eds) *Anti-asthma Xanthines and Adenosine*. Amsterdam, Excerpta Medica, 1985, pp 352–360.
90. Furukawa CT, Shapiro CG, Duhamel T, Weimer L, Pierson WE, Bierman CW: Learning and behaviour problems associated with theophylline therapy. *Lancet* (1985) **I**: 621.
91. Furukawa CT, Duhamel T, Weimer L, Shapiro CG, Pierson WE, Bierman W: Cognitive and behavioural findings in children taking theophylline. *J Allergy Clin Immunol* (1988) **81**: 83–85.
92. Rachelefsky GS, Wo J, Adelson J, *et al.*: Behaviour abnormalities and poor school performance due to oral theophylline use. *Pediatrics* (1986) **78**: 1133–1138.
93. Niemand D, Martiness S, Arvidsson S, *et al.*: Adenosine in the inhibition of diazepam-sedation by aminophylline. *Acta Anaesthet* (1986) **30**: 493–495.
94. Persson CGA: Subdivision of xanthines. In Anderson KE, Persson CGA (eds) *Anti-Asthma Xanthines and Adenosine*. Amsterdam, Excerpta Medica, 1985, pp 23–39.
95. Turner-Warwick M: Study of theophylline plasma levels after oral administration of new theophylline compounds. *Br Med J* (1957) **2**: 67–69.
96. Mitenko PA, Ogilvie RI: Rational intravenous doses of theophylline. *N Engl J Med* (1973) **289**: 600.
97. Maselli R, Casal GL, Ellis EF: Pharmacological effects of intravenously administered aminophylline in asthmatic children. *J Ped* (1970) **76**: 777.
98. Svedmyr K: β_2-Adrenoceptor stimulants and theophylline in asthma therapy. Thesis. *Eur J Respir Dis* (1981) **62**(Suppl 116): 1–48.
99. Billing B, Dahlqvist R, Garle M, *et al.*: Separate and combined use of terbutaline and theophylline in asthmatics. Effects related to serum concentrations. *Eur J Respir Dis* (1982) **63**: 399.
100. Brenner M, Berkowitz R, Marshall N, Strunk RC: Need for theophylline in severe-steroid requiring asthmatics. *Clin Allergy* (1988) **18**: 143–150.
101. Niki Y, Soejima R, Kaware H, Sumi M, Umeki S: New synthetic quinolone antibacterial agents and serum concentration of theophylline. *Chest* (1987) **92**: 663–669.
102. Hemstreet MP, Miles MV, Rutland RO: Effect of intravenous isoproterenol on theophylline kinetics. *J Allergy Clin Immunol* (1982) **69**: 360–364.
103. Shenfield GM: Combination bronchodilator therapy. *Drugs* (1983) **24**/5: 414.
104. Menendez R, Kelly HW: Theophylline therapy. *J Asthma* (1983) **20**: 455.
105. Jordan TJ, Reichman LB: Once-daily versus twice-daily dosing of theophylline. *Am Rev Respir Dis* (1989) **140**: 1573–1577.
106. Siegel D, Sheppard D, Gelb A, Weinberg PF: Aminophylline increases the toxicity by not the efficacy of an inhaled β-adrenergic agonist in the treatment of acute exacerbations of asthma. *Amer Rev Respir Dis* (1985) **132**: 283–286.
107. Littenberg B: Aminophylline treatment in severe acute asthma. A meta-analysis. *JAMA* (1988) **259**(11): 1678–1684.

108. Connelly MS, Jenkins PF: Role of intravenous aminophylline in the management of acute severe asthma. *Thorax* (1990) **45**: 341P.
109. Fanta H, Rossing TH, McFadden Jr ER: Emergency room treatment of asthma. *Am J Med* (1982) **72**: 416.

Anti-allergic Drugs

P. RAFFERTY AND S.T. HOLGATE

INTRODUCTION

In Ishizaka's classical description of mast cell activation,[1] inhaled antigen interacts with specific IgE molecules bound to mast cells, resulting in secondary bridging of IgE-Fc receptors. The subsequent biochemical changes in the membrane phospholipids facilitate the influx of extracellular calcium and mobilize this cation from intracellular stores, coupling the activation signal to the energy-dependent secretion of a wide variety of granule-associated mast-cell mediators including histamine, eosinophil chemotactic factors (ECF), high molecular weight neutrophil chemotactic factor (NCF), heparin, tryptase and other neutral proteases and a number of exoglycosidases. Of these mediators, histamine is the only known bronchoconstrictor agent in man. In addition to releasing preformed mediators, activation of mast cells leads to the mobilization of arachidonic acid from membrane phospholipids. Arachidonic acid is metabolized along two pathways, the 5-lipoxygenase pathway, giving rise to the potent bronchoconstrictors leukotrienes (LTs) C_4, D_4 and E_4 and the leucocyte chemotactant LTB_4, and the cyclooxygenase pathway, resulting in the formation of the bronchoconstrictor prostaglandins PGD_2 and thromboxane A_2 (TxA_2). Additional mediators may also be released from eosinophils, platelets and macrophages, since these cells have been shown to possess low-affinity receptors for IgE.[2] Finally, an array of inflammatory mediators is released as a consequence of primary mediators interacting with secondary effector cells in the airway.

A drug that interferes with any step of the pathway from initial activation of primary effector cells to the end-organ effects of the mediators can therefore be considered 'anti-allergic' (Fig. 35.1). Several important groups of drugs that can directly interfere with the manifestation of the allergic asthmatic response will not be covered in this chapter since they are dealt with in other sections of the book. It is sufficient here to mention

ASTHMA: BASIC MECHANISMS AND CLINICAL MANAGEMENT (2nd Edn)
ISBN 0-12-079026-2

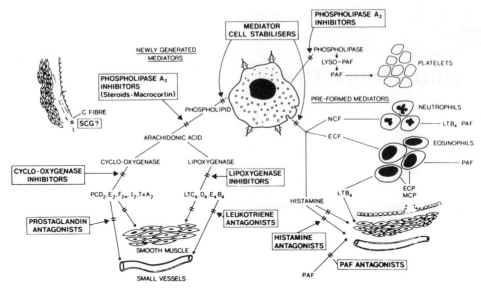

Fig. 35.1 The possible mechanisms of action of anti-allergic drugs.

that, in addition to relaxing airway smooth muscle, β_2-adrenoceptor agonists inhibit the release of mast-cell mediators,[3] theophylline exhibits a variety of actions that could affect the allergic response, including receptor antagonism of adenosine[4] and inhibition of the late-phase reaction,[5] and corticosteroids, in part through the induction of an intracellular protein, lipocortin, can inhibit newly formed mediator release from a variety of pro-inflammatory cells and modify the generation of cytokines that maintain individual inflammatory cells in their microenvironment.[6] However, in this chapter particular attention will be focused on inhibitors of mediator release, inhibitors of arachidonic acid metabolism and antagonists of mediator end-organ effects.

SODIUM CROMOGLYCATE

Sodium cromoglycate was developed following the investigation of an eastern Mediterranean herb used for its bronchodilator properties. An extract from the plant, khellin, is a mixture of cromones, sodium cromoglycate being a synthetic derivative of a bis-cromone. Sodium cromoglycate (SCG) has come to be regarded as a classical mast-cell stabilizing agent and represents a standard against which other non-bronchodilator antiasthma drugs are measured. Initial *in vitro* work has shown that SCG inhibits IgE-mediated release of histamine from rat peritoneal mast cells.[7] Subsequent studies have shown inhibition of mediator release provoked by other mast-cell secretagogues, e.g. calcium ionophore A23187, compound 48/80 and phospholipase A. Sodium cromoglycate exhibits species and organ specificity in its action. At high concentrations, SCG produces a dose-related inhibition of IgE-triggered mediator release from human enzymatically dispersed mast cells,[3] and at 100-fold lower concentrations from mast cells recovered by bronchoalveolar lavage.[8] In contrast, it has no activity against mast cells of human skin or basophils. *In vivo*, SCG inhibits both the early and late bronchoconstrictor reaction following allergen challenge and the accompanying increase in circulating levels of histamine and NCA, provided that the drug is administered before challenge.[9]

While the exact mechanisms underlying bronchoconstriction induced by exercise, cold air, and hyperventilation are still in question, evidence is accumulating that mediator release from mast cells activated by hypertonicity is involved. With exercise, isocapnic hyperventilation and hypertonic saline challenge of asthmatic airways, bronchoconstriction is accompanied by an increase in one or both of histamine and NCA. Sodium cromoglycate inhibits bronchoconstriction and the accompanying rise in mediators following exercise[10,11] and hypertonic saline challenge as well as blocking the responses to cold air and isocapnic hyperventilation.[12] The mechanism of cromoglycate in mast-cell inhibitory action is poorly understood but probably involves the stimulation of a specific cell surface receptor and the activation of a protein by phosphorylation which is involved in the termination of IgE-triggered mediator release.

Despite the inhibitory properties of SCG on mast cells, some doubt has been cast on this mechanism as its major protective action in clinical asthma. Firstly, a large number of pharmaceutical companies have produced compounds which have up to 1000 times greater potency as inhibitors of mast-cell mediator secretion *in vitro* and protect against exercise and allergen provocation, and yet do not exhibit efficacy in the long-term treatment of asthma. Secondly, the β_2-adrenoceptor agonist salbutamol will inhibit mediator release from human mast cells at concentrations 1000 times lower than that of SCG,[3] but is reported not to protect against the late reaction or acquired bronchial hyperresponsiveness with allergen challenge whereas SCG is active against both.[13] More recently the lack of protective activity of β_2-agonists against late-phase responses has been questioned.[14] Finally, there is convincing clinical evidence to suggest that SCG is active against forms of asthma that are not considered to involve IgE-dependent mast-cell activation, e.g. diisocyanate-induced asthma[15] and intrinsic asthma.[16]

One additional mechanism of action of SCG is its role in inhibiting neural reflexes within the lung. In dogs, the stimulation of irritant receptors within the airways by capsaicin (extract of hot pepper) results in the release of substance P and related tachykinins from afferent nerve endings of C-fibres (non-myelinated) which provoke bronchoconstriction.[17] Sodium cromoglycate can effectively inhibit C-fibre excitation at concentrations 10% of those required for mast-cell stabilization. In humans, sulphur dioxide and metabisulphite are also thought to mediate bronchoconstriction via a neurogenic mechanism, and SCG has been found to be more effective than atropine in preventing these reactions.[18] Moreover, SCG also inhibits bronchoconstriction provoked in man by inhaled neurokinin A and bradykinin, peptides that are not considered to be mast-cell secretogogues.

Allergen challenge of atopic subjects results in an early reaction developing within 10 min and slowly resolving over the next 2 h followed by a late reaction with a second fall in FEV$_1$ occurring 6–24 h after challenge. The late response is associated with an inflammatory infiltrate of the airways with eosinophils and neutrophils.[19] Patients developing late reactions show an increased airway responsiveness to a wide variety of irritants which lasts for up to 2–3 weeks from the onset of the reaction.[20] Since SCG is able to block both early and late reactions, it might also be expected to reduce subsequent hyperreactivity. In clinical studies carried out in grass-pollen sensitive subjects during the hay fever season, SCG reduced the symptoms experienced by patients and prevented the development of hyperreactivity seen in the control groups,[15] and Cockcroft and Murdoch have shown that this drug inhibits the acute allergen acquired increase in non-specific airway responsiveness.[21]

Long-term studies with SCG have shown that the addition of SCG can lead to a reduction in concomitant medication.[22] In the study conducted on behalf of the British Medical Research Council, 40% of patients on oral steroid therapy were able to either withdraw steroids completely or reduce the dosage to a minimal level following the addition of SCG to their therapy.[16] In most studies, young atopic asthmatics appear to gain the greatest benefit from SCG, but improvement has also been noted in non-atopic asthmatics. Petty *et al.*[23] reported significant symptomatic improvement in a group of 68 chronic adult asthmatics following the addition of sodium cromoglycate 2 mg daily to their treatment. Few side-effects have been reported with the use of the drug, perhaps the commonest being mild throat infection following use of the dry powder spinhaler. This minor problem has become even less evident now that the standard and high-dose pressurized aerosols have been introduced. Possibly relevant actions of SCG pertinent to its protective activity against hyperresponsiveness include inhibition of eosinophil cyto-toxicity,[24] activation of neutrophils and monocytes by chemotactic factors,[25] and inhibition of platelet-activating factor PAF-induced inflammatory response.[26] The time has now passed for considering SCG as purely a mast-cell stabilizing agent, and multiplicity of its pharmacological effect is more likely to account for its clinical efficacy that any single action.

NEDOCROMIL SODIUM

Since the development of SCG, pharmaceutical companies have sought a drug with similar 'mast-cell stabilizing' properties but with greater potency. Using animal models as the targets for developing drugs of this type, drug after drug failed to reach its clinical expectations. The precise reasons for this have never been clearly explained, but one outcome has been a serious question as to the role of mast cells in asthma pathogenesis. The situation, however, rapidly changed with the discovery of a highly novel compound called nedocromil sodium. Nedocromil sodium has been shown to possess similar activities to SCG in a variety of test systems, but in some has been found to be more potent. *In vitro*, nedocromil has been shown to inhibit IgE-dependent histamine release from rat peritoneal mast cells in a dose-dependent manner.[27] It also prevents passive cutaneous and lung anaphylaxis in rat models, with a potency similar to that of SCG.[27] However, entirely new test systems were developed to evaluate this drug. Macaque monkeys infected with *Ascaris suum* developed eosinophilia and specific IgE antibodies to the parasite, and when challenged via the airways by an extract of the parasite antigen, acute bronchoconstricion occurred similar in time course and in magnitude to the asthmatic early reaction.[28] In bronchoalveolar lavage (BAL) fluid from these infected monkeys up to 20% of the nucleated cells were mast cells and 10% eosinophils, which contrasts with the predominance of macrophages (>95%) normally found in the lavage of these animals. Further experiments showed that when sensitized BAL cells were challenged with *Ascaris antigen*, histamine, LTC_4 and PGD_2 were released primarily from mast cells. Moreover, in this *ex vitro* test system of 'mucosal mast cells', nedocromil sodium was 200 times more potent than SCG at inhibiting the release of all three mediators.[27] Further experiments have shown that nedocromil sodium also inhibits the immediate airway response to *in vivo* provocation of monkey airways with *Ascaris* antigen.[29] Like SCG, nedocromil sodium enhances the production of a 78-KDa protein from mast cells that may act in a negative feedback system to reduce mediator release.[27] In man, nedocromil sodium has been shown to inhibit both the immediate and late bronchoconstricitor reactions following allergen challenge[30] and to reduce the acquired increased airway responsiveness to allergen exposure that develops in grass-pollen sensitive asthmatics during the hayfever season.[31] Several studies of the effect of nedocromil on exercise-induced asthma have shown a reduction in bronchoconstriction when doses of 2–4 mg are given before exercise, and the inhibitory effect has usually been greater than that of a 20-mg dose of SCG.[30,32,33]

Adenosine is a naturally occurring nucleoside released into the circulation under conditions of hypoxia or following allergen challenge. Both adenosine and adenosine 5'-monophosphate (AMP) (from which adenosine is derived) cause bronchoconstriction in asthmatic subjects.[34] Since Marquardt *et al.*[35] have demonstrated that adenosine can enhance mast-cell degranulation with the release of histamine without stimulating the production of newly generated mediators, it has been proposed as a model for *in vivo* mast-cell activation.[36] Nedocromil inhibits AMP-induced bronchoconstriction, presumably by its effect on bronchial mast cells. Furthermore, like SCG, nedocromil inhibits sulphur-dioxide induced bronchoconstriction[37] probably by interfering with neural reflexes at the level of neuropeptide-containing non-myelinated C-fibres in the airways. Nedocromil has also been shown to inhibit PAF-induced contraction with sheep trachea.[38]

In clinical studies, the addition of nedocromil sodium to standard asthma therapy has resulted in reduction of symptoms and improvement in objective measures of lung function. Several studies have been performed in which inhaled steroid therapy was gradually reduced and replaced with nedocromil.[39] In these studies most patients were able to tolerate the change in therapy, but this was often accompanied by deterioration in pulmonary function, albeit to a lesser degree than occurred with placebo. Svendsen *et al.*[40] recently reported an important study comparing the addition of nedocromil 4 mg twice daily or beclomethazone 200 mg twice daily to inhaled bronchodilators in a group of 39 asthmatics. While both treatments brought about significant improvement in lung function and symptom control beclomethasone proved more effective than nedocromil. Goldin and Bateman[41] found that the addition of nedocromil did not have a significant steroid-sparing effect in patients requiring oral prednisolone. Thus it appears unlikely that nedocromil sodium will be able to replace inhaled corticosteroids, although the drug may be complementary. Only minor side-effects have been reported with this drug, the most common being an unpleasant taste and nausea. It seems likely that nedocromil will prove useful for supplementing treatment with inhaled bronchodilators and may benefit those patients whose asthma is not satisfactorily controlled with inhaled corticosteroids. Whether the anti-inflammatory action of nedocromil sodium resides in its ability to inhibit mast-cell mediator release or more upon its action upon secondary effector cells such as eosinophils, neutrophils and monocytes has not been evaluated, despite the demonstration of obvious activities *in vitro* on these cell types.

ANTIHISTAMINES

Histamine was first implicated in the pathogenesis of asthma in 1919 following the demonstration by Sir Henry Dale that an infusion of histamine reproduced the cardo-respiratory features of anaphylaxis in guinea-pigs.[42] Subsequently, Weiss *et al.* were able to induce wheezing in asthmatic patients by the infusion of histamine.[43] Further circumstantial evidence for the role of histamine in asthma was provided in the 1940s and 1950s, when several investigators documented elevated plasma histamine concentrations in patients during exacerbations of their asthma.[44,45] The technique of bronchoscopy and bronchoalveolar lavage has now revealed evidence of increased histamine in the airway of asthmatics in the resting state[46] with further elevation of this histamine level in response to allergen challenge.[47] Histamine is known to cause bronchoconstriction by direct stimulation of smooth muscle and via stimulation of vagal reflexes. Histamine also affects pulmonary vasculature, H_1-receptors mediating vasoconstriction and H_2-receptors producing vasodilation.[48] Other effects of histamine include increased lung permeability[49] and stimulation of leucocyte chemokinesis.[50]

H_1-receptor antagonists

With the increasing evidence for the role played by histamine in human allergic diseases, competitive antagonists have been developed. These drugs are classified according to their chemical structures: ethanolamines, ethylenediamines, alkylamines, piperazines, piperidine and phenylthiazines. In the early 1940s, antihistamines were used with reasonable success in the treatment of hayfever, but in a great many trials in asthma involving in total about 700 patients, subjective improvement was only found in 10–12%, with no objective evidence of any benefit being obtained.[51] However, interest in antihistamines was maintained, since Herxheimer demonstrated that H_1-antihistamines could cause bronchodilation in asthmatics,[52] and Schild *et al.*, using human tracheal rings, demonstrated reduction of histamine and allergen-induced bronchoconstriction by antihistamines.[53] In the early 1970s, Booij-Noord *et al.*[54] reported that intramuscular thiazinium caused bronchodilation, and subsequently similar results were found using a further antihistamine, chlorpheniramine,[55] administered intravenously, and clemastine, administered by inhalation.[56] Furthermore, those patients demonstrating the greatest bronchodilation were those with more severe bronchoconstriction, leading Nogrady *et al.*[57] to suggest that there might be an underlying 'histamine tone' due to the constant background production and release of histamine by activated endobronchial mast cells.

By the late 1970s several studies had shown that inhaled or parenteral antihistamines could offer a degree of protection against bronchoconstriction provoked by inhaled histamine,[58,59] allergen[60,61] or exercise challenge,[62] but the same could not be said for the drugs when administered orally. This apparent discrepancey may have been because many of the older antihistamine preparations caused sedation and systemic side-effects, attributed to their anticholinergic and anti-adrenergic properties, thereby limiting the doses that could be used. In recent years a number of new antihistamines, astemizole, terfenadine and cetirizine, have been developed which appear to be free from the adverse central nervous system and other effects previously associated with this drug class.[63] Astemizole has a slow onset of action because of its hepatic uptake and release from lysozomes as an active metabolite, and its slow dissociation from H_1-receptors. Thus the H_1-blocking activity of astemizole can last for up to 32 days following the last oral dose. Two weeks' treatment with astemizole, 10 mg daily, has been shown to displace the histamine dose–response curve on the airways to the right by a factor of 17-fold,[64] demonstrating that this drug is at least four times as potent as the maximum tolerated doses of the older antihistamine preparations. Astemizole has also been shown to attenuate bronchoconstriction during the first 10–15 min following inhaled allergen by 50%,[64] and in a prolonged study carried out during the hayfever season, significantly reduced the severity of wheezing experienced by seasonal asthmatics.[65]

Terfenadine is a shorter-acting histamine H_1-receptor antagonist whose pharmacological activity reaches a peak within 2–3 h of oral administration, with some activity being retained for up to 12–16 h.[66] Terfenadine undergoes extensive biotransformation to two major metabolites, one of which possesses one-third of the *in vitro* antihistaminic activity of terfenadine. The currently recommended dose in the treatment of allergic rhinitis is 60 mg twice daily, although higher doses have been shown to provide increased protection against histamine-induced bronchoconstriction. In increasing doses of 60, 120 and 180 mg, terfenadine displaced histamine-concentration–response curves to the right by factors of 14, 22 and 35,[67] which compares to only 5–7-fold shifts achieved by the older antihistamine preparations such as chlorpheniramine.[60] Both terfenadine[68] and astemizole are free of anticholinergic activity even at high doses. Three hours after a single oral dose of terfenadine of 180 mg, the immediate bronchoconstrictor response to inhaled allergen was inhibited by 50%.[69] Single doses of 120 and 180 mg of terfenadine significantly inhibit asthma induced by exercise,[70] cold air hyperventilation[71] or hyperresponder saline.[72] In addition to H_1-receptor blockade Nabe *et al.*[73] have recently shown that terfenadine can inhibit the release of histamine from basophils at concentrations from 2–20 μM or inhibit the release of leukotrine LTC_4 from eosinophils at 20 μM.

Azelastine

Azelastine is an oral long-acting phthalazine derivative which is a potent H_1-antihistamine with other 'anti-allergic' properties. In addition to inhibiting allergic reactions in guinea-pigs and rats,[74] it has been shown to prevent the release of histamine from rat peritoneal mast cells stimulated by allergen, phospholipase A_2, compound 48/80 and calcium ionophore, A23187.[75–77] Azelastine inhibits allergen-induced mediator release from rabbit[78] and human leucocytes and fragments of human lung tissue.[79] In these studies azelastine was estimated to be approximately twice as potent as ketotifen on a molar basis. Studies *in vivo* have also demonstrated inhibition of leukotriene-[80] and allergen-induced[74] bronchoconstriction in guinea-pigs. Both azelastine and ketotifen have been shown to inhibit the skin wheal and flare response to the injection of PAF but did not affect PAF-induced bronchoconstriction.[81] Other activities of this compound include prevention of IgE-dependent increases in vascular permeability[82] and inhibition of macrophage chemotaxis.[83]

In clinical studies azelastine administered as 4.4 mg in single and multiple oral doses produced bronchodilation,[84] and reduced exercise-induced asthma[85] and this is in keeping with similar findings using other H_1 histamine-receptor antagonists such as terfenadine.[86] In patients with asthma, a dose of 4.4 mg azelastine displaces the histamine concentration–response curve to the right by a factor of 6, and this increases to 40 when a dose of 17.6 mg is used.[87] Ollier *et al.* reported that prolonged therapy for 3 weeks with azelastine will significantly inhibit allergen-induced bronchoconstriction in man.[84] The most commonly reported side-effects with this drug are those of drowsiness and a metallic taste, although in some studies these symptoms have diminished after the first few weeks of therapy.

Cetirizine

Cetirizine is a novel, potent H_1-receptor antagonist with additional effects on cell migration. A single 15 mg dose of cetirizine has been shown to reduce airway responsiveness to histamine by a factor of 70 while having no effect on the response inhaled LTD_4[88] or methacholine.[89] Skin chamber studies have demonstrated that cetirizine inhibits the migration of neutrophils, eosinophils and basophils into the chamber in response to allergen stimulation and also reduces the release of histamine and PGD_2 *in situ*.[90–92] Cetirizine has not been found to inhibit allergen-induced bronchoconstriction[93] nor to exhibit any consistent effect upon exercise-induced asthma when given orally[93] but is effective by inhalation.

Other H_1-antagonists with mediator inhibitor properties include loratidine and azatidine which have been shown to inhibit the release of leukotrienes,[94] and histamine[95] from sensitized human lung fragments.

Clinical effects of H_1-receptor antagonists

While many short-term studies have demonstrated significant bronchodilation following H_1-antagonist, this response does not appear to be maintained in long-term trials. Taytard *et al.*[96] found that terfenadine 120 mg twice daily resulted in a reduction in patients symptoms with a small increase in peak flow rate. These findings were confirmed in the UK using a higher dose of terfenadine 180 mg three times daily.[97] In this study a group of atopic grass-pollen sensitive patients were treated with 180 mg of terfenadine three times daily and this resulted in a significant reduction in patient symptoms, a small increase in peak flow of approximately 5% and 40% reduction in the use of inhaled β-agonists.

Storms *et al.*[98] reported similar results with azelastine but a dose ranging study by Tinkelman *et al.*[99] using 2, 4, 6 or 8 g of azelastine given twice daily over a 12-week period, reported significant reduction in concomitant medication used with the 4- and 6-mg group only. No significant differences in FEV_1 were observed. In a parallel group study of grass-pollen sensitive patients Bruttman *et al.*[100] found that cetirizine reduced patients asthmatic symptoms, β_2-agonist requirement and prevented the fall in FEV_1 that was observed in the placebo group during the pollen season. From the studies available to date it appears that the patients most likely to benefit from currently available antihistamines are young atopic asthmatics with seasonal symptoms.

H_2-receptor antagonists

The presence of more than one histamine receptor was first demonstrated in 1966 by Ash and Schild,[101] using a variety of histamine analogues. They compared the effects of these analogues with those of histamine on gastric-acid secretion, guinea-pig ileal smooth muscle contraction and inhibition of rat uterine contraction, and found that the different analogues varied in their potency of action in the different test systems. In 1972 Black et al.[102] described the first H_2-antagonist, burimamide, and using this antagonist, Lichtenstein and Gillespie[103] were able to demonstrate that exogenous histamine could inhibit the IgE-dependent release of histamine from leucocyte preparations and that this effect was mediated by H_2-receptors. Subsequently, Dunlop et al.[104] showed that histamine- and antigen-induced bronchoconstriction of sensitized human bronchial strips could be inhibited by H_1-antagonists and enhanced by H_2-antagonists. Clinical studies of H_2-antagonists of asthma provided conflicting results. Whilst some claim that cimetidine increased bronchial responsiveness to histamine,[105,106] many were unable to show any effect.[107–109] Eiser et al. reported a small reduction in the airway responsiveness to inhaled histamine and allergen following cimetidine 400 mg administered intravenously,[110] while Leopold et al. found that the H_2-antagonist exerted no effect on exercise-induced asthma.[111] It seems reasonable to conclude from these studies that H_2-receptor-mediated effects of histamine have little part to play in the pathogenesis of asthma.

H_3-receptors

Most recently a new class of receptors for histamine has been described and designated H_3. Arrang et al.[112] reported that histamine acts via H_3-receptors in the brain to inhibit the release of further histamine. In guinea-pig airways these receptors have been localized to nerve endings and probably serve to downregulate neurotransmitter release.[113]

Ketotifen

Ketotifen is an orally active benzocycloheptathiophine derivative which, amongst its other properties, acts as a non-competitive antagonist of histamine at H_1-receptors[114] and appears to have an inhibitory effect on mast cells akin to that of SCG.[115] In vitro studies using guinea-pig trachea and human bronchus have shown weak inhibition of constriction induced by histamine and acetylcholine.[116] However, studies in vivo using anaesthetized guinea-pigs have demonstrated that intravenous ketotifen can inhibit histamine-induced bronchoconstriction with a potency considerably greater than that of the antihistamine clemastine.[114] Ketotifen inhibits histamine release from rat peritoneal mast cells when the stimulus used is compound 48/80 but not following antigen.[117] However, when human basophils are challenged with rabbit anti-IgE (reversed anaphylaxis) or calcium ionophore (A23187), ketotifen inhibits the release of histamine and slow-reacting substance of anaphylaxis (SRS-A, sulphidopeptide leukotrienes).[118] Using human lung fragments, Ross et al.[119] found effective inhibition of SRS-A release with relatively poor inhibition of histamine release. Like many H_1-antihistamines, ketotifen exhibits weak antiserotonin activity, but this is only seen at concentrations 100 times higher than those showing an antihistaminic effect. Calcium uptake is involved in the release of mediators from mast cells and in smooth muscle contraction. Recent studies have shown that ketotifen inhibits calcium uptake by both mast cells [117] and smooth muscle,[120] and this action may further contribute to its inhibitory action on excitation and contraction coupling.

Clinical studies have demonstrated inhibitory activity of ketotifen when administered orally or by inhalation against single challenges using histamine or allergen.[121] However, there is some doubt over whether ketotifen's effect on allergen provocation extends beyond its H_1-blocking effect. It appears to have inconsistent effects inhibiting exercise-induced bronchoconstriction,[122–125] and is ineffective against bronchoconstriction provoked by inhaled acetylcholine. Morgan et al.[126] noted that while inhaled ketotifen (0.5 mg), SCG (20 mg) and clemastine (0.5 mg) all inhibit allergen-induced broncho-constriction, none of the drugs influenced the associated increase in serum levels of neutrophil chemotactic activity (NCA), which would suggest that simple inhibition of mast-cell derived mediators is not the major mechanism underlying its pharmacological action with allergen challenge.

It has been suggested that many of the actions of ketotifen might be explained by its inhibitory effect against PAF, acetylglyceryletherphosphorylcholine.[127] PAF is an ether-linked phospholipid which is liberated from eosinophils,[128] macrophages[129] and platelets[130] in response to allergen and other forms of cell perturbation. When administered intravenously or by inhalation, PAF produces bronchoconstriction both in animals[131,132] and in man.[133] PAF can also give rise to the other features of the inflammatory airway response seen following allergen challenge, since it increases vascular permeability,[134] promotes accumulation of platelets[135] and stimulates the selective chemotactic migration of eosinophils into the airways.[136] As with bronchoconstriction provoked by inhaled allergen in asthma, inhalation of PAF, at least in non-asthmatic subjects, results in a small increase in bronchial responsiveness to methacholine challenge (an index of increased non-specific bronchial responsiveness) that may persist for several weeks.[137] This effect has proven variable and difficult to reproduce in humans. Ketotifen has been shown to inhibit PAF-induced bronchoconstriction and subsequent hyperresponsiveness in guinea-pigs.[138] In man, ketotifen failed to inhibit PAF-induced bronchoconstriction or increased airway responsiveness but significantly attenuated the skin wheal and flare response to intradermal PAF probably by inhibiting PAF-induced histamine release.[136]

Several long-term clinical studies have been carried out with ketotifen, usually using an oral dose of 1 mg twice daily. In a 6-month parallel group study and a 3-month crossover study with SCG, ketotifen gave only subjective symptomatic improvement.[140] Craps et al.[121] reported a 12-month trial of ketotifen 1 mg twice daily in 29 patients in whom there was a significant improvement in objective measures of airway calibre in addition to subjective improvement. However this trial did not include a control group. Tinkleman et al.[141] conducted a double-blind placebo-controlled trial of ketotifen given during the pollen season. Although the placebo group showed a gradual decline in FEV_1 during the season and the ketotifen group did not, this change failed to reach statistical significance. A similar parallel group study in children resulted in a significant reduction in the number of asthma attacks and the use of concomitant medication.[142] However, other long-term trials in children have failed to show a convincing therapeutic effect in asthma.[143] Lane has demonstrated that the addition of ketotifen to the treatment of corticosteroid-dependent asthmatic patients results in a significant reduction in their corticosteroid requirement, daily prednisolone doses falling from 8.8 to 4.4 mg in the ketotifen group compared to a fall from 7.9 to 6.2 mg in the placebo group.[144] In many studies the beneficial effects of ketotifen only become apparent 6–12 weeks after starting treatment, whereas in challenge studies it has an immediate protective effect. An explanation for this finding has been offered,[145] which is that ketotifen inhibits allergen-induced bronchoconstriction, the late reaction and consequent hyperresponsiveness, these inhibitory effects only become apparent once the existing pathology has regressed over several months as seen following allergen avoidance.

In common with many of the earlier antihistamines, the most common side-effect reported with ketotifen is drowsiness, this being found in up to 23% of patients. This symptom is often short-lived in resolving after 1–2 weeks of therapy. There have been occasional reports of thrombocytopaenia in diabetic patients taking ketotifen and oral hypoglycaemic agents, and therefore ketotifen should not be prescribed to patients in this category.

CYCLOOXYGENASE INHIBITORS

Mast-cell activation results not only in the release of preformed mediators but in the production of newly generated mediators formed as a result of metabolism of arachidonic acid. When this is metabolized along the cyclooxygenase pathway, the main product in man appears to be prostaglandin $(PG)D_2$, a bronchoconstrictor and vasodilator, which in molar terms is 30 times more potent than histamine in causing airway narrowing.[146] Other cyclooxygenases products include thromboxane A_2 (TxA_2) and $PGF_{2\alpha}$, both of which produce bronchoconstriction and also may enhance airway hyperresponsiveness, and PGE_2 and prostacyclin (PGI_2), both of which are bronchodilators and functional antagonists. On the basis of this, it might be expected that cyclooxygenase inhibitors may have a potential role in the treatment of asthma by inhibiting the production of pro-inflammatory bronchoconstrictor prostanoids. However, complex interactions appear to occur between the prostanoids and other mediators, and clinical trials of cyclooxygenase inhibitors in asthma have produced variable results. Dunlop and Smith[147] demonstrated that allergen-induced contraction of the human bronchus was associated with the release of $PGF_{2\alpha}$, and that both $PGF_{2\alpha}$ release and the bronchoconstriction could be reduced by indomethacin. Peters et al.[148] have also shown that indomethacin inhibits anti-IgE-and ionophore A23187-induced release of PGD_2 while having little effect on release of histamine. Adams and Lichtenstein[149] found that indomethacin enhanced both the early reaction to allergen challenge (Schultz–Dale reaction) in human bronchus in vitro and histamine release. Marone et al.[150] reported that PGE_2 inhibited allergen-induced histamine release from basophils but this effect was reversed by indomethacin. Adcock et al.[151] found similar results using chopped human lung cells stimulated with calcium ionophore, suggesting that PGE_2 acts as a negative feedback mechanism for further histamine release from mast cells.

Walters et al.[152] noted that $PGF_{2\alpha}$ increased airway responsiveness to inhaled histamine and found that this response could be reduced in asthmatics but not in normal subjects following the administration of indomethacin orally in a dose of 50 mg four times daily. Studies of the effects of cyclooxygenase inhibition on allergen-induced bronchoconstriction have produced varying results. Smith[153] was unable to show any effect against allergen- or exercise-induced bronchoconstriction after indomethacin

200 mg daily for 1 week. Shepherd et al.[154] documented inhibition of the late reaction to allergen following 4 days treatment with indomethacin, but this had no effect on the early reaction. Similarly, Fairfax et al.[155] and Joubert et al.[156] inhibited the late response with indomethacin but only partially reduced the early reaction in some of their patients.

Some of the variations encountered in these clinical studies may be due to differing degrees of cyclooxygenase inhibition achieved at the level of the bronchial mucosa. We have studied the effects of flurbiprofen (which is 13 times more potent than indomethacin and approximately 5000 times more potent than aspirin) on the inhibition of the cyclooxygenase enzyme system in a number of in vitro systems.[157] In asthmatic subjects, flurbiprofen 50 mg three times daily for 3 days reduced airway responsiveness to histamine, displacing the concentration-dose–response curves three-fold to the right, but did not affect responsiveness to methacholine challenge.[158] In atopic non-asthmatic subjects, the early phase of allergen-induced bronchoconstriction was inhibited by 30% by the same dose of flurbiprofen. Interpretation of the effects of cyclooxygenase inhibitors is made more difficult by the mediator interactions that occur. Thus it might be argued that the effects of cylooxygenase inhibitors may be to reduce contraction of the airway smooth muscle by inhibiting the production of bronchoconstrictor prostanoids PGD_2 and $PGF_{2\alpha}$. However, as a consequence, this treatment might also reduce the production of the antibronchoconstrictor and mast-cell inhibiting prostanoids PGE_2[159] and PGI_2. An alternative explanation is that blockade of the cyclooxygenase pathway may lead to increased metabolism of arachidonic acid along the lipoxygenase pathway, producing increased amounts of the bronchoconstrictor leukotrienes C_4, D_4 and E_4. The development of specific prostaglandin and leukotriene antagonists is helping to clarify the extent of these interactions.

In clinical practice, asthmatics vary in their responses to cyclooxygenase inhibitors. Although the majority are unaffected by aspirin and similar drugs, a small percentage develop severe bronchoconstriction,[160] and fewer still demonstrate a bronchodilating response to these drugs.[161] Szczeklik et al.[162] offer an explanation of these reactions based on a balance of prostanoid concentration present in the airways. Thus in those patients who bronchoconstrict to aspirin, they suggest that the bronchodilatory prostaglandins PEG_2 and PGI_2 are predominant in the airways prior to drug therapy, and that these bronchodilator prostaglandins are removed when the cyclooxygenase pathway is inhibited. However, in those patients who bronchodilate following aspirin, they consider the predominant prostaglandins prior to therapy to have been bronchoconstrictor PGD_2 and $PGF_{2\alpha}$ and thus their influence is diminished by cyclooxygenase inhibition. Diversion of arachidonic acid from the cyclooxygenase along the lipoxygenase pathways to the highly potent contractile mediators LTC_4, LTD_4 and LTE_4, and to the chemotactic factor LTB_4, is an alternative explanation for asthma provoked by cyclooxygenase inhibitors such as aspirin.

LEUKOTRIENE SYNTHESIS INHIBITORS

The leukotrienes are amongst the most potent inflammatory mediators so far described in man. When studied in vitro, LTC_4 and LTD_4 are approximately 1000 times more potent as contractile agonists of human airways than is histamine.[163] Other actions of the sulphidopeptide leukotrienes include increasing vascular permeability[164] and stimulation of mucus secretion.[165] Leukotriene B_4 is known to be a potent chemotactic agent for both neutrophils and eosinophils,[166] and together with PAF may be involved in the development of the last asthmatic reaction and the associated increase in airway responsiveness through the selective recruitment and activation of neutrophils and eosinophils. Thus, drugs with the potential of inhibiting the formation of these agents might prove beneficial in the treatment of asthma.

Piriprost (6,9-diepoxy-6,9-phenylamino-6,8-prostaglandin I_1) is an analogue of PGI_1 and has been found to inhibit leukotriene production by rat peritoneal mononuclear cells,[167] asthmatic lung fragments[168] and dispersed cells,[169] neutrophils[170] and eosinophils.[171] Studies *in vivo* have shown that inhaled piriprost inhibits immediate allergen-induced bronchoconstriction in rhesus monkeys[172] and guinea-pigs.[173] In asthmatic subjects challenged with inhaled allergen, piriprost, 1 mg by inhalation, did not significantly alter either the early or late responses seen.[174]

Sch 37224 is a lipoxygenase inhibitor that has been shown to inhibit the release of LTD_4 and Thromboxane B_2 from anaphylactic guinea-pig lung.[175] It has been found to inhibit LTD_4—and hyperventilation-induced bronchoconstriction in the guinea-pig.[175] In allergic sheep, Sch 37224 has reduced the immediate and late bronchoconstrictor response following allergen challenge and prevented the development of increased airway responsiveness.[176] Recently two studies[177,178] have shown that the 5-lipoxygenase inhibitor A 64077 inhibits the production of LTB_4 without affecting prostaglandin production or thromboxane B_2 synthesis and is effective in reducing the bronchoconstrictor response to cold air as well as the nasal congestion produced by local allergen challenge.

AMOXINOX

Amoxinox (AA-673-2-amino-7-isopropyl-5-oxo-5H(1)-benzylpyrano (2,3-B)pyridine-3-carboxylic acid) is another novel anti-allergic agent that has been shown to inhibit mast-cell mediator release *in vitro*[179] and also to inhibit LTD_4 and PAF-induced bronchoconstriction in guinea-pigs and rats.[180] *In vitro*, amoxinox has been found to prevent calcium ionophore A23187-induced formation of 5-HETE, LTB_4 LTC_4, LTD_4 and 12-HETE in rat peritoneal monocytes without affecting the formation of TxB_2 and 6-keto PGF_1(hydrolysis products of TxA_2 and PGI_2 respectively) in guinea-pig lung, or $PGE_{2\alpha}$ in bovine seminal vesicles, suggesting that it does not inhibit cyclooxygenation of arachidonic acid, but inhibits the lipoxygenase pathway.

LEUKOTRIENE ANTAGONISTS

During the last 5 years a number of leukotriene antagonists have become available. ICI 198 615 has been shown to inhibit LTD_4- and C_4-induced bronchoconstriction in the guinea-pig and reduced antigen-induced contacts of guinea-pig trachea by 45%.[181,182]

In an allergic sheep model WY-48252 was shown to inhibit both the early and late response to inhaled allergen.[183] Two LTD_4/E_4 antagonists have been investigated clinically in man, L-649,923 (Merk Sharp and Dohme) and LY 171883 (Eli Lilly). When administered orally in single doses, L-649,923 displaced LTD_4 concentration–response curves to the right by 3–4-fold[184] and had a minimal inhibitory effect on the later aspects of the early allergen-provoked response in the airways.[185] Unfortunately, this compound caused appreciable gastrointestinal upset. LY 171883 appears to be a more potent LTD_4-antagonist in producing up to 30-fold dose-related displacement of bronchoconstrictor LTD_4 concentration–response curves to the right.[186] In atopic subjects LY 171883 in a dose of 400 mg had no effect on baseline lung function but partially inhibited the early response to inhaled allergen without affecting the late response.[187] At a dose of 600 mg twice daily this compound was found to have a minor effect in preventing cold-air induced bronchoconstriction[188] but over a period of 6 weeks it has been shown to be efficacious in asthma with improvement in symptoms and reduction in bronchodilator usage.[189] This represents an exciting breakthrough and, providing that specificity can be shown for this drug, it provides the first real evidence that sulphido-peptide leukotrienes are involved in asthma pathogenesis. Recently a more potent LTD_4 antagonist, ICI 204,219 has been shown to displace the dose response curve to inhaled LTD_4 by a factor of 117 at 2 h after oral ingests of 40 mg.[190] Recently the LTD_4-receptor antagonist MK 571 has been found to inhibit exercise-induced asthma reducing the maximum fall in FEV_1 by 69%.[191]

PAF ANTAGONIST

In recent years a great deal of interest has surrounded PAF, and its role in asthma, since it has been shown to act as a potent bronchoconstrictor,[133] to increase permeability,[134] to be a chemoattractant for eosinophils, and also to induce airway hyperresponsiveness.[136] The ginkgolides are a class of PAF antagonists that have been isolated from the leaves of a Chinese tree (Ginkgo biloba). An extract from this tree has been used in China for chest complaints for several centuries. Ginkgolide B(BN52021) is the most potent PAF-acether antagonist found in this class, and both in vitro and in vivo studies in animals have shown it to inhibit all the known pharmacological actions of PAF.[192] This has also been demonstrated to reduce allergen-induced bronchoconstriction and airway responsiveness in rabbits[193] and in guinea-pigs to inhibit the eosinophil accumulation and airway hyperresponsiveness following PAF or allergen inhalation.[194] Chung et al. have now shown that a mixture of ginkgolides A, B and C (BN52063) inhibits PAF-induced skin wheal and flare response and platelet aggregation in man.[195] In response to intradermal allergen BN 52063 had no effect on the early wheal and flare response but inhibited the late cutaneous reaction.[196] Interestingly Tomioka et al. using the PAF antagonists YM 461 in allergic sheep, found that although there was no significant effect upon the early bronchoconstriction following allergen inhalation, the late reaction and airway hyperresponsiveness were both reduced.[196]

Extensive investigations have now been reported on WEB 2086. In both in vitro studies and in animal models it has been shown to inhibit PAF- and allergen-induced bronchoconstriction and prevent the increase in airway responsiveness.[198,199] The allergen-induced neutrophilia observed in BAL fluid following challenge was also inhibited by WEB 2086 in an allergic sheep model.[200] A number of other compounds have shown activity as PAF antagonists *in vitro* or in animal studies and these include CV 3988, SDZ 64-412, RO 19-3704 and L-652-731.[201–205]

In normal subjects both BN 52063[206] and WEB 2086[207] have been shown to inhibit PAF-induced bronchoconstriction. If these compounds produce a similar inhibitory effect on the late reaction within the airways as that observed in the skin this may represent a significant form of asthma therapy.

PROSPECTS FOR THE FUTURE

There continue to be a great many drugs under investigation that are of therapeutic potential in the field of asthma. Some of the preliminary results with leukotriene and PAF antagonists have been quite encouraging and it is to be hoped that the 'next generation' of inhibitors of the lipoxygenase pathway and combined inhibitors of both the lipoxygenase and cyclooxygenase pathways will be well tolerated in man permitting further exploration of this area of mediator production. Much attention is being turned to the interaction between cells in the inflammatory process of asthma with particular emphasis on cytokines. With the recognition that interleukins (IL-3, IL-4, IL-5, IL-9, IL-10) and GM-CSF are involved in the isotype switching of IgE (IL-4), mast-cell growth and priming (IL-4, IL-9, IL-10) and eosinophil proliferation and maturation (IL-3, IL-4, IL-5, GM-CSF) pharmacological agents that specifically target these activities will be of considerable interest. Drugs with the ability to antagonize selectively the chemical messengers promoting cell activation may play a useful role.

REFERENCES

1. Ishizaka T: Analysis of triggering events in mast cell for immunoglobulin E-mediated histamine release. *J Allergy Clin Immunol* (1981) **67**: 90–96.
2. Capron A, Dessaint, JP: From protective immunity to allergy: the cellular partners of IgE. *Chem Immunol* (1990) **49**: 236–240.
3. Church MK, Young KD: The characteristics of inhibition of histamine release from human lung fragments by sodium cromoglycate, salbutamol and chlorpromazine. *Br J Pharmacol* (1983) **78**: 671–679.
4. Cushley MK, Tattersfield AE, Holgate ST: Adenosine-induced bronchoconstriction in asthma: Antagonism by inhaled theophylline. *Am Rev Resp Dis* (1984) **129**: 380–384.
5. Pauwels R, Van Renterghern D, Van der Straeten M, Johannesson N, Persson CGA: The effect of theophylline and enprofylline on allergen-induced bronchoconstriction. *J Allergy Clin Immunol* (1985) **76**: 583–590.
6. Blackwell GJ, Carnuccio R, Di Rosa M, *et al.*: Macrocortin: a polypeptide causing the antiphospholipase effect of glucocorticoids. *Nature* (1980) **287**: 147–149.
7. Cox JSC: Disodium cromoglycate (FLP 670) (Intal): A specific inhibitor of reaginic antibody-antigen mechanisms. *Nature* (1967) **216**: 1328.
8. Flint KC, Leung KBP, Pearce FL, Hudspith EN, Brostoff J, Johnson NMcI: Human mast cells recovered by bronchoalveolar lavage: their morphology, histamine release and the effects of sodium cromoglycate. *Clin Sci* (1985) **68**: 427–432.

9. Atkins PC, Norman ME, Zweiman B: Antigen-induced neutrophil chemotactic activity in man: Correlation with bronchospasm and inhibition by disodium cromoglycate. *J Allergy Clin Immunol* (1978) **52**: 149–155.

10. Lee TH, Nagakura T, Papageorgiou N, Cromwell O, Iikura Y, Kay AB: Mediators in exercise-induced asthma. *J Allergy Clin Immunol* (1984) **73**: 634–639.

11. Bierman CW: A comparison of late reactions to antigen and exercise. *J Allergy Clin Immunol* (1984) **73**: 654–659.

12. Breslin FJ, McFadden ER, Ingram RJ: The effect of cromolyn sodium on the airway response to hyperpnoea and cold air in asthma. *Am Rev Resp Dis* (1980) **122**: 11–16.

13. Altounyan REC: Review of clinical activity and mode of action of sodium cromoglycate. *Clin Allergy* (1980) **10**(Suppl): 481–489.

14. Twentyman OP, Finnerty JP, Holgate ST: Salbutamol inhibits the allergen-induced late asthmatic reaction and increase in responsiveness. *Clin Exp Allergy* (1990) **20**(Suppl 1): 94.

15. Butcher BT: Inhalation challenge and pharmacological studies of toluene di-isocyanate (TDI) sensitive workers. *J Allergy Clin Immunol* (1979) **64**: 146–152.

16. Brompton Hospital/Medical Research Council Collaborative Trial: Long-term study of disodium cromoglycate in treatment of severe extrinsic or intrinsic bronchial asthma in adults. *Br Med J* (1972) **4**: 383–388.

17. Dixon M, Jackson DM, Richards IM: The action of cromoglycate on 'C' fibre endings in the dog lung. *Br J Pharmacol* (1980) **70**: 11–13.

18. Harries MG, Parkes PEG, Lessof MH: Role of bronchial irritant receptors in asthma. *Lancet* (1981) **1**: 5.

19. Abraham WM, Sielezut MW, Pearruchoud AP, *et al.*: The role of airway inflammation and mediators in late phase allergic bronchial obstruction, *Am Rev Resp Dis* (1984) **129/4**: 4.

20. Cockcroft DW, Ruffin RE, Dolovich J, Hargreave FE: Allergen-induced increase in non-allergic bronchial reactivity. *Clin Allergy* (1977) **7**: 503–513.

21. Cockcroft DW, Murdoch KY: Protective effect of inhaled albuterol, cromolyn, beclomethasone and placebo on allergen-induced early asthmatic response (EAR), late asthmatic response (LAR) and allergen-induced increase in bronchial responsiveness to inhaled histamine. *J Allergy Clin Immunol* (1986) **77**(Suppl): 122.

22. Godfrey S, Balfour-Lynn L, Keonig P: The place of cromolyn sodium in the long term management of childhood asthma based on a 3–5 year follow-up. *J Pediatr* (1975) **87**: 465–473.

23. Petty TL, Rollins DR, Christopher K, Good JT, Oakley R: Cromolyn sodium is effective in adult chronic asthmatics. *Am Rev Resp Dis* (1989) **139**: 694–701.

24. Moqbel R, Walsh GM, MacDonald AJ, Kay AB: Effect of disodium cromoglycate on activation of human eosinophils and neutrophils following reversed (anti-IgE) anaphylaxis. *Clin Allergy* (1986) **16**: 73–83.

25. Richerson HB, Walsh OM, Walport MJ, Moqbel R, Kay AB: Enhancement of human neutrophil complement receptors: a comparison of the rosette technique with the uptake of radiolabelled anti CRI monoclonal antibody. *Clin Exp Immunol* (1985) **62**: 442–448.

26. Basran JS, Page CP, Paul W, Morley J: Cromoglycate (DSCG) inhibits response to platelet activating factor (PAF-acether) in man: an alternative mode of action for DSCG in asthma? *Eur J Pharmacol* (1983) **86**: 143–144.

27. Eady RP: The pharmacology of nedocromil sodium. *Eur J Respir Dis* (1986) **69**(Suppl 147): 112–119.

28. Richards IM, Eady RP, Jackson DM, *et al.*: Ascaris-induced bronchoconstriction in primates experimentally infected with *Ascaris suum* ova. *Clin Exp Immunol* (1983) **54**: 461–468.

29. Eady RP, Greenwood B, Jackson DM, Orr TSC, Wells E: The effect of nedocromil sodium and sodium cromoglycate on antigen-induced bronchoconstriction in the ascaris sensitive monkey. *Br J Pharmacol* (1985) **85**: 322–325.

30. Crimi E, Brusasco V, Crimi P: Effect of nedocromil sodium on the late asthmatic reaction to bronchial antigen challenge. *J Allergy Clin Immunol* (1989) **83**: 985–990.

31. Dorward AJ, Roberts JA, Thomson NC: Effect of nedocromil sodium on histamine airway responsiveness in grass-pollen sensitive asthmatics during the pollen season. *Clin Allergy* (1986) **16**: 309–317.

32. Roberts JA, Thomson NC: Attenuation of exercise induced asthma by pretreatment with nedocromil sodium and minocromil. *Clin Allergy* (1985) **15**: 377–381.
33. Shaw RJ, Kay AB: Nedocromil, a mucosal and connective tissue mast cell stabilizer inhibits exercise induced asthma. *Br J Dis Chest* (1985) **79**: 385–389.
34. Cushley MJ, Tattersfield AE, Holgate ST: Adenosine antagonism as an alternative mechanism of action of methylxanthines in asthma. *Agents Actions* (1983) **13**(Suppl): 109–131.
35. Marquardt DL, Walker LL, Wasserman SJ: Adenosine receptors on mouse bone marrow-derived mast cells. Functional significance and regulation by aminophylline. *J Immunol* (1984) **133**(2): 932–937.
36. Altounyan REC, Lee TB, Rocchiccioli KMS, Shaw CL: A comparison of the inhibitory effects of nedocromil sodium and sodium cromoglycate on adenosine monophosphate induced bronchoconstriction in atopic subjects. *Eur J Resp Dis* (1986) **69**(Suppl 147): 277–279.
37. Altounyan REC, Cole M, Lee TB: Inhibition of sulphur dioxide induced bronchoconstriction by nedocromil sodium in non-asthmatic atopic subjects. *Ann Allergy* (1985) **55**: 689.
38. Soler M, Manour E, Fernandez A, D'Brot S, Ahmed T, Abraham WM: PAF-induced airway responses in sheep, effects of a PAF antagonist and nedocromil sodium. *J Allergy Clin Immunol* (1990) **85**: 661–668.
39. Holgate ST: Clinical evaluation of nedocromil sodium in asthma. *Eur J Resp Dis* (1986) **69**(Suppl): 149–159.
40. Svendsen UG, Frolund L, Madsen F, Nielsen NH: A comparison of the effects of nedocromil sodium and beclomethasone dipropriate on pulmonary functions, symptoms and bronchial responsiveness in patients with asthma. *J Allergy Clin Immunol* (1989) **84**: 224–237.
41. Goldin JG, Bateman EA: Does nedocromil sodium have a steroid sparing effect in adult asthmatic patients requiring maintenance oral corticosteroids. *Thorax* (1988) **43**: 982–986.
42. Dale HH, Laidlaw PP: Histamine shock. *J Physiol* (1919) **52**: 355.
43. Weis S, Robb GP, Blumgart HL: The velocity of blood flow in health and disease as measured by the effect of histamine on the minute vessels. *Am Heart J* (1928) **4**: 664–691.
44. Randolph TG, Rackemann FM: The blood histamine level in asthma and in eosinophilia. *J Allergy* (1941) **12**: 450–456.
45. De Cara PF: Chemical determination of histamine in blood in health and disease. *J Allergy* (1951) **22**: 429–437.
46. Gravelyn TR, Pan PM, Eschenbacher WL: Mediator release in air isolates airway segment in subjects with asthma. *Am Rev Resp Dis* (1988) **137**: 641–646.
47. Wenzel SE, Fowler III AA, Schwartz LB: Activation of pulmonary mast cells by bronchoalveolar allergen challenge: *in vivo* release of histamine + lyphase in atopic subjects with and without asthma. *Am Rev Resp Dis* (1988) **137**: 1002–1008.
48. Boe J, Boe MA, Simmonsson BG: A dual action of histamine on isolated human pulmonary arteries. *Respiration* (1980) **40**: 117–122.
49. Propst K, Millen JE, Clauser FL: The effects of endogenous and exogenous histamine on pulmonary alveolar membrane permeability. *Am Rev Resp Dis* (1978) **117**: 1063–1068.
50. Seliomann BE, Fletcher MP, Gallin JI: Histamine modulation of human neutrophil oxidative metabolism, locomotion, degranulation and membrane potential changes. *J Immunol* (1983) **130**: 1902–1909.
51. Karlin JM: The use of antihistamines in asthma. *Ann Allergy* (1972) **30**: 342–347.
52. Herxheimer H: Antihistamines in bronchial asthma. *Br Med J* (1949) **2**: 901–905.
53. Schild HO, Hawkins DF, Mongar JL, Herxheimer H: Reactions of isolated human asthmatic lung and bronchial tissue to a specific antigen histamine release and muscular contraction. *Lancet* (1951) **1**: 376–382.
54. Booij-Noord H, Orie NGM, Berg W, De Vries K: Protection tests on bronchial allergen challenge with disodium cromoglycate and thiazinium. *J Allergy* (1970) **46**: 1–11.
55. Popa VT: Bronchodilating activity on an H_1 blocker, chlorpheniramine. *J Allergy Clin Immunol* (1977) **59**: 54–63.
56. Norgrady SG, Bevan C: Inhaled antihistamines—bronchodilation and effects on histamine and methacholine-induced bronchoconstriction. *Thorax* (1978) **33**: 700–704.

57. Norgrady SG, Hartley JPR, Handslip PDJ, Hurst NP: Bronchodilation after inhalation of the antihistamine clemastine. *Thorax* (1978) **33**: 479–482.

58. Curry JJ: The effect of antihistamine substances and other drugs on histamine bronchoconstriction in asthmatic subjects. *J Clin Invest* (1946) **25**: 792–799.

59. Casterline CL, Evans R: Further studies on the mechanism of human histamine-induced asthma: the effect of an aerosolized H_1 receptor antagonist (Diphenhydramine). *J Allergy Clin Immunol* (1977) **59**: 420–424.

60. Popa VT: Effects of an H_1 blocker, chlorpheniramine, on inhalation tests with histamine and allergen in allergic asthma. *Chest* (1980) **78** (3): 442–451.

61. Phillips MJ, Ollier S, Gould CAL, Davies RJ: Effect of antihistamines and antiallergic drugs on responses to allergen and histamine provocation tests in asthma. *Thorax* (1984) **39**: 345–351.

62. Hartley JPR, Norgrady SG: Effect of an inhaled antihistamine on exercise-induced asthma. *Thorax* (1980) **35**: 675–679.

63. Nicholson AN, Stone B: Performance studies with the H_1-histamine receptor antagonists, astemizole and terfenadine. *Br J Clin Pharmacol* (1982) **13**: 199–202.

64. Howarth PH, Holgate ST: Astemizole, an H_1-antagonist in allergic asthma. *J Allergy Clin Immunol* (1985) **75**: 166.

65. Howarth PH, Holgate ST: Comparative trial of two non-sedative H_1 antihistamines, terfenadine and astemizole, for hay fever. *Thorax* (1984) **39**: 668–672.

66. Foster TS, Batenhorst RL: Pharmacokinetic and pharmacodynamic investigation of terfenadine. *J Allergy Clin Immunol* (1985) **75**: 168.

67. Rafferty P, Holgate ST: Terfenadine is a potent selective histamine H_1-receptor antagonist in asthmatic airways. *Am Rev Resp Dis* (1987) **135**: 181–184.

68. Patel KR: Effect of terfenadine on methacholine-induced bronchoconstriction in asthma. *J Allergy Clin Immunol* (1987) **79**: 355–358.

69. Rafferty P, Beasley CR, Holgate ST: The contribution of histamine to bronchoconstriction produced by inhaled allergen and adenosine 5' monophosphate in asthma. *Am Rev Resp Dis* (1987) **136**: 369–373.

70. Weibicke W, Paynter A, Montgomery M, Chjernick V, Pasterkamp H: Effect of terfenadine on the response to exercise and cold air in asthma. *Paediatr Pulmonol* (1988) **4** (4): 255–229.

71. Bewtra AK, Hopp RJ, Nair NM, Townley RG: Effect of terfenadine on cold air induced bronchospasm. *Ann Allergy* (1989) **52**(4): 298–301.

72. Finnerty J, Milmot C, Holgate ST: Inhibition of hypertonic saline-induced bronchoconstriction by terfenadine and flurbiprofen: Endemic for the predominant role of histamine. *Am Rev Resp Dis* (1989) **140**: 593–7.

73. Nabe M, Agmawal DK, Miyagawa H, Townley RG: Histamine and LTC_4 release inhibitor by terfenadine. *Am Rev Resp Dis* (1989) **1239**: 4 A63.

74. Zechel HJ, Brock N, Lenke D, Achterrath-Tuckerman U: Pharmacologic and toxicological properties of azelastine, a novel antiallergic agent. *Arzneim Forsch* (1981) **31**: 1184.

75. Katayama S, Akimoto N, Shionoya H, Morimoto T, Katoh Y: Antiallergic effect of azelastine hydrochloride on immediate type hypersensitivity reactions *in vivo* and *in vitro*. *Arzneim Forsch* (1981) **31**: 1196.

76. Fields DAS, Pillar J, Diamantis W, Perhach JL, Sofia RD, Chand N: Inhibition by azelastine of non-allergic histamine release from rat peritoneal mast cells. *J Allergy Clin Immunol* (1984) **73**: 400–403.

77. Diamantis W, Chand N, Harrison JE, Pillar J, Perhach JL, Sofia RD: Inhibition of release of SRS-A and its antagonists by azelastine, and H_1 antagonist antiallergic agent. *Pharmacologist* (1982) **24**: 200.

78. Diamantis W, Pillar J, Natarajan V, Chand N, Sofia RD: Inhibition of IgE mediated allergic histamine release by azelastine from rabbit basophils. *Fed Proc* (1984) **43/3**: 614A.

79. Little MM, Casale TB: Azelastine inhibits both human lung and basophil degranulation. *J Allergy Clin Immunol* (1987) **79** (1): 204.

80. Chand N, Nolan K, Diamantis W, Perhach JL, Sofia RD: Inhibition of leukotriene (SRS-A) mediated allergic bronchospasm by azelastine, a novel orally effective anti-asthmatic drug. *J Allergy Clin Immunol* (1983) **71**: 149.

81. Lai CKW, Lau CK, Ollier S, Aurich R, Holgate ST: Bronchial and skin responses to platelet activating factor (PAF) in man: effect of azelastine and ketotifen. *Clin Exp Allergy* (1990) **20** (Suppl 1): 96.

82. Tanigawa T, Honda M, Miura K: Effect of azelastine hydrochloride on vascular permeability in hypersensitivity reaction skin site in guinea pig. *Arzneim Forsch* (1981) **31**: 1212–1215.

83. Honda M, Miura K, Tanigawa T: Effect of azelastine hydrochloride on macrophage chemotaxis and phagocytosis *in vitro*. *Allergy* (1982) **37**: 41–47.

84. Ollier S, Gould CAL, Davies RJ: The effect of single and multiple dose therapy with azelastine on the immediate asthmatic response to allergen provocation testing. *J Allergy Clin Immunol* (1986) **78**: 358–364.

85. Magnussen H, Reuss G, Jorres R, Aurich R: The effect of azelastine on exercise induced asthma. *Chest* (1988) **93**: (5) 937–940.

86. Patel KR: Terfenadine in exercise-induced asthma. *Br Med J* (1984) **288**: 1496–1497.

87. Rafferty P, Harrison P, Aurich R, Holgate ST: The *in vivo* potency and selectivity of azelastine as an H_1 histamine receptor antagonist in human airways and skin. *J Allergy Clin Immunol* (1988) **6**: 1113–1118.

88. Ghosh SK, McIlroy I, Patel KR: Effect of cetirizine on histamine and LTD_4 induced bronchoconstriction in mild atopic asthmatics. *Thorax* (1989) **44**: 851.

89. Finnerty JP, Holgate ST, Rihoux JP: The effect of 2 weeks' treatment with cetirizine on bronchial reactivity to methacholine in asthma. *Br J Clin Pharmacol* (1990) **29**: 79–84.

90. Fadel R, Herpin-Richard N, Rihoux JP, Henocq E: Inhibitory effect of cetirizine dihydrochloride on eosinophil migration *in vivo*. *Clin Allergy* (1987) **17**: 373–379.

91. Charlesworth EN, Kagey-Sobotka A, Norman PS, Lichtenstein LM: Effect of cetirizine on mast cell mediator release and cellular traffic during the cutaneous late phase response (LPR) *J Allergy Clin Immunol* (1989) **83**: 905–912.

92. Michel L, De Vos C, Rihoux JP, Burtin C, Benveniste J, Dubertret L: Inhibitory effect of oral cetirizine on *in vivo* antigen induced histamine and PAF-acether release and eosinophil recruitment in human skin. *J Allergy Clin Immunol* (1988) **82**: 101–109.

93. Gong H, Tashkin DP, Dauphinee B, Djahed B, Wu TC: Effects of oral cetirizine, a selective H_1 antagonist, an allergen and exercise induced bronchoconstriction in subjects with asthma. *J Allergy Clin Immunol* (1990) **85**(3): 532–541.

94. Temple DM, McCluskey M: Loratidine, an antihistamine, blocks antigen- and inophores-induced leukotriene release from human lung *in vitro*. *Prostaglandins* (1988) **35**: 549–554.

95. Daniels C, Temple DM: The inhibition by azatedine of the immunological release of leukotrienes and histamine from human lung fragments. *Eur J Pharmac* (1986) **123**: 463–467.

96. Taytard A, Beaumont D, Pujet JC, Sapere M, Lewis PS: Treatment of bronchial asthma with terfenadine. A randomised controlled trial. *Br J Clin Pharmacol* (1987) **24**: 743–746.

97. Rafferty P, Jackson L, Smith R, Holgate ST: Terfenadine, a potent histamine H_1 receptor antagonist in the treatment of grass pollen sensitive asthma. *Br J Clin Pharmac* (1990) **30**: 229–235.

98. Storms W, Middleton E, Dvorin D, *et al*.: Azelastine (Azel) in the treatment of asthma. *J All Clin Immunol* (1985) **75**: 167.

99. Tinkelman DG, Bucholtz GA, Kemp JP, *et al*.: Evaluation of the safety and efficacy of multiple doses of azelastine to adult patients with bronchial asthma over time. *Am Rev Respir Dis* (1990) **141**: 569–574.

100. Bruttman G, Pedrain P, Arendt C, Rihowe JP: Protective effect of cetirizine in patients suffering from pollen asthma. *Ann Allergy* (1990) **54** (2): 224–228.

101. Ash ASF, Schild HO: Receptors mediating some action of histamine. *Br J Pharmacol Chemother* (1966) **27**: 427–434.

102. Black JW, Duncan WAM, Durant CJ, Ganellin CR, Parsons EM: Definition and antagonism of histamine H_2-receptors. *Nature* (1972) **236**: 385–390.

103. Lichtenstein LM, Gillespie E: Inhibition of histamine release by histamine controlled by H_2 receptor. *Nature* (1975) **244**: 287–288.

104. Dunlop LS, Smith AP, Piper PJ: The effect of histamine antagonists on antigen induced contractions of sensitized human bronchus *in vitro*. *Br J Pharmacol* (1977) **59**: 475.

105. Nathan RA, Segall N, Glover GC, Schoclet AL: The effects of H_1 and H_2 antihistamines on histamine inhalation challenges in asthmatic patients. *Am Rev Resp Dis* (1979) **120**: 1251–1258.

106. Schachter EN, Brown S, Lach E, Gerstenhaber B: Histamine blocking agents in healthy and asthmatic subjects. *Chest* (1982) **82**: 143–147.

107. Maconachie JG, Woodbines EP, Richards DA: Effects of H_1 and H_2 receptor blocking agents on histamine-induced bronchoconstriction in non-asthmatic subjects. *Br J Clin Pharmacol* (1979) **7**: 231–236.

108. Thomson NC, Kerr JW: Effect of inhaled H_1 and H_2 receptor antagonists in normal and asthmatic subjects. *Thorax* (1980) **35**: 428–434.

109. Norgrady SG, Bevan C: H_2 receptor blockade and bronchial hyperreactivity to histamine in asthma. *Thorax* (1981) **36**: 268–271.

110. Eiser NM, Mills J, Snashall PD, Guz A: The role of histamine receptors in asthma. *Clin Sci* (1981) **50**: 363–370.

111. Leopold JD, Hartley JPR, Smith AP: Effects of oral H_1 and H_2 receptor antagonists in asthma. *Br J Clin Pharmacol* (1979) **8**: 249–251.

112. Arrang JM, Garbang M, Schwartz JC: Auto-inhibition of brain histamine release mediated by a novel class (H_3) of histamine receptor. *Nature* (1983) **302**: 832–837.

113. Ichinose M, Stretton CD, Schwartz JC, Barnes PJ: Histamine H_3 receptor inhibits cholinergic neurotransmission in guinea-pig airways. *Br J Pharmacol* (1989) **97**: 13–15.

114. Martin M, Romer D: The pharmacological properties of a new orally active antianaphylactic compound: Ketotifen, a benzocycloheptathiopene. *Arznei-mittelforsch/Drug Res* (1978) **28**: 770–782.

115. Martin U, Romer D: Antianaphylactic properties of ketotifen in animal experiments. *Triangle* (1978) **17**: 141–147.

116. Loftus BG, Price JF, Heaton R, Costello J: Effects of ketotifen on *in vivo* bronchoconstriction. *Clin Allergy* (1985) **15**: 465–471.

117. Martin H, Romer D: Ketotifen, a new type of antianaphylactic agent. *Allergol Immunopath* (1977) **5**(Suppl): 5.

118. Tomioka H, Yoshida S, Tanaka M, *et al.*: Inhibition of chemical mediator release from human leucocytes by a new antiasthma drug HC 20-511(Ketotifen). *Monogr Allergy* (1979) **14**: 313.

119. Ross WJ, Harrison RG, Jolley MR, *et al.*: Antianaphylactic agents, 1,2-(acylamine) oxazoles. *J Med Chem* (1979) **22**: 412–417.

120. Lowe DA, Richardson BP: The effects of cyproheptadine, ketotifen and sodium nitroprusside on mechanical activity and calcium uptake in guinea pig taenia coli *in vitro*. *Respiration* (1980) **39**: Suppl 1: 44–46.

121. Craps L, Greenwood C, Radielovic P: Clinical investigation of agents with prophylactic antiallergic effects in bronchial asthma. *Clin Allergy* (1978) **8**: 373–382.

122. Dorward AJ, Patel KR: A comparison of ketotifen with clemastine, ipratropium bromide and sodium cromoglycate in exercise-induced asthma. *Clin Allergy* (1982) **12**(4): 355-61.

123. Petharam IS, Moxham J, Bierman CW, McAllen M, Spiro S: Ketotifen in atopic asthma and exercise-induced asthma. *Thorax* (1981) **36**: 308–312.

124. Kennedy JD, Hashan R, Clay MJD, Jones RS: Comparison of the action of disodium cromoglycate and ketotifen on exercise-induced bronchoconstriction in childhood asthma. *Br Med J* (1980) **2**: 1458.

125. Lilja G, Graff-Lonnevig V, Bevegard S: Comparison of the protective effect of ketotifen and disodium cromoglycate on exercise-induced asthma in asthmatic boys. *Allergy* (1983) **38**: 31–35.

126. Morgan DJR, Moodley I, Cundell DR, Shienman BD, Smart W, Davies RJ: Circulating histamine and neutrophil chemotactic activity during allergen induced asthma: the effect of inhaled antihistamines and antiallergic compounds. *Clin Sci* (1985) **69**: 63–69.

127. Morley J, Page CP, Mazzoni L, Sanjor S: Effect of ketotifen upon responses to platelet activating factor: a basis for asthma prophylaxis. *Ann Allergy* (1986) **56**: 335–340.
128. Gleich GJ, Frigas E, Filley WV, *et al.*: Eosiniphils and bronchial inflammation. In Kay AB, Austen KF, Lichtenstein LM (eds) *Asthma: Physiology, Immunopharmacology and Treatment.* London, Academic Press, 1984, pp 195–207.
129. Joseph M, Capron M: IgE receptors on macrophages; biological significance. *Ag Act* (1985) **16**: 27–29.
130. Morley J, Sanjar S, Page CP: The platelet in asthma. *Lancet* (1984) **2**: 1142–1144.
131. Vargaftig BB, Lefort J, Chignard M, *et al.*: Platelet activating factor induces a platelet dependent bronchoconstriction related to the formation of prostaglandin derivatives. *Eur J Pharmacol* (1980) **65**: 185–192.
132. Mazzoni L, Morley J, Page CP, *et al.*: induction of airway hyperreactivity by platelet activating factor in guinea pig. *J Physiol* (1985) **365**: 107.
133. Gateau O, Arnoux B, Deriaz H, *et al.*: Acute effect of PAF-acether (platelet activating factor) in humans. *Am Rev Resp Dis* (1982) **129**: A3.
134. Mojarad M, Hamasaki Y, Said SI: Platelet activating factor increases pulmonary microvascular permeability and induces pulmonary oedema. *Bull Eur Physiopath Resp* (1983) **19**: 253–257.
135. Page CP, Paul W, Morley J: Platelets and bronchospasm. *Int Arch Allergy Appl Immunol* (1984) **74**: 347–350.
136. Denjean A, Arnoux B, Lockhart A, *et al.*: Modification of alveolar cell population after PAF acether induced bronchoconstriction in baboons. *Am Rev Resp Dis* (1982) **129**: A3.
137. Cuss FM, Dixon CMS, Barnes PJ: Effect of inhaled platelet activating factor on pulmonary function and bronchial responsiveness in man. *Lancet* (1986) **ii**: 189–192.
138. Page CP, Tomiak RHH, Sanjar S, *et al.*: Suppression of PAF-acether response: an antiinflammatory effect of antiasthma drugs. *Ag Act* (1985) **16**: 33–35.
139. Chung KF, Minette P, McCusker M, Barnes PJ: Ketotifen inhibits the cutaneous but not the airway responses to platelet activating factor in man. *J Allergy Clin Immunol* (1988) **81**: 1192–1198.
140. Paterson JW, Yellin RH, Tarola RA: Evaluation of ketotifen (HC20-511) in bronchial asthma. *Eur J Clin Pharmacol* (1983) **25**: 187–193.
141. Tinkelman DG, Webb CS, Vanderppl GE, Carrol S, Spangler DL, Lotner GZ: The use of ketotifen in the prophylaxis of season allergic asthma. *Ann Allergy* (1986) **56**: 213–217.
142. Broberger H, Graff-Lonnevig V, Lilja G, Rylander E: Ketotifen in pollen-induced asthma: a double blind placebo controlled study. *Clin Allergy* (1986) **16**: 119–127.
143. Graff-lonnevig V, Hedlin G: The effect of ketotifen on bronchial hyperreactivity in childhood asthma. *J Allergy Clin Immunol* (1985) **76**: 59–63.
144. Lane DJ: A steroid sparing effect of ketotifen in steroid dependent asthmatics. *Clin Allergy* (1980) **10**: 519–525.
145. Morley J, Page CP, Mazzoni L, Sanjar S: Effects of ketotifen upon responses to platelet activating factor: a basis for asthma prophylaxis. *Ann Allergy* (1986) **56**: 335–340.
146. Hardy CC, Robinson C, Tattersfield AE, Holgate ST: The bronchoconstrictor effect of inhaled prostaglandin D_2 in normal and asthmatic men. *N Eng J Med* (1984) **311**: 209–213.
147. Dunlop LS, Smith AP: Reduction of antigen-induced contraction of sensitized human bronchus *in vitro* by indomethacin. *Br J Pharmacol* (1985) **54**: 495–497.
148. Peters SP, Macglashan DW, Schleimer RP, Hayes EC, Adkinson NE, Lichtenstein LM: The pharmacological modulation of the release of arachidonic acid metabolites from purified human lung mast cells. *Am Rev Resp Dis* (1985) **135**: 367–373.
149. Adams GK, Lichtenstein LM: Indomethacin enhances response of human bronchus to antigen. *Am Rev Resp Dis* (1985) **131**: 8–10.
150. Marone G, Kagey-Sabotka A, Lichtenstein LM: Effects of arachidonic acid and its metabolites on antigen induced histamine release from human basophils *in vitro*. *J Immunol* (1979) **123**: 1669–1677.
151. Adcock JJ, Garland LG, Moncada S, Salmon JA: The mechanism of enhancement by fatty acid hydroperoxides of anaphylactic mediator release. *Prostaglandins* (1978) **16**: 179–187.

152. Walters EH, Parrish RW, Bevan C, Smith AP: Induction of bronchial hypersensitivity: evidence for a role for prostaglandins. *Thorax* (1981) **36**: 571–574.

153. Smith AP: Effect of indomethacin in asthma: evidence against the role of prostaglandins in asthma. *Br J Clin Pharmacol* (1975) **2**: 307.

154. Shepherd EG, Malan L, MacFarlane CM, Mouton W, Joubert JR: Lung function and plasma levels of thromboxane B_2, 6-ketoprostaglandin F_1, and B-thromboglobulin in antigen induced asthma before and after indomethacin pretreatment. *Br J Clin Pharmacol* (1985) **19**: 459–470.

155. Fairfax AJ, Hansen JM, Morley J: The late reaction following bronchial provocation with house dust mite allergen. Dependence on arachidonic acid metabolism. *Clin Exp Immunol* (1985) **52**: 393–398.

156. Joubert JR, Shepherd E, Mouton W, Van Zyl L, Viljoen I: Non-steroidal antiinflammatory drugs in asthma: dangerous or useful therapy? *Allergy* (1985) **40**: 202–207.

157. Crook D, Cullins AJ, Rose AJ: A comparison of the effect of flurbiprofen on prostaglandin synthetase from human rheumatoid synovium and enzymatically active animal tissues. *J Pharm Pharmac* (1976) **28**: 535.

158. Curzen N, Rafferty P, Holgate ST: Effect of a cyclo-oxygenase inhibitor, flurbiprofen and an H_1 histamine receptor antagonist, terfenadine, alone and in combination on allergen induced immediate bronchoconstriction in man. *Thorax* (1987) **2**: 946–952.

159. Peters SP, Schulman ES, MacGlashan DW, Schleimer RP, Newball HH, Lichtenstein LM: Pharmacological and biochemical studies of human lung mast cells. *J Allergy Clin Immunol* (1982) **69**: 150.

160. Szczeklik A: Asthma, aspirin and leukotrienes. *Bull Eur Physiopath Resp* (1983) **19**: 531–538.

161. Szczeklik A, Cryglewski RJ, Nizankowsua E: Asthma relieved by aspirin and by other cyclo-oxygenase inhibitors. *Thorax* (1978) **33**: 664–665.

162. Szczeklik A, Cryglewski RJ, Czerniawska-Mysik G: Relationship of inhibition of prostaglandin biosynthesis by analgesics to asthma attacks in aspirin-sensitive patients. *Br Med J* (1975) **1**: 67–69.

163. Dahlen SE, Hedqvist P, Hammarstrom S, Samuelsson B: Leukotrienes are potent constrictors of human bronchi. *Nature* (1980) **288**: 484–486.

164. Drazen JM, Austen FK, Lewis RA, *et al.*: Comparative airway and vascular activities of leukotrienes C_1 and D *in vivo* and *in vitro*. *Proc Natl Acad Sci USA* (1980) **77**: 4354–4358.

165. Ahmed T, Greenblatt DW, Birch S, Marchette B, Warner O: Abnormal mucociliary transport in allergic patients with antigen-induced bronchospasm—role of slow reacting substance of anaphylaxis. *Am Rev Resp Dis* (1981) **124**: 110–114.

166. Goetzl EJ: Mediators of immediate hypersensitivity derived from arachidonic acid. *N Eng J Med* (1980) **303**: 822–825.

167. Bach MK, Brashler JR, Fitzpatrick FA, *et al.*: In vivo and in vitro actions of a new selective inhibitor of leukotriene C and D synthesis. In Samuelson B, Ramwell PW, Paoletti R (eds) *Advances in Prostaglandin and Thromboxane Research*, Vol. II. New York, Raven Press, 1982, p 39.

168. Dahlen SE, Hedqvist P, Bjorck T, Granstrom E, Dahlen B: Allergen challenge of lung tissue from asthmatics elicits bronchial contraction that correlates with release of leukotrienes C_4, D_4 and E_4. *Proc Natl Acad Sci USA* (1983) **80**: 1712–1716.

169. Robinson C, Holgate ST: Ionophore-dependent generation of eicosanoids in human dispersed lung cells: modulation by 6,8 depoxy 6,9-(phenylimino)-^{6,8}prostaglandin I_1. *Biochem Pharmacol* (1986) **35**: 1903–1908.

170. Smith RJ, Sun FF, Bowman BJ, Iden SS, Smith HW, McGuire JC: Effect of 6-9-deepoxy-6,9-(phenylamine)-^{6,8}prostaglandin I_1 (U-6-,257), an inhibitor of leukotriene synthesis on human neutrophil functions. *Biochem Biophys Res Commun* (1982) **109**: 943–949.

171. Cromwell O, Shaw RJ, Walsh GM, Kay AB: Inhibition of leukotriene C_4 and B_4 generation by human eosinophils and neutrophils. *Br J Pharmacol* (1985) **86**: 427 (Abstract).

172. Johnson HG, McNee ML, Back MK, Smith HW: The activity of a new, novel inhibitor of leukotriene synthesis in rhesus monkeys, *Ascaris* reactions. *Int Arch Allergy Appl Immunol* (1983) **70**: 169–173.

173. Back MK, Griffin RL, Richards IM: Inhibition of the presumably leukotriene- dependent component of antigen-induced bronchoconstriction in the guinea pig by piriprost (U-60,257). *Int Arch Allergy Appl Immunol* (1985) **77**: 264–266.

174. Mann JS, Robinson C, Sheridan AQ, Clement P, Back MK, Holgate ST: Effect of inhaled piriprost (U-60,257) a novel leukotriene inhibitor, on allergen and exercise-induced broncho-constriction in asthma. *Thorax* (1986) **41**: 746–752.

175. Kreutner W, Sherwood J, Sehrine S, *et al.*: Antiallergy activity of Sch 37224, a new inhibitor of leukotriene formation. *J Pharmacol Exp Ther* (1988) **247**: 997–1003.

176. Abraham WM, Stevenson JS, Garrido R: A leukotriene and thromboxane inhibitor (Sch 37224) blocks antigen-induced immediate and late responses and airway hyperresponsive-ness in allergic sheep. *J Pharmacol Exp Therap* (1988) **247**: 1004–1011.

177. Knapp HR: Reduced allergen-induced nasal congestion and leukotriene sythesis with an orally active 5-lipoxygenase inhibitor. *N Eng J Med* (1990) **323** 1745–1748.

178. Israel E, Dermarkarian R, Rosenberg M, *et al.*: The effects of a 5-lipoxygenase inhibitor on asthma induced by cold, dry air. *N Eng J Med* (1990) **323**: 1740–1744.

179. Saijo T, Makino H, Tamura S, *et al.*: The anti-allergic agent Amoxanox suppresses SRS-A generation by inhibiting lipoxygenase. *Int Arch Allergy Appl Immunol* (1986) **79**: 231–237.

180. Saijo T, Kuriki H, Ashida Y, Makino H, Maki Y: Inhibition by amoxanox (AA-673) of the immunologically, leukotriene D_4-or platelet activating factor-stimulated bronchoconstriction in guinea pigs and rats. *Int Arch Allergy Appl Immunol* (1985) **77**: 315–321.

181. Redkar-Brown DG, Aharong D: Inhibitors of antigen-induced contrachea of guinea pig trachea by ICI 198,615. *Eur J Pharmacol* (1989) **165**: 113–121.

182. Patterson R, Harris KE, Bernstein PR, Krell RD, Handley DA, Saunders RN: Effects of combined receptor antagonists of leukotriene D_4 (LTD_4) and platelet activating factor (PAF) on rhesus airway responses to LTD_4, PAF and antigen. *Int Arch Allergy Appl Immunol* (1989) **88**: 462–470.

183. Abraham WM, Stevenson JS, Garrido R: The effect of an orally active leukotriene (LTD_4) antagonist WY-48,252 on LTD_4 and antigen induced bronchoconstriction in allergic sheep. *Prostaglandins* (1988) **35**: 733–745.

184. Barnes N, Piper PJ, Costello JF: The effect of an oral leukotriene antagonist L-649,923 on histamine and leukotriene-induced bronchoconstriction in normal man. *J Allergy Clin Immunol* (1987) **79**: 816–821.

185. Britton J, Hanley SP, Tattersfield AE: The effect of an orally active leukotriene D_4 (LTD_4) antagonist L-649,923 on the airway response to inhaled antigen in asthma. *Thorax* (1987) **42**(3): 219.

186. Phillips GD, Rafferty P, Holgate ST: LY171883 as an oral leukotriene D_4 antagonist in non-asthmatic subjects. *Thorax* (1987) **42**(9): 723.

187. Fuller R, Black PN, Dollery CT: Effects of the oral leukotriene D_4 antagonist LY 171883 on inhaled and intradermal challenge with antigen and leukotriene D_4 in atopic subjects. *J Allergy Clin Immunol* (1989) **83**: 939–944.

188. Israel E, Juniper EF, Callaghan JT, *et al.*: Effect of leukotriene antagonist, LY 171883 on cold air induced bronchoconstriction in asthmatics. *Am Rev Respir Dis* (1989) **40**: 1348–1353.

189. Cloud ML, Enas GC, Kemp J, *et al.*: Efficacy and safety of LY171883 in patients with mild chronic asthma. *J Allergy Clin Immunol* (1987) **79**(1): 256.

190. Smith LJ, Geller S, Ebright L, Glass M, Thyrum PT: Inhibition of leukotriene D_4 induced bronchoconstriction in normal subjects by the oral LTD_4 receptor antagonist ICI 204,209. *Am Rev Resp Dis* (1990) **141**: 988–992.

191. Manning PJ, Watson RM, Margolskee DJ, Williams VC, Schwartz JI, O'Byrne PM: Inhibition of exercise-induced bronchoconstriction by MK-571, a potent leukotriene D_4 receptor antagonist. *N Eng J Med* (1990) **32**: 1736–1739.

192. Braquet P, Guinot P, Touvay C: The role of PAF-acether in anaphylaxis demonstrated by the use of the antagonist BN 52021. In Scmitz-Shumann J, Menz G, Page CP (eds) *Platelets, PAF and Asthma*. Basel, Birkhauser (1987) *Agents Actions* [Suppl] **41**: 97–117.

193. Coyle AJ, Page CP, Atkinson L, Sjoerdsma K, Tonvay C, Metzger WJ: Modification of allergen-induced airway obstruction and airway hyperresponsiveness in an allergic rabbit

model by the selective platelet activating factor antagonist BN 52021. *J Allergy Clin Immunol* (1989) **84**: 960–967.

194. Coyle AJ, Urusin SC, Page CP, Tonray C, Villain B, Braquet P: The effect of the selective PAF antagonist BN52021 on PAF-and antigen-induced bronchial hyper-reactivity and eosinophil accumulation. *Eur J Pharmacol* (1988) **148**: 51–58.

195. Chung KF, Dent G, McClusker M, Guinot PH, Page CP, Barnes PJ: Effect of a ginkgolide mixture (BN 52063) in antagonising skin and platelet responses to platelet activating factor in man. *Lancet* (1987) **1**: 248–251.

196. Roberts NM, Page CP, Chung KF, Barnes PJ: Effect of a PAF antagonist, BN 52063, an antigen-induced, acute and late onset cutaneous responses in atopic subjects. *J Allergy Clin Immunol* (1988) **82**: 236–241.

197. Tomioka K, Garride R, Ahmed A, Stevenson JS, Abraham WR: YM461, a PAF antagonist, blocks antigen-induced late airways responses and airway hyperresponsiveness in allergic sheep. *Eur J Pharmacol* (1989) **170**: 209–215.

198. Pretolani M, Lefat J, Malanchere E, Vargaftig BB: Interference by the novel PAF-acether antagonist WEB 2086 with the bronchopulmonary respects to PAF-acether and to active and passive anaphylactic shock in guinea pigs. *Eur J Pharmacol* (1987) **140**: 311–321.

199. Dixon EJA, Wilsoncroft P, Robertson DN, Page CP: The effect of PAF antagonists on bronchial hyperresponsiveness induced by PAF, propanolol or indomethacin. *Br J Pharmacol* (1989) **97**: 717–722.

200. Soler M, Sielczak MW, Abraham WM: A PAF antagonist blocks antigen-induced airway hyperresponsiveness and inflammation in sheep. *J Appl Physiol* (1989) **67**: 406–413.

201. Takizawa H, Ishll A, Suzuki S, Shiga J, Miyamoto T: Bronchoconstriction induced by platelet activating factor in the guinea pig and its inhibition by CV 3988 a PAF antagonist: serial changes in findings of lung histology and bronchoalveolar lavage cell population. *Int Arch Allergy Appl Immunol* (1988) **85**: 375–382.

202. Ward SG, Westwick J: Antagonisms of the platelet activating factor-induced rise of the intracellular calcium ion concentration of U 937 cells. *Br J Pharmacol* (1988) **93**: 769–774.

203. Havill AM, Van Valen RG, Handley DA: Prevention of non-specific airway hyperreactivity after allergen challenge in guinea pigs by the PAF receptor antagonist SDZ 64-412. *Br J Pharmacol* (1990) **99**: 396–400.

204. Gilfillan A, Wiggan GA, Hqe WR, Patel BJ, Weltan AF: Ro 19-3704 directly inhibits immunoglobulin E-dependent mediated release by a mechanism independent of its platelet activating factor antagonist properties. *Eur J Pharmacol* (1990) **176**: 255–262.

205. Sanjar S, Aoki S, Banbekeur K, *et al.*: Eosinophil accumulation in pulmonary airways of guinea pigs induced by exposure to an aerosol of platelet activation factor: effect of acute asthma drugs. *Br J Pharmacol* (1990) **99**: 267–272.

206. Roberts NM, McCusker M, Chung KF, Barnes PJ: Effect of a PAF antagonist, BN 52063, on PAF induced bronchoconstriction in normal subjects. *Br J Clin Pharmac* (1988) **26**: 65–72.

207. Adamus WS, Huer HO, Meade CJ, Schilling JC: Inhibitory effects of the new PAF acether antagonist WEB-2086 on pharmacologic changes induced by PAF inhalation in human beings. *Clin Pharmacol Ther* (1990) **47**: 456–462.

Glucocorticosteroids

ROGER ELLUL-MICALLEF

HISTORICAL BACKGROUND

One of the earliest reports on the use of 'adrenal substance' appears to be that by Solis-Cohen in 1900,[1] who wrote, 'I believe that we have in this substance a decided addition to therapeutic resources . . ,' and finally commented, 'What the active agent is and how much or how little of that active agent is absorbed, I must leave to laboratory students to determine.' The isolation of this 'active agent', cortisone, originally termed compound E, was first achieved in Kendall's laboratory, but its further characterization and synthesis proved to be a slow process. It took a further 16 years before cortisone was used in rheumatoid arthritis. Within a year, it was administered intramuscularly in bronchial asthma. In an attempt to potentiate the anti-inflammatory effects further and decrease the unwanted mineralocorticoid influence, a number of other glucocorticoids were later synthesized and tried out. The standard oral glucocorticoid remains prednisolone, originally introduced under the name of metacortandrolone, whilst hydrocortisone and methylprednisolone are the preparations predominantly used intravenously.

As glucocorticoids rapidly gained a prominent place in the control of various disease states, it soon became obvious that they were a double-edged therapeutic weapon and could result in undesirable side-effects. As early as 1950, attempts were made to deliver them locally to the airways in order to minimize the risk of their potential hazards. These attempts proved to be largely unsuccessful, as enough of the glucocorticoid was usually absorbed to cause systemic side-effects. Success was first achieved in 1972 with betamethasone valerate and beclomethasone dipropionate (BDP). These were the first topical aerosol glucocorticoids to be used in bronchial asthma without producing any significant side-effect.[2,3] Others have since followed and include the fluorinated compounds, triamcinolone acetonide and flunisolide and the non-halogenated glucocorticoid, budesonide.[4]

ASTHMA: BASIC MECHANISMS AND CLINICAL MANAGEMENT (2nd Edn)
ISBN 0-12-079026-2

PHARMACOKINETICS OF GLUCOCORTICOIDS

Structure–function relationships

The glucocorticoids are a group of C_{21} steroids whose structure is characterized by: (a) a double bond at C-4 and an oxo group at C-3; (b) a side chain at C-17; (c) a hydroxyl or oxo group at C-11; (d) a hydroxyl group at C-17; and (e) a C-21 hydroxyl group with an oxo group at C-20. Substitution at various sites has resulted in the synthesis of a number of such compounds. Thus, the introduction of a 1,2 double bond resulted in prednisolone. This structural alteration results in an increased affinity for the glucocorticoid receptor, enhancing its glucocorticoid potency and reducing its mineralocorticoid effects. The addition of a halogen atom to the nucleus resulted in such potent compounds as triamcinolone, dexamethasone and betamethasone, which owe their marked potency to increased receptor affinity and reduced hepatic inactivation. These compounds did not offer any real advance over prednisolone. Acetonide or ester modifications appear to increase topical activity. Recent structure–activity investigations have shown that optimization of the 16α, 17α-acetal substitution is important to achieve marked topical anti-inflammatory activity. Budesonide is such a 16α, 17α-glucocorticoid without halogen atoms in its structure, whilst BDP is a 17α, 21-diester with a chlorine atom in the 9α position.

General considerations

Glucocorticoids are carried in the body partly bound to transcortin, an α_1-glycoprotein, partly bound to albumin and partly as the free drug. Transcortin has a high affinity but a low capacity, whilst albumin has a low affinity but a much greater capacity for glucocorticoid binding. Compared with transcortin, albumin exhibits a 10^4 times lower affinity for prednisolone binding. Consequently, at low concentrations the glucocorticoid is tightly bound to transcortin and the unbound amount of the circulating drug is low, whilst at high concentrations a greater fraction of the drug is loosely bound to albumin and the unbound fraction increases. As the liver metabolizes the free fraction of the drug, a higher fraction of the dose of administered glucocorticoid is removed during its first pass through the liver when the dose administered is high than when it is low. This would explain the higher systemic availability when the same total amount of glucocorticoid is divided into several small doses instead of being given as a single dose. With the exception of prednisone and prednisolone, synthetic glucocorticoids do not bind appreciably to transcortin, but even so, prednisolone has only half the affinity of hydrocortisone for transcortin. It appears that there is some sort of relationship between plasma glucocorticoid levels and biological effect. Although it is usually stated that it is only the unbound part of the drug that is biologically active, there is still some controversy as to whether unbound plus the albumin-bound and/or transcortin-bound glucocorticoid molecules can penetrate tissues and are therefore active biologically. It has also been suggested that a substantial concentration of hydrocortisone is associated with erythrocytes, and the latter cells may well serve as a major conduit for hydrocortisone transport to the tissues.[5] Very few studies have actually compared the ability of different systemically administered glucocorticoids to penetrate into lung tissue; from those carried out it

seems that hydrocortisone has the highest penetrability,[6] followed by methylprednisolone and finally prednisone and prednisolone.[7,8]

Glucocorticoids may be metabolized via various pathways, and such biotransformation occurs mainly in the liver. The excretion of prednisolone by the kidney is still not
completely understood, but it appears that renal clearance of both total and unbound
prednisolone increases with increasing dose and accounts for only 10–30% of the total
body clearance of prednisolone. Conjugation as glucuronides or sulphides makes them
more water-soluble. In the case of BDP, esterases in the lung begin to hydrolyse it soon
after inhalation, although cleavage of its 17α-ester bond probably occurs principally in
the liver. The rate of metabolic degradation is decreased by the inclusion of a double
bond at C-1 or C-2, or by the inclusion of a fluorine atom in the molecule.

Pharmacokinetic profile of different glucocorticoids

Various studies in both normal subjects and asthmatic patients[9] have indicated that
prednisolone exhibits dose-dependent, non-linear kinetics; this was thought to be due
mainly to its non-linear protein binding over the therapeutic concentration range,[10] but
doubts have since been expressed about this.[11] The dose-dependent pharmacokinetics of
prednisolone offer a partial explanation for the clinical observation that alternate day
administration of this drug results in fewer biological effects. Overall, the effects of age
on the pharmacokinetics of glucocorticoids appear to be variable; there are reports
showing no effect[12] whilst other workers have shown that the renal and non-renal
clearance of both total and unbound prednisolone is much lower in elderly subjects.[13] A
similar increase in half-life ($t_{\frac{1}{2}}$) had been reported earlier in older subjects after intravenous hydrocortisone.[14] In spite of higher free concentrations of prednisolone, the
concentrations of endogenous hydrocortisone were higher in the elderly. This could
point to a blunted response of the hypothalamic–pituitary–adrenal axis to prednisolone
and/or a decrease in metabolic clearance of endogenous hydrocortisone. Gender also
seems to influence pharmacokinetics, as it has been shown that women have free
prednisolone clearances that are about 20% higher than those of males, although others
have found no such difference.[15]

In contrast to the large number of studies on prednisolone, there are very few on the
pharmacokinetics of intravenously administered methylprednisolone or hydrocortisone.
Methylprednisolone has a shorter $t_{\frac{1}{2}}$, a larger volume of distribution to tissues, a faster
clearance and lower bioavailability than prednisolone, when given in approximately
similar doses. Unlike prednisolone, it does not exhibit non-linear pharmacokinetics.[15] It
has been shown that in normals the distribution and elimination characteristics of
hydrocortisone are independent of dose size at low intravenous doses up to 20 mg, but
were dose-dependent after a dose of 40 mg. There seems to be a variation in the rate of
disappearance of this glucocorticoid from plasma following its intravenous administration. The apparent $t_{\frac{1}{2}}$ of exogenous hydrocortisone was reported to be higher in the
morning (8 a.m.) than in the afternoon (4 p.m.). The glucocorticoid-binding capacity of
transcortin has been described as having a diurnal variation, the binding capacity being
highest at night. Unbound prednisolone clearance has been reported to be lower in the
morning, though when the dose administered was high no circadian variation was
detected. A study that took into consideration only total prednisolone levels measured at

two time points (8 a.m. and 8 p.m.) but which was carried out in both normal and asthmatic subjects also failed to detect any circadian variation in prednisolone pharma-cokinetics.[9] It has been suggested that throughout the day there may be two phases of ACTH secretion under different control mechanisms. The nocturnal phase appears to be sensitive to physiological levels of glucocorticoids, whilst a second phase, responsible for the steady basal activity during the day, responds only to large doses of the hormone.[16] In view of the fact that there is some evidence showing that pituitary–adrenocorticol suppression is appreciably shorter when glucocorticoids are administered in the morning than at night, it appears reasonable to prescribe these drugs in the morning. Glucocorticoid dosing is often empirical and, especially in the case of the systemically administered drug, there is no consensus with regard to the appropriate dose. In asthmatic patients, the long-term oral administration of prednisolone at 8 a.m. and 3 p.m. was found to be more effective in controlling the condition and improving airflow than when the same doses were given at 3 p.m. and 8 p.m.[17] Recently, a 'dose-sparing' effect has been claimed for methylprednisolone if this is administered in two divided doses at 8 a.m. and 4 p.m. rather than as a single 8 a.m. dose.[18] Modifications of established dosing patterns need to be further investigated and have to be validated for individual glucocorticoids.

One of the main factors determining the site of aerosol deposition within the lung is aerosol particle size; particles having a diameter of $<5\,\mu$m being the ones best reaching the lower airways. Although it has been shown that only between 10 and 20% of an inhaled dose enters the small airways, glucocorticoid aerosols have become firmly established as one of the principal forms of maintenance therapy in bronchial asthma. This is mostly because of their high bioavailability and the greatly reduced risk of systemic side-effects. Large volume spacer devices facilitate the inhalation of aerosols[19] and result in a reduction in particle size thereby increasing the amount of drug reaching the airways, as well as reducing the incidence of dysphonia and candidiasis. Simple mouth rinsing will further reduce the incidence of these side-effects. Topically active glucocorticoids are rapidly absorbed into the lung; this has been shown with both BDP and flunisolide. BDP is strongly bound to plasma proteins; 87% binding to human plasma proteins has been reported in an *in vivo* investigation. Lung esterases are known to hydrolyse BDP rapidly to beclomethasone-17-α-propionate (BMP) and then more slowly to beclomethasone. Further metabolic breakdown of any BDP and BMP reaching the blood takes place in the liver, the inactive polar metabolites being excreted via the bile.

Of the topical glucocorticoids, budesonide is amongst those whose pharmacokinetics have been best defined. The plasma protein binding of budesonide is reported to be around 90%, with negligible binding to transcortin. This compound has been shown to have a very high affinity for the glucocorticoid receptor. Budesonide has a much higher volume of distribution than most other glucocorticoids with more than 95% of it being tissue bound. The major fraction of the drug deposited within the lung is absorbed within 10–30 min and perhaps redistributed via the microcirculation. This time appears to be sufficient for the full triggering of glucocorticoid receptors. Budesonide is not biotransformed in the lung or blood but is rapidly oxidized by the cytochrome P_{450} system in the liver (biotransformation is two to three times more rapid than BMP). After oral dosing (11–13% oral bioavailability), its first pass metabolism is about 90%.

Budesonide has been reported to have a significantly lower effect in depressing plasma cortisol levels and in changing the total or different white blood cell count than BDP.[20]

Another recently introduced topical glucocorticoid is flucatisone 17α-propionate (fluoromethyl carbothioate 17α propionate). It has been shown to have marked anti-inflammatory activity and virtually negligible systemic effects when inhaled, because of very limited absorption (<1% oral bioavailability) and an almost complete first-pass metabolism. Its main metabolite, 17β-carboxylic acid, is practically inactive.[21] The dose of any glucocorticoid which will completely saturate the glucocorticoid receptors within the lungs is not known; though it is probable that only a very small concentration of drug is required.

Variations in glucocorticoid pharmacokinetics

There is some disagreement in the literature as to whether the pharmacokinetics of glucocorticoids differ between asthmatics and normal subjects. Early workers reported finding that when hydrocortisone was administered to steroid-dependent asthmatics, its metabolic clearance was greater than in healthy volunteers or in asthmatics not receiving glucocorticoids. It had been previously suggested that as glucocorticoids may induce the oxidative metabolism of many drugs, they may be able to stimulate their own metabolism. Recently doubts have been expressed on the designs of this study.[22] On the other hand, in two separate studies from the Brompton Hospital, no change was detected in the metabolic clearance of hydrocortisone when this was administered intravenously in doses of 2–8 mg/kg to healthy volunteers, to asthmatics not previously given glucocorticoids, and to asthmatics who had been receiving more than 100 mg prednisone daily.[23,24] Except for one report showing irregular prednisolone serum concentration profiles following oral doses of 20 mg prednisolone in asthmatics,[25] most studies carried out with oral prednisolone indicate that its $t_{\frac{1}{2}}$, total plasma clearance and steady-state volume of distribution were similar in asthmatic and normal subjects.[26] On the whole, the evidence available indicates that the asthmatic state has no appreciable influence on glucocorticoid pharmacokinetics, nor does a self-induced increase in their metabolism appear likely. The effects of various concomitant conditions that may alter glucocorticoid pharmacokinetics are summarized in Table 36.1.

The differences reported between the studies on inflammatory bowel conditions may have resulted from the fact that the sites and degree of inflammatory involvement may well have differed. It is difficult to predict accurately the clinical consequences of hypoalbuminaemia in any individual patient, even though attempts at adjusting dosage in such circumstances have been made. An increase in the concentration of free glucocorticoid may well be balanced by an increase in the systemic clearance of the drug. It is likewise difficult to predict the effects that changes in renal function might have on the metabolism of prednisolone.[22] Undoubtedly there will be instances, admittedly not many, when bronchial asthma may be present in patients with the above disorders. A knowledge of the alterations in pharmacokinetic profiles may well then be important for therapeutic reasons, as change in dosage may be necessary to achieve the desired results and avoid side-effects.[22] Thus dysphonia has been reported to be commoner, more severe and more persistent in asthmatics with associated hypothyroidism treated with glucocorticoid aerosols.[27]

Table 36.1   Effect of concomitant conditions on glucocorticoid pharmacokinetics.

Condition	Alteration
Inflammatory bowel disease	Decreased bioavailability of prednisolone post-oral administration Decreased plasma protein binding of prednisolone No decrease in bioavailability
Hepatic disorders	Decreased metabolic clearance and increased $t_{\frac{1}{2}}$ of hydrocortisone, dexamethasone and prednisolone Impaired conversion of prednisone to prednisolone Increased free prednisolone levels
Renal conditions	Prolongation of $t_{\frac{1}{2}}$ of hydrocortisone and prednisolone Increased free dexamethasone and prednisolone levels Decreased concentrations of albumin and transcortin but greater affinity of these proteins for prednisolone Reduced renal and non-renal clearance of prednisolone in renal transplant patients
Thyroid disorders Thyrotoxicosis	 Increased metabolic breakdown, increased clearance and decreased free plasma cortisol levels Possible decreased intestinal absorption and enhanced non-renal clearance of prednisolone Impaired hepatic conversion of hydrocortisone to cortisone
Hypothyroidism	Slower clearance

Drug interactions

There are various reports in the literature of drugs influencing glucocorticoid metabolism. The first reports involved the enhancement of hepatic microsomal hydroxylation enzyme activity by phenytoin which resulted in an increased clearance rate of cortisol.

Table 36.2 lists the various interactions of glucocorticoids with other drugs. Perhaps the most relevant interaction is that involving oral contraceptives. The latter have been shown to cause a decrease in free prednisolone clearance varying between 30 and 63% as well as a 73% increase in $t_{\frac{1}{2}}$.[28,29] This is to be kept in mind when asthmatic patients regularly using oral contraceptives require glucocorticoid therapy. One other possible interaction worthy of consideration is the increase in airflow obstruction brought about when intravenous hydrocortisone—but not other glucocorticoids—is administered to patients with aspirin-induced asthma.

Pregnancy and lactation

Studies with both natural and synthetic glucocorticoids carried out mostly in mid- and late-pregnancy have shown that these compounds easily cross the placenta. Cortisol appears to cross the placenta far more rapidly than prednisolone but is quickly converted into the inactive cortisone by foetal enzymes. In a study on women undergoing elective caesarian section, foetal [^{3}H] prednisolone levels were reported to have been

Table 36.2   Interactions of glucocorticoids with other drugs.

Drugs affecting glucocorticoid pharmacokinetics
Accelerate metabolic breakdown and enhance clearance
   Phenytoin
   Primidone
   Phenobarbitone
   Rifampicin
   Ephedrine
   Cimetidine (in patients with chronic hepatic disease)
   Spironolactone (in patients with chronic hepatic disease)
   Theophylline (a small and transient increase in cortisol clearance)
   Carbimazole, methimazole
   Carbamazepine

Reduce clearance
   Oestrogens (increase transcortin levels, bind irreversibly to cytochrome P_{450})
   Macrolide antibiotics (action specific for methylprednisolone)
   Ketoconazole
   Sodium cromoglycate (small and insignificant effect)

Interfere with absorption
   Cholestyramine
   Antacids

Drugs affected by glucocorticoids	
Salicylates	Increased induction of metabolism
Phenylbutazone	Increased excretion of metabolites
Anticholinesterase drugs	Interfere with neuromuscular transmission
Pancuronium	Reversal of neuromuscular blocking effect
Anticoagulants	Inactivation of heparin if mixed outside body with hydrocortisone
	Reduction of oral anticoagulant effect
Theophylline	Serum levels may rise
	Increased elimination
Metronidazole	Increased induction of metabolism, increased renal clearance

---

8–10-fold less than maternal [^{3}H]prednisolone concentration.[30] Dexamethasone has been reported to cross the placenta in high concentrations, achieving levels in the foetus similar to maternal concentrations, but methylprednisolone does not functionally cross the placenta, while betamethasone levels in foetal serum were found to be only one-third of those in maternal serum. It must be emphasized that the use of both systemic and inhaled glucocorticoids in a large number of pregnancies has been reported not to increase the risk of maternal or foetal complications. In particular, no increased incidence of cleft palate has been reported even when the drugs were administered in the first trimester. As potential adverse effects are probably dose-related, it is advisable to give the smallest dose compatible with proper control of the mother's asthmatic state. Neonates whose mothers have been given prednisone or triamcinolone throughout pregnancy were found to have normal cortisol production. Prednisone and prednisolone are only secreted in milk in small amounts, and are not likely to give rise to serious problems in breast-fed infants.

GLUCOCORTICOID ACTION AT THE SUBCELLULAR LEVEL

The glucocorticoid receptor—structure and function

The currently accepted model of glucocorticoid action suggests that these compounds diffuse passively through the cell membrane into the cytoplasm, where they bind non-covalently with high affinity and specificity to soluble receptor proteins (GRs) by hydrophobic and hydrogen ion interactions, activating the receptors prior to their translocation to the nucleus.[31] It is unlikely that the GR traverses nuclear pores by simple diffusion; probably it does so by a facilitated transport mechanism. The GR is the only steroid receptor which, when unbound, is mainly located in the cytoplasm.[32] The cytosolic location of the GR has, at times, been questioned.[33]

The GR was first discovered in thymic lymphocytes just over 20 years ago. Of all the steroid receptors it is the most extensively studied. The human GR (hGR) is known to belong to a super family of ligand-modulated transcription regulatory factors.[34,35] When hormone activated, the hGR interacts in a specific manner with transcriptional enhancer-like sequences in the DNA, termed glucocorticoid response elements (GREs) which are located close to hormone-responsive promoters.[36] Two signals in the GR are said to mediate hormone-dependent nuclear localization.[37] One of these signals has been mapped out to a 28 amino-acid segment that is closely associated, but not coincident, with the GR domain which binds DNA. The other was mapped to the GR domain which binds the hormone. These specific nuclear localization signals perhaps facilitate the diffusion and intranuclear retention of the GR by interacting with putative carriers that may be responsible for the GR transportation to the nucleus. Nuclear translocation appears to be a somewhat rapid process. In intact thymus cells, cortisol–receptor complexes were completely transferred to the nucleus within a minute of hormone addition. Activation of the GR takes 30–60 s and subsequent nuclear binding occurs within 10 s. It has been calculated that the unactivated and nuclear-bound GR complexes reach a steady state by 30 min. This means that within a few minutes mRNA may already be produced. GREs are frequently found clustered with binding sites for other transcription factors.[38] They have been detected as close as 39 base pair and as far as 2.6 kilobase pair downstream from the initiation site. GREs can modulate the expression of heterologous promoters in a distance- and orientation-independent manner.[39] Although various mechanisms have been proposed, it is not known how GREs, which may be located quite far from the site of interaction of RNA polymerase, can influence the rate of transcription.[40] Apparently the number of glucocorticoid-regulated genes in any hormone-responsive cell is unlikely to exceed 30. The GR must probably be able to select on the order of 1 in 1000 genes.[41] The number of potential binding sites is thought to exceed by far the number of GRs in a steroid-responsive cell. Hence it must be a major task for the GR to identify and bind in a stable manner to its proper GREs in the midst of the large excess of DNA present in the nucleus.

It is presently thought that the unliganded, and therefore non-transformed and non-activated, GR complexes exist as 300 kDa phosphoproteins. There is a considerable body of evidence that indicates that these unliganded cytosolic complexes consist of a single 94 kDa glucocorticoid-binding subunit[42] associated with two 90 kDa non-hormone binding subunits.[43,44] The latter have been identified as heat-shock proteins (hsp90).[45] Tight binding between the GR and hsp90 occurs at, or very near, the end of GR translation.[46] It is still uncertain whether the 300 kDa form represents the whole complex or whether other proteins, some of which may be involved in its translocation, are associated with it. It is now being suggested that this inactive receptor complex may well be a core unit derived from a cytosolic higher-order heteromeric complex that contains, besides the GR and an hsp90 dimer, other associated proteins such as a 56-kDa protein (p56)[47] as well as possibly a 23-kDa protein.[48] The manner in which all these proteins interact is unknown but it is possible that the GR becomes associated only with a subclass of hsp90 which is bound to p56. The GR is said to be only able to bind hormone if it is associated with hsp90.[49] The geometry of this heteromeric complex still needs to be unravelled. The p56 may be so oriented as to link the GR with the hsp90 dimer, or it may well be separated from the GR by the hsp90 dimer. This hsp90 dimer appears to interact with the GR within the same region as its ligand.[42,50] Binding of hsp 90 to the hGR could possibly take place at a site encompassing amino acids 477–596. It has been suggested that this region could be involved in transducing the signal of ligand binding into a derepression of the domain required for DNA binding.[50] The DNA-binding and transcriptional activities of the GR seem to be inversely correlated with its association with hsp90.[51] A possible inhibitory function of hsp90 may be the prevention of GR monomers from forming into dimers, a step thought to be necessary in activating GREs.[52,53] It has been shown that hsp90 is associated with tubulin in cytosol and it is thought to be distributed within cells in a pattern similar to that observed for micro-tubules.[54] Hence the unoccupied GR may be associated with elements of the cytoskel-eton; such an organization may well contribute to the formation of a stable heteromeric complex.[55] Interaction between the heteromeric complex and its glucocorticoid ligand results in the dissociation of hsp90 molecules and other possibly associated proteins from the GR, transforming it to its biologically active DNA-binding state.[56] It has been known for some time that an endogenous, heat-stable cytosolic factor also inhibits GR activation, stabilizing the association between the unoccupied GR and the hsp90 dimer. This low molecular weight inhibitor has been termed 'modulator'[57] and proposed to be novel ether aminophosphoglycerides.[58] Other workers have however put forward the idea that this GR stabilizing factor is an endogenous metal anion[59] and glucocorticoid binding promotes the conversion of the GR to its DNA-binding through an effect on this metal anion centre. The metal anion stabilization site has been presumed to be located towards the carboxyl terminus of the steroid-binding domain.

Both sulphydryl and phosphate groups on the GR have been said to be involved in its ability to bind glucocorticoid. Sulphydryl groups are apparently involved in the trans-formation and activation processes of the GR complex by its ligand[60] and may also play a role in the association of the receptor with the nuclear matrix.[61] Different sulphydryl groups are said to be required for ligand binding and DNA binding. Silva and Cidlowski have provided evidence for the formation of both intramolecular disulphide bonds within the GR monomer as well as intermolecular disulphide bonds between the GR and another 40 kDa protein.[62] Formation of intramolecular disulphide bonds within a protein can affect its conformation, transforming it into a more folded globular form. On the other hand reduction of these bonds results in an unfolding of the protein, changing it into a more rod-like state. It is possible that the oxidation–reduction of disulphide bonds could play a role in the mechanism of GR activation to the DNA-binding form; only the reduced forms of the GR being able to bind DNA on exposure of the DNA-binding domain. NADPH-dependent thioredoxin reductase is thought to be responsible for maintaining the GR in a reduced state through thiol-disulphide exchange with thioredoxin.[63]

The GR has been detected in nearly all cell types, including cells from lungs and in inflammatory cells such as eosinophils, neutrophils, macrophages and lymphocytes. Human alveolar macrophages have been found to have on average 12×10^3 GRs per cell.[64] The gene for hGR is said to map to the distal long arm of chromosome 5, being assigned to 5q31–q32.[65] Successful efforts in cloning the hGR cDNA[66–68] led to the complete determination of its amino-acid sequence and have contributed to the understanding of its functional arrangement, revealing discrete sites of important functional domains. Work based on both the rat GR as well as the hGR indicates that the GR protein folds into three distinct functional domains separated by protease-sensitive regions, probably hinge regions within the protein.[69] The hGR consists of 777 amino acids and is made up of an immunogenic or modulatory domain spanning the amino acids 1–420, a central, highly conserved, DNA-binding domain, spanning amino acids 421–486 and a steroid-binding domain, not as precisely defined, but known to encompass a large portion of the receptor protein, and spanning amino acids 528–777. The modulatory domain is located near the amino-terminus ($-NH_2$) half of the molecule. Its precise function remains unknown but it may play a modulatory role in the normal regulation of gene expression by glucocorticoids. It may also enable the GR to differentiate between various target genes through protein–protein interactions with promoter-specific transcription factors.[70] Miesfeld favours the notion that it amplifies basal GR activity which is sometimes required in the induction of certain genes.[71] The glucocorticoid-binding domain is located towards the carboxyl terminus ($-COOH$) of the GR. In the absence of hormone ligand, this domain normally represses the activity of the GR. Hollenberg et al.[72] have provided evidence that the steroid-binding domain has two distinct regions responsible for the repression of GR function. The inhibitory effect of this domain may be mediated by the hsp90 dimer[51] that is now thought to bind to the GR at two independent sites residing within the steroid-binding domain.[50,59] The steroid-binding domain is emerging as a structurally and functionally complex region. Besides its ability to bind glucocorticoids, leading to derepression of the GR, it also seems to have a role to play in nuclear translocation and appears to modulate transactivation and to possess dimerization functions.[73] Hormone binding results in a conformational change probably centred on the hinge region between the steroid-binding and DNA-binding domains.[69] It is often stated that the affinity of binding between a particular glucocorticoid and its receptor is highly correlated with drug potency. However the number of GRs per cell may well also influence the degree of response.

The DNA-binding domain of the hGR spans 66 amino acids and includes two zinc 'fingers'. This domain has nine invariant cysteine residues which, except for the ninth (nearest COOH terminal) are all important for transcriptional activity and DNA-binding.[74] Amino-acid analysis shows that these cysteine residues occur as free thiols.[75] The existence of free thiol groups supports the zinc 'finger' hypothesis of DNA-binding by the GR. This hypothesis presupposes the formation of two zinc 'fingers'[76] each 'finger' having a zinc atom co-ordinated in a tetrahedral manner to four cysteines.[73,77,78] These 'fingers' are thought to be located towards the amino end of the DNA-binding domain. Other critical amino acids have also been localized in the first half of the interfinger region. The two zinc-binding sites of the GR, together with those of other steroid and thyroid receptors, represent a new structural motif for DNA binding and recognition of GREs. It has been suggested that activated GRs bind DNA and then quickly scan over the double helix in search of GREs. The GR is thought to bind to target genes which contain the highest number of GREs or those with 'better' quality GREs.[79] A model is being put forward in which a GR dimer contacts, by means of specific hydrogen bonding, two turns of the DNA double helix over a conserved 15-mer consensus sequence and, in addition, the two flanking turns by electrostatic sequence-independent binding.[80] GR dimer formation at the recognition site seems to enhance binding of the GR to GREs.[81] This binding brings about a change in chromatin structures at the GRE and alterations in the frequency of transcriptional initiation at the nearby promoter. Within minutes of adding glucocorticoid, nuclease-hypersensitive chromatin structures form at GREs, disappearing upon hormone withdrawal.[82] The 15-mer consensus sequence making up the GRE consists of two conserved blocks of six nucleotides each, separated by three non-conserved nucleotides: 5'-GGTACAnnnTGTTCT-3'.[80] The first zinc 'finger' (5' 'finger' or CI) and the region immediately following it appear to be involved in protein–DNA interactions and determine GRE binding specificity.[78,83] The second zinc 'finger' (3' 'finger' or CII) may contribute to non-specific DNA binding and may take part in DNA-binding domain dimerization, involving simple protein–protein interactions. The residues that are actually responsible for specific GRE binding are being said to reside not within the zinc 'finger' but in the root or 'knuckle' of the 'finger' and its immediate vicinity.[73] It has been suggested that two amino acids located between the distal two cysteines in the C-terminal half of the first 'finger' may be the primary determinant of sequence recognition; the rest of the DNA-binding domain will then normally confer structural information which may be necessary for impeding 'promiscuous' hormone-responsive element recognition.[84]

Although GR binding to GREs via its DNA-binding domain (nuclear localization) is an indispensable prerequisite, it does not appear to be sufficient for trans-activation.[73] The DNA-binding domain appears to contribute only a small fraction of the total trans-activation activity of the receptor. Additional trans-activation sites, also referred to as enhancement domains,[85] appear to be located outside the DNA-binding domain. Two such sites have been mapped out, one lying between the steroid- and DNA-binding domains, consisting of a 30 amino-acid peptide and another located in the modulatory domain, consisting of about 200 amino acids.[74] These trans-activation domains may be defined as protein regions which, when combined with a DNA-binding function, enhance productive transcriptional initiation by RNA polymerase II.[74,86] The two sequences mentioned are structurally unrelated and appear to have autonomous trans-activation properties although they probably communicate with each other.[85,87]

Findings from a number of gene transfer experiments indicate that the different GR domains are self-contained units which are modular in nature.[88] A precise spatial array of the different domains does not seem essential for their activity. It is generally being held that the DNA-binding domain serves mainly to position the trans-activation domain in the neighbourhood of a particular promoter. No transmission of information between this domain and other regions of the receptor is thought to be indispensable for trans-activation to occur. It is not yet known how the GR, correctly positioned on the right promoter, actually modulates transcriptional efficiency. It has been suggested that functional interactions with other essential transcriptional factors, perhaps stabilizing the formation of a transcription complex, may be required for this to happen.[89] A participation of chromatin structural features in the mechanism of glucocorticoid gene regulation has also been repeatedly put forward.[90] The binding of glucocorticoid to its receptor accelerates the kinetic parameters of the interaction between the GR and DNA.[91] Such an effect on the kinetics of DNA binding may facilitate the search for GRE sequences.[92]

It has been frequently implied that phosphorylation is involved in the regulation of GR functions but there is still some controversy about this.[93–95] It has been hypothesized that GRs traverse a glucocorticoid-driven phosphorylation–dephosphorylation cycle and it appears that both the GR and the hsp90 proteins are phosphorylated.[96,97] GR complexes appear to be associated *in vivo* with a number of small RNAs at both cytosolic and nuclear sites.[98] A number of possible functional roles for such an interaction have been put forward. These include control of GR transformation to the DNA-binding form, decrease of the ability of the activated GR to bind DNA,[99] as well as the release of GR from genes whose transcription has already been stimulated.[100] RNA association may also mark the GR for degradation.[99]

Glucocorticoids, besides influencing the transcription of specific genes, also appear to exert post-transcriptional effects which are said to result in enhanced processing, nucleocytoplasmic transport and stability of mRNA, as well as splicing of mRNA precursors and control of both protein maturation and secretion. Post-transcriptional glucocorticoid effects do not always need *de novo* protein synthesis. It has also been mentioned that such glucocorticoid post-transcriptional effects, as those controlling the splicing of mRNA precursors and protein translocation across the endoplasmic reticulum, may be partly mediated through an interaction of receptor complexes with small RNAs.[101]

The binding of the GR to GREs ultimately results in either induction or repression of specific gene regulatory networks.[39] Induction of transcription leads to *de novo* synthesis of mRNA which is finally translated by ribosomes into specific proteins. These resulting primary gene products probably influence such cellular functions as phosphorylation, proteolysis and perhaps even the transcriptional regulation of secondary target genes. All these finally lead to the phenotypic response which will of course vary between the different tissues.

Glucocorticoid-induced regulatory proteins

Lipocortins

Glucocorticoids, like other steroid hormones, control the rate of synthesis and also of release of a number of regulatory proteins, by interacting with their receptors. These regulatory proteins appear to inhibit eicosanoid release from arachidonic acid by inhibiting the activity of the enzyme phospholipase A_2 (PLA_2).[102,103] It had originally been shown that glucocorticoids prevented phospholipid deacylation and arachidonic acid release from stimulated cultured fibroblasts.[104] Evidence that glucocorticoid action on eicosanoid release was mediated via regulatory proteins was produced by four independent groups. These groups worked on guinea-pig lung, rat macrophages, rabbit neutrophils and rat cultured renomedullary cells. The regulatory proteins detected were termed 'macrocortin',[105] 'lipomodulin'[106] and 'renocortin'.[107] Further collaborative experiments between the different groups have established that the various proteins are functionally and immunologically identical entities, possibly fragments from a precursor molecule. These regulatory proteins are now known as lipocortins.[108] Two lipocortin genes have been cloned and expressed, both encode homologous 37 kDa proteins. Some *in vivo* studies have reported finding increased levels of mRNA lipocortin 1 following glucocorticoid treatment,[109] but others have failed to detect this.[110] Besides glucocorticoids, the presence of an as yet unidentified cofactor may also be required before the lipocortin 1 gene expression is induced,[111] and this could explain the contradictory findings.

Lipocortins have been purified from various organs and cells, including the lungs, which are an especially rich source, the kidneys, as well as from neutrophils, fibroblasts, macrophages, epithelial and smooth muscle cells.[112,113] In both rat and porcine lungs lipocortin 1 was detected in airway epithelium from nose to bronchioles, in vascular smooth muscle cells and in alveolar macrophages and polymorphonuclear leucocytes.[114] Human Type II alveolar cells, as well as human alveolar macrophages, were also recently shown to be able to produce lipocortin 1.[115,116] Workers from Bath have recently shown that fairly rapid changes in lipocortin 1 levels can occur *in vivo* in man following an intravenous bolus injection of 100 mg hydrocortisone.[117] The rise in lipocortin 1 levels was detected both intracellularly as well as on the cell surface of peripheral mononuclear cells. Increased lipocortin 1 levels have also been shown on the alveolar surface of the lung following glucocorticoid treatment in both normals[115] and in patients with idiopathic pulmonary fibrosis.[116] It has also been said that lipocortin 1 levels are positively correlated to circulating levels of endogenous glucocorticoids.[118]

Lipocortins are now thought to form part of a family of related calcium-dependent phospholipid membrane-binding proteins, sometimes referred to as annexins.[119] Members of this related group of proteins also include the chromobindins, calpactins, calelectrins, calcimedins, endonexins, and placental anticoagulant protein.[120] They appear to have distinct but as yet ill-defined biological functions. Lipocortins 1 and 2 as well as endonexin have been shown to display anti-PLA_2 activity *in vitro*. Besides its anti-PLA_2 activity, there is also *in vitro* evidence that lipocortin 1 inhibits cyclooxygenase synthesis.[121] Lipocortins differ from conventional calcium-binding proteins in that they lack an 'EF-hand' type calcium-binding site.[122] Lipocortin 1 seems to have four Ca^{2+}-binding sites. This group of proteins has been said to comprise at least eight different members, as may be inferred from cDNA sequence analysis, sharing approximately sequence identity.[123] The largest of these proteins, 67-kDa calelectrin contains eight repeats of a 70 amino-acid unit whilst the 38-kDa lipocortins consist of four copies of this unit. This 70 amino-acid consensus sequence is the most conserved between the various proteins. The repeated motifs fold to form a relatively protease-resistant core where the Ca^{2+} and phospholipid-binding sites are located.[124] Besides this C-terminal core domain, each protein has a unique amino terminal segment believed to be essential for its activity, for it appears to regulate binding affinities and to confer functional specificity.[120,125] This N-terminal domain is sensitive to phosphorylation and proteolysis. Lipocortins 1 and 2 each have an N-terminal segment consisting of 30 amino acids. Both lipocortins are highly polar molecules with about a third of their total number of amino acids being charged. The charged amino acids are distributed throughout the molecules, being separated by short stretches of hydrophobic residues. Significant communication appears to take place between the two domains making up the lipocortin molecules. The

N-terminal domain appears to regulate the Ca^{2+}/phospholipid-binding of the C-terminal core domain in a way specific for each lipocortin.

PLA$_2$ is an enzyme thought to play a pivotal role in the production of a whole cascade of pro-inflammatory eicosanoids by releasing arachidonic acid from phospholipids. There is also indirect evidence that it may also be involved in the formation of platelet-activating factor (PAF)-acether, as well as in histamine release from mast cells. The mechanism by which lipocortins may inhibit PLA$_2$ activity remains controversial. It has been thought that lipocortins antagonize the action of PLA$_2$ by binding themselves to it, thereby preventing it from cleaving arachidonic acid from membrane phospholipid stores. Some doubt has however been cast about the specificity of lipocortins as PLA$_2$ inhibitors. It has been suggested that lipocortins exert their anti-PLA$_2$ activity by 'substrate depletion'; through a coating of membrane phospholipids by lipocortins and not by direct interaction with the enzyme itself.[126–127] This hypothesis however fails to explain all the observed facts; thus lipocortins were inactive when tested against a phosphatidylcholine-specific PLA$_2$ derived from human platelets.[128] Residues 97–178 in the second repeat sequence of lipocortin 1 appear to be necessary for PLA$_2$ inhibition; this region is reported to be 70% homologous with the corresponding region in lipocortin 2. Lipocortins have been reported to exist in an active membrane form at high calcium concentrations ($>100\,\mu M$). The presence of Ca^{2+} is required for lipocortin 1 to inhibit eicosanoid synthesis.[102] Glucocorticoid treatment may result in the release of lipocortin into an extracellular milieu where the presence of a higher Ca^{2+} concentration may convert it into an active membrane-binding form. Localization of the lipocortin in cell membranes may allow it to interact with membrane phospholipids and PLA$_2$. The anti-inflammatory action of this regulatory protein may well be related to the intracellular Ca^{2+} concentration, the ratio of the membrane- and non-membrane-binding forms of lipocortin, the extracellular and intracellular concentrations of the protein, and finally its degree of phosphorylation. Phosphorylation interferes with the lipocortin inhibition of eicosanoid production. Lipocortins may be reversibly phosphorylated by tyrosine and serine–threonine kinases. There is also some recent evidence that neutrophil elastase is capable of degrading lipocortin 1 in a dose-dependent fashion.[115]

Certain lines of evidence point to the possibility that lipocortins may play an active role in modulating cell-membrane structure, acting in an opposite manner to that of mellitin or of a functionally related protein, phospholipase activating protein (PLAP).[129] PLAP, whose synthesis is increased by interleukin-1 (IL-I), tumour necrosis factor (TNF) and leukotriene D$_4$ (LTD$_4$), may convert inactive PLA$_2$ to its active form, perhaps through proteolytic activity or by competing for the same regulatory site on PLA$_2$ as lipocortin. The latter may exert a continuous inhibitory tone on PLA$_2$ activity *in vivo*.[102] On the other hand, some research workers have shown that the effects of glucocorticoids in inhibiting PLA$_2$ activity and eicosanoid synthesis may be independent of lipocortin. In a thymic epithelial cell line, dexamethasone decreased PLA$_2$ activity even in the absence of lipocortin 1, pointing to the possible existence of other lipocortin-independent anti-PLA$_2$ mechanisms.[130] A decrease in prostaglandin I$_2$ synthesis, without a detectable parallel increase in lipocortin 1 synthesis, was also shown in human endothelial cells following dexamethasone treatment.[131] In these endothelial cells dexamethasone failed to have any effect on phospholipid deacylation and therefore arachidonic acid liberation. However triacylglycerol concentration was increased. As it is known that triacylglycerol modulates intracellular arachidonic acid concentration, it has been suggested that glucocorticoids might induce the incorporation of arachidonic acid into this neutral lipid. Triacylglycerol might act as a temporary storage site for arachidonic acid when this is present in excess. The effects of glucocorticoids in inhibiting PLA_2 activity and eicosanoid synthesis may be independent of lipocortin.[132] Northup *et al.* have also reported that extracellular lipocortin 1 did not inhibit PLA_2 activity when applied to mouse peritoneal macrophages.[133] Similarly, although dexamethasone was shown to inhibit TNF-mediated cytotoxicity against fibrosarcoma cells, neither lipocortin 1 nor lipocortin 2 had any effects.[134]

These findings have cast some doubt as to the actual roles of lipocortins especially as the lipocortin 1 cDNA sequence does not predict a signal sequence, something expected for a secretory protein. These proteins are present in epithelial cells in concentrations as high as 0.1–0.5% of the total cell protein, suggesting that most of the endogenous lipocortin 1 is biologically inactive as a PLA_2 inhibitor, possibly because it is present in a phosphorlylated or non-calcium-bound form.[135] Lipocortin 1 may on the other hand be involved in a number of other, as yet undefined, physiological processes. Members of this group of regulatory proteins appear to be involved not only in the suppression of inflammation and the immune response but also in blood coagulation, exocytosis, membrane–cytoskeleton interactions as well as cell growth and differentiation.[120,136] Autoantibodies to lipocortin 1 have been detected in some asthmatic patients,[137] though other workers have failed to find any difference in lipocortin 1 autoantibody levels between asthmatics and normal control subjects.[138] The presence of these antibodies does not seem to be related to either severity or duration of asthma, to therapy or to the development of glucocorticoid resistance and their significance remains to be determined. Lipocortin 1 has been shown to inhibit the production of a number of mediators (Table 36.3) as well as to impair the chemotaxis and accumulation of neutrophils in an inflamed site in mice.[139] Most of the data have been derived from *in vitro* work and there is little *in vivo* evidence of lipocortin suppression of inflammatory mediators. Recently, nonapeptide fragments of lipocortin (antiflammins) have been shown to inhibit PLA_2 and PAF synthesis *in vitro* and to have anti-inflammatory effects *in vivo*.[140,141] Whilst lipocortin 1 appears to duplicate glucocorticoid action on carrageenin induced rat-paw oedema,[142] it has no effect on dextran, PAF, bradykinin or serotonin-induced oedema. Glucocorticoids block all these, indicating other possible mechanisms or regulatory proteins.

Table 36.3   Mediators shown to be blocked by lipocortin.

Mediator	System
Recombinant human lipocortin	
PGE$_2$	Human fibroblasts
PGI$_2$	Human endothelial cells
TXA$_2$	Isolated perfused guinea-pig lung
O$_2^-$	Guinea-pig alveolar macrophages
H$_2$O$_2$	Human neutrophils
PGD$_2$, LTC$_4$, serotonin	Rat basophilic leukaemia cells
Mouse lipocortin	
LTB$_4$, PAF	Rat neutrophils
PGE$_2$, LTB$_4$	*In vivo*, in subcutaneous area in mice

Vasoregulin and vasocortin

It is now recognized that lipocortins are not the only anti-inflammatory proteins induced by glucocorticoids. Vasoregulin, a 40-kDa protein, is an example of another anti-inflammatory protein induced in Namalva cells and mouse macrophages by dexamethasone, fluocinolone, prednisolone and hydrocortisone.[143,144] It seems to regulate vascular permeability directly without inhibiting eicosanoid formation and can block both carrageenin- and serotonin-induced paw oedema in mice (Table 36.4). The concentrations of glucocorticoids (10^{-6}–10^{-4} M) required for its induction were somewhat high. Vasoregulin was found to be easily inactivated by the superoxide radical. There is some evidence that glucocorticoids may induce vasoregulin not only directly but also indirectly by causing a rapid increase in ornithine decarboxylase which in turn forms the polyamines, spermine and spermidine. These polyamines may then act in some way as secondary mediators in the synthesis of vasoregulin.[144]

A further anti-inflammatory protein with an apparent molecular weight of 100 kDa has been shown to be released into the rat peritoneal cavity following systemic glucocorticoid administration.[145] This protein, named vasocortin, is distinct from lipocortins and unlike them inhibits dextran-induced oedema. Vasocortin-like proteins were also induced by dexamethasone in rat and bovine aorta rings[146] and selectively inhibit histamine release from rat peritoneal cells and mast cells induced by dextran or concanavalin A.[147,148] Induction of histamine release by compound 48/80 or calcium ionophore A23187 was not affected by vasocortin, thus mimicking the action of glucocorticoids.[149] The synthetic lipocortin nonapeptide fragments antiflammin 1 (His-Asp-Met-Asn-Lys-Val-Leu-Asp-Leu) and antiflammin 2 (Met-Gln-Met-Asn-Lys-Val-Leu-Asp-Leu) have been shown to have no effect on the early phase (1 h) of carrageenin-induced rat-paw oedema but to inhibit the late phase (3–4 h). In contrast vasocortin inhibits the early phase of this oedema but not the late phase. Combining vasocortin with either of the antiflammins resulted in a similar inhibitory profile to that obtained when dexamethasone was administered.[150] Antiflammins have also been shown to inhibit the synthesis of PAF, as well as neutrophil aggregation and chemotaxis.[141] Not surprisingly antiflammins are ineffective against dextran-induced oedema. It has been suggested that dextran-induced oedema as well as the early phase of carrageenin-induced oedema are mainly mediated by the release of histamine and 5-hydroxytryptamine (5-HT) whereas

Table 36.4 Effects of a number of agents on induced paw oedema in rats or mice.

	Carrageenin	Dextran	Histamine	5-HT	Bradykinin	PAF
Glucocorticoids	+	+	+	+	+	+
Lipocortins	+	−	−	−	−	−
Vasoregulin	+	?	+	+	+	?
Vasocortin	(early phase) +	+	?	?	?	?
Antiflammins 1 and 2	(late phase) +	−	?	?	?	?
Cu, Zn Super-oxide disumutase	?	?	+	+	+	?
Polyamines (spermidine, spermine)	+	?	+	+	+	?

+ = Inhibit; − = no effect; ? = not tested.

the late phase of carrageenin-induced oedema is mediated by pro-inflammatory eicosa-noids. It appears that vasocortin may suppress the release of histamine and 5-HT whilst antiflammins and the lipocortins inhibit the generation of eicosanoids.

Clara cell protein (CC10)

Human Clara cell 10-kDa protein is present exclusively in the non-ciliated cells of the surface epithelium of the pulmonary airways.[151] Expression of CC10 mRNA in the lung is said to be regulated by glucocorticoids.[152] This protein has been shown to inhibit pancreatic phospholipase A_2 and therefore could also possibly contribute to the regulation of inflammatory responses in the lung.

When lipocortin was discovered it was at first thought that this regulatory protein lay at the basis of all the anti-inflammatory actions of glucocorticoids. It is becoming increasingly obvious that such an explanation does not account for the wide range of glucocorticoid actions. However, these known glucocorticoid-induced proteins, and perhaps others yet to be discovered, do appear to have a role to play in modulating the inflammatory processes present in bronchial asthma.

Gene inhibition by glucocorticoids

The inhibitory actions of glucocorticoids on the various components of the inflammatory response and their modulatory effects on immunological mechanisms form the pharma-cological basis of their frequent therapeutic use in bronchial asthma. Some of these effects may be brought about by inhibition of expression of a number of genes. It is being increasingly realized that glucocorticoid-induced gene repression may be at least as important a mode of regulation as induction appears to be. It is not yet definitely established whether glucocorticoids induce and repress genes by similar mechanisms or whether different GR domains or dissimilar GREs are involved. Negative regulation by glucocorticoids seems to occur mainly, but not exclusively, at the transcriptional level. The GR may, like other steroid receptors, negatively regulate gene expression by interfering with the activity of other essential transcription factors or by competing with them for binding to their cognate DNA sequences.[79,80,153] It is interesting to note that many of the genes that glucocorticoids repress are induced by a cAMP-dependent mechanism. Repression may be brought about by interference with cAMP-responsive elements. Alternative mechanisms for steroid repression have also been proposed and include the existence of 'negative' GREs (nGRE).[154] Sequences that may function as nGREs have been tentatively identified for a number of genes whose transcription appears to be inhibited by glucocorticoids. Once bound to the nGRE, the GR may be structurally altered in such a way as to prevent it from inducing gene expression.[155,156] This would suggest that GREs and nGREs may act as allosteric ligands being able to change GR structure enabling it either to induce or inhibit transcription. Other data suggest that transcription inhibition is not necessarily mediated by the interaction of GR with DNA, since DNA-binding may not always be required. Oestrogen repression of the prolactin gene could be mediated by receptors which lacked the DNA-binding domain, though the degree of inhibition was not very marked.[157] A 63 amino-acid region immediately adjacent to the DNA-binding domain in the oestrogen receptor appears responsible for the inhibition of the prolactin gene expression. A comparable 45 amino-acid region of the GR was able to replace functionally the oestrogen receptor inhibitory region in a hybrid receptor. These two regions share only 45% homology but have similar hydrophilicity profiles and contain clusters of basic amino acids indicating that structural arrangements rather than primary amino-acid sequences may be the critical determinants of the negative regulatory actions of steroid receptors. Thus steroid receptors may regulate gene transcription in a positive or negative manner via different functional domains. Other workers have also postulated that it is a different form of the GR that interacts with nGREs.[158]

Glucocorticoids are known to inhibit the synthesis and release of a number of specific proteins that have pro-inflammatory activities such as interleukin-1 (IL-1) and interferon (IFNγ) (Table 36.5). These hormones have been shown to inhibit the transcription of both IL-1α and IL-1β genes leading to decreased levels of IL-1α and IL-β mRNA, as well as of the biologically active proteins.[159] Besides an inhibition of transcription, other workers have also shown that glucocorticoids bring about a decrease in stability of IL-1β mRNA.[160] In a monocyte cell line, dexamethasone was shown to block the transcription of IL-1 mRNA as well as post-transcriptional synthesis of IL-1, possibly by increasing cellular cAMP levels.[161] However, other workers using human blood monocytes have failed to detect any effect on LPS-induced IL-1β gene transcription and IL-1β mRNA accumulation on dexamethasone exposure. Low levels of IL-1 gene transcriptional activity normally present in unstimulated cells were also unaffected by dexamethasone. Dexamethasone is now considered to exert its effects on IL-1 production via post-transcriptional mechanisms, mainly through a moderate inhibition of translation of the IL-1β precursor and a more marked repression of the extracellular release of IL-1β.[162] Another LPS-induced cytokine, TNF, also appears to be negatively controlled by dexamethasone, mainly at a post-transcriptional level. However although translational derepression appears to be the predominant mode of glucocorticoid action,[163] some inhibition of TNF gene transcription also occurs.[164] Granulocyte–macrophage colony stimulating factor (GM-CSF) mRNA may also be similarly inhibited through a post-transcriptional mechanism[165] that may involve the induction or activation of a specific RNase which breaks down mRNAs.[166] Glucocorticoids are not the only agents that negatively affect gene expression. PGE$_2$ has also been shown to regulate macrophage-derived TNF gene transcription.[167] Glucocorticoids appear to lower mRNA levels not only for certain cytokines but also for their receptors, as in the case of IL-2.[168] IFNγ production is also reduced following dexamethasone because of a decrease in the level of its mRNA but the regulatory mechanism is as yet uncertain.[169] IL-6 is a potent pleiotropic cytokine which stimulates immunoglobulin production by

Table 36.5 Glucocorticoid inhibitory effects on gene expression.

POMC	GM-CSF
Prolactin	IFN-γ
Glucocorticoid receptor	TNFα
IL-1α and IL-1β	PLA$_2$
IL-2 receptor and IL-2	1a (Class II) antigens
IL-3	IgG
IL-6	Stromelysin
IL-8	Procollagen Type I

B-cells and is even more powerful than IL-1, with which it acts synergistically, in promoting T-cell growth and differentiation. Some workers have shown that in myeloma cells[170] and in human peripheral blood mononuclear cells,[171] glucocorticoids prevented IL-6 gene transcription. However, other workers have shown that dexamethasone could upregulate the number of IL-6 receptors on different human cell lines.[172]

The cytokines IL-1 and TNFα are known to release PLA_2 from a number of cell types, stimulating eicosanoid synthesis.[173] Both cytokines have been shown capable of increasing group II PLA_2 mRNA levels in rat vascular smooth muscle cells leading to enhanced secretion of the PLA_2 enzyme.[174] Downregulation of these polypeptide mediators may well be one of the ways by which these drugs reduce levels of arachidonic-acid derived pro-inflammatory mediators. The mechanism by which glucocorticoids exert an anti-PLA_2 effect is somewhat controversial. As has already been stated, it is uncertain at what level lipocortins actually exert their effect. In rat cultured smooth muscle cells dexamethasone was shown to inhibit the production of group II PLA_2 by blocking the accumulation of PLA_2-encoding mRNA as well as by inhibiting the post-transcriptional expression and release of this enzyme.[175] In endotoxin-treated rats dexamethasone administration also suppressed the accumulation of PLA_2-II mRNA in the tissues; this being reflected in an inhibition in the rise of plasma PLA_2 activity in these animals.[176] Such findings point to another possible mechanism of glucocorticoid-mediated PLA_2 suppression; that exerted through the negative regulation of the PLA_2 gene.

Glucocorticoid receptors are downregulated by their cognate ligand in a dose- and time-dependent manner by about 50–70%.[158] GR autoregulation has been shown to be receptor mediated, requiring a fully functional receptor for the process to occur. Downregulation of hGR mRNA has been shown in a number of different cell lines. The mechanisms underlying this physiological response have not been completely worked out but recent data suggest that the human glucocorticoid receptor contains intragenic regulatory sequences, potentially capable of functioning both transcriptionally and post-transcriptionally, sufficient for its own downregulation.[177] This GR autoregulation is thought to be the result of a reduction in both steady-state levels of GR mRNA[178] as well as in GR protein levels.[179] Thus glucocorticoids may regulate GR mRNA levels both by influencing gene transcription and also, perhaps, by decreasing receptor stability, thereby shortening its $t_{\frac{1}{2}}$.[180] The GR may be degraded by the ubiquitin-dependent proteolytic pathway.[181] Cellular GR concentration is known to be modulated by a number of other factors including cAMP and IL-1. cAMP, probably through the action of cAMP-dependent protein kinase, increases both the cellular amount of GR protein and glucocorticoid responsiveness. cAMP increases the stability of GR mRNA, increasing steady-state levels of GR mRNA by a post-transcription mechanism.[182] On the other hand, IL-1 has been shown to decrease cytosolic GR binding possibly as a result of diminishing cytosolic GR concentrations. IL-1 has been hypothesized to cause altered regulation of expression of the GR gene.[183] IL-1 and glucocorticoids also have opposite effects on the stromelysin gene, glucocorticoids repressing transcription. Stromelysin is involved in the extracellular matrix degradation present in such processes as wound healing and inflammation.

The inhibition of gene induction by glucocorticoids is a somewhat rapid process. Glucocorticoids produced a maximal inhibition rate of the pro-opiomelanocortin (POMC) gene within 20 min of their addition to cell cultures.[184] Of course, glucocorticoids, besides exerting a direct inhibitory effect on gene transcription, mRNA stability and processing, may inhibit mRNA transport and also alter the cell-membrane characteristics to interfere with secretion. The mechanisms by which the GR evokes opposite regulatory effects from specific DNA sequences still remain to be ultimately defined. Although playing a role, the DNA sequence does not appear to be the sole determinant of positive or negative regulation. The GR seems to bring about negative regulation by displacing or inactivating transcriptional enhancement induced by the binding of non-receptor stimulatory factors to the same GRE as that recognized by the GR. Recently, a new class of GRE has been proposed, a 'composite GRE' at which glucocorticoid regulation depends not only on DNA binding by the GR, but also on non-receptor factors with which the receptor interacts via protein–protein interactions. It is being suggested that composite GREs may well be the prevalent mode for regulation by glucocorticoids.[185] It is likely that there exists a threshold level of GR which is required for glucocorticoid-induced transcriptional responses.[186]

Glucocorticoid resistance

Resistance to the action of glucocorticoids in bronchial asthma has been variously defined in different studies making it hard to evaluate and compare findings.[187–189] It is now generally accepted that some asthmatics require larger than usual doses of glucorti-coids to bring their condition under control and a number appear not to respond at all to these drugs. Fortunately, such true glucocorticoid-resistant asthmatics seem to be few in number, although the frequency of glucocorticoid resistance in the normal population has been said to be around 15%.[190] The majority of these patients are mostly to be found amongst the older instrinsic asthmatics but younger extrinsic asthmatic patients have also been detected. This phenomenon although usually unremitting is, in some patients, said to be a transient occurrence lasting only a few months or years and then disappearing spontaneously. One of the earliest reports on glucocorticoid resistance in bronchial asthma is that of Schwartz et al. in 1968. They reported finding a markedly reduced eosinopenic effect following a single intravenous dose of 40 mg hydrocortisone in a group of six asthmatics who were relatively resistant to the effects of oral prednisone.[187] In a later study, glucocorticoid-resistant patients were reported to have had significantly greater airway hyperresponsiveness to metacholine as well as a longer duration of symptoms, more nocturnal wheeze and morning dipping and a more frequent family history of asthma than glucocorticoid-responsive asthmatics.[188] However, none of these features are particularly discriminatory. Over the years a number of mechanisms have been put forward in an attempt to explain this phenomenon. These have ranged from pharmacokinetic changes, such as an increase in plasma clearance, increased plasma protein binding, and impaired diffusion through defective cell membranes, to a decrease in the number of glucocorticoid receptors as well as possible dysfunction of the glucocorticoid–receptor complexes.[187] Glucocorticoid pharmacokinetics in glucocorticoid-resistant patients have, however, proved to be no different than in responsive patients or healthy volunteers.[189,191] Similarly it has been shown that glucocorticoid resistance cannot be explained on the basis of reduced glucocorticoid-receptor numbers or abnormalities in receptor characteristics.[189] Glucocorticoid administration in vivo failed to reduce complement receptor expression (C3b) in monocytes obtained from glucocorticoid-resistant asthmatics.[192] Moreover, in later studies from the same group, it was shown that there was a quantitative relationship between the glucocorticoid responsiveness of colony growth of peripheral blood mononuclear cells (PMBC) *in vitro* and the improvement in FEV_1 following the daily administration of 20 mg prednisolone for a week.[193] T_4- and T_8-lymphocyte colony growth was not inhibited by methylprednisolone when these were co-cultured with monocytes derived from glucocorticoid-resistant patients.[194] These studies point to the existence of a defect in monocyte responsiveness in these patients. This is of obvious importance as macrophages are now thought to be activated in late-phase reactions.

It might be expected that glucocorticoids will fail to inhibit the release of cytokines, such as IL-1, from defective macrophages, allowing activated T lymphocytes to proliferate. Dexamethasone has also failed to inhibit the production of IL-2 and IFNγ from lymphocytes derived from glucocorticoid-resistant asthmatics. Recent work has shown that PMBCs derived from asthmatics produced a 3-kDa peptide that augments neutrophil generation of leukotriene B_4 and superoxide anion when stimulated by the calcium ionophore (A23187) and phorbol myristate acetate respectively.[195] Glucocorticoids suppressed the *in vitro* production of this factor in sensitive asthmatics but not in glucocorticoid-resistant patients.[189] Furthermore no significant differences were detected in values for the dissociation constant for dexamethasone receptor density in monocytes derived from glucocorticoid-resistant or -sensitive asthmatics. This would seem to imply that the mechanism underlying glucocorticoid resistance is to be looked for amongst the post GR-ligand binding events within the monocytes, perhaps at the level of the GREs. Other workers have, however, shown that although no difference in GR numbers could be detected in PBMCs from glucocorticoid-resistant and -sensitive asthmatics, those GRs from resistant patients showed a lower glucocorticoid affinity.[196]

A rare form of inherited primary cortisol resistance was first described in 1976. Cells from these patients showed decreased levels of GR mRNA resulting in a low GR concentration.[197] Other defects reported from different studies have included a decreased affinity in GR binding to its ligand[198] and a decrease in the binding of the GR complex to DNA.[199] In none of the patients with primary cortisol resistance so far studied has bronchial asthma been reported. The mechanism(s) underlying the cellular basis of glucocorticoid resistance in asthmatics is still somewhat obscure. As with a number of other pharmacological agents there is probably a whole spectrum of responsiveness to the action of these drugs. It is important, for obvious reasons, to be able to identify in an easy and reliable manner those asthmatics who are glucocorticoid-resistant. In these patients it may be worth trying oral betamethasone or a parenteral glucocorticoid such as triamcinolone acetonide. These have sometimes been shown to work.[200,201]

MECHANISMS OF ACTION

Anti-inflammatory effect of glucocorticoids

In 1819, Laennec attributed asthma to a contraction of the bronchial smooth muscle fibres,[202] and for a long time it was simply equated with bronchospasm whilst workers

Table 36.6 Glucocorticoid effects on inflammatory cell migration-enhancing factors.

Mediator	Source	Drug effect
PAF-acether	Alveolar macrophages, eosinophils, neutrophils platelets, vascular endothelium	Formation and release of 2-lyso-PAF inhibited
LTB_4	Neutrophils, basophils macrophages, airway epithelium, vascular endothelium	Formation blocked through inhibition of PLA_2 activity
Complement-derived factors, e.g. C5a	Activation of complement system in plasma	Binding of C5a to cell surface blocked. Effect on granulocyte surface charge inhibited
15-HETE	Eosinophils, airway epithelial cells	Formation blocked
PGE_2	Eosinophils, vascular endothelium, epithelium, macrophages	Formation blocked
Thromboxane B_2	Alveolar macrophages	Production inhibited
Histamine	Mast cells. Basophils	No effect. Exocytosis suppressed. H_1-receptor function suppressed
Cytokines		
Interleukin-1	Macrophages, monocytes	Production suppressed. Secretion inhibited
Interleukin-2	T-lymphocytes	Synthesis blocked but no effect on its action
Interleukin-8	Monocytes, T-lymphocytes, fibroblasts, endothelial cells	Inhibit production at pretranslational level
Interferon (IFNγ, macrophage-activating factor)	Alveolar macrophages, T-lymphocytes	Formation inhibited
GM-CSF	T-lymphocytes, macrophages, fibroblasts, endothelial cells, mast cells	Production inhibited

looked for mediators that could cause this phenomenon. The pathophysiological features of asthma have since become better appreciated, although perhaps not yet ultimately defined.[204–207] Inflammation is now generally recognized to be a basic pathological feature of asthma arising as the result of the synergized activity of various primary effector cells in releasing a bewildering spectrum of mediators which directly and through their interactions are capable of further recruiting secondary effector cells responsible for amplifying the inflammatory process (Table 36.6). The therapeutic success of glucocorticoids in the control of the asthmatic state is being increasingly ascribed to their actions on the various components of the inflammatory process. There is no consensus as to which particular inflammatory cells or which released mediators are specifically involved in particular pathological features of asthma. Although mast-cell activation appears to be of importance in the acute responses to allergens and possibly to exercise, it is uncertain whether this cell has any role to play in chronic asthma or airway hyperresponsiveness.

Of the cells involved in inflammatory processes, the eosinophils, monocytes and macrophages are amongst the most glucocorticoid-sensitive cells, whilst the neutrophils, and even more so the mast cells, are the least sensitive to the action of these drugs (Table 36.7). The role of the neutrophils in human asthma remains unclear and they may only be involved in some types of occupational asthma. Similarly there is little evidence proving basophil participation in the inflammatory processes of asthma. However it has been shown recently that histamine-containing cells, recovered in bronchoalveolar lavage (BAL) fluid obtained during the late-phase response to allergen, were baso-phils.[208] Whilst platelets may contribute to such processes, it remains controversial whether they can migrate from blood. They have been detected in BAL fluid together with activated T-lymphocytes and macrophages, 24 h after PAF inhalation.[209] T-lymphocytes are emerging amongst the key players. Not only do they have an important role in organizing the cellular composition of the inflammatory cell infiltrate in the airways, but they are also important in the induction of IgE-dependent responses. Recruited inflammatory cells tend to be somewhat short lived and perhaps it is the resident tissue cells themselves that perpetuate the chronic inflammatory response. The vascular endothelium and the respiratory epithelium are assuming fundamental roles in mediating and modulating the pro-inflammatory activities of a whole array of mediators, being strategically positioned at key interfaces.

Microvascular leakage is a recognized feature of asthma which may lead to submuco-sal oedema.[210] This oedema could contribute to epithelial sloughing, impairment of mucociliary transport, airway narrowing, mucus plug formation and ultimately to hyperresponsiveness. Glucocorticoids can suppress protein leakage through their inhibi-tory actions on various mediators (Table 36.8) as well as by dampening the response of the endothelium to the action of these mediators. Mediators increasing the blood flow of the microcirculation of the lung obviously contribute to protein extravasation via this mechanism. Some mediators may increase leakage both through a direct action on endothelial cells, by opening up postvenular intercellular gap junctions, and indirectly by increasing blood flow. Glucocorticoids exert an effect at this level too (Table 36.9). Besides inhibiting the formation and/or secretion of these mediators, glucocorticoids are also thought to inhibit postcapillary venule endothelial cell separation via a direct action on the endothelial cells.[211,212] These drugs are also able to decrease the excessive respiratory mucus glycoprotein secretion seen in asthma (Table 36.10). Such an effect may be the result of an inhibition of the secretory process and not a reduction in glycoprotein synthesis.[213]

Amongst the many mediators involved in the asthmatic process the ones that are fast emerging as having pivotal roles are the pleotropic cytokines. They are capable of eliciting a complex set of changes in the properties and functions of both resident and recruited cells, thereby initiating and maintaining the inflammatory process, interacting with a host of other mediators. The ability of the glucocorticoids to inhibit the synthesis and/or release of a number of these cytokines (Table 36.5), and sometimes of their receptors as well, appears to be of fundamental importance in the way these drugs exert their antiasthma activities. However the actions of various cytokines are often not

Table 36.7 Effects of glucocorticoids on the various cell components of airway inflammation (besides the reduction in release of mediators and blunting of their effects).

Cell	Drug effect
Primary effector systems	
Alveolar macrophages	Migration to inflammatory site inhibited IgG and complement receptors decreased Induction of Ia antigens necessary for antigen presentation inhibited
Epithelial cells	Increase in permeability reduced Promotion of repair and ciliogenesis
Endothelial cells	Inhibit Class II MHC (Ia) antigen expression Inhibit transendothelial migration *in vitro* Do not prevent expression of surface adherence glycoproteins
Mast cells	Inhibit proliferation of mucosal type of mast cells probably by inhibition of growth factors (IL-3, IL-4, GM-CSF) May decrease histamine content
Basophils	Reduce number of circulating cells selectively, decreasing mainly lower density basophil subtype Local influx to tissue site inhibited Response to immunological stimuli blunted
Secondary recruited effector systems	
Eosinophils	Marked eosinopenia resulting from a reduction in proliferation and differentiation of progenitors, probably through an inhibitory effect of the release of growth factors (e.g. GM-CSF, IL-3, IL-5) Reduction of influx at inflammatory site probably as a result in fall in circulating numbers, reduction of local chemotactic factors, possible inhibition of eosinophil chemotaxis and diapedesis and decreased adherence to endothelium Inhibition of priming and conversion to hypodense phenotype probably by inhibiting release of cytokines (e.g. IL-3, GM-CSF) and other mediators (histamine, PAF) and possibly also by a direct effect on the cells themselves *In vitro* inhibition of degranulation and of superoxide production Decrease in serum ECP levels. Reduction in MBP and ECP levels in nasal lavage fluid Reduction of complement receptors
Monocytes	Marked monocytopenia, especially those bearing the $Fc_\gamma R$, as a result of reduced bone marrow release and a redistribution to extra vascular pool Migration inhibited
Lymphocytes	Transient lymphocytopenia resulting from decreased bone marrow production and release, with a redistribution to extravascular compartments Inhibition of T-lymphocyte proliferation, mainly the helper (CD_4^+) subset, probably by decreasing IL-2 production and inhibiting expression of IL-2 receptors on T-lymphocytes Communications between lymphocytes and cells of the monocyte/macrophage system disrupted by inhibiting release of IL-1 and IFNγ

Table 36.7 Continued.

Cell	Drug effect
Secondary recruited effector systems (continued)	
Lymphocytes	Early events in B-cell cycle (activation, proliferation) may be modulated but no effect on differentiation to immunoglobulin producing state
Neutrophils	Transient neutrophil leucocytosis resulting from an increased bone marrow release, increased recovery from marginated pool and diminished rate of removal
	Some reduction in adherence to inflamed endothelium, possibly by affecting CR3 (adherence molecules) numbers
	Accumulation at inflammatory site inhibited by blocking the release of recruitment factors (PAF, LTB$_4$, IL-1) and possibly by inhibiting diapedesis
	Inhibition of primary factors (e.g. IFN-γ, GM-CSF) and possibly also the priming response
	Activation of such neutrophil responses *in vitro* as chemotactic ability, release of lysosomal enzymes or arachidonate metabolites is not diminished
Platelets	Platelet kinetics normalized

inhibited by glucocorticoids even when these are given in high dosage. Of the many cytokines that may be involved in the inflammatory process, IL-1 is emerging as a key mediator. Together with TNF it exerts important effects on the tissue microenvironment, regulating the recruitment of leukocytes at inflammatory sites. IL-1 and TNF can modulate the process of extravasation and localization of leucocytes at these sites, involving the adhesion and passage through endothelial linings in response to tissue-derived signals. GM-CSF may be produced by respiratory epithelial cells[214] and is known to prolong survival of human eosinophils *in vitro* and to augment eicosanoid mediator release. Glucocorticoids, by blocking the synthesis and/or release of these cytokines, are able to exert powerful anti-inflammatory actions. In spite of considerable *in vitro* data showing glucocorticoid inhibitory action on the release of various mediators, there is very little direct evidence in man that these drugs affect mediator release *in vivo*.[215,216]

Although there is little direct evidence indicating the sort of contribution neurogenic inflammation makes in human airway disease, neurogenic mechanisms may amplify inflammatory processes present in asthmatic airways through the release of a number of neuropeptides from sensory nerves. A membrane-associated enzyme, neutral metalloendopeptidase (NEP), is now known to modulate the actions of neuropeptides by being able to cleave them both at the sites of their release, as well as at the sites of their actions. NEP is present in the plasma membrane of several types of cells present in the airways and besides cleaving tachykinins is also able to cleave bradykinin. Kininase II (ACE) is another tachykinin-degrading enzyme whose expression may also be increased by glucocorticoids.[217] NEP activity can be decreased by viral infections, O$_2$ free radicals and air pollutants, including cigarette smoke. It can be upregulated by glucocorticoids because the latter have been shown to increase gene expression of NEP.[218] Glucocorticoids may thus also modulate the effects of neurogenic inflammation. The tachykinin-

Table 36.8 Glucocorticoid effects on some mediators increasing microvascular leakiness in lung blood vessels.

Mediator	Source	Drug effect
Direct action permeability-increasing mediators (response immediate)		
LTC$_4$, LTD$_4$, LTE$_4$	Eosinophils, macrophages, basophils	Secretion inhibited, formation blocked through anti-PLA$_2$ action
PAF-acether	Alveolar macrophages, eosinophils, neutrophils, platelets, vascular endothelium	Formation and release of 2-lyso-PAF (PAF precursor) inhibited
PGE$_1$	Vascular endothelium, eosinophils	Formation inhibited
PGD$_2$	Mast cells	No effect
	Macrophages, platelets	Possibly, formation blocked
Thromboxane B$_2$	Alveolar macrophages	Production inhibited
Bradykinins	Plasma (via kininogenases activity released from various cells)	Formation inhibited
Histamine	Mast cells	No effect
	Basophils	Release inhibited
O$_2$-derived free radicals	Activated macrophages eosinophils, neutrophils	Formation suppressed
Neutrophil-dependent mediators (response delayed)		
Complement-derived factors (C3$_a$, C5$_a$)	Complement system in plasma	Binding to leucocytes blocked
LTB$_4$ (not yet shown in airways)	Alveolar macrophages neutrophils, airway epithelium	Formation blocked

degrading enzymes NEP and ACE appear to mediate a selective inhibitory effect of glucocorticoids on neurogenic-induced plasma extravasation.[219]

Effect on the late-phase response and airway hyperresponsiveness

Airway hyperresponsiveness (AHR) to many different stimuli is now widely accepted as being a cardinal feature of bronchial asthma and has been reported to be closely related to the frequency of attacks and the severity of asthma, as well as the need for treatment. The precise underlying mechanisms remain to be defined, although a number of possible hypotheses have been put forward. AHR was initially reported to occur only if exposure to a provoking agent had previously induced a late asthmatic response. AHR has however also recently been detected before the development of a late response.[220,221] In some patients AHR has actually been observed to occur in the absence of a late-phase response. It is now becoming apparent that whilst the allergen-provoked late asthmatic response and AHR may develop in parallel, they seem to have different underlying

Table 36.9 Glucocorticoid effects on some mediators increasing blood flow of the microcirculation of the lung.

Mediator	Source	Drug effect
PGE_1, PGE_2	Eosinophils, vascular endothelium, central airway smooth muscle, epithelium	Formation blocked through inhibition of PLA_2
PGD_2	Mast cells Macrophages, platelets	No direct effect Formation blocked
PGI_2	Vascular endothelium, airway epithelium	Formation blocked
Bradykinins	Exuded plasma (kininogenases e.g. tryptase, released from mast cells, basophils, neutrophils and present in plasma)	Formation inhibited Inhibition of PLA_2 and PLC (known to be activated by BK)
Histamine	Mast cells Basophils	No direct effect Exocytosis suppressed H_1-receptor function suppressed
O_2-derived free radicals, e.g. super-oxide ion $(.O_2^-,)$ singlet oxygen $(^1O_2)$	Activated alveolar macrophages, eosinophils, neutrophils	Formation suppressed

Table 36.10 Glucocorticoid effects on some mediators increasing mucus secretion and impairing mucociliary clearance.

Mediator	Source	Drug effect
Mono-HETEs (5, 11, 12, 15-HETE)	Airway epithelium, eosinophils, alveolar macrophages	Formation blocked through anti-PLA_2 activity
LTC_4, LTD_4, LTE_4	Eosinophils, basophils, macrophages, monocytes Mast cells	Formation blocked No effect
PGD_2, $PGF_{2\alpha}$	Macrophages, platelets Mast cells	Formation blocked No effect
Histamine	Mast cells Basophils	No effect Release inhibited
PAF-acether	Macrophages, eosinophils, neutrophils, basophils, platelets, vascular endothelium	Formation and release of 2-lyso-PAF inhibited
O_2-derived free radicals	Activated eosinophils, macrophages, neutrophils	Formation suppressed

Table 36.11   Effect of glucocorticoids on airway hyperresponsiveness.

Drug	Challenge	
	Cholinergic agent	Histamine
Oral cortisone	O	
Oral prednisolone	O	
Oral prednisolone	—	
Oral methylprednisolone	—	
Inhaled BDP	—	—
Inhaled Budesonide	—	—

O = No effect; — = reduced hyperresponsiveness.

mechanisms. It has been known for a long time that glucocorticoids, given either orally in high doses or by inhalation, are able to block very effectively the development of the late response as well as the associated AHR.[222–224] There are also indications that if these drugs are given over an adequate period of time prior to challenge they may likewise affect the immediate response to allergen and exercise, possibly by depletion of mucosal mast cells, perhaps through a reduction of cytokine secretion (e.g. IL-3). Prednisone has also been shown to inhibit the early increase in AHR that occurs soon after the early asthmatic response in a number of dual responders.[225]

A 'special' type of inflammatory response is thought to underlie the pathogenesis of AHR,[226] although other factors may also be operative.[227,228] It is likely that complex interactions between sensory nerves and a whole array of cells, releasing a cascade of mediators, are responsible for the development of AHR; with eosinophils, macrophages and lymphocytes playing key roles against a background of damaged epithelium. The exact relationship between airway inflammation, AHR and asthmatic symptoms still needs to be unravelled. This inflammation may, at times, appear to be associated with symptoms that are responsive to glucocorticoid therapy without there being an increase in AHR or airflow obstruction.[229] AHR is probably as episodic and variable as other clinical and physiological asthmatic features. Although AHR to histamine or metacholine has been said to correlate closely with the presence and degree of diurnal variation of peak expiratory flow rates, asthmatic symptoms need not always be closely related to the degree of AHR.[230] The degree of airway inflammation, as shown by the presence and activity of a number of airway cells in BAL fluid, has been shown by some workers to bear a relationship to the levels of AHR, but not to the severity of asthmatic symptoms. More detailed studies have failed to detect significant correlations between cellular events in the bronchial mucosa and asthmatic symptom scores and AHR.[231] The latter group of workers have, however, obtained direct evidence of an anti-inflammatory effect of inhaled BDP in atopic asthma, relating clinical improvement to reductions in eosinophils and mast cells in the epithelium and submucosa and also to a decrease in AHR.[232] In another study, in which no relationship could be established between the degree of AHR and total or differential cell numbers in BAL fluid, inhaled budesonide failed to decrease significantly eosinophil numbers but reduced the concentration of eosinophil cationic protein.[233] Data acquired from bronchoscopic studies in asthmatics appear beset with difficulties, especially because there are problems in quantifying the condition, and they require careful interpretation.

Some early studies appeared to show a lack of protective effect of glucocorticoids on AHR following cholinergic challenge, irrespective of the route of administration. In some of these studies the doses used were apparently too low.[234] In one report, 4 months' treatment with inhaled BDP did not produce any change in AHR,[235] however the PC_{20} values obtained had not been log-transformed prior to their analysis. A later re-analysis of the data using log-transformed PD_{20} FEV_1 values did actually show an improvement in AHR.[236] Glucocorticoids are perhaps the most important therapeutic agents currently available for preventing and modifying AHR. Inhaled glucocorticoids appear to be more effective in reducing AHR than when they are orally administered.[237,238] There does not appear to be a clear relationship between measured changes in airflow obstruction (e.g. FEV_1) and in AHR (PC_{20} values). Following inhaled glucocorticoids PC_{20} values have been shown to change independently of changes in FEV_1, indicating that improvement in AHR is not simply the result of a change in airway calibre.[239,240] AHR may persist after FEV_1 values have returned to pre-challenge baseline levels. Occasionally, during treatment with glucocorticoids, patients may become symptom-free although they still remain hyperresponsive.[240] On the other hand, in patients undergoing glucocorticoid withdrawal, asthmatic symptoms have been reported to precede increases in AHR and changes in airway function.[241,242] Glucocorticoids not infrequently produce a dramatic reduction in asthmatic symptoms with only a small effect on AHR. Whilst these drugs are highly effective in inhibiting allergen-induced AHR, their effect on basal AHR is much more modest. Frequently, maximum reduction in AHR may only be achieved after months of inhaled therapy,[243] not infrequently the normal range is not attained, even after high doses of glucocorticoids. The improvement in AHR following glucocorticoid treatment appears to be not only time- but also dose-dependent.[240,244] However, some workers have shown that this is not always so.[236,245] A difference in the type and severity of the condition of patients studied could perhaps explain the different results. In one of the few double-blind, randomized, controlled, prolonged (1-year) trials, inhaled budesonide produced a four-fold mean improvement in AHR in non-steroid-dependent asthmatics when compared with those receiving a placebo. Maximum response occurred during the first 3 months but some were still improving slowly after 1 year; just under a third of the patients achieved the normal range. The majority of patients became asymptomatic.[246] Similar results were obtained by the same workers in a group of more severe steroid-dependent asthmatics.[247] A wide individual variation in the degree, as well as in the rate, of improvement in AHR is often seen both in the short term, as well as in the more prolonged trials with glucocorticoids.

There are also differences reported in the duration of effects on AHR once glucocorticoid treatment is reduced or stopped altogether. The Canadian group reported that their patients who had been treated for a whole year maintained their improvement for about 3 months on reduced glucocorticoid use. Symptoms, mainly increased sputum production, preceded increases in AHR. Treatment for shorter periods of time have resulted in earlier deterioration in AHR when glucocorticoids were stopped.[248,249] In children treated for a 2-month period with inhaled budesonide, the protective effect was reported to wear off rapidly once treatment was discontinued.[250]

Glucocorticoids have been repeatedly shown to reduce AHR that had been induced both by directly acting spasmogens (e.g. histamine) as well as by indirect challenges (e.g. exercise, eucapnic dry air hyperventilation, bradykinin).[251,252] This protection, afforded against both direct spasmogens, as well as indirect agents operating through airway nerves and released mediators, argues in favour of action at a central site. This site has been variously suggested to be the airway smooth muscle or the airway wall. It has been suggested that perhaps glucocorticoid action on AHR could be explained by their anti-inflammatory effects on the microenvironment of airway smooth muscle. Events taking place in this microenvironment, probably as a result of microvascular leakage, could possibly lead to the development of hyperreactive airway smooth muscle *in vivo*, in spite of the fact that various *in vitro* studies have failed to detect any intrinsic abnormalities in airway smooth muscle.[253,254] Of course, the increased submucosal oedema *per se*, present in asthmatic airways, may also be the explanation for the underlying AHR. Glucocorticoids probably act directly on endothelial cells in post-capillary venules, inhibiting their separation, thus preventing microvascular leakage.[255]

The relationship between inflammation, as reflected by inflammatory cell numbers, and AHR remains difficult to define. A follow-up of six severe asthmatics, treated daily with inhaled glucocorticoids for 10 years, showed that all patients still had a degree of AHR in spite of biopsy evidence of suppression of inflammation. The increase in AHR could perhaps be explained by the fact that four of the patients still showed epithelial changes, with reduced numbers of ciliated cells, in spite of 10 years' treatment.[256] Overall, there is a strong body of evidence showing that inhaled glucocorticoids can bring about a marked improvement in AHR.

Effects on airway smooth muscle

Glucocorticoids are said to relax airway smooth muscle both directly and via the potentiation of β_2-adrenoreceptor mediation. The direct relaxing effects reported in earlier studies may well have been due to the paraben preservatives present in the drug preparations,[257] and there is no real evidence to support the view that glucocorticoids have a direct relaxant effect on airway smooth muscle. It has recently been shown that a 24-h exposure to dexamethasone inhibited an antigen-induced contractile response of sensitized guinea-pig tracheal ring preparations without altering the response of this tissue to either metacholine or histamine. Such an inhibition was probably the result of a reduced release of inflammatory mediators occurring post-antigen challenge.[258] Pre-treatment with glucocorticoids has attenuated sensitization-induced changes of airway smooth muscle (ASM) cells and also inhibited both the contractile and the electrical responses of these cells to antigen challenge.[259] The duration of exposure of ASM cells to glucocorticoids appeared critical and more important than the actual concentration of the drugs. It has been suggested that glucocorticoid pretreatment attenuates sensitization-induced sodium and calcium influx into ASM cells, thereby preventing changes in the membrane properties of ASM cells. Alternatively glucocorticoids could also interfere with the occupancy of Fc receptors which may be present on the surface of ASM cells. The opening of both sodium and calcium channels has been said to result from the aggregation of Fc receptors. In rabbit ASM methylprednisolone has been shown to potentiate the electrogenic Na^+–K^+ pump.[260] Asthmatic ASM, for as yet undefined reasons, has been shown to have a greater maximal response to contractile agonists, as well as impaired relaxation to β-adrenoreceptor agonists.[261,262] A cellular defect in β-adrenoreceptor function in asthma may perhaps be located at the level of stimulus–receptor coupling. Possibly, inflammatory mediators, by stimulating phosphoinositide (PI) hydrolysis may lead to the downregulation and uncoupling of β-adrenoreceptors from the G_s protein in ASM.[263] This effect on receptors could occur as a result of protein kinase C activation in response to diacylglycerol derived from PI metabolism.[264,265] Glucocorticoids could prevent and reverse such a downregulation and uncoupling of receptors.[266,267] Phospholiphase A_2 also appears to have a role to play in β-adrenoreceptor dysfunction.[268] Hydroperoxyeicosatetraenoic acids (HPETEs) are shown to reduce β-adrenoreceptor binding sites and function in the lung. These cyclo-oxygenase products may also induce uncoupling of the receptor and adenylate cyclase by promoting the phosphorylation of the receptor. Glucocorticoids could exert an effect at this level as well. These drugs have been shown to increase β-adrenoreceptor mRNA levels dramatically a few hours after hamster ASM cells were exposed to them.[269] In cultured human lung cells, induction of new receptors has been reported to occur within 12 h of exposure.[270,271] Besides an increase in β-adrenoreceptor mRNA levels, glucocorticoids also induce the expression of mRNA for both G protein α-[272] and β-subunits.[273] Prolonged β-adrenergic agonist administration may result in subsensitivity as a result of both downregulation and uncoupling of the receptor from the adenyl cyclase system, though whether this subsensitivity is ever important clinically is controversial. Although both *in vitro* and *in vivo* studies clearly show that β_2-adrenoreceptor subsensitivity can be reversed by glucocorticoids, this mode of action does not seem to be particularly significant in the average asthmatic needing these drugs. It may, however, be clinically relevant in a subset of patients in whom subsensitivity to β-agonists may develop.[274] Perhaps a more important effect of glucocorticoids on smooth muscle is their ability to block the formation and/or the release of a number of mediators with smooth muscle constricting properties. Many inflammatory mediators, spasmogens and possibly tachykinins induce PI hydrolysis, leading to impaired β-adrenergic receptor function. Glucocorticoids may exert a positive effect on ASM through their ability to block the formation and/or the release of a number of these mediators.

CHANGES IN RESPIRATORY PHYSIOLOGY INDUCED BY GLUCOCORTICOIDS

Walsh and Grant[275] were the first to introduce the idea of a trial with these drugs in asthma in order to determine responsiveness. The first objective study reporting improvement in lung function appeared in 1971.[276] Further studies soon followed, both from the same group from Edinburgh and Malta[277–279] and from other workers.[280] The acute effects of glucocorticoids in bronchial asthma have been reviewed more recently.[281] The administration of these drugs to chronic asthmatic patients resulted in significant improvement in measurements of dynamic and static lung volumes, body plethysmography and flow–volume curves.[277–279] In a group of adult chronic asthmatics, oral prednisolone resulted in both an improvement in airflow and a concomitant increase in arterial oxygen tension.[282] In contrast, in adult acute asthma, the relief of arterial hypoxaemia appeared to lag behind changes in airflow obstruction.[283] Studies in severely asthmatic children have shown, however, that the addition of glucocorticoids to their therapeutic regimen produced a significant increase in arterial oxygen tension with little change in the rate and degree of improvement in the forced expiratory volume in 1 s

(FEV_1),[284] perhaps suggesting that changes were occurring predominantly in the peripheral airways.

Objective evidence of the usefulness of intravenous hydrocortisone in improving the FEV_1 in acutely asthmatic patients has been provided by a well-controlled clinical trial.[283] A later study comparing the effect of intravenous administration of hydrocortisone, methylprednisolone and dexamethasone in patients with acute asthma has confirmed the improvement in FEV_1 brought about, in a similar fashion, by all three glucocorticoids.[285] The dose that is required to reverse the acute asthmatic state is a matter of some controversy, and there are advocates for low, moderate and high doses of glucocorticoids. Studies have shown that there are no marked advantages in using very high doses in treating severe asthma. This holds true both for children[286] and for adults.[287] There are also claims that intravenous glucocorticoids may not always be required in treating patients with severe asthma.[288] Such claims have not been confirmed and such treatment should not be recommended.

The possible need for the *de novo* synthesis of proteins as the lipocortins and/or the repressive effect on the genetic transcription of certain mediators, explains the observed time lag between the administration of glucocorticoids and the onset of most of their physiological actions. The time taken by glucocorticoids to work in acute asthma is, perhaps understandably, longer. In a number of studies, the time taken for a detectable effect on pulmonary function was at least 6 h and sometimes longer,[24,283,285] and a maximum improvement might require as long as 6 days to occur.[289] Such a difference in time lag between the action of glucocorticoids in the acute and chronic states of the asthmatic condition is probably due to differences in the pathophysiology underlying the two states. In spite of a better understanding of the pathophysiological mechanisms underlying asthma, mortality trends for the condition are a cause for growing concern. The safety in using inhaled glucocorticoids and their widespread anti-inflammatory actions should advocate an earlier employment of these drugs in the treatment regimen of asthma.

REFERENCES

1. Solis-Cohen S: The use of adrenal substance in the treatment of asthma. *JAMA* (1900) **34**: 1164–1166.
2. Clark THJ: Effect of beclomethasone dipropionate delivered by aerosol in patients with asthma. *Lancet* (1972) **1**: 1361–1364.
3. Brown HM, Storey G, George WHS: Beclomethasone dipropionate: A new steroid aerosol for the treatment of allergic asthma. *Br Med J* (1971) **1**: 585–590.
4. Ellul-Micallef R, Hansson E, Johansson SA: Budesonide: A new corticosteroid in bronchial asthma. *Eur J Respir Dis* (1980) **61**: 167–173.
5. Driessen O, Treuren L, Moolenaar AJ, Meijer JWA: Distribution of drugs over whole blood: III. The transport function of whole blood for hydrocortisone. *Ther Drug Monitor* (1989) **11**: 401–407.
6. Braude AC, Rebuck AS: Pulmonary disposition of cortisol. *Ann Intern Med* (1982) **97**: 59–60.
7. Braude AC, Rebuck AS: Prednisone and methylprednisolone disposition in the lung. *Lancet* (1983) **2**: 995–997.
8. Vichyanond P, Irvin CG, Larsen GL, Szefler SJ, Hill MR: Penetration of corticosteriods into the lung: evidence for a difference between methylprednisolone and prednisolone. *J Allergy Clin Immunol* (1989) **84**: 867–873.

9. McAllister WAC, Mitchell DM, Collins JV. Prednisolone pharmacokinetics compared between night and day in asthmatic and normal subjects. *Br J Clin Pharmacol* (1981) **11**: 303–304.

10. Legler UF, Frey FJ, Benet LZ: Prednisolone clearance at steady state in man. *J Clin Endocrinol Metab* (1982) **55**: 762–767.

11. Ferry JJ, Wagner JG: The nonlinear pharmacokinetics of prednisone and prednisolone II. Plasma protein binding of prednisone and prednisolone in rabbit and human plasma. *Biopharm Drug Disposition* (1987) **8**: 261–272.

12. Rose JQ, Yurchak AM, Meikle AW, Jusko WJ: Effect of smoking on prednisone, prednisolone and dexamethasone pharmacokinetics. *J Pharmacokin Biopharm* (1981) **9**: 1–14.

13. Stuck AE, Frey BM, Frey FJ: Kinetics of prednisolone and endogenous cortisol suppression in the elderly. *Clin Pharmacol* (1988) **43**: 354–361.

14. West CD, Brown H, Simons EL, Carter DB, Kumagai LF, Englert E: Adrenocorticol function and cortisol metabolism in old age. *J Clin Endocrinol Metab* (1961) **21**: 1197–1207.

15. Boekenoogen SJ, Szefler SJ, Jusko WJ: Prednisolone disposition and protein binding in oral contraceptive users. *J Clin Endocrinol Metab* (1983) **56**: 702–709.

16. Ceresa F, Angeli A, Buccuzzi G, Molino G: Once-a-day neurally stimulated and basal ACTH secretion phases in man and their response to corticoid inhibition. *J Clin Endocrinol* (1969) **29**: 1074–1082.

17. Reinberg A, Gervais P, Chaussade M, Fraboulet G, Duburque B: Circadian changes in effectiveness of corticosteroids in eight patients with allergic asthma. *J Allergy Clin Immunol* (1983) **71**: 425–433.

18. Reiss WG, Slaughter RL, Ludwig EA, Middleton E, Jusko WJ: Steroid dose-sparing: pharmacodynamic responses to single versus divided doses of methylprednisolone in man. *J Allergy Clin Immunol* (1990) **85**: 1058–1066.

19. Ellul-Micallef R, Moren F, Wetterlin K, Hidinger KC: Use of a special inhaler attachment in asthmatic children. *Thorax* (1980) **35**: 620–623.

20. Johansson SA, Andersson KE, Brattsand R, Gruvstad E, Hedner P: Topical and systemic glucocorticoid potencies of budesonide, beclomethasone dipropionate and prednisolone in man. *Eur J Respir Dis* (1982) **63**(Suppl 122): 74–82.

21. Harding SM: The human pharmacology of fluticasone propionate. *Resp Med* (1990) **84** (Suppl): 25–29.

22. Frey BM, Frey FJ: Clinical pharmacokinetics of prednisone and prednisolone. *Clin Pharmacokinet* (1990) **19**: 126–146.

23. Collins JV, Clark TJH, Harris PWR, Townsend J: Intravenous corticosteroids in the treatment of acute bronchial asthma. *Lancet* (1960) **1**: 1047–1050.

24. Collins JV, Clark TJH, Brown D, Townsend J: The use of corticosteroids in the treatment of acute asthma. *Q J Med* (New Series) (1975) **44**: 259–273.

25. Wilson CG, Ssendagire R, May CS, Paterson JW: Measurement of plasma prednisolone in man. *Br J Clin Pharmacol* (1975) **2**: 321–325.

26. May CS, Caffin JA, Halliday JW, Bochner F: Prednisolone pharmacokinetics in asthmatic patients. *Br J Dis Chest* (1980) **74**: 91–92.

27. Toogood JH, Jennings B, Greenway RW, Chuang L: Candidiasis and dysphonia in complicating beclomethasone treatment of asthma. *J Allergy Clin Immunol* (1980) **65**: 145–153.

28. Gustavson LE, Legler OF, Benet LZ: Impairment of prednisolone disposition in women taking oral contraceptives or conjugated estrogens. *J Clin Endocrinol Metab* (1986) **62**: 234–237.

29. Meffin PJ, Wing LMH, Sallustio BC, Brooks PH: Alterations in prednisolone disposition as a result of oral contraceptive use and dose. *Br J Clin Pharmacol* (1984) **17**: 655–664.

30. Beitens IZ, Bayard F, Ances IF, Kowarski A, Migeon CJ: The transplacental passage of prednisone and prednisolone in pregnancy near term. *J Pediatr* (1972) **81**: 936–945.

31. Gustafsson J-Å, Carlstedt-Duke J, Poellinger L, *et al.*: Biochemistry, molecular biology, and physiology of the glucocorticoid receptor. *End Rev* (1987) **8**: 185–234.

32. Wilkström A-C, Bakke O, Okret S., Brönnegärd M, Gustafsson J-Å: Intracellular localization of the glucocorticoid receptor: evidence of cytoplasmic and nuclear localization. *Endocrinology* (1987) **120**: 1232–1242.

33. King RJB: Receptor structure. A personal assessment of the current status. *J Steroid Biochem* (1986) **25**: 451–454.

34. Evans RM: The steroid and thyroid hormone receptor superfamily. *Science* (1988) **240**: 889–895.

35. Burnstein KL, Cidlowski JA: Regulation of gene expression by glucocorticoids. *Annu Rev Physiol* (1989) **51**: 683–699.

36. Chandler VL, Maler BA, Yamamoto KR: DNA sequences bound specifically by glucocorticoid receptor *in vitro* render a heterologous promoter hormone responsive *in vivo*. *Annu Rev genet* (1985) **19**: 209–232.

37. Picard D, Yamamoto KR: Two signals mediate hormone-dependent nuclear localization of the glucocorticoid receptor. *EMBO J* (1987) **6**: 3333–3348.

38. Schüle R, Muller M, Kaltschmidt C, Renkawitz R: Many transcription factors interact synergistically with steroid receptors. *Science* (1988) **242**: 1418–1420.

39. Yamamoto KR: Steroid receptor regulated transcription of specific genes and gene networks. *Annu Rev Genet* (1985) **19**: 209–232.

40. Serfling E, Jasin M, Schaffner W: Enhancers and eukaryotic gene transcription. *Trends Genet* (1985) **1**: 224–230.

41. Tully DB, Cidlowski JA: Affinity of interactions between human glucocorticoid receptors and DNA: At physiologic ionic strength, stable binding occurs only with DNA's containing partially symmetric glucocorticoid response elements. *Biochemistry* (1990) **29**: 6662–6670.

42. Gehring U, Arndt H: Heteromeric nature of glucocorticoid receptors. *FEBS Lett* (1985) **179**: 138–142.

43. Howard KJ, Distelhorst CW: Evidence for intracellular association of the glucocorticoid receptor with the 90-kDa heat shock protein. *J. Biol Chem* (1988) **263**: 3474–3481.

44. Mendel DB, Orti E: Isoform composition and stoichiometry of the ~90-kDa heat shock protein associated with glucocorticoid receptors. *J Biol Chem* (1988) **263**: 6695–6702.

45. Catelli MG, Binart N, Jung-Testas I, *et al.*: The common 90-kD protein component of non-transformed '8S' steroid receptors is a heat shock protein. *EMBO J* (1985) **4**: 3131–3135.

46. Dalman FC, Bresnick EH, Patel PD, *et al.*: Direct evidence that the glucocorticoid receptor binds to hsp 90 at or near the termination of receptor translation *in vitro*. *J Biol Chem* (1989) **264**: 19815–19821.

47. Sanchez ER, Faber LE, Henzel WL, Pratt WB: The 56–59 kilodalton protein identified in untransformed steroid receptor complexes is a unique protein that exists in cytosol in a complex with both the 70- and 90-kilodalton heat shock protein. *Biochemistry* (1990) **29**: 5145–5152.

48. Bresnick EH, Dalman FC, Pratt WB: Direct stoichiometric evidence that the untransformed Mr 300 000, 9S, glucocorticoid receptor is a core unit derived from a larger heteromeric complex. *Biochemistry* (1990) **29**: 520–527.

49. Bresnick EH, Dalman FC, Sanchez ER, Pratt WB: Evidence that the 90-kDa heat shock protein is necessary for the steroid binding conformation of the L cell glucocorticoid receptor. *J Biol Chem* (1989) **264**: 4992–4997.

50. Pratt WB, Jolly DJ, Pratt DV, *et al.*: A region in the steroid binding domain determines formation of the non-DNA binding, 9S glucocorticoid receptor complex. *J Biol Chem* (1988) **263**: 267–273.

51. Picard D, Salser SJ, Yamamoto KR: A movable and regulable inactivation function within the steroid binding domain of the glucocorticoid receptor. *Cell* (1988) **54**: 1073–1080.

52. Ptashne M: How eukaryotic transcriptional activators work. *Nature* (1988) **335**: 683–689.

53. Wrange Ö, Erikson P, Perlmann T: The purified activated glucocorticoid receptor is a homodimer. *J Biol Chem* (1989) **264**: 5253–5259.

54. Sanchez ER, Redmond T, Scherrer LC, Bresnick EH, Welsh MJ, Pratt WB: Evidence that the 90-kilodalton heat shock protein is associated with tubulin-containing complexes in L cell cytosol and in intact PtK cells. *Mol Endocrinol* (1988) **2**: 756–760.

55. Housley PR: Aluminium fluoride inhibition of glucocorticoid receptor inactivation and transformation. *Biochemistry* (1990) **29**: 3578–3585.

56. Mendel DB, Bodwell JE, Gametchu B, Harrison RW, Munck A: Molybdate-stabilized nonactivated glucocorticoid receptor complexes contain a 90kDa non-steroid binding phosphoprotein that is lost on activation. *J Biol Chem* (1986) **261**: 3758–3763.

57. Goidl JA, Cake MH, Dolan KP, Parchman LG, Litwack G: Activation of the rat liver glucocorticoid-receptor complex. *Biochemistry* (1977) **16**: 2125–2130.

58. Bodine PV, Litwack G: Purification and characterization of two novel phosphoglycerides that modulate the glucocorticoid-receptor complex. *J Biol Chem* (1990) **265**: 9544–9554.

59. Meschinchi S, Sanchez ER, Martell KJ, Pratt WB: Elimination and reconstitution of the requirement for hormone in promoting temperature-dependent transformation of cytosolic glucocorticoid receptors to the DNA-binding state. *J Biol Chem* (1990) **265**: 4863–4870.

60. Tienrungroj W, Sanchez ER, Housley PR, Harrison RW, Pratt WB: Glucocorticoid receptor phosphorylation, transformation and DNA binding. *J Biol Chem* (1987) **262**: 17342–17349.

61. Kaufmann SH, Okret S, Wilkstrom AC, Gustafsson JA, Shaper JH: Binding of the glucocorticoid receptor to the rat liver nuclear matrix. *J Biol Chem* (1986) **261**: 11962–11967.

62. Silva CM, Cidlowski JA: Direct evidence for intra- and inter molecular disulfide bond formation in the human glucocorticoid receptor. *J Biol Chem* (1989) **264**: 6638–6647.

63. Grippo JF, Holmgren A, Pratt WB: Proof that the endogenous, heat-stable glucocorticoid receptor-activating factor is thioredoxin. *J Biol Chem* (1985) **260**: 93–97.

64. Van Hal PTW, Mulder E, Hoogsteden HC, Hilvering C, Benner R: Glucocorticoid receptors in alveolar macrophages: Methodological aspects of the determination of the number of glucocorticoid receptors per cell. *Agents and Actions* (1989) **26**: 128–131.

65. Francke E, Foellmer BE: The glucocorticoid receptor gene is in 5q-q32. *Genomics* (1989) **4**: 610–612.

66. Govindan MV, Devic M, Green S, Gronemeyer H, Chambon P: Cloning of the human glucocorticoid receptor cDNA. *Nucl Acids REs* (1985) **13**: 8293–8304.

67. Weinberger C, Hollenberg SM, Ong ES, et al.: Identification of human glucocorticoid receptor complementary DNA clones by epitope selection. *Science* (1985) **228**: 740–742.

68. Hollenberg SM, Weinberger C, Ong ES, et al.: Primary structure and expression of a functional human glucocorticoid receptor cDNA. *Nature* (1985) **318**: 635–641.

69. Carlstedt-Duke J, Strömstedt PE, Wrange Ö, Bergman T, Gustafsson JA, Jörnvall H: Domain structure of the glucocorticoid receptor protein. *Proc Natl Acad Sci USA* (1987) **84**: 4437–4440.

70. Tora L, Gronemeyer H, Turcotti B, Gaub MP, Chambon P: The N-terminal region of the chicken progesterone receptor specifies target gene activation. *Nature* (1988) **334**: 543–546.

71. Miesfeld RL: The structure and function of steroid receptor proteins. *Crit Rev Biochem Mol Biol* (1989) **24**: 101–117.

72. Hollenberg SM, Giguere V, Evans RM: Identification of two regions of the human glucocorticoid receptor hormone binding domain that block activation. *Cancer Res* (1989) **49**(Suppl): 2292–2294.

73. Beato M: Gene regulation by steroid hormones. *Cell* (1989) **56**: 335–344.

74. Hollenberg SM, Evans RM: Multiple and cooperative trans-activation domains of the human glucocorticoid receptor. *Cell* (1988) **55**: 899–906.

75. Dahlman K, Strömstedt P-E, Rae C, et al.: High level expression in *Escherichia coli* of the DNA-binding domain of the glucocorticoid receptor in a functional form utilizing domain-specific cleavage of a fusion protein. *J Biol Chem* (1989) **264**: 804–809.

76. Miller J, McLachlan AD, Klug A: Receptive zinc-binding domains in the protein transcription factor IIIA from *Xenopus* oocytes. *EMBO J* (1985) **4**: 1609–1614.

77. Friedman LP, Luisi BF, Korszun ZR, Basavappa R, Sigler PB, Yamamoto KR: The function and structure of the metal coordination sites within the glucocorticoid receptor DNA binding domain. *Nature* (1988) **334**: 543–546.

78. Berg JM: DNA binding specificity of steroid receptors. *Cell* (1989) **57**: 1065–1068.

79. Miesfeld RL: Molecular genetics of corticosteroid action. *Am Rev Respir Dis* (1990) **141** (Suppl): 11s–17s.

80. Beato M, Chalepakis G, Schauer M, Slater EP: DNA regulatory elements for steroid hormones. *J Steroid Biochem* (1989) **32**: 737–748.

81. Hard T, Dahlman K, Carlstedt-Duke J, Gustafsson J-Å, Rigler R: Cooperativity and specificity in the interactions between DNA and the glucocorticoid receptor DNA-binding domain. *Biochemistry* (1990) **29**: 5358–5364.

82. Zaret KS, Yamamoto KR: Reversible and persistent changes in chromatin structure accompany activation of a glucocorticoid-dependent enhancer element. *Cell* (1984) **38**: 29–38.

83. Green S, Kumar V, Theulaz I, Wahli W, Chambon P: The N-terminal DNA-binding 'zinc finger' of the oestrogen and glucocorticoid receptors determines gene specificity. *EMBO J* (1988) **7**: 3037–3044.

84. Danielsen M, Henck L, Ringold GM: Two amino-acids within the knuckle of the first zinc finger specify DNA response element activation by the glucocorticoid receptor. *Cell* (1989) **57**: 1131–1138.

85. Godowski PJ, Picard D, Yamamoto KR: Signal transduction and transcriptional regulation by glucocorticoid receptor-Lex A fusion proteins. *Science* (1988) **241**: 812–816.

86. Sigler PB: Acid blobs and negative noodles. *Nature* (1988) **333**: 210–212.

87. Webster NJG, Green S, Jin JR, Chambon P: The hormone-binding domains of the estrogen and glucocorticoid receptors contain an inducible transcription activation function. *Cell* (1988) **54**: 199–207.

88. Green S, Chambron P: Oestradiol induction of a glucocorticoid-responsive gene by a chimaeric receptor. *Nature* (1987) **325**: 75–78.

89. Chalepakis G, Arnemann J, Slater E, Brüller H-J, Gross B, Beato M: Differential gene activation by glucocorticoids and progestins through the hormone regulatory element of mouse mammary tumor virus. *Cell* (1988) **52**: 371–382.

90. Perlman T, Wrange Ö: Specific glucocorticoid receptor binding to DNA reconstituted in a nucleosome. *EMBO J* (1988) **7**: 3073–3079.

91. Schaeür M, Chalepakis G, Willmann T, Beato M: Binding of hormone accelerates the kinetics of glucocorticoid and progesterone receptor binding to DNA. *Proc Natl Acad Sci USA* (1989) **86**: 1123–1127.

92. Arnemann J, Brüggemeier V, Carballo M, *et al.*: Differential gene regulation by steroid hormones. In Ringold G (ed) *Steroid Hormone Action*. New York, Alan R Liss, 1988, pp 185–192.

93. Auricchio F: Phosphorylation of steroid receptors. *J Steroid Biochem* (1989) **32**: 613–622.

94. Munck A, Mendel DB, Smith LI, Orti E: Glucocorticoid receptors and actions. *Amer Rev Respir Dis* (1990) **141** (Suppl): 2s–10s.

95. Mendel DB, Bodwell JE, Munck A: Activation of cytosolic glucocorticoid-receptor complexes in intact WEH1-7 cells does not dephosphorylate the steroid-binding protein. *J Biol Chem* (1987) **262**: 5644–5648.

96. Orti E, Mendel DB, Munck A: Phosphorylation of glucocorticoid receptor-associated and free forms of the 90-kDa heat shock protein before and after receptor activation. *J Biol Chem* (1989) **264**: 231–237.

97. Mendel DB, Orti E, Smith LI, Bodwell J, Munck A: Evidence for a glucocorticoid receptor cycle and nuclear dephyosphorylation of the steroid-binding protein. *Prog Clin Biol Res* (1990) **322**: 97–117.

98. Rossini GP: Glucocorticoid receptors are associated with particles containing DNA and RNA *in vivo*. *Biochem Biophys Res Commun* (1987) **147**: 1188–1193.

99. Tymoczko JL, Anderson EE, Lee KA, Unger AL: The ability to convert the 4S glucocorticoid receptor to the 7–8S form is dependent on both RNA and protein factors. *Biochim Biophys Acta* (1987) **930**: 114–121.

100. Liao S, Smythe S, Tymoczko JL, Rossini GP, Chen C, Hiipakka RA: RNA-dependent release of androgen and other steroid-receptor complexes from DNA. *J Biol Chem* (1980) **255**: 5545–5551.

101. Rossini GP, Wilkström A-C, Gustafsson J-Å: Glucocorticoid-receptor complexes are associated with small RNA *in vitro*. *J Steroid Biochem* (1989) **32**: 633–642.

102. Flower RJ: Lipocortin and the mechanism of action of the glucocorticoids. *Br J Pharmacol* (1988) **94**: 987–1015.

103. Flower RJ: Lipocortin. *Prog Clin Biol Res* (1990) **349**: 11–25.

104. Hong SC, Levine L: Inhibition of arachidonic acid release from cells as the biochemical action of anti-inflammatory steroids. *Proc Natl Acad Sci USA* (1980) **77**: 2533–2536.

105. Blackwell GJ, Carnuccio R, Di Rosa M, Flower RJ, Parente L, Persico P: Macrocortin: a polypeptide causing the anti-phospholipase effect of glucocorticoids. *Nature* (1980) **287**: 147–149.
106. Hirata F, Schiffmann E, Venkatasubramanian K, Solomon D, Axelrod J: A phospholipase A$_2$ inhibitory protein in rabbit neutrophils induced by glucocorticoids. *Proc Natl Acad Sci USA* (1980) **77**: 2233–2236.
107. Cloix JF, Colard O, Rothhut B, Russo-Marie F: Characterization and partial purification of 'renocortins': two polypeptides formed in renal cells causing the anti-phospholipase-like action of glucocorticoids. *Br J Pharmacol* (1983) **79**: 313–321.
108. Di Rosa M, Flower RJ, Hirata F, Parente L, Russo-Marie F: Anti-phospholipase proteins. *Prostaglandins* (1984) **23**: 441–442.
109. Wallner BP, Mattaliano RJ, Hession C, *et al.*: Cloning and expression of human lipocortin, a phospholipase A$_2$ inhibitor with potential inflammatory activity. *Nature* (1986) **320**: 77–81.
110. Bronnegard M, Andersson O, Edwall D, Lund J, Norstedt G, Carlstedt-Duke J: Human calpactin II (lipocortin 1) messenger ribonucleic acid is not induced by glucocorticoids. *Mol Endocrinol* (1988) **2**: 732–739.
111. Browning JL, Ward MP, Wallner BP, Pepinsky RB: Studies on the structural properties of lipocortin-1 and the regulation of its synthesis by steroids. *Prog Clin Biol Res* (1990) **349**: 27–45.
112. Stoehr SJ, Smolen JE, Suchard SJ: Lipocortins are major substrates for protein kinase C in extracts of human neutrophils. *J Immunol* (1990) **144**: 3936–3945.
113. Comera C, Rothhut B, Russo-Marie F: Identification and characterization of phospholipase A$_2$ inhibitory proteins in human mononuclear cells. *Eur J Biochem* (1990) **188**: 139–146.
114. Fava RA, McKanna J, Cohen S: Lipocortin 1 (p 35) is abundant in a restricted number of differentiated cell types in adult organs. *J Cell Physiol* (1989) **141**: 284–293.
115. Smith SF, Tetley TD, Guz A, Flower RJ: Detection of lipocortin 1 in human lung lavage fluid: lipocortin degradation as a possible proteolytic mechanism in the control of inflammatory mediators and inflammation. *Env Hlth Persp* (1990) **85**: 135–144.
116. Ambrose MP, Hunninghake GW: Corticosteroids increase lipocortin 1 in BAL fluid from normal individuals and patients with lung disease. *J Appl Physiol* (1990) **68**: 1668–1671.
117. Goulding NJ, Godolphin JL, Sharland PR, *et al.*: Anti-inflammatory lipocortin 1 production by peripheral blood leucocytes in response to hydrocortisone. *Lancet* (1990) **335**: 1416–1418.
118. Smith SF: A potential mechanism for some anti-inflammatory effects of the glucocorticoids. *Respir Med* (1990) **84**: 435–436.
119. Blackwood RA, Ernst JD: Characterization of Ca^{2+}-dependent phospholipid binding, vesicle aggregation and membrane fusion by annexins. *Biochem J* (1990) **266**: 195–200.
120. Crompton MR, Moss SE, Crumpton MJ: Diversity in the lipocortin/calpactin family. *Cell* (1988) **55**: 1–3.
121. Pash JM, Bailey JM: Inhibition by corticosteroids of epidermal growth factor-induced recovery of cyclooxygenase after aspirin inactivation. *FASEB J* (1988) **2**: 2613–2618.
122. Kretsinger RH, Creutz CE: Consensus in exocytosis. *Nature* (1986) **320**: 573.
123. Moss SE, Crumpton MJ: Alternative splicing gives rise to two forms of the p 68 Ca^{2+}-binding protein. *FEBS Lett* (1990) **261**: 299–302.
124. Pepinsky RB, Sinclair LK, Douglas I, Liang C-M, Lawton P, Browning JL: Monoclonal antibodies as probes for biological function. *FEBS Lett* (1990) **261**: 247–252.
125. Ando Y, Imamura S, Hong Y-M, Owada MK, Kakanuga T, Kannagi R: Enhancement of calcium sensitivity of lipocortin 1 in phospholipid binding induced by limited proteolysis and phosphorylation at the amino terminus as analyzed by phospholipid affinity column chromatography. *J Biol Chem* (1989) **264**: 6948–6955.
126. Davidson FF, Dennis EA, Powell M, Glenney JR: Inhibition of phospholipase A$_2$ by 'lipocortins' and calpactins. *J Biol Chem* (1987) **262**: 1698–1705.
127. Davidson FF, Lister MD, Dennis EA: Binding and inhibition studies on lipocortins using phosphatidylcholine vesicles and phospholipase A$_2$ from snake venom, pancreas and a macrophage cell-line. *J Biol Chem* (1990) **265**: 5602–5609.
128. Pepinsky RB, Tizard R, Mattaliano RJ, *et al.*: Five distinct calcium and phospholipid binding proteins share homology with lipocortin 1. *J Biol Chem* (1988) **263**: 10799–10811.

129. Bomaleski JS, Baker D, Resurreccion NV, Clark MA: Rheumatoid arthritis synovial fluid phospholipase A₂ activating protein (PLAP) stimulates human neutrophil degranulation and superoxide ion production. *Agents-Actions* (1989) **27**: 425–427.

130. Piltch A, Sun L, Fava RA, Hayashi J: Lipocortin-independent effect of dexamethasone on phospholipase activity in a thymic epithelial cell line. *Biochem J* (1989) **261**: 395–400.

131. Hullin F, Raynal P, Ragab-Thomas JMF, Fauvel J, Chap H: Effect of dexamethasone on prostaglandin synthesis and on lipocortin status in human endothelial cells. *J Biol Chem* (1989) **264**: 3506–3513.

132. Bienkowski MJ, Petro MA, Robinson LJ: Inhibition of Thromboxane A synthesis in U937 cells by glucocorticoids. *J Biol Chem* (1989) **264**: 6536–6544.

133. Northup JK, Valentine-Braun KA, Johnson LK, Severson DL, Hollenberg MD: Evaluation of the anti-inflammatory and phospholipase inhibitory activity of calpactin II/lipocortin 1. *J Clin Invest* (1988) **82**: 1347–1352.

134. Beyaert R, Suffys P, Van-Roy F, Fiers W: Inhibition by glucocorticoids of tumor necrosis factor-mediated cytotoxicity. Evidence against lipocortin involvement. *FEBS Lett* (1990) **262**: 93–96.

135. Violette SM, King I, Browning JL, Pepinsky RB, Wallner BP, Sartorelli AC: Role of lipocortin 1 in the glucocorticoid induction of the terminal differentiation of a human squamous carcinoma. *J Cell Physiol* (1990) **142**: 70–77.

136. Klee CB: Ca²⁺-dependent phospholipid- (and membrane-) binding proteins. *Biochemistry* (1988) **27**: 6645–6653.

137. Chung KF, Podgorski MR, Goulding NJ, *et al.*: Circulating autoantibodies to recombinant lipocortin-1 in asthma. *Resp Med* (1991) **85**: 121–124.

138. Wilkinson JRW, Podgorski MR, Godolphin JL, Goulding NJ, Lee TH: Bronchial asthma is not associated with auto-antibodies to lipocortin-1. *Clin Exp Allergy* (1990) **20**: 189–192.

139. Errasfa M, Russo-Marie F: A purified lipocortin shares the anti-inflammatory effect of glucocorticoids *in vivo* in mice. *Br J Pharmacol* (1989) **97**: 1051–1058.

140. Miele L, Cordella-Miele E, Facchiano A, Mukherjee AB: Novel anti-inflammatory peptides from the region of the highest similarity between uteroglobin and lipocortin 1. *Nature* (1988) **335**: 726–730.

141. Camussi G, Tetta C, Bussolino F, Baglioni C: Anti-inflammatory peptides (antiflammins) inhibit synthesis of platelet-activating factor, neutrophil aggregation and chemotaxis, and intradermal inflammatory reactions. *J Exp Med* (1990) **171**: 913–927.

142. Cirino G, Peers SH, Flower RJ, Browning JL, Pepinsky RB: Human recombinant lipocortin 1 has acute local anti inflammatory properties in the rat paw oedema test. *Proc Natl Acad Sci* (USA) (1988) **86**: 3428–3432.

143. Oyanagui Y: Anti-inflammatory effects of polyamines in serotonin and carrageenin paw oedemata—possible mechanism to increase vascular permeability inhibitory protein level which is regulated by glucocorticoids and superoxide radical. *Agents-Actions* (1984) **14**: 228–237.

144. Oyanagui Y, Suzuki S: Vasoregulin, a glucocorticoid-inducible vascular permeability inhibitory protein. *Agents-Actions* (1985) **17**: 270–277.

145. Carnuccio R, Di Rosa M, Guerrasio B, Iuvone T, Sautebin L: Vasocortin: a novel glucocorticoid-induced anti-inflammatory protein. *Br J Pharmacol* (1987) **90**: 443–445.

146. Carnuccio R, Di Rosa M, Iuvone T, Marotta P, Sautebin L: Vasocortin-like proteins induced by glucocorticoids in vascular tissue. *Eur J Pharmacol* (1989) **166**: 535–539.

147. Carnuccio R, Di Rosa M, Ialenti A, Iuvone T, Sautebin L: Selective inhibition by vasocortin of histamine release induced by dextran and concavalin A from rat peritoneal cells. *Br J Pharmacol* (1989) **98**: 32–34.

148. Di Rosa M, Ialenti A: Selective inhibition of inflammatory reactions by vasocortin and antiflammin 2. *Prog Clin Biol Res* (1990) **349**: 81–90.

149. Heiman AS, Crews FT: Inhibition of immunoglobulin, but not polypeptide base-stimulated release of histamine and arachidonic acid by anti-inflammatory steroids. *J Pharmacol Exp Ther* (1984) **230**: 175–182.

150. Ialenti A, Doyle PM, Hardy GN, Simpkin DS, Di Rosa M: Anti-inflammatory effects of vasocortin and nonapeptide fragments of uteroglobin and liportin 1 (antiflammins). *Agents-Actions* (1990) **29**: 48–49.
151. Singh G, Katyal SL, Brown WE, Kennedy AL, Singh U, Wong-Chong ML: Clara cell 10-kDa protein (cc 10): comparison of structure and function to uteroglobin. *Biochim Biophys Acta* (1990) **1039**: 348–355.
152. Hagen G, Wolf M, Katyal S, Singh G, Beato M, Suske G: Tissue-specific expression, hormonal regulation and 5′-flanking gene region of the rat Clara cell 10-kDa protein: comparison to rabbit uteroglobin. *Nucleic Acids Res* (1990) **18**: 2939–2946.
153. Aberblom IE, Slater EP, Beato M, Baxter JD, Mellon PL: Negative regulation by glucocorticoids through interference with a cAMP responsive enhance. *Science* (1988) **241**: 350–353.
154. Drouin J, Sun YL, Nemer M: Glucocorticoid repression of pro-opiomelanocortin gene transcription. *J Steroid Biochem* (1989) **34**: 63–69.
155. Sukai DD, Helms S, Carlstedt-Duke J, Gustafsson JA, Rottman FM, Yamamoto KR: Hormone-mediated repression of transcription: A negative glucocorticoid response element from the bovine prolactin gene. *Genes-Dev* (1988) **2**: 1144–1154.
156. Drouin J, Trifiro MA, Plante RK, Namer M, Eriksson P, Wrange O: Glucocorticoid receptor binding to specific DNA sequence as required for hormone-dependent repression of pro-opiomelanocortin gene transcription. *Mol Cell Biol* (1989) **9**: 5305–5314.
157. Adler S, Waterman ML, He X, Rosenfeld MG: Steroid receptor-mediated inhibition of rat prolactin gene expression does not require the receptor DNA-binding domain. *Cell* (1988) **52**: 685–695.
158. Burnstein KL, Cidlowski JA: Regulation of gene expression by glucocorticoids. *Ann Rev Physiol* (1989) **51**: 683–699.
159. Lew W, Oppenheim JJ, Matsushima K: Analysis of the suppression of IL-1α and IL-1β production in human peripheral blood mononuclear adherent cells by a glucocorticoid hormone. *J Immunol* (1988) **140**: 1895–1902.
160. Lee S, Tsou A-P, Chan H, *et al.*: Glucocorticoids selectively inhibit the transcription of the interleukin 1β gene and decrease the stability of interleukin 1βmRNA. *Proc Natl Acad Sci USA* (1988) **85**: 1204–1208.
161. Knudsen PJ, Dinarello CA, Strom TB: Glucocorticoids inhibit transcriptional and post-transcriptional expression of interleukin 1 in U937 cells. *J Immunol* (1987) **139**: 4129–4134.
162. Kern J, Lamb RJ, Reed JC, Daniele RP, Nowell PC: Dexamethasone inhibition of interleukin 1 beta production by human monocytes. *J Clin Invest* (1988) **81**: 237–244.
163. Han J, Thompson P, Beutler B: Dexamethasone and pentoxifylline inhibit endotoxin-induced cachectin/tumour necrosis factor synthesis at separate points in the signalling pathway. *J Exp Med* (1990) **172**: 391–394.
164. Beutler B, Krochin N, Milsark IW, Luedke C, Cerami A: Control of cachectin (tumor necrosis factor) synthesis: mechanisms of endotoxin resistance. *Science* (1986) **232**: 977–980.
165. Thorens B, Mermod JJ, Vassalli P: Phagocytosis and inflammatory stimuli induce GM-CSF mRNA in macrophages through post-transcriptional regulation. *Cell* (1987) **48**: 671–679.
166. Hamalainen L, Oikarenen J, Kivirikko KI: Synthesis and degradation of Type 1 Procollagen mRNAs in cultured human skin fibroblasts and the effect of cortisol. *J Biol Chem* (1985) **260**: 720–725.
167. Kunkel SL, Spengler M, May MA, Spengler R, Larrick J, Remick D: Prostaglandin E$_2$ regulates macrophage-derived tumor necrosis factor gene expression. *J Biol Chem* (1988) **263**: 5380–5384.
168. Grabstein K, Dower S, Gillis S, Urdal D, Larsen A: Expression of interleukin 2, interferon-γ, and the IL-2 receptor by human peripheral blood lymphocytes. *J Immunol* (1986) **136**: 4503–4508.
169. Gessani S, McCandless S, Baglioni C: The glucocorticoid dexamethasone inhibits synthesis of interferon by decreasing the level of its mRNA. *J Biol Chem* (1988) **263**: 7454–7457.
170. Ishikawa H, Tanaka H, Iwato K, *et al.*: Effect of glucocorticoids on the biologic activities of myeloma cells: Inhibition of interleukin-1β osteoclast activating factor-induced bone resorption. *Blood* (1990) **75**: 715–720.

171. Zanker B, Walz G, Wieder KJ, Strom TB: Evidence that glucocorticoids block expression of the human interleukin-6 gene by accessory cells. *Transplantation* (1990) **49**: 183–185.
172. Snyers L, De-Wit L, Content J: Glucocorticoid up-regulation of high-affinity interleukin 6 receptors on human epithelial cells. *Proc Natl Acad Sci USA* (1990) **87**: 2030–2042.
173. Lyons-Giordano B, Davis GI, Galbraith W, Pratta MA, Arner EC: Interleukin 1β stimulates phospholipase A$_2$mRNA synthesis in rabbit articular chondrocytes. *Biochem Biophys Res Commun* (1989) **164**: 488–495.
174. Nakano T, Ohara O, Teraoka H, Arita H: Group II phospholipase A$_2$mRNA synthesis is stimulated by two distinct mechanisms in rat vascular smooth muscle cells. *FEBS Lett* (1990) **261**: 171–174.
175. Nakano T, Ohara O, Teraoka H, Arita H: Glucocorticoids suppress Group II phospholipase A$_2$ production by blocking mRNA synthesis and post-transcriptional expression. *J Biol Chem* (1990) **265**: 12745–12748.
176. Nakano T, Arita H: Enhanced expression of group II phospholipase A$_2$ gene in the tissues of endotoxin shock rats and its suppression by glucocorticoid. *Cell* (1990) **273**: 23–26.
177. Burnstein KL, Jewell CM, Cidlowski JA: Human glucocorticoid receptor cDNA contains sequences sufficient for receptor down-regulation. *J Biol Chem* (1990) **265**: 7284–7291.
178. Kalinyak JE, Dorin RI, Hoffman AR, Perlman AJ: Tissue-specific regulation of glucocorticoid receptor mRNA by dexamethasone. *J Biol Chem* (1987) **262**: 10441–10444.
179. Hoeck W, Rusconi S, Groner B: Down-regulation and phosphorylation of glucocorticoid receptors in cultured cells. *J Biol Chem* (1989) **264**: 14396–14402.
180. Rosewicz S, McDonald AR, Maddux BA, Goldfine ID, Miesfeld RL, Logsdon CD: Mechanism of glucocorticoid receptor down-regulation by glucocorticoids. *J Biol Chem* (1988) **263**: 2581–2584.
181. Vedeckis WV, Ali M, Allen HR: Regulation of glucocorticoid receptor protein and mRNA levels. *Cancer Res* (1989) **49**: 2295s–2302s.
182. Dong Y, Aronsson M, Gustafsson J-Å, Okret S: The mechanism of cAMP-induced glucocorticoid receptor expression. *J Biol Chem* (1989) **264**: 13679–13683.
183. Hill MR, Stith RD, McCallum RE: Human recombinant IL-1 alters glucocorticoid receptor function in reuber hepatoma cells. *J Immunol* (1988) **141**: 1522–1528.
184. Autelitano DJ, Lundblad JR, Blum M, Roberts JL: Hormonal regulation of POMC gene expression. *Annu Rev Physiol* (1989) **51**: 715–726.
185. Diamond MI, Miner JN, Yoshinaga SK, Yamamoto KR: Transcription factor interactions: Selectors of positive or negative regulation from a single DNA element. *Science* (1990) **249**: 1266–1272.
186. Dong Y, Cairns W, Okret S, Gustafsson J-Å: A glucocorticoid-resistant rat hepatoma cell variant contains functional glucocorticoid receptor. *J Biol Chem* (1990) **265**: 7526–7531.
187. Schwartz HJ, Lowell FC, Melby JC: Steroid resistance in bronchial asthma. *Ann Int Med* (1968) **69**: 493–499.
188. Carmichael J, Paterson IC, Diaz P, Crompton GK, Kay AB, Grant IWB: Corticosteroid resistance in asthma. *Br Med J* (1981) **282**: 1419–1422.
189. Lane SJ, Lee TH: Glucocorticoid receptor characteristics in monocytes of patients with corticosteroid resistant bronchial asthma. *Am Rev Respir Dis* (1991) **143**: 1020–1024.
190. Walker KB, Potter JM, House AK: Interleukin 2 synthesis in the presence of steroids: a model of steroid resistance. *Clin Exp Immunol* (1987) **68**: 162–167.
191. Mortimer Ö, Grettve L, Lindström B, Lönnerholm G, Zetterström O: Bioavailability of prednisolone in asthmatic patients with a poor response to steroid treatment. *Eur J Respir Dis* (1987) **71**: 372–379.
192. Kay AB, Diaz P, Carmichael J, Grant IWB: Corticosteroid resistant asthma and monocyte complement receptors. *Clin Exp Immunol* (1981) **44**: 576–580.
193. Poznansky MC, Gordon ACH, Douglas JG, Krajewski AS, Wyllie AH, Grant IWB: Resistance to methylprednisolone in cultures of blood mononuclear cells from glucocorticoid-resistant asthmatic patients. *Clin Sci* (1984) **67**: 639–645.

194. Poznansky MC, Gordon ACH, Grant IWB, Wyllie AH: A cellular abnormality in glucocorticoid resistant asthma. *Clin Exp Immunol* (1985) **61**: 135–142.
195. Wilkinson JRW, Crea AEG, Clark TJH, Lee TH: Identification and characterization of a monocyte-derived neutrophil-activating factor in corticosteroid-resistant bronchial asthma. *J Clin Invest* (1989) **84**: 1930–1941.
196. Corrigan CJ, Brown P, Kay AB: Characteristics of peripheral blood mononuclear cell corticosteroid (CS) receptors in CS resistant asthmatics. *Thorax* (1989) **44**: 882(A).
197. Linder MJ, Brad Thompson E: Abnormal glucocorticoid receptor gene and mRNA in primary cortisol resistance. *J Steroid Biochem* (1989) **32**: 243–249.
198. Brandon DD, Markwick AJ, Chrousos GP, Loriaux DL: Glucocorticoid resistance in humans and non human primates. *Cancer Res* (1989) **49** (Suppl): 2203–2213.
199. Nawata H, Sekija K, Higuchi K, Kato K-I, Ibayashi H: Decreased deoxyribonucleic acid binding of glucocorticoid-receptor complex in cultured skin fibroblasts from a patient with the glucocorticoid resistance syndrome. *J Clin Endocrinol Metab* (1987) **65**: 219–226.
200. Grandordy B, Belmatoug N, Morelle A, de Lauture D, Marsac J: Effect of betamethasone on airway obstruction and bronchial response to salbutamol in prednisolone resistant asthma. *Thorax* (1987) **42**: 65–71.
201. McLeod DT, Capewell SJ, Law J, MacLaren W, Seaton A: Intramuscular triamicolone acetonide in chronic severe asthma. *Thorax* (1985) **40**: 840–845.
202. Ellul-Micallef R: Asthma: A look at the past. *Br J Dis Chest* (1976) **70**: 112–116.
203. Hogg JC: Is asthma an epithelial disease? *Am Rev Respir Dis* (1984) **129**: 207–208.
204. Barnes PJ: Asthma as an axon reflex. *Lancet* (1986) **i**: 242–245.
205. Persson CGA: Role of plasma exudation in asthmatic airways. *Lancet* (1986) **ii**: 1126–1129.
206. Roche WR, Williams JH, Beasley R, Holgate S: Subepithelial fibrosis in the bronchi of asthmatics. *Lancet* (1989) **1**: 520–524.
207. Editorial: Bronchial inflammation and asthma treatment. *Lancet* (1991) **337**: 82–83.
208. Guo C-B, Liu MC, Galli SJ, Kagey-Sobotka A, Lichetenstein LM: The histamine containing cells in the late phase response in the lung are basophils. *J Allergy Clinical Immunol* (1990) **85**: 172 (Abstract 113).
209. Wilson JW, Lai C, Sjukanovic R, Howarth PH, Holgate ST: The influence of inhaled platelet activating factor (PAF) on bronchoalveolar lavage and peripheral blood leukocytes and platelets. *J Allergy Clin Immunol* (1990) **85**: 187 (Abstract 176).
210. Chung KF, Rogers DF, Barnes PJ, Evans TW: The role of increased microvasclar permeability and plasma exudation in asthma. *Eur Respir J* (1990) **3**: 329–337.
211. Björk J, Goldschmidt T, Smedegard G, Arfors KE: Methylprednisolone acts at endothelial cell level reducing inflammatory responses. *Acta Physiol Scand* (1985) **123**: 221–224.
212. Barnes PJ, Boschetto P, Rogers DF, *et al.*: Effects of treatment on airway microvascular leakage. *Eur Respir J* (1990) **3**: 663s–671s.
213. Schimura S, Sasaki T, Ikeda K, Yamauchi K, Sasaki H, Takishima T: Direct inhibitory action of glucocorticoid on glycoconjugate secretion from airway submucosal glands. *Am Rev Respir Dis* (1990) **141**: 1044–1049.
214. Churchill L, Friedman B, Schleimer RP, Proud D: Granulocyte macrophage colony stimulating factor (GM-CSF) production by cultured human tracheal epithelial cells. *J Allergy Clin Immunol* (1990) **85**: 233 (Abstract 358).
215. Naray-Fejes-Toth A, Rosenkranz B, Frolich JC, Fejes-Toth G: Glucocorticoid effect on arachidonic acid metabolism *in vivo*. *J Steroid Biochem* (1988) **30**: 155–159.
216. Manso G, Baker AJ, Taylor IK, Fuller RW: Effect of glucocorticoids on the human monocyte function *in vivo* and *in vitro*. *Thorax* (1990) **45**: 331P (Abstract).
217. Piedimonte G, McDonald DM, Nadel JA: Neutral endopeptidase and kininase II mediate glucocorticoid-induced inhibition of neurogenic plasma extravasation in the rat trachea. *Clin Res* (1990) **38**: 160 (Abstract).
218. Borson DB, Gruenert DC: Glucocorticoids induce expression of neutral endopeptidase in transformed human tracheal epithelial cells. *Am J Physiol* (1991) **260**: L83–L89.
219. Piedimonte G, McDonald DM, Nadel JA: Neutral endopeptidase and kininase II mediate glucocorticoid inhibition of neurogenic inflammation in the rat trachea. *J Clin Invest* (1991) **86**: 1409–1415.

220. Durham SR, Graneek BJ, Hawkins R, Taylor AJN: The temporal relationship between increases in airway responsiveness to histamine and late asthmatic responses induced by occupational agents. *J Allergy Clin Immunol* (1987) **79**: 398–406.
221. Thorpe JE, Steinberg D, Bernstein IL, Murlas CG: Bronchial reactivity increases soon after the immediate response in dual responding asthmatic subjects. *Chest* (1987) **91**: 15–21.
222. Booij-Noord H, Orie NGM, De Vries K: Immediate and late bronchial obstructive reactions to inhalation of house dust and protective effects of disodium cromoglycate and prednisolone. *J Allergy Clin Immunol* (1971) **48**: 344–354.
223. Fabbri LM, Chiesura-Corona P, Dal Vecchio L, *et al.*: Prednisone inhibits late asthmatic reactions and the associated increase in airway responsiveness induced by toluene diisocyanate in sensitized subjects. *Am Rev Respir Dis* (1985) **132**: 1010–1014.
224. Cockcroft DW, Murdock KY: Comparative effects of inhaled salbutamol, sodium cromoglycate and beclomethasone dipropionate on allergen-induced early asthmatic responses, late asthmatic responses and increased bronchial responsiveness to histamine. *J Allergy Clin Immunol* (1987) **79**: 734–740.
225. Murlas C, Bernstein DI, Bernstein IL, Steinberg DR: Prednisone inhibits the early increase in bronchial reactivity that occurs soon after the immediate response in dual responding asthmatics. *Am Rev Respir Dis* (1987) **135**: 311 (Abstract).
226. Chung KF: Role of inflammation in the hyperreactivity of the airways in asthma. *Thorax* (1986) **41**: 657–662.
227. Snashall PD, Gillett MK, Chung KF: Factors contributing to bronchial hyper-responsiveness in asthma. *Clin Science* (1988) **74**: 113–118.
228. Hopp JR, Townley RG, Biven RE, Bewtra AK, Nair NM: The presence of airway reactivity before the development of asthma. *Am Rev Respir Dis* (1990) **141**: 2–8.
229. Gibson PG, Dolovich J, Denburg J, Ramsdale EH, Hargreave FE: Chronic cough: eosino-philic bronchitis without asthma. *Lancet* (1989) **1**: 1346–1348.
230. Pattemore PK, Asher MI, Harrison AC, Mitchell EA, Rhea HH, Stewart AW: The interrelationship among bronchial hyperresponsiveness, the diagnosis of asthma, and asthma symptoms. *Am Rev Respir Dis* (1990) **142**: 549–554.
231. Djukanovic R, Wilson JW, Britten KM, *et al.*: Quantitation of mast cells and eosinophils in the bronchial mucosa of symptomatic atopic asthmatics and healthy control subjects using immunohistochemistry. *Am Rev Respir Dis* (1990) **142**: 863–871.
232. Howarth PH, Djukanovic RJ, Wilson JW, *et al.*: Influence of inhaled beclomethasone on airway inflammatory cell populations in asthma and the clinical correlates. *Thorax* (1990) **45**: 799 (Abstract).
233. Adelroth E, Rosenhall L, Johansson S-Å, Linden M, Venge P: Inflammatory cells and eosinophilic activity in asthmatics investigated by bronchoalveolar lavage. *Am Rev Respir Dis* (1990) **142**: 91–99.
234. Wolfe JD, Rosenthal RR, Bleecker E, Laube B, Norman PS, Permutt S: The effect of corticosteroids on cholinergic hyperreactivity. *J Allergy Clin Immunol* (1979) **63**: 163(A).
235. Easton JH. Effect of an inhaled corticosteroid on methacholine airway reactivity. *J Allergy Clin Immunol* (1981) **67**: 388–390.
236. Ryan G, Latimer KM, Juniper EF, Roberts RS, Hargreave FE: Effect of beclomethasone dipropionate on bronchial responsiveness to histamine in controlled non steroid dependent asthma. *J Allergy Clin Immunol* (1985) **75**: 25–30.
237. Jenkins CR, Woolcock AJ: Effect of prednisone and beclomethasone dipropionate on airway responsiveness in asthma: a comparative study. *Thorax* (1988) **43**: 378–384.
238. Bosman HG, van Uffelen R: Different effects of inhaled beclomethasone dipropionate and oral prednisone on bronchial hyperresponsiveness in asthma. *Eur Respir J* (1990) **3** (Suppl 10): 134s–135s (Abstract).
239. Svendson UG, Frolund L, Madsen F, Nielsen NH, Holstein-Rothlou NH, Weeke B: A comparison of the effects of sodium cromoglycate and beclomethasone dipropionate on pulmonary function and bronchial hyperreactivity in subjects with asthma. *J Allergy Clin Immunol* (1987) **80**: 68–74.
240. Kraan J, Koëter GH, van der Mark TW, *et al.*: Dosage and time effects of inhaled budesonide on bronchial hyperreactivity. *Am Rev Respir Dis* (1988) **137**: 44–48.

241. Juniper EF, Kline PA, Vanzieleghem MZ, Hargreave FE: Effect of inhaled steroid reduction on airway responsiveness and clinical asthma severity: a double blind, randomized controlled trial. *Thorax* (1989) **44**: 851P (Abstract).

242. Gibson PG, Hepperle MJE, Kline P, *et al.*: The first marker of an asthma exacerbation: symptoms, airway responsiveness, circulating eosinophils and progenitors. *J Allergy Clin Immunol* (1990) **85**: 166 (Abstract).

243. Kerrebijn KF, van Essen-Zandvliet EEM, Neijens HJ: Effect of long-term treatment with inhaled corticosteroids and beta-agonists on the bronchial responsiveness in children with asthma. *J Allergy Clin Immunol* (1987) **79**: 653–659.

244. De Marzo N, Fabbri LM, Crescioli S, Plebani M, Testi R, Mapp CE: Dose-dependent inhibitory effect of inhaled beclomethasone on late asthmatic reactions and increased responsiveness to metacholine induced by toluene diisocyanate in sensitized subjects. *Pulm Pharmacol* (1988) **1**: 15–20.

245. Owen S, Pickering CAC, Woolcock A: Effect of increasing doses of beclomethasone dipropionate on bronchial hyperreactivity in asthma. *Thorax* (1990) **45**: 786 (Abstract).

246. Juniper EF, Kline PA, Vanzieleghem MA, Ramsdale EH, O'Byrne PM, Hargreave FE: Effect of long-term treatment with an inhaled corticosteroid (budesonide) on airway hyperresponsiveness and clinical asthma in nonsteroid-dependent asthmatics. *Am Rev Respir Dis* (1990) **142**: 832–836.

247. Juniper EF, Kline PA, Vanzieleghem MA, Ramsdale EH, O'Byrne PM, Hargreave FE: Long-term effects of budesonide on airway responsiveness and clinical asthma severity in inhaled steroid-dependent asthmatics. *Eur Respir J* (1990) **3**: 1122–1127.

248. Bel HE, Timmers MC, Hermans J, Dijkman JH, Sterk PJ: The long term effects of nedocromil sodium and beclomethasone dipropionate on bronchial responsiveness to metacholine in nonatopic asthmatic subjects. *Am Rev Respir Dis* (1990) **141**: 21–28.

249. Dutoit JI, Salome CM, Woolcock AJ: Inhaled corticosteroids reduce the severity of bronchial hyperresponsiveness in asthma but oral theophylline does not. *Am Rev Respir Dis* (1987) **136**: 1174–1178.

250. De Baets FM, Goeteyn M, Kerrebijn KF: The effect of two months of treatment with inhaled budesonide on bronchial responsiveness to histamine and house-dust mite antigen in asthmatic subjects. *Am Rev Respir Dis* (1990) **142**: 581–586.

251. Vathenen AS, Knox AJ, Wisniewski A, Tattersfield AE: Effect of inhaled budesonide on bronchial responsiveness to histamine, eucapnic dry air hyperventilation and exercise in asthma. *Am Rev Respir Dis* (1989) **139**: A109 (Abstract).

252. Fuller RW, Barnes PJ: Mechanisms of asthma, bronchial hyperresponsiveness and action of glucocorticoids in asthma. In Hargreave FE, Hogg JC, Malo J-L, Toogood JH (eds), *Glucocorticoids and Mechanisms of Asthma*. Amsterdam Excerpta Medica, 1989, pp 5–12.

253. Thomson NC: *In vivo* versus *in vitro* human airway responsiveness to different pharmacologic stimuli. *Am Rev Respir Dis* (1987) **136**: S58–S62.

254. Gustafsson B, Persson CGA: Effect of three weeks' treatment with budesonide on *in vitro* contractile and relaxant airway effects in the rat. *Thorax* (1989) **44**: 24–27.

255. Van de Graaf EA, Out TA, Roos CM, Jansen HM: Respiratory membrane permeability and bronchial hyperreactivity in patients with stable asthma. Effects of therapy with inhaled steroids. *Am Rev Respir Dis* (1991) **143**: 362–368.

256. Lundgren R, Söderberg M, Hörstedt P, Stenling R: Morphological studies of bronchial mucosal biopsies from asthmatics before and after ten years treatment with inhaled steroids. *Eur Respir J* (1988) **1**: 883–889.

257. Geddes BA, Lefcoe NM: Respiratory smooth muscle relaxing effect of commercial steroid preparations. *Am Rev Respir Dis* (1973) **107**: 395–399.

258. Schleimer RP, Undem BJ, Meeker S, *et al.*: Dexamethasone inhibits the antigen-induced contractile activity and release of inflammatory mediators in isolated guinea pig lung tissue. *Am Rev Respir Dis* (1987) **135**: 562–566.

259. Souhrada M, Souhrada JF: Corticosteroids attenuate sensitization-induced membrane changes in airway smooth muscle cells. *Pulm Pharmacol* (1988) **1**: 69–76.

260. Schramm CM, Grunstein MM: Corticosteroid potentiation of the electrogenic Na^+-K^+ pump in rabbit airway smooth muscle. *Am Rev Respir Dis* (1988) **137**: 310 (Abstract).

261. Goldie RG, Spina D, Henry PJ, Lulich KM, Paterson JW: *In vitro* responsiveness of human asthmatic blockers to carbachol, histamine, beta-receptor agonists and theophylline. *Br J Clin Pharmacol* (1986) **22**: 669–676.

262. Bai TR: Abnormalities in airway smooth muscle in fatal asthma. *Am Rev Respir Dis* (1990) **141**: 552–557.

263. Spina D, Rigby PJ, Paterson JW, Goldie RG: Autoradiographic localization of beta-adrenoreceptors in asthmatic human lung. *Am Rev Respir Dis* (1989) **140**: 1410–1415.

264. Grandordy BM, Barnes PJ: Phosphoinositide turnover. *Am Rev Respir Dis* (1987) **136**: S17–S20.

265. Van Amsterdam RGM, Meurs H, Ten Berge REJ, Veninga NCM, Brouwer F, Zaagsma J: Role of phosphoinositide metabolism in human bronchial smooth muscle contraction and in functional antagonism by beta-adrenoreceptor agonists. *Am Rev Respir Dis* (1990) **142**: 1124–1128.

266. Samuelson WM, Davies AO: Hydrocortisone-induced reversal of beta-receptor uncoupling. *Am Rev Respir Dis* (1984) **130**: 1023–1026.

267. Davies AO, Lefkowitz RJ: Regulation of β-adrenergic receptors by steroid hormones. *Ann Rev Physiol* (1984) **46**: 119–130.

268. Taki F, Takagi K, Satake T, Sugiyama S, Ozawa T: The role of phospholipase in reduced beta-adrenergic responsiveness in experimental asthma. *Am Rev Respir Dis* (1986) **133**: 362–366.

269. Collins S, Caron MG, Lefkowitz RJ: Beta-adrenergic receptors in hamster smooth muscle cells are transcriptionally regulated by glucocorticoids. *J Biol Chem* (1988) **263**: 9067–9070.

270. Mano K, Akbarzadeh A, Townley RG: Effect of hydrocortisone on beta-adrenergic receptors in lung membranes. *Life Sci* (1979) **25**: 1925–1930.

271. Fraser CM, Venter JC: The synthesis of β-adrenergic receptors in cultured human lung cells: induction by glucocorticoids. *Biochem Biophys Res Commun* (1980) **94**: 390–397.

272. Chang FH, Bourne HR: Dexamethasone increases adenyl cyclase activity and expression of the α-subunit of G_s in GH$_3$ cells. *Endocrinology* (1987) **121**: 1711–1714.

273. Ros M, Watkins DC, Rapiejko PJ, Malbon CC: Glucocorticoids modulate mRNA for G-protein beta-subunits. *Biochem J* (1989) **260**: 271–275.

274. Ellul-Micallef R, Fenech FF: Effect of intravenous prednisolone in asthmatics with diminished adrenergic responsiveness. *Lancet* (1975) **2**: 1269–1271.

275. Walsh SD, Grant IWB: Corticosteroids in treatment of chronic asthma. *Br Med J* (1966) **2**: 796–802.

276. Ellul-Micallef R, Borthwick RC, McHardy GJR: Time course of response to corticosteroids in chronic airway obstruction. *Scot Med J* (1971) **16**: 534 (Abstract).

277. Ellul-Micallef R, Borthwick RC, McHardy GJR: The time course of response to prednisolone in chronic bronchial asthma. *Clin Sci Mol Med* (1974) **47**: 105–117.

278. Ellul-Micallef R, Fenech FF: Intravenous prednisolone in chronic bronchial asthma. *Thorax* (1975) **30**: 312–315.

279. Ellul-Micallef R, Johansson SA: Acute dose response studies in bronchial asthma with a new corticosteroid—budesonide. *Br J Clin Pharmacol* (1983) **15**: 419–422.

280. Klaustermeyer WB, Hale FC: The physiological effect of an intravenous glucocorticoid in bronchial asthma. *Ann Allergy* (1976) **37**: 80–86.

281. Ellul-Micallef R: The acute effects of corticosteroids in bronchial asthma. *Eur J Respir Dis* (1982) **63**(Suppl 122): 118–125.

282. Ellul-Micallef R, Borthwick RC, McHardy GJR: The effect of oral prednisolone on gas exchange in chronic bronchial asthma. *Br J Clin Pharmacol* (1980) **9**: 479–482.

283. Fanta CH, Rossing TH, McFadden ER: Glucocorticoids in acute asthma: a critical controlled trial. *Am J Med* (1983) **74**: 845–851.

284. Pierson WE, Bierman CW, Kelley VC: A double-blind trial of corticosteroid therapy in *status asthmaticus. Paediatrics* (1974) **54**: 282–288.

285. Sue MA, Kwong FK, Klaustermeyer WB: A comparison of intravenous hydrocortisone, methylprednisolone and dexamethasone in acute bronchial asthma. *Ann Allergy* (1986) **56**: 406–409.

286. Harfi H, Hanissian AS, Crawford LV: Treatment of *status asthmaticus* in children with high doses and conventional doses of methylprednisolone. *Paediatrics* (1978) **61**: 829–831.
287. Haskell RJ, Wong BM, Hansen JE: A double blind randomized clinical trial of methylprednisolone in *status asthmaticus*. *Arch Intern Med* (1983) **143**: 1324–1327.
288. Harrison BDW, Stokes TC, Hart CJ, Vaughan DA, Ali NJ, Robinson AA: Need for intravenous hydrocortisone in addition to oral prednisolone in patients admitted to hospital with severe asthma without ventilatory failure. *Lancet* (1986) **1**: 181–184.
289. Shenfield GM, Hodson ME, Clarke SW, Paterson JW: Interaction of corticosteroids and catecholamines in the treatment of asthma. *Thorax* (1975) **30**: 430–435.

Other Therapies Used in Asthma

PETER J. BARNES AND NEIL C. THOMSON

INTRODUCTION

Several other classes of drug have been used in the therapy of asthma, although none has proved to be of major clinical benefit.[1] Some of these treatments (e.g. antihistamines and cyclosporin) are discussed elsewhere in the book; in this chapter we discuss drugs that have occasionally been used in the treatment of asthma, together with non-pharmacological treatments, such as acupuncture, hypnotism and yoga, which have become popular as alternative therapies.

CALCIUM ANTAGONISTS

Calcium antagonists, which inhibit the entry of calcium ions (Ca^{2+}) into cells via voltage-dependent calcium channels, are widely used in the treatment of cardiovascular diseases, and it was hoped that they would find some application in the treatment of asthma, particularly in dilating or inhibiting the contraction of airway smooth muscle. In practice a number of calcium antagonists, such as nifedipine, verapamil and diltiazem, have been investigated in asthmatic patients. While a weak inhibitory effect on bronchoconstriction induced by spasmogens, such as histamine, methacholine, exercise and cold air, have been reported, there is no evidence that these drugs are bronchodilator or that they have any significant effect on clinical symptoms of asthma.[2,3]

The reasons for the clinical ineffectiveness of calcium antagonists in airway disease stems largely from the mechanisms involved in contraction of airway smooth muscle, as discussed in Chapter 5. Contraction of airway smooth muscle in response to the

ASTHMA: BASIC MECHANISMS AND CLINICAL MANAGEMENT (2nd Edn)
ISBN 0-12-079026-2

endogenous spasmogens released in asthmatic inflammation is mediated largely via phosphoinositide hydrolysis and release of Ca^{2+} from internal stores.[4] Although the maintenance of tone may depend on some calcium entry, this may be via channels that are not sensitive to conventional calcium antagonists. Similarly the release of mediators from inflammatory cells is not mediated via voltage-dependent calcium channels, and there is no evidence that calcium antagonists have a significant effect on either mediator release, activation of inflammatory cells or on the process of inflammation. In guinea-pigs calcium antagonists have a biphasic effect on airway microvascular leakage, with inhibition at low concentrations and increased leakage at high concentrations, presumably due to dilatation of bronchial vessels.[5]

Although calcium antagonists have no obvious beneficial effects in asthma, they are safe to use in asthmatic patients and may be useful in the treatment of concomitant ischaemic heart disease and hypertension.

α-ADRENOCEPTOR ANTAGONISTS

Although α-adrenoceptors, which mediate contraction of airway smooth muscle, have been described in several animal species, there is little evidence that they are important in mediating bronchoconstriction in asthma. There is no convincing evidence that α-receptors which mediate bronchoconstriction are present in human airways *in vitro*, even under conditions in which α-receptor activation has been described in other species or in airways from asthmatic patients (see Chapter 22).[6] The potent selective α_1-adrenoceptor antagonist prazosin has no effect, when given by inhalation, on resting airway tone in asthmatic patients and does not inhibit the bronchoconstrictor effect of histamine.[7] A small protective effect of inhaled prazosin on exercise-induced asthma may be due to an effect on bronchial blood flow. A trial of oral prazosin in chronic asthma provided no evidence of clinical benefit,[8] although occasional case reports of the beneficial effects of α-blockers are reported.

In canine airways the α-receptor which mediates bronchoconstriction is a post-junctional α_2-receptor, which is inhibited by α_2-antagonists such as yohimbine.[9] There is some evidence for a beneficial effect of an α_2-antagonist in asthma, although whether this is mediated via antagonism of α_2-receptors in airways is not yet certain.[10] Indeed other studies have claimed that an α_2-agonist clonidine has some beneficial effect in allergen-induced asthma.[11]

As with calcium antagonists, α-blockers have proved to be disappointing in the management of asthma, although they are safe to use in patients with asthma when used in the management of hypertension.

MUCOLYTICS

Although it is well known that asthmatics have viscid mucus plugs and that mucus plugging is probably common in severe asthmatic patients, there is no convincing evidence that mucolytic therapies have any beneficial effect on either lung function or symptoms of mucus hypersecretion in asthma. It is possible that more effective muco-lytic therapies than acetylcysteine and carbocysteine will be developed in the future, however.

METHOTREXATE

Methotrexate has long been used in the management of other chronic inflammatory conditions such as rheumatoid arthritis and psoriasis, so some beneficial effect in asthma might be expected. In a low dose (15 mg weekly) methotrexate has a sparing effect on the requirements for oral steroids in both children[12] and adults.[13,14] This is equivalent to approximately 7 mg prednisolone, although there is a large interindividual variation, which may be related to the clinical characteristics of the asthma. Even in a low dose, methotrexate has relatively frequent side-effects (nausea, gastrointestinal upset, blood dyscrasias, hepatic dysfunction), and should only be seriously considered as therapy in those patients who require maintenance oral steroids when side-effects (e.g. osteo-porosis, dyspepsia) are a problem. It is advisable to commence treatment with a low dose (5 mg orally), and only increase the dose to 15 mg weekly if there are no problems. If nausea is a major problem, intramuscular injection may be tolerated.[13] Regular blood counts and liver function tests should be carried out. As in the management of other chronic diseases, resistance to the effects of methotrexate may occur after prolonged use. There is no evidence that cyclophosphamide and azathiptrine provide a similar benefit in chronic asthma, although extensive clinical trials with these alternative immunosuppressive therapies have not yet been conducted.

GOLD

Gold salts are also used for treatment of rheumatoid arthritis and have been used in the management of chronic asthma in Japan for many years.[15] An open study suggests that there may be some clinical benefit of an oral gold preparation (auranofin) in asthma with a reduction in airway hyperresponsiveness,[16] but controlled studies are currently underway. In view of the numerous side-effects of gold salts this treatment cannot be recommended until there is convincing evidence for clinical benefit.

TROLEANDOMYCIN

The macrolide antibiotic troleandomycin has been used for the treatment of severe asthma for many years in the USA. It has some steroid-sparing activity, but only in patients taking methylprednisolone rather than prednisolone.[17] It appears to act by increasing the plasma half-life of methyl prednisolone through inhibition of hepatic cytochrome P_{450} activity (and prolongs the half-life of theophylline via the same mechanism).[18]

ALTERNATIVE FORMS OF TREATMENT

A number of non-pharmacological forms of treatment have been employed to treat asthma. The efficacy of these different therapies is often unclear because they have not often been assessed by appropriately controlled randomized studies.

Negative ion generators (ionizers)

Negatively charged air ions have been claimed to improve asthma.[19,20] In some asthmatic children, positively ionized air has been shown to potentiate exercise-induced asthma.[21] In a double-blind placebo-controlled crossover study undertaken over a 6-month period, Nogrady and Furnass[22] failed to demonstrate that the use of a negative ion generator produced any significant improvement in asthma control as assessed by peak flow measurements, symptom score or use of medication.

Yoga

Yoga has been employed to treat asthma in India for many years. A randomized study of yoga treatment found it to be significantly better than standard therapy in the long-term control of asthma.[23] A major defect in the design of this investigation was the fact that patients recruited for the study were all referred for yoga therapy, so the control group may have been adversely affected by being denied a treatment they believed might benefit their asthma. A recently reported double-blind, controlled study employing yoga breathing exercises (pranayama), however, has reported that this type of controlled ventilation resulted in improvements in asthma symptom control, lung function and medication use.[24]

Homoeopathy

Homoeopathic preparations are available for the treatment of asthma, although the efficacy of these substances has not been assessed in randomized placebo-controlled double-blind studies. Interestingly, an investigation employing this type of study design reported that a homoeopathic preparation of mixed grass pollen was more effective than placebo in the treatment of patients with hayfever due to grass pollen.[25] None of the patients in this study had asthma.

Hypnosis

In several poorly controlled studies, hypnosis has been reported to have a beneficial effect in the treatment of asthma.[26-28] Ewer and Stewart[29] undertook a trial of hypnotic technique using a prospective, randomized, single-blind controlled study design. Patients described as having a moderate to high susceptibility to hypnosis showed an improvement in methacholine airway responsiveness, symptom dairy card scores, peak flow recording and use of bronchodilators after 6 weeks of hypnotherapy. No improvement in these measurements occurred in a control group or in patients with low susceptibility to hypnosis. These results suggest that a small percentage of asthmatic patients may obtain some benefit from hypnotherapy although further evidence from controlled studies is required.

Acupuncture

A number of studies have examined the effects of acupuncture in asthma, although the results have often been conflicting.[30–36] A small bronchodilator effect has been reported in some[30,31] but not all[32,33] studies after a single acupuncture session. The bronchoconstrictor response to exercise[27] and methacholine,[34] but not histamine,[30,36] can be partly attenuated by acupuncture. Others have reported no significant effect of acupuncture on exercise-induced asthma.[30] In a carefully controlled study, Tashkin et al.[35] failed to demonstrate any useful effect of acupuncture treatment given for a 4-week period on various indices of asthma control.

Surgical techniques

On the basis that carotid body chemoreceptor may be involved in producing bronchoconstriction,[37] a number of asthmatic patients have been subjected to unilateral and, in some cases, bilateral carotid body excision, in the hope of improving the control of their asthma.[38] There is no convincing evidence that this surgical technique is of any value and it is not without serious side-effects.[38]

Surgical denervation of vagus nerve has been undertaken for the treatment of asthma.[39,40] These operations were uncontrolled, and objective assessments of asthma control were not undertaken.

Physical training

Physical training has been advocated as a method of improving exercise tolerance in asthmatic patients.[41,42] These exercise programmes have been used particularly in children, and it has been suggested that other beneficial effects, including increased self confidence, improved general health and reduction in drug medication, may result from this therapy. Although there are a number of reports describing the value of physical training programmes, only a few trials have examined this treatment by means of randomized single-blind controlled studies.[43,44] Swann and Hanson[43] studied asthmatic children with evidence of exercise-induced asthma, and randomized one group to undergo a graduated physical training programme, the other group taking part in relaxation classes. Both forms of treatment were supervised by a physiotherapist. At 3 months there was no significant difference in peak expiratory flow measurements, diary symptom scores or degree of exercise-induced asthma between the two groups.

Interestingly, both groups showed a decrease in maximal fall in PFR after exercise at 3 months compared to baseline values. This result suggested that the reduction in exercise-induced asthma during the study was not related to the physical training programme. In adult patients with perennial asthma, Bundgaard et al.[44] showed that physical training which improved maximal oxygen consumption produced a small reduction in β_2-agonist usage, whereas physical training which did not alter maximal oxygen uptake did not change drug requirements. More recently, however, Cochrane and Clark[45] found that a submaximal physical exercise programme undertaken over a 3-month period produced improvements in fitness and cardiorespiratory performance of a group of adult asthmatic patients. The main factors influencing an improvement in fitness were the subject's motivation, the initial level of fitness and the symptom score at the time of training.

REFERENCES

1. Barnes PJ: A new approach to asthma therapy. *N Engl J Med* (1989) **321**: 1517–1527.
2. Barnes PJ: Clinical studies with calcium antagonists in asthma. *Br J Clin Pharmacol* (1985) **20**: 289–298S.
3. Löfdahl C-G, Barnes PJ: Calcium channel blockade and asthma—the current position. *Eur J Respir Dis* (1985) **67**: 233–237.
4. Hall I, Chilvers ER: Inositol phosphates and airway smooth muscle. *Pulm Pharmacol* (1989) **2**: 113–120.
5. Boschetto P, Roberts NM, Rogers DF, Barnes PJ: The effect of antiasthma drugs on microvascular leak in guinea pig airways. *Am Rev Respir Dis* (1989) **139**: 416–421.
6. Spina D, Rigby PJ, Paterson JW, Goldie RG: α_1-Adrenoceptor function and autoradiographic distribution in human asthmatic lung. *Br J Pharmacol* (1989) **97**: 701–708.
7. Barnes PJ, Wilson NM, Vickers H: Prazosin, an α_1-adrenoceptor antagonist partially inhibits exercise-induced asthma. *J Allergy Clin Immunol* (1981) **68**: 411–419.
8. Baudouin SV, Aitman TJ, Johnson AJ: Prazosin in the treatment of chronic asthma. *Thorax* (1988) **43**: 385–387.
9. Barnes PJ, Skoogh B-E, Nadel JA, Roberts JM: Postsynaptic α_2-adrenoceptors predominate over α_1-adrenoceptors in canine tracheal smooth muscle and mediate neuronal and hormonal α-adrenergic contraction. *Mol Pharmacol* (1983) **23**: 570–575.
10. Yoshie Y, Iizuka K, Nakazawa T: The inhibitory effect of a selective α_2-adrenergic receptor antagonist on moderate to severe-type asthma. *J Allergy Clin Immunol* (1989) **84**: 747–752.
11. Lindgren BR, Ekström T, Andersson RGG: The effect of inhaled clonidine in patients with asthma. *Am Rev Respir Dis* (1986) **134**: 266–269.
12. Mullarkey MF, Blumenstein BA, Mandrade WP, Bailey GA, Olason I, Wetzel CE: Methotrexate in the treatment of corticosteroid-dependent asthma. *N Engl J Med* (1988) **318**: 603–607.
13. Mullarkey MF, Lammert JK, Blumenstein BA: Long-term methotrexate treatment in corticosteroid-dependent asthma. *Ann Int Med* (1990) **112**: 577–581.
14. Shiner RJ, Nunn AJ, Chung KF, Geddes DM: Randomized, double-blind, placebo-controlled trial of methotrexate in steroid-dependent asthma. *Lancet* (1990) **336**: 137–140.
15. Muranaka M, Miyamoto T, Shida T, *et al.*: Gold salt in the treatment of bronchial asthma. *Ann Allergy* (1978) **40**: 132–137.
16. Bernstein DI, Berstein IL, Bodgenheimer SS, Pietrosko RG: An open study of Auranofin in the treatment of steroid-dependent asthma. *J Allergy Clin Immunol* (1988) **81**: 6–16.
17. Zeiger RS, Schatz M, Sperling W, Simon RA, Stevenson DD: Efficacy of troleandomycin in outpatients with severe corticosteroid-dependent asthma. *J Allergy Clin Immunol* (1980) **66**: 438–446.

18. Szefler SJ, Rose JQ, Ellis EF, Spector SL, Green AW, Jusko WJ: The effect of troleandomycin on methylprednisolone elimination. *J Allergy Clin Immunol* (1980) **66**: 447–451.
19. Jones DP, Connor SA, Collins JV, Watson BW: Effect of long term ionised air treatment on patients with bronchial asthma. *Thorax* (1976) **31**: 428–432.
20. Osterballe O, Weeke B, Albrechesten O: Influence of small atmospheric ions on the airways in patients with bronchial asthma. *Allergy* (1979) **34**: 187–194.
21. Lipin I, Gur I, Amitai Y, Amirav I, Godfrey S: Effect of positive ionisation of inspired air on the response of asthmatic children to exercise. *Thorax* (1984) **39**: 594–596.
22. Nogrady SG, Furnass SB: Ionisers in the management of bronchial asthma. *Thorax* (1983) **38**: 919–922.
23. Nagarathma R, Nagendra HR: Yoga for bronchial asthma: a controlled study. *Br Med J* (1985) **293**: 1129–1132.
24. Singh V, Wisniewski A, Britton J, Tattersfield A: Effect of yoga breathing exercises (pranayama) on airway reactivity in subjects with asthma. *Lancet* (1990) **335**: 1381–1383.
25. Reilly DT, Taylor MA, McSharry C, Aitchison T: Is homoeopathy a placebo response? Controlled trial of homoeopathic potency, with pollen in hay fever as a model. *Lancet* (1986) **2**: 881–886.
26. Diamond HH: Hypnosis in children: complete cure of 40 cases of asthma. *Am J Hypnosis* (1959) **1**: 124–129.
27. Maher-Loughnan GP, MacDonald N, Mason AA, Fry L: Controlled trial of hypnosis in the symptomatic treatment of asthma. *Br Med J* (1962) **2**: 371–376.
28. Aronoff GM, Aronoff S, Peck LW: Hypnotherapy in the treatment of bronchial asthma. *Ann Allergy* (1975) **34**: 356–362.
29. Ewer TC, Stewart DE: Improvement in bronchial hyperresponsiveness in patients with moderate asthma after treatments with a hypnotic technique: a randomized controlled trial. *Br Med J* **293**: 1129–1132.
30. Yu DYC, Lee SP: Effect of acupuncture on bronchial asthma. *Clin Sci* (1976) **51**: 503–509.
31. Virsik K, Kristufek P, Bangha D, Urloan S: The effects of acupuncture on pulmonary function in bronchial asthma. *Pract Resp Res* (1980) **14**: 271–275.
32. Fung KP, Chow OKW: Attenuation of exercise-induced asthma by acupuncture. *Lancet* (1986) **2**: 1419–1422.
33. Chow OKW, So SY, Lam WK, Yu DYC, Yeung CY: Effect of acupuncture on exercise-induced asthma. *Lung* (1983) **161**: 321–326.
34. Tashkin DP, Brester DE, Kreoning RJ, Kerschner H, Katz RL, Coulson A: Comparison of real and stimulated acupuncture and isproterenol in methacholine-induced asthma. *Ann Allergy* (1977) **39**: 379–387.
35. Tashkin DP, Kroening RJ, Bresler DE, Simmons M, Coulson AH, Kershnan H: A controlled trial of real and stimulated acupuncture in the management of chronic asthma. *J Allergy Clin Immunol* (1985) **76**: 855–864.
36. Tandon MK, Soh PFT: Comparison of real and placebo acupuncture in histamine-induced asthma. A double-blind crossover study. *Chest* (1989) **96**: 102–105.
37. Nadel JA, Widdicombe JG: Effect of changes in blood gas tensions and carotid sinus pressure on tracheal volume and total lung resistance of airflow. *J Physiol* (1962) **163**: 13–22.
38. Anderson JA, Chai H, Claman HN: Carotid body resection. *J Allergy Clin Immunol* (1986) **78**: 273–275.
39. Phillips EW, Scott WJM: The surgical treatment of bronchial asthma. *Arch Surg* (1925) **19**: 1425–1430.
40. Dimitrov-Szokodi D, Husvéti A, Balogh G: Lung degeneration in the therapy of intractable bronchial asthma. *J Thorax Surgery* (1957) **33**: 166–184.
41. Oseid S: Physical activity as part of a comprehensive rehabilitation programme in asthmatic children. In Oseid S, Edwards AM (eds) *The Asthmatic Child in Play and Sport*. London, Pitman Press, 1983, pp 237–245.
42. Fitch KD: Sport, physical activity and the asthmatic. In Oseid S, Edwards AM (eds) *The Asthmatic Child in Play and Sport*. London, Pitman Press, 1983, pp 246–258.

43. Swann IL, Hanson CA: Double-blind prospective study of the effect of physical training on childhood asthma. In Oseid S, Edwards AM (eds) *The Asthmatic Child in Play and Sport.* London, Pitman Press, 1983, pp 318–322.
44. Bundgaard A, Ingemann-Hansen T, Halkjear-Kristensen J, Schmidt A, Block I, Andero PK: Short term physical training in bronchial asthma. *Br J Dis Chest* (1983) **377**: 147–152.
45. Cochrane LM, Clark CJ: Benefits and problems of a physical training programme for asthmatic patients. *Thorax* (1990) **45**: 345–351.

Severe Acute Asthma

GRAHAM K. CROMPTON

INTRODUCTION

Severe acute asthma has replaced the old term '*status asthmaticus*' as a description of a life-threatening episode of bronchial asthma. Clinically patients are distressed by dyspnoea, chest tightness and are unable to speak full sentences. They sit or stand with shoulder muscles braced in an attempt to assist their breathing. Ill patients are usually pale and sweaty. Obvious cyanosis indicates severe hypoxaemia. Confusion and drowsiness only accompanies gross hypoxaemia and hypercapnia. Respiratory acidosis should be regarded as evidence of impending death. Children, however, tend to develop acidaemia more readily than adults and this is often due to a combination of respiratory and metabolic acidosis.

Subcutaneous emphysema of the neck and face occurs in some patients with severe asthma and is a reflection of very high intrathoracic pressures but rarely is subcutaneous emphysema associated with pneumothorax.

GENERAL ASSESSMENT AND MANAGEMENT

A rapid clinical appraisal of the features mentioned above usually gives a fairly accurate assessment of disease severity. Auscultation of the chest is of limited value since patients with severe disease are unable to shift enough air to produce rhonchi, but in the absence of a chest radiograph auscultation is essential to ensure that the breath sounds are present over both lungs. Whenever possible a chest X-ray should be performed, especially if mechanical ventilation is necessary, in order to exclude a pneumothorax

ASTHMA: BASIC MECHANISMS AND CLINICAL MANAGEMENT (2nd Edn)
ISBN 0-12-079026-2

which is a rare but potentially fatal complication of severe asthma. Measurement of heart rate and the degree of *pulsus paradoxus*[1] are invaluable in initial assessment and subsequent monitoring of response to treatment. The heart rate is usually rapid and almost invariably over 100–120/min. However, it must be appreciated that severe hypoxaemia can cause progressive bradycardia which can culminate in hypoxaemic cardiac asystole unless hypoxaemia is reversed. A marked degree of *pulsus paradoxus* of 40 mmHg or more is present in some patients. The absence of *pulsus paradoxus* does not, however, exclude severe asthma.

Ventilatory function tests such as the peak expiratory flow (PEF) and the forced expiratory volume in 1 s (FEV_1) are of limited value in the assessment of very seriously ill patients since anxiety and distress make it difficult for them to perform forced expiratory manoeuvres, and values recorded may be inaccurate. However, PEF should be recorded in all patients able to co-operate to provide an objective baseline to allow subsequent rapid assessment of response to treatment. A PEF of <40% of predicted normal or of the best obtainable result if known (<200 litres/min if the best obtainable result is not known) should be regarded as evidence of a potentially life-threatening attack of asthma.[2]

Arterial blood gas analysis is essential in the assessment of disease severity and repeated measurements are necessary to assess response to treatment. Normal blood gas tensions with the patient breathing air exclude life-threatening disease. All ill patients are hypoxaemic. Hypoxaemia plus hypercapnia is only found in severely ill patients.

General measures

Severe acute asthma causes great respiratory distress and most ill patients are terrified because they feel that they are going to die. It would seem logical, therefore, to ease distress and anxiety with a sedative or anxiolytic drug. However, although reports of deaths directly attributable to sedation are few[3,4] sedation must be avoided since it is illogical. Patients with severe acute asthma breathe with the maximum efficient use of their respiratory muscles and in spite of this are unable to maintain normal arterial blood gas tensions. To suppress ventilation with any form of sedation is, therefore, likely to lead to a deterioration in, rather than an improvement of, the basic disease state. Occasionally patients with mild or moderately severe asthma become excessively agitated and this leads to hyperventilation out of proportion to the severity of asthma. These patients usually have near normal arterial oxygen tensions and respiratory alkalosis. The use of diazepam in small doses may be appropriate in such circumstances. However, as a general rule, sedation in severe asthma must be avoided and should never be given without immediate access to facilities for arterial blood gas monitoring and assisted ventilation.[2] Sedation is, of course, mandatory in patients who are being mechanically ventilated (page 672) or being intubated prior to assisted ventilation.

Hydration

Intravenous fluids are rarely necessary for rehydration unless the attack has been of many hours' duration. Prolonged severe asthma does lead to fluid deprivation, since breathless patients avoid drinking as they 'cannot afford the time to swallow'. Hyperventilation associated with severe asthma also leads to an increase in obligatory fluid loss. Although fluid replacement is necessary in only a few patients this should always be kept in mind and it is wise to have an intravenous access in all ill patients, particularly in those who do not rapidly respond to initial nebulized bronchodilator therapy. The intravenous line can be used for fluid replacement when necessary, but its main purpose is to provide immediate intravenous access for the administration of drugs should this be necessary. All ill patients are capable of developing sudden deterioration and if respiratory arrest occurs an *in situ* IV line is invaluable. Electrolyte imbalance can occur in some patients. Hypokalaemia can be induced by β-agonist and corticosteroid therapy, and can be made worse by over-zealous intravenous transfusion of potassium-free solutions.

SPECIFIC TREATMENT FOR SEVERE ACUTE ASTHMA

There is no fixed order for the treatments used for severe asthma since in very ill patients almost all drugs and oxygen will be given at the same time. In less critically ill patients bronchodilator drugs alone may be given and other treatments may not be necessary. In the majority of patients with severe asthma, however, a combination of treatments is usually necessary. Response to treatment must be assessed by measurements of PEF, and arterial blood gas analysis together with careful clinical observations.

Oxygen therapy

All ill patients are hypoxaemic and require oxygen. At one time it was suggested that low inspired oxygen concentrations should be given unless blood gas monitoring was immediately available[5] in order to avoid the precipitation of, or worsening of hypercapnia. However, it is now accepted that there is no risk of causing carbon dioxide retention in an asthmatic who does not also have co-existing chronic obstructive bronchitis. Oxygen should, therefore, be given by face mask in the highest concentration possible. Masks delivering 24 or 28% oxygen are not appropriate.[2] The most comfortable masks for distressed patients are high-concentration Venturi oxygen systems employing the Bernoulli principle. However, the recommended oxygen flow rate for these masks may have to be exceeded to maintain the desired high inspired oxygen tension in patients with rapid breathing frequencies and high tidal volumes.[6]

Hypoxaemia should be treated with oxygen in concentrations as high as is necessary to maintain an arterial oxygen tension (PaO_2) of at least 9 kPa (80 mmHg). When facilities for arterial blood gas analysis are not available, and it is known that the patient suffers from asthma and not chronic bronchitis, high concentrations of oxygen should be given (35–60%). Even when patients are found to have hypercapnia and hypoxaemia, high concentrations of oxygen must be administered (35% or more) since such abnormalities of blood gas tensions reflect severe airflow obstruction, and not a central defect of carbon dioxide responsiveness, which requires oxygen, optimal bronchodilator therapy (page 670) and corticosteroids (page 672). To deny adequate oxygenation of these patients is irrational since deliberate perpetuation of hypoxaemia is dangerous. When hypoxaemia persists and hypercapnia worsens assisted ventilation is required (page 672) and this cannot be avoided by giving low concentration oxygen therapy. In the treatment of patients with uncomplicated bronchial asthma high concentrations of oxygen carry no dangers,[7] and an inspired oxygen concentration of at least 30% should be used in all patients.[8] Most distressed patients dislike closely fitting face masks and should be treated with masks employing the Venturi principle or even nasal prongs providing high flows are used. Oxygen tents may have to be used for young children.

The administration of bronchodilator drugs, particularly when given by the intravenous route, can cause worsening of hypoxaemia. It is, therefore, prudent to treat patients with oxygen before, during and after such treatments. Patients with severe asthma should be given oxygen during the transfer from home to hospital. The general practitioner, or family physician, should give oxygen in the home whenever possible, and ensure that oxygen therapy is administered by the ambulance crew when admission to hospital is necessary.

β_2-Adrenoreceptor agonist therapy

Treatment with selective β_2-adrenoreceptor agonists is now first-line therapy in most hospitals in the UK[9] and other countries. A large dose of one of these drugs nebulized in oxygen is to be preferred to their intravenous administration,[10] since although both routes of treatment are effective,[11–13] high dose inhaled salbutamol has been shown to be more effective than conventional doses of the same drug given intravenously.[14] The dose of intravenous salbutamol necessary to achieve a better response than nebulized treatment causes unacceptable cardiovascular effects.[15] A combination of aerosol and intravenous β_2-adrenoreceptor agonists should be avoided. Salbutamol (2.5–5.0 mg) or terbutaline (5–10 mg) should be nebulized in oxygen whenever possible. Nebulized therapy is unlikely to cause worsening of hypoxaemia,[16] but oxygen therapy should not be interrupted during treatment of hypoxaemic patients. Ultrasonic nebulizers and air compressors to drive jet nebulizers should, therefore, not be used in hospital. Aerosol therapy delivered by intermittent positive-pressure breathing (IPPB) has no advantages over simple jet nebulizer treatment.[17,18] The response to a large dose of nebulized salbutamol is rapid and continued improvement of ventilatory function should not be expected for more than 10–20 min.[16,18] Hence, if a patient remains unwell more than 20 min after a large dose of a β_2-adrenoreceptor agonist, treatment should be repeated or additional therapy with ipratropium bromide (page 671) and in some patients a xanthine derivative (page 671) should be given.

Large volume spacer attachments to the conventional metered-dose inhaler (MDI) provide an alternative to nebulizers as a method of administering high doses of β_2-adrenoreceptor agonists in the treatment of severe asthma.[19] Such devices can be used outside hospital when facilities for nebulization in oxygen are not available. Face masks specially designed for use with large volume holding chambers make administration of drugs to children much easier than via a mouthpiece. Salbutamol (4 μg/kg body weight) or terbutaline (0.25–0.5 mg) can be given by slow intravenous injection, and also by continuous intravenous infusion. Compared with aerosol therapy intravenous administration is associated with more unwanted effects, and is also more likely to cause an increase in the degree of arterial hypoxaemia. Administration of β_2-adrenoreceptor agonists by intramuscular or subcutaneous injection should be avoided whenever possible, since it is difficult to assess response when such drugs are given by these routes.

Anticholinergics

The quarternary ammonium compound ipratropium bromide has little value in the treatment of chronic asthma but has an important role in the management of patients with severe acute asthma. The onset of bronchodilator action of this drug is considerably slower than that of inhaled sympathomimetic bronchodilators, but is as effective as salbutamol.[20,21] Also there is evidence that a combination of ipratropium bromide and an inhaled sympathomimetic is considerably better than either drug given alone[20-23] although this has been questioned.[24] Ipratropium bromide should be nebulized in a dose of 0.1–0.5 mg, but should never be given alone as primary treatment since it has a much slower onset of action than salbutamol and terbutaline and it has been reported to cause bronchoconstriction.[25,26] Most bronchoconstrictor responses were probably caused by the tonicity of and preservative in the original respirator solution[27,28] but since the first report of an adverse reaction was to ipratropium bromide inhaled from a pressured aerosol[26] it is wise to avoid this drug as primary treatment. However, combination of ipratropium bromide and a sympathomimetic bronchodilator is often given when there has not been a satisfactory response to initial treatment with a nebulized β_2-adrenoreceptor agonist and the combination of ipratropium bromide and salbutamol or terbutaline may become first-line treatment for severe asthma.

Xanthine derivatives

Xanthine derivatives (aminophylline, theophylline) by intravenous injection have been used for many years in the treatment of severe asthma. However, intravenous salbutamol has been shown to be at least as effective as intravenous aminophylline[29,30] and since high dose aerosol β_2-agonist therapy is as effective, and has fewer side-effects than intravenous treatment (page 670), nebulized β_2-adrenoreceptor agonists have replaced intravenous theophyllines as first-line treatment of severe asthma.

Aminophylline is recommended as a slow intravenous injection over 20 min (5 mg/kg body weight) followed, if necessary, by a continuous infusion (0.5 mg/kg body weight.[31] An alternative dose recommendation is 0.5–0.9 mg/kg/h without a loading dose. If the weight of the patient is unknown, doses can be estimated depending upon the patient's size (small patients—600–1000 mg/24 h; medium size patients—900–1500 mg/24 h; large patients—1100–1900 mg/24 h).[2] Unwanted effects such as nausea are common and potentially fatal central nervous system toxic effects can occur if serum levels exceed 30 mg/litre. It is, therefore, unwise to give an intravenous loading dose to patients already taking an oral methylxanthine preparation, unless the serum theophylline level is known. Infusions of theophylline should be adjusted to maintain a blood level within the 'therapeutic range' of 10–20 mg/litre[32] unless this is associated with unacceptable side-effects. Aminophylline (theophylline) should be used in patients who do not quickly respond to a nebulized β_2-adrenoreceptor agonist combined with ipratropium bromide. In moribund patients, however, it should be given at once together with nebulized therapy.

Corticosteroids

The value of corticosteroid therapy in the management of severe asthma was first reported in 1949[33] and confirmed by clinical trial in 1956.[34] During the last three decades corticosteroids have been used routinely by most physicians in the treatment of patients with severe asthma, although some paediatricians tend to reserve their use for the most critically ill patients. The value of these drugs in severe asthma has only rarely been questioned[35] and their use should be routine in all patients who do not respond rapidly and substantially to bronchodilator therapy.[36,37] Large doses of intravenous hydrocortisone or methylprednisolone are usually given empirically since short course high-dose corticosteroid treatment is free from serious unwanted effects providing the possibilities of hypokalaemia and fluid retention are borne in mind. Very high doses of hydrocortisone or methylprednisolone are probably not necessary,[38,39] and might cause an acute myopathy.[40] Doses of hydrocortisone which produce blood levels that exceed stress-induced physiological levels have been recommended[41] — 3–4 mg/kg loading dose followed by the same dose by intravenous infusion 6-hourly. However, standard empirical doses of 200 mg 4–6-hourly during the first 24–48 h of treatment are often used. Intravenous corticosteroids are then replaced by prednisolone in doses of 30–60 mg daily. Oral therapy is given initially to patients who do not have life-threatening disease. It has, however, been suggested that intravenous corticosteroid therapy is not necessary if large doses of oral prednisolone, together with a nebulized sympathomimetic drug plus intravenous aminophylline are also used.[42]

ASSISTED VENTILATION

Assisted ventilation is rarely necessary, but has to be instituted in a few patients as a life-saving procedure. In adults a cuffed endotracheal tube is essential and a powerful volume-cycled ventilator must be used.

The indications for assisted ventilation in asthma are difficult to define since some patients have to be electively ventilated because of lack of response to treatment together with the assumption that a crises situation is impending. However, it is generally accepted that assisted ventilation is essential in patients who, in spite of full medical treatment, have:

(1) A $PaCO_2$ of more than 50 mmHg (6.6 kPa) and rising;
(2) A PaO_2 of less than 50 mmHg (6.6 kPa) and falling;
(3) A pH of 7.3 or less and falling;
(4) Intolerable respiratory distress;
(5) Respiratory arrest;
(6) Cardio-respiratory arrest.

Ventilation should also be considered in all patients who have had prolonged severe asthma and who are becoming tired and exhausted. Physical exhaustion associated with systemic hypotension is a dangerous combination. When there is any doubt about whether a patient should or should not be ventilated the safest course of action is to ventilate and not to procrastinate.

It has been suggested that the complications of ventilation of patients with asthma are a consequence of barotrauma caused by high intrapulmonary pressures.[43,44,45] For this reason it has been recommended that inflation pressures of greater than 50 cm of water should be avoided by planned assisted hypoventilation, irrespective of the inevitable perpetuation of respiratory acidosis in some patients.[43] However, this approach to the ventilation of patients with severe asthma has been questioned and the restoration of normal blood gas tensions as quickly as possible, irrespective of the inflation pressures necessary to achieve this objective, has been recommended.[46] The dangers of barotrauma caused by high inflation pressures are claimed to be over-estimated after a review of the literature and an assessment of personal experience.[46] The debate about the advantages and disadvantages of adopting policies of planned hypoventilation or the more aggressive approach of trying to normalize arterial blood gas tensions as quickly as possible will continue. However, there appears to be no doubt that the combination of planned assisted hypoventilation and therapeutic bronchial lavage is associated with unacceptable pulmonary infection and death.[47] Patients treated with planned assisted hypoventilation almost invariably have to be given muscle relaxants to allow them to synchronize with the ventilator, whereas with patients in whom respiratory acidosis is normalized as quickly as possible, sedation with opiates is usually sufficient. In a small minority of patients it is not possible to ventilate mechanically because of extremely high inflation pressures that exceed the pressures most volume-cycled ventilators are capable of generating. In these patients it is always worthwhile trying the effects of the anaesthetic diethyl ether which has long been known to have a relaxant effect on the airways.[48,49] The most effective, more modern, anaesthetic agent with properties similar to diethyl ether is isoflurane which should be given if diethyl ether is not available or cannot be given via a modern anaesthetic apparatus.

MANAGEMENT OF CATASTROPHIC ASTHMA

Some patients suddenly develop catastrophic attacks of asthma perhaps in spite of receiving treatment which controls the symptoms of most other patients. These individuals are, of course, at greatest risk of dying from asthma. Little can be done for the unfortunate patient whose onset of asthma is a devastating attack, except hope that it is not fatal so that appropriate plans for the management of the next anticipated severe attack can be made. All patients who have had one life-threatening episode of asthma must be regarded as high-risk candidates for a recurrence. Not only is the asthmatic who has had one bad attack more likely to have a recurrence than patients who have never experienced a severe episode, but the pattern of future attacks is likely to be similar also. Once recognized, therefore, the catastrophic asthmatic provides a difficult therapeutic challenge since severe attacks of sudden onset can be anticipated in the future and many patients with this type of asthma can die within a short time of the attack starting. There are a number of important issues concerned in the management of patients with catastrophic asthma which can be discussed under separate headings but these are obviously intimately interrelated in clinical practice.

Identification of possible trigger factors

Hypersensitivity reactions are usually easy to recognize even in retrospect. Drug reactions are sometimes more difficult particularly those caused by aspirin, non-steroidal anti-inflammatory drugs (NSAIDS) or combinations containing such drugs. It is unlikely that ingestion of a β-blocker was responsible since this should have been discovered by the general practitioner or the team responsible for resuscitation. Even if no drug cause is obvious, on general principles, aspirin, NSAIDS and all β-blockers should be avoided. A card on which this information is stated should be carried by the patient.

Regular treatment to be taken in order to try to prevent recurrence of the severe episode

It would appear to be prudent for all patients who have experienced a life-threatening episode of asthma to be treated with an inhaled corticosteroid in a dose of at least 800–1000 μg daily. Immediately, after a devastating attack, long-term prednisolone may be given in an initial dose of 10 mg daily with reductions in dose thereafter by 1 mg decrements every month until treatment is withdrawn or symptoms recur.

Recognition of the onset of a potentially life-threatening attack in the future

Most patients have no difficulty in recognizing the onset of a severe episode but sometimes deterioration can take place over hours or even days before the patient is aware of symptomatic deterioration. Patients with catastrophic asthma should, therefore, record their peak expiratory flow (PEF) regularly in order to pick up any deterioration which should allow therapeutic intervention at the earliest possible stage. At the onset of a severe attack large doses of a bronchodilator, e.g. 20–50 doses from a conventional inhaler, should be taken and the patient should seek medical advice immediately.

Self-treatment

As well as being advised to inhale a large dose of a β-agonist, perhaps via a large volume spacer or nebulizer if possible, selected patients should be provided with preloaded syringes containing either terbutaline or adrenaline for subcutaneous or intramuscular injection. A number of such syringes should be provided so that they can be kept in strategic places such as home, brief case, schoolbag, glove compartment of car, office drawer, etc. Oral prednisolone should also be taken in a single dose of 60 mg as soon as the onset of a severe attack has been recognized.

Admission to hospital as soon as possible

Some hospitals run formal self-admission services which have been shown to save lives.[50] If possible arrangements for self-admission should be made for all patients who have experienced a rapid onset episode of life-threatening asthma. Preferably admission should be by ambulance since this will allow nebulized salbutamol or terbutaline in oxygen to be given by the ambulance crew during the journey to hospital.[51] The ambulance crew should alert the receiving hospital of the imminent arrival of a patient with severe asthma in order that the hospital can be prepared for resuscitation and ventilation if necessary.

OTHER MEASURES

Antibiotics

Antibiotics have somehow become almost routine in the treatment of severe asthma even though there is no evidence that they are of any value.[52,53] Patients with severe acute asthma should only be given antibiotic therapy when there is an absolute indication for this treatment, such as pneumonia or overt bronchial infection.

Mucolytics

There is no evidence that the mucolytic drugs presently available have any beneficial effects in any of the diseases for which they are recommended. They are of no value in the treatment of asthma.

Bronchial lavage

The mechanical removal of mucus plugs by lavaging the bronchi with saline via an endotracheal tube or bronchoscope has been recommended in patients who require assisted ventilation. This technique has been reported to be associated with serious bronchopulmonary infection.[47] Therefore, the routine use of bronchial lavage in patients requiring assisted ventilation can no longer be advocated.

Physiotherapy

Patients with severe acute asthma cannot cough efficiently, because of severe generalized airflow obstruction. The physiotherapist has no role in the management of the severely ill patient in terms of assisted coughing and expectoration.[2]

Magnesium sulphate

Magnesium sulphate was first reported to have a bronchodilating action in 1936[54] and recently there has been a resurgence of interest in its possible role in the treatment of severe acute asthma.[55,56] These reports suggest that intravenous magnesium sulphate in doses of 1.2–3.0 g has a beneficial effect in patients with severe asthma and that it is free from serious adverse effects. However, results of assessments of this drug in trials in which larger numbers of patients have been included must be awaited before it can be decided whether or not magnesium sulphate has any useful therapeutic role in the treatment of severe asthma.

SUMMARY

All patients with severe acute asthma should survive if they reach a hospital alive. Unfortunately, many patients die outside hospital or in ambulances travelling to hospital. Every attempt should be made to speed up the admission process for all patients and the organization of more formal self-admission services should be encouraged.[50] Family physicians should be persuaded to treat patients in their own homes with bronchodilators and corticosteroids, and ensure that oxygen in high concentration is administered by the ambulance crew if admission to hospital is necessary. The facility now exists in many regions of the UK for a β_2-adrenoreceptor agonist to be given in ambulances, and full use of this service must be encouraged. Ideally, all ambulances should be equipped with nebulizers and all ambulance personnel trained to administer a nebulized β_2-adrenoreceptor agonist in oxygen.

Hospitals accepting patients with severe acute asthma should be fully equipped for respiratory resuscitation and assisted ventilation.

REFERENCES

1. Knowles GK, Clark TJH: *Pulsus paradoxus* as a valuable sign indicating severity of asthn *Lancet* (1973) **ii**: 1356–1359.
2. British Thoracic Society, Research Unit of the Royal College of Physicians of London, King's Fund Centre, National Asthma Campaign: Guidelines for management of asthma in adults: II Acute severe asthma. *Br Med J* (1990) **301**: 797–800.
3. Benatar SR: Fatal asthma. *N Engl J Med* (1986) **314**: 423–429.
4. Eason J, Markowe HLJ: Controlled investigation of deaths from asthma in hospitals in the North East Thames Region. *Br Med J* (1987) **294**: 1255–1258.
5. Rebuck AS, Read J: Assessment and management of severe asthma. *Am J Med* (1971) **51**: 788–798.
6. Goldstein RS, Young J, Rebuck AS: Effect of breathing pattern on oxygen concentration received from standard face masks. *Lancet* (1982) **ii**: 1188–1190.
7. Flenley DC: In *Respiratory Medicine*. London, Baillière Tindall, 1990, pp 157–158.
8. Emerson P: In Emerson P (ed) *Thoracic Medicine*. London, Butterworth, 1981, p. 495.
9. O'Driscoll BR, Cochrane GM: Emergency use of nebulised bronchodilator drugs in British hospitals. *Thorax* (1987) **42**: 491–493.

10. Crompton GK: Editorial. Nebulised or intravenous beta$_2$ adrenoreceptor agonist therapy in acute asthma? *Eur Respir J* (1990) **3**: 125–126.
11. Fitchett DH, McNicol MW, Riordan JF: Intravenous salbutamol in the management of status asthmaticus. *Br Med J* (1975) **1**: 53–55.
12. Streeton JA, Morgan BE: Salbutamol in *status asthmaticus* and severe chronic obstructive bronchitis. *Postgraduate Medical Journal* (1971) **47**(Suppl 47): 125–128.
13. Bloomfield P, Carmichael J, Petrie GR, *et al.*: Comparison of salbutamol given intravenously and by intermittent positive pressure breathing in life-threatening asthma. *Br Med J* (1979) **1**: 848–850.
14. Swedish Society of Chest Medicine: High dose inhaled versus intravenous salbutamol combined with theophylline in severe acute asthma. A multicentre study of 176 patients. *Eur Respir J* (1990) **3**: 163–170.
15. Cheong B, Reynolds SR, Rajan G, Ward MJ: Intravenous beta agonist in severe acute asthma. *Br Med J* (1988) **297**: 448–450.
16. Douglas JG, Rafferty P, Fergusson RJ, *et al.*: Nebulised salbutamol without oxygen in severe acute asthma: how effective and how safe? *Thorax* (1985) **40**: 180–183.
17. Campbell IA, Hill A, Middleton H, *et al.*: Intermittent positive-pressure breathing. *Br Med J* (1978) **1**: 1186.
18. Fergusson RJ, Carmichael J, Rafferty P, *et al.*: Nebulised salbutamol in life-threatening asthma: is IPPB necessary? *Br J Dis Chest* (1983) **77**: 255–261.
19. Morgan MDL, Singh BV, Frame MH, Williams SJ: Terbutaline aerosol given through pear spacer in acute severe asthma. *Br Med J* (1982) **285**: 849–850.
20. Ward MJ, Fentem PH, Roderick Smith WH, Davies D: Ipratropium bromide in acute asthma. *Br Med J* (1981) **1**: 598–600.
21. Leahy BC, Gomm SA, Allen SC: Comparison of nebulised salbutamol with nebulised ipratropium bromide in acute asthma. *Br J Dis Chest* (1983) **77**: 159–163.
22. Rebuck AS, Chapman KR, Abboud R, *et al.*: Nebulised anticholinergic and sympathomimetic treatment of obstructive airways disease in the emergency room. *Am J Med* (1987) **82**, 59–64.
23. O'Driscoll BR, Taylor RJ, Horsby MG, Chambers DK, Bernstein A: Nebulised salbutamol with and without ipratropium bromide in acute airflow obstruction. *Lancet* (1989) **ii**: 1418–1420.
24. Summers QA, Tarala RA: Nebulised ipratropium in the treatment of acute asthma. *Chest* (1990) **97**: 430–434.
25. Patel KR, Tullet WM: Bronchoconstriction in response to ipratropium bromide. *Br Med J* (1983) **286**: 1318.
26. Connolly CK: Adverse reaction to ipratropium bromide. *Br Med J* (1982) **285**: 934–935.
27. Mann JS, Howarth PH, Holgate ST: Bronchoconstriction induced by ipratropium bromide in asthma: relation to hypotonicity. *Br Med J* (1984) **289**: 469.
28. Beasley CRW, Rafferty P, Holgate ST: Bronchoconstrictor properties of preservatives in ipratropium bromide (Atrovent®) nebuliser solution. *Br Med J* (1987) **294**: 1197–1198.
29. Williams SJ, Parrish RW, Seaton A: Comparison of intravenous aminophylline and salbutamol in severe asthma. *Br Med J* (1975) **4**: 685.
30. Femi-Pearse D, George WO, Ilechukwu ST, *et al.*: Comparison of intravenous aminophylline and salbutamol in severe asthma. *Br Med J* (1977) **1**: 491.
31. British National Formulary, No. 22. London, The Pharmaceutical Press, 1991.
32. Weinberger M, Hendeles L: Use of theophylline for asthma. In Clark TJH, Godfrey S (eds) *Asthma*, 2nd edn. London, Chapman and Hall, 1983, pp 336–357.
33. Bordley JE, Carey RA, Harvey AM, *et al.*: Preliminary observations on the effect of adrenocorticotropic hormone (ACTH) in allergic diseases. *Bull Johns Hopkins Hosp* (1949) **85**: 396–398.
34. Medical Research Council: Controlled trial of effects of cortisone acetate in status asthmaticus. *Lancet* (1956) **ii**: 803–806.
35. Luksza AR: Acute severe asthma treated without steroids. *Br J Dis Chest* (1982) **76**: 15–19.
36. Anonymous: Acute asthma. *Lancet* (1986) **1**: 131–133.
37. Fanta CH, Rossing TH, McFadden ER: Glucocorticoids in acute asthma: a critical controlled trial. *Am J Med* (1983) **74**: 845–851.

38. Britton MG, Collins JV, Brown D, *et al.*: High-dose corticosteroids in severe acute asthma. *Br Med J* (1976) **2**: 73–74.
39. Tanaka RM, Santiago SM, Kuhn GJ, *et al.*: Intravenous methyl prednisolone in adults in status asthmaticus. *Chest* (1982) **4**: 438–440.
40. Shee CD: Risk factors for hydrocortisone myopathy in acute severe asthma. *Respiratory Medicine* (1990) **84**: 229–233.
41. Collins JV, Clark TJH, Brown D, Townsend J: Intravenous corticosteroids in treatment of acute bronchial asthma. *Lancet* (1970) **ii**: 1047–1050.
42. Harrison BDW, Stokes TC, Hart GJ, *et al.*: Need for intravenous hydrocortisone in addition to oral prednisolone in patients admitted to hospital with severe asthma without ventilatory failure. *Lancet* (1986) **i**: 181–184.
43. Darioli R, Perret C: Mechanical controlled hypoventilation in *status asthmaticus. Am Rev Respir Dis* (1984) **129**: 385–387.
44. Karetzky MS: Asthma mortality: an analysis of one year's experience, review of the literature and assessment of current modes of therapy. *Medicine (Baltimore)* (1975) **54**: 471–484.
45. Branthwaite MA: The management of severe asthma. In Baderman H (ed) *Management of Medical Emergencies.* Tumbridge Wells, Pitman Medical, 1978, pp 48–56.
46. Higgins B, Greening AP, Crompton GK: Assisted ventilation in severe acute asthma. *Thorax* (1986) **41**: 464–467.
47. Luksza AR, Smith P, Coakley J, *et al.*: Acute severe asthma treated by mechanical ventilation: 10 years' experience from a district general hospital. *Thorax* (1986) **41**: 459–463.
48. Adriani J, Rovenstine EA: The effect of anaesthetic drugs upon bronchi and bronchioles of excised lung tissue. *Anesthesiology* (1943) **4**: 253–262.
49. Robertson CE, Steedman D, Sinclair CJ, *et al.*: Use of ether in life-threatening acute severe asthma. *Lancet* (1985) **i**: 187–188.
50. Crompton GK, Grant IWB, Bloomfield P: Edinburgh Emergency Asthma Admission Service; Report on 10 years' experience. *Br Med J* (1979) **2**: 1199–1201.
51. Crompton G. The catastrophic asthmatic. *Br J Dis Chest* (1987) **81**: 321–325.
52. Shapiro GC, Eggleston PA, Pierson WE, *et al.*: Double-blind study of the effectiveness of a broad spectrum antibiotic in status asthmaticus. *Pediatrics* (1974) **53**: 867–872.
53. Graham VAL, Milton AF, Knowles GK, Davies RJ: Routine antibiotics in hospital management of acute asthma. *Lancet* (1982) **i**: 418–420.
54. Rosello JC, Pla JC: Sulfato de magnesio en la crisis de asma. *Prensa Med Argent* (1936) **23**: 1677–1680.
55. Skobeloff EM, Spivey WH, McNamara RM, Greenspon L: Intravenous magnesium sulphate for the treatment of acute asthma in the Emergency Department. *JAMA* (1989) **262**: 1210–1213.
56. Noppen M, Vanmaele L, Impens N, Schandevyl W: Bronchodilator effect of intravenous magnesium sulphate in acute severe bronchial asthma. *Chest* (1990) **97**: 373–376.

39

Management of Asthma in Adults

ANN J. WOOLCOCK

INTRODUCTION

This chapter discusses the management of the disease 'asthma' with brief reference to the management of acute episodes of airway narrowing (attacks of asthma). The poor understanding of the causes and natural history of asthma means that there are no accurate documented methods of treatment. Since many approaches to treatment exist, patients receive confusing information from doctors, nurses, pharmacists and asthma educators and conflicting information about drugs and their side-effects exists in the literature. Furthermore, drugs that are widely used in one country appear to be ineffective in another. To try to deal with the existing confusion, management plans for asthma have been written in several countries.[1-3] The purpose of these plans is to provide a basis for a unified approach to management and, eventually, to allow self management by the patient. Hopefully they will also form the basis of studies to determine if management plans are effective in improving long-term outcome.

Management plans are written as 'consensus' documents and are not set out in a way that makes them easy to use by busy doctors. The answers to specific questions frequently asked by doctors, such as when to use which drug, the appropriate doses and criteria for altering the doses, are not addressed. Furthermore, the term 'asthma' is sometimes used to mean both the disease and the episodes of airway narrowing which leads to confusion.

Some of these problems are addressed by presenting a Management Plan with six points, based on that published by the Thoracic Society of Australia and New Zealand.[1] The ways in which the severity of the disease can be reduced using both pharmacological and non-pharmacological measures are described. Details of the ways in which factors that trigger and aggravate the disease can be controlled are outlined and the

ASTHMA: BASIC MECHANISMS AND CLINICAL MANAGEMENT (2nd Edn)
ISBN 0-12-079026-2

drugs commonly used are described. The management of patients with a poor response to conventional treatment is discussed and finally the likely changes in treatment that will occur in coming years are outlined.

There are almost no long-term studies of outcomes in patients with asthma and no trials of specific forms of management that have lasted for more than 2 years. Thus the methods of treatment outlined are largely empirical and in coming years may well be of little benefit. The emphasis of this chapter is mainly on the management of patients with persistent asthma although it is likely that many patients with asthma have episodic or mild disease and need little or no therapy. The criteria for treatment, other than for symptomatic relief, are largely unknown and this lack of knowledge is a serious deficiency in our knowledge about this disease.

CLASSIFICATION OF ASTHMA FOR PURPOSES OF MANAGEMENT

Persistent asthma

The airways narrow too much and too easily in response to a wide variety of provoking stimuli. It varies from mild to life-threatening in severity. Bronchial hyperresponsiveness (BHR) is easily demonstrated and biopsy evidence suggests that these patients, even those with mild disease, have persistent airway inflammation.[4,5]

Episodic asthma (often seasonal)

The airways narrow too much and too easily in response to specific stimuli such as pollen allergens. Between attacks, airway function and bronchial responsiveness are normal. Episodic asthma is more common in children than adults but occurs in some patients who are allergic to pollens, grain dusts and hay during the season of exposure. Some patients, particularly children, have episodes of airway narrowing only during viral respiratory infections. The histological changes present during and between episodes have not been reported.

Occupational asthma

The airways narrow in response to a specific substance to which the patient becomes 'sensitized' at the workplace. Usually it is episodic at first but then becomes persistent. In the overall population, these patients are uncommon but it is important to recognize them at an early stage when the disease is potentially reversible. Pathology of the airways of a patient who died with this disease shows the same changes as seen in other forms of asthma.[6]

Asthma in remission

Asthma well-documented previously, usually in childhood, but no symptoms exist and no medications are required. Such patients rarely present for treatment unless they again develop symptoms—usually after the age of 30. If discovered by chance, they may have a small decrease in lung function, a mild degree of BHR or an increased response to bronchodilator.

AIMS OF MANAGEMENT

(1) To diagnose and classify the disease;
(2) To prevent symptoms;
(3) To prevent the long-term risks, including persistent airflow limitation;
(4) To prevent the side-effects of drugs.

Although these aims seem logical, there are no long-term trials to determine the best ways of achieving them. It is generally agreed that the aims of asthma management are largely related to prevention, yet prevention of the disease and of attacks is hardly ever mentioned in articles and book chapters relating to management, even though there is good evidence that the disease is caused by exposure to allergens.

ASTHMA MANAGEMENT PLAN

Table 39.1 shows the six steps in the Management Plan.[1] The plan stresses assessment of the severity and type of asthma present (when the patient is not having an attack) and indicates ways to monitor and reduce the severity of the disease.

Step 1: Assess severity and type of asthma

All other aspects of treatment depend on this step. The process allows confirmation of the diagnosis, classification of the nature of the disease as well as its severity. At present

Table 39.1 Summary of asthma management.

Assess severity of asthma

Achieve 'target' lung function

Maintain 'target' lung function by:
    Avoiding causes/triggers/aggravators
    Optimal medication
        for asthma—inhaled corticosteroids, cromoglycate, nedocromil
        for symptoms—bronchodilators
        for triggers—cromoglycate, nedocromil, bronchodilator aerosols

Write an action plan

Educate the patient and family

Review regularly

there is no 'gold standard' against which to assess severity. Table 39.2 shows a scoring system that has proved useful. The total score ranges from 1 to 12 with 0–4 for symptoms, 0–4 for bronchodilator use over a 24-h period and 0–4 for variability of peak expiratory flow (PEF) rates. The symptoms are wheeze, chest tightness, breathlessness and cough—alone or in combination. The frequency of symptoms is important and in particular, waking at night regularly with wheezing or coughing is a symptom of severe disease.[7] It is important to include bronchodilator use in the score as many subjects do not have symptoms because they use bronchodilators while others have frequent symptoms but rarely use bronchodilators. The presence of daily symptoms, in spite of frequent bronchodilator use, usually means severe disease.

Daily measurement of PEF and assessment of variability is the mainstay not only of determining the severity of asthma but also of continuing management. Most patients who have moderate or severe disease and who are interested in maintaining control of their disease continue PEF monitoring after the initial period of assessment. The method of determining the variability of PEF measurement is shown in Fig. 39.1 and is based on the methods used by Ryan et al.[8] A week of readings, recorded twice daily, before and after a bronchodilator aerosol (four readings), is usually enough to provide an accurate reflection of the situation—unless the patient is having, or has just had, a severe exacerbation. The mean of seven daily values is calculated and used in the total score.

Those with a score of more than 6 usually have persistent asthma. Those with a score of less than 6 may have mild persistent asthma, episodic asthma or occupational asthma.

Table 39.2 Asthma severity score (not during an exacerbation).

	Score
Symptoms	
None for >6 months	0
< once/week or only with exercise	1
< daily, > weekly	2
Daily symptoms, none at night	3
Waking at night with symptoms	4
Bronchodilator required	
None in last year	0
<1 week	1
< daily	2
1–3 times/24 h	3
>4 times/24 h	4
Variability of PEF	
<6%	0
6–10%	1
11–15%	2
16–25%	3
>25%	4

Maximum possible score = 12

1–5 = Mild, 6–8 = moderate, 9–12 = severe

N.B. >10 suggests that severity may be life threatening

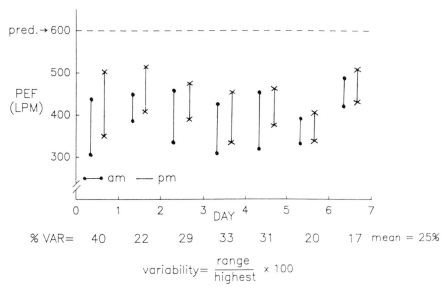

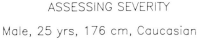

Fig. 39.1   Chart showing daily variability in peak flow (PEF) readings over a period of a week in a male aged 25 years. The lines join values before and after aerosol bronchodilator.

This distinction must be made from the history and from the PEF variability. If PEF is normal and its variability is less than 10% in spite of symptoms, the asthma can be diagnosed as episodic and treatment can be directed at the attacks or trying to find the cause of the attacks. The history from all patients should include details of the work environment. The episodic nature of the disease can be confirmed by a provocation test with histamine or methacholine which in most cases will be normal.

Step 2: Achieve 'target' lung function

This value is needed as a guide to the control of asthma in the future as treatment will be aimed at keeping lung function close to this value. If the patient has not achieved a PEF value close to the predicted value (obtained from the tables for age, sex, height and race) or if variability is marked (greater than 20%), it is possible that the best lung function has not been reached. In such patients, a trial of oral steroids with PEF monitoring, as shown in Fig. 39.2, should be undertaken. Usually 5 days of 0.8 mg/kg/day is enough, but if improvement is still occurring after 5 days the medication can be continued for up to 10 days. The prednisone is then stopped and inhaled corticosteroids are continued. The PEF values over the next few days can be used to determine a 'target' range for lung function. Usually PEF values within 90% of the best value on oral steroids are realistic 'target' values. The patient should be told that the aim of treatment is to try to reach that range each day.

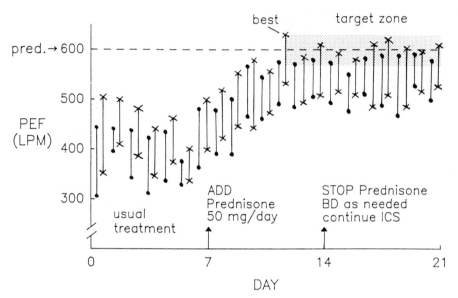

Fig. 39.2 Chart of the same patient as in Fig. 39.1 showing the method of finding the target lung function using oral prednisone.

Step 3: Maintain 'target' lung function

Avoid causes/triggers/aggravators

Causes

These are rarely known except for occupational sensitizers and some seasonal allergens. Once known, every measure should be taken to avoid them before the disease becomes persistent.[9]

Triggers

A. Physical factors. These include exercise, strong smells, cold, changes in the weather, etc. They are usually easily identified by the patient. The effect of most can be minimized by appropriate use of sodium cromoglycate or β-agonist aerosols before a known exposure such as exercise.

B. Allergens. There is no doubt that aeroallergens are important triggers of attacks in most allergic asthmatics. There is also increasing evidence that asthma is caused by exposure to allergens[10] and that avoidance improves the severity of the disease.[11–13] Allergen exposure in the first year of life may be particularly important in causing severe disease in children. These, together with the fact that asthma rarely completely reverses once it becomes persistent, mean that the most rational approach to asthma management is prevention. Allergen avoidance is important for families with a history of allergic disease. The allergens that appear to be important throughout the world are dust, mites, moulds, pollens and animal proteins. Large amounts of these allergens can be found in house dust, particularly in carpets. House dust mites, both alive and dead, present the biggest problem. Present evidence suggests that most mattresses and pillows in the world harbour mites.

It seems likely that allergens are constantly inhaled and this can lead to continuing inflammation of the airways. The most sensible solution for patients is to live in an allergen-free environment as much as possible. However, there is currently no ground swell of public opinion for building allergen-free houses. Houses in many tropical countries are relatively free from allergens and hopefully fashion will not lead to changes such as reduction in ventilation and the widespread introduction of carpets.

C. Recommendations for reducing allergen levels in houses

(1) All wall to wall carpet should be removed from the house. It is almost impossible to make a house in a humid environment allergen free while carpets remain.
(2) If carpet remains, it should be recognized by the patient that no vacuum cleaner removes more than a small percentage of mites (which have sticky legs) from the carpet and that anti-mite sprays must be used frequently and in a quantity that wets the carpet completely.
(3) All bedding (mattress, pillow and doonas (duvets)) that is not able to be washed regularly in hot water, should be encased in allergen-proof covers. Spraying the bedding with anti-mite sprays periodically may be of value. Sunlight is excellent and, whenever practical, bedding should be put in the sun.
(4) Sheep skins should be discarded or washed frequently with water at at least 60°C.
(5) Babies should never be put directly on to a carpet but rather on a cover that can be kept free from mites and allergen by hot washing.
(6) Cats and dogs should be removed from outside and inside the house.
(7) Clothes should be kept in cupboards and washed or dry cleaned frequently.
(8) The humidity in the house should be minimized by good ventilation.

Aggravators. It should be routine to ask for symptoms of rhinitis (nasal obstruction or sneezing), about snoring and interrupted sleep, and about gastric reflux. These problems, when treated, help the overall well-being of patients and though they may have only a small effect on the underlying severity of the asthma, they are well worth undertaking.

Optimal medication

In patients with persistent disease, drug therapy aimed at keeping the airway function in the 'target' zone with the least amount of bronchodilator therapy, is the mainstay of treatment. A suggested scheme for treatment, using the severity score as a guideline, is outlined in Table 39.3. The aim is to reduce the severity by treating the airway inflammation and by minimizing its recurrence using a combination of strategies including appropriate drugs, preventing exacerbations, reducing triggers (allergen avoidance) and treating aggravating factors.

Table 39.3   Asthma management — drugs (adults).

| Classification | For the disease | For symptoms | |
		β-Agonists	Other
Episodic	? Nil	When required	SCG/NS during season
Persistent			
mild	? Nil	When required	SCG/NS before exercise
(1–5)	SCG 20–80 mg/day		and known triggers
	NS 8–16 mg/day		
moderate	SCG 20–80 mg/day	When required	SCG/NS before exercise
(6–8)	NS 8–16 mg/day	When PEF <80% target	and known triggers
	ICS 0.5–1.0 mg/day		
severe	ICS 1–2 mg/day	When required	Theophylline
(9–12)	OCS in low dose?	When PEF <80% target	Atrovent®

Sodium cromoglycate and nedocromil sodium

Mechanisms of action. In spite of their widespread use and a large body of literature, little is known about how these drugs work. While they stabilize isolated mucosal mast cells and reduce the release of mediators,[14] the extent to which they do this *in vitro* is not known. However, their action in blocking the effects of many challenges (allergens, exercise and SO_2) is well documented. It is likely that they act on other inflammatory cells and on afferent nerve endings as well as on mast cells. *In vitro* nedocromil sodium (NS) appears to be more potent in preventing mast-cell degranulation than sodium cromoglycate (SCG), although the clinical efficacy of the two drugs appears to be similar.

Clinical effects. (a) Short term. They prevent exercise-induced attacks in many adults and most children. The degree to which they inhibit the attacks is dose related and is short lived, since the drugs are rapidly removed from the airways during exercise. Taken before an allergen challenge they prevent both early and late reactions.[15] They also inhibit the effects of other 'indirect' provoking stimuli such as SO_2. In this respect, NS is more effective than SCG.

(b) Long term. In patients with episodic asthma they prevent seasonal and 'spontaneous' exacerbations so that the episodes are prevented or decreased in adults and children. These drugs have the reputation of being more effective in children probably because episodic asthma is common in children. Some patients with persistent asthma and documented BHR have fewer symptoms when taking these drugs on a regular basis and in some studies a decrease in BHR has been observed.[16] It appears that the drug must be given in adequate doses for at least 12 weeks. In patients taking inhaled corticosteroids the response to SCG appears less good than those not taking inhaled steroids[16] but there is some evidence that NS improves the overall control of the disease in such patients.[17]

Side-effects. These drugs are amongst the safest drugs used today and have virtually no side-effects. The dry powder form of SCG sometimes causes minor irritation and some patients complain that NS has an unpleasant taste.

Doses and administration. SC is usually administered as 5 mg per puff and NS as 4 mg per puff from metered-dose aerosols although SCG is also available as 20–mg spincaps and 20 mg nebulizer solution. They can be used immediately prior to exposure to known triggers to prevent attacks.

For long-term use, they need to be given in an adequate dose and at regular intervals—initially four times a day. Once control is improved they are used three times a day. In children with moderate disease, e.g. a score of 6, the disease can be usually controlled with SCG alone. In those with a score of 7 or more, experience shows that inhaled corticosteroids (ICS) (see below) are usually needed to obtain control. The question then arises, should SCG or NS be used as well? In long-term management, a trial (adequate doses essential over a period of weeks) is indicated to determine if the overall score is improved while the patient stays on a fixed dose of ICS. In adults with severe disease, high doses of ICS are needed initially (see below). Once the severity is reduced (score of 8 or less), SCG or NS can be introduced and the dose of ICS can be reduced.

Inhaled corticosteroids (ICS)

Mechanism of action. These drugs are effective probably because they have a number of actions.[18] They are topically active and known to cause vasoconstriction in the skin.[19] This action, together with their ability to interfere with the local production of cytokines which lead to inflammatory cell infiltration are probably key elements in their effectiveness. They also induce the synthesis of proteins which interfere with the production of arachidonic acid from cell membranes. This prevents the formation of a number of different mediators, resulting in less vascular leak, less oedema and less infiltration of inflammatory cells. Biopsy studies show that they restore the bronchial epithelium which is commonly shed in patients taking only bronchodilator drugs.[20] Their effects on cells and structures deeper in the airway wall is unknown.

Clinical effects. Unlike SCG and NS, they do not inhibit the early and late phases of allergen challenges when given as acute doses but when given for several days they have some inhibitory effect. In most patients, particularly those who have not taken the drugs previously, there is a dose-related effect in improving the severity of the disease as measured by symptoms, baseline lung function and PEF variability. Improvement may take several weeks to become apparent to the patient and may continue for many months.[18] In some patients they appear to have little effect on BHR.[21,22]

The response appears to be dose related and the drugs can usually be given twice daily. Although these drugs have now been in use for many years, there is little published about their long-term effectiveness in individual patients but clinical experience suggests that relapse occurs when they are stopped. Finding a maintenance dose requires trial and error and the continuing use of diary cards with symptoms and PEF values.

Side-effects. (a) Pharyngeal effects. Some adult patients taking ICS experience dysphonia, which may result from a localized steroid myopathy, and a smaller number develop thrush.[23] These problems can be prevented by the use of a spacer device,[24,25] by reducing the number of inhalations (using high-strength aerosols) and by gargling after use. In some patients antifungal agents are needed to control the local symptoms.

To date refractoriness to these has not been described in the way that refractoriness to oral steroids appears to occur but clinical experience suggests that some patients, who initially have good control, become more difficult to manage even when these drugs are used in high doses. Such patients are usually also taking regular doses of β-agonist aerosols. Since it is possible that β-agonists make asthma worse, apparent refractoriness to ICS may simply be worsening asthma due to other factors.

(b) Systemic effects. The side effects of ICS appear to be less severe than those observed with oral steroids, particularly since the doses needed for control are much less. Biochemical evidence of adrenal suppression rarely occurs on doses of less than 1.5 mg daily. When it is present, it is probably not medically important but indicates that enough drug is being absorbed to have a systemic effect. More important effects are bruising, osteoporosis, and development of cataracts. All of these are likely to develop when these drugs are used for long periods.[26]

Dose and administration. Table 39.3 shows the suggested doses for patients with moderate and severe disease. In general, a higher dose is used in those with severe disease. Nebulized forms (available as budesonide) may be needed initially in those with poor lung function, but the role of this form of the drug in adults is not established. Attention should be paid to patients taking these drugs, adjusting the dose to gain control but to minimize side-effects.

Oral steroids

Mechanism of action. Corticosteroids, when administered systemically, have similar actions to those described for topical steroids although their effect on small vessels in the airways is unknown. Oral forms take 4–6 h to have an effect and will act on all the cells in the body that have steroid receptors.

Clinical effects. In the Management Plan oral steroids are used to find the target lung function in patients whose lung function is low, and to prevent severe exacerbations. In children it has been shown that a single dose (30 or 60 mg) of prednisone as well as nebulized bronchodilator, reduces the need for hospital admission[27] and this also happens in adults although data showing this rapid effect have not been published.

Side-effects. These are well documented and include bruising, osteoporosis, cataracts, hypertension, diabetes and cushingoid features. Some of these effects are potentially reduced by changing the patient to ICS. It takes many months to change patients to the inhaled form and care must be taken to implement all the other steps in the Management Plan at the same time.

Dose and administration. For finding the target lung function, it is usual to use 0.8–1.0 mg/kg body weight per day in divided doses. Trial and error will determine the symptoms and the PEF values that herald an exacerbation and the dose of oral steroid needed to abort a severe attack. Usually 25 mg in divided doses for 1–2 days is sufficient. It is not necessary to reduce the dose slowly when it has been used for less than a week unless experience shows that sudden withdrawal is associated with worsening asthma. The ICS should not be stopped while the patient is on oral steroids. Some patients, usually those who have been on oral steroids before the advent of the inhaled forms, require daily use of oral steroids to control symptoms. During the years before ICS were available, these were given on alternate days. Sometimes this is useful but often results in less control and in more overall steroid administration than the use of 'pulses' of high dose therapy, even if these are necessary at monthly intervals.

β-Agonists

Mechanism of action. These drugs have evolved over the last 30 years to become more selective (β_2-specific) and longer acting. Salbutamol, fenoterol and terbutaline act for 6–8 h while the newer salmeterol and formoterol act for 12 h. Their main action is to relax bronchial smooth muscle. They also stabilize mast cells, preventing release of mediators after mast cells are provoked with different releasing factors. In this respect they are more potent than SCG.[15,28]

Clinical effects. (a) Short term. They bronchodilate maximally within 10 min and last for 4–6 h. When inhaled, but not when ingested, they protect against induced attacks, including the early response after an allergen challenge, for 2–3 h. They do not protect against late allergic reactions and are variably effective in reversing late reactions.
   (b) Long term. It is difficult to demonstrate tachyphylaxis to the bronchodilating effects of salbutamol.[29] Their effect on asthma in the long term is controversial. There is a question about their effect on the severity of asthma when they are used regularly. In children, BHR was shown to increase when terbutaline was used alone in contrast to inhaled steroids which improved the severity.[30,31] Recently a year-long study in New Zealand showed that four times a day use of fenoterol was associated with worsening control of asthma in 40 out of 64 subjects who completed a trial.[32] It is not clear if these observations in adults apply to all β-agonists. However, it is clear that when used alone β-agonists do not improve the overall severity of asthma. Nevertheless, many people with mild disease use them to control symptoms and their asthma remains well controlled. Huge amounts of salbutamol have been used in the last 20 years and there is little objective evidence that the use of this drug has caused any problem.

Side-effects. Tremor and slight tachycardia occur acutely and are well known. These effects usually decrease with time and are rarely a problem unless the drugs are used to excess.[33] Attempts have been made to show tachyphylaxis to the bronchodilating effects of salbutamol in asthmatic airways but this has not been found although it probably occurs in normal people.[29]

Dose and administration. These drugs are usually given in the inhaled form with doses varying from 100–200 μg. Metered-dose inhalers, nebulizing solutions and dry powder forms are available in addition to tablets and syrups. Beta-agonists are used for making the diagnosis (a > 15% increase in lung function within 10 min of an aerosol bronchodilator is diagnostic of asthma), for assessing severity (Table 39.2), for severe symptoms lasting more than 10 min and for reversing low levels of lung function (e.g. when the PEF is less than 60–70% of the target PEF) (Table 39.4). These drugs are not needed on a regular basis except in those patients whose symptoms cannot be controlled by corticosteroid therapy.

Table 39.4   Indications for use of β-agonist aerosols.

Acute severe attacks—these drugs may be life saving
For diagnosis—does lung function improve within minutes?
For assessment of severity—amount required plus PEF variability
For symptoms which are causing distress or anxiety
Before exercise to prevent airway narrowing

Long-acting β-agonists

These act for 12 h[34,35] and, in the case of salmeterol, appear to have actions other than bronchodilation.[36] Their overall place in the management of patients with asthma of different types and severity is not well established.

Other sympathomimetics

Adrenaline, which has both α- and β-effects, is used for acute attacks. It may be given subcutaneously or intravenously (see Chapter 32). It has no place in long-term management. Isoprenaline and ephidrine are largely drugs of the past in countries where longer acting β-agonists are available. They are cheap and still widely used in some countries.

Anticholinergics

The drugs ipratropium bromide and oxitropium are used to block the cholinergic receptors.[37] They are effective bronchodilators and are useful in patients with chronic obstructive pulmonary disease. They have a slower onset than the β-agonists. They are used in the treatment of acute attacks, particularly in children. At present they have little role in long-term management but they may come to have a place in patients in whom β-agonists cause worsening disease and who need regular bronchodilatation.

Theophylline

Mechanism of action. This drug has many actions.[38,39] The mechanism by which it bronchodilates is unknown although it appears to increase intracellular cyclic AMP by a mechanism different from the β-agonists. It may also have some 'anti-inflammatory' effects[40] but the mechanisms are largely unknown. There is no place for theophylline as a second drug when a β-agonist has failed to control the disease. If the patient needs more than occasional β_2-agonist aerosols then either cromoglycate or ICS, not theophylline, is indicated.

Known effects. Theophylline gives symptomatic relief to those with severe airway narrowing. There is a well-recognized group of subjects, usually dependent on long-term or frequent short-term courses of oral steroids, who need theophylline to control their symptoms. Many of these patients need doses above the usual to keep the serum levels in the 'therapeutic' range. These patients apparently metabolize the drug differently which acts on some unknown mechanism to maintain bronchodilation. There are some patients who get immediate symptomatic relief from the drug and use it either intermittently or as a single dose at night.

Side-effects. These are well known and include nausea, headache and hyperreactivity in children. The drug can cause fatal neurological and cardiovascular events. The increasing awareness of side-effects of this drug has led to its decreasing use in some countries. It has been reported to cause learning difficulties in children, perhaps because it interferes with sleep. However, use of the drug in lower doses as an adjunct to other therapy rather than as a primary bronchodilator, can avoid these side effects in most patients. In coming years, it is likely that the exact place of the drug will be defined and the side effects largely avoided.

Dose and administration. When used as a bronchodilator — particularly in treating severe attacks, doses are adjusted to keep the serum levels within the 'therapeutic' range while avoiding toxicity. The slow release forms are most effective in reducing large fluctuations in serum levels. In patients with severe disease, especially those requiring low doses of oral prednisone in addition to ICS, they appear to have a steroid-sparing effect and can be used in lower doses. The effort and expense of monitoring serum levels is not required for low dose treatment.

Other treatments

Other drugs are rarely needed in long-term management. However, a few drugs need to be commented on.

Antihistamines. In general these have no place in the treatment of asthma itself. However, the non-sedating antihistamines have few side-effects and are useful in subjects with other allergic problems that often accompany asthma such as urticaria, allergic reactions to foods and rhinitis. A number of patients with seasonal exacerbations of their asthma find that regular use of antihistamines during 'the season' controls their symptoms.[41]

Ketotifen. Ketotifen is marketed as an antihistamine with antiasthma effects and is widely used.[42] There are no published trials that show that it is effective in reducing the severity of the disease in those with moderate and severe persistent asthma but *in vitro* it has some 'anti-inflammatory' properties and in patients with mild disease it can reduce symptoms to the point where other drugs are not necessary.

Inhaled frusemide. Recently it has been shown that inhaled frusemide has much the same action as SCG and NS in preventing the effects of triggers such as allergen and exercise.[43] Oral frusemide, given in high dose has no effect. The long-term effects of this drug on the severity of the disease are unknown.

Gold salts. These drugs, sometimes used for the treatment of arthritis, are used in some countries for treatment of patients with severe asthma.[44] There has been no trial published of the effects on patients already enrolled in a management plan that maximizes the use of inhaled steroids and other measures aimed at reducing severity.

Methotrexate. This drug is used commonly in the USA in patients who need high doses of oral steroids to control their asthma.[45,46] It has anti-inflammatory actions and in some subjects can be used to reduce the dose of prednisone without causing too many side-effects itself. Discontinuing the methrotrexate usually leads to a relapse. As with gold, there has been no trial in patients who have been treated with a management plan, such as that described here, for several years.

Non-pharmacological treatments

Exercise. Active exercise should be encouraged in all patients. Swimming appears to be particularly beneficial. In patients who have severe disease with panic attacks and hyperventilation, swimming helps to teach them to control their breathing rate. There are numerous studies that show the effectiveness of exercise in improving overall well-being.[47,48] The symptoms can be prevented with either SCG/NS or a bronchodilator aerosol prior to the exercise.[48]

Other measures. Acupuncture, hypnosis, meditation, Chinese herbal medicine, garlic tablets and many other remedies are used frequently by patients with asthma. These measures are almost never successful in reducing the basic severity of the disease but often the patient feels better and patients should be encouraged to explore these treatments, provided that the other measures outlined in the Management Plan are continued.

Step 4: Action plan

Written plan for exacerbations

A written action plan is necessary for all patients who present for treatment, even if they have infrequent attacks. The general aim is to abort a severe attack by increasing the dose of inhaled steroids or starting high dose oral steroids. There is no place for low doses of oral steroids in aborting attacks. A flow chart for writing an action plan is shown in Fig. 39.3 and the written plan for the patient whose PEF values are shown in Table 39.2 are shown. The plan should be written and the subject should be able to recognize an impending attack, know which drugs to take and how to call for help.

Treatment of acute attacks

If, in spite of the written plan or because the plan was not used, the patient has a severe attack, the guidelines outlined by the British Thoracic Society[49] should be followed. The patient should be monitored—with an ear oximeter and PEF measurements and oxygen given. The drugs needed are oral or intravenous steroids in adequate doses, nebulized bronchodilating drugs and, if the response is poor after several hours, parental bronchodilators—usually intravenous salbutamol. Many patients do well with intravenous aminophylline but this is not used actively.

Step 5: Education

There are few reports that show that educating patients with asthma leads to decreased severity or to improved control. However, unless the patient, the family, and in the case

ACTION PLAN

Date: X - Y - Z2

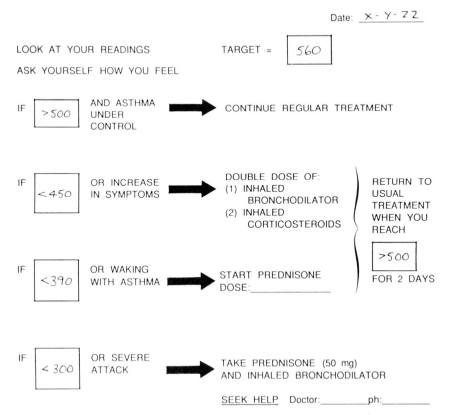

LOOK AT YOUR READINGS   TARGET = [560]

ASK YOURSELF HOW YOU FEEL

IF [>500]   AND ASTHMA UNDER CONTROL ➤ CONTINUE REGULAR TREATMENT

IF [<450]   OR INCREASE IN SYMPTOMS ➤ DOUBLE DOSE OF:
(1) INHALED BRONCHODILATOR
(2) INHALED CORTICOSTEROIDS
} RETURN TO USUAL TREATMENT WHEN YOU REACH [>500] FOR 2 DAYS

IF [<390]   OR WAKING WITH ASTHMA ➤ START PREDNISONE DOSE:_____

IF [<300]   OR SEVERE ATTACK ➤ TAKE PREDNISONE (50 mg) AND INHALED BRONCHODILATOR

SEEK HELP   Doctor:_____ph:_____

Fig. 39.3   Action plan for the patient whose lung function is shown in Fig. 39.2.

of children, the teacher most involved, understand the nature of asthma, the aims of treatment and the Management Plan, it will not be possible to achieve full control of the disease. This is especially important in those with a score of more than 6. Studies of the role of education when a strict Management Plan is used are awaited.

Education takes time which may not be available to all doctors. This means that an education programme should be developed in association with hospitals where asthma is treated. Each doctor needs a kit which includes pictures of airways, drugs and a number of peak flow meters. The latter can be lent until it is decided whether one is needed permanently (score of 6 or more). Figure 39.5 shows a way of illustrating the nature of the problem that can be understood by most people.

Step 6: Review regularly

Asthma is a chronic disease which carries a number of long-term risks including continuing symptoms, altered lifestyle, the development of permanently abnormal lung function, the side-effects of drugs and premature death. In those with moderate or severe persistent asthma (a score of 6 or more), it almost never remits and this means

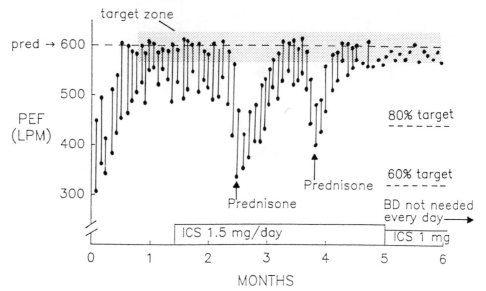

Fig. 39.4 Peak flow chart showing the response to treatment over a period of six months of the patient shown in Fig. 39.2.

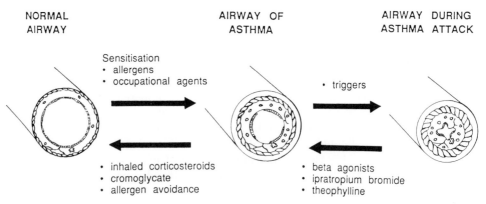

Fig. 39.5 Diagram illustrating the pathology of normal and asthmatic airways with some of the factors that cause the airways to go from one state to another. This diagram is useful in patient education.

continuing care. Regular visits to the doctor, at which the diaries are reviewed, are essential. At these visits a new score (hopefully less) is calculated, treatment changed, the action plan updated, drugs prescribed and education continued. Figure 39.4 shows the progress of the patient shown in Figure 39.2 treated using the management plan for six months. Some patients improve more rapidly than this, others take much longer. This patient attended on 4 occasions over that period. In time, patients can take more responsibility but in the first year of treatment, regular appointments, regardless of symptoms, must be made. Every asthmatic should have one doctor who is committed to her/his care for life.

TREATMENT OF THE PATIENT WITH SEVERE PERSISTENT ASTHMA

Use of the Plan fails to reduce the severity of asthma in some patients. In this group long-term commitment is needed and each step in the Management Plan should be implemented carefully. In addition, it is helpful to ask the following questions:

(1) Does the patient have asthma? Sometimes a diagnosis is assumed in a patient who is hyperventilating, simulating symptoms or who has bronchiectasis or cystic fibrosis. A biopsy is usually diagnostic and can give helpful information.
(2) Is the patient complying with drugs? Some patients deliberately avoid the drugs, others forget, others take them incorrectly. This may be difficult to determine but often explains the lack of improvement. Objective studies of compliance show that the majority of patients fail to take their medications as prescribed.[50]
(3) Have the relevant allergens and aggravators been removed/treated? In particular, does the patient snore or have severe reflux? Treating the rhinitis usually allows the patient to sleep better and treatment of severe snoring is very helpful.[51]
(4) Does the patient respond to high doses of prednisone using objective measures? If so, then adequate doses of inhaled plus oral pulse therapy are needed. If not, the diagnosis should be questioned. The patient may have chronic fixed airway obstruction and not be capable of improvement.
(5) Would a trial of gold salts or methotrexate help? A trial with one of these drugs is indicated if the Management Plan has been implemented and drugs complied with for at least a year. In addition, it should be demonstrated that steroid therapy is effective but needed in amounts that cause excessive side-effects before these potentially toxic agonists are used.
(6) Is the environment a causal factor? If the patient knows that in a different house, region or country, asthma control is improved then a trial of living in a new environment is indicated.
(7) Does the patient have abnormal illness behaviour? Some patients need to be sick and will only respond to asthma management if they develop another illness. A variety of psychological problems occur in patients with severe persistent asthma and the help of a psychiatrist can be of great benefit.

LIKELY CHANGES TO MANAGEMENT

Asthma continues to be managed without the benefit of a systematic approach and without the results of long-term trials of treatment, in which the effect of specific management plans on the outcome of the disease are defined. Until such trials are done, it is unlikely that dramatic progress will be made. The following list outlines some of the likely changes in the overall approach to the management of asthma, based on results of recent studies and on the increasing use of management plans.

(1) More emphasis will be placed on investigation of infants and children at the time of the first wheeze with a view to prevention.

(2) Less emphasis will be placed on the use of presently available β-agonists. As a result of long-term studies now being undertaken these drugs may come to be regarded as causing more harm than benefit if used inappropriately.

(3) Increasing use of long (12-h) acting bronchodilators. These drugs may replace the presently used β-agonists in patients with severe disease—especially those who wake at night. Their role in newly diagnosed patients and in those with mild disease is undefined.

(4) Inhaled corticosteroids will be used more precisely. These drugs are expensive and it is increasingly realized that they have major side effects, and may induce a state of partial refractoriness to higher doses. At present the doses used are largely arbitrary. It is possible to define protocols for determining the dose that is most likely to be effective in the individual patient for both initial control and long-term use. Short courses of high doses may be used for several weeks followed by low doses, together with sodium cromoglycate or nedocromil sodium, allowing control to occur over a period of months and avoiding the side-effects of high doses of inhaled corticosteroids.

(5) Alternatives to metered-dose aerosols that contain chlorinated fluorocarbons will be increasingly used. Dry powder dispensers and mini nebulizers will become more sophisticated. This is likely because of pressure for environmental responsibility and because the technology for delivering dry powders and nebulized solutions successfully will reach a high level of sophistication.

(6) New non-steroidal anti-inflammatory medication will be developed. Although not yet available, it makes sense to develop drugs that help to control the allergic reaction in the airways so that less cytokines are released and inflammation prevented.

(7) Self management by each patient. This is already happening and will continue as management plans become introduced widely.

(8) More emphasis on non-pharmacological treatments. The role of controlling the patient's home environment, of not treating minor attacks, of swimming and exercise programmes and of relaxation will be much more widely accepted. It is possible that not treating some patients with mild, episodic asthma may be beneficial in the long term.

(9) Large population studies of management plans to determine those treatments that lead to the best long-term outcome will be undertaken.

(10) As the cost of drugs increases, patients, doctors and governments will need to be assured that the drugs being used have definite effects to prevent symptoms, to treat symptoms or to reduce the severity of the disease. Thus the introduction of protocols which allow doctors to determine the exact number and doses of drugs needed to obtain predetermined outcomes seems inevitable.

REFERENCES

1. Woolcock AJ, Rubinfield AR, Seale JP, *et al.*: Asthma management plan, 1989. *Med J Aust* (1989) **151**: 650–653.

2. Hargreave FE, Dolovich J, Newhouse MT: The assessment and treatment of asthma: a conference report. *J Allergy Clin Immunol* (1990) **85**: 1098–1111.

3. British Thoracic Society: Guidelines for management of asthma in adults: I—chronic persistent asthma. *BMJ* (1990) **301**: 651–653.

4. Laitinen LA, Heino M, Laitinen A, Kava T, Haahtela T: Damage of the airway epithelium and bronchial reactivity in patients with asthma. *Am Rev Respir Dis* (1985) **131**: 599–606.

5. Beasley R, Roche WR, Roberts JA, Holgate ST: Cellular events in the bronchi in mild asthma and after bronchial provocation. *Am Rev Respir Dis* (1989) **139**: 806–817.

6. Saetta M, Di Stefano A, Rosina C, Thiene G, Fabbri LM: Quantitative structural analysis of peripheral airways and arteries in sudden fatal asthma. *Am Rev Respir Dis* (1991) **143**: 138–143.

7. Martin RJ, Cicutto LC, Ballard RD: Factors related to the nocturnal worsening of asthma. *Am Rev Respir Dis* (1990) **141**: 33–38.

8. Ryan G, Latimer KM, Dolovich J, Hargreave FE: Bronchial responsiveness to histamine: relationship to diurnal variation of peak flow rate, improvement after bronchodilator, and airway calibre. *Thorax* (1982) **37**: 423–429.

9. Chan-Yeung MB: Occupational asthma update. *Chest* (1988) **93**: 407–411.

10. Sporik R, Holgate ST, Platts-Mills TAE, Cogswell JJ: Exposure to house-dust mite allergen (Der p I) and the development of asthma in childhood: a prospective study. *N Engl J Med* (1990) **232**: 502–507.

11. Platts-Mills TAE, Mitchell EB, Noch P, Tovey E, Moszoro H, Wilkins SR: Reduction of bronchial hyperreactivity during prolonged allergen avoidance. *Lancet* (1982) **II**: 675–678.

12. Murray AB, Ferguson AC: Reduction of bronchial hyperreactivity during prolonged allergen avoidance: letter. *Lancet* (1982) **II**: 1212.

13. Dorward AJ, Colloff MJ, MacKay NS, McSharry C, Thomson NC: Effect of house dust mite avoidance measures on adult atopic asthma. *Thorax* (1988) **43**: 98–102.

14. Church MK, Young KD: The characteristics of inhibition of histamine release from human lung fragments by sodium cromoglycate, salbutamol and chlorpromazine. *Br J Pharmacol* (1983) **78**: 671–679.

15. Booij-Noord H, Orie NGM, de Vries K: Immediate and late bronchial obstructive reactions to inhalation of house dust and protective effects of disodium cromoglycate and prednisolone. *J Allergy Clin Immunol* (1971) **48**: 344–354.

16. Hoag JE, McFadden ER: Long-term effect of cromolyn sodium on nonspecific bronchial hyperresponsiveness: a review. *Ann Allergy* (1991) **66**: 53–63.

17. Boulet L-P, Cartier A, Cockcroft DW, *et al.*: Tolerance to reduction of oral steroid dosage in severely asthmatic patients receiving nedocromil sodium. *Respir Med* (1990) **84**: 317–323.

18. Woolcock AJ, Jenkins CR: Clinical responses to Corticosteroids. In Kaliner MA, Barnes PJ, Persson CGA (eds) *Asthma, its Pathology and Treatment. Lung Biology in Health and Disease*, Vol 49. New York, Marcel Dekker, 1991, pp 633–665.

19. Place VA: Precise evaluation of topically applied corticosteroid potency. *Arch Dermatol* (1970) **101**: 531–537.

20. Ollerenshaw SL, Woolcock AJ: Characteristics of the inflammation in biopsies from large airways of subjects with asthma and subjects with chronic airflow limitation. *Am Rev Respir Dis* (1991) (in press).

21. Ryan G, Latimer KM, Juniper EF, Roberts RS, Hargreave FE: Effect of beclomethasone dipropionate on bronchial responsiveness to histamine in controlled nonsteroid-dependent asthma. *J Allergy Clin Immunol* (1985) **75**: 25–30.

22. Frankel D, Latimer K, Ruffin R: Does bronchial hyperresponsiveness improve following hospitalisation for acute asthma? *Aust NZ J Med* (1990) **20**(Suppl): 522.

23. Toogood JH, Jennings B, Greenaway RW, Chuang L: Candidiasis and dysphonia complicating beclomethasone treatment of asthma. *J Allergy Clin Immunol* (1980) **65**: 145–153.

24. Toogood JH, Jennings B, Baskerville J, Newhouse M: Assessment of a device for reducing oropharyngeal complications during beclomethasone treatment of asthma. *Am Rev Respir Dis* (1981) **123**: 113.

25. Toogood JH, Baskerville J, Jennings B, Lefcoe NM, Johansson SA: Use of spacers to facilitate inhaled corticosteroid treatment of asthma. *Am Rev Respir Dis* (1984) **129**: 723–729.

26. Maxwell DL: Adverse effects of inhaled corticosteroids. *Biomed Pharmacother* (1990) **44**: 421–427.

27. Storr J, Barry W, Barrell E, Lenney W, Hatcher G: Effect of a single oral dose of prednisone in acute childhood asthma. *Lancet* (1987) **I**: 879–882.

28. Howarth PH, Durham SR, Lee TH, Kay AB, Church MK, Holgate ST: Influence of albuterol, cromolyn sodium and ipratropium bromide on the airway and circulating mediator responses to allergen bronchial provocation in asthma. *Am Rev Respir Dis* (1985) **132**: 986–992.

29. Harvey JE, Tattersfield AE: Airway response to salbutamol: effect of regular salbutamol inhalations in normal atopic, and asthmatic subjects. *Thorax* (1982) **37**: 280–287.

30. Kerrebijn K, van Essen-Zandvliet EEM, Neijens HJ: Effect of long-term treatment with inhaled corticosteroids and beta-agonists on the bronchial responsiveness in children with asthma. *J Allergy Clin Immunol* (1987) **79**: 653–659.

31. Kraan J, Koeter GH, Mark TW, Sluiter HJ, de Vries K: Changes in bronchial hyperreactivity induced by four weeks treatment with anti-asthmatic drugs in patients with allergic asthma: a comparison between budesonide and terbutaline. *J Allergy Clin Immunol* (1985) **76**: 628–636.

32. Sears MR, Taylor DR, Print CG, *et al.*: Regular inhaled beta-agonists treatment in bronchial asthma. *Lancet* (1990) **336**: 1391–1396.

33. Wong CS, Pavord ID, Williams J, Britton JR, Tattersfield A: Bronchodilator, cardiovascular, and hypokalaemic effects of fenoterol, salbutamol, and terbutaline in asthma. *Lancet* (1990) **336**: 1396–1399.

34. Arvidsson P, Larsson S, Lofdahl C-G, Melander B, Wahlander L, Svedmyr N: Formoterol, a new long-acting bronchodilator for inhalation. *Eur Respir J* (1989) **2**: 325–330.

35. Ullman A, Hedner J, Svedmyr N: Inhaled salmeterol and salbutamol in asthmatic patients. An evaluation of asthma symptoms and the possible development of tachyphylaxis. *Am Rev Respir Dis* (1990) **142**: 571–575.

36. Twentyman OP, Finnerty PJ, Harris A, Palmer J, Holgate ST: Protection against allergen-induced asthma by salmeterol. *Lancet* (1990) **336**: 1338–1342.

37. Chapman KR: The role of anticholinergic bronchodilators in adult asthma and chronic obstructive pulmonary disease. *Lung* (1990) **168**(Suppl): 295–303.

38. Pauwels RA: New aspects of the therapeutic potential of theophylline in asthma. *J Allergy Clin Immunol* (1989) **83**: 548–553.

39. Hendeles L, Weinberger M: Theophylline: a 'state of the art' review. *Pharmacotherapy* (1983) **3**: 2–44.

40. Billing B, Dahlqvist R, Hornblad Y, Leideman T, Skareke L, Ripe E: Theophylline in maintenance treatment of chronic asthma: concentration-dependent additional effect of beta 2 agonist therapy. *Eur J Respir Dis* (1987) **70**: 35–43.

41. Howarth PH: Histamine and asthma: an appraisal based on specific H1-receptor antagonism. *Clin Exp Allergy* (1990) **20**(Suppl): 31–41.

42. Grant SM, Goa KL, Fitton A, Sorkin EM: Ketotifen. A review of its pharmacodynamic and pharmacokinetic properties, and therapeutic use in asthma and allergic disorders. *Drugs* (1990) **40**: 412–448.

43. Bianco S, Pieroni MG, Refini RM, Rottoli L, Sestini P: Protective effect of inhaled furosemide on allergen-induced early and late asthmatic reactions. *N Engl J Med* (1989) **321**: 1069–1073.

44. Klaustermeyer WB, Noritake DT, Kwong FK: Chrysotherapy in the treatment of corticosteroid-dependent asthma. *J Allergy Clin Immunol* (1987) **79**: 720–725.

45. Shiner RJ, Nunn AJ, Chung KF, Geddes DM: Randomised, double-blind, placebo-controlled trial of methotrexate in steroid-dependent asthma. *Lancet* (1990) **336**: 137–140.

46. Mullarkey MF, Lammert JK, Blumenstein BA: Long-term methotrexate treatment in corticosteroid-dependent asthma. *Ann Intern Med* (1990) **112**: 577–581.

47. Svenonius E, Kautto R, Arborelius M Jr: Improvement after training of children with exercise-induced asthma. *Acta Paediatr Scand* (1983) **72**: 23–30.

48. Anderson SD: Exercise-induced asthma: stimulus, mechanism and management. In Barnes PJ, Rodger I, Thomson NC (eds) *Asthma: Basic Mechanisms and Clinical Management.* London, Academic Press, 1988, pp 503–522.

49. British Thoracic Society: Guidelines for management of asthma in adults: II—acute severe asthma. *BMJ* (1990) **301**: 797–800.

50. Horn CR, Clark TJ, Cochrane GM: Compliance with inhaled therapy and morbidity from asthma. *Respir Med* (1990) **84**: 67–70.
51. Chan CS, Woolcock AJ, Sullivan CE: Nocturnal asthma: role of snoring and obstructive sleep apnea. *Am Rev Respir Dis* (1988) **137**: 1502–1504.

Asthma in Children

SØREN PEDERSEN

INTRODUCTION

The reported prevalence rates of childhood asthma in western Europe and the USA vary from 5 to 10%, with an increase in occurrence during the last decades in many countries.[1-4] This makes asthma the most common chronic disease in children in the western world. Furthermore, asthma ranks as one of the most important causes of ill health[5-7] and not only creates a myriad of physical, emotional and social problems for the child and the family but in most countries also creates a financial burden on the family. Finally, there seems to be a clear increase in hospital admissions of children due to acute wheeze[8,9] with an unacceptable number of children still dying from asthma.[10,11]

Although childhood and adult asthma share the same underlying pathophysiological mechanisms, there are some important anatomical, physiological, social, emotional and developmental, age-related differences. Therefore, it is necessary to consider the management of this age group in its own right and not merely extrapolate from experience with adults. The present chapter will try to highlight and discuss some of the features and problems that are distinctive in children and important in the day-to-day management of asthma in this age group.

ANATOMICAL AND PHYSIOLOGICAL FACTORS

There are many reasons why infants and young children are at increased risk to symptomatic airway obstruction, and at times do not respond so well to broncho-

ASTHMA: BASIC MECHANISMS AND CLINICAL MANAGEMENT (2nd Edn)
ISBN 0-12-079026-2

dilators or other inhaled drugs. Compared to adult airways, young children have disproportionally smaller peripheral airways and smaller cross-sectional airway area,[12,13] rendering them more easily obstructed by oedema, secretions, cellular debris and smooth muscle contraction. The chest wall of an infant is more compliant than in later life and there is a relative lack of elastic recoil predisposing to early airway closure even during tidal breathing.[14,15] This in combination with less rigid walls of the bronchi produces ventilation–perfusion mismatching and lower oxygen tensions than in adults.[16]

The collateral channels between the alveoli (pores of Kohn) and the bronchoalveolar communications (Lambert's canals) are decreased in number and size.[17] Therefore, collateral ventilation is less developed and airway obstruction is more likely to cause segmental collapse and atelectasis than in older subjects.

Finally, the angle of insertion of the diaphragm is more horizontal than in adults. This means that during inspiration the infant's diaphragm tends to cause retraction of the compliant rib cage rather than elevation and increased diameter as seen in adults. This makes the diaphragm less efficient and, due to few fatigue-resistant muscle fibres,[18] less suitable to cope with prolonged increased workloads. Therefore, young children more readily tend to develop respiratory failure during acute episodes of asthma.

In infancy, airway smooth muscle is present all the way out to the peripheral airways;[19] it has the ability to contract under provocation[19] and also to bronchodilate under the influence of drugs. However, compared with adults there may be differences in the quantity and area of distribution of the airway smooth muscles.

NATURAL HISTORY

Accurate information about the natural history of childhood asthma is difficult to obtain because it requires that a large totally unselected cohort of children is assessed clinically and then followed prospectively for many years with regular clinical controls and lung function measurements.

It is often anticipated, however, that childhood asthma is a self-limiting disorder which will improve spontaneously during adolescence. This seems to be an oversimplification that only applies to children with mild, episodic symptoms. The majority of children with persistent symptoms in childhood will continue to wheeze and have reduced pulmonary function values into adult life, though many tend to improve somewhat.[20–31] Furthermore, a large proportion of children with apparent remissions in early adolescence will have recurrence of their symptoms when they grow older.[20] Finally, the term 'outgrowing the asthma' may be somewhat misleading since recent studies indicate that many patients who consider themselves symptom-free still have reduced pulmonary functions[22,23,25,31–33] and increased bronchial reactivity to specific and non-specific agents.[26,27,29]

In the clinical situtation it is difficult to differentiate reliably beforehand whether or not an individual patient will eventually grow out of the disease. The presence of atopy, low pulmonary functions and smoking in adolescence usually indicates a less favourable prognosis in terms of outgrowing the asthma.[25,31] Controversy still exists as to the importance of age of onset as a prognostic factor. Some suggest that an early debut indicates a more favourable prognosis, others that it is associated with a poorer prognosis and still others that age of onset has no influence on the ultimate prognosis.[23,28] At present there is no indication that therapy or other measures can alter the natural history of the asthma once it is present. However, controlled long-term studies in this area are still lacking.

PREVENTION

It is well known that atopic children whose parents have asthma are at a high risk of developing the condition themselves.[34–37] Naturally it is the dream of many paediatricians to find measures to prevent or postpone this. In this respect strict breast-feeding and delayed introduction of solid foods have been most thoroughly studied. There have been methodological flaws in many of the reported studies and the data have been conflicting,[38] about half of the studies reporting some protective effect on asthma whereas the other half find no effect. The study by Høst et al. clearly shows how difficult it may be just to control exposure correctly.[39] It appears, however, that at best such measures will only produce a small reduction in asthma frequency or some delay in the development in high risk children.[35,38,40–47] Crowded living, frequent viral infections, high mite- and dander-allergen exposure, parental smoking and gas cooking fumes are all risk factors for frequent wheeze during early childhood,[40–47] and they have been shown to modify the expression of the disease once it has developed. There is no consisting evidence, however, that environmental intervention in these areas will influence the development of reactive airway disease, but the strong association between these risk factors and the occurrence of wheeze calls for further studies.

GROWTH

Children with moderate and severe chronic asthma seem to have a growth pattern that is different from normal children. Many show delayed onset of puberty and pre-adolescent deceleration of growth velocity resembling growth retardation.[48,49–53] This deviant growth pattern is accompanied by a retarded bone age so that the bone age corresponds to the height. The difference in growth pattern seems to be unrelated to the use of inhaled corticosteroids[49,50] but it seems to be more pronounced in the children with the most severe asthma. Generally these children tend to grow for a longer period of time than their peers so that before the age of 20 they will achieve normal height.[49–53] By contrast, growth retardation caused by daily and alternate-day administration of large doses of systemic corticosteroids for extended periods of time may be permanent.[51]

The deviant growth pattern complicates the interpretation of results from studies comparing the heights of asthmatic children treated with inhaled corticosteroids with the heights of normal children. Furthermore it means that case reports of apparently reduced growth in association with an asthma treatment should not lead to conclusions about cause–effect relationships. Only controlled longitudinal studies with carefully selected control groups of asthmatic children can be used to assess the influence of exogenous factors upon growth. Such studies are difficult to conduct. Some attempts have been made, however, to evaluate the influence of inhaled corticosteroids on growth. There have been flaws in the designs but the general conclusions have been that long-term treatment of asthmatic children with normally recommended doses of inhaled corticosteroids does not adversely affect growth.[48,54] Recently, knemometry has made it possible to measure changes in short-term growth within weeks.[55] This may become a valuable adjustment/alternative to traditional growth studies since knemometry allows very controlled designs. However, the clinical implications of knemometry findings still need further study.

PHARMACOKINETICS AND PHARMACODYNAMICS

Only the pharmacokinetics of theophylline have been studied to a satisfactory extent in all age groups of children. It appears, however, that children metabolize most drugs more rapidly than adults and that the clearance of drug varies from age group to age group and from patient to patient.[56–59] Therefore, children often require quite high, individually adjusted doses of oral drugs to achieve a satisfactory effect. This is not always appreciated and consequently many drugs are used in suboptimal or ineffective doses in children. Furthermore, the tablet sizes available often do not allow the dose to be related accurately to the size of the child. This may also contribute to suboptimal therapy. The rapid clearance of drugs means that children must take oral drugs at short intervals or slow release preparations twice daily. The latter is preferable due to an improved compliance with twice-daily dosing. However, the advantages of slow-release products may sometimes be outweighed by inconsistent absorption characteristics of these products when taken in combination with food.[62] Since the various products are influenced in different and unpredictable ways, children should only be treated with slow-release preparations whose absorption characteristics have been found reliable also in the presence of food. As a rule the bioavailability of slow-release β-agonist is lower than the bioavailability of plain tablets and syrup. Therefore, the dose should normally be increased by 30% or more when switching from plain oral β_2-agonist therapy to a slow-release therapy.[60,61] Food also reduces the bioavailability and if the product is normally taken with the meals the dose should be increased by an additional 30%.[60,61]

In day-to-day management, sparse knowledge about the pharmacokinetics and pharmacodynamics of the various drugs may to some extent be compensated for by careful monitoring of the effect and repeated adjustment of dose. This is time consuming but mandatory for a successful therapy.

ASSESSMENT OF THE CLINICAL CONDITION

Before treatment of a child is decided it is important to define the objectives of the treatment (Table 40.1). Though these objectives are achievable in the majority of children and they are probably agreed upon by most physicians, clinical experience and the literature suggest that they are not fulfilled in many children.[6,7] The main reason for

Table 40.1 Treatment objectives.

Make the child symptom free
Normalize pulmonary function
Prevent the development of asthma-related disorders (psychosocial problems)
Prevent irreversible airway obstruction and pulmonary damage
Reduce/abolish number of acute admissions
Reduce/abolish mortality from asthma

this discrepancy seems to be variations in the perception and definition of the terms 'symptom free' and 'normal pulmonary functions'. Since reliable and accurate assessment of the clinical condition presents particular problems in children, this will be discussed before an effective treatment plan is suggested.

History-taking

History-taking forms the basis of the assessment of the child's condition. For many reasons most of the important information about the child is usually obtained by careful questioning of the parents. This complicates the assessment to a great extent: many parents are unaware of important details. In our experience the common assumption that children tolerate various drugs better than adults is a result of problems with accurate history-taking rather than a real difference between children and adults. Further, the majority of children find parental smoking a problem for their asthma. Less than 10% of the parents in our clinic realize that. Another problem is that parents unconsciously or consciously interpret their observations, and present an 'edited' version to the physician. Thus, a question about whether or not the child participates in sport activities is rarely answered by a simple 'yes' or 'no' but with a more plausible explaining answer such as 'he/she is not interested in sports' emphasizing that the problem is not that the child is sick. Furthermore, many parents do not like their child to be in regular medication because they are afraid of side-effects and because it constantly reminds them that they have a sick child (in some countries the costs of medicine also plays an important role in this respect). This also influences their description of the child's symptoms. Finally, most children with chronic asthma have had their symptoms since early childhood. Consequently they have adjusted their life-style to the asthmatic condition and their parents have come to accept a state of chronic invalidism in their child as 'normal'.

Communicating directly with the child is often more useful but not without problems either. Children have a limited vocabulary; they do not readily open themselves to the physician; they are not used to long conversations with adults; they are influenced by the parents' opinion about tobacco smoke; acceptance of a certain symptom's level, etc. and they do not want to disappoint or bother the doctor. Finally, children require some time for their answers and therefore are frequently interrupted by their parents. Inaccurate and unspecific questions such as 'how is your asthma' are of little value since the answer will be 'fine' or 'OK' by 9 out of 10 children in whom subsequent specific and careful questioning will reveal important problems interfering with an unrestricted daily life.

Standardized questionnaires are useful but only to some extent diminish the problems with accurate history-taking. Considering these problems with accurate history-taking it is no wonder that the term 'symptom-free' may represent a large scale of asthma control.

Pulmonary function tests

Since history-taking is difficult and often inaccurate it is important to make objective measurements of pulmonary functions in all children who can co-operate. Most children older than 3 years will be able to give reproducible PEF measurements and this should be done at home from time to time. However, PEF and FEV_1 may be normal in the presence of quite marked small airway obstruction.[22,23,63] Even though the detection of small airway obstruction or hyperinflation in an apparently symptom-free period is not of proven clinical importance, it may be of some help to select the children who may benefit clinically from a more aggressive treatment in spite of an apparently stable condition. A standardized exercise test is also very useful in this respect. A fall in pulmonary function >20% after an exercise test performed without any inhaled premedication strongly suggests the presence of a bronchial hyperreactivity that is incompatible with a normal unrestricted lifestyle in most children, irrespective of what information is gained from the history-taking.

Measured pulmonary functions are normally related to some reference value and expressed in per cent predicted normal. This expression may be deceptive and the per cent predicted normal should alway be evaluated in the light of the substantial interindividual variation that is seen in lung functions in growing children. A pulmonary function of 85% predicted normal may be quite good in one child whereas it may be unacceptable in another since we regularly see children whose best pulmonary functions are around 125% predicted normal. All these problems complicate the assessment of the second objective in Table 40.1. Therefore, it is better to use the best value from each child established during aggressive treatment as a reference value and subsequently aim at pulmonary functions around that level.

Psychosocial behaviour

There do not seem to be any inherited characteristic personality features amongst asthmatic children. Yet, the incidence of emotional disorder is about twice as common as in the general population.[64] Anxiety states, school attendance problems, underachievement, dependency problems, peer-group ridicule and social isolation all seem to contribute to this. In adition all clinics see parents who fail to give the child an opportunity to socialize, learn and separate. The result is family dysfunction with overprotection of and over-involvement with the child or a negative attitude to the child.[65,66] Once developed, such dysfunctions are very difficult to treat and they may adversely affect the child's behaviour for many years. The majority of the problems mentioned above stem from preventable conditions such as lack of information, misunderstanding, ignorance or under-treatment of the disease.[67] Therefore, the preconditions for preventing these inexpedient disorders seem to be an early diagnosis, information and effective treatment. This requires an open, active attitude from the physician and effective management from early childhood. It is time-consuming, but likely to pay off in the long run since these dysfunctions are easier to prevent than to treat.

Irreversible bronchopulmonary and chest damage

It is normally anticipated that childhood asthma does not lead to chronic irreversible airway obstruction or pulmonary damage. However, some children may develop these conditions to a clinically important extent.[22,25,32,33,68–70] Furthermore, chest deformities due to persistent hyperinflation are also quite common. However, it is difficult before-hand to differentiate reliably those individuals who are destined to develop these complications and it is not known whether they are preventable. It is the author's philosophy to treat children with persistent asthma continously with anti-inflammatory drugs in the hope of lessening any irreversible damage.

TREATMENT

Asthma in children is rewarding to treat since the life of the child can usually be radically altered. We still have no cure for asthma so pharmacotherapy is likely to remain the cornerstone of asthma management in children for the next decade. As in adults, the various drugs can be given either systemically or by inhalation. There is much evidence in favour of the inhaled route. The medication is deposited directly at the receptors in the airway allowing for a rapid onset of action. The administered therapeutic dose is small compared with other routes of administration and hence the incidence of side-effects for a given clinical effect is lower.[71,72] Exercise-induced bronchoconstriction which is a troublesome, socially invalidating problem in the majority of asthmatic children, can only be effectively blocked by inhaled therapy. In addition, the drugs available for a safe, effective long-term treatment of the inflammatory component of the disease (inhaled corticosteroids and sodium cromoglycate) can only be given by the inhaled route. For these reasons inhaled therapy should be the mainstay of treatment of childhood asthma. This is not the case in many clinics, perhaps because of the common belief that children tend to over-use their inhalers. There are no indications that this is true. Too frequent use of an inhaler is associated with unpleasant side-effects and therefore there is no incentive for the child to misuse it. During the last 10 years virtually all children in our clinic have received inhaled therapy and the majority of children older than 5 years carry their β_2-agonist inhaler wherever they go. Yet we have not encountered one single case of excessive inhaler use, which has not been due to either ineffective inhalation technique or insufficient asthma control, both of which are preventable conditions.

Inhalation therapy in children is not without problems and pitfalls, however.[73] Since accurate knowledge about the nature and magnitude of these problems and about the age groups that can normally use the various inhalation devices correctly is a precondition for effective asthma treatment in children, the advantages and disadvantages of the most widely used inhalers will be discussed in some detail.

INHALER STRATEGY

Metered-dose inhalers

Virtually all children's difficulties with the metered-dose inhaler (MDI) are related to the high velocity of the aerosol particles (100 km/h) leaving the mouthpiece, e.g. problems with correct co-ordination of actuation and inhalation, stop of inhalation when the cold aerosol particles reach the soft palate, actuation of the aerosol into the mouth followed by inhalation through the nose, and a rapid inhalation.[74,75] All these mistakes are associated with a reduced effect. As a consequence more than 50% of children receiving inhalation therapy with an MDI can be expected to gain reduced or no benefit from the prescribed medication.[75,76] Therefore, conventional MDIs cannot normally be recommended for children if alternative devices are available. If this is not the case, all prescriptions of an MDI should be accompanied by repeated, thorough tuition of correct inhaler use followed by the child's demonstration of inhalation technique. Such instruction will take at least 10–20 min.[74] Even if this is done, most pre-school children will not be able to learn effective MDI use.[74,77]

Use of a breath-actuated MDI (Autohaler) will reduce tuition time and abolish the co-ordination difficulties. The remaining problems are unaffected, however, and this inhaler should be reserved for children older than 6–7 years.[77]

Spacers

Attachment of a spacer to the mouthpiece of an MDI ensures that the drug particles due to evaporation of the propellants become smaller and move more slowly when they are inhaled. This leads to reduced impaction on the posterior wall of the pharynx and a reduced oropharyngeal deposition of drug.[78,79] Consequently, the dose swallowed is markedly diminished, and therefore the total body dose is less following administration by such devices.[70,71] This may be of particular importance when high doses of inhaled corticosteroids are used since spacers in such circumstances will reduce the risk of a systemic effect.[81–83] Therefore, spacers are indicated at all ages for treatment with inhaled corticosteroids — particularly so when high doses are used.

Spacers are easy to use, particularly if they have a valve system like the Nebuhaler, Volumatic or Aerochamber. Virtually all schoolchildren can learn the use of these devices and also use them effectively during attacks of acute bronchoconstriction.[84] Between 18 months and 4 years of age it is also possible to train children to use them for prophylactic administration of all appropriate antiasthma medications.[85–87] During episodes of acute wheeze, however, many may not be able to open or close the valve system properly. In such situations nebulizers are the best alternative. Problems with opening and closure of the valve may also be a problem in some younger children not suffering from acute wheeze. It may be reduced by attaching a face mask to the spacer mouthpiece and tilting the spacer inhaler upwards during the inhalations.[87] The inhalation technique of these young age groups is often quite poor. As a result a substantial part of the dose can be recovered from the spacer after the inhalation. This has to be compensated by using somewhat higher doses, otherwise therapy may fail.

The problem with spacers is that they are bulky and difficult to carry about. They are more suitable for prophylactic treatment given at home, morning and evening. Due to their many advantages, a variety of new spacer systems is being launched every year. Though deceptively similar in appearance there may be marked differences in the amount of drug retained in them. Therefore, uncritical use of any new spacer device is not recommended until its value has been documented in controlled trials.

Dry powder inhalers

For many years dry powder inhalers have been single-dose inhalers and therefore less convenient than the MDI. Furthermore, some children have difficulties with correct loading and splitting of the capsules when using the single-dose inhalers, particularly during episodes of acute wheeze.[87,89] Several recent studies have shown that the new multiple-dose powder inhalers are easier to use and more convenient, so these inhalers are to be preferred to the single-dose inhalers.

The effect of powder inhalers increases with increasing inspiratory flow rates.[87,90,91] Therefore, children should be taught to inhale rapidly through these inhalers. Many young children and some older children with severe wheeze cannot generate a sufficient inspiratory flow rate to benefit optimally from a powder inhaler.[87,90,91] Therefore, these inhalers should not be routinely prescribed for children younger than 5 years just as some older children on powder inhaler therapy may need a spacer inhaler during episodes of severe acute wheeze. Apart from a rapid inspiration, dry powder inhalers can be used with a very simple inhalation technique.[88,90,92] This is another advantage since tuition becomes easy. Thus virtually all children over 4 years can be taught correct use of the multiple-dose dry powder inhaler Turbuhaler in less than 5 min.

Nebulizers

For many years nebulizers have been extremely popular among paediatric patients and therefore widely used. Such widespread use is not now justified since alternative devices can be used with the same efficacy.[84] Compared with other devices nebulizers are expensive, bulky, inconvenient, time-consuming, inefficient delivery systems. Therefore, their use should be limited to children who cannot be trained to use another device correctly. In clinical practice this means some children younger than 3–4 years and mentally retarded older children. The vast majority of school children who claim that they need a nebulizer for home treatment are under-treated and once their asthma treatment has become optimized the requirement of a nebulizer disappears. In our clinic no child older than 4 years has a nebulizer at home.

Remarkably few controlled nebulizer studies have been carried out in the age groups that require nebulized treatment. Therefore our knowledge about dose requirement and optimal nebulizer systems for the young age groups is rather limited. Recent studies in our own clinic have shown that it is not justified simply to transfer the doses in milligrams per kilogram recommended for older children to the young age group since their inhalation technique, tidal volume breathing and anatomy of the upper airways are different. Very young children often require much higher doses to achieve the same clinical result. Thus most adults and school children will require 500–1000 μg nebulized budesonide per day to achieve effective asthma control whereas young infants require 1500–2000 μg budesonide per day to control the disease.[93,94] This finding may also to some extent explain why nebulized beclomethazone is normally not very effective in young children.[95–97] Due to the low concentration of beclomethasone in the nebulizer solution it is difficult and time-consuming to give this drug in doses higher than 400–600 μg/day.

In addition, we still do not know which nebulizer is best for young children. A powerful compressor capable of a dynamic flow rate of at least 10 litres/min and a volume fill of 4 ml will produce the best output of respirable budesonide particles in an acceptable nebulization time and this combination therefore may be advantageous.[98] However, in wheezy young children with a minute ventilation of around 2 litres/min, a dynamic flow of 10 litres/min may be too high because of air entrainment.[99] Such flow will result in a substantial waste of drug as compared with an adult or older child with higher minute ventilations. These problems are complicated and not sufficiently elucidated, so at present nebulized therapy to young children has to be based on a few clinical studies and empirical experience.

In the same way the assumption that β_2-agonists are ineffective in young children may have to be re-evaluated in the light of the new findings with corticosteroids. The claimed lack of effect may be due to an insufficient dose of drug being delivered to the airways rather than a lack of effect of the nebulized drug. The results from recent studies using higher doses, other delivery systems or routes of administration indicate that β_2-agonists may have some effect also in the very young infants.[100–103]

Though spacers, powder inhalers and nebulizers are apparently easy to use, careful and repeated tuition is required every time one of these inhalers is prescribed otherwise the therapeutic result will not be satisfactory.

The inhaler strategy we at present find most useful is summarized in Table 40.2. Children younger than 2 years use nebulizers. The age groups from 2 to 5 years use a large-volume spacer with a valve system except when they are severely obstructed, in which case many use a nebulizer. Older children by routine are prescribed a multiple-

Table 40.2 Inhaler strategy in children.

(A) Multiple-dose dry powder inhalers	β_2-agonists in children >5 years
(B) Large-volume valved spacers	Inhaled corticosteroids in children >2 years β_2-agonists in children 2–5 years (+ severe attacks in some older children) Sodium cromoglycate
(C) Nebulizers	Children <2 years Children who cannot use other devices (corticosteroids require special compressors and nebulizers)
(D) Single-dose dry powder inhalers	Obsolete, if (A) is available. Otherwise as (A) + sodium cromoglycate in children >5 years
(E) Breath-actuated metered-dose inhaler (Autohaler)	Children >7 years if dry powder inhalers are not available/feasible
(F) Metered-dose inhaler	Obsolete if alternative devices are available

dose powder inhaler for their β_2-agonists and a large-volume spacer for the administration of inhaled corticosteroids morning and evening. With this approach children can be taught effective inhaler use with a minimum of instructional time. Once the inhalation technique has been learned by the child it is rarely forgotten if the inhaler is used regularly.[75] Finally, it must be remembered always to consider the child's wishes since prescription of an inhaler which the physician but not the child likes is likely to reduce compliance.

DRUG STRATEGY

The correct way to treat a child requiring daily medication is controversial and important differences in strategy exist between the USA, where slow-release theophylline is recommended as first line therapy, and Europe where inhaled therapy is preferred. The arguments for inhaled therapy have already been discussed.

In most paediatric clinics it is traditional to build up the treatment gradually starting with inhaled β_2-agonists, then adding theophylline or oral β_2 or disodium cromoglycate (DSCG), and if all these drugs are not sufficient then adding inhaled corticosteroids (or in the USA alternate-day oral steroids) as the last resort before daily oral steroids are used.[104,105]

Due to the many problems with severity assessment and estimation of optimal control this strategy carries a substantial risk of ending up at a treatment level at which the child is treated suboptimally. Since all the drugs mentioned have been shown to be effective, they are likely to improve the condition to some extent. Everybody will be pleased with the treatment initiated and it will therefore continue. Most parents and children will not be prepared to try a more aggressive treatment because they do not want to change a treatment that has proved to be useful. The major problem with this approach is that the condition after initiation of treatment is always compared with the situation where no, or less, treatment was given.

It is the author's suggestion that treatment should instead be much more outcome oriented. This is in agreement with the recommendations of a recent conference report.[106] Instead of building up the treatment it is important first of all to establish a condition of optimal control. That can only be achieved by a period of aggressive treatment such as high-dose inhaled corticosteroids (800–1000 μg/day) in combination with inhaled β_2-agonists for 4–6 weeks. After this period the smallest amount of medication needed to maintain optimal control is determined by gradually reducing the dose of inhaled corticosteroid every 4–6 weeks until unacceptable symptoms/decrease in pulmonary function appear. Then the dose of inhaled corticosteroid may be increased a little or additional treatment added, whichever is more acceptable (Figure 40.1). Since symptoms do not normally correlate well with changes in pulmonary function, the clinical condition at each treatment level should be monitored closely both with home PEF recordings and diary recordings of symptoms.

This strategy is a change in the traditional way of treating childhood asthma since it uses inhaled corticosteroids and inhaled β_2-agonists as a first line therapy instead of a last resort after everything else has been tried. The advantage of early use of inhaled corticosteroids is that it allows both the asthmatic child, its family and the physician to experience how the child's life may be during optimal treatment. That offers a much better basis for deciding the final therapy. With the traditional building up of the treatment there is a substantial risk that the optimal condition may not be achieved in many children.

Since we have adopted the strategy outlined in Figure 40.1 we have realized that many of our apparently optimally treated children could actually improve markedly, and after a period of high-dose inhaled corticosteroids most children and their parents were not prepared to accept the previous control level which both they and we were pleased with. Often it is the general well-being and the mood of the child and the ability to socialize rather than changes in pulmonary functions that show the most marked improvements. In addition to improvements in quality of life and a reduced morbidity, the effect of the change in management plan is also reflected in the number of acute admissions among the patients regularly seen in our out-patient clinic. This has been reduced from around 65 per year to less than 10 per year in children older than 4 years.

In the majority of children the asthmatic condition will be sufficiently controlled with doses of inhaled corticosteroids of 400 μg/day or less plus inhaled β_2-agonists p.r.n. Such doses of inhaled corticosteroids have been shown to be at least as effective as—or even more effective than—any other asthma therapy. Therefore, we continue with low-dose inhaled corticosteroids rather than switching to other treatments which in many of these patients controlled on 200–300 μg inhaled corticosteroid per day would be equally effective. This also implies the advantages of twice-daily dosing and the use of a limited number of drugs in most patients. The only argument for replacement of low-dose inhaled corticosteroids with other therapy would be fear of side-effects. At present low

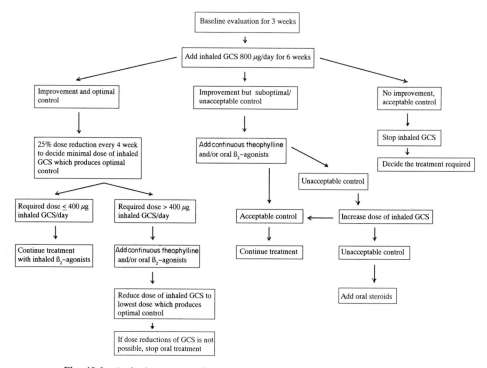

Fig. 40.1 Author's suggestion for treatment strategy. GCS = glucocorticosteroids.

doses of inhaled corticosteroids have been used in children for more than 15 years. During this time many controlled studies and clinical experience reports have evaluated the risk of systemic side-effects. So far there are no controlled data indicating that long-term use of low doses of inhaled corticosteroids in children is associated with any serious side-effects. The vast majority of studies indicate that such treatment is as safe as other treatments.[48] Finally, the long-term prognosis of the children who are controlled on low doses of inhaled corticosteroids is normally good. Therefore, the majority will only require continuous treatment for a limited number of years.

Apart from oral steroids, which are associated with unacceptable side-effects if they are used in the doses required to control the asthmatic condition, high-dose inhaled corticosteroids is the most effective treatment available and they cannot be replaced by any other drug. However, since experience with long-term high-dose therapy is at present rather limited, such treatment should be reserved for patients who are not controlled on lower doses of inhaled corticosteroids in combination with oral bronchodilators or the new inhaled long-acting β_2-agonists formoterol and salmeterol.

No matter which strategy is chosen it is important that the child itself and the family are involved in the therapeutic decisions, otherwise compliance is likely to become poor. Scrutiny and strict control will not improve compliance, only collaboration with the child and its parents will do so. This means that they must be educated in preventing and controlling symptoms, The child must be able to detect initial symptoms and know the appropriate action to take. This is best achieved by using self-management programmes.[107] When the child and the parents get the feeling of being equal partners management normally becomes quite easy.

When the treatment level has been decided each child should be supplied with a written personal management plan for early treatment of exacerbations. This plan should include criteria to introduce or increase a treatment, criteria to reduce the increased treatment to the normal level and criteria to indicate when the patient should contact his/her physician or emergency department. Since no children are alike the criteria and the action to take need to be tailored individually to each patient. Valuable alternatives are the addition of an oral bronchodilator, the increase in the dose of inhaled corticosteroids, the addition of oral steroids or a combination of these. It is important though, that the instructions are simple and in writing—perferably with illustrations—otherwise the risk of misunderstandings is too high.[108]

Special problems in young children

The best treatment strategy in children younger than 2 years is not certain. Oral bronchodilators are widely used but their effectiveness is often disappointing. For oral β_2-agonists it is not known whether this is due to the use of insufficient doses as controlled clinical trials are lacking. It is the author's experience that oral terbutaline in doses from 0.5 to 1.0 mg/kg/day may sometimes produce some effect. Though young children are normally said to be poorly responsive to inhaled β_2-agonists administered by nebulizer, such drugs are still worthy of a trial, even allowing for the fact that they may produce temporary deterioration in lung function.[109,110] This is probably important only when the child is critically ill. However, recent studies with large-volume spacers strongly suggest that inhaled β_2-agonists may produce significant bronchodilatation in most children in this age gorup.[110,111] Furthermore, such therapy may also have a prophylactic role.[101]

Nebulized ipratropium bromide has been shown to relieve brochial obstruction in 40% of β_2-agonist-resistant young wheezers.[113,114] However, clinical trials evaluating the value of ipratropium bromide in the day-to-day management have been disappointing.[115] In contrast to other therapies, inhaled corticosteroids have been found very effective in young children. However, the results with nebulized beclomethazone dipropionate have been discouraging.[95–97] Therefore this drug plays a limited role in the routine management. In contrast, high-dose nebulized budesonide or inhaled corticosteroids given through spacers seem very effective in reducing morbidity and the number of acute admissions.[86,93,116] However, the safety of long-term treatment still remains to be settled. Until that has been done this therapy should be reserved for the more severe cases.

It is the author's experience that it often takes 6–10 weeks (considerably longer than in older children) before nebulized budesonide therapy reaches its maximum effect. If a quicker effect is desired, the nebulized therapy has to be combined with oral prednisolone during the first 10 days of treatment.

SEVERE ACUTE ASTHMA

Generally, principles and modalities of emergency treatment are the same as in adults. The situation denotes a prolonged episode of severe bronchial obstruction which is temporarily refractory to the patient's usual therapy. Since it is a life-threatening condition that requires immediate and correct action all physicians dealing with childhood asthma should be familar with the paediatric doses of medications used in these situations (Table 40.3). The optimal dose of the various drugs shows marked interindividual differences. Therefore, the recommended doses should always be individualized upon the basis of the response and—for theophylline—on serum level monitoring.

Quite often inappropriate investigations and treatments are initiated. This is unfortunate since the severity cannot be assessed accurately by clinical examination alone.[117] Wheeziness correlates poorly with airway obstruction and the physician should always be aware of 'the danger of the silent chest'. Objective monitoring of the clinical condition at arrival and at regular intervals thereafter is crucial for an effective treatment. The key parameters to monitor are respiration rate, degree of hyperinflation, use of accessory muscles, pulse rate, colour, peak flow rate, blood gases and oxygen saturation. Standardized forms for these recordings are strongly recommended. PCO_2 is particularly important.[118] It can be measured transcutaneously in young children. If such equipment is not available a capillary blood sample is reliable. Thus difficulty with artery puncture is not an excuse for not measuring PCO_2. As in adults, PCO_2 is normally low. A normal or high PCO_2 in a wheezy child indicates that the condition is so severe that it requries close monitoring.

Nebulized β_2-agonists and systemic steroids are the cornerstones of the emergency treatment. When normal therapy fails it is often due to a marked inflammation and mucus plugging in the airways. Therefore, it is better to initiate systemic steroids early rather than to 'wait and see how the condition develops'.[119] If the severity was milder

Table 40.3 Doses of drugs most commonly used during the first 2 h in the treatment of acute severe asthma/*status asthmaticus* in children at the author's department. After the initial treatment the various doses should be adjusted individually according to the clinical effect/side-effects. Increase of theophylline dose requires measurement of serum theophylline concentration.

Nebulized β_2-agonists	≤5 years 3–5 mg
	>5 years 5–10 mg
Intravenous methylprednisolone	
Loading dose	1 mg/kg
Continuous	1 mg/kg/8 h
Prednisolone	
Loading dose	1 mg/kg
Continuous	0.7 mg/kg/8 h
Intravenous β_2-agonists	
Loading dose	2–5 μg/kg during 5 min
Continuous	5 μg/kg/h
Intravenous theophylline (in children not given theophylline prior to admission)	
Loading dose	6 mg/kg during 10 min
Continuous	≤11 years 1 mg/kg/h
	>11 years 0.8 mg/kg/h

than anticipated on arrival the steroid treatment can always be stopped. There are no studies on children that evaluate the doses or preparations to be used in true *status asthmaticus*. The author prefers methylprednisolone because of its favourable penetration into the lungs[120,121] and its less mineralocorticoid effect on fluid and electrolytes. The duration of steroid treatment depends upon the rate of recovery. Sometimes a few days' treatment is sufficient, but when the child responds slowly steroids should be administered for 10–15 days and then tapered off according to the clinical condition assessed by PEF measurements and clinical scoring.

Inhaled oxygen is an important part of emergency treatment and the inhaled β_2-agonists should be nebulized with oxygen. The inhaled β_2-doses given in Table 40.3 are the ones used in the author's department. Many other regimens are recommended in the literature.[122–124] Though large-volume spacers are valuable alternatives to nebulizers outside hospital[84] the large doses of freon and lubricant (irritants) that goes with them,[84] their inferiority in oxygen delivery and problems with opening and closure of the valve systems make them less suitable than nebulizers in hospital settings. The reasons for the relatively high doses in young children have been discussed earlier.

The recommended doses of intravenous β_2-agonists are partly emperical and partly derived from other studies[124–127] of which only one is a dose–response study.[127] Undoubtedly, due to systemic absorption of drug from the lungs and gastrointestinal tract, nebulized therapy alone will be able to produce therapeutic plasma levels of β_2-agonists if sufficiently high doses and frequent administrations are used. However, at present it is not known whether nebulized therapy can totally replace the intravenous route in children.

Normally plasma levels of β_2-agonists are not measured. The dose has to be adjusted upon the basis of the clinical response. It seems, however, that optimal clinical effect is rarely achieved until the child experiences some side-effects such as tremor, palpitations or headache.[127] The criteria for admittance to the intensive care unit and ventilation are similar to those in adults. As soon as the child does not have to stay in bed, it can be assumed that the absorption of oral drugs will be reliable and the intravenous therapy can be switched to oral therapy.

Fortunately full recovery after *status asthmaticus* in children is the rule. It is, however, important to realize that the return to a completely normal state is very slow. After 1–2 days' treatment children may clinically appear deceptively well. This should not lead to a premature cessation of treatment. Normally it takes at least 1 month until the bronchial hyperreactivity has returned to normal. Therefore, it is important that these children monitor PEF and clinical symptoms in a diary for some weeks after discharge and that they are all treated with high-dose inhaled corticosteroids during the recovery phase, otherwise the risk of relapse or many weeks with an uncontrolled disease is too high.[118]

IMMUNOTHERAPY

This issue is discussed in detail in a separate chapter. Therefore only some considerations particular for childhood asthma will be mentioned.

A subcommittee of the European Academy of Allergology and Clinical Immunology recently recommended that hyposensitization should not normally be used in children under 5 years.[128,129] Furthermore, it should only be initiated when a clear, important and unavoidable allergic factor has been identified by a bronchial challenge since a positive skin prick test and/or RAST test do not accurately define the importance of the allergy for the asthma disease.

Immunotherapy seems most beneficial in children with mild and moderate asthma, a condition which is normally safely and effectively treated with DSCG or low doses of inhaled corticosteroids.[128,129] Furthermore, these groups of children seem to have the best prognosis for outgrowing their asthma. Once initiated immunotherapy must be continued for as long as any other form of prophylactic treatment. For these reasons its role in the treatment of childhood asthma still remains controversial.

GENERAL MEASURES

Environmental control

Removal of important allergens and irritants such as cigarette smoke is an important requisite for good management of childhood asthma. This topic is discussed elsewhere. However, when such measures are considered in children it must always be remembered to balance the potential benefits against the psychologic consequences of the recommendations given. The asthmatic child is an integrated part of a family and the various advice may have an important impact upon the family relations since the restrictions often involve subjects who are not sick. Removal of the father's sporting dog, banning cigarette smoking or moving the asthmatic child to a sibling's room because it is bigger, more easy to clean or seems to have a better indoor climate, may create negative tensions and adverse effects that counterbalance the beneficial effects upon the asthma. Therefore, the physician should supply the family with knowledge and discuss the problems rather than just ordering various measures. It is up to the family to make the decisions. What is best for one family may not be good for another. Such policy is more likely to preserve a good physician–patient relationship.

Young children in day-care institutions tend to get viral upper airway infections much more frequently than their peers.[43] This increases the likelihood of recurrent wheeze and it may be tempting to advise these children to stay away from the crowded day-care centres. Though likely to be beneficial, such an intervention has a heavy impact not only upon the child's social development but also upon the life of the parents who may not be able to work full time if the child has to be isolated from contact with other children. Therefore, such advice should be reserved for the very severe cases who cannot be controlled on regular therapy with bronchodilators and inhaled corticosteroids.

Exercise

Participation in sport and play is important for a normal growth and psychosocial development in children. Therefore, exercise-induced asthma is an even bigger problem in children than in adults. 'Our sense of identity is rooted in our physical being' (Freud) and children with asthma should be encouraged to participate in play and all physical activities. Much effort should be put into stimulating enjoyable, balanced physical activities to build up fitness and self-confidence in the child's own environment. Many asthmatic children are physically unfit[130] and therefore may require a short physical training programme to break the vicious circle of exercise-induced asthma and unfitness. Such a programme does not have any direct effect upon the asthma but it is likely to improve physical fitness, exercise tolerance, the child's ability to cope with the asthma, neuromuscular co-ordination and self-confidence,[130–132] all of which are important for a normal integration of the child with his/her peers. It is important that this aspect of asthma management is not forgotten. Often a 6–8 weeks training course is sufficient.[130–132]

Prophylactic medication with inhaled β_2-agonists or DSCG just prior to exercise is the most widely recommended treatment. However, often children do not know beforehand when they are going to be physically active. Furthermore, experience shows that many children are reluctant, or forget, to take their medication before their exercise. Instead they choose not to participate wholeheartedly in the physical activity. Therefore, to be effective, it is better to treat this socially invalidating symptom with drugs that do not require premedication immediately prior to the exercise. In this respect continuous treatment with inhaled corticosteroids[132–134] and/or an inhalation of a long acting β_2-agonist such as formoterol or salmeterol in the morning is very effective.[135]

REFERENCES

1. Dodge RR, Burrows B: The prevalence and incidence of asthma and asthma-like symptoms in a general population sample. *Am Rev Respir Dis* (1980) **112**: 567–575.

2. Dowse GK, Turner KJ, Stewart GA, *et al.*: The association between *Dermatophagoides* mites and the increasing prevalence of asthma in village communities within the Papua New Guinea highlands. *J Allergy Clin Immunol* (1985) **75**: 75–83.

3. Mitchell EA: Increasing prevalence of asthma in children. *NZ Med J* (1983) **96**: 463–464.

4. Fleming DM, Crombie DL: Prevalence of asthma and hay fever in England and Wales. *Br Med J* (1987) **294**: 279–283.

5. Schiffer CG, Hunt EP: Illness among children. In *Childrens' Bureau Publication No. 405*. Washington DC, US Department of Health Education and Welfare, 1963, p 14.

6. Speight ANP, Lee DA, Hey EN: Underdiagnosis and undertreatment of asthma in childhood. *Br Med J* (1983) **286**: 1253–1256.

7. Anderson HR, Bailey PA, Cooper JS, *et al.*: Morbidity and school absence caused by asthma and wheezing illness. *Arch Dis Child* (1983) **58**: 777–784.

8. Anderson HR: Increase of hospitalisation for childhood asthma. *Arch Dis Child* (1978) **53**: 295–300.

9. Anderson HR, Bailey P, West S: Trends in the hospital care of acute childhood asthma 1970–8: a regional study. *Br Med J* (1980) **281**: 1191–1194.

10. Inman WHW, Adelstein AM: Rise and fall of asthma mortality in England and Wales in relation to use of pressured aerosols. *Lancet* (1968) **2**: 279–285.

11. Sly RM: Increases in deaths from asthma. *Ann Allergy* (1984) **53**: 20–25.

12. Hislop A, Muir DCF, Jacobsen M, Simon G, Reid L: Postnatal growth and function of the pre-acinar airways. *Thorax* (1972) **27**: 265–274.

13. Hogg J, Williams J, Richardson J, *et al.*: Age as a factor in the distribution of lower airway conductance and in the pathologic anatomy of obstructive lung disease. *N Engl J Med* (1970) **232**: 1283–1287.

14. Bryan AC, Mansell AL, Levison H: In Hodson WA (ed) *Development of the Lung*. New York, Marcel Dekker, 1977, p 445.

15. Helms P: Chest wall mechanics. In Warner JO, Metha MH (eds) *Scoliosis Prevention*. New York, Praeger, 1985, pp 184–189.

16. Newth CJL: Respiratory disease and respiratory failure: implications for the young and the old. *Br J Dis Chest* (1986) **80**: 209–217.

17. Boyden EA: Notes on the development of the lung in infancy and early childhood. *Am J Anat* (1967) **121**: 749–762.

18. Keens TG, Bryan AC, Levison H, Ianazzo CD: Development pattern of muscle fibre types in human ventilatory muscles. *J Appl Physiol* (1978) **44**: 909–913.

19. Prendiville A, Green S, Silverman M: Bronchial responsiveness to histamine in wheezy infants. *Thorax* (1987) **42**: 92–99.

20. McNicol KN, Williams HE: Spectrum of asthma in children. Clinical and physiological components. *Br Med J* (1973) **4**: 7–11.

21. Blair H: Natural history of childhood asthma. 20 years follow-up. *Arch Dis Child* (1977) **52**: 613–619.

22. Friberg S, Bevegård S, Graff-Lonnevig V: Asthma from childhood to adult age. *Acta Pædiatr Scand* (1988) **77**: 424–431.

23. Gerritsen J, Koëter GH, Postma DS, Schouten JP, Knol K: Prognosis of asthma from childhood to adulthood. *Am Rev Respir Dis* (1989) **140**: 1325–1330.

24. Balfour-Lynn L: Childhood asthma and puberty. *Arch Dis Child* (1985) **60**: 231–235.

25. Kelly WJH, Hudson I, Raven J, *et al.*: Childhood asthma and adult lung function. *Am Rev Respir Dis* (1988) **138**: 26–30.

26. Davé NK, Hopp RJ, Biven RE, *et al.*: Persistence of increased nonspecific bronchial reactivity in allergic children and adolescents. *J Allergy Clin Immunol* (1990) **86**: 147–153.

27. Foucard T, Sjöberg O: A prospective 12-year follow-up study of children with wheezy bronchitis. *Acta Pædiatr Scand* (1984) **73**: 577–583.

28. Martin AJ, Landau LI, Phelan PD: Predicting the course of asthma in children. *Aust Paediatr J* (1982) **18**: 84–87.

29. Gerritsen J, Koëter GH, Monchy JGR, Campagne JGL, Knol K: Change in airway

responsiveness to inhaled house dust from childhood to adulthood. *J Allergy Clin Immunol* (1990) **85**: 1083–1089.

30. Martin AJ, McLennan LA, Landau LI, Phelan PD: The natural history of childhood asthma to adult life. *Br Med J* (1980) **280**: 1397–1400.

31. Kelly WJW, Hudson I, Phelan PD, Pain MCF, Olinsky A: Childhood asthma in adult life: a further study at 28 years of age. *Br Med J* (1987) **294**: 1059–1062.

32. Martin AJ, Landau LI, Phelan PD: Lung function in young adults who had asthma in childhood. *Am Rev Respir Dis* (1980) **122**: 609–616.

33. Blackhall M: Ventilating function in subjects with childhood asthma who have become symptom free. *Arch Dis Child* (1970) **45**: 363–366.

34. Kjellman N: Atopic disease in seven-year-old children: Incidence in relation to family history. *Acta Pædiatr Scand* (1977) **66**: 465–471.

35. Horwood LJ, Fergusson DM, Hons BA, Shannon FT: Social and familial factors in the development of early childhood asthma. *Pediatrics* (1985) **75**: 859–868.

36. Lubs M-LE: Empiric risks for genetic counseling in families with allergy. *J Pediatr* (1972) **80**: 26–31.

37. Luoma R, Koivikko A, Viander M: Development of asthma, allergic rhinitis, and atopic dermatitis by the age of five years. *Allergy* (1983) **38**: 339–346.

38. Kramer MS: Does breast feeding help protect against atopic disease? Biology, methodology, and a golden jubilee of controversy. *J Pediatr* (1988) **112**: 181–190.

39. Høst A, Husby S, Østerballe O: A prospective study of cow's milk allergy in exclusively breast-fed infants. *Acta Pædiatr Scand* (1988) **77**: 663–670.

40. Wright AL, Holberg CJ, Martinez FD, Morgan WJ, Taussig LM: Breast feeding and lower respiratory tract illness in the first year of life. *Br Med J* (1989) **299**: 946–949.

41. Welliver RC, Sun M, Rinaldo D, Ogra PL: Predictive value of respiratory syncytial virus-specific IgE responses for recurrent wheezing following bronchiolitis. *J Pediatr* (1986) **109**: 776–780.

42. Weiss ST, Tager IB, Munzo A, Speizer FE: The relationships of respiratory infections in early childhood to the occurrence of increased levels of bronchial responsiveness and atopy. *Am Rev Respir Dis* (1985) **131**: 573–578.

43. Bisgaard H, Dalgaard P, Nyboe J: Risk factors for wheezing during infancy. *Acta Pædiatr Scand* (1987) **76**: 719–726.

44. Ownby DR, McCullough J: Passive exposure to cigarette smoke does not increase allergic sensitization in children. *J Allergy Clin Immunol* (1988) **82**: 634–638.

45. Lau S, Falkenhorst G, Weber A, *et al.*: High mite-allergen exposure increases the risk of sensitization in atopic children and young adults. *J Allergy Clin Immunol* (1989) **84**: 718–725.

46. Martinez FD, Antognoni G, Macri F, *et al.*: Parenteral smoking enhances bronchial responsiveness in nine-year-old children. *Am Rev Respir Dis* (1988) **138**: 518–523.

47. Sporik R, Holgate ST, Platts-Mills TAE, Cogswell JJ: Exposure to house-dust mite allergen (Der p I) and the development of asthma in childhood. *N Engl J Med* (1990) **323**: 502–507.

48. Pedersen S: The safety of inhaled steroids in children. In *Controversies in Inhaled Steroid Therapy* (*a satellite symposium of SEPCR '89*). Ipswich, WS Cowell, 1989, pp 29–37.

49. Balfour-Lynn L: Effect of asthma on growth and puberty. *Pediatrician* (1987) **14**: 237–241.

50. Balfour-Lynn L: Growth and childhood asthma. *Arch Dis Child* (1986) **61**: 1049–1055.

51. Martin AJ, Landau LI, Phelan PD: The effect on growth of childhood asthma. *Acta Pædiatr Scand* (1981) **70**: 683–688.

52. Hauspie R, Susanne C, Alexander F: Maturational delay and temporal growth retardation in asthmatic boys. *J Allergy Clin Immunol* (1977) **59**: 200–206.

53. Shohat M, Shohat T, Kedem R, Mimouni M, Danon YL: Childhood asthma and growth outcome. *Arch Dis Child* (1987) **62**: 63–65.

54. Hughes IA: Steroids and growth. *Lancet* (1987) **295**: 683–684.

55. Wolthers O, Pedersen S: Short term linear growth in asthmatic children during treatment with prednisolone. *Br Med J* (1990) **301**: 145–148.

56. Hendeles L, Weinberger M: Drugs in perspective. Theophylline. A 'State of the Art' Review. *Pharmacotherapy* (1983) **3**: 2–44.

57. Hendeles L, Iafrate RP, Weinberger M: A clinical and pharmacokinetic basis for the selection and use of slow release theophylline products. *Clin Pharmacokin* (1984) **9**: 95–135.

58. Pedersen S, Steffensen G, Ekman I, Tönnesson M, Borgå O: Pharmacokinetics of Budesonide in children with asthma. *Eur J Clin Pharmacol* (1987) **31**: 579–582.

59. Hultquist C, Lindberg C, Nyberg L, Kjellman B, Wettrell G: Kinetics of terbutaline in asthmatic children. *Eur J Respir Dis* (1984) **65**(Suppl 134): 195–203.

60. Nyberg L, Kennedy B-M: Pharmacokinetics of terbutaline given in slow-release tablets. *Eur J Respir Dis* (1984) **65**(Suppl 134): 119–139.

61. Davies DS: The fate of inhaled terbutaline. *Eur J Respir Dis* (1984) **65**(Suppl 134): 141–147.

62. Pedersen S: Effects of food on the absorption of theophylline in children. *J Allergy Clin Immunol* (1986) **78**: 704–709.

63. Cooper DM, Cutz E, Levison H. Occult pulmonary abnormalities in asymptomatic asthmatic children. *Chest* (1977) **71**: 361–365.

64. Mattson A: Psychologic aspects of childhood asthma. *Pediatr Clin North America* (1975) **2**: 77–78.

65. Pinkerton P: Childhood asthma. *Br J Hosp Med* (1971) **9**: 331–338.

66. Liebman R, Minuchin S, Baker L: The use of structural family therapy in the treatment of intracable asthma. *Am J Psychiat* (1974) **131**: 535–540.

67. Reddihough D, Landau L, Jones H, Richards W. Family anxieties in childhood asthma. *Aust Pediatr J* (1977) **13**: 295–298.

68. Burrows B, Knudson RJ, Lebowitz MD: *Am Rev Respir Dis* (1977) **115**: 751.

69. Loren ML, Leung PK, Cooley RL, *et al.*: *Chest* (1978) **74**: 126.

70. Brown PJ, Greville HW, Finucane KE: *Thorax* (1984) **39**: 131.

71. Thiringer G, Svedmyr N: Comparison of infused and inhaled terbutaline in patients with asthma. *Scand J Respir Dis* (1976) **57**: 17–24.

72. Williams SJ, Winner SJ, Clark TJH: Comparison of inhaled and intravenous terbutaline in acute severe asthma. *Thorax* (1981) **36**: 629–631.

73. Pedersen S: Inhaler use in children with asthma. MD thesis. *Danish Med Bull* (1987) **34**: 234–249.

74. Pedersen S, Østergaard PA: Nasal inhalation as a cause of inefficient pulmonary aerosol inhalation technique in children. *Allergy* (1983) **38**: 191–194.

75. Pedersen S, Frost L, Arnfred T: Errors in inhalation technique and efficiency in inhaler use in asthmatic children. *Allergy* (1986) **41**: 118–124.

76. Pedersen S: Aerosol treatment of bronchoconstriction in children, with or without a tube spacer. *N Engl J Med* (1983) **308**: 1328–1330.

77. Pedersen S, Mortensen S: Use of different inhalation devices in children. *Lung* (1990) (Suppl): 653–657.

78. Newman SP, Moren F, Pavia D, Little F, Clarke SW: Deposition of pressurized suspension aerosols inhaled through extension devices. *Am Rev Respir Dis* (1981) **124**: 317–320.

79. Newman SP: Deposition and effects of inhalation aerosols. Thesis, Lund, Rahms Tryckeri (1983).

80. Lindgren SB, Larsson S: Inhalation of terbutaline sulphate through a conventional actuator or a pear-shaped tube: effects and side effects. *Eur J Respir Dis* (1982) **63**: 504–509.

81. Prahl P, Jensen T: Decreased adreno-cortical suppression utilizing the Nebuhaler for inhalation of steroid aerosols. *Clin Allergy* (1987) **17**: 393–398.

82. Farrer M, Francis AJ, Pearce SJ: Morning serum cortisol concentrations after 2 mg inhaled beclomethasone dipropionate in normal subjects: effect of a 750 mg spacing device. *Thorax* (1990) **45**: 740–742.

83. Brown PH, Blundell G, Greening AP, Crompton GK: Do large volume spacer devices reduce the systemic effects of high dose inhaled corticosteroids? *Thorax* (1990) **45**: 736–739.

84. Fuglsang G, Pedersen S: Comparison of Nebuhaler and nebulizer treatment of acute severe asthma in children. *Eur J Respir Dis* (1986) **69**: 109–113.

85. Gleeson JGA, Price JF: Controlled trial of budesonide given by the Nebuhaler in preschool children with asthma. *Br Med J* (1988) **297**: 163–166.

86. Bisgaard H, Munck SL, Nielsen JP, Petersen W, Ohlsson SV: Inhaled budesonide for treatment of recurrent wheezing in early childhood. *Lancet* (1990) **336**: 649–651.

87. Bisgaard H, Ohlsson S: PEP-spacer: an adaptation for administration of MDI to infants. *Allergy* (1989) **44**: 363–364.

88. Pedersen S: How to use a Rotahaler. *Arch Dis Child* (1986) **61**: 11–14.

89. Pedersen S: Treatment of acute bronchoconstriction in children with use of a tube spacer aerosol and a dry powder inhaler. *Allergy* (1985) **40**: 300–304.

90. Pedersen S, Steffensen G: Fenoterol powder inhaler technique in children: influence of inspiratory flow rate and breathholding. *Eur J Respir Dis* (1986) **68**: 207–214.

91. Pedersen S, Hansen OR, Fuglsang G: Influence of inspiratory flow rate upon the effect of a Turbuhaler. *Arch Dis Child* (1990) **65**: 308–319.

92. Hansen OR, Pedersen S: Optimal inhalation technique with terbutaline Turbuhaler. *Eur Respir J* (1989) **2**: 637–639.

93. Pedersen S: Studies with nebulized budesonide. In Godfrey S (ed) *Budesonide. Nebulising Suspension.* Oxford, Henry Ling, Dorset Press, 1989, pp 25–29.

94. de Jongste JC, Duiverman EJ: Nebulised budesonide in severe childhood asthma. *Lancet* (1989) **335**: 1388.

95. Webb MSC, Milner AD, Hiller EJ, Henry RL: Nebulised beclomethasone dipropionate suspension. *Arch Dis Child* (1986) **61**: 1108–1110.

96. Maayan C, Itzhaki T, Bar-Yishay E, *et al.*: The functional response of infants with persistent wheezing to nebulized beclomethasone dipropionate. *Pediatr Pulmonol* (1986) **2**: 9–14.

97. Storr J, Lenney CA, Lenney W: Nebulised beclomethasone dipropionate in preschool asthma. *Arch Dis Child* (1986) **61**: 270–273.

98. Clay MM, Pavia D, Newman SP, Lennard-Jones T, Clarke SW: Assessment of jet nebulisers for lung aerosol therapy. *Lancet* (1983) **2**: 592–594.

99. Collis GG, Cole CH, Le Souëf PN: Dilution of nebulised aerosols by air entrainment in children. *Lancet* (1990) **336**: 341–343.

100. Kraemer R, Birrer P, Schöni MH: Dose–response relationships and time course of the response to systemic beta adrenoreceptor agonists in infants with bronchopulmonary disease. *Thorax* (1988) **43**: 770–776.

101. Prendiville A, Green S, Silverman M: Airway responsiveness in wheezy infants: evidence for functional beta adrenergic receptors. *Thorax* (1987) **42**: 100–104.

102. Bentur L, Kerem E, Canny G, *et al.*: Response of acute asthma to a β_2-agonist in children less than two years of age. *Ann Allergy* (1990) **65**: 122–126.

103. Mallol J, Barrueto L, Girardi G, *et al.*: Use of nebulized bronchodilators in infants under 1 year of age: analysis of four forms of therapy. *Pediatr Pulmonol* (1987) **3**: 298–303.

104. Warner JO, Göetz M, Landau LI, *et al.*: Management of asthma: a consensus statement. *Arch Dis Child* (1989) **64**: 1065–1079.

105. Canny GJ, Levison H: Childhood asthma: a rational approach to treatment. *Ann Allergy* (1990) **64**(5): 406–418.

106. Hargreave FE, Dolovich J, Newhouse MT: The assessment and treatment of asthma: A conference report. *J Allergy Clin Immunol* (1990) **85**: 1098–1111.

107. Lewis CE, Rachalefsky G, de la Sota A, *et al.*: A randomized trial of asthma care training for kids. *Pediatrics* (1984) **74**: 478–486.

108. Pedersen S: Ensuring compliance in children. *Lung* (1991) in press.

109. Prendiville A, Green S, Silverman M: Paradoxical response to nebulised salbutamol in wheezy infants, assessed by partial expiratory flow-volume curves. *Thorax* (1987) **42**: 86–91.

110. Prendiville A, Rose A, Maxwell DL, Silverman M: Hypoxaemia in wheezy infants after bronchodilator treatment. *Arch Dis Child* (1987) **62**: 997–1000.

111. Lodrup KC, Carlsen KH: The effect of inhaled nebulised racemic adrenaline upon lung function in infants with bronchiolitis. *European Paediatric Respiratory Society 1990 Meeting.* London, 1990, Abstract No. 22.

112. Aebischer CC, Wirz C, Frey U, Kraemer R: Response of a beta adrenoreceptor agonist in infants with bronchopulmonary disease. Comparison of three routes of administration. *European Paediatric Respiratory Society 1990 Meeting.* London, 1990, Abstract No. 28.

113. Hodges IGC, Groggins RC, Milner AD, Stokes GM: Bronchodilator effect of inhaled ipratropium bromide in wheezy toddlers. *Arch Dis Child* (1981) **56**: 729–732.
114. O'Callaghan C, Milner AD, Swarbrick A. Spacer device with face mask attachment for giving bronchodilators to infants with asthma. *Br Med J* (1989) **298**: 160–161.
115. Henry RL, Hiller EJ, Milner AD, Hodges IGC, Stokes GM: Nebulised ipratropium bromide and sodium cromoglycate in the first two years of life. *Arch Dis Child* (1984) **59**: 54–57.
116. Greenough A, Pool J, Gleeson JGA, Price JF: Effect of budesonide on pulmonary hyperinflation in young asthmatic children. *Thorax* (1988) **43**: 937–938.
117. Canny GJ, Levison H: Pulmonary function abnormalities during apparent clinical remission in childhood asthma. *J Allergy Clin Immunol* (1988) **82**: 1–4.
118. Weiss EB, Segal MS, Stein M (eds) *Status Asthmaticus*, 2nd edn. Baltimore, University Park Press, 1985, pp 1–408.
119. Storr J, Barrel E, Barry W, Lenney Hatcher G: Effect of a single oral dose of prednisolone in acute childhood asthma. *Lancet* (1987) **1**: 879–882.
120. Wichyanond P, Irvin CG, Larsen GL, Szefler SJ, Hill MR: Penetration of corticosteroids into the lung: Evidence for a difference between methylprednisolone and prednisolone. *J Allergy Clin Immunol* (1989) **84**: 867–873.
121. Harfi H, Hanissian AS, Crawford LV: Treatment of *status asthmaticus* in children with high doses and conventional doses of methylprednisolone. *Pediatrics* (1978) **61**: 829–831.
122. Rubin BK, Marcushamer S, Priel I, App EM: Emergency management of the child with asthma. *Pediatric Pulmonol* (1990) **8**: 45–57.
123. Schuh S, Parkin P, Rajan A, *et al.*: High- versus low-dose, frequently administered, nebulized albuterol in children with severe, acute asthma. *Pediatrics* (1989) **83**: 513–518.
124. Edmunds AT, Godfrey S: Cardiovascular response during severe acute asthma and its treatment in children. *Thorax* (1981) **35**: 745–750.
125. Hambleton G, Stone MJ: Comparison of IV salbutamol with IV aminophylline in the treatment of severe, acute asthma in childhood. *Arch Dis Child* (1979) **54**: 391–402.
126. Bohn D, Kalloghlian A, Jenkins J, Edmonds J, Barker G: Intravenous salbutamol in the treatment of *status asthmaticus* in children. *Cri Care Med* (1984) **12**: 892–896.
127. Fuglsang G, Pedersen S, Borgström L: Dose-response relationships of intravenously administered terbutaline in children with asthma. *J Pediatr* (1989) **114**: 315–320.
128. Warner JO: Immunotherapy: Yesterday's treatment. In Reed CE (ed) *Proc XII International Congress of Allergology and Clinical Immunology*. CV Mosley, 1986, pp 323–326.
129. Warner JO, Kerr JW: Hyposensitisation. *Br Med J* (1987) 1179.
130. Henriksen JM, Nielsen TT: Effect of physical training on exercise-induced bronchoconstriction. *Acta Pædiatr Scand* (1983) **72**: 31–36.
131. Oseid S, Edwards AM: *The Asthmatic Child in Play and Sport*. London, Pitman, 1983.
132. Østergaard PA, Pedersen S: The effect of inhaled disodium cromoglycate and budesonide on bronchial responsiveness to histamine and exercise in asthmatic children: a clinical comparison. In Godfrey S (ed) *Glucocorticosteroids in Childhood Asthma*. Amsterdam, Excerpta Medica, 1987, pp 69–76.
133. Henriksen JM, Dahl R: Effects of inhaled budesonide alone and in combination with low-dose terbutaline in children with exercise-induced asthma. *Am Rev Respir Dis* (1983) **128**: 993–997.
134. Henriksen JM: Effect of inhalation of corticosteroids on exercise induced asthma: randomised double blind crossover study of budesonide in asthmatic children. *Br Med J* (1985) **291**: 248–249.
135. Ruggins NR, Milner AD: The prolonged effect of salmeterol hydroxynaphthoate on exercise induced bronchoconstriction (EIB) in asthmatic children. *European Paediatric Respiratory Society 1990 Meeting*. London, 1990, Abstract No. 35.

Education and Compliance

MARTYN R. PARTRIDGE

INTRODUCTION

Consensus-type conferences have produced clear guidelines on the good management of asthma in both adults and children.[1-5] Such guidelines are of little value if the treatments that they recommend are prescribed but not taken by the patient. This chapter is concerned with compliance and with an evaluation of methods of giving information and altering behaviour.

As treatments become more effective it is more important that they are used.

COMPLIANCE

Compliance is often defined as action in accordance with a command, but a less proscriptive wording is 'the extent to which a patient's behaviour coincides with medical advice'. In the context of asthma this emphasizes that compliance involves both compliance with drug treatment and compliance with the seeking of medical attention at appropriate times.

Compliance with drug therapy

Measurement

A physician's ability to predict compliance just by familiarity with the patient has been shown to be unreliable.[6] Some form of planned assessment is therefore necessary. Compliance may be inferred by assessing outcome (well-controlled disease) or drug

ASTHMA: BASIC MECHANISMS AND CLINICAL MANAGEMENT (2nd Edn)   Copyright © 1992 Academic Press Limited
ISBN 0-12-079026-2

taking may be monitored. This may involve measurement of drug levels in urine, plasma or saliva or be by prescription monitoring or by the counting of tablets or weighing of aerosols.[7] Microprocessors may be fitted to the lids of bottles[8] or to aerosols[9] and these may be programmed to record time intervals between doses and total doses used.

Such extreme measures may be necessary in clinical trials but these methods each have limitations and are often not applicable to a day-to-day clinical setting. Assays may not be available for the drug in question and pill counting may reveal an appropriate reduction in numbers without the tablets necessarily having been taken. Weighing of aerosols or the use of attached microprocessors may give misleading results if the patient habitually test fires the inhaler before use. Forewarning the patient of such monitoring of compliance may lead to further subterfuge, and secret testing of patients' honesty is correctly abhorrent to many physicians. A suitable compromise may be the use of written or verbal questioning. Written questionnaires have been used in some studies[11] and in one[12] the patients were simply asked to record their current medication and then asked to select an option which most closely approximated to their current compliance. The options ranged from 'I can honestly say I have never missed a dose' through, 'I usually miss 5–6 doses per week' to 'When I'm well I stop the treatment altogether'. Such studies almost certainly still over-estimate compliance and verbal questioning has been shown to do so by up to 30%.[13] However in routine clinical practice an awareness of the size of the problem and the use of simple verbal questions may still be useful and reveal unexpected non-compliance. Questions such as 'How often do you find you remember to take the medicines?' are more likely to provoke realistic answers than 'You are taking the medicines aren't you?' This approach is also more likely than secret testing to proceed to a solving of the problems behind the patient's non-compliance.

Factors affecting compliance

Therapeutic regimes and demographic factors. Complicated therapeutic regimes are more likely to lead to non-compliance than simple schedules that fit in with activities of daily living. In one study observing 3428 patient days of anti-epileptic therapy, compliance was 87% with once-daily regimes, 81% with twice-daily treatment, 77% with three-times daily and 39% with q.d.s. regimes.[8] Other studies have not shown that once-daily regimes are necessarily any better than twice-daily and the latter permits treatment to be conveniently taken on rising and on going to bed.[14,15] Side-effects of medication may lead to problems but some studies have apparently shown that imagined side-effects may lead to greater non-compliance than genuine complications.[16]

Older patients are generally thought to be more compliant with therapy than the young and adolescents have been said to complain particularly of the futility of regular treatments which do not cure the condition. Minority ethnic groups may not comply because of cultural prejudices about conventional medicine or routes of administration, or there may be problems associated with communication or the need for strict fasting during religious festivals. In one study 50% of Asians fasted at some stage for such reasons and yet health professionals were rarely asked to advise about the use of medication at these times.[17]

Communication failure and compliance. 'Non-compliance' implies a defect in patient behaviour but it may equally reflect inadequacy on the doctor's behalf. A patient may omit therapy because of inadequate advice on how to take it. Over half of all verbal information is forgotten within 5 minutes of a consultation. Supporting written information is helpful but an average British adult reading age of 9 years and the use of 150 different languages in the UK alone may make it difficult to write clear instructions suitable for everyone. Misunderstanding probably explains only a part of this problem. A study by Korsch and Negrette[18] showed a direct relationship between patient satisfaction with communication and compliance with treatment. Of the patients who were satisfied with the communication aspects of the consultation, 54% complied totally whereas in the dissatisfied group the equivalent figure was 16%. Subsequent studies have confirmed the importance of the patient/physician relationship and the physician's belief in the efficacy of the treatment.

Types of non-compliance with treatment

Patients may fall into one of three categories: (a) total compliers; (b) partial compliers; and (c) non-compliers. Some may regard total compliance as being an almost abnormal trait and in practice partial compliance is probably more usual. The degree of compliance will vary and the factors involved in determining compliance may be very different according to type. Forgetfulness is the likely explanation for not taking the occasional dose of a medication, whereas rebellion, mistrust of drugs, fear of side-effects or a feeling of lack of efficacy may be the factors more likely to be involved in total non-compliance. Compliance is unlikely to be a steady state. Mood and one's attitude to ill health may vary with time and it is possible that frequency of symptoms may either reinforce the need to comply with treatment or alternately lead to rejection of therapy as being ineffective. Compliance may also be greater where the consequences of omitting therapy are immediate rather than distant.

The size of the problem

Where compliance has been specially measured, rates of between 4 and 93% have been reported.[19] Rates of compliance are usually lower in the treatment of chronic conditions than in short-course treatment and mean non-compliance rates of 37.5% have been reported in 20 studies of the taking of antituberculosis chemotherapy, 48.7% in eight studies of antibiotic use, and 38.6% in nine studies of psychotropic medication. An overall range of compliance of between 29 and 59% was reported in another review.[20]

Specific studies in asthma often relate to the use of theophyllines because of the wide availability of an assay for that medication but Horn et al.[7] have reported studies using a urinary salbutamol assay. Fifty-one adult patients in a general practice who said they had taken 200 mcg salbutamol from a pressurized aerosol gave a urine sample. Results showed that five of the 51 had urine salbutamol levels much lower than expected and 11 had much higher than expected levels. The results could not be related to technique of aerosol usage. Thus with inhaled bronchodilators, patients can be demonstrated to both under comply and to over use the drug. The same authors have also studied compliance with prophylatic therapy and reported 50% non-compliance rates with inhaled treatments, in general practice.[28] An identical figure has been reported for overall compliance in a study in a hospital asthma clinic.[21] Surprisingly even amongst children with asthma compliance rates of only 54%[11] and 68%[22] have been reported.

Table 41.1   Factors associated with non-compliance with therapy.

Drug factors
   Problems with inhaler devices
   Complicated regimes leading to forgetfulness
   Side-effects

Patient/physician problems
   Poor communication/poor relationship
   Misunderstanding/lack of information
   Inappropriate expectations about the condition and its treatment (and lack of opportunity to
      discuss such expectations)
   Attitude towards ill health of patient and family/personality/mood
   Age/sex/ethnic factors

The difficulty with most of these studies however is the lack of longitudinal data and the lack of data relatable to individual drug therapies. It is thus difficult to determine the relative size of the problem of partial and total non-compliance and there are few clues as to the relative importance of the several potential causes of non-compliance with asthma therapy. The possibilities are listed in Table 41.1.

Specific drug-related problems. Extrapolation from compliance studies in other diseases would suggest that preventative therapies involving four times daily administration (e.g. sodium cromoglycate) may be more problematical than those involving morning and evening dosing (e.g. nedocromil sodium and inhaled steroids). Nausea with xanthines, palpitations or tremor with β-agonists, the bitter taste of nedocromil, or hoarseness or candidiasis with inhaled steroids may all contribute to non-compliance by some patients.

Lack of information. Problems using inhalers are a well-recognized cause of non-compliance[24] but lack of instruction may extend to a failure to explain the differences between relieving therapies and regular treatment to prevent asthma. Fourteen per cent of patients in one study[24] and 11% in another[26] thought that inhaled steroids should be used for immediate relief. At the time of diagnosis of asthma a quarter of patients interviewed in a National Asthma Campaign/Mori Poll of 1490 members did not understand that treatment would need to be taken regularly and 46% had received no written instructions.[27] Sixty-two per cent lacked understanding of the condition and 59% wanted more information. Even amongst patients attending a hospital asthma clinic 22% felt they had had too little information about their condition or its treatment.[26]

Expectations. The patient with asthma may have an expectation that the doctor will be able to provide a cure or be able to provide a list of circumstances that should be avoided to prevent attacks. This expectation can rarely be met and if the patient is instead given, without adequate explanation, a steroid inhaler to take for ever, then non-compliance is the likely result. The patient may also have a false expectation of side-effects and the patient needs to be given adequate time to air his or her fears and expectations. Low expectations as to what treatment may achieve may also lead to an over-reliance on bronchodilator therapy and non-compliance with regular preventative treatment.

Sixty-four per cent of patients in one study put up with waking at least three nights per week because of their asthma and received only brochodilator treatment.[28]

Attitudes to ill health. In a study of 210 patients with asthma, 26% admitted to feeling different to other people and 38% were angry, 32% depressed and 13% felt somehow to blame for their condition. Thirty-nine per cent felt that they could not enjoy a full life.[29] In another survey 11% felt extremely frustrated at having to take regular medication and 21% were embarrassed about taking medication in public.[27] The effect of such stigmatization on compliance may be difficult to predict. A study by Sibbald[29] has suggested that bronchodilator usage is greater the greater the stigma felt by the patient and this is not related to morbidity. There are no comparable studies on how stigma affects long-term compliance with preventative therapy, but it is possible that feeling stigmatized may reduce the patient's receptiveness to instruction and this may have an effect upon compliance.

Compliance with the seeking of medical attention

The decision as to whether to seek medical attention in the event of deteriorating asthma involves the patient in making a correct risk vs. benefit assessment of the situation. To do this he/she needs to have been taught how to recognize the signs of deteriorating asthma, both subjectively and objectively and it is probably important for the patient to know the consequences of non-compliance. When asked whether people could die from asthma, 82% of the patients attending a hospital asthma clinic knew that that was a possibility whilst 8% denied that it happened and 10% left this question, but not the majority of others, unanswered.[26] In another study 28% of the patients did not think it was possible to die during an asthma attack.[30] The patient needs to have been told what action to take in the event of deteriorating asthma and yet in one survey 35% of patients had had no prior discussion with their doctor on this subject.[27] Asked to explain the action they would take, 14% of asthmatics attending a hospital clinic described inappropriate self help without resort to medical advice.[26] In another study in general practice, 80 patients using drug therapy were asked what they would do if their usual medication was having no effect. Three patients said that they would go straight to hospital, 46 said that they would contact their doctor immediately and 21 said that they would wait and see if their condition improved—perhaps trying relaxation and deep breathing—and if it did not then they would contact their doctor.[31]

A patient's response to such a situation may not just reflect adequacy of preceding training and it is likely to be modified by previous experience. Chronic symptoms may induce a sense of stoicism or complacency, and inconvenience, fear of hospitalization or previous experience of inexpert painful arterial blood gas sampling may all interfere with the patient's risk vs. benefit analysis. In one study 22% of patients expressed a fear of hospital admission as a reason for delay in seeking help.[29] In assessing patients' responses to a set of deteriorating circumstances no connection was shown between response and age, sex, social class, psychiatric morbidity or duration of asthma. However those with the highest morbidity in the preceding 6 months were those who would delay longest before self treatment or seeking medical attention.[29] In the face of a rising death rate from asthma this subject merits further attention.[32]

How do we overcome the problems of non-compliance and can better education alter behaviour?

EDUCATION

In this section it is important to appreciate that we are dealing with two important components — (a) giving information and (b) changing behaviour.

How may we give information and does it alter behaviour?

Patients may receive information about their condition and its treatment verbally or by means of written information, audio tapes or video recordings. These would usually be directed to the patient by a health professional but information is increasingly available to patients in magazines, on television programmes and via self-help groups. Patients exposed to all of these methods have been reported to express a preference for receiving information from the doctor[26] but the effectiveness of the doctor compared with a nurse has not been formally assessed in asthma management although nurse educators have been evaluated and shown to be successful.[33]

The sender of the information is only one aspect of effective communication and the message and the recipient are probably of greater importance. The messages that need to be given should be decided in advance and given in small quantities. At initial consultation it may thus be decided that the important facts to give are the diagnosis and then explain the difference between relieving and preventing therapies, and highlight the symptoms that suggest deteriorating asthma. The early messages are likely to be the best understood and retained and simple words, short sentences and lack of jargon increase recall. Advice should be as specific and detailed as possible, and information should be repeated by different methods if possible. Verbal communication has the advantage of being potentially interactive.

The third component of successful communication is the recipient. Unfortunately the passage of information sometimes involves the doctor sending a didactic message that the patient may or may not wish to receive and the fears, concerns or questions which the patient has may not be aired. This may be avoided by the use of prepared written questions — 'Please write down your expectations of this consultation and list your questions/concerns', or preferably the patient should be allowed to set the agenda and encouraged to communicate by the liberal use of open-ended questions — 'I expect that you have been concerned to be told you have asthma?' or 'The thought of taking steroids worries some people, how do you feel about them?' The same format is adopted during subsequent consultations and recall is checked and misunderstandings clarified before further information is offered according to need and abilities. Simple written information outlining the name of the preventor and reliever therapies and the doses aids recall and is followed by detailed personal instruction in the use of inhaler devices. The patient may then be given booklets of general information or loaned audio tapes or watch video recordings.

How effective are these methods of giving information? In general improved consultation skills are helpful and Ley[34] has instructed general practitioners in these skills and found that as a result their patients recalled a statistically significantly increased amount. He also demonstrated that patient compliance increased with recall. In reviewing the subject of written information Weinman[35] has concluded that patients have an overwhelming desire for such material and that they do read it. The use of prescription information leaflets has been shown to increase patients' knowledge about their medicines, including side-effects, and those who received such leaflets were significantly more satisfied than those who did not.[36] However in a study of hospital out-patients only 14% of patients had been given written information about their treatment and few patients requested information on their own initiative.[39] Others have suggested that such information should be prescribable.[38] Such information is provided in the USA and under European Community Directive 89/341 all medicinal products marketed by EC member states have been accompanied by a package insert since 1st January 1992. These contain information regarding indications, contraindications, interactions, and instructions for use and side-effects.

Written information about the diseases themselves has been evaluated in other studies and positive results, for example, demonstrated in hypertension.[39] In another study a health education booklet describing six common symptoms had no effect on knowledge but a paradoxical reduction in the number of new requests for medical attention for the symptoms described in the book.[40] However the symptoms that were covered were mainly due to short-lived problems and the same may not apply in a chronic condition like asthma and it is essential to know whether giving information actually alters patient behaviour or morbidity.

In one study[41] a questionnaire was given to 339 patients to assess knowledge of asthma, self-management and morbidity. A third of the patients then underwent maximal education with initial interviews being followed by a posted booklet and treatment card. They had a 10–15-min structured consultation with encouragement to ask questions and . . . 6–8 weeks later were given a 35-min audio tape of asthma information for a 2-week period. They subsequently had 3-monthly consultations with their doctor for a 12-month period. A second group received only a booklet and treatment card whilst the third group acted as a control. Results showed that knowledge about mechanisms of asthma and drug action (but not side-effects) was significantly better in the maximum education group but the intervention programmes had no significant effect on self-management of attack, stated drug compliance or inhaler technique (or its overuse). Intervention did not reduce evaluable morbidity other than by the parameter of a reduction in emergency attendance at hospital in both the extensive and limited-intervention group.

Jenkinson et al.[42] have looked in greater depth at a comparison between the value of booklets and audiotapes. Patients received either a book, a tape, book and tape or neither. All the intervention groups demonstrated increased knowledge about drugs and this persisted after 12 months. Use of the tape was associated with the greatest improvement in knowledge but despite this the patients paradoxically preferred the book. Video recordings are similarly liked by patients[26] and have been shown to be an effective methods of instructing patients in inhaler usage[43] but these studies demonstrate that preference does not necessarily equate with effectiveness.

The message from most of these interventional studies is that knowledge may be increased by all methods of giving information but morbidity is not necessarily reduced. To test the hypothesis that this may be because the information given is rather general, several other workers have used more intensive regimes and specific instruction to try and alter behaviour. Does giving patients control of their own disease reduce morbidity? Reviews of the studies up to 1988[44,45] have shown such a variation in types of intervention that it is difficult to conclude whether such attempts at self-management work. Subsequently Beasley et al.[46] have assessed the effect of very detailed management plans upon adult patients. Thirty-six out-patients were treated with bronchodilators and inhaled steroids to achieve a maximal peak expiratory flow (PEF). PEF was then monitored and doses of inhaled steroid or introduction of oral steroids were adjusted by the patient according to predetermined levels of PEF. In the 30 patients who completed the study it was possible to compare morbidity and drug usage in the 6 months before and after the introduction of self-management plans. As a result of the plans there was a significant improvement in both subjective and objective measurements of asthma severity, with less night-time symptoms, less work absence and a significant improvement in baseline lung function. Interestingly despite self-treatment with oral steroids being one of the options open to the patients, they used less after introduction of the plan than before. This suggests either that the option of doubling inhaled steroids at the onset of deterioration was responsible for the avoidance of lots of attacks or that giving patients control of their disease improved compliance, or both. This study did not have a control group, but a similar self-management plan was used in conjunction with easy access to an asthma clinic in another study which involved patients who had previously required multiple hospital admissions for asthma.[47] The results demonstrated a threefold reduction in hospitalization in the intervention group. Again there was a significant reduction in oral steroid usage. These authors were unable to determine which were the most useful components of intervention and the exact role of the peak flow meter in monitoring was uncertain.

A general practice study by Charlton et al. compared the effect of self-management plans based on peak flow readings with plans where intervention was based on symptoms or diminishing effect of bronchodilators.[48] Both groups of patients had careful supervision in a nurse-run asthma clinic and comparison of morbidity during the study with that recorded previously showed that both groups had reduced need for doctor consultations, less emergency use of nebulized bronchodilators and less use of oral steroids. There was no significant difference between the group whose self-management plans were based upon peak flow readings and those based upon symptoms. However other studies[49] have shown that up to 20% of patients may not be able to perceive significant deterioration in airway calibre and self-management plans should probably continue to include treatment changes based on both subjective and objective parameters.

The contribution of regular supervision in an asthma clinic to the favourable outcome of both the general practice[48] and the hospital[47] study cannot be discerned. In the UK such clinics are increasing in number and the use of nurses to run such clinics has been costed and shown to lead to a potential saving in medical costs.[50] Within these clinics or during routine consultations the patients require their self-management plans to be written down and carefully explained. The plans include information about usual doses of relieving bronchodilator and preventative therapies and list the level of peak expiratory flow or symptoms at which the patient should (a) increase preventative treatment; (b) start/increase oral steroids; and (c) seek medical attention. Such information may be entirely written or included in partially preprinted cards.

CONCLUSION

Non-compliance with therapy and delay in seeking medical attention is likely to be a contributory factor in the persisting high levels of morbidity and mortality from asthma. The size of the problem of non-compliance can be estimated but which of many potential causes are the most important remains unknown. However there appear to be defects in both the giving of information and in basic communication between physician and patient, and the patient's attitude to his or her own health may be an important factor in some cases.

Giving information to the patient increases knowledge about his or her condition and its treatment and this increases satisfaction and confidence but by itself has only a very small effect on changing the patient's behaviour. There is little to choose between the different methods of giving such information and the patient's preference may not equate with effectiveness. Modifying behaviour involves giving the patient detailed and specific instructions as to what action to take in the event of certain symptoms or certain readings of peak expiratory flow. It is likely that part of the success of such self-management plans reflects their issue within an asthma clinic where regular supervision is also possible. Giving the patient greater control of his or her own condition seems to be beneficial; this may be as a result of improved compliance.

REFERENCES

1. Woolcock A, Rubinfeld AR, Seale JP, et al.: Asthma management plan, 1989. Med J Australia (1989) **151**: 650–653.
2. British Thoracic Society, Research Unit of Royal College of Physicians, Kings Fund Centre, National Asthma Campaign: Guidelines for management of asthma in adults: I: chronic persistent asthma. Br Med J (1990) **301**: 651–653.
3. British Thoracic Society, Research Unit of Royal College of Physicians, Kings Fund Centre, National Asthma Campaign: Guidelines for management of asthma in adults: II—acute severe asthma. B Med J (1990) **301**: 797–800.
4. Hargreave FE, Dolovich J, Newhouse MT: The assessment and treatment of asthma: a conference report. J Allerg & Clin Immunol (1990) **85**: 1098–1111.
5. Warner JO, Gotz M, Landau LI, et al.: Management of asthma: a consensus statement. Arch Dis Childhood (1989) **64**: 1065–1075.
6. Mushlin AI, Appel FA: Diagnosing partial non compliance. Arch Intern Med (1977) **137**: 318–321.
7. Horn CR, Essex C, Hill P, Cochrane GM: Does urinary salbutamol reflect compliance with aerosol regimes in patients with asthma? Resp Med (1989) **83**: 15–18.
8. Cramer JA, Mattson RH, Prevey MC, Scheyer RD, Ovellette VL: How often is medication taken as prescribed? JAMA (1989) **261**: 3273–3277.
9. Spector SL, Kinsman R, Mawhinny H, et al.: Compliance of patients with asthma with an experimental aerosolized medication. Implications for controlled clinical trials. J Allergy Clin Immunol (1986) **77**: 65–70.
10. Pullar T, Kumar S, Tindall H, et al.: Time to stop counting the tablets? Clin Pharmacol Ther (1989) **46**: 163–168.
11. Smith NA, Seale JP, Ley P, et al.: Effects of intervention on medication compliance in asthmatic children. Med J Aust (1986) **144**: 119–122.
12. Partridge MR: Problems with the delivery of asthma care. In Mitchell D (ed) Recent Advances in Respiratory Medicine: 5. Edinburgh, Churchill Livingstone, 1991, pp 61–67.

13. Editorial: Are you taking the medicine? *Lancet* (1990) **i**: 262–263.
14. Pullar T, Birtwell AJ, Wiles PG, *et al.*: Use of a pharmacologic indicator to compare compliance with tablets prescribed to be taken once, twice or three times daily. *Clin Pharmacol Ther* (1988) **44**: 540–545.
15. Taggart AJ, Johnson GD, McDevitt DG: Does the frequency of daily dosage influence compliance with digoxin therapy? *Br J Clin Pharmacol* (1981) **1**: 31–34.
16. Sbarbaco JA: The patient–physician relationship: compliance revisited. *Ann Allerg* (1990) **64**: 325–331.
17. Wiggins H: Meeting the needs of minority ethnic groups. *Br J Pharmaceutical Practice* (1990) **12**: 170–177.
18. Korsch BM, Negrette VF: Doctor patient communication. *Scientific American* (1972) **227**: 66–72.
19. Greenberg RN: Review of patient compliance with medication dosing: a literature review. *Clin Ther* (1984) **6**: 5.
20. Evans L, Spelman N: Problems of non compliance with drug therapy. *Drugs* (1983) **25**: 63–76.
21. Horn CR: Compliance by asthmatic patients—how much of a problem? *Res and Clin Forums* (1986) **8**: 47–53.
22. James PNE, Anderson JB, Prior JG, *et al.*: Patterns of drug taking in patients with chronic airflow obstruction. *Postgrad Med J* (1985) **61**: 7–10.
23. Smith NA, Seale JP, Shaw J: Medication compliance in children with asthma. *Aust Paediatr J* (1984) **20**: 47–51.
24. Crompton CK: Problems patients have using pressurized aerosol inhalers. *Eur J Respir Dis* (1982) **63**: 101–104.
25. Ellis ME, Friend JAR: How well do patients understand their asthma? *Br J Dis Chest* (1985) **74**: 43–48.
26. Partridge MR: Asthma education: more reading or more viewing? *JR Soc Med* (1986) **79**: 326–328.
27. National Asthma Campaign: Mori Poll survey of members, National Asthma Campaign, Providence House, Providence Place, London N1 0NT, UK, (1990) personal communication.
28. Turner-Warwick M: Nocturnal asthma: a study in general practice. *J Roy Coll Gen Pract* (1989) **39**: 239–243.
29. Sibbald B: Patient self care in acute asthma. *Thorax* (1989) **44**: 97–101.
30. Ellis ME, Friend JAR: How well do asthma clinic patients understand their asthma? *Br J Dis Chest* (1985) **79**: 43–48.
31. Harding JM, Modell M: How patients manage asthma. *J Roy Coll Gen Pract* (1985) **35**: 226–228.
32. Burney PGJ: Asthma mortality in England and Wales: evidence for a further increase, 1974–84. *Lancet* (1986) **ii**: 323–326.
33. Maiman LA, Green LW, Gibson C, *et al.*: Education for self treatment by adult asthmatics. *JAMA* (1979) **241**: 1919–1921.
34. Ley P: Towards better doctor–patient communications. Contributions from social and experimental psychology. In Bennett AF (ed) *Communications in Medicine*. London, Oxford University Press, for the Nuffield Provincial Hospital Trust, 1976, p. 33.
35. Weinman J: Providing written information for patients: psychological considerations. *JR Soc Med* (1990) **83**: 303–304.
36. Gibbs S, Waters WE, George CF: Communicating information to patients about medicine. *JR Soc Med* (1990) **83**: 292–297.
37. McMahon T, Clark CM, Bailie GR: Who provides patients with drug information? *Br Med J* (1987) **294**: 355–356.
38. Clayton S: Prescribing information to patients. *Br Med J* (1986) **292**: 1368.
39. Laher M, O'Malley K, O'Brien E, *et al.*: Educational value of printed information for patients with hypertension. *Br Med J* (1981) **282**: 1360–1361.
40. Anderson JE, Morrell DC, Avery AJ, Watkins CJ: Evaluation of a patient education manual. *Br Med J* (1980) **281**: 924–926.
41. Hilton S, Sibbald B, Anderson HR, Freeling P: Controlled evaluation of the effects of patient education on asthma morbidity in general practice. *Lancet* (1986) **i**: 26–29.

42. Jenkinson D, Davison J, Jones, Hawtin P: Comparison of effects of a self management booklet and audio cassette for patients with asthma. *Br Med J* (1988) **297**: 267–270.

43. Mulloy EMT, Albazzaz MK, Warley ARH, Harvey JE: Video education for patients who use inhalers. *Thorax* (1987) **42**: 719–720.

44. Klingelhofer EL, Gershwin ME: Asthma self management programs: Premises, not promises. *J Asthma* (1988) **25**: 89–101.

45. Howland J, Bauchner H, Adair R: The impact of pediatric asthma education on morbidity — assessing the evidence. *Chest* (1988) **94**: 965–969.

46. Beasley R, Cushley M, Holgate ST: A self management plan in the treatment of adult asthma. *Thorax* (1989) **44**: 200–204.

47. Mayo PH, Richman J, Harris HW: Results of a program to reduce admissions for adult asthma. *Ann Intern Med* (1990) **112**: 864–871.

48. Charlton I, Charlton G, Broomfield J, Muller MA: Evaluation of peak flow and symptoms on self management plans for control of asthma in general practice. *Br Med J* (1990) **301**: 1355–1357.

49. Rubinfield AR, Pain MCF: The perception of asthma. *Lancet* (1976): **ii**: 882–884.

50. Charlton I, Charlton G: A nurse run asthma clinic — (1): Setting up: dealing with some of the problems. *Practice Nurse* (April 1990) (Suppl): 2–7.

Future Trends in Therapy

PETER J. BARNES, NEIL C. THOMSON AND IAN W. RODGER

INTRODUCTION

There is evidence for increased morbidity and mortality from asthma, despite increases in the amount of treatment prescribed. This suggests that currently available therapy may be contributing to these statistics or that it is not being used optimally. Despite considerable efforts by the pharmaceutical industry there have been no new types of drug introduced for asthma therapy over the last 20 years. It may be important to understand more about the mechanisms of asthma and also how the currently used drugs work before rational improvements in therapy can be expected. Advances in smooth muscle and receptor pharmacology have opened the way to the development of new classes of bronchodilator, and the further understanding of inflammatory mechanisms in asthma has encouraged exploration of new mediator antagonists, anti-inflammatory and immunomodulatory drugs. Advances in delivery systems are also important for inhaled drugs.

There are two main approaches to the development of new antiasthma treatments — either improvement in an existing class of effective drug, or development of novel compounds.

NEW BRONCHODILATORS

Bronchodilators are presumed to act by reversing contraction of airway smooth muscle, although some may have additional effects on mucosal oedema or inflammatory cells. The biochemical basis of airway smooth muscle relaxation has been studied extensively,

ASTHMA: BASIC MECHANISMS AND CLINICAL MANAGEMENT (2nd Edn)
ISBN 0-12-079026-2

Table 42.1 New bronchodilators.

Improvement in existing drugs	
β_2-Agonists	Inhaled long-acting β_2-agonists (salmeterol, formoterol)
Methylxanthines	Enprofylline
Anticholinergics	M_3-selective antagonists
Novel drugs	
Guanylate cyclase activators	Atrial natriuretic peptide, nitro dilators
Selective PDE inhibitors	SK&F 94120, zardaverine
K^+ channel openers	Lemakalim

yet few new classes of bronchodilator have had any clinical impact. The molecular basis of bronchodilation may involve an increase in intracellular cyclic AMP and a reduction in cytosolic calcium ion concentration ($[Ca^{2+}]$). In addition recent studies suggest that the rise in cyclic AMP is linked to the opening of Ca^{2+}-activated K^+ channels in airway smooth muscle.[1,2] All of these mechanisms may be amenable to pharmacological manipulation. New bronchodilators are shown in Table 42.1.

β_2-Agonists

β_2-Agonists remain the most widely used and effective bronchodilators in clinical practice (see Chapter 32). This is because they act as functional antagonists and reverse airway smooth muscle contraction irrespective of the spasmogen. They are equally effective on large and small airways, and may have effects on cells other than airway smooth muscle, such as mast cells, to prevent mediator release, or microvascular leak, on cholinergic neurotransmission and on release of epithelial factors. Many selective β_2-agonists are now available and there has been a search for β-agonists which have even greater selectivity for β_2-receptors. However it is unlikely that any greater selectivity would be an advantage clinically, since when the drugs are given by inhalation a high degree of functional β_2-selectively is obtained. Furthermore, many of the side-effects of β-agonists (tremor, tachycardia, hypokalaemia) are mediated via β_2-receptors.

    The most important recent advance has been the introduction of inhaled β_2-agonists with a long duration of action, such as salmeterol and formoterol, which give broncho-dilation and protection against bronchoconstriction for over 12 h.[3] They are highly effective in preventing nocturnal asthma and in controlling 'brittle' asthma. Clinical trials show that both of these long-acting β_2-agonists are highly effective in controlling chronic asthma, have no significant side-effects and (perhaps surprisingly) tachyphyl-axis (tolerance) does not develop.[4] It is difficult to imagine that any future drug could be more effective than a β_2-agonist as a bronchodilator, but doubts have recently been expressed about the role of inhaled β-agonists in the control of asthma. Regular use of inhaled β-agonists appears to give worse control of asthma than the use of β-agonists 'as required' for symptom control.[5] It is probable that β-agonists do not have a significant anti-inflammatory effect on the chronic inflammatory component of asthma. It has even been suggested that their mast-cell stabilizing action may be deleterious by inhibiting the release of heparin, which would counteract the effects of eosinophil basic proteins.[6]

Drugs which increase cyclic AMP

Further understanding of the molecular mechanism of β-agonists has prompted a search for other drugs that might increase intracellular cyclic AMP concentrations in airway smooth muscle (Fig. 42.1). Of course such drugs might also be effective in inhibiting the activation and secretion of inflammatory cells. Several other receptors on airway smooth muscle, other than β-receptors, may activate adenylyl cyclase via a stimulatory G-protein (G_s).

Vasoactive intestinal peptide

Vasoactive intestinal peptide (VIP) is a potent relaxant of human bronchi *in vitro*,[7] yet it has no action in asthmatic subjects, when given by inhalation,[8] probably because of

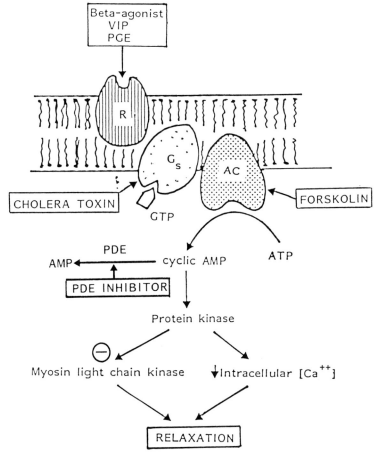

Fig. 42.1 Mechanisms of bronchodilatation. Stimulation of surface receptors ($β_2$-adrenergic, vasoactive intestinal peptide or prostaglandin E receptors) activates adenylyl cyclase (AC) via a G-protein (G_s), resulting in an increase in intracellular concentration of cyclic AMP, which leads to relaxation of airway smooth muscle via activation of protein kinase A. Cyclic AMP is rapidly broken down by phosphodiesterases (PDE). There are several mechanisms of bronchiodilatation based on an increase in cyclic AMP concentration.

problems with diffusion and degradation by airway enzymes, such as mast-cell derived tryptase. When given by infusion the cardiovascular effects preclude the giving of a dose which causes bronchodilatation.[9]

Prostaglandins

PGE stimulate adenylyl cyclase, yet have not proved to be very effective as bronchodilators, and may even lead to constriction and coughing in asthmatics since they also stimulate sensory receptors in airways.[10]

G-protein/adenylyl cyclase stimulation

Receptor-mediated stimulation of adenylyl cyclase involves activation of G_s, which may be stimulated irreversibly by cholera toxin. Less toxic compounds which stimulate G_s are under investigation. Forskolin directly activates the catalytic subunit of adenylyl cyclase, and increases cyclic AMP in airway smooth muscle, but has not proved to be very effective as a bronchodilator *in vitro*, however,[11] possibly because there is a compartmentalization of cyclic AMP stimulated by certain receptors.

Selective phosphodiesterase inhibitors

By inhibiting the breakdown of cyclic AMP by phosphodiesterase (PDE), it should be possible to increase intracellular concentrations and thereby relax airway smooth muscle and also potentiate the bronchodilator effect of β-agonists. It is now recognized that there are several isoenzymes of PDE and several selective inhibitors have recently been developed.[12,13] The isoenzymes that are involved in relaxation of airway smooth muscle (Types III and IV) make up <5% of the total enzyme activity.[14,15] Selective inhibitors of these isoenzymes, such as SK&F 94836 which inhibits Type III isoenzyme, may therefore be useful as bronchodilators. Evidence now suggests that Type IV isoenzyme may be important in inflammatory cells such as mast cells, eosinophils and macrophages,[13,16] and that Type IV isoenzyme inhibitors, such as rolipram and denbufylline, may be useful anti-inflammatory drugs in asthma. Drugs that inhibit both Type III and Type IV enzymes, such as AH 21-132 and zardaverine,[17,18] may be both bronchodilator and anti-inflammatory, and are therefore of particular interest for future development. The main problem with PDE inhibitors appears to be the profile of side-effects. Type III inhibitors are associated with cardiovascular side-effects, whereas the major problem with Type IV inhibitors is nausea and vomiting.

Methylxanthines

Theophylline has remained an important treatment in asthma for over 50 years, yet its mode of action is still unknown (Chapter 34). It now seems unlikely that bronchodilation plays an important role in the antiasthma effect of theophylline, and increasingly likely that some anti-inflammatory or immunomodulatory effect is important. Several molecular mechanisms have been proposed to explain the actions of theophylline, but perhaps the most likely is that it non-selectively inhibits PDE. There is little doubt that theophylline has a critical role in the management of more severe asthma and it is important that its mode of action in these patients is elucidated. The currently used 'therapeutic concentration' of plasma theophylline is derived from the belief that theophylline is a bronchodilator, but it is likely that the other antiasthma effects of theophylline might be achieved at lower plasma concentrations, thereby avoiding the problems of toxicity and side-effects that currently limit the use of this drug.

The development of slow-release formulations has made it possible to achieve 'therapeutic concentrations' with twice-daily and even once-daily dosing. The twice-daily formulations are probably most useful, since they may be given in the evening in a single daily dose, giving therapeutic concentrations overnight to protect against nocturnal asthma.

The major problem with theophylline has been the frequency of side-effects, several of which may be due to adenosine receptor antagonism. The development of enprofylline (3 propylxanthine), which retains the bronchodilator and PDE-inhibitory effect but is not an adenosine antagonist is therefore an advance. Enprofylline is an effective bronchodilator[19] and shares other antiasthma properties of adenosine, but is not an adenosine antagonist at therapeutic concentrations.[20] Side-effects, such as diuresis, seizure and cardiac arrythmias, are less common than with theophylline, although headache is a problem. Although enprofylline is not being developed because of toxicological problems, other related drugs are under invesigation.

Drugs that increase cyclic GMP

Atrial natriuretic peptide (ANP) when given by intravenous infusion produces a significant bronchodilator response and reduces the bronchoconstrictor response to inhaled histamine and fog challenge (see Chapter 22). It is likely that the effects of ANP on airways are mediated by stimulation of particulate quanylyl cyclase and subsequent generation of cyclic GMP.[21] Nitro compounds such as isosorbide dinitrate, glyceryl trinitrate (GTN) and sodium nitroprusside are thought to activate soluble quanylyl cyclase. A dose-dependent relaxant effect of various nitro compounds has been demonstrated on airway smooth muscle in a number of animal studies, and this effect appears to be mediated via stimulation of soluble quanylyl cyclase and subsequent generation of cyclic GMP.[21,22] Intravenous GTN relaxes human tracheal smooth muscle in normal subjects undergoing cardiac surgery.[23] Sublingual GTN and isosorbide dinitrate have been reported to have a bronchodilator effect in patients with asthma[24,25] and to inhibit exercise-induced asthma.[26] Others have not confirmed the beneficial effects of nitro dilators, however.[27,28] These studies suggest that bronchodilators with an alternative intracellular mechanism of action to β_2-agonists may be possible and further investigation is warranted, particularly with inhaled formulations in order to avoid vasodilator side-effects.

Selective anticholinergics

Recently it has been established that there are several distinct subtypes of muscarinic receptor, which have differing physiological roles in the airway (see Chapters 22 and 33).[29] Muscarinic receptors which inhibit the release of acetylcholine have been described in airway cholinergic nerves of animal and are classified as M_2-receptors, which are clearly different from the receptors on airway smooth muscle (M_3-receptors). Non-selective antagonists, such as ipratropium bromide, will inhibit prejunctional M_2-receptors and thus increase the amount of acetylcholine released as vagal stimulation which may then overcome the postjunctional blockade of M_3-receptors, and may therefore not be as effective against reflex bronchoconstriction. Selective M_3-antagonists which block only postjunctional receptors on smooth muscle should be more effective, but have proved difficult to develop for clinical use.

Calcium antagonists

Contraction of airway smooth muscle and release of inflammatory mediators results from an increase in intracellular $[Ca^{2+}]$ and subsequent activation of calmodulin. Several important advances have been made in understanding the regulation of intra-cellular $[Ca^{2+}]$ and many new types of drug are under development. Drugs that block calcium entry through voltage-dependent calcium channels (VDC), such as nifedipine, verapamil and diltiazem, have not proved effective in asthma, as discussed in Chapter 37. This suggests that Ca^{2+} entry via VDCs is not important in human airway smooth muscle contraction. Calcium entry via receptor-operated channels (ROCs) may be more important in airway smooth muscle, and drugs that act on these channels are currently under development.

Release of Ca^{2+} from intracellular stores is probably the most important source of calcium for contraction of airway smooth muscle. Drugs that inhibit calcium release, such as TMB-8, may have effects in airway smooth muscle, but they lack selectivity and will probably be too toxic for clinical use. Most spasmogens contract airway smooth muscle by stimulating phosphoinositide (PI) hydrolysis.[30] Drugs that inhibit PI turn-over or effects may, therefore, be of potential use in asthma. Inositol (1,4,5)trisphos-phate (IP_3) generated by PI hydrolysis, causes release of intracellular calcium by binding to specific binding sites on endoplasmic reticulum. Heparin is a potent competi-tive inhibitor of IP_3 binding in airway smooth muscle,[31] but is not of therapeutic use since it does not penetrate cells. Analogues of IP_3 are currently under development.

Breakdown of PI also leads to the function of diacylglycerol which activates protein kinase C (PKC). This enzyme regulates many cellular events, including slow contractile responses. Antagonists of PKC, such as staurosporine, might be useful, but currently available PKC antagonists lack specificity. The recognition that there are several isoenzymes of PKC may make it possible to develop blockers selective to certain cell types of functions in the future.[32]

K^+ channel activators

K^+ channels play an important role in the recovery of excitable cells after activation and in maintaining cell stability. Opening of K^+ channels therefore results in relaxation of smooth muscle and inhibition of secretion. Many different types of K^+ channel have now been recognized electrophysiologically and with the discovery of several selective toxins and drugs. Drugs that selectively activate a K^+ channel in smooth muscle, such as BRL3491 (cromakalim), have been developed for the treatment of hypertension.

These drugs inhibit spontaneous and induced tone in airway smooth muscle *in vitro* and might, therefore, have a role in normalizing 'hyperreactive' airway smooth muscle. K^+ channel activators are currently under investigation as potential antiasthma compounds.[33] The active enantiomer of cromakalim, BRL38227 (lemakalim), is a relatively effective relaxant of human bronchi *in vitro* and appears equally active against several spasmogens.[34] *In vivo* it has no bronchodilator effect or protective effect against bronchoconstrictor challenge at maximally tolerated oral doses,[35] but has been shown to have a small protective effect against the fall in lung function at night in asthmatic patients.[36] Side-effects include headache, flushing and postural hypotension, due to vasodilatation. It will therefore be necessary to develop these drugs for inhalational use in order to avoid these effects, although it may be possible to develop K^+ activators that are more selective for airway than vascular smooth muscle, in view of the diversity of K^+ channels.

The future success of these compounds in asthma will probably depend on whether they have any additional effects not shared with β-agonists. K^+ channel activators inhibit the release of neuropeptides from sensory nerves and modulate neurotransmission in the airways,[37] but whether they have effects on inflammatory cells is not certain. Many different types of K^+ channel have now been characterized; cromakalim and related drugs appear to open a low affinity ATP-dependent channel. Relaxation of airway smooth muscle in response to β-agonists and theophylline appears to involve another type of channel, a calcium-activated K^+ channel which is selectively blocked by charybdotoxin.[1,2] Development of activators of this channel may therefore be an important area for future development.

ANTI-INFLAMMATORY DRUGS

There are several new types of treatment designed to reduce features of airway inflammation in asthma (Table 42.2).

Corticosteroids

Corticosteroids are the most efficacious treatment currently available for the long-term management of asthma. Steroids of high topical potency, such as budesonide and beclomethasone, are highly effective when given by inhalation. Future developments will depend upon the development of inhaled steroids of even higher topical potency or which are metabolized locally ('hit and run' steroids), so that the local dose of steroids in the airways will be increased without the systemic effects that currently limit dose.[38] Perhaps steroids that are 'targeted' to key inflammatory cells such as macrophages would also be useful, and the use of liposomes to deliver steroids to specific sites may be considered.

Because steroids are so effective in the control of asthma, an important goal of research is to identify the particular cellular and molecular mechanisms which are of critical importance in asthmatic inflammation. This may then lead in the future to non-steroidal drugs that mimic the beneficial effects, without the side-effects that are due to the other actions of steroids.

Table 42.2   New anti-inflammatory drugs.

Improvement in existing drugs	
Corticosteroids	Increased topical potency
	Increased first pass metabolism
	Increased local metabolism
Cromoglycate	Increased potency (nedocromil sodium)
	Frusemide-related drugs?
Novel drugs	
Mediator antagonists	LTD$_4$ antagonists (ICI 204,219)
	PAF antagonists (WEB 2086)
Enzyme inhibitors	5-LO inhibitors (zileuton, MK-886)
	Phospholipase A$_2$ inhibitors
Immunomodulators	Cyclosporin A, FK 506
	Cytokine synthesis inhibitors/receptor antagonists
Neuropeptide inhibitors	Release inhibitors (BW 443C)
	Tachykinin antagonists (CP-96,345)
Adhesion blockers	?
IgE synthesis inhibitors	IL-4 antagonists?

Lipocortin

Steroids stimulate the production of a protein, lipocortin, which inhibits phospholipase A$_2$ (PLA$_2$),[39] the enzyme which leads to the generation of arachidonic acid and platelet-activating factor (PAF). Recombinant human lipocortin is now available, but there might be problems in delivering such an agent, and it may be degraded at inflammatory sites. The presumed advantage of lipocortin might be reduction in glucocorticoid side-effects. However, there are doubts as to whether many of the effects of steroids are mediated via PLA$_2$ inhibition.

Mediator antagonists

Many different inflammatory mediators have now been implicated in asthma (as discussed in Chapters 14–21), and several specific receptor antagonists and synthesis inhibitors have been developed which will prove invaluable in working out the contribution of each mediator (Table 42.3). As many mediators probably contribute to the pathological features of asthma, it seems unlikely that a single antagonist will have a major clinical effect, compared with non-specific agents such as β-agonists and corticosteroids. However, until such drugs have been evaluated in careful clinical studies, it is not possible to predict their value.

Lipid mediators may play an important role in asthmatic inflammation. Several potent leukotriene, PAF and thromboxane antagonists have now been developed and are currently undergoing clinical trials in asthma. Initial results appear to suggest that potent leukotriene antagonists, such as MK-571 and ICI 204,219, have a significant protective effect against some constrictor challenges, such as exercise and allergen,[40,41]

Table 42.3 Mediator antagonists.

Mediator	Antagonist
Histamine	Terfenadine, astemizole
Thromboxane	Vapiprost
Leukotriene D_4	ICI 204,219, MK-571
Platelet-activating factor	WEB 2086, UK 80,067
Bradykinin	Hoe 140
Adenosine	Theophylline

and long-term clinical trials are now underway, with preliminary encouraging results. It seems rather unlikely that antagonizing a single mediator will ever be as useful as less specific therapies, but such therapies may have the advantage of fewer side-effects and oral administration. Certain types of asthmatic patient may respond much better to these more specific therapies.

Enzyme inhibitors

An alternative to antagonists of mediator receptors are drugs that inhibit the enzymes involved in mediator synthesis. Since PLA_2 appears to be of critical importance in the generation of all lipid mediators, it is a suitable target for inhibitory drugs. Drugs other than steroids that inhibit PLA_2, such as mepacrine, might be expected to share the beneficial effects of steroids, but this drug is weak and non-specific. Perhaps more potent and selective PLA_2 inhibitors, such as manoalide, derived from a sponge, may be useful leads in developing such inhibitors in the future.[42] Inhibition of phospholipase C, which is the enzyme leading to PI breakdown, could also be useful, as discussed above.

Cyclooxygenase inhibitors, which inhibit the formation of prostaglandins and thromboxane, are of no obvious therapeutic value in asthma, and in a small group of asthmatics with aspirin-sensitive asthma they may cause a deterioration in asthma.

5-Lipoxygenase (5-LO) is the critical enzyme involved in the generation of leukotrienes. Several drugs have been developed that inhibit 5-LO, although most of these compounds are very weak. Thus zileuton, the most effective of these drugs available for clinical use, has only a trivial inhibitory effect on allergen-induced responses and leukotriene production.[43] Zileuton, as most other 5-LO inhibitors, appears to work as a redox inhibitor of the enzyme, but more recently a novel inhibitor MK-886 has been developed, which appears to bind to a 5-LO activating protein (FLAP) in the cell membrane, to which cytosolic 5-LO must bind in order to be active.[44] There is a theoretical advantage to the use of 5-LO inhibitors compared with leukotriene antagonists since the formation of LTB_4 and other 5-LO products, as well as sulphidopeptide leukotrienes will be also be inhibited.

Inhibitors of neurogenic inflammation

Neuropeptides, which may be released from sensory nerves in airways in asthma via an axon reflex, might amplify the inflammatory response (see Chapter 23). There are several approaches to inhibiting these local reflexes.[45] Antagonists of sensory neuropeptides, such as substance P, neurokinin A and calcitonin-gene related peptide, are currently under development. Most of the inflammatory effects of tachykinins are mediated by NK_1-receptors and several selective antagonists have been developed. A potent non-peptide NK_1-antagonist, CP-96,345, has recently been been described, which may prove to be a very useful lead compound which avoids all the problems associated with the development of peptide antagonists.[46] Another approach is to inhibit the release of these peptides from C-fibres rather than to block their effects, since several peptides are likely to be released from sensory nerves. Opioids markedly inhibit sensory neuropeptide release and have been shown to block neurogenic plasma exudation, mucus secretion and bronchoconstriction in guinea-pigs and neurogenic mucus secretion in human airways.[8] Opioids that act peripherally, such as the opioid peptide BW443C, may be effective in reducing neurogenic inflammation in asthma (and also the associated sensory symptoms such as cough).[47] Several other agonists act on prejunctional receptors on sensory nerves in airways to inhibit neuropeptide release; these include α_2-agonists, γ amino butyric acid, and histamine H_3-agonists, which all appear to open a common K^+ channel that is blocked by charybdotoxin.[8]

A third possibility is to inhibit activation of sensory nerves. This may be achieved by drugs such as sodium cromoglycate and nedocromil sodium, that appear to stabilize unmyelinated nerves in airways.[48] Another drug which has a similar profile of activity is the loop diuretic frusemide.

Frusemide

Inhaled frusemide protects against 'indirect' bronchoconstrictor challenges, such as exercise, fog, allergen, sodium metabisulphite and adenosine, but has no effect against direct bronchoconstrictor challenges such as histamine, methacholine and $PGF_{2\alpha}$.[49] These effects mimic those of sodium cromoglycate but, in addition, inhaled frusemide inhibits certain types of induced cough.[50] The mechanism of action of frusemide in asthma is not certain, but it is ineffective systemically, suggesting that it is acting at the airway surface. Frusemide works as a diuretic by inhibiting the $Na^+/K^+/Cl^-$ co-transporter in renal tubular cells, but the more potent inhibitor bumetanide is ineffective in the same challenges.[51] Some effects of frusemide are mediated by the release of PGE_2, but cyclooxygenase inhibition does not abolish the antiasthma effect. The most likely possibility is that frusemide blocks a certain type of Cl^- channel that is necessary for the activation of inflammatoy cells and sensory nerves. Indeed frusemide is effective in blocking eosinophil activation and airway sensory nerves, and its actions are mimicked by Cl^- channel-blocking drugs.[52] Frusemide itself causes diuresis when inhaled in high concentrations, but it is possible that derivatives with less diuretic potency or that selective Cl^- channel blockers may be developed for use in asthma in the future.

Immunomodulators

T lymphocytes may play a critical role in initiating and maintaining the inflammatory process in asthma via the release of cytokines (see Chapter 9). Methotrexate has a steroid-sparing effect in asthma, probably acting as a non-specific immunosuppressive or anti-inflammatory agent.[53,54] The side-effects of methotrexate (particularly nausea and blood dyscrasias) preclude its use in all but the most severe asthmatic patients who have problems with oral steroids.

More specific immunomodulators, such as cyclosporin A, which have an inhibitory effect on T-lymphocyte function, might be more useful in controlling asthma, and there is some evidence that low-dose cyclosporin A improves lung function in steroid-dependent asthmatics.[55] The nephrotoxicity of cyclosporin A would limit its widespread use but derivatives with less nephrotoxicity are now being developed. Other immuno-modulators such as FK506 appear to be more potent and less toxic. Since CD4$^+$ lymphocytes appear to play an important role in the maintenance of eosinophilic inflammation in the airways, it is possible that monoclonal or chimaeric antibodies directed against CD4 may be useful in the treatment of severe asthma, as these antibodies have been useful in the control of other chronic T-lymphocytic diseases.

Gold injections have been used for many years in Japan for the treatment of chronic asthma, but cannot be recommended for use until controlled trials define any beneficial effect.[56] Controlled trials of an oral gold preparation (auranofin) are now underway.

Cytokine inhibitors

There is increasing evidence that cytokines may participate in the inflammatory response in asthma. Interleukin (IL)-1, IL-8 tumour necrosis factor and GM-CSF from macrophages, and IL-3, IL-4 and IL-5 from CD4$^+$ T-lymphocytes may all be involved in the chronic inflammation in asthmatic airways, together with additional cytokines (GM-CSF, IL-6, IL-8) that may be released from epithelial cells of the airways. Drugs that interfere with the production or action of these cytokines may therefore prove to be of benefit in asthma. Indeed corticosteroids may be effective in asthma by suppressing cytokine synthesis in inflammatory cells.[57] It may prove difficult to develop specific receptor antagonists for cytokines, since they are large peptides and have a very high affinity for their receptors. Strategies such as antisense nucleotides, which would inactivate the specific mRNA encoded by cytokine genes may be a more optimistic approach.[58] A naturally occurring antagonist of IL-1 has been isolated, and similar antagonists of other cytokines may be discovered which could lead to the development of future antagonists. Specific antibodies to various cytokines have now been developed, but while these may be suitable for revealing the roles of various cytokines,[59] they would not be suitable for chronic administration.

Cell adhesion blockers

It is now recognized that the infiltration of inflammatory cells into tissues is dependent on adhesion of blood-borne inflammatory cells to endothelial cells prior to migration to the inflammatory site.[60] This depends upon specific glycoprotein adhesion molecules (integrins) on both leucocytes and lymphocytes and on endothelial cells, which may be upregulated, or expressed on the cell surface in response to various stimuli such as cytokines or mediators such as PAF or leukotrienes. Monoclonal antibodies that inhibit these adhesion molecules therefore may prevent inflammatory cell infiltration. Thus a monoclonal antibody to ICAM-1 on endothelial cells prevents the eosinophil infiltration into airways and the increase in bronchial reactivity after allergen exposure in sensitized primates.[61] Synthetic peptides with the sequence that is critical for adhesion may have therapeutic potential. Thus some integrins bind to a tripeptide sequence Arg-Gly-Asp (RGD), which may therefore inhibit leucocyte adhesion. Another possibility is to inhibit the expression of adhesion molecules on the cell surface. For example, 3-deazoadenosine inhibits cytokine-mediated induction of ICAM-1.[62]

IgE suppression

Since release of mediators in asthma may be IgE-dependent, an alternative approach may be to inhibit the synthesis of IgE. Suppressor factors that inhibit IgE synthesis, and that are related in structure to the IgE receptor have been described, but have proved disappointing *in vivo*. IgE synthesis by B-lymphocytes is dependent on IL-4, so that IL-4 synthesis inhibitors or receptor antagonists would be useful in allergy suppression.[63]

Allergen control

It is now well established that house dust mites are an important cause of asthma, and recent studies have demonstrated that vigorous house dust mite avoidance measures can produce improvements in asthma control and reductions in non-specific airway hyper-responsiveness (see Chapter 31). The aim in the future will be to establish the most practical, safe and effective methods of reducing house dust mite levels.

Dietary measures

Fish oil contains the long chain polyunsaturated fats eicosapentanoic acid and docosa-hexanoic acid. These substances may have anti-inflammatory properties.[64] They have been shown to reduce the chemotactic activity of neutrophils and monocytes, to decrease LTB_4 and PAF production by these cells, and to have inhibitory effects on the cyclooxy-genase pathway. Dietary supplementation with fish oils can partially attenuate the late asthmatic response to allergen.[65] Clinical studies have demonstrated a slight improvement in symptom control in atopic dermatitis but not in mild asthma.[66] Whether treatment of more severe asthma with higher doses of fish oil might produce clinical benefit is unknown.

CONCLUSIONS

Many different therapeutic approaches to the treatment of asthma may be possible, yet there have been few new drugs. β_2-Agonists are by far the most effective bronchodilator drugs and lead to rapid symptomatic relief. Now that inhaled β_2-agonists with a long duration of action have been developed it is difficult to imagine that more effective bronchodilators could be discovered. Similarly, inhaled corticosteroids are extremely effective as chronic treatment in asthma and suppress the underlying inflammatory process. It follows that a combination of inhaled steroids and β-agonists is required and combined inhalers would seem to be a sensible development, since they will improve the compliance of inhaled steroids (which is poor because of the lack of immediate bronchodilator effect). The ideal drug for asthma would probably be a tablet that can be administered once daily to improve compliance. It should have no side-effects and this means that it should be specific for the abnormality of asthma (or allergy).

Future developments in asthma therapy should be directed towards the inflammatory mechanisms and perhaps more specific therapy may one day be developed. The possibility of developing a 'cure' for asthma seems remote, but when more is known about the genetic abnormalities of asthma it may be possible to search for such a therapy. Advances in molecular biology may aid the development of drugs that can specifically switch off relevant genes, but more must be discovered about the basic mechanisms of asthma before such advances are possible.

REFERENCES

1. Jones TR, Charette L, Garcia ML, Kaczorowski GJ: Selective inhibition of relaxation of guinea-pig trachea by charybodotoxin, a potent Ca^{++}-activated K^+ channel inhibitor. *J Pharmacol Exp Ther* (1990) **225**: 697–706.
2. Miura M, Belvisi MG, Stretton CD, Yacoub MH, Barnes PJ: Role of potassium channels in bronchodilator responses in human airways. *Am Rev Respir Dis* (1992) in press.
3. Löfdahl CG, Chung KF: Long-acting β_2-adrenoceptor agonists: a new perspective in the treatment of asthma. *Eur Resp J* (1991) **4**: 218–226.
4. Ullman A, Hedner J, Svedmyr N: Inhaled salmeterol and salbutamol in asthmatic patients. An evaluation of asthma symptoms and the possible development of tachyphylaxis. *Am Rev Respir Dis* (1990) **142**: 571–575.
5. Sears MR, Taylor DR, Print CG, et al.: Regular inhaled beta-agonist treatment in bronchial asthma. *Lancet* (1990) **336**: 1391–1396.
6. Page CP: One explanation for the asthma paradox: inhibition of rational anti-inflammatory mechanism by β-agonists. *Lancet* (1991) **337**: 717–720.
7. Palmer JBD, Cuss FMC, Barnes PJ: VIP and PHM and their role in nonadrenergic inhibitory responses in isolated human airways. *J Appl Physiol* (1986) **61**: 1322–1328.
8. Barnes PJ, Dixon CMS: The effect of inhaled vasoactive intestinal peptide on bronchial reactivity to histamine in man. *Am Rev Respir Dis* (1984) **130**: 162–166.
9. Palmer JBD, Cuss FMC, Warren JB, Barnes PJ: The effect of infused vasoactive intestinal peptide on airway function in normal subjects. *Thorax* (1986) **41**: 663–666.
10. Walters EH, Davies BH: Dual effect of prostaglandin E_2 on normal airways smooth muscle *in vivo. Thorax* (1982) **37**: 918–922.
11. Waldeck B, Widmark E: Comparison of the effects of forskolin and isoprenaline on tracheal, cardiac and skeletal muscles from guinea-pig. *Eur J Pharmacol* (1985) **112**: 349–353.
12. Beavo JA, Reifsnyder DH: Primary sequence of cyclic nucleotide phosphodiesterase isoenzymes and the design of selective inhibitors. *Trends Pharmacol Sci* (1990) **11**: 150–155.
13. Nicholson CD, Challiss RAJ, Shahid M: Differential modulation of tissue function and therapeutic potential of selective inhibitors of cyclic nucleotide phosphodiesterase isoenzymes. *Trends Pharmacol Sci* (1991) **12**: 19–27.
14. Torphy TJ: Selective inhibitors of phosphodiesterase as bronchodilators. In Barnes PJ (ed) *New Drugs for Asthma*. London, IBC Publications, 1989, pp 66–77.

15. Torphy TJ, Undem BJ: Phosphodiesterase inhibitors: new opportunities for the treatment of asthma. *Thorax* (1991) **46**: 499–503.

16. Dent G, Giembycz MA, Rabe KF, Barnes PJ: Inhibition of eosinophil cyclic nucleotide PDF activity and opsonized zymosan-stimulated respiratory burst by 'type IV' PDE inhibitors. *Br J Pharmacol* (1001) **103**: 1330 1316.

17. Giembycz MA, Barnes PJ: Selective inhibition of high affinity type IV cyclic AMP phosphodiesterase in bovine trachealis by AH 21-132. *Biochem Pharmacol* (1991) **42**: 663–677.

18. Dent G, Evans PM, Chung KF, Barnes PJ: Zardaverine inhibits respiratory burst activity in human eosinophils. *Am Rev Respir Dis* (1990) **141**: A392.

19. Chapman KP, Boucher S, Hyland RH, *et al.*: A comparison of enprofylline and theophylline in the maintenance therapy of chronic reversible obstructive airway disease. *J Allergy Clin Immunol* (1990) **85**: 514–521.

20. Persson CGA: Development of safer xanthine drugs for the treatment of obstructive airways disease. *J Allergy Clin Immunol* (1986) **78**: 817–824.

21. Ishii K, Murad F: ANP relaxes bovine tracheal smooth muscle and increase cGMP. *Am J Physiol* (1989) **256**: C495–500.

22. Gruetter CA, Childers CC, Bosserman MK, Lemke SM, Ball JG, Valentovic MA: Comparison of relaxation induced by glyceryl trinitate, isosorbide dinitrate and sodium nitroprusside in bovine airways. *Am Rev Respir Dis* (1989) **139**: 1192–1197.

23. Byrick RJ, Hobbs EG, Martineau R, Noble WH: Nitroglycerin relaxes large airways. *Anesth Analg* (1983) **62**: 421–425.

24. Hirschleiter L, Arora Y: Nitrates in the treatment of bronchial asthma. *Br J Dis Chest* (1991) **39**: 275–283.

25. Okayama M, Sasaki H, Takishima T: Bronchodilator effect of sublingual isosorbide dinitrate in asthma. *Eur J Clin Pharmacol* (1984) **26**: 151–155.

26. Tullet WM, Patel KR: Isosorbide dinitrate and isoxsuprine in exercise-induced asthma. *Br Med J* (1983) **286**: 1934–1935.

27. Kennedy T, Summer WR, Sylvester J, Robertson D: Airway response to sublingual nitroglycerine in acute asthma. *J Am Med Soc* (1981) **246**: 145–147.

28. Miller WC, Shultz TF: Failure of nitroglycerin as a bronchodilator. *Am Rev Respir Dis* (1979) **120**: 471–472.

29. Barnes PJ: Muscarinic receptors in airways: recent developments. *J Appl Physiol* (1990) **68**: 1777–1785.

30. Hall I, Chilvers ER: Inositol phosphates and airway smooth muscle. *Pulm Pharmacol* (1989) **2**: 113–120.

31. Chilvers ER, Challiss RAJ, Willcocks AL, Potter BUL, Barnes PJ, Nahorski SR: Characterisation of stereospecific binding sites for inositol 1,4,5-trisphosphate in airway smooth muscle. *Br J Pharmacol* (1990) **99**: 297–302.

32. Nishizuka Y: Studies and perspectives of protein kinase C. *Science* (1986) **233**: 205–212.

33. Black JL, Barnes PJ: Potassium channels and airway function: new therapeutic approaches. *Thorax* (1990) **45**: 213–218.

34. Black JL, Armour CL, Johnson PRA, Alouan LA, Barnes PJ: The action of a potassium channel activator BRL 38227 (lemakalim) on human airway smooth muscle. *Am Rev Respir Dis* (1990) **142**: 1384–1389.

35. Kidney JC, Wordsell YM, Lavender EA, Chung KF, Barnes PJ: The effect of an ATP-dependent potassium channel activator BRL 38772 in asthmatics. *Am Rev Respir Dis* (1991) **143**: A423.

36. Williams AJ, Lee TH, Cochrane GM, *et al.*: Attenuation of nocturnal asthma by cromakalim. *Lancet* (1990) **336**: 334–336.

37. Ichinose M, Barnes PJ: A Potassium channel activator modulates both noncholinergic and cholinergic neurotransmission in guinea pig airways. *J Pharmacol Exp Ther* (1990) **252**: 1207–1212.

38. Brattsand R: Glucocorticosteroids for inhalation. In Barnes PJ (ed) *New Drugs for Asthma*. London, IBC Technical Services, 1989, pp 117–130.

39. Flower RJ: Lipocortin and the mechanism of action of the glucocorticoids. *Br J Pharmacol* (1988) **94**: 987–1015.
40. Manning PJ, Watson RM, Margolskee DJ, Williams VC, Schwartz JI, O'Byrne PM: Inhibition of exercise-induced bronchoconstriction by MK-571, a potent leukotriene D$_4$-receptor antagonist. *New Engl J Med* (1990) **323**: 1736–1739.
41. Taylor IK, O'Shaughnessy KM, Fuller RW, Dollery CT: Effect of cysteinyl-leukotriene receptor antagonist ICI 204,219 on allergen-induced bronchoconstriction and airway hyper-reactivity in atopic subjects. *Lancet* (1991) **337**: 690–694.
42. Lombardo D, Dennis EA: Cobra venom phospholipase A$_2$ inhibition by manoalide: a novel type of phospholipase inhibitor. *J Biol Chem* (1985) **260**: 7234–7240.
43. Hui KP, Taylor IK, Taylor GW, *et al.*: Effect of a 5-lipoxygenase inhibitor on leukotriene generation and airway response after allergen challenge in asthmatic patients. *Thorax* (1991) **46**: 184–189.
44. Miller DK, Gillard JW, Vickers PJ: Identification and isolation of a membrane protein necessary for leukotriene production. *Nature* (1990) **343**: 278–281.
45. Barnes PJ, Belvisi MG, Rogers DF: Modulation of neurogenic inflammation: novel approaches to inflammatory diseases. *Trends Pharmacol Sci* (1990) **11**: 185–189.
46. Snider RM, Constantine JW, Lowe JA, *et al.*: A potent nonpeptide antagonist of the substance P (NK$_1$) receptor. *Science* (1991) **251**: 435–437.
47. Posner J, Dear K, Jeal S, *et al.*: A preliminary study of the pharmacodynamics and pharmacokinetics of a novel enkephalin analogue [Tyr-D.Arg-Gly-Phe (4NO$_2$)·Pro·NH$_2$] (BW 443C) in healthy volunteers. *Eur J Clin Pharmacol* (1988) **34**: 67–71.
48. Jackson DM, Norris AA, Eady RP: Nedocromil sodium and sensory nerves in the dog lung. *Pulm Pharmacol* (1989) **2**: 179–184.
49. Chung KF, Barnes PJ: Loop diuretics and asthma. *Pulm Pharmacol* (1992) in press.
50. Ventresca GP, Nichol GM, Barnes PJ, Chung KF: Inhaled furosemide inhibits cough induced by low chloride content solutions but not by capsaicin. *Am Rev Respir Dis* (1990) **142**: 143–146.
51. O'Connor BJ, Chung KF, Chen-Wordsell YM, Fuller RW, Barnes PJ: Effect of inhaled furosemide and bumetamide on adenosine 5'-monophosphate and sodium metabisulphite-induced bronchoconstriction. *Am Rev Respir Dis* (1991) **143**: 1329–1333.
52. Perkins RS, Dent G, Chung KF, Barnes PJ: Effects of anion transport inhibitors and chloride ions on eosinophil respiratory burst activity. *Am Rev Respir Dis* (1991) **143**: A331.
53. Mullarkey MF, Lammert JK, Blumenstein BA: Long-term methotrexate treatment in corticosteroid-dependent asthma. *Ann Int Med* (1990) **112**: 577–581.
54. Shiner RJ, Nunn AJ, Chung KF, Geddes DM: Randomized, double-blind, placeo-controlled trial of methotrexate in steroid-dependent asthma. *Lancet* (1990) **336**: 137–140.
55. Alexander A, Barnes NC, Kay AB: Cyclosporin A in chronic severe asthma: a double-blind placebo-controlled trial. *Am Rev Respir Dis* (1991) **143**: A633.
56. Bernstein DI, Berstein IL, Bodgenheimer SS, Pietrosko RG: An open study of Auranofin in the treatment of steroid-dependent asthma. *J Allergy Clin Immunol* (1988) **81**: 6–16.
57. Guyre PM, Girard MT, Morganelli PM, Manginiello PD: Glucocorticoid effects on the production and action of immune cytokines. *J Steroid Biochem* (1988) **30**: 89–93.
58. Colman A: Antisense strategies in cell and developmental biology. *J Cell Sci* (1990) **97**: 399–409.
59. Coffman RL, Seymour BWP, Hudak S, Jackson J, Rennick D: Antibody to interleukin-5 inhibits helminth-induced eosinophilia in mice. *Science* (1989) **245**: 308–310.
60. Albelda SM: Endothelial and epithelial cell adhesion molecules. *Am J Resp Cell Mol Biol* (1991) **4**: 195–203.
61. Wegner CD, Gundel L, Reilly P, Haynes N, Letts LG, Rothlein R: Intracellular adhesion molecule-1 (ICAM-1) in the pathogenesis of asthma. *Science* (1990) **247**: 456–459.
62. Jurgensen CH, Huber BC, Zimmermann TP, Wolberg G: 3-Deazoadenosine inhibits leuko-cyte adhesion and I CAM-I biosynthesis in TNF-stimulated human endothelial cells. *J Immunol* (1990) **144**: 653–661.
63. Ricci M, Rossi O: Dysregulation of IgE responses and airway allergic inflammation in atopic individuals. *Clin Allergy* (1990) **20**: 601–609.

64. Lee TH, Arm JP: Prospects for modifying the allergen response by fish oil diets. *Clin Allergy* (1986) **16**: 89–100.
65. Arm JP, Horton CE, Eiser NM, Clark TJH, Lee TH: The effects of dietary supplementation with fish oil lipids on asthmatic responses to allergen, *Am Rev Respir Dis* (1989) **139**: 1395 1400.
66. Arm JP, Horton CE, Mencia-Huerta, JM, House F, *et al.*: Effect of dietary supplementation with fish oil lipids on mild asthma. *Thorax* (1988) **43**: 84–92.

Index

751